P9-CKV-752

Clinical Pharmacy and Therapeutics

Third Edition

Clinical Pharmacy and Therapeutics

Third Edition

edited by

Eric T. Herfindal, Pharm.D., M.P.H.

Clinical Professor and Chairman
Division of Clinical Pharmacy
School of Pharmacy
Director
Department of Pharmaceutical Services
University of California, San Francisco
San Francisco, California

Joseph L. Hirschman, Pharm.D.

Associate Clinical Professor
School of Pharmacy
University of California, San Francisco
San Francisco, California
General Manager
American Druggist Blue Book Data Center
The Hearst Corporation
Burlingame, California

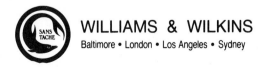

WILLIAMS & WILKINS
Baltimore • London • Los Angeles • Sydney

Editor: John P. Butler
Copy Editor: William G. Vinck
Design: Joanne Janowiak
Illustration Planning: Lorraine Wrzosek
Production: Raymond E. Reter

Copyright ©, 1984
Williams & Wilkins
428 East Preston Street
Baltimore, MD 21202, U.S.A.

All rights reserved. This book is protected by copyright. No part of this book may be reproduced in any form or by any means, including photocopying, or utilized by any information storage and retrieval system without written permission from the copyright owner.

Accurate indications, adverse reactions, and dosage schedules for drugs are provided in this book, but it is possible that they may change. The reader is urged to review the package information data of the manufacturers of the medications mentioned.

Made in the United States of America

Library of Congress Cataloging in Publication Data

Main entry under title:

Clinical pharmacy and therapeutics.

   Bibliography: p.
   Includes index.
   1. Chemotherapy. 2. Therapeutics. I. Herfindal, Eric T. II. Hirschman, Joseph L.
[DNLM: 1. Drug therapy. 2. Therapeutics. WB 330 C641]
RM262.C5 1984   615.5′8   83-16795
ISBN 0-683-03962-8

Composed and printed at the
Waverly Press, Inc.

87 88 89
10 9 8 7 6 5

Foreword

When the first edition of this text appeared in 1975, its title and contents served abrupt notice to the nation that a different kind of pharmacist had arrived on the health care scene. It was entitled *Clinical Pharmacy and Therapeutics*, and what a strange and alien combination of words these were. Never before had "pharmacy" and "therapeutics" appeared together on the cover of a textbook because prior to the late 1960s, few persons within the profession saw any connection between them. Until that time, the majority of practicing pharmacists would have firmly declared that their primary professional task was the filling of a prescription "exactly as ordered by the physician." They would have argued that therapeutics—the act of selecting the right drug for the right patient at the right time—was the sole responsibility of the physician and others who were authorized to prescribe. The pharmacist was not a member of this select group, *ergo* he or she had no place in therapeutics.

But this changed, albeit somewhat slowly in the beginning. By the early 1970s, pharmacists had already begun to assume the responsibility of assuring that patients received optimum drug therapy. This, in turn, led to changes in the curricula of pharmacy schools, including therapeutics courses and clinical clerkships that enabled students to apply these principles to patient care. These newer concepts of practice came to be known as clinical pharmacy, and the text you now hold in your hand was the very first attempt by a team of editors and authors—all of them clinical pharmacists—to meet the information needs of pharmacy students wishing to assume these new roles.

Yet, even when the book first appeared, there were still many within the profession of pharmacy who felt that clinical pharmacy was simply a shooting star on a wishful horizon, destined to blaze gloriously for the briefest of moments, but destined also to destroy itself in the process. There is and can be no future role beyond the distribution of drugs, they said, because physicians will never allow pharmacists to assume important roles in drug therapy.

That was nearly 10 years ago, and as I write these words, history has rather resolutely proven the doomsayers wrong. In the interim, clinical pharmacy has traded in its starburst for an eternal flame which it effectively uses to burn down the barricades of resistance. Today, pharmacists are assuming roles totally unheard of or unthought of as few as 5 years ago. Furthermore, the clinical pharmacy faculties of the nation have become as productive as their counterparts in other health professions, and they have had a marked impact on the practice of drug therapy in the United States.

As shall always be the case, however, the sages of doom are with us still. They speak now of computers and cost containment. There is no future, they say, because that which the pharmacist does can be captured on a piece of plastic or metal: a computer disk. Furthermore, they add, the advent of prospective payment schemes and other cost-control measures will result in serious cutbacks in the number of pharmacists, thereby minimizing or totally eliminating their impact on drug therapy.

But I disagree, as do the many dedicated practitioners who have been responsible for the several editions of this book. The future will challenge us, yes, but its winds will bear no doom unless we pay undue heed to the words of the doomsayers and cower before them. Winston Churchill once said that "frightfulness is not a remedy known to the *British Pharmacopeia*." Nor is it a remedy that has a place in our profession.

Jere E. Goyan
April, 1984

Preface

In the dozen years since the original concept for this book was developed, pharmacy has continued to evolve toward a clinical profession. Pharmacists are assuming larger roles as disseminators of drug information, patient educators, therapeutic consultants and direct providers of care. Concomitantly, technology has introduced many new drug entities and dosage forms, and the volume of biomedical information has greatly increased. We realize that the mastery of the knowledge necessary to fully function as an effective health care provider cannot be achieved through a book. However, a book can serve as a starting point. Combined with access to skilled teachers, clinical facilities and recent biomedical literature, the properly motivated student can master the field of clinical pharmacy.

This edition of *Clinical Pharmacy and Therapeutics*, like earlier editions, is based on the concept that pharmacists must be able to make therapeutic judgments as a matter of course.

Indeed, many patients and other health professionals now expect it. The success of the earlier editions of this book indicates that our approach is effective in helping prepare the pharmacist and pharmacy student for this responsibility.

Some chapters contained in previous editions have been dropped, and several new chapters have been included. There has also been an attempt to include more pharmacokinetic information where it is relevant. The selection of contributors continues to be based upon the same criteria used for previous editions, i.e., clinically experienced in the subject discussed.

We cannot mention here everyone who assisted us but we are, nevertheless, grateful to all of them. Our particular thanks, however, go to the participating authors who have put out an extraordinary effort.

E.T.H.
J.L.H.

Contributors

DONALD P. ALEXANDER, Pharm.D.
Assistant Professor of Clinical Pharmacy, University of Utah, Department of Pharmacy Practice, College of Pharmacy, Salt Lake City, Utah

STEVEN L. BARRIERE, Pharm.D.
Associate Professor of Pharmacy, College of Pharmacy, University of Michigan, Ann Arbor, Michigan

CONSTANTINE G. BERBATIS, M.Sc., F.P.S.
Clinical Pharmacist, Fremantle Hospital, Fremantle, Western Australia

LINDA R. BERNSTEIN, Pharm.D.
Assistant Clinical Professor, School of Pharmacy, University of California, San Francisco, California

C. A. BOND, Pharm.D.
Clinical Associate Professor, Assistant Dean for Professional and Student Affairs, University of Wisconsin School of Pharmacy, Madison, Wisconsin

R. KEITH CAMPBELL, B.Pharm., M.B.A.
Professor of Clinical Pharmacy, Coordinator of Off Campus Programs, Washington State University College of Pharmacy, Pullman, Washington

JANNET M. CARMICHAEL, Pharm.D.
Assistant Professor, Department of Family and Community Medicine, Department of Internal Medicine, School of Medicine, University of Nevada, Reno, Nevada

DOUGLAS G. CHRISTIAN, B.S.Pharm., M.B.A.
Product Marketing Documentation Manager, IVAC Corporation, San Diego, California

RICHARD GRANT CLOSSON, Pharm.D.
Associate Clinical Professor, Division of Clinical Pharmacy, School of Pharmacy, University of California, San Francisco, California

WILLIAM A. CORNELIS, Pharm.D.
Director, Department of Pharmaceutical Services, Hutzel Hospital, Detroit, Michigan

RICHARD F. DE LEON, Pharm.D.
Director of Pharmacy Services, Associate Professor of Pharmacy, Associate Dean for Clinical Sciences, The University of Michigan Hospitals, and College of Pharmacy, Ann Arbor, Michigan

RICHARD J. DE MEO, Pharm.D.
Director of Pharmacy Operations, Pharmacy Enterprises, Inc., Orange, California

BETTY J. DONG, Pharm.D.
Associate Clinical Professor, Division of Clinical Pharmacy, School of Pharmacy, University of California, San Francisco, California

MICHAEL N. DUDLEY, Pharm.D.
Assistant Professor of Pharmacy, University of Rhode Island, College of Pharmacy, The Roger Williams, General Hospital, Department of Pharmacy Services, North Kingstown, Rhode Island

ROBERT M. ELENBAAS, Pharm.D.
Associate Professor, Schools of Pharmacy and Medicine, University of Missouri-Kansas City, Clinical Pharmacist, Department of Emergency Health Services, Truman Medical Center, Kansas City, Missouri

PETER J. FORNI, Pharm.D.
Director of Health Care Industry Marketing, The Mastercare Corporation, San Mateo, California

CLARENCE L. FORTNER, M.S.
Chief, Drug Management and Authorization Section, Investigations Drug Branch, Cancer Therapy Evaluation Program, National Cancer Institute, Bethesda, Maryland

MARK A. GILL, Pharm.D.
Assistant Professor of Clinical Pharmacy, University of Southern California, School of Pharmacy, Los Angeles, California

DICK R. GOURLEY, Pharm.D.
Professor and Chairman, Department of Pharmacy Practice, University of Nebraska Medical Center, College of Pharmacy, Omaha, Nebraska

WILLIAM R. GROVE, M.S..
Director, Clinical Research Pharmacy Services, University of Maryland Cancer Center, University of Maryland Hospital, Baltimore, Maryland

ARTHUR F. HARRALSON, Pharm.D.
Director, Pharmacokinetics Service, Memorial Hospital Medical Center, Assistant Clinical Professor, School of Pharmacy, University of California, Long Beach, California

JOHN W. HILL, Ph.D.
Associate Professor, Counseling and Special Education Director, Learning Disabilities, Meyer Children's Rehabilitation Institute, University of Nebraska Medical Center, Omaha, Nebraska

ROBERT J. IGNOFFO, Pharm.D.
Associate Clinical Professor, School of Pharmacy, University of California, San Francisco, California

MARTIN J. JINKS, Pharm.D.
Associate Professor of Clinical Pharmacy, College of Pharmacy, Washington State University, Pullman, Washington

PAUL M. JUST, B.Sc., Pharm.D.
Adjunct Assistant Professor of Pharmacy, University of Illinois, Department of Pharmacy Services, Mercy Hospital and Medical Center, Chicago, Illinois

STANLEY G. KAILIS, Ph.D., F.P.S..
Principal Lecturer in Pharmaceutical Biology and Clinical Pharmacy, School of Pharmacy, Division of Health Services, Western Australian Institute of Technology, Bentley, Western Australia

STEVEN R. KAYSER, Pharm.D.
Associate Clinical Professor of Pharmacy, Clinical Pharmacist-Cardiology, School of Pharmacy, University of California San Francisco, San Francisco, California

DONALD T. KISHI, Pharm.D.
Clinical Professor and Vice Chairman, Divison of Clinical Pharmacy, School of Pharmacy, Associate Director of Pharmaceutical Services, University of California San Francisco, Department of Pharmaceutical Services, San Francisco, California

WENDY KLEIN-SCHWARTZ, Pharm.D.
Assistant Director, Maryland Poison Center, Assistant Professor, University of Maryland, School of Pharmacy, Baltimore, Maryland

PETER J. S. KOO, Pharm.D.
Assistant Clinical Professor of Pharmacy, University of California, School of Pharmacy, San Francisco, California

WAYNE A. KRADJAN, Pharm.D.
Associate Professor, Pharmacy Practice, University of Washington School of Pharmacy, Seattle, Washington

ANDREW L. LEEDS, Pharm.D.
Adjunct Lecturer, Clinical Pharmacist, Division of Clinical Pharmacy, School of Pharmacy, University of California, San Francisco, San Francisco, California

ROBERT H. LEVIN, Pharm.D.
Clinical Professor of Pharmacy, University of California, School of Pharmacy, Director, Clinical Pharmacy Services, San Francisco General Hospital, Medical Center, San Francisco, California

ARTHUR G. LIPMAN, Pharm.D.
Professor of Clinical Pharmacy, Chairman, Department of Pharmacy Practice, College of Pharmacy, University of Utah, Salt Lake City, Utah

PAUL W. NIEMIEC, JR., Pharm.D.
Clinical Pharmacy Coordinator, Surgery-Critical Care Division, Department of Pharmacy Services, The Johns Hopkins Hospital, Baltimore, Maryland

JEAN K. NOGUCHI, Pharm.D.
Assistant Professor of Clinical Pharmacy, University of Southern California, School of Pharmacy, Los Angeles, California

GARY M. ODERDA, Pharm.D., M.P.H.
Associate Professor, Director, Maryland Poison Center, University of Maryland, School of Pharmacy, Baltimore, Maryland

WILLIAM A. PARKER, Pharm.D., M.B.A.
Associate Professor and Coordinator of Clinical Pharmacy, Clinical Pharmacist, Dalhousie University, College of Pharmacy, Halifax, Nova Scotia, Canada

PETER M. PENNA, Pharm.D.
Professional Coordinator for Pharmacy Services, Group Health Cooperative of Puget Sound, Renton, Washington

ROBERT W. PIEPHO, Ph.D., F.C.P.
Professor and Associate Dean, University of Colorado, School of Pharmacy, Denver, Colorado

ELAINE OBSTARCZYK REALE, Pharm.D.
Assistant Clinical Professor, University of California, School of Pharmacy, Division of Clinical Pharmacy, San Francisco, California

DANIEL C. ROBINSON, Pharm.D.
Assistant Professor Clinical Pharmacy, School
of Pharmacy, University of Southern California, Los Angeles, California

MICHAEL L. RYAN, Pharm.D.
Assistant Clinical Professor of Pharmacy, University of Michigan College of Pharmacy, Acting Director of Drug Information Services, University of Michigan Hospitals, Ann Arbor,
Michigan

SAM K. SHIMOMURA, Pharm.D.
Clinical Professor, Vice Chairman, Division of
Clinical Pharmacy, School of Pharmacy, Uni-
versity of California, Irvine, California

JOHN K. SIEPLER, Pharm.D.
Staff Clinical Pharmacist, Department of Pharmacy, University of California Davis, Sacramento Medical Center, Sacramento, California

GARY H. SMITH, Pharm.D.
Associate Professor of Pharmacy Practice, Assistant Head and Director for Drug Information, University of Arizona, College of Pharmacy, Tucson, Arizona

GLEN L. STIMMEL, Pharm.D.
Associate Professor of Clinical Pharmacy, Psychiatry and the Behavioral Sciences, University of Southern California, Schools of Pharmacy and Medicine, Los Angeles, California

DAVID S. TATRO, Pharm.D.
Assistant Director Pharmacy Services, for Drug
Information and Educational Services, Stan-
ford University Hospital, Stanford, California

THEODORE G. TONG, Pharm.D.
Professor of Pharmacy Practice, Department of
Pharmacy Practice, College of Pharmacy, Uni-
versity of Arizona, Tucson, Arizona

WALTER L. TRUDEAU, B.M., B.Ch.
Associate Clinical Professor of Medicine, Chief
of Clinical Gastroenterology, Department of
Medicine, University of California Davis, Sacramento Medical Center, Sacramento, California

TIMOTHY W. VANDERVEEN, Pharm.D., M.S.
Clinical Services Manager, IMED Corporation,
San Diego, California

ROBERT T. WEIBERT, Pharm.D.
Associate Clinical Professor, School of Phar-
macy, University of California Medical Center,
San Diego, California

Contents

SECTION 1
General

SECTION 2
Infectious Disease

SECTION 7
Renal Disease

SECTION 8
Rheumatic Diseases

SECTION 9
Diseases of the Blood

SECTION 10
Neurological and Psychological Disorders

SECTION 11
Diseases of the Eye

SECTION 12
Skin Diseases

SECTION 13
Neoplastic Diseases

SECTION 1
General

CHAPTER 1

Clinical Toxicology

GARY M. ODERDA, Pharm.D., M.P.H.
WENDY KLEIN-SCHWARTZ, Pharm.D.

INTRODUCTION

Clinical toxicology deals with the assessment and medical management of persons exposed acutely or chronically to a potentially harmful agent. Because of the diverse nature of the substances involved in poisonings as well as the wide range of clinical manifestations and their treatment, optimal management of the poisoned patient is achieved through an interdisciplinary approach to patient care. Expertise provided by physicians, nurses, pharmacists, social workers and paraprofessionals contributes greatly to the care of these patients.

In order to function effectively as a contributor to the clinical toxicology team, pharmacists must be trained in the retrieval of poison information and be familiar with the basic principles of the treatment of poisoning. Poisoning calls are frequently received by poison centers, community pharmacies and hospital pharmacies. A poisoning call from another health professional, or a frantic parent, can be traumatic, but rewarding, to the pharmacist equipped to handle such a medical emergency. Many pharmacists who receive these calls, however, are not prepared to handle them. It is the purpose of this chapter to provide pharmacy students and pharmacists with the basic knowledge necessary to deal with these poisoning calls.

GENERAL INFORMATION

Poisoning, be it accidental or intentional, is a serious problem in the United States today. The National Clearinghouse for Poison Control Centers processes approximately 150,000 reports of ingestions per year (1). This figure in no way reflects the actual number reported to poison centers since reporting to the National Clearinghouse is voluntary and most large centers do not report. Since there are no legal reporting requirements for poisoning, it is difficult to be certain of the true magnitude of the problem. It is estimated, however, that each year 3.5 million poison exposure cases occur nationally (1), with accidental poisoning from liquids, solids and gases accounting for 4,900 deaths in 1979 (2).

Poisoning is the most common pediatric medical emergency. Eighty percent of acute poisonings occur in children, with approximately 75% of these poisonings occurring in children less than 5 years of age. Most childhood poisonings are accidental and occur via the oral route. Children's natural curiosity can at times have disastrous consequences. They are exposed to thousands of drugs and hundreds of thousands of chemicals and household products. Although some children learn by their past poisoning experiences, a significant number of children are "repeaters," i.e., they ingest more than once. The most common substances involved in poison exposures in children less than 5 years of age are drugs, household products, personal care products and plants. In our experience the drugs most commonly involved are analgesics and antipyretics, antihistamines/cough and cold products, vitamins and topical preparations.

For years, aspirin was the leading cause of accidental poisoning and poisoning deaths in children under 5 years of age. This is no longer the case, as there has been a progressive decline in both ingestions and deaths since the mid-1960s (3). The percentage of ingestions due to aspirin in those under 5 years of age has decreased steadily from around 25% in 1966 to 3.9% in 1979 (4). Many factors are responsible for this decrease, and among them are an increased awareness on the part of the general public of the dangers of aspirin. The safety closure requirement for all products containing aspirin, and all liquid preparations containing methyl salicylate, is largely responsible for the decline. Hopefully, safety packaging will further decrease the number of intoxications from other products on which these closures are now required. The limit of 36 tablets (each 81 mg) per bottle of children's aspirin has helped reduce the severity of the ingestions which still occur. Working toward preventing poisoning is the most logical approach to this problem. The old cliche "an ounce of prevention is worth a pound of cure" obviously applies here.

Approximately 20% of poisonings occur in adults and are often the result of an intentional exposure (suicide or drug abuse) but may also be accidental (e.g., industrial exposure). While poison prevention activities may decrease the number of pediatric exposures and minimize the severity of childhood intoxications, these efforts have almost no impact on adult poisoning. In fact, many clinical toxicologists feel that poisonings in adults are responsible for more significant morbidity and mortality today.

ROLE AND STATUS OF POISON CENTERS

Since the first poison center was established in Chicago in 1953, the number of poison centers in the United States has increased dramatically. According to the National Clearinghouse for Poison Control Centers the number of official centers peaked at approximately 590 centers in 1970 and has decline to 466 in 1980 (5).

Official centers exist in most major U.S. metropolitan areas and are most commonly staffed by physicians, nurses and pharmacists. The 1980 survey of poison control centers conducted by the National Clearinghouse for Poison Control Centers found that, of the 275 operating centers that responded, 81% are poison information and treatment centers, 13% are poison information centers, and 4% are treatment centers only. While 88% of the centers are located in hospitals, 10% are found in educational institutions. Sixty-four percent of the poison centers are affiliated with the emergency department, 13% are located in the pharmacy and 13% are affiliated with both the emergency department and other departments. Ninety-five percent of the respondent centers are open 24 hours per day, 365 days per year and 96% of them answer calls from the general public and health professionals. These figures indicate an increase in the percentage of centers that respond to both types of callers since in a 1970 survey this number was only 78%. In 1979 30% of the centers

received less than 500 calls, 43% received over 1000 calls, 15% received over 10,000 calls and 6% received over 25,000 calls annually. Toll-free numbers exist for 17% of these centers and 21% of the centers are linked to 911 emergency systems.

Even today many centers listed in the National Clearinghouse directory are small centers located in hospital emergency rooms whose primary function is to treat poisoned patients who come in. Recently, however, the concept of regionalization of poison centers has developed in an attempt to more efficiently and effectively meet the needs of the poisoned patient. Many large centers serve as regional centers and provide information to a large population or geographic area. This may involve a major metropolitan area, a portion of a large state, an entire state, or several states. The distribution depends primarily upon population and geography. It is not unusual for these regional centers to handle 15,000 to 30,000 or more calls per year. It is the current feeling that development of 50 to 100 top notch regional poison centers could adequately serve the entire United States. In this way one avoids duplication of information sources and staff. In addition, this allows regional poison center staff to handle large numbers of cases and develop expertise in this area.

The American Association of Poison Control Centers has developed standards for regional poison centers and is presently an organization that certifies regional centers. According to their criteria regional programs should provide the following services (6):

1. A regional poison information service including 24-hour a day availability, toll-free telephone access, comprehensive information sources, management protocols and access to regional treatment facilities for patient referral and transport.

2. A regional system for providing poisoning care, with at least one comprehensive poisoning treatment center.

3. An outreach health profession education program.

4. An outreach public education program.

5. A regional data collection and reporting system.

Ideally, the medical director of the center should be a board certified medical toxicologist. As the number of these individuals is limited, however, the medical director is often selected on the basis of interest, training and experience. Clinical pharmacists or nurses are often administratively responsible for the day to day operation of the center as well as providing professional input into the management of the poisoned patient. Poison information specialists, usually pharmacists or nurses, are responsible for providing primary telephone consultations.

Poison information is also provided by "unofficial" poison centers. Most drug information centers also provide some poisoning information. It is important to note, however, that these two types of centers (drug information versus poison) differ. Poison centers usually provide services both to professionals and to the general public, whereas drug information centers usually provide information only to health professionals. In addition, poison centers specialize in providing poison information, whereas with drug information centers this is usually a sideline. At present several combined poison information-drug information centers exist. Since there is an overlap in both staffing and information sources, more of these combined centers may be expected in the future. It is essential that the pharmacist be acquainted with available centers in the local area so as to be able to refer those problems that are either beyond his or her ability or reference sources. A list of poison centers is included in the *Physicians Desk Reference* and the *Drug Topics Red Book*.

ROLE OF THE PHARMACIST

Pharmacists, because of their extensive background in biopharmaceutics and pharmacokinetics, drugs interactions, chemistry, pharmacognosy, pharmacy, and therapeutics, can become valuable resources in poison centers. In addition, pharmacists have as much, or more, didactic pharmacology training than any other health discipline. Many pharmacy schools provide specific toxicology coursework.

The community pharmacist may be the first professional contacted after ingestion of a toxic compound, especially when a drug is involved. Pharmacists must be able to determine whether home treatment is advisable or whether the person should be referred to an emergency room. Hospital pharmacists may be involved in the selection, stocking and supplying of drugs used to manage poisoned patients.

Kinnard (7) suggests that pharmacists could be involved in an acute poisoning case in many ways, including: (a) being the initial patient contact in a poison center, or a pharmacy; (b) serving as a clinical pharmacist in an emergency room or poison center to provide therapeutic consultation; (c) being involved in the identification of the ingested materials both via gross examination and chemical analysis of the agent and body fluids; (d) preparing intravenous fluids the patient may require; (e) serving as a member of the cardiac arrest team that may treat a poisoned patient; (f) in some cases being the individual who directly administers drugs; and (g) providing poison information as a staff member, or director, of a drug information center.

Pharmacists can be involved in providing information on toxicokinetics as well as in researching the kinetics of drugs in overdose situations. Toxicokinetics is the study of the absorption, distribution, metabolism and elimination of drugs from the body in the overdose situation. Each of these parameters may be altered following the ingestion of a large dose of some drugs. Absorption may be delayed and various transport and metabolic processes may be saturated. An awareness of the toxicokinetics of specific drugs allows for an educated prediction of the time course of the intoxication in an individual patient.

Pharmacists already serve in many of these roles. Knowledgeable pharmacists in any setting may perform many of these roles with little additional training.

POISON PREVENTION

According to the 1980 National Clearinghouse survey, 78% of the respondent poison centers conduct poison prevention education activities. The types of educational activities include distribution of pamphlets, newspaper articles, radio and TV spots, videotapes, slide shows, special school programs, speakers' bureaus, and poison warning labels. The two most common activities are distribution of pamphlets and newspaper and magazine articles. Most centers produce and/or distribute their own materials.

Pharmacists can also play an important role in poison prevention. This should be a year round project with an increase in activity during National Poison Prevention Week.

The FDA approves the nonprescription sale of appropriately labeled 1-oz quantities of ipecac syrup. Pharmacists should stock syrup of ipecac and be familiar with its use for the management of acute poisoning including indications and dosing.

Pharmacists can be influential in promoting the distribution of syrup of ipecac. Local pharmaceutical organizations have provided ipecac free of charge to families with young children through community pharmacies. If this service is not available, pharmacists can display ipecac, provide information, and urge that families with young children purchase a 1-oz container. Parents should be cautioned to contact their physician, pharmacist or poison center before giving the ipecac. In this way a health professional can evaluate the situation and determine the appropriateness of administering an emetic and if necessary call an ambulance, physician or an emergency room. If syrup of ipecac is indicated, the health professional can review dosing with the caller, follow-up on the call to determine if the person has vomited and provide additional instructions regarding the side effects of ipecac and/or symptoms to watch for which might indicate the need for additional evaluation and treatment. If ipecac is not indicated the health professional can discourage its administration and recommend modalities of treatment if necessary.

Many other poison prevention activities are possible. An important first step is to see that the pharmacy is poison proof. Since children can ingest products stored on low shelves in pharmacies, these shelves should be stocked with articles with a low potential for toxicity. All prescription drugs required to be dispensed in safety containers should be so dispensed. In those few instances where a patient requires a nonsafety container, be certain to warn the patient to store the container properly to avoid an accidental poisoning. Elderly patients who require nonsafety containers may not have young children of their own, but many have young grandchildren who come to visit. Poison prevention posters that make customers aware of the danger of poisoning should be displayed. Fliers discussing poison dangers may be distributed. Pharmacists can act as speakers to discuss poisoning dangers with parents of young children. Points to be stressed include: (a) keeping harmful substances out of reach of children, (b) not calling medicine candy or taking medicine in front of children, (c) using safety closures, (d) keeping medicines and household products in their original containers, (e) disposing of unused portions/cleaning out the medicine cabinet, (f) reading labels and precautionary statements, (g) keeping syrup of ipecac in the house, and (h) having the phone number of the poison center in a readily accessible place.

Since the most active ingestors are unable to read, a warning on a product label has no effect on the child. Some toxicologists feel that the traditional warning symbol, the skull and crossbones, is not an effective warning symbol. It has been suggested that many young children think of pirates and adventure, and not poison when they see this symbol (8). In addition, the skull and crossbones is required only on the most dangerous products. Many commonly ingested agents that have the potential for producing fatality, automatic dishwasher detergent, petroleum distillates, and drugs for example, do not carry this warning. Poison warning symbols such as Mr. Yuk and Officer Ugg have been developed to warn young children to stay away from dangerous products.

ANALYSIS OF A POISONING SITUATION—TYPES OF QUESTIONS ASKED

Unfortunately in many poisoning calls, the caller does not volunteer enough information for the pharmacist to adequately answer all pertinent questions. The history is also often incomplete in cases where the patient is discovered in a coma from an unknown cause, a child ingests an unknown amount of tablets or capsules from an unmarked container, or an unidentified plant has been ingested. Generally, the caller is trying to determine the potential toxicity or lethality of the substance. Some examples: A mother calls and say, "My son took four of my birth control pills. Should I make him vomit?" A suicide prevention worker calls and says, "Mr. X took 100 secobarbital, should I call an ambulance for him?" A physician in an emergency toom asks: "Mr. Y took 10 pentazocine, is this a dangerous dose in this patient and what treatment is appropriate?" A family physician calls and asks, "Mrs. Smith's 4-year-old son took four or five green and white capsules with Lilly H69 on them. What are they and what should I do?"

Most of the above questions can be answered with relative ease. Examples of questions more difficult to answer include a physician calling and saying, "Mrs. Jones was found comatose at her home with an empty bottle of amitriptyline, pargyline and diazepam lying next to her. At present she has the following symptoms ... How should I treat her?"

And more of a challenge, "Mrs. Doe was brought into the emergency room by friends who claim she took an unknown number of tablets of an unidentified drugs and is showing the following symptoms ... do you know what it might be and what I should do about it?"

Often only incomplete information is available, and the pharmacist working in poison control must be ready to ask appropriate questions to extract all of the facts from the caller. Occasionally a poisoning situation can be uncovered only by persistent, clever questions. For example, questions such as "What is a small yellow tablet with MSD 45 on it?" can be easily answered, "Elavil 25 mg." By asking the question, "Why do you need this information?" one might determine that an ingestion has occurred and be of further assistance in recommending appropriate treatment.

Even more confusing is the situation where there is no history of a poisoning in a person who presents with signs or symptoms which suggest a poisoning (9, 10). Or manifestations which are initially thought to be due to some other disease process may turn out to be poison-related. A poisoning should be considered in the differential diagnosis whenever there is an abrupt onset of illness with multiple organ system involvement, especially if the patient is a child under 5 years of age or has a history of a previous ingestion.

When a poisoning is suspected, what questions should the pharmacist ask? The following is a discussion of the minimum amount of information necessary to "analyze" a poisoning situation. Most poison centers record this information on an ingestion reporting form. Thus written documentation of each call is available for use statistically and otherwise.

1. *Name of Product Ingested.* If known, this information is usually volunteered. From the name of the product one must identify the ingredients and their percentages, if available, to determine the potential toxicity.

2. *Amount Ingested.* This piece of information is often difficult to determine. Paracelsus (1493–1541) said, "All substances are poisons, there is none which is not a poison. The right dose differentiates a poison and a remedy." The ingestion of 4 children's aspirin by a 2-year-old is clearly a different situation than a 2-year-old who has taken 36 adult aspirin tab-

lets. In determining the amount ingested, the following points must be kept in mind: (a) careful questioning is important. Often a parent will say, "My child ate one red berry off the green bush in our front yard, what should I do?" When asked, how do you know the child ate one berry, the reply is often, "He wasn't alone very long, therefore he couldn't have eaten many." This information is unreliable. In many cases children eat things adults consider unappetizing. In addition, a child can eat a fairly large number of berries, or tablets, in a short period of time. (b) If an accurate determination of the amount ingested is impossible, and the product is potentially toxic, one must assume that a potentially toxic amount was ingested or that the total amount originally in the container was ingested. For example, if two children are found with an empty container of vitamins with iron which originally contained 50 tablets and it is impossible to determine the number of tablets taken, the most appropriate initial recommendation is to assume that each child might have taken 50 tablets. Treatment should initially be based on this assumption since it would be dangerous to assume that the two children had split the tablets evenly amongst themselves.

3. *Time Since Ingestion.* The time since ingestion gives you a great deal of information. By knowing about the onset, duration of action and the elimination of the ingested compound, one can determine whether the symptoms the patient is showing are appropriate for the amount ingested and the time since ingestion. In addition, treatment recommendations, such as whether or not to empty the stomach, may be influenced by the length of time since ingestion.

4. *Symptoms.* This is one of the most important pieces of information and one that is commonly missed. The majority of treatment is symptomatic and supportive. Support of vital functions, including attention to the respiratory and cardiovascular systems, is the primary concern. One important questions that must be asked is—do the symptoms "fit" the poison? If not, one must ask why not? Was another agent ingested? Symptoms may serve as a contraindication to treatment, e.g., emetics are contraindicated in the comatose patient.

5. *Age and Weight of the Patient.* In many instances the toxicity of an agent is described in a dose per weight basis, e.g., 1 g/lb or 5 ml/

kg. Thus the determination of toxicity would depend on the patient's weight. Some antidotes, and other drugs used in treatment are likewise administered on a mg/kg of body weight basis or by dose/year of age basis.

The above constitutes the minimum amount of information necessary to deal with most poisoning situations. In addition, one would like to know:

1. *The Patient's Name, Location and Phone Number.* Nothing is more frustrating than being cut off from the caller and not being able to call back. In addition, this information allows you to "follow-up" on the call.

2. *Other Drugs Administered.* Is the patient taking any other drugs therapeutically? Were other drugs taken at the same time? If so, what effect would these agents have?

3. *Patient History.* Is there anything in the patient's medical history that would influence the intoxication or treatment prescribed?

4. *Prior Therapy.* Was any other therapy done previously? It is not unusual that a parent will have administered a home remedy before calling for help, which may complicate therapy. One must then evaluate how this previous treatment will influence your recommendations.

Now that the baseline data has been obtained, how does one determine what treatment, if any, is necessary? This is an extremely difficult question to answer. It is clear that a child who has taken a subtoxic dose of a drug for which there is a great deal of human toxicity information, e.g., aspirin, and who is showing no symptoms would require no treatment. Many cases where minimal toxicity is expected, i.e., no severe or life-threatening symptoms that would require emergency treatment, may be treated at home. Often ipecac syrup is indicated. All potentially serious intoxications must be referred to an emergency treatment facility. It is critically important that all patients for whom you are unsure of the expected toxicity be referred for treatment. Treatment for severe intoxications depends upon symptomatology and the agent ingested. To be proficient at making the judgments described in this paragraph takes special training and a great deal of personal experience. In all cases where a pharmacist is called for poison information, and is uncertain as to what should be done, it is imperative that a local poison center be contacted for guidance. The information may be given directly to the pharmacist who may play an integral role in the treatment of that individual or in some cases it will be recommended that the caller directly contact the poison center.

INFORMATION SOURCES

The next step in the assessment of a poisoning situation is to consult appropriate information sources. The major toxicologic information sources are designed to allow rapid retrieval of toxicity and management information. If one is looking for specific information on a particular agent and time is not critical, it is suggested that the current literature, i.e., journals, be consulted for the most up to date information.

Below is a list of general references that are commonly used in handling poisoning cases. The references are strictly toxicology oriented and do not include other important references, such as pharmacology texts, drug interaction texts, etc., that would be expected to be found in both pharmacies and poison centers.

Poisindex. (B. Rumack, editor, published by Micromedex, Englewood, Colorado, new edition published 4 times yearly). This system is a computer-generated microfiche system with information on over 160,000 products. For each product, the manufacturer's name, the type of product, ingredients, percentages (if available), and tablet imprint are listed on the compound data cards. In many cases specific toxicity information is also included. For all products the user is referred to the appropriate management protocols which are shown on a separate fiche. Some managements are preceded by "overviews" which contain emergency treatment information on one microfiche frame (see Fig. 1.1) eliminating the need to scan several microfiche frames initially. The overview is followed by the extended management which includes information on available forms, pharmacology, clinical effects, kinetics, range of toxicity laboratory (blood levels, etc.), treatment, and major references. The major advantages of this system are: (a) ease of use; (b) it stores a large amount of materials in a small space; (c) it is up to date; (d) the management protocols are well thought out, up to date, provide specific information and are reviewed by an editorial board. The editorial board is comprised of individuals actively involved with poisoning and poison centers throughout the United States; (5) the data base includes information on drugs, chemicals,

OVERVIEW: SALICYLATES

AN OVERVIEW OF DIAGNOSIS AND TREATMENT

Life Support:

This overview assumes that basic life support measures have been instituted.

Characteristic Signs/Symptoms:

GASTROINTESTINAL: Nausea, vomiting, and dehydration.

NEUROLOGIC: Lethargy, tinnitis, tachypnea, convulsions, and coma.

METABOLIC: Fluid-electrolyte disturbances, dehydration, fever, hypoglycemia (child), metabolic acidosis (child), respiratory alkalosis (adult). Chronic salicylate poisoning characteristically results in metabolic acidosis regardless of the age.

Treatment Overview:

ORAL EXPOSURE

1. Emesis should be initiated, unless the patient is comatose, convulsing, or has lost the gag reflex. If any of these contraindications are present, endotracheal intubation should precede gastric lavage with a large-bore tube.
2. Administer activated charcoal (Adult: 60–100 g; Child: 30–60 g).
3. Administer a cathartic. Magnesium sulfate (Adult: 30 g; Child: 250 mg/kg).
4. DETERMINE SERUM SALICYLATE level at 6 hr postingestion and compare it to the Done nomogram to assess the severity of intoxication.
5. DEHYDRATION: Initially administer 88 mEq/L sodium bicarbonate (2 amps) in 0.45 NaCl, or similarly appropriate solution, at a rate of 10–15 ml/kg/hr over 1–2 hr until a good urine flow is obtained. To avoid pulmonary edema, do not overhydrate.
   SUBSEQUENT HYDRATION and HYPOKALEMIA may be treated with 20–40 mEq KCl/L and 44–88 mEq NaHCO$_3$ (1–2 amps)/L in D5W at a rate of 4–8 ml/kg/hr until salicylate level is therapeutic. Place patient on a CARDIAC MONITOR while adiministering KCl. Do NOT administer potassium to oliguric patients.
6. ALKALINIZE the urine (only after adequate rehydration) with a maintenance solution of 20 mEq/L sodium bicarbonate and 20 mEq/L KCl in D5W at a rate of 2–3 ml/kg/hr to achieve a urine pH of 7–8 and urine flow of 3–6 ml/kg/hr. Additional sodium bicarbonate (1 to 2 mEq/kg/hr) and KCl (20–40 mEq/L) may be needed to achieve an alkaline urine.
7. ACIDOSIS: Administer IV sodium bicarbonate. Monitor blood gases and pH to guide bicarbonate therapy. About 1–2 mEq/kg is an appropriate starting dose.
8. FEVER: Hyperpyrexia should be treated with external cooling. DO NOT USE ASPIRIN OR ACETAMINOPHEN.
9. HEMODIALYSIS: Consider hemodialysis for intoxications refractory to conventional therapy. INDICATIONS: Hemodialysis is recommended in those patients with high blood salicylate levels (greater than 130 mg/dl at 6 hr postingestion), refractory acidosis (pH < 7.1), progressive clinical deterioration despite appropriate therapy (hydration, alkalinization, etc.), pulmonary edema or renal failure. If these clinical effects exist hemodialysis may be useful regardless of the serum salicylate level.

Range Of Toxicity:

1. ACUTE INGESTION: Ingestion of 150 mg/kg to 300 mg/kg can produce mild to moderate intoxication. Ingestion of greater than 300 mg/kg may produce severe intoxication.
2. CHRONIC INGESTION: Ingestion of greater than 100 mg/kg/24 hr over 2 days may produce toxicity.

Laboratory:

1. Obtain CBC, electrolytes, blood gases and blood glucose.
2. Obtain serum salicylate level at 6 or more hours postingestion and compare to the Done nomogram.

MORE DETAILED INFORMATION APPEARS ON NEXT FRAMES

Figure 1.1. Example of *Poisindex* microfiche. (Courtesy of B. Rumack, Micromedex, Englewood, Col., 1982.)

household products, food poisoning, mushrooms, snakes, and drug imprint codes; and (6) the product information is cross referenced. Because of the cost of subscribing to this system, *Poisindex* is generally limited to poison centers. For further information contact Micromedex, Inc., 2750 South Shoshone Street, Englewood, Colorado 80110.

Toxifile. This is another microfiche system that originally contained National Clearinghouse cards and the updates for *Clinical Toxicology of Commercial Products.* Information on more than 100,000 products is included, some of which has been obtained directly from manufacturers. Managements are compiled from information in the current literature and are reviewed by an editorial board from the University of Illinois Colleges of Pharmacy and Medicine. To use the system, one looks up the product in a printed directory and is then referred to an appropriate microfiche card and location. Some preliminary information is presented including ingredients, amounts, toxicity and treatment and depending on the product, one might then be referred to a generic management section, e.g., salicylates or propoxyphene for more detailed toxicity and treatment information. For further information contact: Chicago Micro Corporation, 3157 West Lawrence Avenue, Chicago, Illinois 60625.

Poison Control Cards. At one time the National Clearinghouse for Poison Control Centers provided a complete set of approximately 10,000 cards free of charge to poison centers. While these cards are no longer available, most existing centers still have access to these cards. For each particular product the manufacturer, ingredients, amounts, toxicity information, symptoms and findings, recommended treatment and a list of sources of information are listed on one card. Major disadvantages include: (a) cards are easily lost or misfiled, (b) information is often sketchy and incomplete, (c) data base often does not contain information one is looking for, and (d) information is frequently out of date. In some cases new cards were issued for 15 to 20 years. Obviously, this will become more of a problem now that the system has been discontinued and cards will not be updated.

Many poison centers develop a card file of their own in order to maintain information obtained by calling manufacturers about individual products for which there is insufficient information in other existing resources.

Clinical Toxicology of Commercial Products (M. N. Gleason, R. E. Gosselin, H. C. Hodge, and R. P. Smith, Ed. 4, Williams & Wilkins, Baltimore, Maryland, 1976). This text is divided into seven sections: 1) First Aid and General Emergency Treatment, 2) Ingredients Index, 3) Therapeutics Index, 4) Supportive Treatment, 5) Trade Name Index, 6) General Formulations, and 7) Manufacturers Names and Addresses. For those unfamiliar with using the text, a guide describing how it should be used is included in the front. Most commonly one looks up the name of a product in the trade name index and is provided with the names of the ingredients and in most instances their percentage in the product. One then looks up each ingredient in the ingredients index where specific toxicity information is included. The therapeutics index has detailed toxicity and treatment information in general categories such as antihistamines. The general formulations index is very useful in those situations where a brand is unavailable. If for example you are dealing with a child who drank an unknown brand of furniture polish, one could find the ingredients generally included in furniture polishes. Although this is obviously not as useful as knowing the exact ingredients, it is still helpful.

Toxicology of the Eye (W. G. Grant, Ed. 2, Charles C Thomas, Springfield, Illinois, 1974). This text is an excellent resource that covers the effects of various agents upon contact with the eye. In addition, those agents for which systemic intoxication produces ocular effects, e.g., methanol, are included. Specific human information is discussed where available. A separate treatment section is included.

Industrial Hygiene and Toxicology (F. A. Patty, editor, Ed. 3, Interscience Publishers, New York, 1981). This series is published in three volumes. Volume I discusses general principles, Volume IIA and IIB specific toxicology information and Volume III industrial hygiene practice. Poison centers would find Volume IIA and IIB the most useful. Included in this text are chemicals to which industrial workers would commonly be exposed. Since many of these chemicals find their way out of industrial areas, the information is valuable. Both chronic and acute exposures are described. For each chemical the following information is provided: (a) source, use and industrial exposure; (b) physical and chemical properties; (c) determination in the atmosphere; (d) physiological response; (e) hygiene standard of permissible exposure; (f) flammability, and (g) odor and warning properties.

Toxicology—The Basic Science of Poisons (L. Cassarett, and J. Doull, Macmillan, New York, 1980). Although this book is designed primarily as a textbook for toxicology courses it also is quite useful as a reference text. The book is divided into five units: 1) General Principles of Toxicology; 2) Systemic Toxicology, a discussion by organ system of the effect of toxic agents; 3) Toxic Agents, a discussion of various groups of toxic agents, e.g., pesticides, and their effects; 4) Environmental Toxicology, and 5) Applications of Toxicology. The book's strength is in its discussion of mechanisms of toxicity of the various agents and its weakness is the discussion of treatment.

MANUFACTURERS' INFORMATION

Several manufacturers provide toxicological information for their products on request. In emergency situations most pharmaceutical manufacturers will accept phone calls and provide toxicology information on their products. This is sometimes true of manufacturers of household products for which ingredients are not normally released.

TREATMENT—GENERAL

The treatment of poisoning is complicated, requiring a background of information as well as the ability to analyze situations quickly and carefully, applying and modifying basic principles to each individual case. One must consider all the ramifications of an ingestion. If the intent was suicidal, psychiatric counseling is also essential. If the incident was, in fact, accidental, care must be taken to avoid a recurrence.

In general there are three major areas of therapy for an acute ingestion. They are: (a) supportive care, (b) measures to decrease absorption or hasten elimination of the ingested agent, and (c) specific measures to counteract the ingested agents effects.

Supportive Care

Support of vital functions is the single most important component of treatment. Searching for an antidote, a toxicology textbook or the poison center phone number are obviously not the first priority when an apneic narcotic overdose patient is brought into the emergency room. Treatment of many intoxications is largely symptomatic and supportive. In most poisoning situations, if the patient's vital functions are supported and symptoms that develop are treated, most patients will detoxify themselves and recover. Morelli (11) has stated, "Treat the patient, then his poison."

This is a critical point! Assessment of respiratory, central nervous system and cardiovascular status with provision of symptomatic and supportive care are the cornerstones of therapy.

Many drugs produce CNS depression and depending on the quantity ingested may produce symptoms ranging from lethargy and sedation to grade IV coma. The first priority in treating the unconscious patient is to ensure a patent airway and adequate ventilation. The airway may become obstructed by secretions, the tongue or laryngeal edema. Removal of secretions and insertion of an artificial airway may be required. Next the adequacy of ventilation is assessed by observing respiratory rate and depth and by analysis of arterial blood gases. Depending on the situation, therapy may include administration of oxygen, initiation of mouth-to-mouth resuscitation, and provision of assisted ventilation using a mechanical respirator. Continued monitoring of the patient's respiratory status is essential.

Another possible manifestation of drug overdose is seizures, which may be produced directly by the ingested agent or indirectly via the production of systemic disturbances (e.g., hypoglycemia, hypoxia) (11, 12). Initial efforts should be geared toward prevention of injury during the seizure. If the seizure is caused by other than a direct drug effect, therapy should be aimed at correcting the etiology (e.g., administration of glucose). Otherwise, termination of the convulsion using intravenous diazepam or a barbiturate should be attempted. Once the patient has stopped seizing, consideration should be given to the continued administration of anticonvulsants to prevent seizures if the likelihood of recurrence is high.

Cardiovascular complications of poisoning are frequent and include hypotension and shock, hypertension, and arrhythmias. The picture can be further complicated by the effects of hypoxia and acidosis on myocardial and vascular function. Hypotension may be due to many different effects of the ingested agents on cardiac output and peripheral vascular resistance (13). Minor degrees of hypotension are well tolerated and the critical issue is the adequacy of tissue perfusion (11–13). The sensitive indicator of hypoperfusion is urine output; other parameters to be monitored in the hypotensive patient may include fluid intake and output, presence of acidosis and signs of sympathetic nervous system overactivity, direct measurement of intra-arterial blood pressure, central venous pressure or pulmonary capillary wedge pressure, etc. The clinical status of the patient will dictate which of these measures is warranted. Intravenous fluids should be administered to achieve adequate intravascular volume. The patient is placed in the Trendelenburg position in order to minimize venous pooling in the lower extremities. If hypotension with hypoperfusion persists, vasopressors may be administered. In most cases dopamine has become the pressor agent of choice because of its effects on renal blood flow (13).

Hypertension may also occur with drug overdose and can result in complications such as cerebrovascular accidents. Depending on the severity of the blood pressure elevation and the nature of the ingested agent, different antihypertensive drugs may be indicated.

Arrhythmias may be produced directly by the ingested agent or may be secondary to systemic disturbances such as hypoxia, acid-base or electrolyte abnormalities. Therapy may include antiarrhythmic drugs such as lidocaine or propranolol, electrical cardioversion, or temporary intracardiac pacing depending on the clinical situation. Severely intoxicated patients and patients who have ingested drugs with a high propensity for cardiac arrhythmias should be placed on a cardiac monitor in an intensive care setting.

Hypothermia may occur following the ingestion of most CNS depressant drugs and can usually be managed with warming blankets. Hyperthermia is seen with salicylates, atropine-like drugs, amphetamines, and phencyclidine and is managed with tepid sponge baths and cooling blankets (14).

Cerebral edema can be seen as a complication of many types of poisonings and is managed with the intravenous administration of hypertonic mannitol or urea as well as steroids such as dexamethasone. Pulmonary edema can also be a complication and may be related to increased pulmonary capillary permeability and/or overzealous fluid therapy. Therapy may include restricting intravenous fluids and the use of mechanical ventilation with PEEP (13).

Close attention must also be paid to acid-base and electrolyte status of the patient. Similarly, therapeutic maneuvers to prevent the complications of coma and immobility should be considered. Chest physiotherapy and suctioning, and turning the patient to prevent decubiti are all essential components of the supportive care required by the comatose patient.

Local Exposure

Various chemicals such as strong acids and bases are quite toxic when they come in direct contact with the skin, eyes, or mucous membranes. In the majority of instances, damage is caused by a direct effect of the chemical on the exposed tissue. There are a number of compounds, however, that are capable of producing systemic toxicity via percutaneous absorption. Examples of these agents include the carbamate and organophosphate insecticides and the halogenated hydrocarbons.

The clinician treating a topical or inhalation exposure must consider and treat all body areas exposed to the chemical agent. If, for example, a patient is in an enclosed area and exposed to a toxic gas, the patient must be removed to fresh air. Oxygen administration and/or artificial respiration may be necessary following prolonged exposure to some toxic gases. Additionally, care must be taken to decontaminate all exposed areas such as the nose, mouth, eyes, and skin.

A skin exposure should be terminated by immediate irrigation with large volumes of water. The two most important considerations are the amount of fluid and time. Large amounts of fluid must be used as quickly after the exposure as possible. Time should not be wasted looking for a specific agent that will neutralize the chemical. Large amounts of water can be delivered by using a faucet, hose or shower. Vinegar or baking soda or other acids and bases should not be used for neutralization of base or acid exposure, respectively. Neutralization may cause additional tissue damage as a result of heat released from this exothermic reaction and thus is not recommended. Other liquids that have been used in emergency situations when water has not been available include soft drinks, beer or even urine (15).

Topical exposure to agents that can be absorbed and produce systemic toxicity (e.g., chlorinated and organophosphate insecticides) requires both local and systemic therapy. Mechanical washing as described previously will reduce any local irritation as well as reduce the amount available for further absorption.

With many of the fat-soluble compounds, soap and water is useful for removing the agent and decreasing absorption. Two areas are commonly missed that may provide a reservoir for further absorption: the clothes and the hair. All exposed clothing must be removed. If the hair is exposed it too must be thoroughly washed. Care must also be taken by members of the treatment team to avoid exposure to the chemical. As these chemicals are percutaneously absorbed, all persons directly involved in decontaminating the patient should wear gloves. Further treatment must also be aimed toward the systemic sequelae resulting from percutaneous absorption in the patient.

Exposure of the eye to caustic chemicals can cause burns of the cornea and conjunctiva. Instillation of a specific neutralizing agent into the eye is generally considered detrimental. An exception to this rule is treatment of Lewisite burns with BAL (9). The basic first-aid treatment for an eye exposure is to immediately flood the eye with copious amounts of water for at least 10 to 15 min. Industrial areas where exposure is likely to take place are commonly provided with foot-operated eye baths. If this is not the case, usually the most efficient washing procedure is to directly place the patient's head underneath a faucet. Cool or lukewarm water is then run directly from the bridge of the nose into the eye(s). The eyelids should be held open throughout the washing procedure. Any exposure of the eye to chemicals must be considered quite serious. In all but the least harmful exposures, an ophthalmologist should be seen, preferably within 2 hours of exposure. Note that the use of topical corticosteroids is contraindicated in alkali burns.

Decreasing Absorption

If absorption of the ingested agent from the gastrointestinal tract can be minimized one can decrease the toxic potential of an ingestion. This may be accomplished by emptying the stomach, administering an absorbent and inducing catharsis. These modalities of therapy are indicated when a toxic amount of a potentially toxic substance has been ingested within a reasonable time period. For most substances, this time period is within the past 4 hours. Exceptions include salicylates which delay gastric emptying, anticholinergics which decrease GI motility and phenytoin which is slowly and erratically absorbed from the GI tract. For drugs such as these emptying the GI tract may be warranted 10 to 12 hours post-ingestion.

The stomach may be emptied by inducing emesis or performing gastric lavage. The trend in management has favored emesis over lavage, since studies have generally indicated a more efficient removal of stomach contents through the induction of emesis (16–20).

Probably the most descriptive analysis of the efficacy of ipecac syrup-induced emesis was reported by Boxer et al. (19) in 1969. They examined 20 patients between 12 and 20 months of age who had ingested salicylates. Lavage was performed and emesis induced on each patient and the amount of salicylates returned by each method was measured. Approximately one half of the patients were lavaged first and the other half were given syrup of ipecac first. Overall, ipecac removed significantly more salicylate than lavage, even when emesis was induced after lavage was completed. They concluded that "ipecac-induced emesis is superior to gastric lavage for emptying the stomach per os of unwanted contents ... and ipecac-induced emesis leaves little or no salicylate which could potentially be removed by lavage."

Goldstein (20) reported two acute overdoses in adults seen 10 to 15 min after ingestion. Each patient was lavaged with 3 liters of normal saline through a 20 French tube. Both patients were then given ipecac and vomited successfully. In one case 25 tablets were found in the vomitus and in the other 10 to 15 tablets. This was after lavage had been completed.

It must be pointed out that, in many of these studies including the two described above, either the size of the lavage tube is not mentioned or it is smaller than is currently recommended. The smaller tubes, including Levine tubes and urethral catheters that have been used in the past, are clearly too small to remove large particles of tablets, whole tablets, or groups of tablets clumped together. Lavage with a large Ewald tube, 28 to 36 French or larger, should more efficiently empty the stomach and may in fact be as effective as emesis.

Another important clinical consideration is that the percentage return with both emesis and lavage is low. In 14 humans given magnesium hydroxide and then ipecac, a mean return of 28 ± 7.0% was found with a range of

0 to 78% (21). Arnold et al. (18) showed under optimal conditions dogs that had been given sodium salicylate would return 38% (range 2 to 69%) after lavage and 45% after ipecac-induced emesis. When the administration of ipecac was delayed until 30 min postingestion and lavage was not performed until 1 hour postingestion, only 13% (range 0 to 40%) was removed by lavage and 39% (range 5 to 74%) by emesis (18). It is important to note that a small tube, 16 French was used for lavage. In a similar study in dogs with barium sulfate 29 ± 10%, with a range of 10 to 62%, was returned with gastric lavage, 19 ± 9%, with a range of 2 to 31%, with ipecac and 74 ± 5% with a range of 54 to 87% with apomorphine (22).

It is clear that neither emesis nor lavage completely empty the stomach. This fact underscores the importance of the administration of an absorbent and a cathartic following either emesis or lavage. Until more data are available the choice between emesis and lavage is a difficult one. It is our opinion that emesis with syrup of ipecac should routinely be the procedure of first choice. In those cases where emetics are contraindicated, e.g., the CNS depressed patient, lavage with a large bore tube is preferred. Lavage should also be performed if induction of emesis with ipecac fails.

Emetics

Emetics (Table 1.1) are agents that induce vomiting (emesis). Although emetics can act locally on the GI tract and/or centrally through stimulation of the chemoreceptor trigger zone and the vomiting center, vomiting can be produced only if medullary centers are still responsive. Emetics are absolutely contraindicated in the following situations: (a) patients with significant CNS depression manifested by severe lethargy, loss of gag reflex or unconsciousness. In this instance, the emetic may not produce vomiting and if it does, the risk of aspiration of the vomitus into the lungs, a potentially fatal consequence, is significant; (b) patients who are seizing or in whom seizures are imminent since aspiration is a significant risk in these patients as well; and (c) patients who have ingested a caustic since strong acids and bases may produce severe burns of the mucous membranes of the mouth and esophagus. By inducing emesis these tissues will be reexposed to the caustic and further damage may occur. In addition, the force of vomiting may cause perforation of the damaged esophagus.

The question often arises as to whether emetics should be administered following an antiemetic overdose. Theoretically, because of their antagonistic pharmacologic effects, the antiemetic may block the action of the emetic. Although this issue has been addressed in the literature, it remains controversial. Two studies have concluded that antiemetics do not significantly interfere with the effectiveness of emetics (23, 24). Both studies are plagued by insufficient data, however, since neither study

Table 1.1.
Comparison of Emetics (Arbitrary Values 0 to 4)

	Ipecac Syrup (30 ml limit)	Apomorphine Hydrochloride	Copper Sulfate	Zinc Sulfate	Antimony and Potassium Tartrate	Salt Water	Mustard Powder	Mechanical
Effectiveness	4	4	3	2	2	1	1	1
Speed of action:								
Home	3	0[a]	0[a]	0[a]	0[a]	2	2	2
Hospital	3	4	1	1	1	1	1	4
Safety	4	3	1	1	1	1	4	4
Lack of need for antidote	4	2	1	1	1	4	4	4
Ready availability:								
Home	2	1	1	1	1	4	2	4
Hospital	4	3	1	1	1	3	1	4
Low cost	4	1	4	4	4	4	4	4
Acceptance by patient	4	1	1	1	1	1	1	1

[a] Generally not available. Numbers used consider ready availability in each area. (Adapted from T. M. Cashman and H. C. Shirkey: Emergency management of poisoning, *Pediatric Clinics of North America, 17:*525, 1970).

addresses the issues of the amount ingested and the time between ingestion and emesis nor quantities through laboratory analysis whether a sufficient quantity of the ingested agent was present to produce an antiemetic effect. For example, in the retrospective study by Thomas and Verhulst (23), 94.5% of the patients who ingested antiemetics vomited compared with 96.2% of those who ingested antiemetic as well as other drugs. The failure rate for ipecac syrup in 166 patients who had taken phenothiazines was 7.83%. If, however, one compares the figures for phenothiazines vs. all drugs other than phenothiazines the failure rates are 7.83% (13/153) and 2.68% (21/184), respectively. Although these investigators conclude that there is not a significant difference, we feel that emetics must be used cautiously in phenothiazine ingestions. This concern is substantiated by the fact that three of the cases of serious toxicity related to ipecac administration involve patients who ingested a phenothiazine, failed to vomit with ipecac and developed cardiac toxicity (25, 26). We, therefore, suggest that ipecac be reserved for asymptomatic patients who have just ingested the antiemetic, e.g., within the past hour. If ipecac is used, and vomiting does not occur, lavage is indicated.

Another controversial issue involves the use of emetics in petroleum distillate (e.g., kerosene, gasoline) exposures. For years, emetics were considered to be contraindicated in petroleum distillate ingestions since it was believed that inducing vomiting would increase the likelihood of aspiration. Petroleum distillates, because of their low viscosity, low surface tension and high volatility are extremely likely to be aspirated and produce significant pulmonary toxicity. When aliphatic hydrocarbons are ingested, emptying the stomach is unnecessary. In those situations, however, where a potentially dangerous chemical in a petroleum distillate base, e.g., pesticides, has been ingested the stomach should be emptied. In a retrospective study of cases reported to the National Clearinghouse for Poison Control Centers, Molinas (27) found that the highest incidence of aspiration pneumonitis following the ingestion of a petroleum distillate occurred in those with spontaneous vomiting (13.3%). In the same series, 136 patients were given syrup of ipecac with no cases of aspiration. Of a total of 244 cases in which syrup of ipecac was given only two cases of pneumonitis oc-

curred. Three percent of those who were lavaged developed aspiration pneumonitis, the same percentage seen in those where the stomach was not emptied or that information was not provided. Similar findings were seen in turpentine ingestions. In a more recent study Ng et al. (28) showed that aspiration pneumonitis was seen on the initial radiograph of 28% of patients treated with ipecac and 56% of those who were lavaged. In addition, the pneumonitis that developed was more severe in those who were lavaged than in those who were given syrup of ipecac. On the basis of these studies and recent clinical experience, most clinicians would agree that an emetic such as syrup of ipecac can be administered in a petroleum distillate ingestion, although many feel that emetics should not be given in petroleum distillate ingestions unless the patient is supervised by a health professional. There is still considerable disagreement over the indications for removal of hydrocarbons from the stomach.

As Table 1.1 indicates, there are many potential emetics which could be considered to empty the stomach in a poisoning. The majority of these agents are not recommended, however, because of a lack of effectiveness or because of toxicity. As a result, syrup of ipecac is considered the emetic of choice.

Syrup of ipecac, a local and centrally acting emetic, should not be confused with fluid extract of ipecac which is 14 times stronger. Ipecac syrup is available without prescription in appropriately labeled 15- and 30-ml vials. The value of ipecac as an emetic has been known for hundreds of years but its use diminished as gastric lavage gained popularity. During the 1950s, the dosage of ipecac was increased and it was shown to be more effective than previously believed, especially when it was given with adequate fluid. Analysis of reports from various sources suggests that syrup of ipecac is almost 100% effective in producing emesis when 15 ml or more are given (29, 30). Unfortunately, very little work has been done to analyze the efficacy of the ipecac-induced expulsion. Only a few individuals have measured the amount of return from ipecac-induced emesis. It is common knowledge, however, that emesis induced with ipecac is more forceful (and presumably more efficient) than mechanically induced emesis but less forceful than following apomorphine (Table 1.1).

Vomiting usually occurs about 18 min after administration of a 15- to 30-ml dose. As the average time between ingestion and delivery of the patient to the hospital is somewhat greater than 1 hour, the long onset time for ipecac as compared with apomorphine (3 to 5 min) becomes less important (31).

The dose of syrup of ipecac is 10 ml in children under 1 year of age, 15 ml in older children and 15 to 30 ml in adolescents and adults. Fluid administration is important since induction of vomiting may not be successful if the stomach is near empty. Since milk significantly increases the time for vomiting to occur when given with syrup of ipecac, any other fluid, e.g., water or fruit juice, is preferred (32). At least 6 to 8 oz are recommended in children and 12 to 16 oz in adults. If vomiting does not occur in 15 to 20 min, the initial dose may be repeated one time.

The most common side effects of therapeutic doses of ipecac are diarrhea and mild drowsiness. The latter may be secondary to vomiting and not a direct pharmacologic effect. Toxic reactions to large amounts of syrup of ipecac or due to the inadvertent use of the fluid extract of ipecac have been reported with the most frequent complications being gastrointestinal and cardiovascular. In large doses, ipecac is a specific cardiotoxin and has been shown to cause reversible depression of T waves, bradycardia, atrial fibrillation and hypotension. Death has been reported following ingestion of as little as 10 ml of the fluid extract in a 4-year-old child (33).

If a child ingests 1 oz of the syrup (the largest amount available without prescription) no real danger exists. If 1 oz is administered to a child and the child does not vomit, the decision as to whether the child should be lavaged would be based primarily on the condition of the child and the potential danger of the ingested agent and not on the fact that the ipecac remains in the stomach.

Apomorphine is a morphine derivative that produces emesis through a central mechanism. It acts very quickly, usually within 3 to 5 min when given subcutaneously. Apomorphine is successful in producing evacuation of large particle of food, enteric-coated tablets and a reflux of contents from the upper intestinal tract. Animal and human studies have shown apomorphine to cause a more violent emesis and a more efficient evacuation than ipecac. Despite these advantage, apomorphine is not considered the emetic of choice. Since it must be administered parenterally, apomorphine is available only in a hospital setting and thus its use is more limited than the readily available ipecac (21). Apomorphine is unstable in solution and must be prepared from a hypodermic tablet immediately prior to use. In addition, apomorphine may produce protracted vomiting as well as CNS, respiratory and cardiovascular depression. In several recent reports, significant respiratory and/or CNS depression has developed in patients who had been given apomorphine which did not respond to naloxone (34).

Therefore, because apomorphine's potential for toxicity outweighs the benefit of a faster onset of action, we feel that apomorphine should not be used in the management of the poisoned patient.

Copper and zinc sulfate work by direct irritation of the gastric mucosa. Although vomiting usually occurs within 5 to 10 min, these agents do not reliably empty the stomach. In addition, gradual absorption from the bowel may occur and cause systemic poisoning. The toxicity of these compounds includes widespread capillary damage and kidney and liver injury. Because of their toxicity and the availability of better agents, these drugs are not recommended.

Salt water and mustard water (made from dry mustard powder) are both unreliable emetics. Since they are both so unpalatable, much time is wasted in coaxing a child to drink these solutions. When salt water is administered, significant quantities of sodium chloride can be absorbed producing hypernatremia and convulsions. Since salt water has produced fatalities in young children and adults, it should never be used (35–38). Mustard water is not routinely recommended since it is ineffective.

Mechanically induced emesis or gagging by stroking the pharynx with either a blunt object or a finger is ineffective and should not be used. Although this method is universally available, the percentage of people who vomit after this procedure is quite low and the mean volume of vomitus is low as compared with other methods. This was probably best illustrated by Dabbous et al. (31) who studied 30 children in the emergency room. The children were gagged at home by their parents and only two vomited with an average volume of vomitus of 50 to 60 ml. All 30 patients were gagged in the emergency room by a nurse. Two of these vomited with a mean volume of vomitus of 90 ml. All 30 were then given syrup of ipecac. All vomited with an average volume of 380 ml with a range of 30 to 1000 ml.

Gastric Lavage

Gastric lavage is a procedure in which a tube is inserted into the stomach via the esophagus. The patient is placed in the left lateral decubitus position with the head forward and down. The tube may be inserted via the nose (nasogastric) or the mouth (orogastric). The contents of the stomach are first aspirated through this tube. Fluid is then instilled into the tube, allowed to mix with gastric contents, and then removed via the same tube. The process is repeated until the gastric washing are clear. The procedure usually takes 20 to 30 min to complete. In contrast with emesis, lavage can be performed only by medical personnel.

Lavage may be performed on patients with significant CNS depression including coma. It is important, however, that the patient's airway be protected by prior insertion of a cuffed endotracheal tube to prevent aspiration. Patients with convulsions may be lavaged once their seizures have been controlled with an anticonvulsant. Lavage is contraindicated in caustic ingestions since the lavage tube may produce additional esophageal and gastric damage as it is being passed. Initial management of a caustic ingestion is limited to dilution with milk or water followed by an evaluation of the extent and degree of burns.

The size of the lavage tube is one of the most important factors determining the effectiveness with which the stomach will be emptied. Optimally a 36 French (12 mm or about ½ inch in diameter) or larger Ewald or Lavacuator tube should be used by the oral route in adults. Nasogastric tubes usually are smaller and therefore less effective. Smaller tubes (16 to 18 French) must be used in children, markedly limiting the effectiveness of the procedure.

The lavage solution is usually tap water or a saline solution. In children, however, it is safer to use normal or one-half normal saline instead of water due to the child's limited tolerance of electrolyte-free solution. Water intoxication, tonic and clonic seizures, and coma can result from an increase of 5% of body water from electrolyte-free solutions. Each wash is approximately 200 to 300 ml in adults or 10 ml/kg (usually 50 to 100 ml) in children. The procedure usually requires several liters of fluid in adults.

In some cases, solutions which chemically inactivate or detoxify the unabsorbed poison can be used. An example of this is the use of sodium bicarbonate solution with overdoses of ferrous salts. Theoretically, this produces the less corrosive and more insoluble ferrous carbonate. Most previously recommended special gastric lavage fluids, e.g., potassium permanganate and tannic acid, have not scientifically been shown to be superior to saline or water. In addition, with many of these solutions the time it takes to find, or make up the solutions, is long. This fact coupled with the possible additional toxicity from the tannic acid, or other agent used, make it difficult to recommend these agents.

When lavage is completed, it is usually a good idea to instill activated charcoal and a cathartic via the tube before it is pulled.

Local Antidotes

Following emesis or lavage, an adsorbent should be administered to bind any of the ingested agent remaining in the GI tract. Activated charcoal, a nonspecific adsorbent, is recommended because of its efficacy as well as it lack of toxicity.

Activated charcoal is an odorless, tasteless, fine black powder that is an effective nonspecific adsorbent of a wide variety of drugs and chemicals. Two characteristics are necessary for activated charcoal to be effective: (a) small particle size and thus large surface area and (b) low mineral content (vegetable origin). For these reasons neither burnt toast nor charcoal tablets are effective. Activated charcoal should be stored in tightly sealed glass or metal containers. Prolonged exposure to vapors of the atmosphere will decrease adsorptive capability.

Activated charcoal has been compared to several other adsorbents—attapulgite, Arizona montmorillonite and evaporated milk. All four of these compounds are somewhat effective. Activated charcoal has, however, been shown to have the broadest spectrum of adsorptive activity (39, 40). Arizona montmorillonite suffers from a poor affinity for anions and organic acids. In its favor, however, is a large surface area and greater esthetic appeal than activated charcoal. Attapulgite is much less effective than activated charcoal in limiting absorption of sodium salicylate. Evaporated milk is not as effective an adsorbent as activated charcoal. It does have the advantage, however, of greater availability. At this time we recommend continued use of activated charcoal.

When given in adequate dosage, activated charcoal is highly effective. Some say it is an effective antidote for virtually all organic and inorganic compounds and cite cyanide as the only exception. Recent evidence, however, does not support this. Activated charcoal also has been shown to be relatively ineffective with ethanol, methanol, caustic alkalis and mineral acids (41). It is, however, quite effective for most other agents. Charcoal should be given in an amount approximately 10 times the amount of the ingested agent. Thus if 3 g of a barbiturate were taken, 30 g of activated charcoal should be administered. Since this does not take into account tablet excipients or food which may bind to the charcoal decreasing its adsorptive capacity it is a good idea to give an excess of charcoal. If the amount taken is unknown, 30 to 60 g (1 to 2 oz) in adults or 1 g/kg in children, should be given. One level measuring tablespoonful of activated charcoal contains between 5 and 6 g. Thus, 1 oz of activated charcoal is 5 to 6 tablespoonfuls. It is a good idea for the pharmacy to prepackage weighed charcoal since the density of charcoal products may vary.

Activated charcoal is mixed with water to the consistency of a slurry and is administered to the patient either orally or by lavage tube. Charcoal does not mix well with water and must be shaken vigorously. To overcome this problem, Manes and Mann (42) tested a suspension of activated charcoal, water, and several thickeners including sodium carboxymethyl cellulose (CMC), sodium alginate, carrageenan, bentonite and gelatin. CMC appeared the most promising and in vitro it did not interfere with the adsorptive capacity of the charcoal. Subsequent in vivo tests have been inconclusive. Gwilt and Perrier (43) have shown that a 2% CMC in charcoal slurry did not significantly affect adsorptive capacity, whereas Mathur et al. (44) demonstrated a reduction in adsorptive capacity for aspirin of a 3.5% CMC in charcoal slurry. Additional studies must be done to determine which agents can be used to increase the lubricity and palatability of the charcoal without affecting the adsorptive capacity. Until that time we do not recommend the addition of suspending agents or flavoring agents to the activated charcoal slurry.

Activated charcoal effectively adsorbs ipecac. Thus if syrup of ipecac is given after charcoal, vomiting will not occur and the adsorptive capacity will be reduced. If these agents are to be used together, the activated charcoal must be given after successful vomiting from ipecac has occurred.

The universal antidote is universally useless. This preparation consists of activated charcoal, an antacid (usually magnesium oxide) and a supposed precipitator of alkaloids (usually tannic acid). The two latter agents not only fail in large part to serve their avowed functions but instead inactivate the single useful ingredient—activated charcoal. Also important is the fact that tannic acid is a hepatotoxin. Activated charcoal alone should be used in place of the universal antidote. The home remedy consisting of burned toast, tea, and milk of magnesia is equally useless.

Acids and bases have been suggested to neutralize orally ingested bases and acids, respectively. Since these mixtures may produce an exothermic reaction they may produce even worse burns. Following the ingestion of a caustic, administration of milk, or water, as soon after the ingestion as possible, is preferred.

Cathartics

Cathartics are used in poisoning cases to further decrease the absorption of the ingested agent from the GI tract. This is especially true if an adsorbent, e.g., activated charcoal, has been used. By speeding the travel of gastric contents, absorption is decreased. Although there are no clinical studies in overdose patients to document that this is indeed the case, an animal study demonstrated that sodium sulfate enhanced the effect of activated charcoal in preventing the absorption of the drugs tested (45).

Saline cathartics are the agents of choice. Irritant cathartics such as aloes or cascara and oil-based cathartics such as castor oil, are generally not recommended.

Magnesium sulfate and sodium sulfate are the two major saline cathartics used. Magnesium sulfate is available as Epsom's salts or as a sterile 10% or 50% solution. The solutions are more commonly available in emergency rooms. The absorbed magnesium is rapidly excreted by normal kidneys. Absorbed magnesium accumulates in patients with decreased renal function and may produce magnesium toxicity. Sodium sulfate is available as Glauber's salt. This agent is not generally available in emergency rooms. The dose for either agent is the same, 250 mg/kg or approximately 15 to 20 g in an adult administered in approximately a 10% concentration. Magnesium citrate is available commercially and may be used in a dose of 200 ml in adolescents and adults. Thirty milliliters of the sodium phosphate-biphosphate solution in Fleet's enema may be diluted 1:4 with water and administered *orally* as a saline cathartic in poisoning.

It is critical to understand that these agents must be administered orally or via lavage tube. The onset of action is within 3 hours and these agents may be repeated in 4 to 6 hours if needed. If charcoal has been administered the appearance of a charcoal stool indicates that the charcoal (and hopefully the toxic agent) has transited the GI tract.

Hastening Excretion

If a poison has been absorbed in potentially dangerous quantities, it becomes necessary to examine mechanisms of minimizing the toxic effects by hastening elimination. Procedures such as forced diuresis, alteration of urine pH, dialysis and hemoperfusion may be considered in the moderately to severely intoxicated patient. These procedures, however, will not be warranted in the majority of poisoned patients and should in no way supplant good supportive care.

Some drugs are resecreted into the stomach or undergo biliary secretion. Recently advantage has been taken of these two factors in an attempt to augment excretion of these drugs via the GI tract. Since phencyclidine, a weak base, is resecreted into the stomach acid, management of a severely intoxicated patient can include continuous or intermittent gastric suction or repeated doses of activated charcoal (46). Similarly since tricyclic antidepressant and their active metabolites undergo enterhepatic recycling, many clinicians recommended repeated administration of activated charcoal every 6 to 8 hours to bind the drug and prevent its absorption.

Forced Diuresis and Alteration of Urine pH

Enhancing the renal elimination of drugs for which this route is the predominant pathway of elimination has been a component of managing the poisoned patient for years. The composition of urine is determined by a combination of ultrafiltration, active tubular secretion and tubular reabsorption. Tubular reabsorption can be either an active or a passive process. Essential compounds, such as glucose and sodium, are actively reabsorbed, whereas foreign substances such as poisons, are generally passively reabsorbed. Since passive tubular reabsorption is determined by the volume and pH of the tubular fluid, retention of water in the filtrate and alteration of urine pH may decrease the gradient for reabsorption of some weak acids and bases. Forced diuresis depresses tubular reabsorption and is accomplished by administering fluid and a diuretic such as mannitol or furosemide. The goal is a urine output of a 3 to 6 ml/kg/hour (47). Care must be taken that too much fluid is not administered producing cerebral or pulmonary edema. Forced diuresis is specifically recommended for alcohol, amphetamines, bromide, phenobarbital, isoniazid, salicylates and strychnine.

Only the unionized form of weak acids and bases is capable of crossing membranes and thus being reabsorbed. Weak acids will be ionized in an alkaline pH while weak bases will be ionized in an acidic medium. By adjusting the pH of the tubular filtrate, for some drugs it is possible to increase the amount of drug in the ionized form, thereby decreasing tubular reabsorption. Clinically, the effectiveness of urine pH alteration will depend on the pKa of the drug and the extent of renal elimination of active drug. Examples where pH manipulations are thought to be effective include phenobarbital (not useful for short acting barbiturates, e.g., pentobarbital and secobarbital) isoniazid, and salicylate (alkalinization) and amphetamines, phencyclidine and strychnine (acidification). The urine is acidified with ammonium chloride (75 mg/kg per day in 4 doses orally or slowly IV) or ascorbic acid (usually 4 to 6 g per day up to 12 g per day in 4 to 6 doses orally or slowly IV). Although ascorbic acid is less effective it is often tried initially because of its lack of toxicity. The goal is a urine pH of 4.5 to 5.5. Urinary alkalinization is accomplished through the use of sodium bicarbonate (usually in adults 7 g is added to the first liter of IV fluid with a total dose of 10 to 15 g per day; 2 mEq/kg is added to initial IV fluids in the pediatric patient and infused over an hour). The goal is a urine pH of 7.0 to 8.0. Alkalinization of the urine in salicylate poisoning is controversial and is no longer recommended by some clinicians (48). Although tromethamine and acetazolamide have been recommended as alkalinizing agents in the past these are no longer recommended because of their potential toxicities which may worsen the course of the intoxication. When one attempts to either acidify or alkalinize the urine, the patient's acid base status must be carefully monitored.

Dialysis and Hemoperfusion

In the severely intoxicated patient dialysis or hemoperfusion may be considered to rapidly remove certain toxins from the blood.

Dialysis refers to the therapeutic procedure whereby unwanted solutes in the plasma are allowed to diffuse across a dialysis membrane into a solution. This solution, the dialysate, is replaced continuously, or intermittently, with fresh solution of carefully defined composition, so the diffusional transport is allowed to continue. In preparing solutions suitable for dialysis, all diffusible solutes should, in theory, be present in concentrations approximating those in an ultrafiltrate of normal plasma. Two basic types of dialysis are used. They are extracorporeal hemodialysis (the "artificial kidney") and peritoneal dialysis.

Hemodialysis, in which drugs are removed from the blood by diffusion across a synthetic semipermeable membrane, is more efficient than peritoneal dialysis. This is a specialized technique and one not available at all hospitals.

Peritoneal dialysis, in which dialysate is instilled into the peritoneum, is less effective than hemodialysis. Generally, peritoneal dialysis will remove the same material as extracorporeal hemodialysis but requires much more time to do so. Peritoneal dialysis does offer the advantages of being adaptable to any hospital setting, requiring less experience and training, and eliminating the need for elaborate equipment. Contraindications for its use are infections of the peritoneal cavity and recent or extensive abdominal surgery. Effectiveness is diminished in the presence of hypotension and vasoconstriction. In some situations, effectiveness may be enhanced by altering the pH or adding albumin to the dialysate.

The use of dialysis in poisoning cases is limited. To be considered, the ingested agent must both be dialyzable and removed at a rate significantly higher than by normal metabolism and renal excretion. Because a drug is dialyzable does not mean that dialysis is indicated, e.g., penicillin.

Dialysis may be considered in those patients who are severely intoxicated with a dialyzable drug and are not responding to conservative therapy. One may also consider dialysis in those situations where the agent ingested is not dialyzable but the procedure is necessary to support the patient, i.e., (a) hyperosmolarity not easily corrected by fluids and (b) severe acid base or electrolyte abnormalities not responding to therapy (47).

Two examples of situations where dialysis may be indicated immediately are methanol and ethylene glycol ingestion. In both cases these agents are metabolized to compounds more toxic than the originally ingested agent. Methanol is metabolized to formaldehyde and ethylene glycol to oxalic acid. If the methanol and ethylene glycol can be removed via dialysis before metabolism, toxicity will be reduced.

Hemoperfusion involves pumping blood from the patient through a cartridge containing coated activated charcoal, uncoated activated charcoal in a fixed-bed system, or a resin such as Amerlite XAD-4. The use of hemoperfusion in the management of poisoning is relatively new compared with dialysis. To be effective not only must the toxin be adsorbed by the material in the column but the amount removed by hemoperfusion must significantly reduce the total body burden of the ingested agent. For some drugs which are effectively adsorbed, a large volume of distribution results in a relatively small proportion of the total body burden being eliminated even if the blood is completely cleared of the drug after passing through the column. Theophylline is an example of a drug for which hemoperfusion has been found to be extremely effective, producing a marked drop in blood levels and a rapid improvement in clinical picture (49).

Early studies of hemoperfusion in animals found embolization of charcoal particles as a potential complication of the procedure. On necropsy of all perfused rabbits, Hagstam et al. (50) found no macroscopic abnormalities but microscopic examination revealed charcoal particles in the lungs of all the hemoperfused animals, in the spleen of 66% and in the kidneys of 25% of treated animals. This problem has been minimized through the use of more effective filters as well as coating or fixing the charcoal. Other potential complications include bleeding, destruction of blood cells including a significant drop in the platelet count immediately following the procedure, removal of plasma proteins and hypothermia (51).

As is the case with dialysis, hemoperfusion should be limited to those severely intoxicated patients who have ingested an hemoperfusable drug who are not responding to conservative therapy. In most situations, aggressive supportive care should be adequate to maintain the patient until his own body is able to detoxify and eliminate the toxin.

Systemic Antidotes

Systemic antidotes are available for only a few commonly ingested agents. These agents may act by a variety of mechanisms to antagonize the effects of a systemically absorbed toxin. Most poisons do not have a specific antidote.

When the use of an antidote is considered, several things must be kept in mind. Antidotes are an addition to other treatment modalities and not a replacement for them. The use of an antidote does not normally replace the need for supportive measures, emptying the stomach, etc. If an antidote is available for a particular intoxicant, it is not always necessary that it be used. Thus, there are specific indications for the use of an antidote.

Included in Table 1.2 is a list of major systemic antidotes. Three of the most important of these: (a) naloxone, (b) deferoxamine and (c) physostigmine, are discussed below in detail. For further information on antidotes the reader is referred to specific management protocols for the agent involved to determine whether an antidote is available. These managements are available in the poison information sources discussed previously.

NALOXONE

Naloxone (N-allynoroxymorphone) is a pure narcotic antagonist possessing no narcotic agonist properties. Previously used narcotic antagonists, nalorphine and levallorphan, have narcotic agonist and antagonist properties. The agonist activity became clinically important when nalorphine or levallorphan were given to patients who were intoxicated with drugs other than narcotics. In a comatose, apneic patient making the distinction between narcotic and non-narcotic ingestions may be difficult. If nalorphine or levallorphan is given to a patient who had taken barbiturates, for example, CNS and respiratory depression could be produced or worsened. With naloxone one does not have this problem. If a narcotic is involved, one would see an immediate reversal of narcotic agonist effects. If a narcotic is not involved, no effect will be observed. For this reason nalorphine and levallorphan should not be used and naloxone is considered the narcotic antagonist of choice.

Naloxone directly competes with the narcotic for the receptor site reversing CNS and respiratory depression. The antagonistic effects usually last at most from 1 to 4 hours. It is important to note that the antagonistic action of naloxone will likely be shorter than the duration of action of the ingested agent. This is especially true when drugs like methadone and diphenoxylate that have a very long duration of action have been taken. It is very important that these patients be watched carefully and that naloxone be readministerd as needed.

Naloxone antagonizes those drugs that one commonly thinks of as narcotics, e.g., heroin, morphine, codeine, and meperidine. In addition, naloxone reverses the effects of propoxyphene, pentazocine, diphenoxylate, and dextromethorphan. Naloxone should be used in severe intoxications with CNS and respiratory depression thought to be caused by narcotics. Thus a patient, seen in the emergency room and who by history has taken codeine but is awake and alert with stable vital signs, need not be given naloxone until his clinical status requires it.

Naloxone should be given at a dose of 0.01 mg/kg intravenously and repeated as needed. The usual adult dosage is 0.4 to 0.8 mg. If no response is seen with the first dose of naloxone, 2 to 4 mg can be administered to both pediatric and adults patients (52). In patients who have ingested a long acting narcotic, such as methadone, a continuous infusion of naloxone in a concentration of 4 mg/liter at a rate of 0.4 mg/hour can be considered after the initial bolus dose of naloxone reverses the narcotic effects.

DEFEROXAMINE

Deferoxamine is a chelating agent that binds with ferric iron. The iron-deferoxamine complex is less toxic and more easily excreted than

Table 1.2.
Major Systemic Antidotes

Antidote	Poison	Usual Dosage and Route	Comments
Atroptine	Carbamate insecticides Organophosphate insecticides Other anticholinesterase	Test dose of 2 mg IV in an adult and 0.05 mg/kg in a child up to 2 mg; anticholinergic symptoms will be seen only if poisoning is not present. Doses are repeated as needed (up to 2000 mg/day in severe cases) with the endpoint being cessation of secretions	In severe organophosphate ingestions usually given in combination with pralidoxime
BAL	Arsenic, gold, mercury, lead	Given by deep IM. Dosage variable depending on the agent being chelated and severity of intoxication. Usually 3–5 mg/kg/dose	Contraindicated in iron, cadmium, or selenium since complex is toxic. For lead used in combination with other agents and only in acute lead poisoning in children
Cyanide antidote kit Amyl nitrite Sodium nitrite Sodium thiosulfate	Cyanide	Amyl nitrite-breathe 30 sec of each 60 sec until sodium nitrite is ready. For adults 300 mg of sodium nitrite (10 ml) is usually given IV followed by 12.5 g of sodium thiosulfate IV. If symptoms persist one half the above dosage of sodium nitrite is repeated. The dose for children depends on the hemoglobin level and is included in the package literature	Overzealous administration of sodium nitrite in children can produce a severe methemoglobinemia.
Deferoxamine	Iron	In children 90 mg/kg IM up to 1 g every 8 hr. In adults an initial dose of 1.0 g followed by 0.5 g every 4 hr for 2 more doses. Additional 0.5-g doses may be given every 4 hr as needed. A maximum of 6.0 g in either children or adults/24 hr should not be exceeded. If the patient is in shock the above doses should be given at a rate not to exceed 15 mg/kg/hr IV	Pink-red urine indicates the presence of the deferoxamine-iron chelate
Diphenhydramine	Phenothiazine-induced extrapyramidal symptoms	Adults 50 mg IV. Children 1–2 mg/kg up to a total of 50 mg IV	
D-Penicillamine	Copper, gold mercury, lead arsenic	Children 20–40 mg/kg/day Adults 1–1.5 g/day	Avoid in patients with penicillin allergy. Inhibits enzymes that are pyridoxal dependent thus pyridoxine usually given concurrently (10–25 mg/day)

Table 1.2—*continued*

Antidote	Poison	Usual Dosage and Route	Comments
Ca-EDTA	Lead, zinc, cadmium, manganese, copper	75 mg/kg per day IV or IM given in 3–6 divided doses for up to 5 days. May repeat course after at least 2 days	May produce renal tubular necrosis. If decreased renal function present dialysis may be necessary to remove chelate
Ethanol	Ethylene glycol, methanol	Ethanol is given to maintain a 100 mg/dl blood level. Loading dose (oral) is 0.8 ml/kg of 95% ethanol given over 30 min followed by an average maintenance dose of 0.15 ml/kg/hr PO. Loading dose (IV) of 10% ethanol is 7.6 ml/kg IV over 30–60 min followed by an average maintenance dose of 1.4 ml/kg/hr IV. Monitor blood levels of ethanol and adjust dose accordingly	Chronic drinkers may require higher doses and nondrinkers may require lower doses. Dosage must be adjusted if dialysis. Glucose usually simultaneously administered
Methylene blue	Nitrates and nitrites	0.2 ml/kg IV over 5 min of a 1% solution	
N-Acetylcysteine	Acetaminophen	140 mg/kg orally diluted 1:3 with Coke, Fresca, grapefruit juice or water as a loading dose. Then 70 mg/kg every 4 hr for a total of 17 maintenance doses	Investigational. Call Rocky Mountain Poison Center (303-534-0312) for further information
Naloxone	Narcotics	0.005–0.01 mg/kg/dose IV; 0.4–0.8 mg in adults. If no response, give 2–4 mg IV (see text)	Should be given several times if no effect before ruling out narcotics as the cause of symptoms. Short duration of action. Levallorphan and nalorphine are no longer recommended
Physostigmine	Anticholinergics, including tricyclic antidepressants	Pediatric dose: 0.5 mg slow IV. If no response and no cholinergic symptoms given 0.5 mg every 5 min until a response is seen or 2 mg is reached. Repeat lowest effective trial dose if severe symptoms recur. Adults: 1–2 mg slow IV. May repeat up to 4 mg total if no response and no cholinergic symptoms. 1–4 mg may be repeated as needed for severe symptoms	Short duration of action. Atropine should be available to reverse cholinergic effects should they occur. Must be given slowly
Pralidoxime	Organophosphates and severe carbamate ingestions, but not carbaryl	Adult: 1 g IV over 2 min. Pediatrics: 25–50 mg/kg slow IV. Either dose may be repeated every 8–12 hr as needed.	Given in combination with atropine. Little benefit if administered more than 36 hr after poisoning.

iron alone. Since this complex relies on the kidneys for its excretion, deferoxamine is normally contraindicated in the anuric patient unless dialysis can be performed.

Deferoxamine should be given in iron intoxications when free iron is present in the serum. This usually occurs at serum iron levels of 350 to 500 μg/100 ml or greater. Free iron is present when the serum iron is greater than the iron-binding capacity. In iron-intoxicated patients whose clinical status suggests a severe iron intoxication (severe vomiting, hematemesis, hypotension, etc.) the use of deferoxamine should be considered before laboratory results are available.

Deferoxamine is generally given intramuscularly to children at a dose of 90 mg/kg up to 1 g every 8 hours for 3 doses. In severe cases, deferoxamine may be administered for up to 36 hours. If the patient is in shock, deferoxamine may be administered intravenously at the rate of 15 mg/kg per hour as a drip up to 90 mg/kg per 8 hours. Adults should be given an initial 1.0-g dose followed by 0.5 g every 4 hours for 2 doses. Additional 0.5-g doses can be given every 4 hours as needed. If given intravenously the rate should not exceed 15 mg/kg per hour. Neither children nor adults should be given more than 6 g per day.

The most common adverse reactions to deferoxamine include generalized erythema, urticaria and hypotension. These are usually related to too rapid intravenous administration.

PHYSOSTIGMINE

Physostigmine is an anticholinesterase agent that is useful in anticholinergic poisonings. By inhibiting acetylcholinesterase, physostigmine inhibits the breakdown of acetylcholine. Thus, acetylcholine accumulates at cholinergic receptors, competes with the anticholinergic agent and reverses the anticholinergic symptoms. Physostigmine is preferred over neostigmine and other quaternary agents since it enters the CNS and will reverse central anticholinergic symptoms. Anticholinergic poisoning is produced by atropine and scopolamine as well as jimson weed, antihistamines, phenothiazines and tricyclic antidepressants.

Physostigmine should be considered in severe anticholinergic poisonings. In these intoxications specific indications for the use of physostigmine include: (a) convulsions, (b) severe hallucinations, (c) hypertension and (d) arrhythmias (53). Although physostigmine will reverse anticholinergic coma, it should not be used solely to keep a patient awake. Physostigmine may be given diagnostically and if anticholinergic symptoms improve and no cholinergic symptoms are produced, it is likely that the patient ingested an anticholinergic agent. In children, a therapeutic trial of 0.5 mg is given slowly (over 2 min) intravenously. If toxic effects persist and cholinergic symptoms are not seen, this dose may be repeated at 5-min intervals up to a maximum of 2 mg (53). The lowest effective total trial dose should be repeated as life-threatening symptoms recur. It is important to note that physostigmine has a very short duration of action (usually 30 to 60 min) and dosage must be repeated as needed. In adults the therapeutic trial dose is 2 mg. An additional 1 to 2 mg may be given in 20 min if reversal of symptoms has not occurred. The therapeutic dose in adults is 1 to 2 mg. A recent report suggests the use of physostigmine for barbiturate and other nonanticholinergic intoxications (54). This is similar to using analeptics in sedative hypnotic ingestions and is not to be recommended. Since there is no pharmacologic rationale for this use and the evidence for its use is purely anecdotal, it should not be recommended unless the ingestion of an agent that produces an anticholinergic type of poisoning is suspected and severe anticholinergic symptoms are present.

References

1. Personal Communication: National Clearinghouse for Poison Control Centers.
2. Anon: Accident facts. National Safety Council, 1980.
3. Done AK: Aspirin overdosage: incidence, diagnosis and management. *Pediatrics* (suppl) 62:890, 1978.
4. Anon: Tabulation of 1979 Reports. *Natl Clgh Poison Control Cent Bull* 25:1, 1981.
5. Schaeffer JH, Lavengood SJ: 1980 survey of poison control centers summary of results. *Natl Clgh Poison Control Cent Bull* 26:2, 1982.
6. Anon: AAPCC regionalization designation. *Natl Clgh Poison Control Cent Bull* 24:7, 1980.
7. Kinnard W: The role of the pharmacist in the control of acute poisoning. *Clin Toxicol* 4:659, 1971.
8. Moriarty R: Personal communication.
9. Arena JM: General considerations of poisoning. In *Poisoning*, ed 4 Springfield, Ill.: Charles C Thomas, 1979, pp 3–125.
10. Mofenson HC, Greensher J: The unknown poison. *Pediatrics* 54:336, 1974.
11. Morelli HF: Rational therapy of poisoning. In Melmon KL, Morelli HF: *Clinical Pharmacology: Basic Principles in Therapeutics*, ed 2. New York: Macmillan, 1978, pp 1028–1051.
12. Done AK: Pharmacologic principles in the treat-

ment of poisoning. *Pharmacol Physicians* 3:1, 1969.

13. Benowitz NL, Rosenberg J, Becker CE: Cardio-pulmonary catastrophes in drug-overdoses patients. *Med Clin North Am* 63:267, 1979.

14. Lovejoy FH: Aspirin and acetaminophen: a comparative view of their antipyretic and analgesic activity. *Pediatrics* (suppl) 62:904, 1978.

15. Cashman TM, Shirkey HC: Emergency management of poisoning. *Pediatr Clin North Am* 17:525, 1970.

16. Yaffe SJ, Sjoquist F, Alvan G: Pharmacologic principles in the management of accidental poisoning. *Pediatr Clin North Am* 17:495, 1970.

17. Abdallah AH, Tye A: A comparison of the efficacy of emetics and stomach lavage. *Am J Dis Child* 113:471, 1967.

18. Arnold FJ Jr, Hodges JB Jr, Barta RA Jr: Evaluation of the efficacy of lavage and induced emesis in treatment of salicylate poisoning. *Pediatrics* 23:286, 1959.

19. Boxer L, Anderson FP, Rowe DS: Comparison of ipecac-induced emesis with gastric lavage in the treatment of acute salicylate ingestion. *J Pediatr* 74:800, 1969.

20. Goldstein L: Emesis vs. lavage for drug ingestion, *JAMA* 208:2162, 1969.

21. Corby D, Decker W, Moran M, et al: Clinical comparison of pharmacologic emetics in children. *Pediatrics* 42:361, 1968.

22. Corby D, Lisciandro R, Lehman R, et al: The efficacy of methods used to evacuate the stomach after acute ingestions. *Pediatrics* 40:871, 1967.

23. Thomas M, Verhulst H: Ipecac syrup in antiemetic ingestions. *JAMA* 195:147, 1966.

24. Manoguerra AS, Krenzelok AP: Rapid emesis from high-dose ipecac syrup in adults and children intoxicated with antiemetics and other drugs. *Am J Hosp Pharm* 35:1360, 1978.

25. Bourianoff G: No time for ipecac. *Emerg Med* 3:5, 1971.

26. MacLeod J: Ipecac intoxication—use of a cardiac pacemaker in management. *N Engl J Med* 268:146, 1963.

27. Molinas S: A note on the use of syrup of ipecac by poison control centers. *Natl Clgh Poison Control Cent Bull* (March–April) 1966.

28. Ng R, Darwish H, Stewart D: Emergency treatment of petroleum distillate and turpentine ingestion. *Can Med Assoc J* 111:537, 1974.

29. Robertson W: Syrup of ipecac—a slow or fast emetic? *Am J Dis Child* 103:136, 1962.

30. MacLean W: A comparison of ipecac syrup and apomorphine in the immediate treatment of ingestion of poison. *J Pediatr* 82:121, 1973.

31. Dabbous IA, Bergman AB, Robertson WO: The ineffectiveness of mechanically induced vomiting. *J Pediatr* 66:952, 1965.

32. Varipapa RJ, Oderda GM: Effect of milk on ipecac induced emesis. *N Engl J Med* 296:112, 1977.

33. Bates B, Grunwaldt E: Ipecac poisoning. *Am J Dis Child* 103:01, 1962.

34. Schofferman J: A clinical comparison of syrup of ipecac and apomorphine use in adults. *JACEP* 5:22, 1976.

35. Laurence B, Hopkins B: Hypernatremia following a saline emetic. *Med J Aust* 1:1301, 1969.

36. DeGenaro F, Nyhan W: Salt—a dangerous antidote. *Pediatrics* 78:1048, 1971.

37. Barer J, Hill L, Hill R, et al: Fatal poisoning from salt used as an emetic. *Am J Dis Child* 125:889, 1973.

38. Robertson W: A further warning on the use of salt as an emetic agent. *J Pediatr* 79:877, 1971.

39. Chin L, Picchioni AL, and Duplisse BR: Comparative antidotal effectiveness of activated charcoal. Arizona montmorillonite and evaporated milk. *J Pharm Sci* 58:1353, 1969.

40. Atkinston JP, Azarnoff DL: Comparisons of charcoal and attapulgite as gastrointestinal sequestrants in acute drug ingestions. *Clin Toxicol* 4:31, 1971.

41. Picchioni AL: Activated charcoal—a neglected antidote. *Pediatr Clin North Am* 17:535, 1970.

42. Manes M, Mann J: Easily swallowed antidote charcoals. *Clin Toxicol* 7:355, 1974.

43. Gwilt PR, Perrier D: Influence of "thickening" agents on the antidotal efficacy of activated charcoals. *Clin Toxicol* 9:89, 1976.

44. Mathur LK, Jaffe JM, Colaizzi JL, et al: Activated charcoal-carboxymethylcellulose gel formulation as an antidotal agent for orally administered aspirin. *Am J Hosp Pharm* 33:717, 1976.

45. Chin L, Picchioni AL: Charcoal and saline laxatives for treatment of poison ingestion. *Vet Hum Toxicol* 21:132, 1979.

46. Done AK: Ion trapping in pathogenesis and treatment of poisoning. *Vet Hum Toxicol* 22(suppl 2):2, 1980.

47. Rumack BH (ed): General or unknown. In: *Poisindex*. Englewood, Col.: Micromedex, 1982.

48. Elenbaas RM: Critical review of forced alkaline diuresis in acute salicylism. *Crit Care Q* 4:89–95, 1982.

49. Russo M: Management of theophylline intoxication with charcoal-column hemoperfusion. *N Engl J Med* 300:24, 1979.

50. Hagstam KE, Larsson LE, Thysell H: Experimental studies on charcoal hemoperfusion in phenobarbital intoxication and uremia, including histopathological findings. *Acta Med Scand* 180:593, 1966.

51. Pond S, Rosenberg J, Benowitz NL, et al: Pharmacokinetics of hemoperfusion for drug overdose. *Clin Pharmacokinet* 4:329, 1979.

52. Rumack BH (ed): Opiates. In: *Poisindex*. Englewood, Col.: Micromedex, 1982.

53. Rumack BH (ed): Anticholinergic poisoning. In *Poisindex*. Englewood, Col.: Micromedex, 1982.

54. Brashares Z, Conley W: Physostigmine in drug overdoses. *JACEP* 4:46, 1975.

CHAPTER 2

Parenteral Nutrition

TIMOTHY W. VANDERVEEN, Pharm.D., M.S.
PAUL W. NIEMIEC, JR., Pharm.D.

There is no pathophysiological process which can be expected to respond more favorably to specific therapeutic endeavors when the patient is in a state of malnutrition than when he is well nourished.

S. DUDRICK, 1979

INTRODUCTION

During the past two decades, the need for aggressive nutritional support of both ambulatory and hospitalized patients has become more widely recognized. Multiple studies have documented a high incidence of protein and energy malnutrition in general patient populations (1, 2). Malnutrition may be present on admission to a hospital, or may develop as a consequence of prolonged hospitalization and inadequate nutritional support. Hospitalized patients may have greater nutritional demands related to increased requirements in the healing process and depletion of nutrient stores secondary to illness. Chronic debilitating diseases such as tuberculosis and cancer frequently cause anorexia and gastrointestinal disturbances which hinder an adequate dietary intake. Acute conditions such as trauma, sepsis, surgical procedures and disease treatment may aggravate or precipitate malnutrition and may increase an individual's energy and protein requirements. Effective nutritional support can enhance wound healing and immunocompetence, increase tolerance to treatment procedures, and significantly decrease morbidity and mortality.

Aggressive nutritional support consists of providing utilizable forms of enteral or parenteral nutrients in amounts sufficient to promote tissue anabolism. Parenteral nutrition (PN) is indicated only when adequate nutritional intake cannot be provided by the gastrointestinal (GI) tract. Patients suffering GI disease or injury, those requiring complete bowel rest, and patients who refuse enteral support are potential candidates for PN therapy. The provision by vein of all nutrients necessary to sustain life and promote growth is a complex therapeutic modality that is considered a major medical breakthrough. PN therapy frequently accompanies multiple drug therapy, vital organ system support, and diagnostic as well as treatment procedures which lend to the overall complexity of patient care. Consequently, multidisciplinary nutrition support teams have evolved which foster the safe and efficacious application of nutrition support principles. These teams bring together physicians, nurses, pharmacists and dietitians to provide a coordinated approach to nutritional assessments, support recommendations, and monitoring of prescribed therapy (3).

The purpose of this chapter is to provide the reader with basic principles and concepts relating to applied parenteral nutrition support in the adult patient. Pharmacists involved with the procurement and preparation of PN solutions and the monitoring of their use will find emphasis placed upon the unique contributions that pharmacists can make on a nutrition support team.

PROTEIN-ENERGY MALNUTRITION

Protein-energy malnutrition (PEM) describes a spectrum of clinical conditions with varying features and biochemical findings. At one end is marasmus (protein-calorie malnutrition), a syndrome related to chronic dietary restriction of energy, protein and other nutrients. Marasmus is associated with diseases such as anorexia nervosa, GI cancer, chronic illness and old age. Marasmic patients often appear cachectic due to a slow, progressive loss of adipose and muscle tissue. At the other end, kwashiorkor (protein malnutrition) develops due to a prolonged deficit of dietary protein intake accompanied by adequate energy intake. Dietary intake is primarily in the form of carbohydrates. Kwashiorkor is associated with fad diets, partial obstruction of the upper GI tract, and prolonged use of protein-free dextrose intravenous solutions. Patients presenting with protein malnutrition may not appear malnourished and may actually be obese. Kwashiorkor may be overlooked unless a careful assessment of laboratory data is made. Table 2.1 provides generally accepted findings that differentiate these two basic types of malnutrition (4).

Between these two extremes are many mixed disorders that have features characteristic of both marasmus and kwashiorkor. A mixed disorder represents a transition of degrees of protein and energy deficiencies in addition to depletion of electrolytes, minerals and vitamins. It frequently is the result of a stressful event being superimposed upon chronic undernutrition and necessitates aggressive nutritional support. Thus, PEM is a complex pathological process that requires a comprehensive approach to accurately assess nutritional status and plan for nutritional intervention.

NUTRITIONAL ASSESSMENT

Assessment of nutritional status includes a comprehensive appraisal of medical, dietary and medication histories, patient appearance upon physical examination, pertinent laboratory indices, and anthropometric measures of body composition. Evaluation and correlation of these parameters will substantiate PEM, with early indicators of patients at nutritional risk including (a) patients with histories of alcoholism and chronic disease, (b) patients experiencing ≥10% weight loss from premorbid weight, and (c) patients who are NPO (nothing by mouth) or receiving standard intravenous fluids for 5 or more days. Anthropometric measurements such as triceps skin fold and midarm muscle circumference relate subcutaneous fat stores and lean body mass to known standards for healthy individuals of comparable sex and age. Laboratory indices such as serum albumin and transferrin, in conjunction with determinations of nitrogen balance comparing nitrogen intake to urea nitrogen excretion serve as biochemical markers of nutritional status and metabolic expenditure. Screening patients for drug-induced taste disorders and drug-induced nutrient deficiencies will complete the assessment profile. Examples of drug-induced nutrient deficiencies are reviewed extensively in a publication by Roe (5). A thorough nutritional assessment will provide the foundation from which to plan nutrition support and evaluate the need for a more aggressive approach. A recent article by Grant et al. (6) provides an excellent review of the benefits and limitations associated with current nutritional assessment techniques.

INDICATIONS FOR NUTRITIONAL SUPPORT

Aggressive nutritional support is utilized in patients when normal dietary intake is not

Table 2.1.
Protein-Energy Malnutrition[a]

	Marasmus	Kwashiorkor
Clinical setting	↓Calorie, ↓protein intake	↓Protein intake
Time course to develop	Months to years	Weeks to months
Clinical features	Starved, wasted appearance Depressed weight for height Limited fat reserves Decreased muscle mass	Well-nourished appearance Hair easy to pluck out Edema
Laboratory findings	Serum albumin >2.8 g/100 ml Depressed creatinine height index	Serum albumin <2.8 g/100 ml Serum transferrin <150 mg/ml Total lymphocyte count <1200 mm^3 Nonreactive to skin tests
Clinical course	Tolerate short-term stress reasonably well Low mortality rate	Impaired wound healing Reduced immunocompetence Increased infection rate

[a] Adapted from C. E. Butterworth and R. L. Weinsier (4).

possible. Nutritional therapy via the parenteral route may be indicated in the following situations:

> Patients who cannot eat: examples include patients who are comatose or suffer head injury, pre- and postoperative patients;
> Patients who will not eat: examples include patients with chronic disease and certain psychiatric disorders;
> Patients who should not eat: examples include patients with esophageal obstruction, inflammatory bowel disease and GI fistulas;
> Patients who cannot eat enough: examples include patients with burns or cancer.

Questions such as the following are helpful as a starting point in assessing the eventual need for aggressive nutrition support:

1. How long has food intake been suboptimal?

2. When will normal dietary intake be established?

3. What does a thorough nutritional assessment indicate?

4. What are the patient's caloric and protein goals?

5. Does the patient require an aggressive approach to nutrition support?

For example, a more aggressive approach may be desired in the patient who presents with a history of chronic undernutrition, or when adequate dietary intake cannot be established within 5 to 7 days due to physical or mechanical reasons. Assessment of a patient's current nutritional status and establishment of projected caloric and protein goals are helpful in characterizing the severity of malnutrition and planning appropriate therapy to meet the patient's individual needs. In general, nutrition support is provided by enteral means (oral, feeding tube) when GI function is intact and use of this route is not contraindicated. When adequate nourishment cannot be provided by the enteral route, consideration is given to the use of PN therapy. Table 2.2 lists some of the diseases or conditions where PN therapy may be indicated.

COMPONENTS OF PN SOLUTIONS

To maintain energy balance and tissue synthesis, human beings require adequate sources of protein, carbohydrates, fats, electrolytes, vitamins, minerals and water. Any total feeding concept must account for these seven basic categories. Components of PN solutions are listed in Table 2.3 and reflect commercially available sources of the required nutrients.

Water is basic to these solutions, with a patient's daily fluid requirements dependent

Table 2.2.
Indications for Parenteral Nutrition

GASTROINTESTINAL DISORDERS
  GI cancer
  Gastric outlet obstruction
  Enterocutaneous fistulas
  Short bowel syndrome
  Inflammatory bowel disease
  Acute or chronic pancreatitis
  Bowel obstruction
  Radiation enteritis
INCREASED NUTRITIONAL DEMAND
  Thermal burns
  Sepsis
  Trauma
PSYCHIATRIC DISORDERS
  Anorexia nervosa
MISCELLANEOUS
  Renal failure
  Hepatic failure
  Cardiac cachexia
  Cancer
  Prolonged unconsciousness

Table 2.3.
Nutrient Substrates in Parenteral Nutrition Solutions

	Source
Energy	Dextrose; intravenous fat emulsions
Nitrogen	Crystalline amino acids, protein hydrolysates
Electrolytes	Injectable salts of sodium, potassium, magnesium, calcium, chloride, phosphate, acetate
Vitamins	Injectable fat-soluble vitamins (A, D, E, K) and water-soluble vitamins (B_1, B_2, B_6, B_{12}, C, nicotinic acid, pantothenic acid, biotin, folic acid)
Trace minerals	Commercially available or extemporaneous preparations including iron, zinc, copper, manganese, chromium, iodide, selenium
Water	Sterile water for injection, USP

upon renal and hepatic function, as well as GI, skin and pulmonary losses. Energy is supplied in the form of glucose and fat emulsions. Fat emulsions also serve as a source of essential fatty acids. Sources of nitrogen include synthetic crystalline amino acids and protein hydrolysates. In addition, PN solutions generally contain electrolytes, vitamins and trace minerals and are compounded to meet specific patient requirements. The hospital pharmacist should assume responsibility for the compounding of these solutions to insure an accurately labeled, sterile, compatible and stable solution.

ENERGY PROVISION DURING PN

The provision of sufficient energy is critical to the success of PN therapy. Following an initial assessment of a patient's energy requirements, a therapeutic regimen can be established to meet this goal. For adult patients, energy requirements may be estimated by using the derived formulas of Harris and Benedict (7) which calculate basal energy expenditure (BEE) in kilocalories (kcal) based upon a patient's age (yr), weight (Wt) (kg), height (Ht) (cm) and sex.

$$\text{Men: BEE (kcal/24 hr)} = 66.5$$
$$+ (13.75 \times \text{Wt})$$
$$+ (5.00 \times \text{Ht}) - (6.76 \times \text{age})$$
$$\text{Women: BEE (kcal/24 hr)} = 655$$
$$+ (9.56 \times \text{Wt})$$
$$+ (1.85 \times \text{Ht}) - (4.68 \times \text{age})$$

Since these formulas estimate daily basal energy requirements, an anabolic factor of 1.75 is multiplied by BEE to estimate the energy requirements of adult patients on PN therapy

who require repletion of body energy stores and tissue synthesis (8). The provision of 45 kcal/kg may also be utilized to estimate anabolic requirements of the adult PN patient. Figure 2.1 illustrates both examples of estimating caloric requirements for an anabolic prescription.

A typical adult patient has an estimated BEE ranging from 1500 to 2000 kcal/day, with parenteral anabolic requirements of 2600 to 3500 kcal/day. This empiric approach requires frequent assessment of progress and may necessitate reestablishment of goals based upon patient weight gain, wound healing, laboratory indices and other objective parameters. Prospective monitoring of tolerance to caloric supplementation will further help to individualize therapy.

GLUCOSE AS AN ENERGY SOURCE

Glucose (dextrose) is the most commonly used energy substrate for PN. It offers the advantages of being readily available, inexpensive, and efficiently metabolized in most patients. Glucose monohydrate provides 3.4 kcal/gram (g), thus 3 liters of 5% dextrose in water provide only 510 kcal/day, an amount that falls far short of providing the basal or anabolic energy requirements of seriously ill and stressed adult patients. Patients receiving standard intravenous therapy with dextrose-saline solutions and poor dietary intake are, in effect, starving.

Glucose may serve as the only nonprotein source of calories during PN. It is generally well tolerated when administered continuously at infusion rates of up to 5 mg/kg/min

---

Patient Data:
    Male
    36 years
    180 cm
    70 kg

Basal Energy Expenditure (BEE):
$$\text{BEE} = 66.5 + (13.75 \times 70) + (5 \times 180) - (6.76 \times 36)$$
$$= 1686 \text{ kcal/24 hr}$$

Anabolic Goals
  Based on BEE:
$$\text{BEE} \times 1.75 = \text{anabolic goal}$$
$$1686 \text{ kcal/24 hr} \times 1.75 = 2951 \text{ kcal/24 hr}$$
  Based on 45 kcal/kg:
$$70 \text{ kg} \times 45 \text{ kcal/kg} = 3150 \text{ kcal/24 hr}$$

Figure 2.1. Energy requirement calculations.

(9). The primary problem associated with high glucose intakes is hyperglycemia (10). Patients with a history of diabetes mellitus, renal failure, critically ill patients who are stressed by sepsis or trauma, and those receiving corticosteroid therapy may exhibit glucose intolerance and require insulin or a modified approach to PN therapy. PN therapy should initially be monitored by continuous 6-hour urine glucose determinations and daily blood sugars. Regular insulin may be administered by admixture and continuous infusion with the PN solution, or by intramuscular and subcutaneous injections in an attempt to maintain serum glucose levels <200 mg/dl. If hyperglycemia fails to respond to insulin therapy and adequate potassium replacement, it may be advisable to reduce glucose intake by reducing the concentration of the PN solution or by slowing the rate of PN infusion. Caution should be exercised in interpreting urine glucose test results in patients receiving medications known to interfere with a specific test (i.e. cephalosporins with Clinitest). Hyperglycemic, hyperosmolar, nonketotic dehydration (HHND) is a preventable complication of PN therapy related to excessive infusion of concentrated glucose and/or glucose intolerance. For instance, a patient presenting with diabetes would be susceptible to HHND unless PN solutions are continuously infused at a rate that does not exceed the patient's capacity for glucose metabolism. Thus, careful monitoring of blood and urine glucose, daily urine output and weight change, and rate of PN infusion are mandatory in this patient example. Likewise, rebound hypoglycemia may be related to inappropriate fluctuations in PN infusion rate. Patients receiving PN without an electronic rate controlling device or infusion pump set correctly to the desired rate of infusion are at risk for the above complications.

Recently Askanazi et al. (11) demonstrated that stressed and septic patients exhibit altered metabolism of energy substrates. When glucose is administered as the sole energy source to provide caloric requirements, critically ill patients may continue to oxidize endogenous fat stores for energy. This may result in glucose intolerance, insulin resistance, hyperglycemia, increase in carbon dioxide production and hepatic fat deposition. It has been suggested that critically ill patients may be more appropriately supported by providing both glucose and fat calories to achieve energy require-

ments while minimizing the above complications associated with the use of glucose as the sole energy substrate. Diabetics and renal failure patients who respond poorly to insulin therapy may also benefit from receiving fat as a part of the calorie source.

Dextrose concentrations ranging from 5 to 70% are commercially available to facilitate the compounding of PN solutions. Table 2.4 lists the caloric value of these solutions. The final dextrose concentrations of PN solutions following admixture rarely exceeds 50%, and most adult standard formulas are 25% dextrose.

FAT AS AN ENERGY AND ESSENTIAL FATTY ACID SOURCE

Fat is a concentrated caloric source providing 9 kcal/g. In the 1920s the Japanese experimented with fat emulsions consisting of butter fat and cod liver oil. Investigators (12) in the United States used intravenous fats in the 1940s, and a commercially available fat emulsion of cottonseed oil for parenteral administration was first marketed in the 1950s. This product was subsequently withdrawn from the market in the early 1960s due to a high frequency of toxic reactions. In 1961, Schuberth and Wretlind (13) developed a nontoxic soybean oil emulsion for intravenous use. This product has been available in the United States for 8 years. Commercially available intravenous fat emulsions are compared in Table 2.5. Each emulsion contains significant amounts of the essential fatty acid, linoleic acid, and can be used as a source of calories and essential fatty acids.

Clinical signs of essential fatty acid deficiency (EFAD) include dry, scaly skin and sparse hair growth, with other changes including increased capillary membrane fragility and permeability, impaired wound healing, and

Table 2.4.
Caloric Equivalents of Intravenous Dextrose Solutions

Solution	Kilocalories/Liter
D_5W	170
$D_{10}W$	340
$D_{20}W$	680
$D_{25}W$	850
$D_{30}W$	1020
$D_{40}W$	1360
$D_{50}W$	1700

reduced resistance to stress and infection (14). Despite the presence of adequate fat stores, continuous infusion of high concentrations of glucose during PN therapy appears to block fatty acid release from adipose tissue and predisposes to EFAD.

Although the exact amount of linoleic acid necessary to prevent or treat EFAD is not known, it is generally recommended to supply at least 5% of the total weekly caloric intake as fat calories during PN (15). In the average adult patient, this is equivalent to providing 2 to 3 bottles of 500 ml of 10% fat emulsion per week.

In addition to providing a source of fatty acids, fat may also serve as an alternate energy source. It has the advantage of a high caloric density (9 kcal/g). Since commercial fat emulsions are rendered isotonic by the addition of glycerin, they may be administered by peripheral vein. The caloric density of the emulsions is between 1.1 and 2.0 kcal/ml. Maximum recommended daily intake of fat calories is 60% of the total infused calories (maximum 2.5 g/kg/day in adults). Because of the physical nature of fat emulsions and the likelihood that divalent cations such as calcium and magnesium will interfere with emulsion stability, it is generally recommended that fat emulsions not be combined with PN solutions in the same container (16). It is acceptable to "piggyback" the PN solution and fat emulsion together using a distal intravenous tubing injection site or "Y" set. If a final in-line filter is being used for PN solution administration, fat emulsion must be "piggybacked" below the filter since emulsion particle size exceeds filter pore size. Special admixture equipment and techniques to provide fat, amino acids, dextrose and elec-

trolytes in one container are available in Europe and Canada, and they have recently been released by the FDA for use in this country.

Fat clearance and metabolism can be monitored by checking serum turbidity for lipemia 4 hours after completing a fat infusion, and by determining serum free fatty acid and triglyceride levels. Fat infusion is contraindicated in lipid metabolism disorders and acute pancreatitis if accompanied by lipemia (16). Fat calories may be administered in chronic pancreatitis with monitoring of serum amylase and triglyceride levels after infusion.

NITROGEN IN PN SOLUTIONS

Nitrogen is an essential component of every tissue and organ system. Proper organ function depends upon the availability of a complete complement of functional proteins. For protein synthesis (anabolism) to occur, the diet must contain adequate nitrogen, usually in the form of protein. Oral ingestion of protein results in digestion to individual amino acids. These amino acids may then be utilized as building blocks for new proteins. Failure to meet nitrogen requirements may accelerate catabolism (protein degradation), induce a negative nitrogen balance (nitrogen intake < output), and interfere with vital body functions. Muscle wasting, impaired wound healing, and decreased immune response may result from prolonged nitrogen intake below requirements. Adults generally require approximately 0.8 to 1.5 g of protein/kg of body weight (8). Thus a 70-kg adult may require between 56 and 105 g of protein each 24 hours in order to prevent negative nitrogen balance. One gram of nitrogen is contained in each 6.25 g of protein or amino acids. A 70-kg adult will

Table 2.5.
Intravenous Fat Emulsions

	Liposyn 10%	Liposyn 20%	Travamulsion 10%	Intralipid 10%	Intralipid 20%
Oil	Safflower	Safflower	Soybean	Soybean	Soybean
Fatty acid content (%)					
Linoleic	77	77	56	54	50
Oleic	13	13	23	26	26
Palmitic	7	7	11	9	10
Linolenic	0.1	0.1	6	8	9
Stearic	2.5	2.5	—	—	—
Egg yolk phospholipids (%)	1.2	1.2	1.2	1.2	1.2
Glycerin (%)	2.5	2.5	2.25	2.25	2.25
Calories/ml	1.1	2.0	1.1	1.1	2.0
Osmolarity (mOsm/L)	300	340	270	280	330

require between 9 and 17 g of nitrogen per 24 hours. The actual protein requirements will depend upon factors such as age. degree of stress, and organ function.

Since PN solutions are delivered into the venous system, the protein must be administered in a form that can be readily utilized. The first solutions utilized for intravenous nutrition were hydrolysates of naturally occurring proteins (fibrin, casein). However, due to incomplete hydrolysis resulting in a large concentration of di- and tripeptides, poor utilization of the nitrogen, and a high incidence of elevated blood ammonia levels, these solutions are infrequently utilized for PN today.

Crystalline or synthetic amino acid solutions have replaced the earlier hydrolysates. Crystalline amino acids provide in a concentrated form a physiological ratio of biologically utilizable substrates for protein synthesis. The three major manufacturers of intravenous solutions market crystalline amino acid solutions containing a combination of essential (40 to 50%) and nonessential (50 to 60%) amino acids. These solutions differ in their concentrations (from 3 to 10%) and individual amino acid profiles. Table 2.6 compares representative amino acid solutions from major manufacturers. The wide range of concentrations available facilitates compounding of PN solutions to meet individual patient needs. It should also be noted that the electrolyte profile of each amino acid solution varies (see Table 2.7).

Other crystalline amino acid solutions are indicated for acute renal failure. These solutions contain no or low concentrations of nonessential amino acids and high concentrations of essential amino acids. Table 2.8 compares the amino acid profile of formulas for renal failure. The expense of these solutions and the lack of conclusive evidence that they offer a significant advantage over combinations of essential and nonessential amino acid solutions may limit their utilization.

Investigational studies continue on special amino acid formulations for liver failure patients. While the exact etiology of altered mental status and encephalopathy in hepatic patients is not known, Fischer and Bower (17) have demonstrated alteration in plasma amino acid patterns in these patients. It is now hypothesized that hepatic patients have elevated

Table 2.6.
Comparison of Amino Acid (AA) Formulations

	Aminosyn 8.5%[a]	Travasol 8.5%[b]	Freamine III 8.5%[c]
ESSENTIAL AA (mg/100 ml)			
L-Isoleucine	620	406	590
L-Leucine	810	526	770
L-Lysine acetate	624	492	620
	(Free base)	(HCl salt)	(Free base)
L-Methionine	340	492	450
L-Phenylalanine	380	526	480
L-Threonine	460	356	340
L-Tryptophan	150	152	130
L-Valine	680	390	560
NONESSENTIAL AA (mg/100 ml)			
L-Alanine	1100	1760	600
L-Arginine	850	880	810
L-Histidine	260	372	240
L-Proline	750	356	950
L-Serine	370	—	500
L-Tyrosine	44	34	—
L-Aminoacetic acid	1100	1760	1190
Cysteine	—	—	<20
Total nitrogen (g/100 ml)	1.34	1.42	1.25
Essential AA (%)	47.5	39.3	47.7
Branched chain AA (%)	24.8	15.5	22.5
Aromatic AA (%)	6.7	8.4	7.2

[a] Other Aminosyn concentrations = 3.5%, 5.0%, 7.0%, 10%.
[b] Other Travasol concentrations = 3.5%, 5.5%, 10%.
[c] Other Freamine III concentrations = 3.0%, 10%.

Table 2.7.
Electrolyte Content of Crystalline Amino Acid (CAA) Products[a]

Electrolyte (mEq/L)	Aminosyn 8.5%		Travasol 8.5%		Freamine III 8.5%
	Without electrolytes	With electrolytes	Without electrolytes	With electrolytes	
Sodium	—	70	—	70	10
Potassium	5.4	66	—	60	—
Magnesium	—	10	—	10	—
Chloride	35	98	34	70	<2
Acetate	90	142	52	135	74
Calcium	—	—	—	—	—
Phosphate (mmol/L)	—	30	—	30	10

[a] Content expressed as mEq/L of pure CAA product, to be adjusted appropriately when compounded with dextrose injection.

Table 2.8.
Amino Acid Solutions for Acute Renal Failure

	Aminosyn-RF 5.2%	Nephramine 5.4%	RenAmin
AMINO ACIDS (mg/100 ml)			
L-Arginine	600	0	630
L-Leucine	726	880	600
L-Isoleucine	462	560	500
L-Phenylalanine	726	880	490
L-Histidine	429	250	420
L-Methionine	726	880	500
L-Threonine	330	400	380
L-Valine	528	640	820
L-Lysine	535	640	450
L-Tryptophan	165	200	160
L-Cysteine HCl-H$_2$O	0	<20	0
Glycine	0	0	300
Proline	0	0	350
Alanine	0	0	560
Serine	0	0	300
Tyrosine	0	0	40
CHARACTERISTICS			
pH	5.2	6.5	6.0
Osmolarity (mOsm/L)	475	440	600
Sodium (mEq/100 ml)	0	0.6	0
Potassium (mEq/100 ml)	0.54	0	0
Acetate (mEq/100 ml)	10.5	4.4	6.0
Total nitrogen (mg/100 ml)	787	650	1000
Total nitrogen (g/container)	2.36	1.63	2.50, 5.00
Total protein (g/container)	15.68	14	16.25, 32.5
Dose units (per container)	2	2	1–2
Volume (ml/container)	300	250	250,500

serum concentrations of the aromatic amino acids, tyrosine and phenylalanine. These amino acids, along with octopamine, may serve as false neurotransmitters in the brain. Additionally, it has also been shown that these patients have low serum levels of the branched chain amino acids, valine, leucine and isoleucine. By substituting amino acid mixtures low in aromatic amino acids and high in branched chains, certain hepatic patients may respond favorably to nutritional support. A parenteral formulation containing amino acids in this configuration is now commercially available. Until additional experience reports are published, most clinicians will utilize low concentrations of conventional amino acid formulations for hepatic failure patients, due in large part to the high cost of these special formulas.

Nitrogen metabolism is generally monitored by serial blood urea nitrogen (BUN), serum ammonia, and 24-hour nitrogen balance studies. The nitrogen balance studies require 24-hour urine collections to compare nitrogen output to nitrogen intake. Serum protein levels may also be determined periodically and compared to baseline pretreatment levels to assess changes in visceral protein status. Albumin, transferrin, and occasionally prealbumin are utilized as these protein markers.

ENERGY-NITROGEN RATIO

The provision of calories and nitrogen to patients should not be looked upon as separate entities. Rather, the ratio of administered calories to grams of nitrogen should promote optimum nitrogen utilization for synthesis of protein. It is generally felt that adult patients with normal renal and hepatic function require 12 to 16% of total administered calories in the form of protein (recall that protein supplies approximately 4 kcal/g). In terms of calorie to nitrogen ratio, the nonprotein calories to grams of nitrogen ratio is generally 127 to 175:1. Thus, a liter of 25% dextrose/4.25% amino acids will provide 1020 calories (based on 3.4 kcal/g for glucose, 4 kcal/g of amino acids), 850 nonprotein calories, and 6.8 g of nitrogen. The protein calorie percentage of this solution is 16.6, and the nonprotein calorie to gram of nitrogen ratio is 125:1. Figure 2.2 reviews the calculations involved in these determinations. Other common examples of energy-nitrogen ratios are listed in Table 2.9.

ELECTROLYTE CONSIDERATIONS DURING PN

Electrolytes must be administered concurrently to patients receiving PN to supply daily metabolic needs and correct any deficits. The electrolytes normally provided in PN therapy include sodium, potassium, chloride, acetate, phosphate, magnesium, and calcium. Modification of PN solution electrolyte content is dependent upon respective serum levels, renal and extrarenal losses (such as vomiting, diarrhea, fistulas, nasogastric suctioning). Quantitation of the extent of daily electrolyte loss in body fluids by urinary or gastric fluid analysis may be necessary in some cases to optimize electrolyte replacement.

Electrolyte requirements are based upon the patient's cardiovascular, renal, hepatic and fluid status. Intracellular electrolytes (potassium, phosphate, magnesium) are especially important in PN therapy, since they are incorporated with nitrogen into tissue formation during nutritional repletion and adequate quantities are necessary for the effective utilization of glucose as an energy substrate. The need for intracellular electrolytes is particularly great when initiating PN in severely malnourished patients, and potentially rapid declines in serum levels require daily monitoring and appropriate supplementation. Figure 2.3 provides a schematic representation of a simplified approach that aids in the interpretation of factors affecting serum electrolyte levels.

Table 2.10 illustrates the typical electrolyte content of an adult PN solution based upon the patient receiving 2000 to 3000 ml of formula per day. A standard electrolyte formula

---

25% DEXTROSE/4.25% AMINO ACIDS
KILOCALORIES/LITER

$$250 \text{ g dextrose/liter} \times 3.4 \text{ kcal/g} = 850 \text{ kcal/L}$$
$$42.5 \text{ g amino acids/liter} \times 4.0 \text{ kcal/g} = \underline{170} \text{ kcal/L}$$
$$1020$$

NITROGEN/LITER
$$\frac{42.5 \text{ g amino acids/L}}{6.25 \text{ g amino acids/g g nitrogen}} = 6.8 \text{ g nitrogen/L}$$

NONPROTEIN CALORIES/GRAMS NITROGEN
$$\frac{850 \text{ kcal/L}}{6.8 \text{ g nitrogen/L}} = 125 \text{ kcal/g nitrogen}$$

PROTEIN CALORIE PERCENTAGE
$$\frac{170 \text{ kcal/L} \times 100}{1020 \text{ kcal/L}} = 16.6\%$$

Figure 2.2. Energy-nitrogen ratio calculations.

will provide the daily requirements of most adult patients with relatively normal renal, cardiovascular and hepatic function. When calculating electrolyte addition to PN solutions, the inherent electrolyte content of the crystalline amino acid solution must be included (Table 2.7). In general, the ratio of sodium to chloride should be maintained 1:1 unless the patient has excessive chloride loss or metabolic alkalosis. When hyperchloremic or other metabolic acidoses occur during PN, sodium and potassium may be added as the acetate or lactate salts rather than chloride to provide readily metabolized bicarbonate precursors. On the other hand, high acetate concentrations may favor metabolic alkalosis, especially in patients with carbon dioxide retention and compensatory metabolic alkalosis. A modified formula adjusting for concurrent acetate and chloride content may minimize fluctuations in acid-base balance. Close monitoring of electrolyte status and organ function is mandatory during PN therapy in addition to recognition of the factors impacting upon electrolyte balance. Renal, cardiac, and hepatic failure patients generally require modified formulas, and standard electrolyte additions cannot be used.

Table 2.9.
Energy-Nitrogen Ratio

	Protein-Calorie %	kcal/g Nitrogen[a]
Normal adult	16	131
Pediatric	12	183
Renal failure (acute)	8	287
Renal failure (chronic)	16	131
Liver failure	6	391

[a] Based on dextrose monohydrate.

IMPLEMENTING PN BY CENTRAL VEIN

PN by central venous catheter requires access to the vena cava. A catheter is placed via a percutaneous puncture into the subclavian vein and advanced to the level of the vena cava. This technique is performed by a skilled physician or surgeon utilizing strict sterile technique. Following the line insertion, x-ray verification is necessary to establish correctness of catheter tip placement. PN should not begin until placement is known, since catheters do not always advance into the vena cava, but rather may pass directly into another vein (e.g. opposite subclavian, internal jugular). The vena cava placement is essential to provide high blood flow rates to rapidly dilute the hypertonic PN solution, as the osmolarity of these solutions may exceed 2000 mOsm/liter.

PN therapy generally commences with a regimen that will supply per 24 hours approximately 25 to 33% of the patient's calculated energy and protein requirements. Following each 24-hour period, the therapy is advanced as tolerated. Thus, the average adult patient will receive 100% of the estimated goal for energy and nitrogen at the end of the third or fourth day. By slowly increasing the infusion of substrates, marked fluctuations in serum glucose and electrolytes may be avoided.

With the wide variety of PN component concentrations available from the various manufacturers, compounding of patient-specific formulas is feasible. However, in practice most clinicians find that standardized formulas can facilitate PN solution ordering from the pharmacy. Table 2.11 lists a typical standard PN formula. There are two basic methods of initiating PN therapy during the initial few

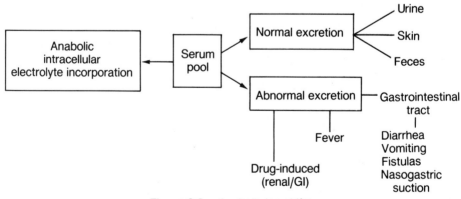

Figure 2.3. Anabolic ion shifts.

days as tolerance is established and substrate infusion is advanced toward the preestablished goals. In the first method (Method I), the rate of infusion of the PN solution is held constant while the formula concentrations are slowly advanced. The second method (Method II) holds the concentrations of glucose and amino acids constant, and varies the rate of infusion. Both methods utilize the same ingredients and arrive eventually at the same goal. Examples of both methods follow.

PN Method I

If a patient requires approximately 2000 to 3000 ml of fluid per 24 hours and is not receiving intravenous (IV) drugs or other IV fluids, the central vein PN may be utilized to provide both fluid and nutritional support. The patient would typically be started on a 10% dextrose ($D_{10}W$) with 1% amino acids (AA_1) at 80 to 120 ml/hour. If this initial infusion is tolerated, the concentration can be increased daily while the

rate is held constant. Electrolytes, vitamins, and trace minerals can be added and adjusted as necessary. An example of this method follows:

Patient A—Requirements/24 hr: 2000 ml, 2000 kcal, 85 g protein

Day 1 — $D_{10}W/AA_1$ @ 85 ml/hr
Day 2 — $D_{15}W/AA_2$ @ 85 ml/hr
Day 3 — $D_{20}W/AA_3$ @ 85 ml/hr
Day 4 — $D_{25}W/AA_{4.25}$ @ 85 ml/hr

After 96 hours, Patient A will receive 2040 ml, 2080 kcal, and 86.7 g protein/24 hours. The protein-calorie percentage on the fourth day will be 16.7. Generally two 500-ml units of intravenous fat would be given per week to provide essential fatty acids.

PN Method II

Method II is generally utilized in patients who are taking in fluids via the GI tract or who must remain on peripheral vein infusions for drug therapy. This method differs from the one above in that the PN dextrose/amino acid/electrolyte formula is held constant, but the infusion rate is slowly increased. An example follows:

Patient B—Requirements/24 hr: 2000 ml, 2000 kcal, 85 g protein

Day 1 — $D_{25}/AA_{4.25}$ @ 25 ml/hr
Day 2 — $D_{25}/AA_{4.25}$ @ 45 ml/hr
Day 3 — $D_{25}/AA_{4.25}$ @ 65 ml/hr
Day 4 — $D_{25}/AA_{4.25}$ @ 85 ml/hr

Table 2.10.
Typical Parenteral Nutrition (PN) Formula Electrolytes

Ingredient	Adult Requirements/Day during PN
Sodium (mEq)	60–150
Potassium (mEq)	70–180
Chloride (mEq)	60–150
Phosphate (mmol)	7–10 mmol/1000 kcal
Acetate (mEq)	25–160
Magnesium (mEq)	10–30
Calcium (mEq)	4–30

Table 2.11.
Typical Standard Adult Parenteral Nutrition (PN) Formula

	Ingredient/Liter	Adult Requirements/Day during PN
Dextrose (g)	250.0	500–750
Crystalline amino acid (g)	42.5	60–120
Sodium (mEq)	40.0	60–150
Potassium (mEq)	40.5	70–180
Chloride (mEq)	33.5	60–150
Phosphate (mmol)	10.0	7–10 mmol/1000 kcal
Acetate (mEq)	40.0	25–160
Magnesium (mEq)	8.0 (as sulfate)	10–30
Calcium (mEq)	5.0 (as gluconate)	4–30
Multiple vitamins (ml)	10.0 (once per day)	
Vitamin K (mg)	1.0	
Zinc (mg)	1.0	2–6
Copper (mg)	0.25	0.5–1.0
Chromium (μg)	5.0	10–15
Manganese (mg)	0.1	0.15–0.8

In this method, following Day 4 Patient B will be receiving exactly the same number of calories and grams of protein from the PN as Patient A. Intravenous fat would generally be given as in Method I. However, in this method a peripheral intravenous solution may be necessary to provide adequate fluid and electrolyte intake during the first 3 to 4 days. This method finds its greatest usefulness in situations where fluid intake must be restricted or where other therapy (e.g. antibiotics) must be given via a peripheral vein. For example, patients with renal failure and severe fluid restriction may receive a 40 to 50% dextrose solution along with a reduced amino acid concentration of 2 to 3%. Although the concentrations are different, the same gradual increase in infusion rate can be utilized to ultimately reach caloric and protein goals.

IMPLEMENTING PN BY PERIPHERAL VEIN

Peripheral vein PN differs from the central vein approach in two basic ways. First, the peripheral veins can only tolerate solutions of low osmolarity, with 900 mOsm/liter as the generally accepted maximum limit. Exceeding this osmolarity will increase the likelihood of venous thrombosis and associated complications. The high concentrations of dextrose in central vein PN raise the osmolarity to 1500 to 2500 mOsm/liter, thus necessitating infusion into the larger central veins where rapid dilution will occur. Second, the peripheral PN system requires that a large percentage of total calories be provided in the form of fat emulsions. Since fat emulsions are approximately isotonic in both 10% and 20% concentrations, they can be infused simultaneously with the dextrose/amino acid/electrolyte solution via a "Y" infusion set. The fat emulsion reduces the combined osmolarity of the two infusions while at the same time it increases the caloric density. This system is more complex than central PN and it is often more expensive. However, in patients for whom a central approach is not indicated, this method may provide an acceptable alternative for nutritional support. An example of peripheral vein PN follows.

Patient C—Requirements/24 hr: 3000 ml, 1900 kcal, 60 g protein

Day 1 — $D_{10}W/AA_3$ @ 40 ml/hr; and
F_{10} @ 20 ml/hr

Day 2 — $D_{10}W/AA_3$ @ 60 ml/hr; and
F_{10} @ 30 ml/hr

Day 3 — $D_{10}W/AA_3$ @ 80 ml/hr; and
F_{10} @ 40 ml/hr

In this method of PN, Patient C will receive approximately the predetermined fluid, energy and protein goals beginning on the third day. The dextrose/amino acid mixture has a caloric density of 0.46 kcal/ml with the 10% fat emulsion (F_{10}) having a density of 1.1 kcal/ml. On Day 3 the patient will receive 1939 kcal, 57.6 g of protein, and 2880 ml, with 54% of the calories from fat. Electrolytes, vitamins, and trace metals would be provided via the dextrose/amino acid mixture.

The peripheral system is very flexible and dextrose/amino acid and fat emulsions can be combined in many combinations depending on venous status, patient goals, and response to therapy. With this method, patients must be able to tolerate large fluid volumes. The percentage of total calories from fat should not exceed 60% of total caloric intake.

VITAMINS IN PN

Vitamins are normally obtained from food, however, in patients who are dependent on PN, the enteric source for vitamins is not available. Consequently, parenteral vitamin supplementation is necessary.

The vitamins normally recognized as being essential are divided into the four fat-soluble vitamins: A (retinol), D (cholecalciferol and ergocalciferol), E (α-tocopherol) and K_1 (phylloquinone); and 9 water-soluble vitamins: B_1 (thiamine), B_2 (riboflavin), B_6 (pyridoxine), niacin (nicotinic acid), pantothenic acid, folacin, B_{12} (cyanocobalamin), biotin, and C (ascorbic acid).

Guidelines for vitamin supplementation in PN have recently been established by the Nutrition Advisory Group of the American Medical Association [18]. Products have been formulated to supply 12 vitamins as a single addition to PN solutions. Generally, 1 ampule per day of the multivitamin preparation in conjunction with vitamin K supplementation will meet the needs of most adult patients. However, patients with severe PEM, cancer or stress may require monitoring of serum vitamin levels and additional supplementation of specific vitamins such as A and C.

TRACE MINERALS IN PN

Trace minerals known to be essential for man include zinc, copper, iron, chromium, manganese, iodine, and selenium. These minerals are available in adequate quantities in the normal diet. PN therapy with highly purified components, however, limits trace mineral supplementation from mineral contamination. Consequently, patients with preexisting deficiencies, pathological states associated with increased trace mineral losses, or on long-term PN therapy may develop signs or symptoms characteristic of the specific deficiency. For example, zinc deficiency is associated with skin rash, poor wound healing, and diarrhea. Copper deficiency has been associated with hematologic abnormalities, and low chromium levels have been linked to glucose intolerance.

Recently the pharmaceutical industry has marketed sterile intravenous solutions of zinc, copper, manganese, chromium, and selenium. Additionally, the Nutrition Advisory Group of the American Medical Association has established guidelines for trace metal supplementation in PN (19). These guidelines provide recommended dosages for both pediatric and adult patients. For a more complete review of the subject, the reader is referred to this publication.

MONITORING PN THERAPY

Central and peripheral PN therapy can be extremely effective in restoring and/or maintaining the nutritional status of patients who cannot receive their nourishment via the GI tract. When PN therapy is administered by clinicians who are knowledgeable in its use, the benefits far outweigh the inherent risks. PN is a complex form of treatment, and failure to carefully administer and monitor PN therapy may lead to serious and potentially fatal complications. Table 2.12 lists many of the potential complications of PN. However, when skilled physicians or surgeons place PN catheters and specially trained nurses maintain the integrity and sterility of the catheter and related administration equipment, the incidence of catheter related complications can be reduced to an acceptable frequency. Likewise, careful PN compounding by the pharmacist will decrease the likelihood of infections related to the PN solutions. Metabolic aberrations may be minimized or prevented by systematic monitoring of the therapy. Table 2.13 lists clinical and laboratory data that are necessary to monitor therapy. Daily rounding, maintenance of PN flow sheets, appropriate PN formula modification, and close communication between the nutrition support team and the primary care physician will help to ensure safe and effective therapy.

HOME PN THERAPY

PN is generally utilized for short-term nutritional support until adequate oral intake can be maintained. However, increasing sophistication and technical improvements have enabled prolonged and occasionally lifelong PN to be extended to home patients (20). Home PN patients generally fit into two categories. The first group consists of patients who receive PN because of extensive small bowel resection due to inflammatory bowel disease or mesenteric infarction. Home PN is also utilized in patients with nonfunctioning bowels due to radiation therapy, malignancy, and scleroderma with GI involvement. It may also be

Table 2.12.
Potential Complications of Parenteral Nutrition

Catheter Insertion	Postinsertion (Catheter Related)	Metabolic
Hydrothorax	Sepsis	Hyper-/hypoglycemia
Pneumothorax	Thrombosis	Hyperosmolar dehydration
Catheter embolism	Septic thrombophlebitis	Hyperglycemia
Arterial puncture		Nonketotic coma
Air embolism		Azotemia
Myocardial perforation		Hyperammonemia
		Hypokalemia
		Hypomagnesemia
		Hypophosphatemia
		Hypocalcemia
		Hypovitaminosis
		Acidosis/alkalosis
		Fatty acid deficiency
		Hypertriglyceridemia
		Trace mineral deficiency

Table 2.13.
Parenteral Nutrition Monitoring Data

Daily	Twice Weekly	Weekly/Biweekly
Nutritional intake	Phosphorus	24-hr urine
Calories	Calcium	Urea nitrogen
Protein	Magnesium	Creatinine
Fluid	Liver function tests[a]	Transferrin
Electrolytes	Alkaline phosphatase	Albumin
Serum electrolytes	Bilirubin	Total proteins
Sodium	SGOT	Complete blood count
Potassium	SGPT	Clotting studies[b]
Chloride	LDH	PT
Bicarbonate	Creatinine	PTT
Serum glucose		Platelets
Urine glucose (6 hr)		Arterial blood gases
Blood urea nitrogen (BUN)		Trace minerals
Body losses		
Urine		
Gastrointestinal		
Vital signs		
Temperature		
Pulse		
Respirations		
Body weight		

[a] SGOT = serum glutamic-oxaloacetic transaminase; SGPT = serum glutamic-pyruvic transaminase; LDH = lactate dehydrogenase.
[b] PT = prothrombin time; PTT = partial thromboplastin time.

utilized as an adjuvant for patients receiving aggressive chemotherapy.

Hospital and home PN are very similar and the components and techniques are essentially identical. The most significant difference is the necessity for the patient or family members to handle all aspects of the home therapy. Compounding as well as administration of the PN solutions may be performed by the patient. Monitoring of biochemical indices is an important aspect of the patient's self-care, but close medical supervision is necessary to ensure safe and effective therapy. Nutritional support teams, often in concert with private industry, must assume responsibility for identifying candidates for home PN, training the patient in all aspects of self-care, providing necessary supplies, and monitoring the patient's response to treatment. Reimbursement is also a component of home PN therapy, as this therapy may cost in excess of $25,000 per patient per year. Home parenteral nutrition is often the only alternative for nutritional support of some patients. While complete and accurate records on the number of patients on home therapy are not available, presently there are over 2000 patients on partial or complete home PN.

COMPATIBILITY CONSIDERATIONS DURING PN

The complex composition of PN solutions renders them highly susceptible to compatibility problems pertaining to nutrient and drug admixture. Numerous papers have been published since 1974 addressing compatibility considerations in these solutions. It is now becoming better appreciated that factors such as amino acid concentration, solution pH and temperature play key roles in admixture compatibilities.

Typical PN solution components as illustrated in Table 2.11 are considered to be compatible for 24 hours. Compatibility concerns in these solutions have traditionally centered around sodium bicarbonate and calcium-phosphate salts. With the availability of acetate and lactate salts which act as in vivo bicarbonate precursors, it now appears that PN admixture of sodium bicarbonate should be avoided, due to interaction with acidic solutions and calcium and magnesium salts. The compatibility of calcium and phosphate salts in PN solutions is a conditional one, with outcome dependent upon a complex set of interrelationships among factors that affect calcium phosphate solubility (21). In general, 5 mEq of calcium as the gluconate salt may be added per liter of adult PN solution without difficulty.

A developing role may be emerging for PN solutions to serve as drug-delivery vehicles in select patients with severe fluid restriction or limited venous access sites. Few medications may actually be suitable for admixture consideration, though, when accounting for dosing and administration requirements. Aminophylline and cimetidine have demonstrated chemical stability in typical adult PN formulations. When assessing nutrient or drug stability in PN solutions, guide books to intravenous admixtures as well as original published studies should be consulted.

PHARMACOTHERAPEUTIC CONSIDERATIONS DURING PN

Since medication therapy and PN are often administered simultaneously, it is essential to recognize drug-nutrition interrelationships and provide each modality in a safe, compatible and efficacious manner. Medications may have a significant impact upon the interpretation of response to PN therapy as well as necessitate therapeutic maneuvers to avoid conflicts. Therapeutic maneuvers to anticipate include electrolyte supplementation in excess of anabolic requirements, aggressive monitoring of serum and urine electrolytes, and modification of PN formulas and rate of administration. Major classes of "interacting" medications include synthetic penicillin antibiotics, diuretics, corticosteroids, antacids and chemotherapy. Table 2.14 presents a compilation of medication-induced changes observed during PN therapy. The drugs may induce alterations in fluid, electrolyte and acid-base balance as well as interfere with glucose and protein metabolism.

In addition to the physiologic processes that affect electrolyte balance, (previously discussed under "Electrolyte Considerations during PN"), medications may significantly alter renal and GI electrolyte excretion. Synthetic penicillins induce a dose-related renal tubular

Table 2.14.
Medication-induced Changes during Parenteral Nutrition

	Clinical Observation[a]
ELECTROLYTE IMBALANCES	Altered renal/GI excretion; inherent drug content
Antibiotics	
Ampicillin, carbenicillin, ticarcillin	↓Serum K
Amphotericin B	↓Serum K, Mg
Diuretics	
Furosemide, ethacrynic acid	↓Serum Na, K, Mg, Ca, Zn, Cl
Thiazides	↓Serum K, Mg, Zn; ↑serum Ca
Spironolactone	↑Serum K
Corticosteroids	↓Serum K, Ca, PO_4; ↑serum Na
Antacids	
Mg-containing	↑Serum Mg (severe renal failure)
Al-containing	↓Serum PO_4
Cisplatin	↓Serum Mg
Glucose/insulin	↓Serum K, Mg, PO_4
ALTERATION OF GLUCOSE METABOLISM	Altered cellular uptake and insulin effectiveness
Corticosteroids	Hyperglycemia, glucosuria
Diuretics	Hyperglycemia
ALTERATION OF PROTEIN METABOLISM	Antianabolic effects
Corticosteroids	↑BUN, ↑UUN; negative nitrogen balance
Diuretics	Factitious ↑BUN with hypovolemia
ALTERATION OF ACID-BASE BALANCE	Function of electrolytes and acid lost in daily fluid losses
Corticosteroids	Metabolic alkalosis
Diuretics (furosemide, ethacrynic acid)	Metabolic alkalosis
Cimetidine	Inhibitory effect upon gastric acid secretion decreases volume and acid loss secondary to nasogastric suction blunting tendency to metabolic alkalosis

[a] BUN, UUN = blood and urinary urea nitrogen, respectively.

potassium wasting that results in persistent urinary potassium losses and hypokalemia, thus requiring aggressive supplementation and monitoring. Amphotericin B therapy is frequently accompanied by renal tubular wasting of potassium and magnesium. Aggressive therapy with potent diuretics such as furosemide and ethacrynic acid may induce a dramatic urinary excretion of sodium and potassium, thus precipitating severely low serum levels of these electrolytes during PN. The extent of diuretic-induced potassium loss varies with diuretic potency and clinical status of the patient. Patients with malnutrition, ascites, and hyperaldosterone-like states such as hepatic cirrhosis and congestive heart failure who are treated aggressively with potent diuretics are particularly prone to severe hypokalemia requiring potassium supplementation. Potassium sparing diuretics such as spironolactone may cause an insidious increase in serum potassium levels over 3 to 5 days in conjunction with compromised renal function and/or co-administration of potassium supplements. In addition, magnesium and zinc depletion may be observed in patients treated chronically with thiazide diuretics, furosemide and ethacrynic acid.

Corticosteroids can have a profound effect upon nutritional assessment and PN therapy, since they influence carbohydrate, protein and fat metabolism as well as fluid and electrolyte balance. They stimulate hepatic gluconeogenesis and interfere with insulin-mediated peripheral glucose uptake. This results in hyperglycemia, glucosuria and a need for careful monitoring during PN therapy. A cautious approach to attaining energy requirements accompanied by judicious use of insulin and potassium supplements will minimize glucose intolerance. Corticosteroids induce amino acid mobilization from muscle for energy purposes, and concurrent steroid-PN therapy may result in increases in blood urea nitrogen (BUN), urinary urea nitrogen (UUN), and a persistent negative nitrogen balance. Increases in PN solution protein-calorie percentage may temper corticosteroid-induced negative nitrogen balance. Corticosteroids possessing significant mineralocorticoid activity act on the distal renal tubules to enhance sodium retention as well as potassium and hydrogen ion excretion. This may result in edema, hypokalemia and metabolic alkalosis. Patients may require potassium supplements and low sodium feedings.

Furthermore, interpretation of anthropometric measurements in patients receiving chronic steroid therapy must be modified due to muscle wasting, fat redistribution and a realization that anthropometric standards have not been established for steroid-treated patients. Patients receiving concurrent steroid-PN therapy require close monitoring of fluid status and weight change, serum and urine electrolytes and glucose, and nitrogen balance.

Cimetidine has been reported to significantly decrease gastric acid output and volume of gastric secretions. Consequently, patients on concurrent cimetidine-PN therapy with simultaneous nasogastric suction will be less predisposed to metabolic alkalosis related to acid loss or use of high acetate-containing PN formulas. Patients predisposed to metabolic acidosis (i.e. renal failure, neonates) may require admixture of bicarbonate precursor salts such as acetate or lactate to PN solutions during cimetidine therapy.

PHARMACOKINETIC CONSIDERATIONS IN MALNUTRITION

The diverse pathophysiologic changes that can occur during PEM are listed in Table 2.15. These changes support the contention that drug response and drug kinetics may be altered during malnutrition (22). Numerous alterations in GI physiology collectively favor a decrease in rate and extent of oral drug absorption. Changes in lean body mass and extracellular fluid compartments, fat distribution and the circulating protein pool may alter a drug's volume of distribution and modify the intensity of pharmacologic response. Although alterations upon metabolic enzyme systems and hepatic drug clearance are anticipated, the overall effect of PEM upon hepatic function and drug clearance is complex and difficult to quantitate. In addition, manipulation of dietary components may induce or alter hepatic enzyme function and drug metabolism. Non-uniform changes in renal function have also been observed in varying patient populations during malnutrition.

Despite evidence suggesting altered drug kinetics in malnutrition, there is a distinct lack of systematic, well-controlled studies relating to drug disposition and drug response in humans with PEM. Supportive documentation is needed to establish clinical significance and

Table 2.15.
Pathophysiological Changes in Malnutrition which May Alter Drug Pharmacokinetics

GASTROINTESTINAL CHANGES
  Anorexia, nausea, vomiting and diarrhea
  Mucosal and villous atrophy
  Hypochlorhydria
  Delayed stomach emptying
  Altered intestinal motility
  Pancreatic exocrine dysfunction
  Malabsorption and maldigestion
BODY COMPOSITION CHANGES
  Increased total body water
  Increased extracellular water
  Decreased somatic protein and body fat
  Electrolyte deficiencies (K^+, Mg^{2+}, PO_4^{2-})
VISCERAL PROTEIN CHANGES
  Depressed levels of albumin, transferrin, preal-
    bumin, and retinol-binding protein
  Decreased lipoprotein
  γ-Globulin changes:
    Increased α
    Normal β
    Reduced γ
HEPATIC CHANGES
  Altered hormone metabolism
  Altered microsomal enzyme levels and micro-
    somal protein concentrations
  Altered enzyme activity
RENAL CHANGES
  Altered blood flow
  Altered glomerular filtration
  Reduced tubular secretion
CARDIOVASCULAR CHANGES
  Reduced cardiac output
  Hypotension and bradycardia
  Circulatory insufficiency

correlate pharmacokinetic changes with the type and extent of malnutrition. Furthermore, interpretation of estimated creatinine clearance and therapeutic drug serum levels may have to be qualified in this patient population, as the hypoalbuminemic patient may present with "normal" drug serum levels (sum of protein-bound and free drug) but a larger than normal free fraction of drug.

CONCLUSION

Aggressive nutritional support with parenteral nutrition affords tremendous opportunities for clinical pharmacy involvement. The pharmacist may participate in establishing nutritional needs, formula design and compounding, and assist in the delivery and monitoring of the therapy. Additionally, the clinical pharmacist's knowledge of drug therapy can be invaluable when the complex interrelationships between drugs and nutritional therapy are evaluated. With an ever increasing number of hospitalized patients receiving PN therapy, the opportunities for pharmacy involvement are almost unlimited.

References

1. Bistrian BR, Blackburn GL, Scrinshaw NS: Protein status of general surgical patients. *JAMA* 230:858, 1974.
2. Bistrian BR, Blackburn GL, Vitale J: Prevalence of malnutrition in general medical patients. *JAMA* 235:1567, 1976.
3. Skoutakis VA, Martinez DR, Miller WA, et al: Team approach to total parenteral nutrition. *Am J Hosp Pharm* 32:693, 1975.
4. Butterworth CE, Weinsier RL: Malnutrition in hospitalized patients: assessment and treatment. In *Modern Nutrition in Health and Disease*, ed 6. Philadelphia: Lea & Febiger, 1980, p 670.
5. Roe DA: *Drug-induced Nutritional Deficiencies.* Westport, Conn.: AVI Publishing Company, 1976.
6. Grant JP, Custer PB, Thurlow J: Current techniques of nutritional assessment. *Surg Clin North Am* 61:437, 1981.
7. Harris JA, Benedict FG: Biometric studies of basal metabolism in man. *Carnegie Inst Wash Publ* No. 279, 1919.
8. Blackburn GL, Bistrian BR, Maini BS, et al: Nutritional and metabolic assessment of the hospitalized patient. *JPEN* 1:11, 1977.
9. Derr RF, Ziere L: Etiology of hyperalimentation coma. *N Engl J Med* 288:1080, 1973.
10. Dudrick SJ, MacFadyen BV, Van Buren CT, et al: Parenteral hyperalimentation—metabolic problems and solutions. *Ann Surg* 176:256, 1972.
11. Askanazi J, Rosenbaum SH, Hyman AI, et al: Respiratory changes induced by large loads of total parenteral nutrition. *JAMA* 243:1444, 1980.
12. McKibbin JM, Pope A, Thayer BA: Parenteral nutrition: studies on fat emulsions for intravenous alimentation. *J Lab Clin Med* 30:488, 1945.
13. Schuberth O, Wretlind A: Intravenous infusion of fat emulsions, phosphotides, and emulsifying agents. *Acta Chim Scand Suppl* 278:1021, 1961.
14. Caldwell MD: Human essential fatty acid deficiency: a review. In *Fat Emulsions in Parenteral Nutrition*. Chicago: American Medical Association, 1976, p 24.
15. Elwyn DH: Nutritional requirements of adult surgical patients. *Crit Care Med* 8:9, 1980.
16. Anon: *Prescribing Information for Liposyn 10% Intravenous Fat Emulsion*. Chicago: Abbott Laboratories, Inc., 1980.
17. Fischer JE, Bower RH: Nutritional support in liver disease. *Surg Clin North Am* 61:653, 1981.
18. Anon: Multivitamin preparations for parenteral use in a statement by the nutrition advisory group. *JPEN* 3:258, 1979.

19. Anon: Guidelines for essential trace element preparations for parenteral use—a statement by the nutrition advisory group. *JPEN* 3:263, 1979.

20. Schneider PJ, Mirtallo JM: Home parenteral nutrition programs. *JPEN* 5:157, 1981.

21. Eggert L, Rusho W, MacKay M: Calcium and phosphorus compatibility in parenteral nutrition solutions for neonates. *Am J Hosp Pharm* 39:49, 1982.

22. Kirshnaswamy K: Drug metabolism and pharmacokinetics in malnutrition. *Clin Pharmacokinet* 3:216, 1978.

CHAPTER 3

Pediatrics

ROBERT H. LEVIN, Pharm.D.

Pediatrics is that branch of medicine which deals with humans from birth through adolescence. Specific terminology is used for different age groups (Table 3.1). Within pediatrics there are as many medical specialties as there are in adult internal medicine. A number of pediatric primary care providers are involved in the care of children, including pediatricians, family practice physicians, and pediatric nurse practitioners. There are many pharmacists active in this field as pediatric specialist's in pediatric clinics, inpatient wards and nurseries. This specialization by pharmacists has led to an enhancement of pediatric reserch with a concomitant increase in knowledge concerning drug use in children (1, 2).

Neonates, infants and children have many unique drug-related considerations. Major age-related differences in body organ function alter the biopharmaceutics and pharmacokinetics of drugs. In infants, particularly in neonates, differences in drug absorption, distribution, excretion, metabolism and sensitivity affect the utilization and dosing of drugs. Pediatric dosing also involves a knowledge of various methods of calculating doses and a consideration of appropriate drug formulations. The child's family or caretakers also must be included in any discussion of medical treatment for administration of drugs to the child. The entire issue of compliance to therapeutic regimens rests on the families willingness to assist in the child's medical care.

The healthy growth and development of children is the major focus for preventative "well baby" clinics. During these visits to the health care provider the parents are counseled about proper nutrition. Considerations involving breast-feeding, maternal diet and avoidances of drugs are stressed. The implementation of synthetic infant formulas, baby foods and table food are also discussed. The prevention of disease is stressed through proper nutrition and the use of prophylactic agents such as immunizations. The advantages and possible adverse effects of each immunization is thoroughly discussed by the physician. Most physicians inquire about and purchase these immunizations from pharmacists. Additionally, many mothers, whether breast-feeding or formula-feeding their infants, will purchase medications, infant formulas and other products from pharmacies. Therefore, it becomes incumbent for the pharmacist to be knowledgable in each of these important childhood areas.

DRUG ABSORPTION

The most frequent route of drug administration in children is the oral one. Newborns and infants have a greater potential for altered absorption due to a faster transit time in the gut, a decreased production of gastric acid, and a lack of hydrolytic enzymes. A significant effect of this lack of hydrolytic enzymes is the inability of infants to split palmitic acid from chloramphenicol palmitate suspension. Oral phenytoin may also be inadequately absorbed in infants less than 6 months of age and doses greater than normal (15–20 mg/kg/day) may be needed to produce therapeutic blood levels (3).

The rectal route is employed more frequently in young children than in adults, since children more frequently have difficulty in swallowing medications. No specific physiologic differences have been shown to influence rectal absorption of medication in children; however, problems have been documented with certain suppository dosage forms. Outdated suppositories or those exposed to air may have erratic melting characteristics and produce decreased and unpredictable drug absorption, e.g. outdated aminophylline suppositories. Foil wrapping of suppositories helps protect suppositories during storage and allows for a more predictable drug release. There has been appropriate therapeutic effects with foil-wrapped suppositories of aspirin, acetaminophen, prochlorperazine, promethazine, glycerine and others. An aqueous retention enema of theophylline is available and should be utilized instead of the suppositories if rectal administration is necessary.

Ointments, lotions and creams are commonly utilized for topical treatment of localized skin lesions. These lesions are usually located in the diaper area in infants and the trunk, limbs and face in children. A number of factors should be considered before selecting a topical agent. Infants compared to older children have a larger skin surface area which is capable of absorbing more topical drugs especially in the groin and facial areas. Inflammation increases the amount of drug absorbed as does occlusion occurring with plastic coated diapers. Infant's skin is very sensitive so that a number of chemicals frequently cause local irritation, e.g., parabens, methyl salicyclate and others.

The parenteral route, frequently used in hospitalized children, is seldom needed for medication administration in ambulatory children. However, it is routinely used for required immunizations such as intramuscular (IM) diphtheria-pertussis-tetanus (DPT) and subcutaneous (SC) measles-mumps-rubella (MMR). Infants have a small muscle mass which requires that routine IM injections be given in the lateral thigh rather than the arm or buttocks. Absorption from IM sites in neonates is slower and more erratic due to a smaller muscle mass and blood supply. Therefore, intravenous is the preferred parenteral route in neonates.

DRUG DISTRIBUTION

Most drugs are primarily distributed in the aqueous portion of the body. In neonates, whose body weight is composed of about 75% water, the volume of distribution is increased. For example, the volume of distribution of theophylline is approximately 1 liter/kg compared to 0.48 liter/kg in a 6-year-old. In addition, the total body water of neonates is 56% extracellular fluid into which many drugs are primarily distributed. Body water composition gradually falls to 40% extracellular and 60% intracellular water and 60% total body water by 1 year of age (Table 3.2) (4). Many drugs are also less avidly bound to plasma proteins which are also lower in neonates. This produces a higher unbound fraction of drugs such as phenytoin and sulfasoxizole leading to their increased clearance and decreased half lives.

DRUG METABOLISM

The liver primarily acts to terminate drug effects by conversion of active lipid soluble drugs to inactive water soluble metabolites. These water-soluble metabolites bind less to serum albumin, penetrate lipid cell membranes less readily and are therefore excreted readily by the kidney.

Liver metabolism is the predominant organ for in vivo drug transformation. Liver enzymes are present at birth and are stimulated to proliferate by the build up of endogenous substrate. Each of the enzyme systems matures at a different rate but is sufficient at 3 days postpartum, in a full term infant, to adequately metabolize endogenous bilirubin. Bilirubin is a by-product of hemoglobin and is one of the major products which requires metabolism through the glucuronyl transferase pathway. This pathway slowly matures so that by 1 to 2

Table 3.1.
Pediatric Definitions

Category	Age
Premature	<38 weeks of gestation
Newborn, neonate	Birth to 1 month old
Infant, baby	1–24 months
Small child	1–5 years
Older child	6–12 years
Adolescent	13–18 years

Table 3.2.
Percentages of Body Water[a]

Age	Extracellular Water (%)	Intracellular Water (%)	Total Body Water (%)
Premature baby (1.5 kg)	60	40	83
Full term baby (3.5 kg)	56	44	74
5-month-old (7.0 kg)	50	50	60
1-year-old (10.0 kg)	40	60	59
Adult male	40	60	60

[a] Developmental changes from birth through adults. The extracellular and intracellular water are expressed as a percentage of total body water. Total body water is expressed as a percentage of body weight. (Data from B. Friis-Hansen (4).)

weeks of neonatal age it is also capable of glucuronidating exogenous substances. It is at this time drugs dependent on this pathway can be safely utilized. If chloramphenicol were to be given to an infant less than 1 week old, at the usual dosage for children of 100 mg/kg/day, the drug would accumulate and cause cardiovascular collapse and cyanosis—this is known as "the gray baby syndrome" (5). If required, chloramphenicol, in a dose of 25 mg/kg/day, can be used in the first week of neonatal life.

Bilirubin itself can be toxic to the newborn. The unconjugated, unmetabolized, protein bound fraction of bilirubin partitions into the brain very readily. With serum bilirubin levels of 12 to 20 mg/dl bilirubin crossing the blood brain barrier will cause a yellow staining of the brain called kernicterus. Kernicterus may progress to irreversible brain damage and death with bilirubin levels greater than 21 mg/dl. Irreversible brain damage can also occur at lower bilirubin serum levels of 12 to 20 mg/dl if drugs such as sulfasoxizole, aspirin, or caffeine are given to the neonate. These drugs displace the bilirubin from albumin sites and allow it to pass into the brain. Bilirubin levels over 12 mg/dl are usually treated by putting the infant under fluorescent lights. The light metabolizes the bilirubin in the skin to harmless metabolites which are excreted by the kidney. Other forms of treatment are phenobarbital, which induces liver enzymes, or blood transfusions.

EXCRETION

The predominant method the body uses to eliminate both metabolized and unmetabolized drugs is through the renal system. Drugs are also excreted through the gastrointestinal tract, lungs and sweat glands. With most drugs that achieve therapeutic serum levels these latter pathways are of only limited significance. Neonatal kidney function matures rapidly from parturition. At birth, a full term newborn has approximately 33% of the glomerular filtration rate and renal tubular excretion capacity of the adult kidney. This capacity is about 15% or less in premature infants. The capacity to excrete solute load quickly improves in the first few weeks of life to about 50% of adult levels at 1 month of age. Improvement is reflected in the decreasing half-lives of penicillin and carbenicillin in neonates (Table 3.3). Drugs which are dependent to a large degree on renal excretion, e.g. aminoglycosides and penicillins, must therefore be adjusted for the neonate. Doses based on the neonate's age and weight have been elaborated for antibiotics and other drugs and should be the only ones utilized. Drugs for normal infants and older children are administered in the usual therapeutic doses with no adjustment needed for renal function. At about 9 to 12 months of age the infant kidney is functioning at adult levels.

DRUG SENSITIVITY

Neonates and infants are more sensitive to the effect of many drugs due to the immaturity of their bodily organs. The central nervous system matures slowly until it reaches adult levels at about 8 years of age. Because of this and the increased permeability of the blood brain barrier, the neonate appears to be especially sensitive to the depressant effects of drugs like phenobarbital, morphine sulfate, chloral hydrate, meprobamate and chlorpromazine. Codeine and meperidine, however, do not produce this exaggerated effect in neonates.

The cardiovascular system usually functions adequately in the neonate and infant. However, in times of stress, exaggerated responses

Table 3.3.
Age-dependent Half-life of Antibiotics in Serum

Age Group (days old)	Study A[a]		Study B[b]	
	No. of patients	Average half-life carbenicillin (hr)	No. of patients	Average half-life penicillin (hr)
1–3	13	5.7	—	
4–7	23	4.2	7 (avg. age 3.7)	3.21
8–14	13	3.4	13 (avg. age 9.5)	1.74
15–21	2	2.2	6 (avg. age 18.5)	1.4
22–45	4	1.5		

[a] J. D. Nelson and G. M. McCracken (6).
[b] G. H. McCracken et al. (7).

may occur due to its immaturity. General anesthetics may cause exaggerated cardiovascular depression. Diuretics and/or antihypertensives in normal doses may induce severe hypotention.

The body temperature regulating system is unstable and immature in the neonate and infant. Many drugs can cause wide fluctuations in temperature and have exaggerated responses in neonates and infants. Drugs in therapeutic doses that normally lower temperature, like aspirin and acetaminophen, can also raise the temperature when taken in toxic doses (Table 3.4 and 3.5). The skin, in addition to its immature thermal regulatory effects, increased permeability and area, is also more sensitive to drug effects. This drug sensitivity may be either allergic in nature or a toxic adverse effect and occur throughout infancy and childhood. The allergic reactions are the most common and may be the immediate onset type such as urticaria, angioneurotic edema, anaphylaxis or the delayed onset types such as erythema multiforme or fixed drug eruption. These drug-induced reactions mimic skin eruptions caused by other pathological processes. The most commonly used pediatric drugs leading to skin reactions are: sulfas, tetracyclines, penicillins, isoniazid, cephalosporins, barbiturates, phenytoin, chloral hydrate, phenothiazines, narcotics, aspirin, indomethacin, phenylbutazone, iodides, griseofulvin, and topical antihistamines. There are a number of other adverse drug effects which occur in children: 1) growth suppression with tetracycline and adrenocorticosteroids; 2) sexual precocity with androgens; 3) neurotoxicity with hexachloraphene; 4) prepubertal effects with levodopa; 5) intracranial hypertension with adrenocorticosteroids, nalidixic acid and nitrofurantoin; 6) jaundice with novobiocin, sulfonamides and vitamin K_3; and, 7) a bulging fontanel and tooth staining with tetracycline (9).

DOSING

As can now be readily appreciated, children are not small adults. Doses for neonates must be tailored for their age and weight with due consideration for decreased liver and kidney function. Doses given on a mg/kg basis which have been tested and found to be therapeutic in neonates, infants and children can be found in a number of sources (10, 11). Drugs which are very toxic such as cancer chemotherapeu-

Table 3.4.
Drugs Causing Hyperthermia[a]

Drug	Comment
Salicylates[b]	Increase temperature with toxicity and cause sweating and dehydration

Dinitrophenols
  Herbicides, fungicides
  Nitrophenols
  Miscellaneous pesticides
  Insecticides
	Increased temperature up to 2 days after heavy exposure, whether inhaled, ingested, or by skin contact

Anticholinergics
  Atropine
  Scopolamine
  Belladonna
  Cogentin
  Probanthine, etc.
	High temperature can result from large doses or repeated therapeutic doses

Sympathomimetics
  Amphetamine and congeners
  Ephedrine
  Epinephrine
  Benzedrex inhalers, etc.
  Cocaine
	Large doses cause chills and fever

p-Aminophenols[b]
  Acetaminophen
  Tempra, Tylenol
  Phenacetin
	Large doses cause sweating and chills and probably fever

Antihistamines
  Benadryl
  Vistaril, etc.
	Large doses will cause fever

Boric acid	Large doses cause fever

Thyroid preparations
  Synthroid
  Proloid, etc.
	Large doses cause fever

Alcohol[b]	Large doses cause fever
Chlorpromazine[b] Possibly other phenothiazines	May initially cause fever that can last a few days

[a] From R. H. Levin and H. E. Maltz (8).
[b] Drug in both lists (see Table 3.5).

tic agents, should be, for better accuracy, dosed on a mg/m^2 basis. Using body surface area takes into account the child's height and weight and is especially useful for children who are not normal for their age in either height or weight. If necessary, the body surface area can be calculated from a child's height and weight, or a suitable nomogram can be utilized (Fig. 3.1). If a dose for a drug cannot be found in appropriate texts or current publications, one has to consider the fact that the drug may not be suitable for pediatric use. This should be evaluated carefully before any dose is calculated. There are many formulas to calculate doses by the child's weight, age, surface area or height; however, none is very accurate or useful and should not be used.

COMPLIANCE

Most compliance studies of adult ambulatory patients reveal that 50 to 70% of patients fail to complete a course of therapy. In addition, a surprising 90% of patients make at least some error in taking their medication such as a forgotten dose or a dose taken at the incorrect time. In pediatrics, which has similar compli-

ance problems, the parents' or child's adherence to a medication regimen is often incomplete, especially when the child is very ill and unwilling to take medications. Becker et al. (12), in an effort to predict compliance in parents, studied mothers whose children had otitis media and were treated with oral penicillin. Mothers who were most diligent in completing drug therapy had the following traits: 1) they were concerned about the child's health and current illness, 2) they felt the illness was a significant threat to the child's health and welfare, 3) they had confidence in the child's physician and the prescribed medication, 4) they had a more satisfactory experience with their pediatric clinic, 5) they actively endeavored to keep the child healthy and prevent future illness, and 6) they were better able to manage the every day problems of life. In contrast, those mothers who complied less

Table 3.5.
Drugs Causing Hypothermia[a]

Drug	Comment
Salicylates[b] Aspirin Sodium salicylate Methyl salicylate (oil of wintergreen)	Lower fever in therapeutic doses
p-Aminophenols[b] Phenacetin Acetaminophen Tylenol Tempra	Therapeutic doses will lower fever
Phenylbutazone Indomethacin Colchicine	Usually used for arthritis and gout but can be used to lower temperature
Chlorpromazine and thorazine[b] Other phenothiazines also	Lower fever
Cholinergic agents Physostigmine Pilocarpine Neostigmine Urecholine, etc.	Large doses or repeated small doses cause profuse sweating and cold extremities
Topical agents Water Alcohol[b] Volatile oils Menthol, etc.	Local cooling causes lower temperature

[a] From R. H. Levin and H. E. Maltz (8).
[b] Drug in both lists (see Table 3.4).

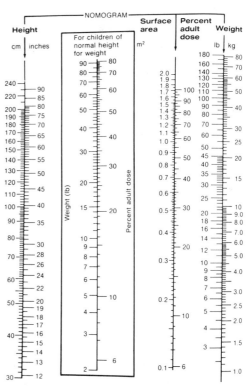

Figure 3.1. Pediatric drug therapy nomogram. (Reproduced with permission from S. M. Kegel and M. I. Singer: Critical care of infants and children after the neonatal period. In D. A. Zschoche (ed.): *Mosley's Comprehensive Review of Critical Care*, The C. V. Mosby Co., St. Louis, 1976. Modified from W. E. Nelson: *Textbook of Pediatrics*, Ed. 8, W. B. Saunders, Philadelphia, 1964.)

well with the medication regimen had opposite attitudes to the above categories. Additionally, these latter mothers thought their health was bad and concerned themselves with their own health problems rather than their child's. To achieve maximum success with medication regimens, therefore, it is appropriate for health care personnel to emphasize and reinforce those traits mentioned that lead to increased compliance. Mattar et al. (13) reported that by emphasizing verbal and written patient instructions and providing calibrated measuring devices and calendars, pharmacists were able to achieve compliance levels of 51% in a cohort of 33 patients being treated with antibiotics for otitis media. In comparison, only 8.5% of 200 control patients were compliant.

A verbal contract between the pharmacist and patient to take the most appropriate medication should improve the patient's understanding and willingness to undertake the course of treatment. It is better to fully explain the disease or illness and its drug treatment to the child and parent and get a "true" informed consent. The pharmacist is in an excellent position to recommend and provide the appropriate dosage formulation for any particular patient considerations. To further increase compliance the pharmacist can recommend the drug which 1) has the least amount of side effects, 2) is taken only once or twice a day, 3) is easy to swallow and palatable, 4) is less expensive, and 5) is easy to use, carry and store. The pharmacist should encourage the parent giving these medications to approach the child with firmness but gentleness. A provocative, angry or punishing parental attitude will increase the child's hostility and defensive medication avoidance behavior. This adversary behavior between parent and child affects compliance and interferes with good parent-child relationships even in adolescents. The adolescent has all the compliance considerations of the child plus those of the adult, therefore, an adolescent needs to be knowledgable about and in control of their medications. Adolescents who feel they have control over their destiny and affairs should achieve good compliance with medications.

INFANT NUTRITION

The practicing pharmacist is often called upon to recommend nutritional infant formulas, dietary supplements, and vitamins and minerals. There are currently a vast array of pediatric preparations available both for normal growing children and those with nutritional deficiency states.

Human breast milk is the most healthy and complete dietary food for the full term infant. It should be the only source of nutrition for infants up to 6 months of age. Breast-feeding is usually supplemented with food in the child over 6 months old. In the United States over 50% of infants are breast-fed until at least 3 months of age. This decreases to 25% in 6-month-old infants and less than 5% in 9- to 12-month-old infants still breast-feeding. In some cultures, however, children at 4 to 6 years of age are still breast-feeding to gain needed protein. There are other advantages to human milk; it is less expensive than infant formulas, the breast is an antiseptic environment, it has better biological value of proteins and curds which are easier to digest; it produces better fat absorption, and it contains immunoglobulins, lysozymes, antistreptococcal agents, complement components, lactoferrin and macrophages which decrease infections.

There are disadvantages to breast-feeding. The mother must want to nurse in order for it to be satisfactory and rewarding for her and the infant. The breasts must be prepared for nursing during the last trimester of pregnancy. There is sometimes pain, inconvenience, engorgement, and minor infections and inflammation associated with breast-feeding. The mother should maintain an adequate diet and must be careful about taking drugs which are excreted in breast milk. The mother should not breast-feed if she has active, untreated tuberculosis, breast cancer or a serious infection. In many cases, active support and encouragement by health care personnel will overcome most, if not all, of the maternal apprehension due to these disadvantages. Even the maternal use of medications can be carefully directed in order to least affect the breast-feeding infant.

NORMAL BREAST PHYSIOLOGY

The breast is composed of glandular, fibrous and adipose tissue and rests on a bed of connective tissue. The glandular tissue is composed of 15 to 20 lobes arranged radially around the nipple. Strands of fibrous tissue connect the lobes, and adipose tissue occupies the space between and around the lobes. Each lobe is divided into several lobules and connected by alveolar tissue, blood vessels and ducts (Fig. 3.2a). Each lobule contains a small lactiferous duct. Eventually these lactiferous

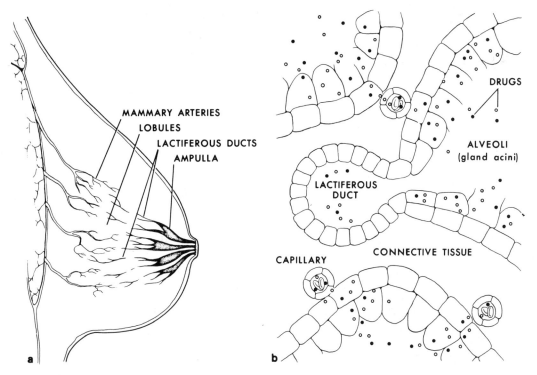

Figure 3.2. (a) Cross section of breast. (b) Magnified cross section of lobule depicting drugs entering alveoli from capillaries. (Adapted from J. Arena (14).)

ducts unite and form a single main canal for each lobe. These 15 to 20 main canals each become dilated and form a reservoir (sinus lactiferous) for milk storage and finally merge and pass through the nipple.

The functioning part of the breast is the alveoli or acini (sacs) in the lobule (Fig. 3.2b). It is in the acini epithelium that milk is produced and secreted into the lactiferous ducts. Drug transition from the blood occurs in capillary beds, through the acini epithelium into the lactiferous ducts.

NORMAL COMPOSITION OF MILK

The composition of milk is determined by the mammary gland with little or no external bodily control (15, 16). The milk occurs in three forms: colostrum, transitional or mature milk. Colostrum, which serves as a precursor of milk, may be expressed from the breasts as early as the 4th month of pregnancy, but it usually appears after parturition. It is scanty the first few days after birth, becomes well established on the 3rd or 4th day and usually continues no more than 5 days. It has, however, been known to continue for as long as 10 days. Colostrum is a transudate consisting primarily of serum albumin (3 to 5%) and cast off epithelium (colostrum corpuscles) which have undergone fatty degeneration. It has a higher specific gravity than mature milk (1.030 to 1.060 compared with 1.026 to 1.036) and also a higher average pH (7.7 compared with 6.8). It is richer in vitamin A, sodium, potassium and other minerals but lower in sugar and fat. Colostrum will be quickly modified by the mammary gland into transitional milk.

Transitional milk is produced within the first week of breast-feeding. It usually lasts for a few weeks during which time it achieves a moderate increase in fat and sugar and a gradual decrease in proteins and minerals. Milk finally takes on a stable or mature character near the end of the first month of lactation.

Mature milk has between 0.9 and 1.6% protein, 2 to 6% fat, and 6.5 to 8% lactose. The composition of milk at the beginning of a feeding is highest in protein and lowest in fat. This is reversed toward the end of the feeding. What effect this might have on excretion of drugs is unknown.

Once established, mature milk will vary little in composition (15, 16). Providing the mother has an adequate nutritional food intake, her diet can be quite varied without affecting milk composition or volume. A deficiency in maternal diet will first cause a decrease in milk quantity but will not affect milk composition unless the mother's tissue stores are depleted. A decreased water intake will cause maternal thirst before it affects milk production.

CONTROL OF MILK PRODUCTION

The initiation and maintenance of milk production has not been adequately studied. The evidence regarding the roles of physiological and endocrine factors in lactation is contradictory (14, 17–19). As previously mentioned, lactation usually begins about the time of birth or shortly thereafter. Its inhibition during pregnancy is assumed to be the result of the occurrence of high estrogen and/or progesterone levels. The effects of estrogen on milk secretion are dose-dependent. At low endogenous levels occurring postpartum, milk secretion occurs, whereas at high doses (diethylstilbestrol or parenteral estrogens given postpartum), lactation is inhibited. In most women, low dose oral contraceptives do not decrease lactation even when given immediately postpartum (20). It is thought that estrogens may work partly by affecting prolactin (lactogenic factor) which is secreted from the anterior pituitary.

Prolactin is presently under extensive investigation in an effort to delineate its true role during pregnancy and lactation (17, 18). During pregnancy, prolactin along with estrogen, progesterone and human growth hormone aids in breast development. It achieves high concentrations during pregnancy and during breast-feeding, but it is in low concentration after birth in the absence of breast-feeding. Interestingly enough, if breast-feeding is total, successful and unrestricted the high levels of prolactin achieved have been reported to be contraceptive (21). This contraceptive effect is seen only in primitive societies and has not been observed in America, where formula supplements are frequently given.

The posterior pituitary, in addition to the anterior pituitary, is involved in and stimulated by an infant breast feeding.

Infant nursing →
stimulation of nerves in nipple →
→ *anterior pituitary* → prolactin production
→ lactation (milk production)
→ *posterior pituitary* → oxytocin release
→ "letdown" reflex

The release of oxytocin by the posterior pituitary initiates the "letdown" reflex (Fig. 3.3). Oxytocin stimulates the expression or ejection of milk from the breast whereas prolactin stimulates milk production. The letdown reflex is responsive to other internal and external factors. The actions and sounds associated with nursing can initiate this reflex. In contrast, distractions such as fright, pain and emotional distress can inhibit milk expression. It is hypothesized that high levels of the catecholamines, adrenaline and norepinephrine produced in the latter circumstances cause a vasoconstriction in the mammary circulation which prevents oxytocin from reaching the contractile cells (19). Medications, in excessive doses which also release endogenous catecholamines, e.g., amphetamines and most decongestants, may interfere with milk secretion.

QUANTITY OF MILK PRODUCED

The quantity of milk produced is dependent upon the demands of the infant. If the infant's demand is increasing, milk supply will adjust accordingly within 2 days and vice versa. The actual secretion of milk is a discontinuous process. During feeding there is increased milk secretion due to the depletion of milk stores. In all probability, drugs would also be excreted into milk in larger amounts when the milk is being actively secreted. To derive the total quantity of drug ingested (measured as mg per 100 ml or mg%), it is necessary to know the quantity of milk ingested by the infant. This is dependent on the age and weight of the infant (Table 3.6).

DRUGS EXCRETED IN MILK

Medications ingested by the mother may be passed to a nursing infant through the breast milk. In this way, the infant may be exposed to a wide variety of foods and medications. The excretion of drugs in breast milk has been reviewed elsewhere (22–36). However, caution is warranted in interpreting the subjective report by Mary White of the La Leche League

---

Infant nursing → stimulates nerves in nipple → afferent stimuli through nerves → posterior pituitary → release of oxytocin → efferent stimuli via blood → mammary blood circulation → contraction of minute contractile cells of alveoli → express milk into ducts → lactiferous sinus → available to infant

Figure 3.3. Letdown reflex.

Table 3.6.
Quantities of Milk Ingested

Amount at Each Feeding[a] (ml)	Age (wk)
20–45	1
30–90	2
40–140	4
60–150	6
75–165	12
90–175	16
120–225	24

[a] Feedings are usually every 3 to 4 hours; quantity consumed dependent on infant's weight.

(37). This extensive listing is documented by numerous personal communications. Interpretations of data tend to favor, with few exceptions, only reports concerning the safety and harmlessness of drugs in breast milk. This oversimplification tends to dismiss the problems associated with drugs in breast milk as unimportant and not harmful in order to promote breast-feeding at all costs.

There is a decided lack of information concerning the excretion of drugs into milk. This is probably due to the difficulty in carrying out experimental observations in nursing mothers, the complicated analytical procedures required on many drugs and a general lack of interest in this subject by most researchers. Furthermore, the majority of scientific data available are generally from uncontrolled, unsophisticated studies. Most original work was done over 20 years ago and consists largely of case reports. Within the last few years, however, there have appeared original articles (listed in Tables 3.7 and 3.8) regarding drugs excreted in breast milk. Many animal studies have been done, but it is difficult to extrapolate these results to humans. What information, then, can the pharmacist utilize to form meaningful judgments concerning the safety of drugs in the nursing mother?

Unless contrary information exists, it can be assumed that any drug orally administered to and absorbed by the mother will be excreted in milk. For a majority of drugs and foods the usual concentration achieved in the milk is insufficient to elicit clinical symptoms in the infant. There are some drugs, however, that are excreted in sufficient quantities to cause observable and sometimes serious effects in the infant. The excretion of drugs is dependent on the following physiological characteristics:

the pH gradient between the plasma and milk, the pK_a or the degree of ionization of the drug, the lipid-water solubility characteristics of the drug, the distribution of the drug by body transport mechanisms and the concentration gradient of diffusable drug between placenta and milk.

The normal pH of blood ranges between 7.35 and 7.45 with an average of 7.4. The average pH of milk is 6.8 with a range of 6.5 to 7.4. The pK_a is the negative log of the dissociation constant of an acid. The more a compound dissociates to release hydrogen ions the more acidic it is and the smaller will be the value of its pK_a. A strong acid such as salicylic acid has a pK_a of 3.0 whereas a weak acid such as phenobarbital has a pK_a of 7.4. The relationship of pH and pK_a is represented by the Henderson-Hasselbach equation:

$$pH = pK_a \text{ (of acid)} + \log \text{(salt)/(acid)}$$

for acidic compounds, and

$$pH = pK_a \text{ (of base)} + \log \text{(base)/(salt)}$$

for basic compounds. This formula is also used when determining physiological acid-base balance where

$$pH \ (7.4) = pK_a \ (6.1) + \log \ (HCO_3^-)/(H_2CO_3)$$

This equation is reduced to the familiar ratio, $HCO_3^-/H_2CO_3 = 20:1$. It is important to remember that when $pH = pK_a$ the concentration of salt and acid in solution is equal. Since the pH and pK_a have logarithmic relationships, each one change of pH reflects a 10-fold change in relative concentrations of acid and salt forms. When exposed to body fluids of differing pH separated by a physical membrane, an acid or base will accumulate in the fluid in which it is most ionized and where most soluble. Serum concentrations of erythromycin with pK_a of 8.8 will have about 15 times more salt (ionized) than base (un-ionized). When erythromycin is excreted into milk with a pH of 6.8, the ratio of ionized to un-ionized molecules is 100:1. Therefore, the concentration of erythromycin in milk should be 6 times its concentration in serum, and in fact this relationship has been shown experimentally (23). In general, basic drugs are excreted in higher concentration in milk, whereas acidic drugs are less concentrated in milk.

Diffusion across a concentration gradient also plays a role in drug excretion. A drug with a high lipid solubility will diffuse very poorly

Table 3.7.
Drugs Excreted in Breast Milk (Substantiated Data)[a]

Drug	Quantity — Maternal dose	Route[b]	Effects in Infants	Comments	Significance[c]
Acetaldehyde	0.6 g/kg ethanol	PO	No effects	Authors feel that acetaldehyde (a metabolite of alcohol) is inhibited from excretion into breast milk (see alcohol) (38)	0
Acetylsalicylic acid (aspirin)	300–600 mg	PO	Infant should have an injection of vitamin K at birth then a risk of bleeding is minimal with normal doses (29). Salicylism occurs only with doses used for treatment of rheumatoid arthritis	Usual analgetic doses (300–600 mg) are probably safe while breast-feeding (39)	+
Alcohol (ethanol)	0.6 g/kg ethanol	PO	None reported	Maternal serum levels correspond to about 80–90 mg/100 ml (or moderate levels) (38), low to moderate amounts taken by mother produce little if any effects, large ingested amounts by alcoholic mothers can produce alcohol effects in infants (41, 42). Maternal doses greater than 1 g/kg may inhibit milk ejection reflex and doses greater than 2 g/kg may completely block oxytocin release by the posterior pituitary (43)	2+
	750 ml/day port wine		Drunkenness Intoxication		
Aldrin		—		An insecticide which should be avoided (44)	2+
Aloe	15 mg aloin	PO	Increased bowel activity in 33% (11/33) with mother receiving normal adult dose; increased bowel activity in 10% (1/11) in same study and included also a chemical analysis of milk which 8/11 were positive for aloin	Detectable in most samples. In usual dose, probably will not cause adverse effects; however, with higher doses, will probably cause increased bowel activity (45)	+
Amitriptyline	25–50 mg	PO	None reported	One dose achieves low levels, and may take chronic use to get good representative milk levels (46)	+
Ampicillin	500 mg every 6 hr × 3 days	PO	None reported; possibility exists of causing skin rash and/or diarrhea	Considerable range of values (47)	+

Drug	Maternal toxicity	Dose	Route	Comments	Rating
Arsenicals (arsphenamine)	None reported	Not reported	IV	The first drug to introduce the concept of chemotherapy but not used now (48)	0
Barbital	None reported	325–650 mg	PO	(See Phenobarbital) (49)	+
Bendroflumethiazide	No adverse effects reported (26); possibility of idiosyncratic reactions occurring (29) including thrombocytopenia	5 mg b.i.d. × 5 days	PO	This is a member of the thiazide diuretics (50). Lactation was suppressed in all tested women and has also been reported elsewhere (51) from thiazide diuretics secondary to causing dehydration. Probably has little or no effect on lactation in women who do not get a diuresis and dehydration	2+
B.H.C. (organochlorine compound)	No effects reported			Present but has caused no problems (52)	+
Bromide, sodium	Drowsiness occurs in significant number of infants with two cases of bromide rash (53, 54)	1000 mg 5 × day × 3 days / 960 mg every 4 hr × 3–5 days	PO	Most samples contained a total of 2 mg bromide. This drug should not be used by nursing mothers. Very few products remain with this compound (53, 54)	3+
Bromocryptine	None reported	2.5 mg b.i.d.—t.i.d.	PO	An investigational drug which appears to inhibit lactation more than estrogens (55–57)	3+
Butabarbital	None reported	8 mg b.i.d. × 7 doses	PO	Very small amounts in milk with little chance of causing problems in infants. May be a problem if larger doses are used (58)	+
Caffeine	No effects	Coffee	PO	Very small quantities excreted in breast milk (59)	+
Calomel	7 infants thought to have an increase in bowel activity	160 mg (2½ gr)	PO	Small series, none found in milk but 50% of infants had increased stools. Need more studies in this little used compound (45)	2+
Carbamazepine	No toxicity reported	8 mg/kg/d for 30 days	PO	Infant plasma level after 3rd day was equal to the concentration in milk. Mother also was on phenytoin 6 mg/kg/day which increases the metabolite of carbamazepine but the infant handled this without an increase in its serum concentration of metabolite (60)	+
Carrots	Yellow discoloration of skin	2–3 carrots per day or 2–3 lb per week	PO	No toxicity reported and this is the only case history (61)	0

Table 3.7.—Continued

Drug	Effects in Infants	Quantity Maternal dose	Route[b]	Comments	Significance[c]
Cascara	4/12 (33%) in one group and 6/10 (60%) in another had increased bowel activity	4 ml of fluid extract	PO	Small series but this is an anthraquinone agent and can cause significant increase in infant bowel activity with normal maternal doses so should not be used (45)	3+
Cefoxitin	None reported	1 g	IV	Reaches about same level in breast milk as serum. Only one level drawn on one woman and unlikely a woman on IV anti-biotics would be breast-feeding (62)	0
Cephalothin	None noted	Unknown	IV	Very small amounts excreted so that less than 0.08% of daily dose would appear in milk (63)	0
Chloral hydrate	None reported Drowsiness	1.33 g Hypnotic dose	PR PO	Both chloral hydrate (64) and metabolite tri-chlorethanol measured, infant could get enough for sedative dose if fed at peak milk concentration (65)	3+
Chloramphenicol	Refusal of breast, falling asleep during feeding and vomiting after feeding (66)	1 g dose	PO	Levels in milk not sufficient to produce "gray baby syndrome" and remote possibility of causing marrow suppression (67)	+
	None reported	250–500 mg every 6 hr for 7–10 days	PO	Probably should avoid breast feeding while taking chloramphenical (68)	
		250 mg q.i.d. (2 pa-tients)	PO	Chemical tests run on breast milk show twice the concentration because they also mea-sure inactive metabolite (69)	
Chloroquine	None reported	20, 30, and 45 mg/day	PO	Assay probably not as accurate as todays, so hard to interpret data (70)	+
	None reported	100–400 mg/day × 3 days	PO	Difficult to interpret with old assays (71)	
Chlorothiazide	None reported	500 mg	PO	Very small quantities and pharmacologically, insignificant, however (see Bendroflume-thiazide) (72)	+
Chlorpromazine	No adverse effects (46)	1200 mg	PO	Possibility of causing gynecomastia (73) in males and galactorrhea in females (26, 74)	+
		600 mg b.i.d.	PO	Large doses given and very little passes into milk (73)	

Drug	Reported effects	Dose	Route	Comments	Rating
Chlortetracycline	None reported	2–3 g/day for 3–4 days	PO	Given with an antacid (Amphogel) which could have lowered levels (see Tetracycline) (75)	2+
Clindamycin	None reported	600 mg every 6 hr	IV	Peak IV levels in 30 min with small amount in milk (reported erroneously as blood levels in original report) (76)	+
Codeine	No effects	300 mg every 6 hr; 65 mg × 1 or 65 mg × 2 or 32 mg × 6	PO PO	Levels small even with IV use. Very low levels and probably will cause no infant effects in these doses (49)	0
Contraceptives, oral (estrogen/progestin combinations and as individual estrogens and progestins)	Breast enlargement in 2 male infants (77, 78) and proliferation of vaginal epithelium in female infants (79) have been attributed to oral contraceptives but this is not established (80). Breast milk jaundice reported with prior contraceptive use (81) but not proven (82)	Usually one daily for 21 days each month	PO	High doses will suppress lactation (83) though not uniformly, whereas low doses usually will not affect lactation (20, 84), especially if well established (80), progestins alone do not appear to affect lactation (85, 86). Some studies show decrease in protein (86–89), fat and minerals (88) but this has not been confirmed (84–89)	+
Cesium-137	None reported	Dietary	PO	Highest levels in spring (90), 10% of a single dose is excreted in a 2-week pooled milk supply. Another study (91) showed a large amount was excreted and was dependent on dietary intake	+
Cyclophosphamide	None reported	500 mg	IV	Because of the presence of drug in the breast milk and the severe problems that could ensue, antimetabolites are considered to be contraindicated if breast feeding (92)	3+
Cycloserine	No adverse effects	250 mg q.i.d.	PO	Achieves milk levels that can be equal concentration to serum levels (93)	+
DDT	None reported	Unknown	PO or inhalant	Finnish babies, close correlation with smoking and increased DDT levels since tobacco is treated with DDT (94)	+
	No adverse effects	Unknown		Rural American blacks (95) and urban American whites. WHO recommends maximum for cows milk at 0.05 ppm which was excreted by most of these women, especially the rural blacks who have a higher exposure rate to insecticides	

Table 3.7.—Continued

Drug	Effects in Infants	Quantity		Route[b]	Comments	Signifi- cance[c]
		Maternal dose				
Demeclocycline (demethylchlor- tetracycline)	No effects	Unknown			Also found in significant amounts in another study (96). Donors were from 7 U.S. cities; mean here was 3 × the WHO recom- mended amount (52, 97, 98)	
	None reported	300–2700 mg/day		PO	Only doses of 600 mg or more achieved a concentration in milk (see Tetracycline); long acting which accounts for amounts excreted up to 3 days (99)	2+
Diazepam	After 3rd day, lethargy and weight loss (170 g), EEG consistent with sedation, symptoms stopped when drug stopped	10 mg t.i.d. × 3 days		PO	Active metabolite oxazepam found in infants' urine. Sufficient drug excreted in milk with normal doses to cause sedative effects in infants (100)	3+
	Possibility of neonatal jaundice secondary to competitive inhibi- tion of metabolism of bilirubin by diazepam	10 mg t.i.d. × 6 days		PO	Infant serum levels initially high due to long half life in neonates secondary to de- creased metabolism (101, 102). Must be watchful of accumulation (102)	
		5 mg × 3 doses over 4 hr		IV	See Ref. 58	
Dichloralphenazone	Possibility of causing sedation	10 mg/day × 6 days 1300 mg h.s.		PO	See Ref. 103 Measured active metabolite trichlorethylalco- hol (65)	+
Dicumarol	Most have normal PT time, no ad- verse effects	200 mg × 1 dose then titrated		PO	Possibility with chronic use enough could en- ter breast milk to cause problems (see Ethyl-biscoumacetate) (104)	+
Dieldrin	None reported	Environmental		PO or inhaled	Insignificant quantities are excreted in milk and no effects on infants would be ex- pected (52). High concentrations are, how- ever, found in maternal adipose tissues	0
Digoxin	None stated	Not stated		PO	Serum and milk levels very close but total excreted in milk is very small (105). Mother should feed infant about 3–4 hr after taking a dose to achieve low milk level	0

Drug	Effect on infant	Dose	Route	Comments	Rating
Dihydrostrepto-mycin	None reported	1 g	IM	Present for long periods in small amounts (106). Possible risk and should probably avoid. Also in the presence of maternal renal failure the concentration in breast milk increases 25 times (107)	+
Diphtheria anti-bodies	None reported	0.5 ml	IM	Traced only in first week of life (108). Very small amounts and not significant	0
Doxycycline	None reported	200 mg and 100 mg 24 hr later	PO	(See Tetracycline) (109)	+
Egg protein	None reported	2 raw eggs	PO	Possibility of transmitting allergy (110)	0
Ergonovine	None reported	200-μg dose	PO	Caused a lowering of prolactin levels in breast feeding patients and with larger doses could cause a significant enough prolactin inhibition to decrease lactation (see Ergot alkaloids) (111)	3+
Ergot alkaloids	90% of infants developed ergotism (vomiting, diarrhea, weak pulse, unstable blood pressure and convulsions)	Unspecified	PO	Used liquid extract of ergot and infants were affected (112). Many other ergot alkaloids can suppress lactation and possibly could cause ergotism. This drug should be avoided while breast-feeding (113)	4+
Erythromycin	None reported	400 mg every 8 hr	PO	See report (27)	0
	None reported	2 g/day	PO	All reported increased levels of erythromycin in milk greater than serum. Animal studies also show higher milk levels. Probably safe drug for infants even in these quantities (114, 115)	
Ether	None reported	170 and 250 g	—	Probably should be avoided since general anesthetics can cause severe depression in infants (116)	2+
Ethinyl estradiol	None reported	500 μg, 1 dose	PO	Used radioactive tagged drug and measured both active and metabolized product (117). Also ran biologic assay which showed no estrogenic activity. Probably no problems with low doses, however high doses may cause problems to infants (see Contraceptives, oral)	+
Ethosuximide	None reported	Not specified	PO	Possibility of adverse effects with normal dosage is small (58)	+

Table 3.7.—Continued

Drug	Effects in Infants	Quantity — Maternal dose	Route[b]	Comments	Significance[c]
Ethyl-biscoumacetate	Hemorrhage of umbilical stump and cephalohematoma	300 mg t.i.d.	PO	Because of bleeding problems one should not breast feed and use oral anticoagulants which achieve milk levels (27)	3+
	No adverse effects in these infants or another 22 infants	600–1200 mg day for 6–19 days	PO	13/38 samples contained drug (118)	
Fava beans	Hemolysis occurred in all 4 G6PD deficient patients	Not given	PO	If beans are cooked well, favism does not occur but with oral ingestion of raw beans severe hemolysis can occur (119–122)	3+
Fluoride	None reported	Variable (average 1.13 ppm) dietary	PO	Need approximately 1 ppm to prevent cavities so supplementation would be needed (123–125)	0
Flufenamic	None reported	200 mg t.i.d. × 4 days	PO	Infants serum also was tested and smaller amounts than in breast milk were found (126)	+
Flunitrazepam	None noted	2 mg	PO	Concentrations in breast milk were 1–2 ng/ml which are very low and unlikely to cause effects in the infant (127)	0
Folate	None reported	Dietary (India) 100–200 μg daily	PO	Adequate amounts present in milk to prevent megaloblastic anemia in infant even if mother is deficient (128)	3+
Gallium-67 citrate	None reported	3 mCi	IV	Authors report that significant amounts are excreted of this radioactive compound and it retains its activity sufficiently to preclude breast feeding indefinitely (129, 130)	4+
Glutethimide	May cause sedation	500 mg dose	PO	Ninety samples used for average values. Very small amounts excreted in milk probably because of high lipid solubility of drug (131)	+
Gold	Trace amounts found in serum and red cells—a potential cause of skin rashes	135 mg dose	IM	Study used auriothioglucose, a very large gold molecule and probably better to not breast feed while using this compound (132)	2+
Haloperidol	None reported	A mean of 29 mg daily for 6 days	PO	Breast milk concentration of 5 ng/ml, 11 hr from last dose. This level is very low and an infant is unlikely to ingest more than 0.01 mg/day much less than a therapeutic dose (133)	0

Drug	Reported in mother	Amount/Dose	Route	Comments	Rating
Heptachlorepoxide	None reported	Unknown		53 breast milk samples (44). Measurable amounts and above WHO standards but have caused no problems in infants (117)	+
Heroin (diacetyl-morphine)	Prolonged habituation; 13 infants had withdrawal symptoms	2–45 mg daily	IV	Appears in milk and can prolong intrauterine habituation in breast fed infants (134). Infant should be withdrawn first before breast feeding started, but possibility exists habituation could recur with breast feeding	3+
Hexachloroben-zene	Some severe skin disease, generalized dystrophy, anemia and porphyria and infant deaths	Ingested food (wheat)	PO	Mothers ate poisoned wheat and significant quantities passed into breast milk (135)	4+
Hexachlorocyclo-hexane (Lindane)	None reported	Through food	PO	Measured in banked milk (96). This can also pass into milk secondary to topical application as a lotion (gamma benzene)	+
Hexachlorophene	None reported	Not reported	Topical	Levels are low and probably pose no hazard to infants (136). Significant levels can occur if large quantities are applied to abraded or inflamed skin and left on the skin	+
^{125}I-labeled albumin	None reported	6 and 10 μCi	IV	Authors conclude this to be a significant milk level and recommend either avoiding this compound or stop breast feeding for at least 10 days after using it (137)	4+
^{131}I (radioactive)	Can cause thyroid suppression and with high doses causes destruction of the thyroid gland, may increase the risk of developing thyroid cancer by as much as 10-fold	100 μCi dose; 10 and 30 μCi each one dose	PO PO	Authors (138) recommend breast feeding is contraindicated after these large doses (138, 139). Authors recommend breast feeding should be withheld for at least 24 hr with small doses (140)	4+
^{131}I-labeled ma-croaggregated albumin	None reported	200-μCi dose	IV	Peak probably 24 hr after dose (141). Authors recommend discontinuing breast feeding for 10–12 days after receiving compound [see ^{131}I (radioactive)]	4+
^{131}I hipparate	None reported	12–20 μCi	IV	Authors recommend discontinuing breast feeding for 1 day after receiving compound. May cause problems if larger doses used (142)	3+
Iodide (potassium, sodium)	Possibility of hypothyroidism and/or goiter	325–650 mg t.i.d.	PO	Does pass through and could cause thyroid suppression and allergic reactions (26, 29, 49)	3+

Table 3.7.—Continued

Drug	Effects in Infants	Quantity — Maternal dose	Route[b]	Comments	Significance[c]
		10 gr (0.6 g)	PO	Reported 15% of dose excreted in milk in 3 days (143)	2+
Iopanoic acid	No adverse effects	300–600 mg	PO	Has iodine in it which could cause problems (see Iodide, sodium) (144)	3+
Iron	None reported, milk can probably prevent iron deficiency anemia in infants less than 1 yr old	Dietary (Denmark)	PO	Small amount of iron (0.5–1.5 mg/L) is in milk but it is adequate due to better utilization (145). Supplemental iron probably would not appreciably change the milk concentration	
Isoniazid	None reported	5–10 mg/kg	PO	Since INH reaches milk levels equal to serum levels care should be taken with this drug (146)	+
Kanamycin	None reported	2 g 1 g	PO IM	PO peak 3 hr after dose, and only 2/4 subjects had a measurable milk level (147). IM peak at 1 hr and milk conc > serum at 8 hr. Not well absorbed orally so even though it passes in milk it causes no systemic problems	0
Labetalol	None	320–1200 mg daily	PO	Peak breast milk level ranged from 29–600 ng/ml which are low levels (148)	+
Lead	None reported Toxicity, after infant ingested lead off of breast	Dietary Lead acetate ointment and lead breast shields	PO Topical	Samples taken in white middle class American women who should have lower levels (149). These levels are lower than those found in canned milk and formulas. Should not use lead ointments on breast	+
Lincomycin	No adverse effects	500 mg every 6 hr × 3 days	PO	Can reach higher levels in milk than serum so should be avoided during breast feeding (150)	+
Lithium carbonate	None reported	—	PO	Also reached infant serum concentration equal to milk level (151). Crosses in sufficient quantity that breast feeding should be avoided while taking medication (56, 151, 152)	3+

Drug	Adverse effects	Dose	Route	Comments	Rating
Mandelic acid	No adverse effects	3 g q.i.d.	PO	Mandelic acid compromises 50% of methenamine mandelate concentrations and are high enough to account for about one half a therapeutic dose in infants (153)	+
Mefenamic acid	None reported	500 mg × 1 then 250 mg t.i.d. × 4 days	PO	Not significant with these therapeutic doses (154)	0
Mercury	Cerebellar gliosis, cerebral neuronal degeneration, cerebral palsy, mental retardation	Through fish	PO	Passage of mercury through breast milk documented in animals (155) and Japanese fish contaminated with mercury and ingested by mothers (156). Probably reaches high levels and if mothers serum level high or symptomatic should not breast feed. Need more studies, this one is not definitive	2+
Mestranol	None reported	150 μg every day	PO	Used radioactive tagged drug which measured active and metabolized products, but did not differentiate between them. No biologic assay so, no clear significance emerged (see Contraceptives, oral) (157)	+
Methadone	Prolong infant habituation unless newborn withdrawn first	10–40 mg per day	PO	Methadone also in amniotic fluid (158)	3+
		50–80 mg day	PO	Infant should be withdrawn first then breast feeding could be continued if mother on a low dose of methadone (<40 mg) (158)	
Methotrexate	None reported	22.5 mg daily	PO	In 12 hr 320 ng was excreted (159). Authors conclude little hazard however, dose is low and drug is potentially very toxic (see Cyclophosphamide)	2+
Methyl ergonovine	None reported	200 μg t.i.d. for 7 days	PO	No change in prolactin levels but problems have occurred with ergot derivatives (see Ergot alkaloids) (160)	3+
Metoclopramide	None reported	10 mg t.i.d. × 7–10 days	PO	Reported to increase milk flow in women whose volume had diminished (161)	2+
Metronidazole	No adverse effects reported	200 mg	PO	Peaks at 4 hr, carcinogenic effects reported in bacteria with possible effects in humans. Until proven safe it probably should be avoided while breast feeding (162)	2+

Table 3.7.—Continued

Drug	Effects in Infants	Quantity	Route[b]	Comments	Significance[c]
		Maternal dose			
Milk of magnesia	No effect	Not specified	PO	Poorly absorbable saline laxatives appear to cause no problems with infants since they do not achieve any measurable level in breast milk (163)	0
Mineral oil	No effect	15 ml	PO	Not absorbed so it would not achieve milk levels (163)	0
Minocycline	None reported	200 mg	PO	This was only a report (not referenced data) (164) (see Tetracycline); 18 μg were excreted in the milk in 12 hr which is a very small amount. Since this drug does cause many side effects it should be avoided	2+
Monosodium glutamate	None reported	6-g dose	PO	This is a common chemical which is put into many foods as a flavor enhancer (165). It has been purported to cause "Chinese restaurant syndrome." Probably little or no effect on infant if mother uses small amounts	+
Morphine	Prolong habituation in infant not withdrawn after birth	16 mg × 1 and 128 mg/day 16 mg	IM IM IM	All levels taken considerably after dose and drug has a short half-life (2–3 hr) and the levels would be low this long after a dose (166). Probably in high enough concentration to prolong withdrawal in an infant habituated during gestation (49)	3+
Nalidixic acid	Hemolytic anemia developed	1 g q.i.d.	PO	Mother also taking amobarbital (167). One case only so caution advised. There was no enzyme deficiencies found in the infant, who improved with bottle feeding	2+
Nicotine (cigarettes)	No adverse effects 1 case of restlessness and circulatory disturbance in heavy smoker and may also cause diarrhea, tachycardia and vomiting	½–1½ packs per day	Inhaled Inhaled	Concentrations found only in smokers milk and varied throughout day; not enough to cause problems in infants. Mostly old data but probably significant amount passes in women who smoke 1 pack per day (168–170)	2+

Nitrofurantoin	Possibility of hemolysis in G6PD deficient infants	100 mg q.i.d. × 3–4 days	PO	Very small quantities excreted (171). Use with caution in G6PD deficient infants to avoid hemolysis (172)	2+
Norethynodrel	None reported	100 mg every 6 hr 5 mg 5 mg × 3 days	PO PO PO	Both studies (117, 173) used radioactive tagged drug and found traces of active and metabolized drug but were unable to differentiate between (174). Estrogenic activity also tested for in milk and found in 4 samples (see also Contraceptives, oral)	+
Novobiocin	None reported	250–500 mg every 6–8 hr	PO	Delayed peak milk level reported at 53–56 hr (27). Unexplained why peak was so extended	2+
	Possibilities of causing hyperbilirubinemia in neonates	500 mg then 250 mg every 6 hr for 4 doses	PO	Does reach small levels with a possibility, although remote, of causing kernicterus in neonates (175)	+
Oxyphenbutazone (hydroxyphenbutazone)	None reported	300 mg b.i.d.	PO	Very small quantities reported in 2/55 samples (176). Manufacturer (Poulenc) states it is in small concentration in 2/24 patients (25). Potent drug which possibly should be avoided with breast feeding	+
Oxytocin	None reported	40 IU/ml as nasal spray prior to each feeding	Nasal	Drug appeared to increase volume of milk excreted (177). This is to be expected since it endogenously initiates the "letdown" reflex	2+
Pantothenic acid	None reported	Dietary (India)	PO	Higher levels were correlated with a higher socioeconomic class in India. This is a normal constituent of breast milk (178)	3+
PBB (polybrominated biphenyls)	None noted	Unknown	PO	In the lower peninsula of Michigan 53 samples of women's breast milk were analyzed and 96% had detectable levels of PBB with a medium range of 0.068 ppm (179)	+
PCB (polychlorinated biphenyls)	None noted	Unknown	PO	Of 1,038 U.S. samples studied by the EPA, 94% had some contamination and 6% had levels above 0.1 ppm (180) which exceeds the FDA daily allowable intake. There has been no reported infant toxicities from these levels	+
Penicillin G	None reported	100,000 units (benzathine)	IM	Insufficient quantities in breast milk to treat infection but could cause allergic reaction (181)	+

Table 3.7.—Continued

| Drug | Quantity | | Effects in Infants | Comments | Significance[c] |
	Maternal dose	Route[b]			
	200,000–600,000 units (benzathine)	IM	None reported	Milk and serum levels somewhat correlated (182)	+
	2.4 million units (procaine)	IM	6 hr after maternal injection child developed febrile and localized reactions which persisted for 10 hr	Infant also received 10 units of PCN directly so hard to interpret this case (183)	
Penicillin V	125–250 mg	PO	None reported	Levels higher than those achieved with penicillin G but any effects would be like penicillin G (27)	+
Pentobarbital	100 mg × 3 days	PO	Probably sedation with hypnotic doses	(see Phenobarbital) Sedative doses in the mother would probably not affect the infant (58)	2+
Phenindione	50 mg every am and 25–50 mg alternating 4 weeks	PO	Incisional and scrotal hemorrhage, PT was 1.4 above and PTT 1.9 above controls	Infant should be given daily doses of phytonadione 1 mg IM (184) (see Ethyl biscoumacetate)	3+
	25, 50 or 75 mg × 1 dose	PO		Only 26% of samples with 25 mg doses contained detectable milk amounts (185)	
Phenobarbital	30 mg q.i.d. 100 mg/ dose and 200 mg/ day	PO	Drowsiness in infants of mothers taking higher doses (100 mg)	Infant sedation occurs when mother consumes hypnotic dose and breast feeds soon after (186). Smaller sedative doses do not seem to cause problems. Probably enough passing through to stimulate liver enzymes and possibly alter the metabolism of other drugs or bilirubin (58). Short acting barbiturates preferable to long acting ones because they appear in lower concentration in milk	2+
Phenolphthalein	30–800 mg	PO	16/39 in a study had purported increase in bowel activity (45); no effects in other studies (49, 187)	Very little found in milk to account for 40% incidence of increased bowel activity (45, 49, 187)	+
Phenylbutazone	750 mg	IM	No adverse effects reported	Appears in small quantities and could cause the blood dyscrasias reported for this drug (188, 189)	2+
	600 mg	IM			

Drug	Amount	Effect on infant	Route	Comments	Rating
Phenytoin (diphenylhydantoin)	400 mg/day	Cyanosis, methemoglobinemia on 4th postpartum day and again on 9th postpartum day with milk rechallenge	PO	Mother also taking phenobarbital 390 mg/day, but reaction thought to be due to phenytoin (190)	3+
	Not specified		PO	Significant amounts (191) probably ingested by infants to cause side effects and possibly enzyme induction	
	100 mg t.i.d.		PO	See report (58, 192)	
Polio virus oral vaccine (OPV)	None	Infants given 3 doses of trivalent oral polio vaccine with no adverse effects, serum levels of polio antibody equal in breast fed infants and bottle fed infants all indicated an adequate response	—	In endemic polio areas mothers who have high polio antibody levels can excrete enough antibody in colostrom to inactivate an oral polio vaccine in neonates if given within 6 hr of a feeding (193–195). If vaccine given to 6-week-old infant in this country it is highly unlikely enough polio antibody will be in breast milk to inactivate the vaccine (196, 197)	+
Prednisilone	5 mg	None reported	PO	This is the active metabolite of prednisone. Low dose radioactive tagged drug was used in this study (198) and dose in milk was very small, however (see Prednisone)	2+
Prednisone	10 mg	None reported	PO	Low dose used in this study—comparable with physiological levels (199). No data on concentrations in milk with high dose steroids. If maternal dose is 2 or more times physiological level then breast feeding probably should be avoided	2+
Pregnane-3-α,20β-diol	Endogenous metabolite	Hyperbilirubinemia or "breast milk jaundice"	PO	Abnormal metabolite of progesterone thought to inhibit glucuronyl transferase (metabolizes bilirubin) so causes increase in unconjugated bilirubin (200). Unknown cause but may be hereditary (201). Also, abnormally high free fatty acids in milk may also contribute to problem (202)	2+
Propranolol	20–160 mg dose	No effects	PO	Very small amounts excreted in milk even with relatively high doses (203–205). This is probably due to the rapid maternal metabolism of this drug	0

Table 3.7.—Continued

Drug	Effects in Infants	Quantity Maternal dose	Route[b]	Comments	Significance[c]
Pyramethamine	Enough excreted in 2 days to treat malaria in 6-month-olds, can also be used for prophalaxis (207) through breast feeding	50–75 mg single dose	PO	Detectable 48 hr after last dose (206). Significant quantities excreted	3+
Pyrazolone (anti-pyrin)	None reported	1200 mg	PO	Little used drug and should be avoided (208)	+
Pyridoxine	None reported	150–200 mg t.i.d.	PO	One study (209) showed a suppression of lactation greater than with DES while the other two (55, 210) showed no better effects than placebo. This is normal constituent of breast milk	3+
Quinine sulfate	Possibility of causing thrombocytopenia	600–1300 mg	PO	Very small quantity excreted even with high dose used so very little chance of adverse effects in infant (166)	0
Rh antibodies	None reported			Any antibodies present in the milk are inactivated in the infants' GI tract and pose no problems (211)	0
Rhubarb	No effects reported	10 ml syrup	PO	Old time drug now in insignificant quantities in some proprietary laxatives (45)	+
Rubella vaccine (Cendehill strain)	None reported	0.5–0.7 ml	SC	Apparently no transfer of live virus through milk (212). Probably would not propagate in GI tract even if it were passed in milk	0
Salicylate sodium	No effects reported	325–650 mg every 4 hr for 2–6 doses	PO	Levels may have been higher if samples collected at 1, 2, or 3 hr after dose but were still small amounts transmitted with low doses (49)	+
Senna	5/10 had increased stools in spite of little showing up in breast milk	4 g 4 ml fluid extract 100 mg Senakot 1 tsp Senakot granules	PO PO PO	With high doses may get problems with salicylism (see Acetylsalicylic acid) (31) Older preparations with higher doses (45). Larger than usual doses of Senakot may cause increase in infant bowel activity where usual doses are probably safe to use (163, 213)	+
Sodium chloride	None reported	65 mg dose	PO	Radioactive tagged compound (214). A normal constituent of breast milk and unlikely to cause adverse effects	0

Drug	Adverse effects	Dose	Route	Comments	Rating
Spironolactone	None reported	25 mg q.i.d.	PO	Very small quantities excreted of canrenone (metabolite), and assuming an infant ingested 1 liter of breast milk this concentration would present the infant with only 0.2% of the maternal daily dose, much lower than a pharmacological level (215)	0
Streptomycin	No adverse effects reported	1 g	IM	Same kinetics as dihydrostreptomycin and would expect same problems (116) (see Dihydrostreptomycin)	+
Strontium-89 and strontium-90	None reported	Dietary intake	PO	Inhibited from excretion into milk probably by calcium (91, 216, 217). Infant probably will receive very little through milk	0
Sulfamethoxypyridazine	—	2 g then 1 g/day × 2 days	PO	Detectable levels in infants after 2 days because of long half-life of this drug (218)	3+
	Caused hemolysis and jaundice in G6PD deficient neonate who was breast fed		PO	Crosses in sufficient quantities to cause hemolysis in G6PD deficient neonates (219). Also will displace enough bilirubin from albumin binding sites to cause jaundice. Should not be used in neonates	
Sulfanilamide	None reported	1.6–5 g/day in divided doses	PO	Compilation of four old studies on this now little used drug. Less than 2% of dose (54–100 mg) excreted in milk after 5 days (see Sulfamethoxypyridazine) (220–223). Also present in infants blood and urine. Reported both as active drug and metabolite	+
Sulfapyridine	None reported	3 g/day	PO	Sufficient quantity to cause problems (224) (see Sulfamethoxypyridazine)	+
Sulfathiazole	None reported	3–6 g/day	PO	Less water soluble so lower milk levels would be expected (see Sulfamethoxypyridazine (225). Infant received about 4 mg total, a very small quantity	+
99mTcO4	None reported	4 mCi dose	IV	Concentrates in milk (226)	—
		10 mCi dose	IV	Concentrates (175) and should not breast feed for 32–72 hr after receiving compound (141)	3+
99mTcO4-labeled macroaggregated albumin	None reported	12 mCi dose	IV	Concentrates with variable rates (141)	—
		2 mCi dose	IV	Has decreasing concentration over 24 hr so authors conclude breast feeding can be resumed after 24 hr (227)	3+

Table 3.7.—Continued

Drug	Effects in Infants	Quantity Maternal dose	Route[b]	Comments	Significance[c]
Tetracycline	No effects, and infant serum levels less than milk levels	500 mg q.i.d. × 3 days 1.5–2.5 g 275 mg/day	PO PO IM	Concentration in milk averages 70% of serum concentrations (228). Possibility (27) of tooth staining and inhibition of bone growth exists, no data available as to whether it is significantly bound by calcium or how available it is for absorption (229). Given as IM pyrrolidino-methylform and achieved milk levels	2+
Theobromine	No adverse effects reported	113 g Hershey's milk chocolate (240 mg theobromine)	PO	If a mother ate 4 oz chocolate every 6 hr and the infant ingested a liter of milk daily the total amount the infant would get would be about 10 mg of theobromine or 1–2 mg/kg/day (230). This could be enough in neonates, because of its long half-life to cause adverse effects	+
Theophylline	Irritability and difficulty with sleeping	4.25 mg/kg dose or 200 mg q.i.d.	PO	Rapid but somewhat delayed equilibration between serum and breast milk (231). Caution should be observed since a significant quantity can pass through breast milk	2+
Thiamine	None reported	Dietary (India)	PO	Levels were not correlated with socioeconomic levels in India (178). Authors recommend that severely deficient women should not breast feed (232). A normal constituent in breast milk	2+
Thiopental sodium	None reported	1,125 mg over 35 min	IV	Old report says very small quantities found (233). Since drug is very lipid soluble it would not be expected to reach significant levels in milk (see Phenobarbital)	0
Thiouracil	Probably would suppress thyroid function in infants and possibility of agranulocytopenia and goiter	1 g dose	PO	Significant level and probably should not be used during breast feeding (234). The other thyroid suppressants, i.e., propylthiouracil, methimazole, also should not be used since they behave much like thiouracil	3+
Tolbutamide	None reported	500 mg dose	PO	Probably not in high enough concentration in milk to cause problems (235). Has caused	+

Drug	Side effects reported	Dose	Route	Comments	Significance
				problems during gestation and does not get into milk (236)	2+
Trimethoprim	None reported	160 mg b.i.d.–t.i.d.	PO	Peak at 2–3 hr (237). This drug is available in the U.S. as a combination with sulfamethoxazole. It should probably be avoided in nursing mothers	+
Tuberculin reactive T cells	8/13 infants born to positive mothers who had positive antibodies after 4 weeks of breast feeding	PPD	ID	The results suggested that breast fed infants may possibly acquire T-cell responsiveness to a specific antigen by ingestion of breast milk from positive mothers (238)	
	No infants of negative mothers had any reactive cells after breast feeding	PPD	ID		
	1 had reactive cells after 4 weeks of breast feeding	PPD	ID		
Vitamin B$_{12}$	None reported	Dietary (India)	PO	Higher socioeconomic class (178) had higher levels with variability probably secondary to variable intake (239). A constituent in breast milk	0
Vitamin D	Possibility of hypercalcemia	Dietary (U.S.) Dietary (Russian) 50,000 units/day	PO PO	Very high doses used here and possibility of high levels in milk leading to hypercalcemia in infants (240). Vitamin D is a constituent in breast milk	+
Vitamin K	Infant prothrombin times not effected until 3rd day after dose	40 mg	PO	Both phytonadione and menadiol sodium diphosphate used (241). Used high doses here. Would not expect any effects in normal infants	0
Warfarin	None reported	Loading dose of 30–40 mg then maintenance of 5–11 mg 2–12 mg	PO PO	Very potent drug which from the literature (242) appears to be safe to use in studied maintenance doses (243, 244). Very small quantities in breast milk which could not be measured within the sensitivity of the instrument	+

[a] Adapted from R. H. Levin and L. A. Pagliaro (40).
[b] PO, orally; ID, intradermal; IM, intramuscular; IV, intravenous; PR, rectally; SC, subcutaneous.
[c] 0, insignificant; +, possibly significant; 2+, probably significant; 3+, significant; 4+, very significant.

Table 3.8.
Drugs Excreted in Breast Milk (Unsubstantiated Data)[a]

Drug	Effects on Infants	Maternal Dose	Route[b]	Comments	Significance[c]
Alphaprodine	Sedation	Not stated	Not stated	This is a personal communication from Hoffman-La Roche and not a published study (25). They also state this drug could impair feeding	3+
Amantadine	Manufacturer claims it can cause vomiting, urinary sedation and skin rashes in infants	Not stated	PO	No published documentation but manufacturer (Dupont) suggests it should not be administered (30)	+
Amikacin	None reported	Not reported	IM	Authors report no knowledge concerning its passage in breast milk and warn against its use (245)	+
Atropine	Possibility of causing anticholinergic side effects	Not stated	PO	No good evidence available to substantiate any claims about this drug. Some authors (29, 246) report it could possibly decrease milk production secondary to its anticholinergic effects. Knowles (23) reports a maternal dose of 600 mg (1000 times the normal dose) and a milk level of 0.1 mg/g (3 times the therapeutic dose of an infant) and references (166) which is a study of morphine and quinine and does not mention atropine. It is probable these values represent quinine, not atropine.	+
Bethanechol	Possibility of causing cholinergic effects	Not stated	Not stated	Manufacturer (MS&D) recommends avoidance of breast feeding if drug taken on a regular basis (25)	+
Carbenicillin disodium	None reported	1 g	IV	Manufacturer (Beecham) reports unpublished data and feels it is insignificant in this dose (30). Higher doses may pose problems and have not been studied	+
Carisoprodol	None reported but possible CNS depression or GI upset	Not stated	PO	Manufacturer (Wallace) recommends not to administer this to breast feeding mothers (30)	2+
Cephalexin	None reported	Not reported	PO	Manufacturer (Lilly) reports all cephalosporins are excreted in milk and should not be used during breast feeding. This is contrary to other reports (24)	+

Drug	Effect on Infant		Route	Comments	Rating
Cephalothin	None reported	Not reported	IV	Manufacturer (Lilly) reports all cephalosporins are excreted in breast milk and should not be used during breast feeding. This is contrary to other reports (24)	+
Chlordiazepoxide	None reported	Not stated	Not stated	Manufacturer (Hoffmann-La Roche) states drug is excreted in breast milk in minimal amounts (26)	+
Chlormadione	None reported	Not stated	PO	Present and possible effects of estrogen on infant, should be considered (174)	+
Chloroform	Sedation and/or deep sleep for 8 h	Not stated but used for anesthesia	Inhalation	Mother received for after pains as anesthetic (26, 247). Poorly documented report, however, general anesthetics do cause significant depression in neonates	2+
Chlorotrianisene	None reported	Not stated	PO	Manufacturer (Merrell) suggests avoiding breast feeding while on this compound (see contraceptives, oral) (30)	+
Chlorthalidone	None noted	—	PO	Drug administrated 3–10 hr before delivery if due to long half-life was still detectable 3 days after delivery. Was in highest concentration at 0.86 μg/ml (248)	+
Cimetidine	None	—	PO	Mothers with level of 5–6 μg/ml in milk so that an infant might ingest up to 6 mg/day (249)	2+
	None reported	Not reported	PO	Authors report it is excreted and recommend not to use while breast feeding (250)	+
Clorazepate, Dipotassium	None reported but may cause drowsiness	Not stated	PO	Manufacturer (Abbott) recommends not to utilize while breast feeding (30)	+
Colchicine	None reported	Not stated	PO	"May pass into the milk," which is a very old statement in a text book (251). Not studied and cannot really interpret the data	+
Corticotropin	None reported	Not given	IM	Not well studied. Authors report a decrease in sodium and increase in potassium in milk (27). Would expect this to correlate directly with serum levels. Also this is reported to be destroyed in the stomach (26)	+
Cyclamate	None reported	Not stated	PO	Manufacturer (Abbott) claims it is present in small quantities and will not effect infant (30)	0
Cycloheptenyl ethyl barbituric acid	None reported	Not stated	PO	Not well studied and large doses should be avoided (115, 252). Probably in low doses will cause little problems	+

Table 3.8.—Continued

Drug	Effects on Infants	Maternal Dose	Route[b]	Comments	Significance[c]
Danthron (1,8-dihydroxyanthroquinone)	Increased bowel activity	Not specified	PO	Manufacturer (Riker) reports excretion (23). Drug is a synthetic anthroquinone derivative and should behave like a natural anthroquinone (see Cascara, Table 3.7)	3+
Deserpidine		Not stated	PO	See Methylcothiazide and deserpidine	
Desipramine	None reported	Not stated	PO	Manufacturer (Lakeside) claims it is not found in breast milk (30). However, this is a potent drug and caution is advised	+
Dextroamphetamine	None reported and study looked for stimulation or insomnia	Not stated	PO	Manufacturer (SK&F) states it is very difficult to extract the drug with solvents from breast milk (23). A large number of mothers were studied here but the data was not published. It is not clear what would happen to the neonate if large maternal doses are taken. It may also decrease lactation with large doses	+
Dextrothyroxin	None reported	Not stated	PO	Manufacturer (Trovenal) states that not enough is present to harm infant (see Thyroxine) (30)	0
Diflunisol	None noted	—	PO	Concentrations in milk were 2–7% of plasma (253)	+
Dihydrotachysterol	None reported	Not stated	PO	Possibility of causing infant hypercalcemia and secondary calcification of internal organs (28). Only actual data is in rats where it did cause organ calcification after glucocorticoid challenge	+
Diphenhydramine	May cause sedation	Not stated	PO	Manufacturer (PD&Co) reports it is present in breast milk (23)	+
Ethisterone	None reported but may cause skeletal problems	Not stated	PO	Probably should be avoided (173)	2+
Fenoprofen	None	—	PO	Reaches milk levels of 1–2% of serum levels (254)	+
Flufenamic acid	None reported	Not stated	PO	Manufacturer (PD&Co) has no recommendation but states it is excreted in small amounts (30)	+
Foods—onions, eggs, chocolate, beans, celery, flaxseed, cotton seed, wheat	Changes in bowel habits, colic, skin rashes, other allergic manifestations	Dietary	PO	Many foods can potentially pass through breast milk and cause problems in infants (27, 42). Mother should avoid eating only those that disagree with her infant	+

Drug		Dose	Route	Comments	
Furosemide	None reported	Not stated	PO	Reports it is not present, however manufacturer warns not to use while breast feeding (24). Can be potent diuretic causing dehydration in mother with subsequent decrease in lactation	2+
Guafenisin (glyceryl guiacolate)	None known	Not stated	PO	Manufacturer (Dow) has not tested this compound but feels even if excreted does not constitute any danger to infant (25)	0
Guanethidine	None reported	Not stated	PO	Manufacturer (Ciba) states it is present but will not affect infant (24). This is a potent drug and caution should be advised until more data is available	+
Heparin	None	Not stated	IV, SC	Does not appear in milk because it is a large ionized protein and passes cell membranes very poorly (93). Not well studied	0
Hydrochlorothiazide	None reported	Not stated	PO	Manufacturer (MS&D) reports drug does appear in milk and may cause toxicities (25)	+
Imipramine	None	200 mg every 8 hr	PO	Breast milk concentration ranged from 4–35 ng/ml so that this dose unlikely infant would ingest enough to cause side effects (255)	+
Indomethacin	None reported	Not stated	PO	Manufacturer (MS&D) feels the drug does not appear in significant doses (24). However, this is a potent drug with adverse effects reported in children and caution is advised	+
Indoprofen	None	200 mg every 6 hr	PO	Breast milk levels peaked at 488 ng/ml (256)	+
Lyndiol	None reported	Not stated	PO	Should be avoided since it caused a decrease in milk protein and fat (88)	2+
Medroxyprogesterone acetate	None reported	Not stated	IM	Potent drug which can alter lactation and probably should be avoided (85). This drug has very few indications in the U.S.	2+
Mepenzolate bromide	None reported	Not reported	PO	Not detected but caution should be observed in its use (257). Data not very good	+
Meperedine	None reported	Not reported	Not stated	Manufacturer (Warren Teed) reports it is excreted in milk but does not get significant levels (30). Should be treated like other narcotics	+
Meprobamate	None reported	800 mg	PO	Manufacturer's unpublished data (46). Does reach high levels and probably should be avoided	2+
Mesoridazine besylate	None reported	Not stated	PO	Manufacturer (Sandoz) claims it does not appear in significant quantities (30)	+

Table 3.8.—Continued

Drug	Effects on Infants	Maternal Dose	Route[b]	Comments	Significance[c]
Metamucil	No effect	Not specified	PO	Nonabsorbable bulk forming and stool softening laxatives cause no increase in bowel activity in breast fed infants (31)	0
Methacycline	None reported	Not reported	PO	Present and should be treated as other tetracyclines (183)	2+
Methenamine (Hexamine)	No effects	Not stated	PO	Peak level at 1 hour not present in sufficient quantities to harm infant (258, 259). These are very old references with very little data	+
Methocarbamol	None reported	Not stated	PO	Probably is not significant in therapeutic doses but not well studied (260)	+
Methotrimeprazine	Does not appear to have adverse effect	Not stated	Not stated	No published data only a manufacturer's (Poulenc Ltd.) statement to the effect it appears in breast milk (25)	+
Methyclothiazide and deserpidine	None reported	Not reported	PO	Manufacturer (Abbott) recommends caution with this combination (30)	+
Methyldopa	None noted	—	PO	Concentration in breast milk too low to effect infant (261)	0
Methyprylon	Possibility of causing sedation	Not reported	PO	Manufacturer (Hoffmann-La Roche) states it crosses into breast milk and may cause problems (25)	+
Metoprolol	None noted	—	PO	Concentrations in breast milk about 3.5 times higher than plasma. Concentration, however, is very low in milk so that it is unlikely a neonate would ingest more than 0.3 mg daily (262)	+
Naproxen	None noted	—	PO	Breast milk concentration is about 1% of serum concentrations (263)	0
Norethindrone	None reported	Not reported	PO	Potent progestin and probably should be avoided (173)	+
Norethisterone ethanate	None reported	Not stated	IM	Potent progestin and probably should not be used (85)	+
D-Norgestrel	None noted	30 µg	PO	Undetected in milk in this dose. Estimate is about 0.1% of dose appears in milk so that infant receives about 1 µg/month which is very low (264)	0
Nortriptyline	None reported	25 mg	PO	According to manufacturer (Lilly) does get into breast milk (46)	+

Drug	Adverse effects	Dose	Route	Comments	Rating
Oxacillin	Possible penicillin allergy	1 g	PO	This was a communication from the manufacturer (Bristol) stating that they did not find it in breast milk (23)	0
Oxytetracycline	None reported	1.5–2 g/day	PO	Excreted in small amounts (27)	2+
Para-amino salicylic acid (PAS)	None reported	Not stated	PO	Manufacturer (Mallincrodt) reports it is not excreted in breast milk (30)	0
Pentazocine	Not reported	Not stated	PO	No published data but probably is excreted in milk (25)	+
Phenformin HCl	None reported	Not stated	PO	Manufacturer (USV) states it does not exert a hypoglycemic effect on infants (30). This drug is now not available in the U.S. and if it were it should not be used	2+
Piperacetazine	None reported	Not stated	PO	Manufacturer (Dow) states this drug may have a great potential for excretion in high levels in milk (30)	2+
Primidone	None reported but may cause sedation or somnolence	Not stated	PO	Manufacturer (Ayerst) cautions about the use of this drug (30). This drug is partially metabolized to phenobarbital	2+
Probucol	None reported	Not stated	PO	Authors report no knowledge of whether it is excreted in breast milk and warn against its use (265)	+
Prochlorperazine	None reported	Not stated	PO	Manufacturer (SK&F) reports it is excreted both in humans and in animals but probably not in significant levels (30)	+
Propantheline bromide	None reported	Not stated	PO	Manufacturer (Searle) claims drug is not excreted in milk. More study needed (30)	0
Propoxyphene, dextro	No adverse effects reported	Not specified, average dose 65–130 mg	PO	Very small quantities excreted according to manufacturer (Lilly) in two studies (25, 26). The data reported here was from a suicidal attempt as also reported by the manufacturer	+
Propylthiouracil	May cause thyroid suppression	Not stated	PO	No studies have been done on this compound but it is closely related to thiouracil so that levels may be significant to cause effects with high doses (29)	3+
Quinidine	None noted	600 mg	PO	Concentrations in milk close to serum levels and ranged from 6.4–8.2 mg/L at 3 hr after the dose (266)	+

Table 3.8.—Continued

Drug	Effects on Infants	Maternal Dose	Route[b]	Comments	Significance[c]
Reserpine	Significant nasal stuffiness and some increase in tracheobronchial secretions in newborns may produce diarrhea and lethargy	Not specified but probably >0.5 mg	PO, IM	No documented evidence of adverse effects (14, 27, 32)	+
Scopolamine (Hyoscine)	None reported	Not stated	PO	Rapidly destroyed in maternal tissues (247) (see Atropine). Old report says there should be no danger in prescribing it for a nursing mother. Needs more study	+
Secobarbital	None reported	Not specified	PO	Hypnotic doses would probably cause infant sedation (58)	+
Sodium fusidate	None reported	Not stated	PO	Not significant in tested doses to affect child (24). Not well documented and more studies are needed	0
Sotalol	None noted	—	PO	Mean serum concentration of 2.3 mcg/ml corresponds to a mean milk concentration of 10.5 μg/ml which could amount to a significant ingestion (267)	2+
Sulfasalazine	None noted	—	PO	About 30% of serum level appears in breast milk which would be a daily dose for an infant of about 4 mg (268, 269)	+
Sulfisoxazole	None reported but possible hyperbilirubinemia	Not stated	PO	Manufacturer (Hoffmann-La Roche) recommends avoiding this drug during the neonatal state to prevent hyperbilirubinemia and kernictirus (30)	3+
Tetrachloroethylene	Obstructive jaundice, hepatomegaly	—	Inhaled	Exposure of mothers at dry cleaning plant produced symptoms in nursing infant. Milk level 1 hr after exposure was 1 mg/dl (270)	3+
Thioridazine	None reported but may cause jaundice	Not stated	PO	Probably not in significant levels but may cause problems (201)	+
Thyroxine (thyroid)	None reported	Not stated	PO	Utilized ^{131}I-labeled thyroxine (27). Thyroxine is a thyroid extract and synthetic T_4 and T_3 probably can be used without problems and may even increase milk production as happens in animals. Manufacturer (Armour) states no problems with therapeutic doses	0

Tobramycin	None noted	80 mg	IM	Breast milk levels recorded were 0.6 μg/ml at 1 hr and 0.85 μg/ml at 8 hrs after the dose (271)	+
Tranylcypromine	None reported	Not stated	PO	Manufacturer (SK&F) states it does not appear in significant amounts (30). However, caution is advised with this very potent drug	2+
Trimeprazine tartrate	None reported	Not stated	PO	Manufacturer (SK&F) claims it is excreted but not in significant amounts to affect infant (30)	+
Valproic Acid	None noted	—	PO	Reaches 5–10% of serum levels in breast milk. These are low levels and do not appear to be enough to cause infant effects (272, 273)	+

[a] Adapted from R. H. Levin and L. A. Pagliaro (40).
[b] PO, orally; ID, intradermal; IM, intramuscular; IV, intravenous; PR, rectally; SC, subcutaneous.
[c] 0, insignificant; +, possibly significant; 2+, probably significant; 3+, significant.

in breast milk but will attain a high level of concentration in fat deposits. A highly ionized large molecule such as heparin, insulin or protamine will also diffuse extremely poorly across cell membranes. To achieve optimal partition, a drug must have a molecular structure which has a balanced lipophilic and hydrophilic nature. Un-ionized nonprotein-bound balanced molecules like alcohol will achieve milk levels equal to their serum levels. Protein binding will decrease the partition of drugs. There is some active transport of drugs but, because of lack of knowledge, the importance of this factor is unknown. Finally, there seems to be a rough correlation between the dialyzability of drugs and their excretion in milk. Generally speaking, the more easily a drug can be dialyzed the greater the concentration it will achieve in milk.

Predicting or calculating the quantities of drugs in breast milk for research purposes has become much more sophisticated. Wilson et al. (36) have developed equations based on a three-compartment open model. The first compartment is the central compartment primarily consisting of blood and extracellular fluids. The second compartment is interstitial and intracellular spaces and the third compartment is the breast milk. This third compartment is considered a deep compartment until the infant feeds when it turns into a infant-modulated zero order rate of excretion compartment. Drugs will transition, in both directions through all three compartments with variable rate constants. Pharmacological factors may also play a significant role in altering the concentration of a drug. Drugs dependent on renal clearance will achieve higher serum and milk levels in a mother with renal insufficiency. Those medications dependent on liver metabolism may have altered half-lives if there is severe hepatic impairment in the mother. Severe impairment of other organs such as the gastrointestinal tract, heart, circulation or lungs may also alter drug absorption, distribution or excretion. Any of these factors which results in increased plasma levels of drugs as compared to normal will also produce elevated drug concentrations in breast milk.

Medications in Breast Milk

It is extremely important for the breast-feeding mother, the pharmacist and the physician to be aware of and avoid those substances which are toxic to the infant. Tables 3.7 and 3.8 are a compilation of the available data on drugs excreted in breast milk. Table 3.7 lists those drugs that have documented, substantiated data while Table 3.8 lists the remaining drugs which have been reported but not adequately documented. Unless otherwise noted, all comments are those of the author of this chapter and reflect a personal interpretation of the literature.

A lactating mother, fortunately, generally does not consume many medications. The most commonly used medications are analgesics, barbiturates, diuretics, antimicrobials, laxatives, antinauseants and antacids. There are a number of drugs within these pharmacological groups that when taken in therapeutic doses by the mother will cause adverse effects in the infant. For example, infant sedation can be expected with excessive doses of narcotics, hypnotic doses of some barbiturates and large doses of alcohol, chloral hydrate, bromides, diazepam and methyprylon. Infant exposure to large doses of reserpine will cause nasal stuffiness. Tetracyclines will cause tooth staining and decreased bone growth. Cascara and danthron will increase bowel activity and possibly cause diarrhea. Medications with strong anticholinergic properties such as antihistamines, phenothiazines and atropine-like compounds may decrease lactation without having any appreciable effect on the infant. There are other less frequently used drugs that also cause problems. Drugs affecting thyroid function such as iodide salts, radioactive I^{131} and propylthiouracil have had adverse effects on infant thyroids. Heavy metals such as mercury, lead and arsenicals have caused toxicities. Ergotrate maleate, given postpartum to enhance uterine contraction, has caused ergotism in a high percentage of infants. Finally, potential risks would seem to exist with maternal ingestion of antimetabolites.

There is very little data regarding the risks of using social drugs such as alcohol, tobacco or other drugs of abuse. Excessive quantities of alcohol have produced infant sedation and smoking of more than 20 regular tobacco cigarettes a day has caused nicotine effects in the infant. Stimulants, depressants, narcotics and psychedelics when taken in high doses as abuse drugs would be expected to achieve high milk concentrations. Although no studies have been undertaken to measure abuse drug levels, it seems prudent for the mother to avoid them.

In general, with the exception of the preceding drugs, the infant will be unlikely to encounter adverse effects from maternally ingested drugs unless taken in excessive quantities. If a mother must consume a medication and is able to safely continue breast-feeding, she should consume the drug about 15 min after nursing or 3 to 4 hours before the next feeding (36). This allows enough time for many medications to clear the maternal serum and result in a relatively low milk concentration. Conversely, medications taken 30 to 60 min prior to a feeding often achieve peak serum and milk concentrations during nursing. If a mother must consume a new or untested medication, breast-feeding should be temporarily stopped. Fortunately, very few mothers have to discontinue breast feeding because of the consumption of medication.

In summary, breast-feeding women should avoid the use of abuse drugs, tetracyclines, cascara, danthron, antithyroid medication, antimetabolites and ergot alkaloids. If these medications are needed they should be utilized in the lowest possible dose. If there are no adverse effects in the infant, breast-feeding could continue. Excessive doses of any drug or new and untested drugs should be avoided. Finally, a lactating woman with decreased renal or hepatic function is likely to predispose herself and the infant to drug toxicity unless the dose is appropriately adjusted.

NUTRITIONAL PRODUCTS

If the woman cannot breast-feed, prepared infant formulas are the best substitute. In the United States they are available as sterile concentrated solutions or powders and if carefully reconstituted are nutritious and will not predispose the child to infections. However, in poor, underdeveloped countries, and in areas with inadequate sanitation and polluted water, breast-feeding is clearly the most hygienic and nutritional source of food. The infant formulas diluted with polluted water, and usually prepared in unnutritious concentrations, lead to a high incidence of infant malnutrition, as well as morbidity and mortality from infections. In the United States the formulas are nutritious and can be utilized as an adequate replacement for breast milk if they are manufactured properly to include all the necessary nutrients in the remcommended quantities, and are utilized correctly by the consumer.

There are disadvantages to using formulas

besides the previously mentioned increased infection rate and malnutrition problems. Infants do gain weight faster on formulas compared to breast-feeding probably due to an increased calorie intake (274). This weight gain has been reported to predispose to obesity in adulthood by producing more fat cells in the infant (275). Advantages of using standard infant formulas are that they: (a) are made to closely resemble breast milk, (b) are as sterile and nutritious as breast milk, (c) are easy to prepare, (d) are convenient to buy and use, and (e) are relatively inexpensive.

The standard infant formulas such as Enfamil and Similac are prepared to simulate human breast milk and are to be used for the first 6 months of life (Table 3.9). Foman (274) has reported that during the first year of life the infants caloric intake should be between 100 and 120 kcal/kg per day of which 5 to 15% should be from protein; 35 to 55% from fat and 35 to 65% from carbohydrate. The standard formulas containing 20 calories per ounce utilize cow's milk for protein which is composed of casein and bovine lactalbumin. Cow's milk is also frequently utilized for the fat source in butterfat, and the carbohydrate source in lactose. Vitamins and minerals are then added to the cow's milk base formulas to bring them up to the recommended dietary allowances (RDA) for infants.

There are a large number of "therapeutic formulas" for infants who have specific needs. The most common of these are used for infants who cannot tolerate cow's milk derived formulas. Those infants with acquired lactase deficiency, commonly due to severe diarrhea, cannot digest lactose. Usually a sucrose-containing formula such as Isomil or Soyalac will suffice. If there is a total disaccharidase deficiency, a carbohydrate-free formula such as RCF (Ross Carbohydrate Free) formula base can be utilized and a monosaccharide like dextrose can be added when needed. There are also infants born with a rare form of lactase deficiency who develop severe diarrhea with any form of lactose. Infants may also exhibit allergy to the casein and bovine lactalbumin in cow's milk. This manifests as severe diarrhea, intestinal cramping, anemia and poor growth. The soy protein base formulas (Isomil, Soyalac) are usually the first alternatives tried. In most cases, the soy formulas correct both of the previously mentioned cow's milk problems. There are, however, a small percentage of infants allergic to soy protein who require a

change in formula. For these infants, meat base, lamb base, or goat's milk are other alternatives for protein. If these cannot be used, a less allergenic amino acid preparation such as Pregestimil or Nutramigen (casein hydralosate with 65% amino acids) or Vivonex (100% amino acids) is utilized.

There have been incidents where necessary nutrients have been inadvertently omitted or were present in inadequate quantities in commercial formulas, leading to infant morbidity (chloride deficiency leading to hypochloremia, diarrhea and dehydration, and vitamin E deficiency leading to neonatal hemolytic anemia). It is important to consider that infant formulas are usually the only source of nutrition for the growing infant. What are the consequences to future generations if some vital ingredient contained in breast milk is not present in formulas? Are we, in fact, by using synthetic infant formulas conducting the largest uncontrolled human experiment in history? Would it not be better for health care providers to recommend that formulas be utilized only when breast feeding cannot be used?

Infants with fat intolerance can be given products with easily digested medium chain triglycerides such as Portagen or Pregestimil. Premature infants who require a higher caloric and protein content formula can be given Premature Formula (Mead Johnson). Infants who are sodium restricted can be given Lonalac and those with restricted intake of phenylalanine are given Lofenalac. Infants with diarrhea can be given a complete formula like Probana or a supplement to replace only diarrheal losses of electrolytes and carbohydrate, e.g. Lytren or Pedialyte. In these infants a major concern is for the formula's osmolarity, osmolality and renal solute load. These terms are frequently confused or misused. Osmolality, the preferred and most accurate measurement, should be determined directly by measuring the formula's freezing point depression or vapor tension, and is expressed as mOsm/kg water. Osmolarity is calculated from osmolality as mOsm/liter of formula and with concentrated infant formulas may be as much as 20% lower than the osmolality. Both of these values are related to the carbohydrate and mineral content of the formulas. Hypertonic solutions, greater than 400 mOsm/kg H_2O drain fluid into the GI tract and may lead to infant diarrhea and dehydration. Renal solute load is related to the protein (converted to urea in the

Table 3.9.
Infant formulas

Product (Manufacturer)[a]	Calories Per 30 ml	Calories Per 100 ml	Protein (g/100 ml)	Source of Protein	Fat (g/100 ml)	Type of Fat	Carbohydrate (g/100 ml)
STANDARD FORMULAS:							
Advance (Ross)	16	54	2.0	Cow's milk, soy protein	2.7	Soy, corn oils	5.5
Breast milk	22	75	1.1	Human milk	4.5	Human milk fat	6.8
Cow's milk, whole, fortified	21	69	3.5	Cow's milk	3.5	Butterfat	4.9
Evaporated milk, diluted 1:1, fortified	21	69	3.5	Cow's milk	4.0	Butterfat	4.9
Goat's milk, fresh	21	69	3.6	Goat's milk	4.0	Goat's milk fat	4.6
Enfamil (Mead Johnson)	20	66	1.5	Cow's milk	3.7	Soy, coconut oils	7.0
Enfamil with Iron (Mead Johnson)	20	66	1.5	Cow's milk	3.7	Soy, coconut oils	7.0
Similac (Ross)	20	68	1.55	Cow's milk	3.6	Soy, coconut oils	7.23
Similac with Iron (Ross)	20	68	1.55	Cow's milk	3.6	Soy, coconut oils	7.23
SMA Improved (Wyeth)	20	68	1.5	Demineralized whey	3.6	Safflower oil (blend) soy, coconut oils	6.9
THERAPEUTIC FORMULAS:							
Milk Allergy							
Isomil (Ross)	20	68	2.0	Soy protein	3.6	Soy, coconut oils	6.80
i-Soyalac (Loma Linda)	20	66	2.1	Soy	3.75	Soy oil	6.65
Meat Base Formula (1:1 dilution) (Gerber)	20	65	2.8	Beef heart	3.3	Sesame, beef fat	6.2
Nursoy (Wyeth)	20	67.6	2.3	Soy isolate	3.6	Safflower oil (blend)	6.8
Nutramigen (Mead Johnson)	20	66	2.2	Hydrolyzed casein	2.6	Corn oil	8.8
Pro-Sobee (Mead Johnson)	20	66	2.5	Soy isolate	3.4	Soy oil	6.8
Soyalac (Loma Linda)	20	66	2.1	Soy	3.8	Soy oil	6.65
Electrolyte Imbalance							
Lytren (Mead Johnson)	9	30	None	None	None	None	7.6
Pedialyte (Ross)	6	20	None	None	None	None	5.0
Medium Chain Triglyceride Requirement							
Portagen (Mead Johnson)	20	66	2.4	Casein	3.2	Corn, MCT[e] oils	7.8
Carbohydrate and/or Fat Restriction							
RCF Ross Carbohydrate Free	Std Dil 12	40.5	2	Soy	3.6	Soy and coconut oils	0
Pregestimil (Mead Johnson)	20	66	2.2	Hydrolyzed casein	2.8	Corn, MCT oils	8.8
Skim milk, fortified, market average	11	36	3.6	Cow's milk	Trace	None	5.3

Type of Carbohydrate	Sodium (mEq/ 100 ml)	Potas- sium (mEq/ 100 ml)	Chloride (mEq/ 100 ml)	Calcium (mg/100 ml)	Phospho- rus (mg/ 100 ml)	Iron (mg/ 100 ml)	Osmo- larity[b] (mOsm/L)	Osmolality[e] (mOsm/kg H2O)	Renal So- lute[d] Load (mOsm/L)
Corn syrup, lac- tose	1.3	2.2	1.6	51.0	39.0	1.2	190	210	130
Lactose	0.7	1.3	1.1	33.6	16.0	0.15	273	300	77
Lactose	2.5	3.6	2.7	120.0	96.0	0.05	290	300	228
Lactose	2.8	3.9	3.2	134.6	102.5	0.05	600	—	512
Lactose	1.4	4.6	4.5	128.0	104.9	0.1	—	—	240
Lactose	1.2	1.8	1.5	55.0	46.0	Trace	260	290	102
Lactose	1.2	1.8	1.5	55.0	46.0	1.2	260	290	102
Lactose	1.1	2.0	1.5	51.0	39.0	Trace	260	290	108
Lactose	1.1	2.0	1.5	51.0	39.0	1.2	260	290	108
Lactose	6.5	1.4	1.0	44.0	33.0	1.3	270	300	90
Sucrose, corn syrup	1.3	1.8	1.5	70.0	50.0	1.2	228	250	126
Sucrose	1.8	1.9	2.6	63.4	52.8	1.6	202	225	129
Sucrose, modified tapioca starch	0.8	1.0	0.6	98	65.0	1.37	—	280	—
Sucrose, corn syrup	0.87	1.9	1.0	63	44	1.3	185	241	130
Sucrose, arrow- root starch	1.4	1.7	1.3	63	47	1.2	400	450	160
Sucrose, corn syrup solids	1.8	1.9	1.2	79	53	1.2	180	235	130
Sucrose, dex- trose, maltose, dextrins	—	2.0	1.3	63.4	52.8	1.6	202	225	129
Corn syrup, solids, glucose	3.0	2.5	2.5	7.9	8.6	None	275	290	106
Dextrose	3.0	2.0	3.0	8.0	None	None	390	410	80
Corn syrup solids, sucrose	1.4	3.2	1.6	63.0	17	1.2	237	357	150
None	1.3	1.8	1.5	70	50	1.2	60	64	126
Glucose, tapioca, starch	1.4	1.7	1.3	63	47	1.2	297	338	125
Lactose	2.3	3.6	3.0	122.7	98.0	Trace	270	—	228

Table 3.9.—*Continued*

Product (Manufacturer)[a]	Calories		Protein (g/ 100 ml)	Source of Protein	Fat (g/100 ml)	Type of Fat	Carbohy- drate (g/ 100 ml)
	Per 30 ml	Per 100 ml					
High Protein and/or Caloric Require- ment							
Premature Formula (Mead Johnson)	24	81	2.4	Cow's milk	4.1	MCT, coconut corn oils	8.9
Probana (Mead Johnson)	20	66	4.2	Cow's milk, ca- sein hydroly- sate	2.2	Butterfat, corn oil	7.9
Similac PM 60/40 (Ross)	20	68	1.58	Demineralized whey, casein	3.5	Corn, coconut oils	6.8
Special Care (Ross)	24	81	2.2	Whey, casein	4.4	MCT, coconut and corn oils	8.6
SMA Preemie (Wyeth)	24	81	2	Whey, casein	4.4	Oleo, coconut, oleic, soy, MCT	8.6
Sodium Restricted							
Lonalac (Mead Johnson)	20	66	2.2	Casein	2.7	Coconut oil	8.8
Phenylketonuria							
Lofenalac (Mead Johnson)	20	66	3.4	Hydrolyzed casein	3.5	Corn oil	4.8

[a] Values are based on ready-to-use strength and were obtained with cooperation of the Dietary
[b] Osmolarity = mOsm/L = mg/MW/L.
[c] Osmolality = mOsm/kg H_2O = mg/MW/kg H_2O.
[d] Renal solute load = protein (g) × 4 + [Na(mEq) + K(mEq) + Cl(mEq)].
[e] MCT = medium chain triglycerides.

body) and mineral content of the formula. This important value represents the osmotic gradient presented to the kidney. It is especially important because high renal solute loads are detrimental in infants with kidney or liver disease.

Patients who are over 6 months old usually do not require the standard formulas with 20 cal/oz so that a reduced 16 cal/oz formula such as Advance was developed. Cow's milk plus baby food will also provide adequate nutrition for this age group. If cow's milk is utilized the daily intake should be kept to 1 quart or less. Greater than 1 quart per day can lead to milk intolerance, diarrhea, and iron deficiency anemia secondary to the large intake of protein which may cause an enteropathy. Reducing the intake of milk to less than a quart and supplementing with iron-rich infant food will help resolve the entropathy and its sequelae. The infant foods utilized should be those with the least possible added salt, sugar and monosodium glutamate (MSG). These substances are added to improve the taste for increased adult acceptability. The added sodium from salt and

MSG has been casually implicated in predisposing susceptible infants to developing hypertension as adults (276). MSG has caused "Chinese restaurant syndrome" in adults and its inclusion in infant food seems unwarranted. The added sugar, as stated before, may be implicated in predisposing to obesity by increasing the total number of fat cells. The daily intake of infant foods for the 6-month-old should consist of 2 or more servings of meat, 4 or more servings of vegetables, 1 or more servings of citrus fruits and 4 or more servings of bread or cereal. Serving sizes will increase as the child grows. The use of infant foods may also start as early as 2 to 3 months of age with cereals and with the addition of vegetables, fruits and meats added as tolerated. Junior foods, which contain small chunks of solid food, are usually begun at 8 to 12 months of age. Adult table food is usually begun at 1 year of age. If the child receives a normal, varied diet which contains the required nutrients, no added supplements are needed. Giving a normal child additional vitamins and minerals adds nothing to his health, is an un-

Type of Carbohydrate	Sodium (mEq/ 100 ml)	Potassium (mEq/ 100 ml)	Chloride (mEq/ 100 ml)	Calcium (mg/100 ml)	Phosphorus (mg/ 100 ml)	Iron (mg/ 100 ml)	Osmolarity[b] (mOsm/L)	Osmolality[e] (mOsm/kg H2O)	Renal Solute[d] Load (mOsm/L)
Lactose, corn syrup solids	1.4	2.3	1.9	94	47	Trace	264	300	220
Dextrose, lactose	2.7	3.1	2.1	116	89	Trace	639	—	250
Lactose	0.7	1.5	0.7	40.0	20.0	0.26	239	260	92
Lactose, corn syrup solids	1.5	2.6	1.8	144	72	3	260	300	147
Lactose, maltose dextrans	1.4	1.9	1.5	75	40	0.3	245	268	—
Lactose	1.4	1.7	1.3	63	47	Trace	200	241	200
Corn syrup, tapioca starch	0.1	2.6	1.7	113	103.3	1.2	454	—	140

Service, Shands Hospital, Gainesville, Florida, and manufacturers.

needed monetary expense, and should only be used if nutritional deficiencies have been documented.

IMMUNIZATIONS

The use of active immunizing agents has prevented millions of children from acquiring certain communicable diseases. The incidence of diphtheria, tetanus, pertusis, and polio is so low in the United States that many practicing pediatricians have never seen these diseases (277). Morbidity and mortality from measles, mumps, and rubella have been greatly decreased (277, 278). Smallpox has been totally eradicated from the world. Research scientists continue to study and develop more effective vaccines to prevent diseases such as hepatitis, herpes, chickenpox and meningitis.

Immunizations or vaccines produce active immunity. That is, the antigenic substance in the vaccine induces the host to elaborate a lymphocyte-produced antibody. The lymphocytes then form the repository for the person's production of antibody against the disease. These lymphocytes generate clone cells which act to produce immunity for extended periods varying from a few years to a lifetime. Generally speaking, the live attenuated vaccines produce the longest sustained and highest antibody titers.

Whenever possible, live vaccines are preferred, but for various reasons, killed whole or partial bacterial or viral products are also utilized. There are both live bacterial and live viral vaccines (Table 3.10). Bacillus Calmette-Guérin (BCG) vaccine developed to prevent tuberculosis is the only live bacterial vaccine available in the United States. The tuberculosis bacteria are attenuated by cultivation on a special bile-containing media at a controlled temperature to decrease virulence but maintain antigenicity. This produces a stable low virulent variant of the tubercle bacillus. All the remaining live vaccines are viral and include: measles, mumps, rubella, oral polio, rabies (HDCV), yellow fever and smallpox. These vaccines are attenuated by successive passages through live cell medias, for example, measles and mumps on chick embryo, and rabies on duck embryo or human diploid cell

Table 3.10.
Immunologic Agents

	Type[a]	Culture Media[b]	Special Indications for Prophalactic Use[c]	Age for Recommended Routine Prophalactic Immunization Schedule[d]					
				2 mo	4 mo	6 mo	15 mo	18 mo	4–6 yr
ACTIVE IMMUNIZA-TION									
Vaccines—Bacterial									
BCG	Live	Special bile	×						
Mixed respiratory	Killed	Standard	×						
Meningitis polysaccharides	Killed	Standard	×						
Cholera	Killed	Agar or broth	×						
Plague	Killed	Standard	×						
Typhoid	Killed	Standard	×						
Pneumococcal (polysaccharide)	Killed	Standard	×						
Pertussis[e]	Killed	Standard		×	×	×		×	×
Vaccines—Viral									
Measles[f]	Live	Chick embryo					×		
Mumps[f]	Live	Chick embryo					×		
Rubella[f]	Live	Human diploid cells					×		
Sabin poliomyelitis (TOPV)	Live	Monkey kidney		×	×	×		×	×
Salk poliomyelitis (TOPV)	Killed	Monkey kidney	×						
Influenza	Killed	Chick embryo	×						
Smallpox	Live	Calf lymph	×						
Yellow Fever	Live	Chick embryo	×						
Hepatitis B	Killed	Chick embryo	×						
Rabies	Live	Human diploid cells	×						
Toxoids									
Tetanus[g] absorbed	Inactivated	Standard		×	×	×		×	×
Diphtheria[g] absorbed	Inactivated	Standard		×	×	×		×	×
Staphylococcus	Inactivated	Standard	×						
In Vivo Diagnostic Agents									
Tuberculin—purified protein; derivative[h]	Inactivated	Standard					×[h]		
Coccidioidin[i]	Inactivated	Standard							
Histoplasmin, diluted[i]	Inactivated	Standard							
Mumps skin test[i] antigen	Killed	Chick embryo							
PASSIVE IMMUNITIES									
Immune Serums		All obtained from pooled human sera high in specific antibodies and used prophylactably to prevent or ameliorate disease. Equine derived antitoxins are also available for many diseases							
Rabies immune globulin human (RIG)									
Immune globulin intramuscular (ISG)									
Immune globulin intravenous									

Table 3.10.—Continued

	Type[a]	Culture Media[b]	Special Indications for Prophalactic Use[c]	Age for Recommended Routine Prophalactic Immunization Schedule[d]					
				2 mo	4 mo	6 mo	15 mo	18 mo	4–6 yr
Pertussis immune globulin (PIG)									
Hepatitis B immune globulin (HBIG)									
Tetanus immune globulin (TIG)									
Varicella-zoster immune globulin (VZIG)									
RHO-(D) immune globulin									

[a] Whether the product is live and attenuated or killed and inactivated.

[b] Standard indicates it is the unspecified usual media the organism is grown on.

[c] Not used for routine immunization practices in the United States. Used only for particular indications, to prevent or treat specific diseases or for travelers to epidemic regions.

[d] The American Academy of Pediatrics recommended immunization schedule for Infants and Children from *Report of the Committee on Infectious Diseases*, 1982. Consult this reference for the schedule of primary immunizations for children not immunized in infancy.

[e] Available only in combination as diphtheria and tetanus toxoids and pertussis vaccine (DPT).

[f] Can be used individually but usually given as combined triple vaccine MMR.

[g] Can be used individually but usually used as triple combination with Pertussis Vaccine as DPT. Also available as DT pediatric and Td adult combinations (see text) Tetanus or Td is given every 5–10 years as a booster dose.

[h] The initial test should be at the time of or preceding the MMR immunization. Repeated tests are dependent on the childs risk of exposure to tuberculosis.

[i] Not used for routine testing only for individual diseases or for immunocompetency testing.

cultures (Table 3.10). The viruses are also propagated and incubated at 0°C to further aid in the attenuation process.

The bacteria from the available killed vaccines are first propagated to produce antigenic substances and then killed or inactivated with heat, ultraviolet light or formaldehyde. The killed pertussis bacteria are utilized intact, or purified through extraction processes to produce a vaccine with less side effects. The vaccines for cholera, plague and typhoid and mixed respiratory vaccine (MRV) commonly utilize whole killed bacteria, while meningitis and pneumococcal vaccines utilize only the purified polysaccharide bacterial coating. The diphtheria and tetanus bacteria produce an exotoxin which is responsible for each disease's systemic effects. This toxin is inactivated with formaldehyde to form the toxoid, which is the immunizing material. The viruses used to produce the killed viral vaccines for polio, influenza, hepatitis, and rabies are initially allowed to propagate, then inactivated with heat or ultraviolet light, and finally utilized as whole viruses or purified extracts of antigenic material.

In contrast to the preceding immunizations which achieve active immunity, there are a number of immunologic materials which are used to produce passive immunity. Passive immunity is conferred on a person through the administration of preformed antibody as a human immune globulin or animal-derived antitoxin. An immediate antibody titer is achieved which lasts for only 4 to 8 weeks. This short duration is a result of rapid elimination of the administered antibody by the recipient—hence passive immunity. To form animal-derived diphtheria and tetanus antitoxin, horses are immunized with the appropriate toxins, their blood collected and purified for antibodies against diphtheria or tetanus. To form pertussis and tetanus immune serums, humans are respectively hyperimmunized and their serums are pooled and concentrated to obtain the appropriate antibodies. To produce hepatitis and varicella zoster immunoglobulin, serum is pooled from donors who are now well but have had the diseases and developed a high antibody titer.

Infants and children receive a number of vaccines as a routine prophylactic measure to prevent disease. The vaccines employed are diphtheria, pertussis, tetanus, measles, mumps, rubella, and oral polio. Each of these immunizations, which will be covered in detail below, is given to healthy infants and children on a routine schedule which has been elaborated by the American Academy of Pediatrics (Table 3.10). Any immunization will be deferred if the infant, child or adolescent has an acute febrile illness, a childhood exanthem or an exacerbation of a chronic illness. In addition, there are further contraindications to live vaccines; pregnancy, severe sensitivity to the culture media (duck, chick embryo), an active malignancy, an altered immune state (immunodeficiency disease, recent use of corticosteroids) or active untreated tuberculosis.

DIPHTHERIA, PERTUSSIS AND TETANUS (DPT)

The three immunizations are considered together because they are usually given as the combined DPT immunization. This combination has been used for over 35 years and is a widely advocated and very effective immunization. It achieves serum protective levels for 85% of recipients for diphtheria, 90% for pertussis and 100% for tetanus. Each of these diseases is a very serious disease with a high incidence of morbidity and mortality and difficult to treat, so that prevention is the key to success. According to the Center for Disease Control (CDC) there were 3 cases of diphtheria, 1,730 cases of pertussis and 95 cases of tetanus in 1980 (278). Diphtheria is an acute infection of the throat, nose, mucous membranes or skin. A gray adherent pseudomembrane is found most often in the pharynx or nasopharynx and occurs along with a sore throat, nasal discharge, hoarseness, and fever. The diphtheria toxin may also produce peripheral neuritis and myocarditis. Penicillin or erythromycin is somewhat effective for treatment. Diphtheria antitoxin is most useful if given to exposed individuals before they develop active disease.

Pertussis or whooping cough has a high mortality in infancy and 75% of the deaths occur in less than 1-year-olds. There is a prodromal catarrhal stage for 1 to 3 weeks, followed by cough, coryza and occasional vomiting. The cough is characterized by a series of paroxysmal expiratory coughs finally ending with a high pitched inspiratory "whoop." Death, when it occurs, usually is a complication of respiratory failure. Erythromycin, if used early in the disease, will prevent transmission to other susceptible persons. Pertussis antitoxin is also effective if used at the time of exposure before the child develops systemic symptoms.

Tetanus has a very high mortality rate of between 68 and 75%. The tetanus bacteria, *Clostridium tetani*, is a ubiquitous anaerobe, and is found as spores in soil and dust. The spores multiply under anaerobic conditions in necrotic tissue and can be found in infected decubitis, varicose ulcers, infected tumors, burns, frostbite, dental abscesses, gangrenous extremities, chronic skin ulcerations and in neonates with infected umbilici. It can also be introduced into the body through deep lacerations, punctures or other forms of traumatized tissue destruction. Tetanus produces local muscle spasm, trismus (lockjaw), convulsions, and death through cardiac and respiratory failure. Penicillin and tetracycline are effective as is tetanus antitoxin, or preferably tetanus immunoglobulin, when used early in the disease. Prevention of infection, however, is the recommended course. All wounds should be thoroughly washed and exposed to air, all necrotic tissue removed and the wounds kept clean. The prevention of tetanus infection depends on the state of prior immunity to injury. The patient may need no immunization, toxoid only or toxoid and immune globulin (Table 3.11).

To prevent these diseases, the combined diphtheria and tetanus toxoids along with pertussis (DPT) is started in infants at 2 months of age (Table 3.10). After the immunizing series is completed at 18 months of age, boosters are given at 4 to 6 years of age and then every 10 years. Pertussis vaccine is eliminated from the combination after the child reaches 6 years of age because of the decreasing incidence of the disease and unwarranted side effects from the pertussis vaccine. The tetanus, diphtheria combination (Td) used for boosters is the adult strength which contains the full amount of tetanus but only about 15% of the diphtheria antigen present in DPT. This reduced amount is used because of the increased incidence of side effects in children over 6 years of age with the full strength diphtheria preparation. A combined tetanus, diphtheria combination (DT) for pediatric use in under 6-years-old is available for children who had adverse reac-

Table 3.11.
Tetanus for Wounds[a]

Immunization Status	Immunization Treatment[b]		
	Low risk wound	Tetanus prone wounds	Wounds neglected >24 hr
Unimmunized, uncertain or incomplete (1 or 2 doses of toxoid)	1 dose Td or DT then complete immunization[c]	1 dose Td or DT plus 250–500 U TIG[d] then complete immunization[c]	1 dose Td or DT plus 250–500 U TIG[d] then complete immunization[c]
Full primary immunization with booster dose within 10 yr of wound	None	>5 yr since last dose use 1 dose Td otherwise no toxoid	1 dose Td plus 250–500 U TIG
Full primary immunization with no booster doses or last booster dose >1 yr from wound	1 dose Td	1 dose Td	1 dose Td plus 250–500 U TIG

[a] Recommendations from *Report of the Committee on Infectious Diseases*, 1982, American Academy of Pediatrics and from the Center for Disease Control.

[b] Tetanus prone wounds are those which yield anaerobic conditions or were incurred in circumstances with probability of exposure to tetanus spores, e.g. severe necrotizing machinery injuries, puncture wounds, wounds heavily contaminated with excreta, etc. All others are considered to be low-risk from the standpoint of tetanus. Neglected wounds have an increased risk for tetanus.

[c] A complete immunization for children or adults is 2 doses of tetanus toxoid or Td, 4–6 weeks apart, then a third dose 1 year after the second dose, followed by a dose every 10 years thereafter.

[d] Use a separate syringe and site of injection (preferably one in each arm or leg) for TIG (tetanus immune globulin) and toxoid. TIG is preferred in almost all instances and tetanus antitoxin should only be used when absolutely necessary.

tions to the pertussis portion of the vaccine. The vaccines are available as the fluid solutions or adsorbed suspensions. The alum-adsorbed suspensions confer a faster and better immunity, under all circumstances, and should be the only preparation employed. The suspensions are given intramuscularly and rarely lead to any significant local or systemic effects. There is usually a small area of erythema and irritation around the injection site. This may lead to a transient increase in temperature usually less than 102°F, within 12 to 48 hours after the injection. Rarely, severe fever, convulsions and encephalitis occur and are usually due to the pertussis portion of the DPT (279).

MEASLES (RUBEOLA), MUMPS (PAROTITIS), GERMAN MEASLES (RUBELLA)

These three diseases will also be considered together because of the common practice of using the triple combined MMR II (measles, mumps, rubella) vaccine. This combination live attenuated vaccine is over 95% effective in producing protective antibody for all three

viruses. In contrast to the use of DPT which is well accepted, the appropriate use of MMR still involves controversy (280).

There is no question that infants should be vaccinated against measles. The controversy arises as to the optimal age. Most infants have adequate amounts of maternal measles antibody to confer immunity until the currently recommended immunization age of 15 months. There are some infants born with little or no maternal antibodies who would benefit from earlier use of the immunization. Currently this is administered as early as 6 to 12 months of age during measles epidemics. The CDC reported 13,506 cases of measles in 1980, some of which may cause serious morbidity. There is usually a 3-day period of fever, conjuctivitis, coryza, photophobia and a barking harsh cough. This is followed by a typical maculopapular confluent rash beginning at the hairline and then spreading down to the face and body over a 3-day period. There is also a 1:1,000 incidence of encephalitis and a 1:10,000 incidence of death. The only treatment is symptomatic in nature.

Mumps contracted in early childhood (CDC reported 8,576 U.S. cases in 1980) is associated with unilateral or bilateral parotid gland swelling. There is pain and discomfort secondary to the swelling although 30 to 40% of the cases are asymptomatic. Aseptic meningitis and seizures can occur but are unusual. The primary reason to give the vaccine in early childhood is to prevent the disease in postpubertal adolescents, especially boys. Pubescent boys contracting mumps can develop pancreatitis, abdominal pain, fever, chills and orchitis. Although the unilateral or bilateral testicular involvement is very painful, there is seldom permanent damage and less than a 1% incidence of sterility. Infected adolescent girls may also experience painful pancreatitis, abdominal pain, and oophoritis. The only treatment of mumps is symptomatic in nature.

Rubella is a very mild disease in young children (CDC reported 3,904 U.S. cases in 1980) and is often confused with a 3-day cold, accompanied by a rash, lymphodenopathy and mild fever. In female adolescents, however, more severe symptoms of arthralgias, arthritis and joint swelling may occur and can incapacitate the patient for a week or more. Aside from these disease symptoms, the main reason to give rubella vaccine is to prevent congenital rubella syndrome (CDC reported 50 U.S. cases in 1980). Fetuses infected with rubella virus in the first trimester of pregnancy are likely to be born with a number of congenital anomalies: neonatal purpura, heart disease, cataracts, glaucoma, mental retardation and deafness. The only treatment for the disease or congenital rubella syndrome is symptomatic. In relation to this immunization, controversy revolves around the need to give an infant rubella vaccine in order to stop the transmission of rubella to a pregnant woman. There is also uncertainty as to whether the immunity will last from infancy to child-bearing age and whether there would have to be a reimmunization program for adolescent females. The current recommendation is not to reimmunize because of recent studies showing adequate ongoing protection in immunized children (280). The recommendation remains to use MMR at 15 months of age and to try and immunize all current adolescent females who have inadequate immunity.

The MMR II vaccine is a more potent, refined combination compared to the original MMR. It contains the live more attenuated line of measles virus from Enders' attenuated Edmonston strain grown in chick embryo; the Jeryl Lynn (B level) mumps strain also grown in chick embryo; the Wistar Institute RA 27/3 strain of rubella virus propagated in human diploid cell (WI 38) culture. There is no recommendation for booster doses of MMR. The individual measles, mumps and rubella vaccines should be used if immunity is lacking to an individual disease. Side effects usually associated with the vaccine are a mild rash and fever (102°F) occurring 7 to 10 days after the injection. There may be localized erythema, irritation and tenderness at the injection site. Adolescent females who are given the rubella vaccine may also experience arthralgia and arthritis-like symptoms.

POLIO

Polio is a serious paralytic disease that occurred in 8 U.S. patients in 1980 and may be caused by any one of the three types of polio viruses. The disease can cause muscle weakness, headache, stiff neck, fever and spinal paralysis. The extent of paralysis depends on the level of the spine that is involved and can be as little as a mild decrease in limb function to full paralysis of the whole body with a loss of respiration. Care is symptomatic in nature. The only way to prevent the disease is through active immunization. There is an ongoing controversy as to whether the live Sabin trivalent oral polio vaccine (TOPV) or the trivalent Salk inactivated polio vaccine (IPV) should be used (280).

The TOPV is easy to use orally, confers 95% immunity both in the gastrointestinal tract and serum, and needs no boosters after the primary immunizations. Its main drawback is its propensity to produce cases of paralytic polio (incidence of 1:3,000,000) in vaccine recipients and susceptible contacts. There are law suits pending concerning liability for these types of cases. The IPV does not cause any cases of paralytic polio, may induce lifelong immunity without boosters, and is given parenterally and could be combined with DPT. Its disadvantages are that there is no proven lifelong immunity and no gastrointestinal immunity so that wild polio virus could propagate in the intestines and a person could act as a carrier.

Until more data are available the current recommendation is to give routine TOPV starting at the second month of life and continued as listed in Table 3.10. Routine immunization of adults is unnecessary (Table 3.10). IPV should be reserved for high risk individuals, e.g. adults over 18 years old in epidemic areas, or immunodeficient contacts or patients. The TOPV causes no significant side effects other than the previously mentioned incidence of paralytic polio. The IPV can cause localized swelling and irritation at the injection site.

Other available vaccines are not used for routine preventative immunization in normal infants and children, but only with special considerations and under certain circumstances. When entering an endemic area or under epidemic conditions children should be immunized with vaccines for meningitis, cholera, plaque, typhoid, typhus, yellow fever or smallpox. Polyvalent pneumococcal polysaccharide vaccine is indicated for children over 2 years of age who are susceptible to pneumococcal infections. These are children who have sicklemia, have undergone splenectomy or have congenital absence of the spleen, nephrotic syndrome or B-cell deficiency. Influenza vaccine, reformulated yearly, is used prior to the impending influenza season. It usually contains a mixture of influenza type A and type B antigens. Those children who should routinely be immunized against influenza are those with heart disease, heart failure, chronic bronchopulmonary disease, or chronic renal, metabolic, hematologic or immunologic disorders. Hepatitis B vaccine, only recently released, will probably be given to children who receive large numbers of blood transfusions or blood products (hemophiliacs, thalassemics), children in institutions with endemic hepatitis B, those requiring hemodialysis, drug abusers, and sexually promiscuous youth. In the future, ongoing trials may produce a live varicella vaccine appropriate for children with leukemia; or an H influenza vaccine appropriate for children under 6 years of age.

References

1. Batey SR, Wright HH: Psychoactive drug use before treatment in a child psychiatry clinic. *Am J Hosp Pharm* 39:1675, 1982.
2. Goldman AG, Rich DS, Jeffrey LP: System for monitoring children with attention-deficient disorders. *Am J Hosp Pharm* 39:2126, 1982.
3. Watson PD, Powell JR, Mimakt T: Anticonvulsant usage. In Jaffe ST: *Pediatric Pharmacology and Therapeutic—Principles in Practice*. New York: Grune & Stratton, 1980, pp 195–212.
4. Friis-Hansen B: Body composition during growth. *Pediatrics* 47:264, 1971.
5. Nelson JD: Antimicrobial drugs. In Jaffe SJ: *Pediatric Pharmacology and Therapeutic—Principles in Practice*. New York: Grune & Stratton, 1980, p 187.
6. Nelson JD, McCracken GM: Clinical pharmacology of carbenicillin and gentamicin in the neonate and comparitive efficacy with ampicillin and gentamicin. *Pediatrics* 52:801, 1973.
7. McCracken GH, Ginsberg C, et al: Clinical pharmacology of penicillin in newborn infants. *J Pediatr* 82:692, 1973.
8. Levin RH, Maltz HE: Fluid balance in drug therapy. In Waechter EH, Blake JB: *Nursing Care of Children*, ed 9. Philadelphia: J. B. Lippincott, 1976, p 102.
9. Tatro DA: Adverse drug reactions in children. In Pagliaro LA, Levin RH: *Problems in Pediatric Drug Therapy*. Hamilton, Ill.: Drug Intelligence Publications, 1979.
10. Zenk KE: Neonatal and pediatric dosing. In Pagliaro LA, Levin RH: *Problems in Pediatric Drug Therapy*. Hamilton, Ill.: Drug Intelligence Publications, 1979.
11. Levin RH, Zenk KE: Medication table. In Rudolph AM: *Pediatrics*, ed 17. Norwalk, Conn.: Appleton-Century-Crofts, 1982.
12. Becker MH, Drachman RH, Kirscht JP: Predicting mothers' compliance with pediatric medical regimens. *J Pediatr* 81:843, 1972.
13. Mattar ME, Markello J, Jaffe SJ: Pharmaceutical factors affecting pediatric compliance. *Pediatrics* 55:101, 1975.
14. Arena J: Contamination of the ideal food. *Nutr Today* 5:2, 1970.
15. Holt LE: Feeding techniques and diets. In Barnett HL: *Pediatrics*, ed 15. New York: Meredith Corp., 1972, p 148.
16. Jelliffe DB, Jelliffe EFP: The volume and composition of human milk in poorly nourished communities—a review. *Am J Clin Nutr* 31:492, 1978.
17. Sherwood LM: Current concepts—human prolactin. *N Engl J Med* 284:774, 1971.
18. Tysor JE, Friesen HG, Anderson JJ: Human lactional and ovarian response to endogenous prolactin release. *Science* 177:897, 1972.
19. Vorherr H: To breast feed or not to breast feed. *Postgrad Med J* 51:127, 1972.
20. Gambrell R: Immediate postpartum oral contraception. *Obstet Gynecol* 36:101, 1970.
21. Jelliffe DB, Jelliffe EFP: Lactation, conception, and the nutrition of the nursing mother and child. *J Pediatr* 81:829, 1972.
22. Anderson PO: Drugs and breast feeding—a review. *Drug Intell Clin Pharm* 11:208, 1977.
23. Knowles JA: Excretion of drugs in milk—a review. *J Pediatr* 66:1068, 1965.
24. Takyi BW: Excretion of drugs in human milk. *J Hosp Pharm* 28:317, 1970.
25. Shore MF: Drugs can be dangerous during pregnancy and lactation. *Can Pharm J* 103:358, 1970.
26. Catz CS, Giacoia GP: Drugs and breast milk. *Pediatr Clin North Am* 19:151, 1972.
27. Knowles JA: Drugs in milk (Ross Laboratories). *Pediatr Currents* 21:28, 1972.
28. Knowles JA: Breast milk; a source of more than nutrition for the neonate. *Clin Toxicol* 7:69, 1974.

29. Anon: Drugs in breast milk. *Med Lett* 16:25, 1974.

30. O'Brien TE: Excretion of drugs in human milk. *Am J Hosp Pharm* 31:844, 1974.

31. Levin RH: Teratogenicity and drug excretion in breast milk (maternogenicity). In Herfindal ET, Hirschman JL: *Clinical Pharmacy and Therapeutics.* Baltimore: Williams & Wilkins, 1979, pp 40–65.

32. Vorherr H: Drug excretion in breast milk. *Postgrad Med* 56:97, 1974.

33. Savage RL: Drugs and breast milk. *Adverse Drug Reaction Bull* No. 61, 212, 1976.

34. Anderson PO: Drugs and breast feeding. *Semin Perinatol* 3:271, 1979.

35. Edwards A: Drugs in breast milk—a review of the recent literature. *Aust J Hosp Pharm* 11:27, 1981.

36. Wilson JT, Brown RD, et al: Drug excretion in human breast milk—principles, pharmacokinetics, and projected consequences. *Clin Pharmacokinet* 5:1, 1980.

37. White M: Breast feeding and drugs in human milk. La Leche League International, Inc. (July) 1977.

38. Kesaniemi YA: Ethanol and acetaldehyde in the milk and peripheral blood of lactating women after ethanol administration. *J Obstet Gynaecol Br Commonw* 81:84, 1974.

39. Putter J: Quantitative analysis of the main metabolites of acetysalicylic acid. Comparative analysis in the blood and milk of lactating women. *Z Geburtshilfe Perinatol* 178:135, 1974. [Abstract per *Int Pharm Abstr* 12:320 (Abstr 1982)(Jan. 30)1975.]

40. Levin RH, Pagliaro LA: Drugs excreted in breast milk. In Pagliaro LA, Levin RH: *Problems in Pediatric Drug Therapy.* Hamilton, Ill.: Drug Intelligence Publications, 1979.

41. Burn JH: Excretion of drugs in milk. *Br Med Bull* 5:190, 1947–1948.

42. Illingworth RS: Abnormal substances excreted in human milk. *Practitioner* 171:533, 1953.

43. Cobo E: Effect of different doses of ethanol on the milk-ejecting reflex in lactating women. *Am J Obstet Gynecol* 115:817, 1973.

44. Larsen AA, Robinson JM, Schmitt N, et al: Pesticide residues in mother's milk and human fat from intensive use of soil insecticides. *HSM HA Health Rep* 86:477, 1971.

45. Tyson RM, et al: Drugs transmitted through breast milk; Part I. Laxatives. *J Pediatr* 11:824, 1937.

46. Ayd FJ: Excretion of psychotropic drugs in human breast milk. *Int Drug Ther Newslett* 8:33, 1973.

47. Lohmeyer H, Halfpap E: Pharmakokinetische Under Behandlung von Infektionen des Urogenitaltrakts der Frau. *Z. Geburtshilfe Gynaekol* 164:184, 1965.

48. Paterson D, Smith JF: *Modern Methods of Feeding in Infancy and Childhood.* London: Cassell, 1938.

49. Kwit NT, Hatcher RA: Excretion of drugs in milk. *Am J Dis Child* 49:900, 1935.

50. Healy M: Suppressing lactation with oral diuretics. *Lancet* 1:1353, 1961.

51. Reiher KM: Unterdruckung der Laktation durch Anregung dur Diurese. *Zentralbl Gynaekol* 85:188, 1963.

52. Egan H, Goulding R, Roburn JOG, et al: Organochlorine pesticide residues in human fat and human milk. *Br Med J* 2:66, 1965.

53. Tyson RM, et al: Drugs transmitted through breast milk; III. Bromides. *J Pediatr* 14:91, 1938.

54. van der Bogert F: Bromine poisoning through mother's milk. *Am J Dis Child* 21:167, 1921.

55. Canales ES, et al: The influence of pyridoxine on prolactin secretion and milk production in women. *Br J Obstet Gynaecol* 83:387, 1976.

56. del Re RB, et al: Prolactin inhibition and suppression of puerperal lactation by a Br-ergocryptine (CB 154). *Obstet Gynecol* 41:884, 1973.

57. Utian WH, et al: Effect of bromocriptine and chlorotrianisene on inhibition of lactation and serum prolactin; a comparative double-bind study. *Br J Obstet Gynaecol* 82:755, 1959.

58. Horning MG, et al: Identification and quantification of drugs and drug metabolites in human breast milk using GC-MS-COM methods. *Mod Prob Paediatr* 15:73, 1975.

59. Schilf E, Wohing R: Über das Vorkommen von Caffein in der Frauenmilch nach Genuss von Kaffee. *Arch Gynaekol* 134:201, 1928.

60. Pynnonen S, Sillanpää M: Carbamezepine and mother's milk. *Lancet* 2:563, 1975.

61. Thomson ML: Carotinaemia in suckling. *Arch Dis Child* 18:112, 1943.

62. Geddes AM, Schnurr LP, et al: Cefoxitin; a hospital study. *Br Med J* 1:1126, 1977.

63. Yoshioka H, Cho K, Takimota M, et al: Transfer of cefazolin into human milk. *J Pediatr* 94:151, 1979.

64. Bernstine JB, et al: Maternal blood and breast milk estimation following the administration of chloral hydrate during the puerperium. *J Obstet Gynaecol Br Emp* 63:228, 1956.

65. Lacey JH: Dichloralphenazone and breast milk. *Br Med J* 4:684, 1971.

66. Havelka J, Frankova A: Study of side effects of maternal chloramphenicol therapy in newborns. *Cesk Pediatr* 21:31, 1972.

67. Smadel JE, et al: Chloramphenicol (Chloromycetin[R]) in the treatment of Tsutsugamushi disease (scrub thyphus). *J Clin Invest* 28:1196, 1949.

68. Brocházka J, et al: Excretion of chloramphenicol in human milk. I. *Cas Lek Cesk* 103:378, 1964.

69. Havelka J, et al: Excretion of chloramphenicol in human milk. *Chemotherapy* 13:204, 1968.

70. Soares R, et al: Da concentracào e eliminacà da cloroquina através da circulacáo placentaria e do leite materno, de paccientes sob regime do sal cloroquinado. *Rev Bras Malariol Doencas Trop* 9:19, 1957.

71. Merland R, Creste M: Recherche de l'élimination de la nivaquine et son dosage dans le lait de femme. *Med Trop* 11:793, 1951.

72. Werthmann MW, Krees SV: Excretion of chlorothiazide in human breast milk. *J Pediatr* 81:781, 1972.

73. Blacker KH, et al: Mother's milk and chlorpromazine. *Am J Psychiatry* 119:178, 1962.

74. Hooper JH, et al: Abnormal lactation associated

with tranquilizing drug therapy. *JAMA* 178:506, 1961.

75. Guilbeau JA, et al: Aureomycin in obstetrics: therapy and prophylaxis. *JAMA* 143:520, 1950.

76. Smith JA, et al: Clindamycin in human breast milk. *Can Med Assoc J* 112:806, 1975.

77. Curtis EsM: Oral-contraceptive feminization of a normal male infant. *Obstet Gynecol* 23:295, 1964.

78. Marriq P, Oddo G: La gynécomastie induite chez le nouveau-né par le lait mataernel? *Nouv Presse Med* 3:2579, 1974.

79. Lauritzen C: On endocrine effects of oral contraceptives. *Acta Endocrinol* 124 (suppl):87, 1967.

80. Anon: Contraceptive steroids in breast milk. *Br Med J* 4:731, 1970.

81. Wong YK, Wood BSB: Breast-milk jaundice and oral contraceptives. *Br Med J* 4:403, 1971.

82. Gould SR, et al: Influence of previous oral contraception and maternal oxytocin infusion on neonatal jaundice. *Br Med J* 3:228, 1974.

83. Llewellyn-Jones D: Inhibition of lactation. *Drugs* 10:121, 1975.

84. Vorherr H: Contraception after abortion and post partum. *Am J Obstet Gynecol* 117:1002, 1973.

85. Karim M, et al: Injected progestogen and lactation. *Br Med J* 1:200, 1971.

86. Sammour MB, et al: Effect of chlormadinone on the composition of human milk. *Fertil Steril* 24:301, 1973.

87. Toaff R, et al: Effects of oestrogen and progestagen on the composition of human milk. *J Reprod Fertil* 19:475, 1969.

88. Kader MMA: Clinical, biochemical and experiemental studies on lactation; III. Biochemical changes induced in human milk by gestagens. *Am J Obstet Gynecol* 105:978, 1969.

89. Barsivala VM, Virkar KD: The effect of oral contraceptives on concentrations of various components of human milk. *Contraception* 7:307, 1973.

90. Aarkrog A: Caesium-137 from fall-out in human milk. *Nature* 197:667, 1963.

91. Calapaj GG, Ongaro D: Sul "rapporto osservato" SR^{90}/Ca e Cs^{137}/k fra dieta e latte umano. *Nuovi Ann Ig Microbiol* 18:383, 1967.

92. Wiernik PH, Duncan JdH: Cyclophosphamide in human milk. *Lancet* 1:912, 1971.

93. Morton RF, et al: Studies on the absorption, diffusion and excretion of cysloserine. *Antibiot Ann* pp 169–172, 1955–1956.

94. Vuori E, Tyllinen H, et al: The occurrence and origin of DDT in human milk. *Acta Pediatr Scand* 66:761, 1977.

95. Woodard BT, et al: DDT levels in milk of rural indigent blacks. *Am J Dis Child* 130:400, 1976.

96. Luquet FM, et al: Pollution of human milk in France with organochlorine insecticide residues. *Pathol Biol* (Paris) 23:45, 1975.

97. Kroger M: Insecticide residues in human milk. *J Pediatr* 80:401, 1972.

98. Wilson J, Locker DJ, Ritzen CA, et al: DDT concentrations in human milk. *Am J Dis Child* 125:814, 1973.

99. Von Kobyletzki D, Strauch D: Zur Frage der Diaplazentaren Passage und Ausscheidung mit der Muttermilch von Demethylchlortetracyclin. *Z Geburtshilfe Gynaekol* 161:292, 1964.

100. Patrick MJ, et al: Diazepam and breast-feeding. *Lancet* 1:542, 1972.

101. Erkkola R, Kanto J: Diazepam and breast feeding. *Lancet* 1:1235, 1972.

102. Cole AP, Hailey DM: Diazepam and active metabolite in breast milk and their transfer to the neonate. *Arch Dis Child* 50:741, 1975.

103. Brandt R: Passage of diazepam and desmethyldiazepam into breast milk. *Arzneim Forsch* 26:454, 1976.

104. Brambel CE, Hunter RE: Effect of dicumarol on the nursing infant. *Am J Obstet Gynecol* 59:1153, 1950.

105. Levy M, Granit L, Laufer N: Excretion of drugs in human milk. *N Engl J Med* 297:789, 1977.

106. Fujimori H, Imai S: Studies on dihydrostreptomycin administered to the pregnant and transmitted to their fetuses. *J Jpn Obstet Gynecol Soc* 4:133, 1957.

107. Fujimori H, Imai S: *Int Abstr Surg* 1960, pp 111–289, in *Surg Gynecol Obstet* (Sept.) 1960.

108. Valquist B, Hogstedt C: Minute absorption of diphtheritic antibodies from the gastrointestinal tract in infants. *Pediatrics* 4:401, 1949.

109. Morganti G, et al: Comparative concentrations of a tetracycline antibiotic in serum and maternal milk. *Antibiotica* 6:216, 1968.

110. Donnally HH: The question of the elimination of foreign protein (egg white) in women's milk. *J Allergy* 1:78, 1929.

111. Shane JM, Naftolin F: Effect of ergonovine maleate on puerperal prolactin. *Am J Obstet Gynecol* 120:129, 1974.

112. Fomina PI: Untersuchunger uber den Ubergang des Aktiven Agens des Mutterkorns in die Milch Stillender Mutter. *Arch Gynaekol* 156:275, 1934.

113. Floss HG, et al: Influence of ergot alkaloids on pituitary prolactin and prolactin-dependent processes. *J Pharm Sci* 62:699, 1973.

114. Rassmussen F: *Studies on the Mammary Excretion and Absorption of Drugs.* Copenhagen: Carl Fr. Mortensen, 1966, pp 25–39.

115. Kobyletzki D: Original investigations of pharmacodynamics during partuition and lactation. *Trans Med Welt* 19:2010, 1968.

116. Gramen K: Bestimmungen über den über gang des äthers in die Müttermilch. *Acta Chir Scand* (Suppl I):83, 1922.

117. Pincus G, et al: Radioactivity in the milk of subjects receiving radioactive 19-norsteroids. *Nature* 212:924, 1966.

118. Illingworth RS, Finch E: Ethyl biscoumacetate (Tromexan^R) in human milk. *J Obstet Gynaecol Br Commonw* 66:487, 1959.

119. Casper J, Schulman T: Bilateral cortical necrosis of the kidneys in an infant with favism. *Am J Clin Pathol* 26:42, 1956.

120. Emanuel B, Schoenfeld A: Favism in a nursing infant. *J Pediatr* 58:263, 1961.

121. Joannides CC: Favism in Cyprus. *Cyprus Med J* 5:795, 1952.

122. Taj ES: Favism in breast fed infants. *Arch Dis Child* 46:121, 1971.

123. Bercovici B, et al: Fluorine in human milk. *Obstet Gynecol* 16:319, 1960.

124. Ericsson Y: Fluoride excretion in human saliva and milk. *Caries Res* 3:159, 1969.

125. Ericsson Y, et al: Pilot studies on the fluoride metabolism in infants on different feedings. *Acta Pediatr Scand* 61:459, 1972.

126. Buchanan RA, et al: The breast milk excretion of flufenamic acid. *Curr Ther Res* 11:533, 1969.

127. Kanto J, Aaltonen L, Kangos L, et al: Flunitrazepam. *Curr Ther Res* 26:539, 1979.

128. Ramasastri BV: Folate activity in human milk. *Br J Nutr* 19:581, 1965.

129. Metz J, et al: Folic acid binding by serum and milk. *Am J Clin Nutr* 21:289, 1968.

130. Larson SM, Schall GL: Gallium-67 concentration in human breast milk. *JAMA* 218:257, 1971.

131. Curry SH, et al: Disposition of glutethimide in man. *Clin Pharmacol Ther* 12:849, 1971.

132. Blau SP: Metabolism of gold during lactation. *Arthritis Rheum* 16:777, 1973.

133. Seward RB, et al: Haloperidol excretion in human milk. *Am J Psychiatry* 137:849, 1980.

134. Cobrinik RW, et al: The effect of maternal narcotic addiction on the newborn infant. *Pediatrics* 24:288, 1959.

135. Cam C: Une nouvelle dermatose épidémique des enfants. *Ann Dermatol Syphiligr* 87:393, 1960.

136. West RW, et al: Hexachlorophene concentrations in human milk. *Bull Environ Contam Toxicol* 13:167, 1975.

137. Bland EP, et al: Radioactive iodine uptake by thyroid of breast-fed infants after maternal blood-volume measurements. *Lancet* 2:1039, 1969.

138. Nurenberger CE, Lipscomb A: Transmission of radioiodine (I[131]) to infants through human maternal milk. *JAMA* 150:1398, 1952.

139. Miller H, Weetch RS: The excretion of radioactive iodine in human milk. *Lancet* 2:1013, 1955.

140. Weaver JC, et al: Excretion of radioiodine in human milk. *JAMA* 173:872, 1960.

141. Wyburn JR: Human breast milk excretion of radionuclides following administration of radiopharmaceuticals. *J Nucl Med* 14:115, 1973.

142. Schwartz KD, et al: The excretion of I[131] in breast milk in isotope nephrography performed with I[131], hippurate post partum. *Radiobiol Radiother* 9:259, 1968.

143. Maurer E, Ducrue H: *Munch Med Wochenschr* 75:249, 1928.

144. Holmdahl KH: Cholecystography during lactation. *Acta Radiol* 45:305, 1956.

145. Saarinen UM, Siimes MA, Dallman PR: Iron absorption in infants-high bioavailability of breast milk iron as indicated by the extrinsic tag method of iron absorption and by the concentration of serum ferritin. *J Pediatr* 91:36, 1977.

146. Ricci G, Copaitich T: Modalita di eliminazione dell'sioniazide somministrata per via orale attraverso il latte di donna. *Rass Int Clin Ter* 209:53, 1954–1955.

147. Chyo N, et al: Clinical studies of kanamycin applied in the field of obstetrics and gynecology. *Asian Med J* 5:265, 1962.

148. Michael CA: Use of labetalol in the treatment of severe hypertension during pregnancy. *Br J Clin Pharmacol* 8:2115, 1979.

149. Dillon HK, et al: Lead concentration in human milk. *Am J Dis Child* 128:491, 1974.

150. Medina A, et al: Absorption, diffusion and excretion of a new antibiotic, lincomycin. *Antimicrob Agents Chemother* 1963:189, 1964.

151. Schou M, Amdisen A: Lithium and pregnancy; III. Lithium ingestion by children breast-fed by women on lithium treatment. *Br Med J* 2:138, 1973.

152. Sykes PA, Quarrie J, Alexander FW: Lithium carbonate and breast feeding. *Br Med J* 2:1299, 1976.

153. Berger H: Excretion of mandelic acid in breast milk. *Am J Dis Child* 61:256, 1941.

154. Buchanan RA, et al: The breast milk excretion of mefanamic acid. *Curr Ther Res* 10:592, 1968.

155. Fujita E: Experimental studies on organic mercury poisoning, on the behavior of the Minamata disease causal agent in maternal bodies and its transfer to their infants via either placenta or breast milk. *Kumamoto Med Soc J* 43:47, 1969.

156. Matsumoto H, et al: Fetal Minamata disease. *J Neuropathol Exp Neurol* 24:563, 1965.

157. Wijmenga HG, van der Molen HJ: Studies with 4-^{14}C-mestranol in lactating women. *Acta Endocrinol* 61:665, 1969.

158. Blinick G, et al: Methadone assays in pregnant women and progeny. *Am J Obstet Gynecol* 121:617, 1975.

159. Johns DG, et al: Secretion of methotrexate into human milk. *Am J Obstet Gynecol* 112:978, 1972.

160. del Pozo E, et al: Lack of effect of methylergonovine on postpartum lactation. *Am J Obstet Gynecol* 123:845, 1975.

161. Sousa PLR: Metoclopramide and breast feeding. *Br Med J* 1:512, 1975.

162. Gray MS, et al: Further observations on metronidazole (Flagyl[R]). *Br J Vener Dis* 37:278, 1961.

163. Baldwin WF: Clinical study of senna administration to nursing mothers-assessment of effects on infant bowel habits. *Can Med Assoc J* 89:566, 1963.

164. Brogden RN, et al: Minocycline—a review. *Drugs* 9:251, 1975.

165. Stegink LD, et al: Monosodium glutamate-effect on plasma and breast milk amino acid levels in lactating women. *Proc Soc Exp Biol Med* 140:836, 1972.

166. Terwilliger WG, Hatcher RA: The elimination of morphine and quinine in human milk. *Surg Gynecol Obstet* 58:823, 1934.

167. Belton EM, Jones RV: Hemolytic anemia due to nalidixic acid. *Lancet* 2:691, 1965.

168. Ferguson BB, Wilson DJ, Schaffner W: Determination of nicotine concentrations in human milk. *Am J Dis Child* 130:837, 1976.

169. Hatcher RA, Crosby HJ: The elimination of nicotine in the milk. *J Pharmacol Exp Ther* 32:1, 1927.

170. Perlman HH, et al: The excretion of nicotine in breast milk and urine from cigaret smoking. *JAMA* 120:1003, 1942.

171. Hosbach RE, Foster RB: Absence of nitrofurantoin from human milk. *JAMA* 202:1057, 1967.

172. Varsano I, et al: The excretion of orally ingested nitrofurantoin in human milk. *J Pediatr* 82:886, 1973.

173. Laumas KR, et al: Radioactivity in the breast milk of lactating women after oral administration of ^{3}H-norethynodrel. *Am J Obstet Gynecol* 98:411, 1967.

174. Laumas V, et al: The possibility of estrogenic activity in the human and goat milk after administration of oral gestagens. *Contraception* 2:331, 1970.

175. Teixeria GE, Scott RB: Further clinical and laboratory studies with Novobiocin; I. Treatment of staphylococcal infection in infancy and childhood; II. Novobiocin concentrations in the blood of newborn infants and in the breast milk of lactating mothers. *Antibiot Med* 5:577, 1958.

176. Strobel VE, Herrmann B: Zur Frage des Überganges von Osyphenbutazon in den Fetalen Kreislauf und die Muttermilch. *Arzneim Forsch* 12:302, 1962.

177. Luhman LA: The effect of intranasal oxytocin on lactation. *Obstet Gynecol* 21:713, 1963.

178. Deodhar AD: Effect of socioeconomic status on the vitamin content of milk. *J Pediatr* 54:34, 1959.

179. Brilliant LB, Wilcox K, Van Amburg G, et al: Breast-milk monitoring to measure Michigan's contamination with polybrominated biphenyls. *Lancet* 2:643, 1978.

180. Savage EP: National study to determine levels of chlorinated hydrocarbon insecticides in human milk: 1975–1976 and supplementory report to the national milk study: 1975–1976. A National Technical Information Service, Richmond, Virginia, 1977.

181. Greene HJ, et al: Excretion of penicillin in human milk following parturition. *Am J Obstet Gynecol* 51:732, 1946.

182. Rozansky R, Brezezinsky A: The excretion of penicillin in human milk. *J Lab Clin Med* 34:497, 1949.

183. Wagner JG: *Biopharmaceutics and Relevant Pharmacokinetics.* Hamilton, Ill.: Drug Intelligence Publications, 1971, pp 392–394.

184. Eckstein HB, Jack B: Breast feeding and anticoagulant therapy. *Lancet* 1:672, 1970.

185. Goguel M, et al: Thérapeutique anticoagulante de allaitement-étude du passage de la phényl-2-dioxo, 1,3-indane dans le lait maternel. *Rev Fr Gynecol Obstet* 65:409, 1970.

186. Tyson RM, et al: Drugs transmitted through breast milk; II. Barbiturates. *J Pediatr* 14:86, 1938.

187. Fantus B, Dyniewicz JM: Phenolphthalein administration to nursing women. *Am J Dig Dis Nutr* 3:184, 1936.

188. Leuxner E, Pulver R: Verabreichrung von Irgapyrin bei Schwangeren und Wochnerinnen. *Munch Med Wochenschr* 98:84, 1956.

189. Strobel S, Leuxner E: On the advisability of administering butazolidin to pregnant and post partum patients. *Med Klin* 39:1708, 1957.

190. Finch E, Lorber J: Methemoglobinemia in the newborn probably due to phenytoin excreted in human milk. *J Obstet Gynaecol Br Emp* 61:833, 1954.

191. Svensmark E, et al: 5,5-Diphenylhydantoin (Dilantin^R) blood levels after oral or intravenous dosage in man. *Acta Pharmacol Toxicol* 16:331, 1960.

192. Rane A, et al: Plasma disappearance of transplacentally transferred diphenylhydantoin in th newborn studied by mass fragmentography. *Clin Pharmacol Therap* 15:39, 1974.

193. *Report of the Committee on Infectious Diseases,* ed 17. Evanston, Ill.: American Academy of Pediatrics, 1974, pp 54–55.

194. Warren RJ, et al: The relationship of maternal antibody, breast feeding and age to the susceptibility of newborn infants to infection with attenuated polioviruses. *Pediatrics* 34:4, 1964.

195. Katz M, Patkin SA: Oral polio immunization of the newborn infant; a possible method for overcoming interference by ingested antibodies. *J Pediatr* 73:267, 1968.

196. Deforest A, et al: The effect of breast feeding on the antibody response of infants to trivalent oral poliovirus vaccine. *J Pediatr* 83:93, 1973.

197. John RJ, et al: Effect of breast feeding on seroresponse of infants to oral poliovirus vaccination. *Pediatrics* 57:47, 1976.

198. McKenzie SA, et al: Secretion of prednisolone into breast milk. *Arch Dis Child* 50:894, 1975.

199. Katz FH, Duncan BR: Entry of prednisone into human milk (letter). *N Engl J Med* 293:1154, 1975.

200. Arias IM, et al: Prolonged neonatal unconjugated hyperbilirubinemia associated with breast feeding and a steroid, pregnane-3(alpha),20(beta)-diol, in maternal milk that inhibits glucuronide formation in vitro. *J Clin Invest* 43:2037, 1964.

201. Arias IM, Gartner LM: Jaundice in breast-fed neonates. *JAMA* 218:746, 1971.

202. Foliot A, et al: Breast milk jaundice-in vitro inhibition of rat liver bilirubin-uridine diphosphate glucuronyltransperase activity and Z porotein-bromosulfophthalein binding by human breast milk. *Pediatr Res* 10:594, 1976.

203. Levitan AA, Manion JC: Propranolol therapy during pregnancy and lactation. *Am J Cardiol* 32:247, 1973.

204. Anderson PO, Salter FJ: Propranolol therapy during pregnancy and lactation. *Am J Cardiol* 37:325, 1976.

205. Karlberg B, et al: Excretion of Propranolol in human breast milk. *Acta Pharmacol Toxicol* 34:222, 1974.

206. Clyde DF, et al: Transfer of pyramethamine in human milk. *J Trop Med Hyg* 59:277, 1956.

207. Clyde DF: Prolonged malaria prophylaxis through pyramethamine in mother's milk. *E Afr Med J* 37:659, 1960.

208. Gensichen E, Klingmüller V: The pattern of concentration of phenylbutazine and isopyrin in serum, umbilical cord serum, and womens' milk. *Arch Exp Pathol* 246:52, 1963.

209. Foukas MD: An antilactogenic effect of pyridoxine. *J Obstet Gynaecol Br Commonw* 80:718, 1973.

210. Macdonald HN, et al: The failure of pyridoxine

in suppression of puerperal lactation. *Br J Obstet Gynaecol* 85:54, 1976.

211. Janeway CA, Diamond LK (Co-Chairmen): Seventh M. R. Pediatric Research Conference: Erythroblastosis Fetalis, 1954, p 55.
212. Farquhar JD: Follow-up on rubella vaccinations and experience with subclinical reinfection. *J Pediatr* 81:460, 1972.
213. Werthmann MW, Krees SV: Quantitative excretion of Senokot in human breast milk. *Med Ann DC* 42:4, 1973.
214. Pommerenke WT, Hahn PF: Secretion of radioactive sodium in human milk. *Proc Soc Exp Biol Med* 52:223, 1943.
215. Phelps DL, Karim A: Spironolactone; relationship between concentration of dethioacetylated metabolite in human serum and milk. *J Pharm Sci* 66:1203, 1977.
216. Jarvis AA, et al: Strontium-89 and strontium-90 levels in breast milk and in mineral supplement preparations. *Can Med Assoc J* 88:136, 1963.
217. Straub CP, Murthy GK: A comparison of Sr^{90} component of human and cows' milk. *Pediatrics* 36:732, 1965.
218. Sparr RA, Pritchard JA: Maternal and newborn distribution of sulfamethoxypyridazine ($Kynex^R$). *Obstet Gynecol* 12:131, 1958.
219. Harley JD, Robin H: "Late" neonatal jaundice following maternal treatment with sulfamethoxypyridazine. *Pediatrics* 37:855, 1966.
220. Adair FL, Hesseltine HC, Hac LR: Experimental study of behavior of sulfanilamide. *JAMA* 111:766, 1938.
221. Hac LR, Adair FL, Hesseltine HC: Excretion of free and acetylsulfanilamide in human breast milk. *Am J Obstet Gynecol* 38:57, 1939.
222. Stewart HL, Pratt JB: Sulfanilamide excretion in human breast milk and effect on breast-fed babies. *JAMA* 111:1456, 1938.
223. Hepburn JS, Paxson NF, Rogers AN: Secretion of ingested sulfanilamide in human milk and in urine of infant. *J Biol Chem* 123:54, 1938.
224. Hawking F, Lawrence JS: *The Sulfonamides.* New York: Grune & Stratton, 1951, pp 95–96.
225. Rieben G, Druey J: Die Ausscheidung der Sulfanilamide insbesondere des Sulfathiazols (Cibazol) durch die Muttermilch und ihre Bedeutung für den Säugling, *Schweiz Med Wochenschr* 72:1376, 1942.
226. Spencer RP, et al: Breast secretion of ^{99m}Tc in the amenorrhea-galactorrhea syndrome. *J Nucl Med* 11:467, 1970.
227. Vagenakis AG, et al: Duration of radioactivity in the milk of a nursing mother following ^{99m}Tc administration. *J Nucl Med* 12:188, 1971.
228. Posner AC, et al: Further observation on the use of tetracycline hydrochloride in prophylaxis and treatment of obstetric infections. *Antibiot Ann* pp 594–598, 1954–1955.
229. Graf VM, Riemann S: Untersuchungen über die Konzentration von Pyrrolidino-Methyl-Tetracyclin in der Müttermilch. *Dtsch Med Wochenschr* 84:1694, 1959.
230. Resman BM, Blumenthal HP, Jusko WJ: Breast milk distribution of theobromine from chocolate. *J Pediatr* 91:477, 1977.

231. Yurchak AM, Jusko WJ: Theophylline secretion into breast milk. *Pediatrics* 57:518, 1976.
232. Fehily L: Human milk intoxication due to B_1 avitaminosis. *Br Med J* 2:590, 1944.
233. Mayo CC, Schlicke CP: Appearance of a barbiturate in human milk. *Proc Staff Meet Mayo Clin* 17:87, 1942.
234. Williams RH, et al: Thiouracil; its absorption, distribution and excretion. *J Clin Invest* 23:613, 1944.
235. Moiel RH, Ryan JR: Tolbutamide (Orinase) in human breast milk. *Clin Pediatr* 8:480, 1967.
236. Anon: Congenital malformations associated with tolbutamide. *J Pediatr* 77:457, 1970.
237. Arnauld R, et al: Étude du passage de la triméthoprime dans le lait maternel. *Ouest Med* 25:959, 1972.
238. Schlesinger JJ, Covelli HD: Evidence for transmission of lymphocyte responses to tuberculin by breast feeding. *Lancet* 2:529, 1977.
239. Collins RA, et al: The folic acid and vitamin B_{12} content of the milk of various species. *J Nutr* 43:313, 1951.
240. Goldbert LD: Transmission of a vitamin-D metabolite in breast milk. *Lancet* 2:1258, 1972.
241. Dyggve HV, et al: Influence on the prothrombin time of breast fed newborn babies of one single dose of vitamin K_1 or Synkavite given to the mother within 2 hours after birth. *Acta Obstet Gynaecol Scand* 35:440, 1956.
242. Baty JD, et al: May mothers taking warfarin breast feed their infants? *Br J Clin Pharmacol* 3:969, 1976.
243. deSwiet M, Lewis PJ: Excretion of anticoagulants in human milk (letter). *N Engl J Med* 297:1471, 1977.
244. Leorme M, Lewis PJ, et al: May mothers given warfarin breast feed their infants. *Br Med J* 1:1564, 1977.
245. Schiffman DO: Evaluation of amikacin sulfate (Amikin)—a new aminoglycoside antibiotic. *JAMA* 41:1547, 1977.
246. Stander HJ: *Williams Obstetrics*, ed 8. New York: Appleton, 1941.
247. Sapeika N: The excretion of drugs in human milk—a review. *J Obstet Gynaecol Br Emp* 54:426, 1947.
248. Mulley BA, Pan GD, Pan WK, et al: Placental transfer of chlorthalidone and its elimination in maternal milk. *Eur J Clin Pharmacol* 13:129, 1978.
249. Somogyi A, Gugler R: Abstract. *Br J Clin Pharmacol* 7:627, 1979.
250. Clayman CB: Evaluation of cimetidine (Tagamet)—an antagonist of hydrochloric acid. *JAMA* 41:1289, 1977.
251. Garrod AE, et al: In Paterson D: *Diseases of Children.* Baltimore: Williams & Wilkins, 1929.
252. Kobyletzki D: The influence on breast fed infants of drugs administered to mothers. *Geburtshilfe Frauenheilkd* 24:606, 1964.
253. Tempro KF, Cirilla VJ, Steelman SL: Diflunisol: a review of pharmacokinetic and pharmacodynamic properties, drug interactions and special tolerability studies in humans. *Br J Clin Pharmacol* 4:31, 1977.

254. Anon: Editorial comparison of anti-inflammatory agents. *Hosp Pharm* 13:178, 1978.
255. Sovner R, Orsulah PJ: Excretion of imipramine and desipramine in human breast milk. *Am J Psychiatry* 136:451; and reply to letter 136:1483, 1979.
256. Lakings DB, Lizarraga C, Haggerty WJ, et al: Human milk. *J Pharm Sci* 68:1113, 1979.
257. Posner C, Konicoff N, et al: Tetracycline in obstetric infections. *Antibiot Ann* pp 345, 1955–1956.
258. Sollmann T: *Manual of Pharmacology*. Philadelphia: W. B. Saunders, 1942.
259. Rieder H: Über de quantitative Ausscheidung von Urotropin in der Frauenmilch. *Monatsschr Kinderheilkd* 11:80, 1912.
260. Campbell AD, Coles FK, Eubanmk LL, et al: Distribution and metabolism of methocarbamal. *J Pharmacol Exp Ther* 311:18, 1961.
261. Jones HMR, Cummings AJ: A study of the transfer of methyldopa to the human fetus and newborn infant. *Br J Clin Pharmacol* 6:432, 1978.
262. Sandstrom B, Regardh CG: Abstract. *Br J Clin Pharmacol* 9:518, 1980.
263. Fritz WL, Paxino J, Gall EP: Rational use of new non-steroidal anti-inflammatory drugs. *Drug Ther* 8:36, 1978.
264. Nilsson S, Nygren KG, Johansson EDB: D-Norgestrol concentration in maternal plasma, milk and child plasma during administration of oral contraceptives to nursing women. *Am J Obstet Gynecol* 129:178, 1977.
265. Murphy BF: Probucol (Lorelco) in treatment of hyperlipemia. *JAMA* 41:2537, 1977.
266. Hill LM, Maikasion GD: The use of quinidine sulphate throughout pregnancy. *Obstet Gynecol* 54:366, 1979.
267. O'Hare MF, Russell CJ, Leahey WJ, et al: Sotalol in the management of hypertension complicating pregnancy (abstract). *Br J Clin Pharmacol* 8:390, 1979.
268. Khan AKA, Truelove SD: Placental and mammary transfer of sulphasalozine. *Br Med J* 2:1553, 1979.
269. Jarnerat G, Into-Malmbery MB: Sulphasalazine treatment during breast feeding. *Scand J Gastroenterol* 14:869, 1979.
270. Bagnell PC, Ellenberger HA: Obstructive jaundice due to a chlorinated hydrocarbon in breast milk. *Can Med Assoc J* 117:1047, 1977.
271. Brogden RN, Pinder RM, Sawyer PR, et al: Tobramycin: a review of its antibacterial and pharmacokinetic properties and therapeutic use. *Drugs* 12:166, 1976.
272. Alexander FW: Sodium valproate and pregnancy. *Arch Dis Child* 54:240. 1979.
273. Dickinson RG, Harland RC, Lyman RK, et al: Transmission of valproic acid across the placenta: half-life of the drug in mother and baby. *J Pediatr* 94:832, 1979.
274. Fomon S: *Infant Nutrition*, ed 2. Philadelphia: W. B. Saunders, 1974, p 79.
275. Vohecky JS, Demers PP, Shapcott D: Western Hemisphere Nutrition Congress VI, Los Angeles, 1980.
276. *Sodium Intake by Infants in the United States*, Committee on Nutrition. Evanston, Ill: American Academy of Pediatrics, 1979.
277. Rudolph AM: *Pediatrics*, ed 7. Norwalk, Conn.: Appleton-Century-Crofts, 1982.
278. Center for Disease Control, Annual Summary, 1980: Reported Morbidity and Mortality in the United States. *Morbidity and Mortality Weekly Report*, 29(54), 1981.
279. Cody CL, et al: Nature and rates of adverse reactions associated with DTP and DT immunizations in infants and children. *Pediatrics* 68:650, 1981.
280. Fulgineti VA: Immunizations: current controversies. *J Pediatr* 101:487, 1982.

CHAPTER 4

Obstetrics and Gynecology

JANNET CARMICHAEL, Pharm.D.

The rational approach to the medical management of common gynecologic problems requires an understanding of the hormones and gonadotropins which regulate the menstrual cycle. The section of this chapter that deals with hormonal birth control will present a rational approach to the selection of oral contraceptive products and the management of patients using these medications. The discussion of mechanical birth control which follows will present alternative methods for contraception.

The other gynecologic complaints and problems that will be considered in this chapter include dysmenorrhea, toxic shock syndrome, endometriosis, the medical management of common forms of vaginitis, pregnancy testing, the menopausal syndrome, and teratogenicty.

HORMONAL BIRTH CONTROL

Paralleling man's search for the liquid that would give eternal youth and the alchemists' endeavor to find a method of turning base metal to gold, there has been a search for an effective oral contraceptive. In fact, considering the tremendous variety of plant materials used, it seems incredible that no natural product for safe and effective oral contraception was found in a period of more than 4000 years.

The use of female sex hormones to prevent development of the female egg was suggested as early as 1940. But it was not until 1956, after the serendipitous discovery of norethynodrel, that field trials were begun on what we now know as birth control pills ("the pill"). In 1960 the U.S. Food and Drug Administration (FDA) first gave approval for the use of the combination pill. There has been much modification and combination of synthetic steroids for contraception since those early days. Today 25 to 50 million women worldwide use oral contraceptive products (1). Despite widespread adverse publicity, the pill remains a safe and acceptable contraceptive method for many women. The popularity of the pill undoubtedly

relates to both its theoretical effectiveness and use effectiveness (Table 4.1). In order to understand the many aspects of hormonal birth control, it is necessary to review the physiology of the menstrual cycle and the development of estrogens and progestins used in contraceptive products.

THE MENSTRUAL CYCLE

The average menstrual cycle (Fig. 4.1) lasts 28 days. Several organ systems are involved in this cycle and must be included in the discussion. First, the changes that occur at the ovaries during this 28-day cycle can be divided into three phases:

The follicular phase occupies about the first 14 days of the cycle. At the beginning of this phase several follicles, each containing an oocyte, began to enlarge in response to pituitary follicle stimulating hormone (FSH). After 5 to 6 days one of the follicles begins to develop more rapidly. The granulosa cells of this follicle multiply and, under the influence of pituitary luteinizing hormone (LH), synthesize estrogens and release them from the ovary at an increasing rate. The estrogens appear to inhibit FSH before midcycle (a negative feedback inhibition system), however, the high level and rate of increase of estrogens stimulates a surge of LH at the end of this phase, which in turn causes final stage growth and rupture of the mature graafian follicle and release of the ovum (ovulation).

The ovulatory phase ordinarily occurs at midcycle, on day 14 or 15. At the time of ovulation the granulosa cells of the follicle begin to secrete progesterone.

The luteal phase follows. Under the influence of LH the ruptured follicle fills with blood and the surrounding theca and granulosa cells proliferate and replace the blood to form the corpus luteum. The cells of this structure produce estrogens and progesterone for the remainder of the cycle unless pregnancy occurs. If pregnancy does not occur during this cycle,

Table 4.1.
Method Effectiveness: Theoretical and Actual Use Rates, Number of Pregnancies during the First Year of Use per 100 Nonsterile Women Initiating Method
(Reprinted with permission from R. A. Hatcher et al.: *Contraceptive Technology, 1980–1981.* New York: Irvington Publishers Inc., 1980 (1).)

Method	Used Correctly and Consistently	Average U.S. Experience Among 100 Women Who Wanted No More Children
	THEORETICAL EFFECTIVENESS	ACTUAL USE EFFECTIVENESS
Abortion	0	0 +
Abstinence	0	?
Hysterectomy	0.0001	0.0001
Tubal Ligation	0.04	0.04
Vasectomy	0.15	0.15 +
Oral Contraceptive (combined)	0.34	4[a]-10[b]
I.M. Long-Acting Progestin	0.25	5-10
Condom + Spermicidal Agent	Less than 1[c]	5
Low Dose Oral Progestin	1-1.5	5-10[b]
IUD	1-3	5[a]
Condom	3	10[a]
Diaphragm (with spermicide)	3	17[a]
Spermicidal Foam	3	22[a]
Spermicidal Suppository	3	20-25
Coitus Interruptus	9	20-25
Fertility Awareness[f] (natural family planning)		
Calendar Only	13	21[a]
BB Temperature Only	7	20
BBT-no intercourse before ovulation	1	—
Cervical mucus only[g]	2	25
Lactation for 12 months[d]	15	40
Chance (sexually active)	90[e]	90[e]
Douche	?	40[a]

[a] Ryder, Norman B., "Contraceptive Failure in the United States," *Family Planning Perspectives* 5:133-142, 1973.

[b] Oral contraceptive failure rates may be far higher than this, if one considers women who become pregnant after discontinuing oral contraceptives, but prior to initiating another method. ORAL CONTRACEPTIVE DISCONTINUATION RATES AS HIGH AS 50-60% in the first year of use are not uncommon in family planning programs.

[c] Data are normally presented as Pearl indices. For conversion to the form used here, the Pearl index was divided by 1300 to give the average monthly failure rate n. The proportion of women who would fail within one year is then 1-(1-n).[13]

[d] Most women supplement breast feedings, significantly decreasing the contraceptive effectiveness of lactation. In Rwanda 50% of non-lactating women were found to conceive by just over 4 months postpartum. It might be noted that in this community sexual intercourse is culturally permitted from about 5 days postpartum on (Bonte, M., and van Balen, H., *J. BioSoc. Sci* 1:97, 1969).

[e] This figure is higher in younger couples having intercourse frequently, lower in women over 35 having intercourse infrequently. For example, MacLeod found that within 6 months 94.6% of wives of men under 25 having intercourse four or more times per week conceived. Only 16.0% of wives of men 35 and over having intercourse less than twice a week conceived (MacLeod, *Fertility and Sterility* 4:10-33, 1953).

[f] *Periodic Abstinence.* Population Report, Series I, Number 1, June 1974. Johns Hopkins University, Population Information Program, Hampton House, 624 North Broadway, Baltimore, MD 21205.

[g] Klaus et al. *Fertility and Sterility* 28:1038-1043, 1977.

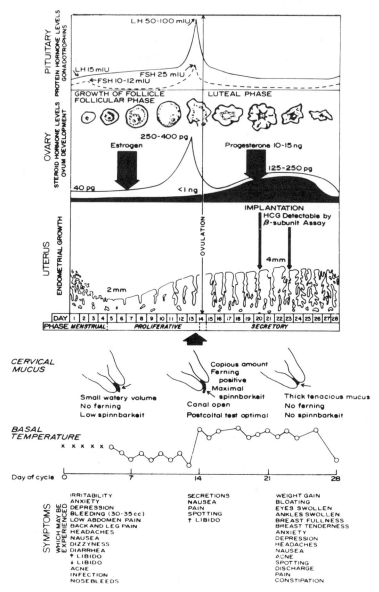

Figure 4.1. Menstrual cycle. (Reproduced with permission from R. A. Hatcher: *Contraceptive Technology, 1980–1981.* New York: Irvington Publisher Inc., 1980 (1).)

the corpus luteum begins to degenerate and ceases hormone production. This drop in serum level of estrogens and progesterone results in endometrial shedding (menstruation) and the beginning of a new cycle. If pregnancy does occur, the corpus luteum remains active because it is stimulated by human chorionic gonadotropin (HCG) derived from the developing placenta, thus maintaining the high levels of progesterone and estrogens necessary for pregnancy.

The changes that occur in the uterus over this 28-day cycle can also be divided into three phases:

1. The menstrual phase starts on day 1 of the menstrual cycle with the sloughing of the old endometrium and the onset of vaginal bleeding. This phase lasts 3 to 6 days.
2. The proliferative phase is a period of growth of the endometrial lining lasting from day 6 to day 14. Estrogens from the developing follicles are responsible for this growth as well as for the growth of

uterine glands and the proliferation of uterine vessels.

3. The secretory phase is primarily under the influence of progesterone. During this phase, the endometrium becomes thicker and is held in place, the uterine glands branch, and the secretory function of these glands begins. The endometrium would be prepared for implantation if pregnancy occurred.

THE ESTROGENS

The major natural estrogens produced by women are estradiol, estrone and estriol. Estradiol is the major secretory product of the ovary. Some estrone is also produced although most of it (and estriol) is formed in the liver from estradiol or converted in the peripheral tissues.

Several synthetic estrogens have been manufactured. Compared to natural estrogens, synthetic estrogens have increased biopotency when administered orally. Only two synthetic estrogens are used in all of the various oral contraceptives on the U.S. market—ethinyl estradiol and mestranol. Ethinyl estradiol is estradiol with an ethinyl group at the 17α position. Mestranol, in addition, has a methyl group at the 3α position (Fig. 4.2).

Ethinyl estradiol is 1.7 to 2 times as potent as mestranol (2, 3). Mestranol is metabolized in the liver to ethinyl estradiol. The amount

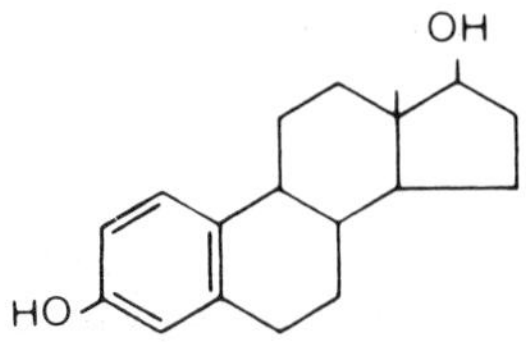

ESTRADIOL

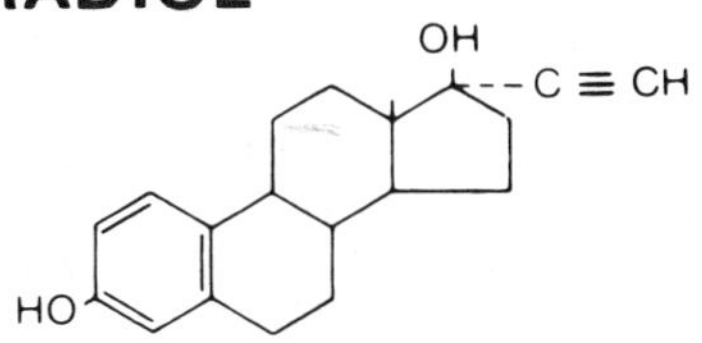

ETHINYL ESTRADIOL

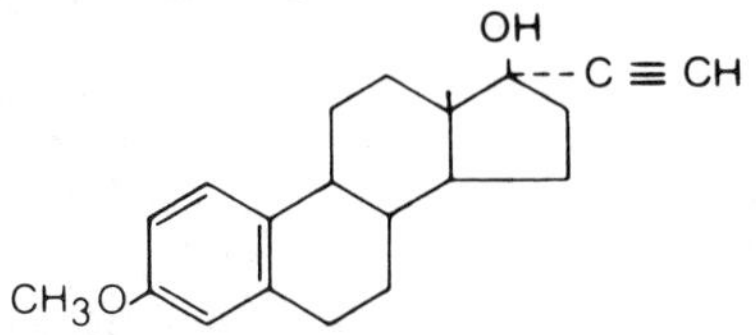

MESTRANOL

Figure 4.2.   Structures of estrogens.

and extent of this metabolism may vary from patient to patient.

THE PROGESTINS

Progesterone is the most important progestin and also serves as a precursor to the estrogens, androgens and adrenocortical steroids. Progesterone is rapidly absorbed following parenteral administration but is poorly absorbed when given orally. Its half-life in the plasma is from 3 to 90 min (4). As is the case with estrogens, it is partially stored in body fat and is almost completely metabolized in one passage through the liver. To overcome these problems, synthetic progestins were developed for use in oral contraceptives.

The five synthetic progestins available in U.S. oral contraceptives are 19-norandrogens derived from testosterone (Fig. 4.3). These agents have different progestational biopotency even though they possess equivalent biologic effects on pituitary LH production and on the cervix and the uterus (Table 4.2). Some progestins with a lower total weight of steroids are actually more potent than other compounds containing a greater amount of less active steroids.

In addition, there are considerations other than the progestational activity when selecting a progestin. Some progestins are metabolized to estrogens or possess estrogenic effects and some progestins exhibit antiestrogenic action and some exhibit androgenicity (Table 4.2). Of the two tests that are used to represent progestational potency, the subnuclear vacuolization test is influenced very little by the estrogenic and androgenic action of the progestogen and therefore correlates most closely with progestational potency observed clinically.

THE "PILL"

Three basic types of preparations have been developed for use as oral contraceptives: (a) combination pill, (b) sequential pill, and (c) mini pill. The combination pill contains a fixed ratio of estrogen and progestin given daily for 21 days beginning on day 5 of the menstrual cycle. Menstrual bleeding usually begins 1 to 4 days after cessation of the medication. The patient then resumes the same dosage exactly 7 days after the last "pill." "Twenty-eight day pills" have placebo tablets to mark these 7 days for the patient.

The combination pill is effective for several of the following reasons. 1) ovulation is in-

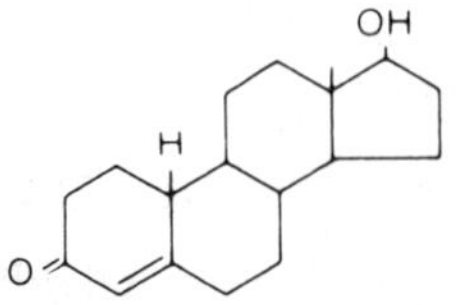

19 NORTESTOSTERONE

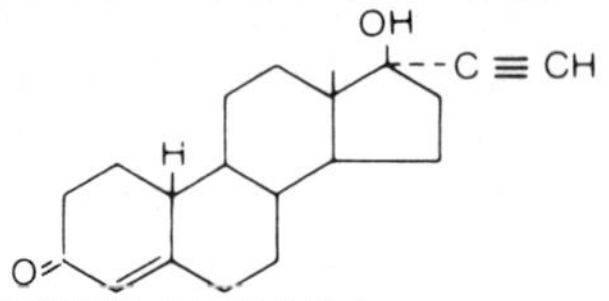

NORETHINDRONE

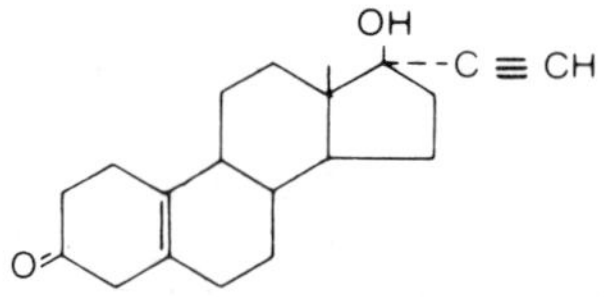

NORETHYNODREL

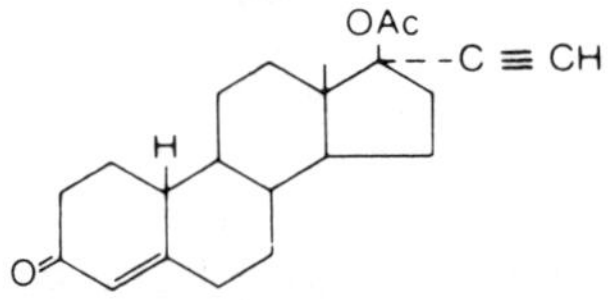

NORETHINDRONE ACETATE

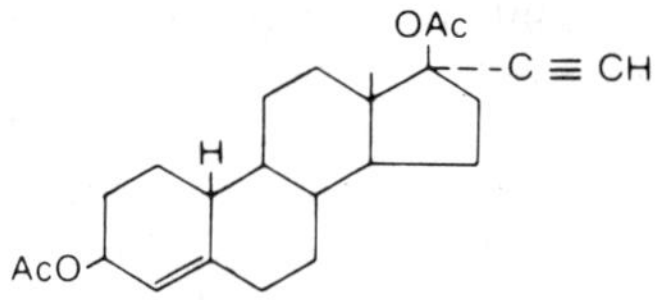

ETHYNODIOL DIACETATE

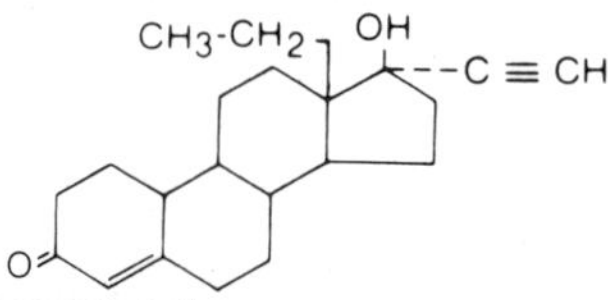

NORGESTREL

Figure 4.3. Structures of progestins.

hibited by the negative feedback inhibition that estrogens have on the hypothalamus and the subsequent suppression of FSH and LH production. Progestogens in sufficient doses also possess the ability to inhibit ovulation through suppression of the preovulatory LH surge. Without FSH and LH the ovarian follicle fails to grow and ovulation does not occur. The success of combination products to inhibit ovulation is a synergistic action of estrogen and progestogen at the level of the hypothalamus. Nevertheless, in combination products containing 50 μg or less of estrogen ovulation is probably suppressed only 95 to 98% of the time (1). The 99+% efficacy of these agents then must be attributed to the progestin. Progestins alone may inhibit ovulation due to a subtle alteration in hypothalamic-pituitary-ovarian function and the midcycle changes of FSH and LH. Additional nonovulatory mechanisms may also add to the pill's effectiveness; 2) progestins cause a thick, tenacious cervical mucus that is very resistant to sperm migration and reduces sperm survival; 3) progestins alter fallopian tube secretions, thereby indirectly affecting the motility of the ovum and sperm; and 4) an atrophic endometrium often results from this dose of progestins. Implantation of the blastocyst is not satisfactory in an atrophic endometrium. All these effects combine to make the combination pill the most popular and effective oral contraceptive on the market.

In an attempt to document the contraceptive effect of estrogen alone, the sequential agent was developed. Estrogen was given alone for 15 days beginning on day 5. Estrogen and progestin were then given together daily for the following 5 to 6 days. The purpose of the estrogen was to inhibit ovulation while the progestin was added at the end of the cycle to produce a more physiologic endometrium and normalize menstruation. The intent of this dosage regimen was to mimic the normal physiologic hormonal condition in the female.

For several reasons, the sequential products (Oracon, Norquens and Ortho-Novum SQ) were voluntarily withdrawn from the U.S. market in 1976 upon recommendation of the FDA. Because these products relied principally on estrogen for their contraceptive effect, the amount of estrogen per dose was higher than required in the combination pills. Since estrogens are responsible for many of the dangerous side effects of pill use, the sequential products would be expected to produce more side effects than the combination product. In addition, the sequential products had a use efficacy rate somewhat below the combination products, especially if pills were missed. Combination products have the added contraceptive protection of a progestational agent throughout the cycle instead of just at the end. Therefore, sequential products offered no real advantage in most patients, and in fact were potentially harmful for many patients who did as well on a lower dose estrogen product.

The third type of oral contraceptive is the "mini pill." Progestin only is given for 28 days continuously. These pills contain a smaller

Table 4.2.
Progestogen Potency
(Reproduced with permission from R. P. Dickey: *International Journal of Gynaecology and Obstetrics*, 16:547, 1979 (51).

| Compound | Progestational | | Androgenic | Estrogenic | |
	Delay of Menses	Subnuclear Vacuolization	Ventral Prostate	Vagina Epithelium[a]	Antiestrogenic
Norgestrel	1.000	1.00	7.6	0.00	18.5
Ethynodiol diacetate	0.500	0.53	1.0	0.86	1.0
Norethindrone acetate	0.067	0.45	2.5	0.38	25.0
Norethindrone	0.050	0.38	1.6	0.25	2.5
Norethynodrel	0.036	0.13	0.0	2.08	0.0

[a] *Ethinyl estradiol = 100%.*

amount of progestin than most combination pills and no estrogen (Table 4.3). Although ovulation may be inhibited in some women, approximately 40% of women will ovulate consistently, 40% will have anovulatory cycles and the other 20% will sporadically ovulate (1). The aforementioned progestin effects contribute to the mini pill's effectiveness. It is less effective than combination oral contraceptive products, especially if one or more tablets are missed. The mini pill, however, may be a good choice in lactating women or patients who are unable to take estrogens. Estrogen related side effects which may indicate a switch to mini pills include hypertension, chloasma, cyclic weight gain, nausea, and headache.

ORAL CONTRACEPTIVE AND CARDIOVASCULAR DISEASE

Hypertension, impaired glucose tolerance, and hyperlipidemia are the three major atherogenic risk factors believed to influence the occurrence of cadiovascular disease (CVD) (5). Oral contraceptives worsen these risk factors to some degree in almost all women and become significant in women with underlying disease or those who have specific susceptibility. Although laboratory values may remain within normal limits, the whole distribution of these risk factors is shifted upward. The implication of these risk factors will now be examined.

Hypertension

There seems to be no doubt that estrogen-progestogen combination oral contraceptives induce a small rise in blood pressure in most patients (6, 7). This rise in blood pressure is noted to occur in previously normotensive women and to aggravate existing hypertension. The average increase noted varies with age, becoming substantial in women about 35 or older. The time of onset and extent of increase varies between individuals. The hypertensive effect may increase with duration of oral contraceptive use (8). It has been estimated that 5% of oral contraceptive users will develop frank hypertension within 5 years. This is an incidence 3 to 6 times greater than in nonusers (9, 10). In addition to producing overt hypertension in some women, oral contraceptives elevate pressure to some extent in almost all women (11) (on the average 1 mmHg diastolic, 5 mmHg systolic). Emphasis, however, should be placed on women 35 or older, smokers, and those with a history of hypertension.

The mechanism of oral contraceptive associated hypertension may involve volume and vasoconstrictive effects of estrogen induced increases in renin (12, 13). Peripheral resistance is elevated through renin substrate activation of plasma angiotensin II levels. Most researchers report that these changes are not related to progestogens, but rather to the estrogen component of oral contraceptives. However, a direct relationship between the amount of norethindrone acetate in oral contraceptives and hypertension has been reported (14). In addition, it must be kept in mind some progesterones are converted to estrogen.

Hypertension associated with birth control pills is reversible. After discontinuing oral contraceptives, a return to normal blood pressure

Table 4.3.
Potency of Oral Contraceptives (A = Estrogen Only, B = Estrogen and Progestogen); * = Estimated, NA = Not Available)[a]
(Reproduced with permission from R. P. Dickey: *International Journal of Gynaecology and Obstetrics*, 16:547, 1979 (51).)

Name	Estrogenic Potency[b]		Progestational Potency[c]	Androgenic Potency[d]	Breakthrough Bleeding and Spotting[e]
	A	B			
Therapeutic indication only					
Enovid 10	100	438	0.94	0.00	4.0
Enovid 5	50	240	0.48	0.00	7.4
Norinyl/Ortho-Novum 10	40	NA	3.71	3.35	3.8
Ortho-Novum 5	50	76	1.90	1.67	3.0
Contraceptive-combination (more than 50 μg of estrogen)					
Enovid E (21)	67	80	0.25	0.00	10.9
Ortho-Novum 0.5	67	68	0.53	0.21	7.7
Ovulen (21)	67	46	0.74	0.67	6.1
Ovulen 0.5	53	42	0.38	0.34	4.8
Norinyl/Ortho-Novum 2	67	64	0.26	0.10	28.8
Norinyl/Ortho-Novum 1/80	67	77	0.19	0.17	7.2
Contraceptive-combination, (50 μg of estrogen)					
Ovcon 50	50	50*	0.38	0.34	11.9
Ovral	50	42	0.50	0.80	4.5
Norlestrin 1/50	50	39	0.44	0.52	13.6
Norinyl/Ortho-Novum 1/50	37	32	0.38	0.34	10.6
Demulen	50	26	0.53	0.21	13.4
Norlestrin 2.5	50	16	1.02	1.25	5.1
Contraceptive-combination (less than 50 μg of estrogen)					
Brevicon/Modicon	35	42	0.19	0.17	14.6
Ovcon 35	35	40*	0.15	0.14	19.0
Lo-Ovral	30	25	0.30	0.48	9.8
Loestrin 1.5/30	30	14	0.65	0.79	25.2
Loestrin 1/20	20	13	0.44	0.52	30.9
Contraceptive-progestogen only					
Nor Q.D./Micronor	0	6	0.80	0.16	42.3
Ovrette	0	0	0.10	0.16	34.9

[a] Pills and manufacturers (in parentheses) include the following: Ovcon 35 and 50 (Mead Johnson Laboratories, Evansville, IN, USA); Micronor, Modicon, Ortho-Novum 0.5, 1/50, 1/80, 2, 5 and 10 (Ortho Pharmaceutical Corp, Raritan, NJ, USA); Loestrin 1.5/30 and 1/20, Norlestrin 2.5 and 1/50 (Parke, Davis & Co, Detroit, MI, USA); Demulen, Enovid E (21) 5 and 10, Ovulen (21) and 0.5 (Searle Laboratories, Chicago, IL, USA); Brevicon, Norinyl 1/50, 1/80, 2 and 10, Nor Q.D. (Syntex Laboratories, Inc, Palo Alto, CA, USA); and Lo-Ovral, Ovral, Ovrette (Wyeth International, Philadelphia, PA, USA).

[b] Micrograms of ethinyl estradiol equivalents per day.

[c] Milligrams of norgestrel equivalents per day.

[d] Milligrams of methyl testosterone equivalents per 28 days.

[e] Information submitted to the FDA by the manufacturer on incidence in third cycle of pill use. These rates are derived from separate studies conducted by different investigators in several population groups and therefore a precise comparison cannot be made.

may take from 3 to 4 months. The patients blood pressure should be monitored at the initiation of oral contraceptive therapy and periodically thereafter. If a large rise in blood pressure is detected, oral contraceptives should be discontinued.

Lipid Metabolism

Although lipid levels generally remain within usual limits, all estrogen-containing oral contraceptives appear to stimulate a significant increase in fasting serum triglyceride levels, very low density lipoproteins (VLDL) and low density lipoproteins (LDL) (15). Very rarely, hyperlipidemic crisis with pancreatitis has been reported (16). Hepatic lipolytic activity (clearance of lipids) is significantly depressed by estrogens but not by progestogens. Indeed high levels of progestogens alone tend to increase the rate of clearance of triglycerides from the plasma (17).

Low levels of serum high density lipoprotein (HDL) cholesterol are a major risk factor for CVD (a decrease in HDL appears to accelerate atherogenesis). The estrogen component has been found to increase the HDL cholesterol, and the progestogen decreases it (18). The net effect of oral contraceptives on lipoprotein levels then, depends on their specific content. Those combination preparations which contain progestins which are strongly antiestrogenic (i.e., norethindrone acetate and norgestrel) decrease HDL cholesterol perhaps by overpowering the estrogen effects (18).

Little is known about the long-term effects estrogen will have by increasing VLDL, LDL and triglycerides. However, even a small decrease in HDL has been shown to contribute to CVD. This affect of the progestins needs further study.

Carbohydrate Metabolism

Women taking combination oral contraceptives show a mild worsening in glucose tolerance curves (an average serum glucose increase in 11 mg/dl in 1 hour). Many women have shown elevations in plasma insulin responses to glucose and worsening of prediabetic type responses. It would appear that these changes are due to a complex synergy between the progestin and estrogenic components of oral contraceptives (19). The mechanism of these changes are uncertain. However, one possibility is a relative deficiency of vitamin B_6 (pyridoxine), which disturbs tryptophan catabolism and leads to the accumulation of diabetogenic agents. This is substantiated by the finding that some women who develop abnormal glucose tolerance tests while taking oral contraceptives are found to revert to normal when given pyridoxine supplements (20). This, however, represents only one possibility and can not explain all cases.

Although the above effects of oral contraceptives on blood pressure carbohydrates and lipid metabolism may appear minor from a clinical standpoint, from an epidemiologic viewpoint, this combination of atherogenic traits has obvious implications. A direct link between altered metabolism and increased mortality and morbidity are largely hypothetical. Circumstantial evidence is strong, however, that these factors may explain the pathologenesis of myocardial infarction and stroke attributed to the long-term past use of oral contraceptive preparations.

Myocardial Infarction and Stroke

It has been shown that oral contraceptives increase the risk of myocardial infarction (MI) and stroke. The risks seem to increase substantially with age, and the presence of such risk factors as cigarette smoking or hypertension (21, 22). Overall, oral contraceptives have been found to multiply the effects of age and other risk factors for MI and stroke, rather than just add to them (22).

Several findings have been identified in recent case controlled studies. First, the risk from MI in an age group 25 to 49 is approximately 3 to 4 times greater than among comparable women who never used oral contraceptives. Second, the risk for short-term users (less than 5 years) after stopping oral contraceptives does not increase. A third new finding indicates that risk among long-term users, (5 years or more) ages 40 to 49, is about 2 times greater than comparable women who never used oral contaceptives. Further, these effects persist for up to 10 years after oral contraceptives have been discontinued (23).

Several studies have shown the risk of thrombotic stroke to be increased among current users of oral contraceptives, but not among past users (22, 24). However, two studies have found the risk of stroke to be increased among both current and past users (25, 26). These findings are based on a small number of cases, the majority of which occurred in women 35 or older. Therefore, the risk of stroke is probably increased in both current and past users of oral contraceptives, but this increase in risk largely applies to women 35 years of age or older.

Although conclusive evidence is lacking, among current users the risk of MI and stroke appears to be directly related to both the progestin and estrogen content of oral contraceptives. This is evidenced by the fact that if you compare old (1970) data with more recent

(1980) data, one sees a decrease in estrogen content of oral contraceptives accompanied by a decrease in the risk of MI and stroke (27). Further, it has been observed that the risk of MI or stroke appears to be 1.5 to 2 times greater among women using the pill with a fixed dose of estrogen and either 3 to 4 mg norethindrone acetate or 1 to 2 mg norethindrone acetate (28).

In addition to the effects of age discussed earlier, other factors appear to effect the risk of MI and stroke associated with oral contraceptive use. Major factors which have been identified to multiply these effects include cigarette smoking (especially 15 or more cigarettes per day), diabetes mellitus, hypertension or history of preeclamptic toxemia, and type II hyperlipidproteinemia. Because cigarette smoking is far more prevalent among women of reproductive age than any of these other risk factors, it becomes by far the most important. In fact, the risk of MI that is attributed to oral contraceptives increases from about 4 cases per 100,000 current users per year among women 30 to 39 years of age who do not smoke cigarettes heavily, to 185 cases per 100,000 current users per year among women 40 to 44 who smoke heavily (29).

The pathogenesis of MI and stroke attributable to oral contraceptives appears to involve two components. The first is the effect of past use that is directly related to the duration of use and persists when oral contraceptives are discontinued. The second effect is that which is unrelated to duration of use and disappears when oral contraceptives are discontinued. The pathogenesis of the first component (long-term past use) has not been well investigated. Circumstantial evidence is strong, however, that the pathogenesis may be related to the atherogenic components discussed earlier (i.e., hypertension, hyperlipidemia, glucose tolerance). The risk associated with current oral contraceptive use is most likely related to the thromboembolic phenomenon associated with oral contraceptive use to be discussed next.

Venous Thromboembolic Disease

Combination oral contraceptives have been found to increase the risks of venous thromboembolic disease during the first month of oral contraceptive use (24). Although continuous data beyond 3 years are not available this effect remains constant regardless of the duration of use and after discontinuation of therapy this risk seems to decline within 1 month to the level found among women who have never used the drug (30).

The most reliable source of information regarding the magnitude of risks for overt venous thromboembolic disease comes from two British cohort studies, that were started in 1968 (31, 32). The relative risk of thromboembolic disease in current users compared to nonusers was found to be approximately 3 times for ideopathic superficial venous thrombosis, in the range of 4 to 11 times for deep vein thrombosis or pulmonary embolism, and the range of 1.5 to 6 times for venous thrombosis or pulmonary embolism in women with conditions that predispose to the development of thromboembolic disease.

Although oral contraceptives have been shown to increase the risk of death from thromboembolic disease, this effect is very rare. During over 450,000 women years of follow-up, these studies observed only 5 fatalities from venous thromboembolic disease.

It is the estrogen component that has been found to increase this risk of thromboembolic disease. Further, this effect appears to be dose related, as evidenced by a drop of one-half to two-thirds fatal or nonfatal pulmonary embolism when the dose of mestranol or ethinyl estradiol was reduced from 100 to 150 μg to 50 to 80 μg per tablet (27).

Oral contraceptives appear to cause structural and histochemical vascular changes in veins and arteries (33). A large number of changes in the process of blood coagulation have been noted, including an increase in platelet stickiness, possible elevation of platelet count, a rise in prothrombin and an increase in factors 7, 8, 9 and 10 (34, 35).

Antithrombin III, an enzyme that inactivates thrombin, has been found to be nearly normal in women using oral contraceptives. However, antithrombin III *activity* has been found to be substantially decreased (36). In addition, oral contraceptives containing 75 to 150 mg of mestranol or ethinyl estradiol, appeared to decrease antithrombin III activity to a greater extent than do oral contraceptives containing only 50 mg (37).

Antithrombin III levels have been shown to be lower in nonuser women of blood type A, B and AB (especially type A) than in women of blood type O (38). This may account for the increase in risk from idiopathic deep venous thromboembolic disease among users and non-oral contraceptive users of blood type A, B or AB (39).

TUMORIGENIC ASPECTS

Because the normal breast is hormone dependent, it should come as no surprise that women who use oral contraceptive tablets may develop some mammary abnormalities. The relationship between the consumption of oral contraceptives and the development of breast disease is by no means a simple one. Oral contraceptives have been known to reduce two common benign forms of breast disease, fibroadenoma and fibrocystic disease.

To date there is no study that directly relates the pill to breast cancer, nor is there evidence that the incidence in breast carcinoma increases with oral contraceptive use. However, certain existing breast cancers may be worsened by the estrogen in oral contraceptive preparations. In spite of widespread oral contraceptive use and extensive observation, no increased incidence of cancer has been observed.

Hepatomas may occur in women taking oral contraceptives. A wide array of different types of benign liver tumors have been reported, the most common of which are focal nodular hyperplasia and liver cell adenomas. In comparing pre- and post-contraceptive use cases of focal nodular hyperplasia, it was revealed that there was little or no change with respect to incidence, age, range, location, and microscopic features of the lesion (40). One important difference, however, was noted. Before oral contraceptives, no serious hemorrhages had been reported. Since the introduction of oral contraceptives, this tumor is sometimes fatal with death usually due to sudden hepatic rupture and hemorrhage.

There has been an increase, however, in the incidence of a formerly rare liver cell adenoma. Numerous cases of this adenoma, which were rarely reported before 1960, have now been reported.

It is generally agreed that the risk of developing a hepatoma is equally shared with the use of products containing mestranol and ethinyl estradiol. Increased clinician and patient awareness of the possibility of this tumor in women with a long history of oral contraceptive use, and careful palpitation of the the abdomen to detect small masses should be a part of oral contraceptive user evaluation.

BREAKTHROUGH BLEEDING

Spotting or midcycle bleeding is a common occurrence among pill users. Patients may expect some degree of breakthrough bleeding the first several months of contraceptive use until the body becomes accustomed to the synthetic hormones. If spotting continues after 3 months of use, the dose of estrogen or progestogen may need to be adjusted. One rule of thumb indicates that if spotting occurs before midcycle, the estrogen component should be increased. If spotting occurs after midcycle, the progestogen potency should be increased. Clearly this recommendation should be evaluated, keeping in mind the hormone potency of the product the patient is now taking.

GALLBLADDER DISEASE

Use of oral contraceptives increases the incidence of gallstones and cholecystitis by at least 2-fold (8). Estrogens alter the composition of the bile. It has been suggested that a rise in cholesterol saturation of gallbladder bile may account for the greater increase in gallbladder disease (41).

DEPRESSION

The incidence of depression among oral contraceptive users is approximately 5 to 6%. The symptoms noted include lethargy, loss of libido, irritability and crying. Because of the subjective nature of depression, much controversy exists as to the etiology. Proponents of a biochemical theory offer evidence that brain amine metabolism is altered as a result of an abnormal tryptophan metabolism. An increased requirement of vitamin B_6 (pyridoxine), an agent which is a cofactor in the metabolism of the amino acid tryptophan to serotonin, has been postulated. In one double-blind crossover study, daily adminstration of vitamin B_6 to pyridoxine-deficient oral contraceptive users was found to relieve the symptoms of depression (42).

DRUG INTERACTIONS

In the last several years, reports of pregnancies which have occurred when oral contraceptives were taken concurrently with other drugs have appeared. It has been shown that there is an increase in plasma clearance of estrogen directly attributable to the enzyme-inducing properties of rifampin (43). This enhanced metabolism is clearly a major contributory factor to contraceptive failure in patients on rifampin. If rifampin therapy is necessary another form of birth control is advised.

Reported pregnancies and patients who experienced breakthrough bleeding have been reported for patients taking oral contraceptives and ampicillin. It appears that ampicillin may eliminate gut microflora which is necessary for enterohepatic circulation of steroid (44). This ultimately will reduce the amount of steroid available for contraception. There is reason to believe that other antibiotics may also cause problems when taken concurrently with oral contraceptives. Case reports of pregnancy attributable to the interaction between tetracycline and oral contraceptives have also been reported (45). If these antibiotics are prescribed for oral contraceptive users, especially during days 1 to 14, barrier contraception should be added for the remainder of the cycle.

OTHER SIDE EFFECTS

Tests which monitor thyroid function may be affected by oral contraceptives. It should be noted that thyroid function is not changed— merely the laboratory tests used to measure thyroid function. Estrogens increase the thyroid binding globulin, therefore tests which are used to measure thyroid function such as protein-bound iodine, T_4 by column and T_4 by Murphy Pattee test will be elevated, and T_3 resin uptake will be decreased (see Chapter 26, "Thyroid and Parathyroid Disorders"). These laboratory values will return to normal 2 to 4 weeks after the discontinuation of oral contraceptives.

Nausea and vomiting appears to be related to the estrogen dose of oral contraceptives. It is a common side effect and may decrease with continued use. Pharmacokinetic data suggest that the majority of estrogen is absorbed within 2 hours after oral administration. It would be wise to repeat the dose if vomiting occurs during the absorption period. Management of pill-associated nausea includes (a) use of low dose estrogen-containing oral contraceptives, (b) reassurance if temporary nausea can be tolerated, and (c) taking the pill at bedtime so the patient will be asleep during peak concentrations.

Weight gain with oral contraceptives has been divided into two categories: (a) persistent weight gain and (b) cyclic weight gain. Persistent acyclic weight gain is thought to be secondary to the anabolic testosterone-like pro-

gestogen increase in appetite or decrease in activity. Cyclic weight gain, on the other hand, is thought to be an estrogen-related side effect, secondary to water retention.

An increase in the incidence of headache (both tension and migraine) has been noted to occur as a side effect of oral contraceptive use. Because headaches are common among all women of reproductive age and because of poor literature documentation, it is difficult to determine the etiology of birth control pill-associated headaches. There is evidence that falling estrogen levels may incite the cerebral-vascular system to respond by producing migraine headaches. It has been estimated that one third of the patients with migraine headaches will be worse on oral contraceptives (8); however, some studies have noted an improvement while taking the medication (46). Patients who develop migraine (vascular headaches) while taking oral contraceptives should discontinue the pill (see Chapter 40, "Headache").

There is no evidence that seizure activity in general becomes worse on oral contraceptives. Their use, therefore, is not contraindicated in epileptic patients unless a primary increase in seizure severity or frequency is noted. The drug interaction noted between oral contraceptives and anticonvulsants is much less clear. Breakthrough bleeding and failure on contraceptive therapy have been noted in patients taking anticonvulsant drugs (44). In contrast, it has been proposed that estrogens may inhibit phenytoin metabolism, thus causing phenytoin toxicity (47). Although information is scanty, clinicians should be aware of the possibility of increased seizure activity or anticonvulsant drug toxicity.

Increased corneal sensitivity, particularly contact lens discomfort, has been noted in about 1 of 5 women who take oral contraceptives (48). Changes in corneal curvature and decreased tear secretion have been blamed for this side effect in oral contraceptive users, as well as pregnant patients. A variety of ocular changes have been attributed to the pill, ranging from retinal vascular accidents to decrease in visual acuity and color changes (49). However, repeated prospective and retrospective studies can find no correlation between the use of birth control pills and many of these abnormalities which are found normally in a population of women of reproductive age. However, caution should be exerted in prescribing oral contraceptives to women with known ophthalmologic disorders.

Erythema nodosum, erythema multiforme, urticaria are hypersensitivity reactions that are occasionally seen with oral contraceptive therapy. They are a rare event, occurring in at most 1 in 1000 users. Oral contraceptives should be discontinued at once. This reaction usually is attributed to the progestin component of the pill, and seems to regress when patients are taken off the pill (8).

Oral contraceptives have been associated with rare flare-ups of systemic lupus erythematosus (SLE) (50). However, it is more common to see SLE and antinuclear antibody (ANA) preparations turn positive in patients using oral contraceptive drugs and revert to negative on discontinuation. The significance of this is unknown.

Megaloblastic anemia has been reported in oral contraceptive users for two reasons: (a) a relative folic acid deficiency may exist because of increased binding of folic acid and (b) a rare decrease in serum vitamin B_{12}, another type of megaloblastic anemia. It is likely that oral contraceptives contribute to, but do not produce this anemia in otherwise healthy women. This anemia, however, responds to appropriate replacement therapy.

Fewer women on oral contraceptives have iron deficiency anemia. This probably reflects a decrease in menstrual flow secondary to the use of oral contraceptives, with subsequent raises in serum iron and iron binding capacity.

Other side effects which have been attributed to pill use include acne, chloasma (skin hyperpigmentation), teratogenicity, abnormal hair growth, changes in libido, increased vaginal infections, breast tenderness, galactorrhea, post-pill amenorrhea, photosensitivity, exacerbation of acute intermittent porphyria, exacerbation of Wilson's disease, and ischemic colitis. Some of these side effects have been attributed to a particular component of birth control pills, or lack thereof, and are listed in Table 4.4.

The absolute contraindications for the use of oral contraceptives include:

1. Estrogen dependent neoplasm
2. Impaired liver function or past history of cholestatic jaundice
3. Deep vein thrombosis, pulmonary embolism, stroke or history of thromboembolic disorders
4. Previous myocardial infarction

Table 4.4.
If These Side Effects Occur, Adjust the Estrogen/Progestogen Balance

Estrogen Excess	Progestogen Excess
Nausea, bloating	Increased appetite
Cervical mucorrhea, polyposis	Persistent weight gain
	Tiredness, fatigue
Hypermenorrhea	Hypomenorrhea
Hyperpigmentation	Acne, oily scalp
Uterine or leg cramps	Hair loss
Hypertension	Depression
Migraine headache	Hirsutism
Breast tenderness	Breast regression
Dizziness, vertigo	Changes in libido
Cyclic weight gain	
Fibroid growth	
Cervical eversion	

Estrogen Deficiency	Progestogen Deficiency
Irritability, nervousness	Late breakthrough bleeding
Early and/or midcycle breakthrough bleeding	Amenorrhea
	Hypermenorrhea weight loss
Increased spotting	
Hot flushes	
Hypomenorrhea	
Amenorrhea	
Dyspareunia	

5. Pregnancy
6. Undiagnosed abnormal genital bleeding

The relative contraindications for the use of oral contraceptives include:

1. Diabetes mellitus
2. Hypertension or history during pregnancy
3. Migraine
4. Depression
5. Glaucoma
6. Systemic lupus erythematosus
7. Acute intermittent porphyria
8. Epilepsy
9. Smoking
10. Obesity

THE SELECTION OF AN ORAL CONTRACEPTIVE PRODUCT

When selecting a combination oral contraceptive product for a patient, there are several very important things to keep in mind: (a) select a product with the lowest effective dose of estrogen and progestin. Nearly all patients do well on products containing 50 μg or less of estrogen; (b) select a product with the minimum side effects acceptable to the patient; (c) consider any special problems or concomitant disease states the patient may have and be willing to adjust to minimize these problems; and (d) consider the age of the patient; an effort should be made to discontinue oral contraceptives by age 35 since the incidence of side effects increases greatly after this point. It is important to understand that oral contraceptives play the role of temporary contraception in family planning, to be used for delaying the first birth and spacing children. Once the family is complete surgical sterilization is the safest plan.

In addition to the above criteria, it is important to have an understanding of the relative estrogen and progestogen potencies of oral contraceptive products. These potencies are reflective of the total amount of estrogen and progestogen as well as the effects they have on each other. For example, if the progestogen in a combination product is metabolized to an estrogen the product will be more estrogenic than the total microgram amount of the estrogen would indicate. Likewise, if the progestin is antiestrogenic the product will be less estrogenic than the amount of estrogen would indicate (Table 4.3, column B).

Table 4.5 lists the common products on the U.S. market and their relative estrogenic and progestogenic potencies. Because of the large number of products available, it is important to be able to recommend a more or less potent product when an estrogen or progestogen-related side effect occurs.

As explained earlier, the ovarian and the uterine cycles are superimposed for 28 days to form the menstrual cycle. When estrogens and progestins in the form of oral contraceptive pills are added to this cycle, an attempt is made to alter the ovarian cycle without affecting the

Table 4.5.
Oral Contraceptive Content in Order of Decreasing Estrogen Potency

Trade Name	Progestogen	Estrogen
Enovid 10	Norethynodrel 10 mg	Mestranol 150 μg
Enovid 5	Norethynodrel 5 mg	Mestranol 75 μg
Enovid-E	Norethynodrel 2.5 mg	Mestranol 100 μg
Ortho Novum 2 mg and Norinyl 2 mg	Norethindrone 2 mg	Mestranol 100 μg
Ovulen	Ethynodiol diacetate 1 mg	Mestranol 100 μg
Norlestrin 2.5 mg	Norethindrone acetate 2.5 mg	Ethinyl estradiol 50 μg
Ovcon 50	Norethindrone acetate 1.0 mg	Ethinyl estradiol 50 μg
Norlestrin 1 mg	Norethindrone acetate 1 mg	Ethinyl estradiol 50 μg
Demulen	Ethynodiol diacetate 1 mg	Ethinyl estradiol 50 μg
Ovral	Norgestrel 0.5 mg	Ethinyl estradiol 50 μg
Ortho Novum 1/80 and Norinyl 1 + 80	Norethindrone 1 mg	Mestranol 80 μg
Ortho Novum 1/35	Norethindrone 1 mg	Ethinyl estradiol 35 μg
Ortho Novum 10/11	Norethindrone 0.5 mg	Ethinyl estradiol 35 μg-10 days
	Norethindrone 1 mg	Ethinyl estradiol 35 μg-11 days
Modicone/Brevicon	Norethindrone 0.5 mg	Ethinyl estradiol 35 μg
Ovcon 35	Norethindrone 0.4 mg	Ethinyl estradiol 35 μg
Lo-Ovral	Norgestrel 0.3 mg	Ethinyl estradiol 30 μg
Nordette	1-Norgestrel 0.15 mg	Ethinyl estradiol 30 μg
Loestrin (Fe) 1.5/30	Norethindrone acetate 1.5 mg	Ethinyl estradiol 30 μg
Ortho Novum 1/50 and Norinyl 1 + 50	Norethindrone 1 mg	Mestranol 50 μg
Loestrin (Fe) 1/20	Norethindrone acetate 1 mg	Ethinyl estradiol 20 μg
Micronor and Nor-Q.D.	Norethindrone 0.35 mg	—
Ovrette	Norgestrel 0.075 mg	—

uterine cycle. However, since these synthetic agents are not identical to the naturally produced hormones, some changes from the "normal" are likely to occur, i.e., a decrease in menstrual flow, occasional spotting, or a missed period.

It is important to note that a woman relies on her normal monthly menstrual bleeding as a crucial sign to indicate she is not pregnant. If pregnancy has been ruled out the patient should be reassured if concern is expressed over the above changes.

To properly select a pill for a woman it is helpful to take a menstrual history including amount of menses and menstrual discomfort. Women who have light flow and mild or no cramps, will do very well on low dose pills of estrogen and progestin. Women with average flow and average cramps do well on the intermediate strength pill. On the other hand, women with very heavy flow and severe menstrual cramps require higher progestational-androgen potency pills.

In addition, women who have symptoms indicating small amounts of endogenous estrogens, such as small breasts, scant menses, and midcycle spotting, should be given low estrogen-containing pills. Attempts to override these effects with large amounts of estrogen may result in undesirable side effects (51). Women with excess androgen effects, such as hirsutism, acne and oily skin, are best treated with oral contraceptives containing higher progestational potency, but low androgen potency (Table 4.2).

By using the information acquired from the patient's menstrual history, as well as hormone characteristics of the patient, informed product selection can be accomplished. This, coupled with information known about side effects caused by excessive or deficient estrogen and progestogen potency (Table 4.4), will allow rational product adjustment.

RISK-BENEFIT RATIO

For the first time in history we are taking normal healthy people and giving them a potent medication over a long period of time. It is increasingly important to discuss the risk of this therapy with the patient, especially when the lay press which is read most by women tends to emphasize these risks.

The pharmacist is in an excellent position to discuss these risks with the patient and put them in the proper perspective. Perhaps some perspective can be gained if we compare the risk of taking oral contraceptives with other common risks of mortality (Fig. 4.4).

MISSED PILLS

As a practical matter it is important to know what to tell patients when birth control pills are missed. Certain information should be obtained before any advice is given:

1. What oral contraceptive product is the patient taking?
2. How long has the patient been taking oral contraceptives?
3. On which days of the menstrual cycle were pills missed?
4. How many pills were missed?

As pointed out earlier, ovulation is not always suppressed in products containing 50 µg or less of estrogen. The more estrogen and progestin in a product, the more reliable it will be. It is logical then, that for a patient taking a high dose product, one missed pill would be of less consequence than for a patient taking a low dose pill. In addition, the progestin content of the low dose pill makes a significant contribution to the contraceptive effect and must be present daily.

Modest fluctuation in the levels of FSH and LH among pill users has been observed. This might indicate that follicular development may proceed to a greater extent in some women, resulting in more breakthrough ovulation. Because women who have taken oral contraceptives for a long period of time have ovaries in a semidormant state, they are less likely to experience breakthrough ovulation as a result of a missed pill. On the other hand, women who are short-term oral contraceptive users are more likely to have mature follicles ready for ovulation; they may be more affected by a missed pill or by missing the usual dosing

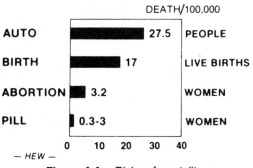

Figure 4.4. Risks of mortality.

time by several hours. Oral contraceptives should be taken at the same time each day.

The first 5 pills of the cycle are the most important for inhibiting ovulation. A high level of hormones early in the cycle is necessary at the level of the hypothalamus for suppression of FSH and LH. Therefore, missing pill number 2, for example, would be more likely to result in a pregnancy than missing pill number 20.

Many clinicians believe that if a patient misses one pill, that missed pill should be taken as soon as it is remembered; the next day's pill should be taken at the regular time (2 pills may be taken at the same time). If 2 consecutive pills are missed, the medication should be doubled for the following 2 consecutive days. Barrier methods of contraception should be started immediately and used the rest of the cycle.

The above information should be evaluated with care. If for example, a patient has been taking a product which contains 80 μg of estrogen for 3 years and missed pill number 18, she probably would not get pregnant. On the other hand, if a patient misses pills 2 and 3 of her 2nd pack of 30-μg pills she is likely to ovulate.

THE MORNING AFTER PILLS

The implantation of the blastocyte is inhibited by high doses of estrogen. Synthetic, natural, and conjugated estrogens have been administered as "morning after" pills. The most frequently used postcoital interceptive agent is diethylstilbestrol (DES), a nonsteroidal synthetic estrogen. It is not recommended for routine use, but rather for cases of rape, incest, or mechanical contraceptive failure near midcycle. The interval between conception and implantation is approximately 6 days. When high risk unprotected intercourse has occurred, it is important to begin estrogen therapy within 72 hours. The dose for DES is 50 mg daily for 5 days. Ethinyl estradiol has been used at doses varying from 2 to 5 mg daily for 5 days. In addition, conjugated estrogens at dosages of 10 mg, administered 3 times daily for 6 days, have also been used with good success. Nausea and vomiting are complications of this high dose estrogen therapy. The patient should experience withdrawal bleeding within 10 days of administration.

Although DES is an effective postcoital contraceptive agent, failures can occur. Cases of vaginal adenosis, vaginal adenocarcinoma and cervical adenocarcinoma in young female offspring of women, who took DES during pregnancy, have been reported. This teratogenic effect of DES appears to occur at the 9th week of pregnancy (52). Thus, no evidence of teratogenicity has been demonstrated in association with the failure of postcoital estrogens. However, abortion should be a first consideration if these agents fail.

THE "SHOT"

Medroxyprogesterone acetate (MPA) has been used in other countries around the world as an injectable contraceptive agent. The drug suppresses the preovulatory surge of LH and thus inhibits ovulation; it also produces the progestin mucus changes and endometrial growth changes discussed earlier.

The dose of MPA is 150 mg IM every 90 days. Women using this form of contraceptive experience very irregular menstrual bleeding patterns; amenorrhea is to be expected 2 to 12 months after beginning use of the medication. The average length of time for return of fertility after discontinuation of this drug is about 8 to 10 months.

The same contraindications exist for MPA as for the "pill" although it is not presently known if thromboembolic disorders increase as a result of MPA use.

MECHANICAL BIRTH CONTROL

The four common mechanical birth control devices are the intrauterine device, diaphragm, condom, and foam. The efficacy of these products in theory and in use can be seen in Table 4.1.

Intrauterine Device

The idea of inserting a foreign body into the uterus to prevent pregnancy is not new. Many years ago natural fibers such as silkworm gut as well as stones and wires containing silver and copper were used as intrauterine contraceptive devices. After World War II, manmade fibers and various types of polythene were available and were molded in many ways as intrauterine devices (IUD) (Fig. 4.5). The copper-containing IUD regained popularity in the 1960s and an IUD which slowly releases progesterone is an innovative development of the 1970s. The mechanism of action of an IUD is still unclear. Ovulation seems to be unim-

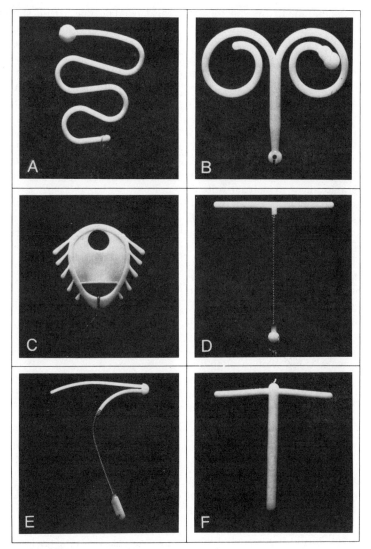

Figure 4.5. Different types of IUDs: (A) Lippes Loop, (B) Saf-T-Coil, (C) Dalkon Shield, (D) Copper T, (E) Cu-7, and (F) Progestasert.

paired in the presence of an IUD. All the postulated mechanisms of action are at the level of the uterus. It is possible any or all of the following mechanisms may be operative.

1. Changes in tubal motility and uterine motility produced by the IUD have been shown in animal studies. The ovum, normally fertilized in the fallopian tube, may be propelled through the genital tract too rapidly for proper implantation to occur. It is questionable whether this effect occurs in humans.

2. The stretching or distortion of the uterus by these devices may have a contracep-

tive effect. However, most of the newer devices have been designed to avoid this distention. It has also been postulated that a mechanical dislodging of the implanted blastocyst may occur.

3. The presence of the device results in the mobilization of polymorphonuclear leukocytes into the endometrium. The local inflammatory responses causes the release of prostaglandins and may increase phagocytic activity against sperms and blastocysts.

4. For devices containing copper it is postulated that interference with enzyme

systems in the endometrium, specifically copper may compete with zinc in the carbonic anhydrase reaction.

Theoretically, the IUD is about 97 to 99% effective. Its use effectiveness is approximately the same since very little compliance is required on the part of the patient.

The only absolute contraindications for the insertion of an IUD in a normal healthy woman are active pelvic infection and pregnancy. However, a number of complications may follow insertion. For instance, there may be an increase in the amount of menstrual flow as well as pain associated with the IUD, particularly for the first several months following IUD insertion. This increased blood loss may cause anemia in some patients. Spotting may also occur. Moreover, all types of IUD may be expelled through the cervix. Obviously the device can be of no value when it is absent. Patients should be taught to check for the IUD string in the vagina to ensure the device is in place. Uterine perforation is most likely to occur at the time of insertion; however, IUDs may gradually work their way through the uterine wall and may need to be removed from the abdominal cavity by use of laparoscopic procedures.

Most serious complications from IUDs are related to infections, including sepsis and in some cases death. IUD use is associated with about a 3-fold increased incidence of developing acute salpingitis (pelvic inflammatory disease, PID) in comparison with users of oral contraceptives and diaphragms. The Dalkon shield has been withdrawn from the market due to several deaths from septic spontaneous abortions. If pregnancy occurs with an IUD in place, there is a 3-fold increased risk of spontaneous abortion with a 10-fold increased risk of ectopic pregnancy (53).

The Diaphragm

The diaphragm ranges in diameter from 55 to 100 mm. It is inserted into the vagina and blocks the opening to the uterus. The diaphragm must be fitted by a clinician for each woman and should be refitted if she delivers a baby, aborts, or gains or loses 10 lb or more.

It was thought that the mechanical barrier of the diaphragm would prevent sperm migration into the uterus; however, it has been shown that the diaphragm moves about during coitus (1). Therefore, its primary mechanism is to hold the spermicidal agent near the cervical os. The diaphragm should not be used without spermicidal jelly or cream. These agents also aid insertion with their lubrication property.

At least a teaspoonful of spermicidal jelly or cream should be spread around the inside of the rim before insertion. It takes 6 to 8 hours for the spermicidal agent to work, therefore, the diaphragm must remain in place at least 8 hours. Another applicatorful of spermicide should be inserted in the vagina leaving the diaphragm in place before each subsequent coitus.

The key to successful diaphragm use is motivation. Many clinicians fail to recognize the diaphragm as a viable contraceptive alternative. However, because of its mechanical action it represents a method of contraception practically devoid of side effects. The diaphragm has come back into vogue over the last several years, and will probably continue to do so, as more and more women of childbearing age become concerned over systemic side effects of other forms of birth control.

The Condom

Condoms are latex rubber that are worn over an erect penis during coitus. This mechanical barrier prevents transmission of the male semen into the vagina. It may also be effective in preventing the transmission of venereal disease from either partner.

Condoms are marketed rolled or unrolled, lubricated or unlubricated, ribbed, or may have reservoir ends to collect the semen. When the condom is put on, one-half inch of empty space should be left at the tip if the condom does not have a reservoir end. A condom should be used only once.

Petroleum jelly should never be used to lubricate a condom (this causes the latex to deteriorate). K-Y jelly, contraceptive foam, or saliva are good lubricants.

Spermicidal Agents

Contraceptive foam is marketed in an aerosol can or bottle with an applicator or as a tablet. The foam is the medium which holds the spermicidal agent against the cervical os. Nonoxynol-9 is the spermicidal agent used in most of these over the counter (OTC) preparations. Two full applicators of foam should be inserted high in the vagina no earlier than 30 min before each ejaculation.

Although contraceptive foam is fairly effective alone, it can be used in conjunction with a diaphragm or condom to produce a very effective method of birth control. Vaginal spermicides marketed to be used with a diaphram are usually less potent, have a different consistency, but the same active ingredient.

If a particular brand of foam is irritating to either partner, the couple should try another brand. Foam is often confused with "feminine hygiene" products. To confuse the issue further, a variety of other insertable spermicides are marketed. There are tablets that are supposed to foam, creams and jellies that are supposed to spread, and suppositories that are supposed to melt; sometimes they do not.

Douching may force sperm in the uterus and is not recommended for at least 8 hours after intercourse when using a diaphragm or foam for contraception.

DYSMENORRHEA

Many women of reproductive age suffer from some degree of primary dysmenorrhea (painful menstruation). Secondary dysmenorrhea, which is due to a definite primary pelvic lesion, may be caused by intrauterine devices, endometriosis, or pelvic adhesions. However, primary dysmenorrhea is thought to be due to an excess of prostaglandins causing uterine hyperactivity (54). Oral contraceptives, by suppression of ovulation, can lower plasma and endometrial prostaglandins and thus prevent symptoms of primary dysmenorrhea. Recently other drugs that inhibit prostaglandin synthesis, such as the nonsteroidal anti-inflammatory agents, have been used as effective treatment for this condition. Ibuprofen, naproxen sodium, mefenamic acid, and indomethacin have been shown to be effective for relief of dysmenorrhea. Other prostaglandin inhibitors, such as fenoprofen, sulindac, and tolmetin sodium have not been studied as extensively for use in dysmenorrhea. Although large comparative trials are lacking, these agents appear to offer an advantage over weaker inhibitors of prostaglandin synthesis, such as aspirin and acetaminophen.

TOXIC SHOCK SYNDROME

Billions of tampons have been produced and used by millions of women throughout the world over the past several decades. In the last several years, a circumstantial relationship has existed between the use of tampons and several disease entities.

The first cases of toxic shock syndrome (TSS) were described in 1978 (55). Since then a wide variety of clinical symptomatology has been described. TSS generally affects previously healthy young women of childbearing age during an otherwise normal menstrual period. It usually begins with a sudden high fever (greater than 102°F) and may be accompanied by severe headache, sore throat, vomiting and diarrhea. Progressive hypotension may be present which may proceed to shock. Palmar erythema is frequent and a diffuse sunburn-like rash has been described. A nonpurulent conjunctivitis is described at the disease onset, and a superficial desquamation of skin on the palms and soles often follows within 2 to 3 weeks of the onset of the disease.

TSS is associated with the use of tampons as well as associated with isolation of coagulase-positive *Staphylococcus aureus* from the vagina or from focal infections of infected patients. The presence of exotoxin of a S. *aureus* infection could certainly account for the number of clinical symptoms identified with this disease. Clinicians should be aware of the possibility of TSS in any menstruating woman with sudden onset of febrile illness. Prompt removal of tampons as well as symptomatic treatment including support of blood pressure may be critical. Use of β-lactimase-resistant penicillins have been shown to lower risk of the recurrence (56). In addition patients with TSS should be instructed to permanently discontinue the use of the tampons.

ENDOMETRIOSIS

It has been estimated that 25% of all women in the third or fourth decade will have endometriosis to some degree. Endometriosis is a disorder which is characterized by the growth of displaced endometrial tissue. This endometrial tissue has been found to proliferate in a variety of unusual sites—ovary, peritoneal cavity, bladder and ureters, appendix, gallbladder, lungs, and elbow. The endometrial plaques respond to fluctuations in estrogen and progesterone levels, similar to normal endometrium.

The site of the disease leads to a wide variety of symptomatology which does not always correlate well with the extent of the disease. Common complaints include infertility, dysmenorrhea, menstrual problems, and pelvic pain. In general, three methods of treatment have been identified for endometriosis (a) surgery, (b) the use of oral contraceptives to induce a "pseudo-pregnancy," and (c) the use of danazol to induce a "pseudo-menopause."

The indications for surgery will not be discussed here. The goal of oral contraceptive therapy is to produce a static endometrium with no cyclic growth and bleeding. The duration of treatment with oral contraceptives is suggested to be 6 months, preferably as long as 12 months. Dosage regiments generally start with 1 oral contraceptive tablet daily, increasing to 1 tablet as needed to prevent breakthrough bleeding (57).

It is unclear whether danazol produces a pseudo-menopause state by acting at the level of the pituitary to inhibit LH and FSH secretion or at the level of the gonads to inhibit estrogen synthesis or both. Although symptoms are relieved earlier, 6 months of danazol therapy is often recommended. Daily dosages of from 200 to 800 mg have been used with good success. Danazol has no progestational or estrogenic effects, but it is weakly androgenic and anabolic. Androgenic side effects associated with danazol therapy include hirsutism, voice changes, clitoral hypertrophy and oily skin or hair. In addition, weight gain and edema have frequently been reported which seems to diminish after the completion of therapy. In the only comparative studies to date, danazol appears to be more effective than oral contraceptives in the relief of dyspareunia, dysmenorrhea and menstrual abnormalities, as well as an improvement in fertility rate after discontinuation of therapy (58).

VAGINITIS

Vaginitis is any inflammation of the vagina; inflammation due to irritation, infections, malignant tumor process, or estrogenic imbalance that alters normal physiology. It is caused by anything that interferes with the protective mechanism normally present in the vagina or lowers nutrition of the vaginal epithelium.

Basic Anatomy and Physiology

The vagina is a musculomembranous canal which connects the vulva, or external area of the genitalia, with the uterus. The vagina is lined by stratified squamous epithelial cells. The thickness of these cells is directly under the influence of estrogenic hormone. When there are low levels of this hormone, as in the case prior to puberty and after menopause, the vaginal mucosa is found to be thin and most vulnerable to infection.

There are four characteristics of the average healthy adult vaginal tract. When all are present, they create a vaginal environment that is resistant to most infection.

1. The pH of the normal vagina from puberty to menopause ranges from 4.5 to 5.5. A change from the normal pH of the tract generally leaves the structures susceptible to infection. This alteration in pH may be the result of physical, chemical, mechanical, or allergic imbalance, or the influence of a vaginal tumor.
2. The vagina has a thick, protective epithelium.
3. The epithelium is maintained by estrogen support. The blood supply is diminished and the nutrition of the epithelial cells is affected as the amount of estrogen is decreased.
4. The vagina has a bacterial flora that maintains the normal level of acidity. The acid is produced from the breakdown of glycogen (present in the epithelial cells) to lactic acid by the bacterial flora. The normal flora usually consists of Doderlein's bacilli (*Lactobacillus* sp.), *Staphylococcus epidermidis*, diphtheroids, bacteroides, peptococci and peptostreptococci. The "normal" flora of asymptomatic women may contain a wide variety of anaerobic as well as aerobic bacteria, any of which may become pathogenic.

The vagina will have some degree of vaginal discharge under normal conditions. This fluidity is due to mucous secretions, transudation through the vaginal wall, and from Bartholin glands. Normal vaginal discharge is generally acidic, odorless, nonbloody, and colorless.

An increased vaginal discharge (leukorrhea) is usually associated with a simple infection of the vagina; but it also may accompany an inflammation or tumor of the Bartholin glands and Skene's ducts, cervix, uterus or fallopian tubes. Vaginal discharge is one of the principal complaints of women with vaginitis. It is estimated that 30% of the women in the United States present with this complaint. In addition, pain, itching and burning are the most common clinical complaints of vaginitis. One or more of these symptoms is almost always present. The patient may also complain of painful urination (dysuria) and painful coitus (dyspareunia).

The different types of vaginal infections are generally classified and diagnosed on the basis of distinguishing and characteristic discharge, pain, itching and burning. An evaluation of these symptoms aid the clinician in differentiating the cause. Nevertheless, microscopic or cultural confirmation is always desirable and often essential for effective therapy because more than one organism may be involved in a given case. The most common mistake made in the management of vaginal infections is the institution of treatment based on the appearance of the discharge without definite diagnosis.

As was stated earlier, the child as well as the postmenopausal adult patients lack the degree of estrogen support to maintain optimum protective epithelium. Their bacterial flora is also more mixed in type than those of menstruating patients. The vaginal pH of these patients tends toward alkalinity.

During pregnancy increased levels of vaginal glycogen may predispose the patient to candidiasis. Diabetic patients also have a much higher incidence of candida infections than the normal population. These patients have a higher nutrient content in the blood and urine which may predispose them to the invasion and growth of yeast fungi.

Menstruation itself may provide a favorable culture medium to stimulate the growth of pathogens. This may result in symptoms several days after menstruation in an individual who was previously asymptomatic. This points to the necessity of instructing the patient to continue whatever medication is prescribed during menstrual flow.

Vaginal infections are common, occurring in about ⅓ of the women of childbearing age. In more than 95% of the cases the organisms involved are (59):

1. Trichomonas
2. Certain yeast fungi (most noteably monilia or *Candida albicans*).
3. *Gardnerella vaginalis* (formerly called *Corynebacterium vaginale* or *Haemophilus vaginalis*).

Basically three factors must be kept in mind in making a diagnosis of vaginitis. First, all of the aforementioned organisms can be isolated from the vagina of women who do not have vaginitis. Second, although each of these three types of vaginitis is associated with definitive clinical symptoms, classical presentations do not occur in all patients. Finally, simultaneous infection with two or more organisms is not uncommon.

Trichomonas Vaginitis

This infection is extremely common. In a report of 5712 obstetrical and gynecological patients examined routinely for trichomonas 24.6% of the smears were positive (60).

The chief symptoms of "trich" are a profuse malodorous vaginal discharge almost always associated with vaginal itching and soreness. The discharge may be thin or thick and has been reported as white, yellow, green, or gray. When the patient is examined with a speculum the discharge at the cervix may be foamy or bubbly. As might be expected, dyspareunia is a frequent complaint. The pH of the vagina is usually found to be 5.0 to 7.5. A pH lower than 5 almost rules out trichomonas as the causative agent. The classic description of the reddened granular or "strawberry-like" appearance is present in only a few cases. Similar hemorrhagic spots may be seen in atropic vaginitis and rarely in severe bacterial vaginitis.

The diagnosis is made by observing the trichomonas under the microscope. A smear of cervical pus is made on a microscope slide and diluted with normal saline to avoid rapid drying thus killing the organism. Microscopy will show the protozoan to be a highly motile, pear-shaped, unicellular flagellate about twice the size of a leukocyte. This procedure is known as a hanging drop or wet mount. Several samples from different areas of the genital tract may be required to demonstrate the trichomonas as they may colonize only certain areas.

Although the source of many trichomonal vaginal infections is uncertain there is little doubt that the organism is usually transmitted through coitus. Trichomonas is considered a sexually transmitted disease venereal disease. Simultaneous treatment of the sexual partner is strongly recommended because this reduces the recurrence rate from 30.6 to 8.5% (59).

Elimination of the protozoan from the vagina is a relatively simple task; however, in addition to the vagina the organism may infect the urethra, vulvovaginal glands and occasionally the bladder. Once sheltered by these sites the trichomonads become almost inaccessible with topical treatment.

Many well-documented clinical studies have shown metronidazole to be the systemic medication of choice. The manufacturer's recommended dose is 250 mg 3 times daily for 7 days in both the female and male. A 5-day regimen of metronidazole has also been shown to be effective (61). In addition simultaneous treatment of all partners with a single 2-g dose is equally effective, less expensive, and requires less compliance.

In a letter (October 22, 1974) to the Commissioner of the U.S. Food and Drug Administration that apparently received wide circulation among physicians, the Health Research Group of Washington, D.C., urged the FDA "to take prompt action against the use of metronidazole for the treatment of trichomonas vaginitis because the drug causes cancer, gene mutations, and birth defects."

Metronidazole has been shown to cause pulmonary, mammary, and hepatic tumors in laboratory mice given high doses (62, 63). No tumors have been shown in hamsters. No human studies have been able to show an increased incidence of cancer in patients previously exposed to metronidazole. Studies done to date are small, however, and only exclude a large risk of cancer in association with small trichomonicidal doses of metronidazole. Metronidazole still remains the drug of choice primarily because there are no other effective systemic agents for trichomonas currently available in the United States.

The single 2-g dose deserves additional comment. The efficacy of the single dose treatment compares well with the standard treatment because it is the peak blood level that eradicates the organism rather than a sustained blood level. A great advantage in compliance is also gained. However, in cases where the drug is to be given to more than 2 partners, it is unlikely that all partners will receive the 2-g dose at the same time. This makes reinfection more likely. In such cases it may be wise to consider conventional therapy.

Metronidazole is reported to cause an Antabuse or disulfiram-type reaction when taken with alcohol. The interaction seems to be vastly overrated, and the reaction probably does not occur in a significant number of patients. The average person taking metronidazole could in no way be expected to exhibit a disulfiram-like reaction after the ingestion of alcohol. A well-controlled study on the amount of alcohol needed to produce the reaction (if at all) is also lacking.

Although no teratogenic effects have been attributed to metronidazole, most obstetricians believe it is wise to delay therapy with metronidazole during the first trimester of pregnancy when risk of structural fetal damage is highest. Only after topical therapy has failed should metronidazole therapy be considered during pregnancy. In addition, if used during pregnancy a divided dosing schedule would be recommended to prevent fetal circulation of the higher peak levels seen with a single 2-g dose.

Monilia Vaginitis (Mycotic, Candida)

In 1940 Hesseltine stated that 10% of nonpregnant and 33% of pregnant women harbor fungi of the yeast group. Because of the increased use of birth control pills and broad spectrum antibiotics the figures have risen to much higher levels. Depending on the patient population, in many areas monilial infections occur more frequently than any other.

The chief symptoms of "yeast" infection are usually intense pruritus which may or may not be associated with leukorrhea. There is usually a marked reddening of the entire vaginal or vulvovaginal mucous membrane associated with thrushlike patches on the vagina, vulva, or both.

Profuse discharge and a disagreeable odor are not features of this disease; however, secretions (usually curdy) are thick and white. The pH of the vaginal secretion is usually found to be 3.8 to 5.0. Therefore, acidifying agents such as vinegar douches would be of little value here as *Candida* thrives in an acid vagina.

A positive diagnosis can usually be made by microscopic demonstration of the fungi. A smear is made of the vaginal exudate on a microscopic slide to which 1 or 2 drops of 10 to 20% potassium hydroxide is added. This is known as a KOH preparation. Although the yeast can also be seen on a Gram stain or hanging drop preparation, the KOH preparation rids the slide of epithelial cells and other cells which might interfere with recognition. *C. albicans* fungi appear in the form of long threadlike fibers of mycelia, to which are attached the tiny buds or conidia. A simple office culture using Nickerson's medium can be performed to confirm the organism.

Because candida is part of the normal flora of the vagina, any vaginal imbalance may cause it to become pathogenic. Reports of the sexual infectivity of vaginal candidiasis have been studied. In one study more than 1 in 10 of the husbands of the 225 affected women had candida balanoposthitis (60). At this time it is not routinely recommended that sexual partner be treated; however, if recurrent monilia is a problem, the possibility of reinfection by the sexual partner should be explored.

The clinical incidence of monilia infection is also related to the widespread use of oral contraceptive medications. It has been reported that women given oral contraceptive medications have an increase in the incidence of vulvovaginal candidiasis as contrasted to a similar group of women not given one of the "pills." Other reports fail to show the existence of this relationship.

Preparations containing gentian violet, proprionic acid, arsenical compounds, chlordantoin, nifuroxime, and a variety of other compounds have been used. Disadvantages of these preparations are numerous.

Nystatin vaginal suppositories inserted high into the vagina 1 to 2 times daily for 2 weeks or longer is effective therapy. However, miconazole nitrate 2% cream has been shown to be superior (cure rates 100% vs. 82.6%) (64). These drugs are reported to be safe for use in the 2nd and 3rd trimesters of pregnancy.

Another report showed miconazole and nystatin creams (5 g each day for 6 days) to be superior to clotrimazole tablets (0.1 g each day for 6 days) (65). This may have been due to the weaker fungicidal effect of clotrimazole, shorter duration of therapy, or tablet formulation.

If reinfection occurs after several trials of therapy, several possibilities should be explored: (a) a fasting blood sugar could be done to rule out diabetes mellitus; (b) the patient could be reinfected by her sexual partner in which case nystatin ointment or miconazole cream may be prescribed for application to the penis, especially if uncircumcised; (c) the patient may be reinfecting herself from intestinal fungus. An oral dose of 500,000 units nystatin suspension taken 3 times daily for 14 days is considered effective in conjunction with vaginal therapy; and (d) in a small percentage of women recurrent infections do not clear up until oral contraceptive medication is discontinued.

Gardnerella vaginalis Vaginitis

An abnormal vaginal discharge that is not caused by C. albicans, trichomonas vaginalis, or Neisseria gonorrhoeae was for many years termed nonspecific vaginitis (NSV). In 1955, Gardner and Duke (66), associated NSV with a single organism which they called Haemophilus vaginalis. Controversy has surrounded the etiology, diagnosis and therapy of NSV ever since.

Under two previous misclassifications the organism has been known as Haemophilus vaginalis and Corynebacterium vaginale. Due to several unusual characteristics the organism and subsequent disease state has been named after its discoverer and is called Gardnerella vaginalis vaginitis. The form of vaginitis, however, is probably caused by a complex aerobic-anaerobic bacterial infection of the vagina that is usually but not always associated with G. vaginalis.

Chief complaints are usually a malodorus discharge with or without pruritus and burning. G. vaginalis is a surface bacteria and therefore rarely produces gross changes in the vaginal mucosa of vulva. The discharge is homogenous and yellow to gray in color with a pH of 5 to 5.5. The leukorrhea may be scant or heavy.

Laboratory findings must be correlated with clinical examination to confirm the diagnosis. The examination of a wet mount shows infrequent pus cells and a few lactobacilli present. Many epithelial cells have a stripped or grandular appearance owing to the adherence of many G. vaginalis on their surfaces. These are called "clue cells." A Gram stain of the vaginal smear will show small Gram-negative bacilli. Other bacteria may also be present in small numbers. In addition, the presence of a fishy odor on the addition of 10% potassium hydroxide to vaginal discharge on a glass slide is helpful in confirming the diagnosis.

It has taken much time to understand why antibiotics such as ampicillin and tetracycline which show how high activity against G. vaginalis seem to be ineffective in treating clinical cases of this disease. In addition G. vaginalis is almost totally resistant to sulfas, and yet triple sulfa vaginal cream at one point was the drug of choice for this condition (67).

Recently, metronidazole 500 mg given twice daily for 7 days has been shown to eliminate both G. vaginalis and NSV from affected women (68). However G. vaginalis is not particularly sensitive to metronidazole in vitro. Several possibilities exist that may explain this dichotomy. It has been postulated that aerobic bacteria in the vagina may provide certain factors that support the growth of *G. vaginalis*. The inhibition of these anaerobes by metronidazole may decrease the concentration of *G. vaginalis* and thus the symptoms of the disease (68).

Metronidazole therapy in humans is a concern, because of its role as a mutagen and a potential carcinogen as discussed earlier. However, once again we are left with few good therapeutic alternatives in the treatment of this disease.

Atropic Vaginitis (Senile)

The atrophy which takes place normally at the time of menopause makes the vaginal mucosa prone to infection. The epithelium is thin, the blood supply is diminished, and the amount of glycogen available is lessened. The pH changes from acid to neutral or alkaline.

The chief complaints are again leukorrhea, itching, and burning. The rugae, or folds of the vaginal mucosa, flatten out and appear smooth and glistening. It is of note that the symptoms may be present without a bacterial, monilial, or flagellate infection. However, microscopic examination is advisable since the mucosa is less resistant to infection; and it is not uncommon for various infective states to accompany this form of vaginitis. The mucosa may appear reddened, and pinpoint hemorrhagic areas may be seen. The blood from the denuded surface is often mixed with a vaginal discharge.

The management of this form of vaginitis involves the replacement of estrogen or its derivatives directly to the vaginal mucosa or by the oral route. The oral conjugated estrogen in a dose of 0.3 to 1.25 mg daily for 3 weeks, combined with a progesterone for the last 7 to 10 days, skip 1 week and repeat, is very popular for the "menopause syndrome." It has been found, however, in order to obtain relief and satisfactory vaginal cornification, in cases with marked atropic vaginitis, that it is necessary to give doses of oral estrogens at levels considerably higher than that required for improvement of systemic manifestations. It must also be remembered that high estrogen therapy may produce uterine bleeding. When estrogen creams are administered topically they are readily absorbed and produce plasma levels which are near or above physiologic levels, depending on the dose and type of estrogen used (69). Thus, the same cautions would apply to topical as well as oral administration of estrogens.

The local application of conjugated estrogen vaginal cream or dienestrol cream is recommended initially in a dose of one full applicator at bedtime for 1 to 2 weeks or until relief of symptoms. Following this reduce the dosage by one-half for a similar period. The use of these creams 2 to 3 times per week may be sufficient for maintenance. Diethylstilbestrol (0.5 mg) vaginal suppositories may also be used at bedtime until epithelial restoration takes place, then 3 to 4 times per week for maintenance.

Other Vaginitis

Other types of vaginal infections including gonorrhea vaginitis in children and postmenopausal adults, pneumococci vaginitis in children, chlamydia, genital herpes, venereal warts, tuberculosis, anerobic infections, pinworms, trematodes (flukes), cestodes (tapeworms), and nematodes (roundworms) have also been reported.

Traumatic Vaginitis

Due to the availability of legal abortions, self-dosage with abortifacients, such as potassium permanganate tablets, has decreased dramatically. The resulting erosion and ulceration was often followed by scarring and contracture.

Injury from chemical irritation as well as mechanical or allergic sensitization may also result in traumatic vaginitis. Chemical irritation from iodine, phenol, and menthol in prescribed medication may cause sensitization. Allergic sensitization may also occur with many of the products mentioned as well as tight fitting undergarments, generally nylon. The logical solution is to discontinue the sensitizing agent.

Foreign bodies high in the vagina are often the cause of vaginitis. Many times the removal of a long forgotten tampon, diaphragm, button or clip may "cure" this type of vaginitis.

A foreign body is one of the common causes of "nonspecific" childhood vaginitis, as is poor perineal hygiene and intestinal parasites. Less commonly, vaginitis may be secondary to respiratory, skin and urinary tract infections. Involvement of the vaginal mucosa with inflammation and edema may occur as a complication of scarlet fever or measles. Also, the eruptions of chickenpox and smallpox may be spread to the vulva and vagina. Vulvovaginitis in children is seen fairly frequently because the immature epithelium is thin and easily traumatized.

DOUCHING

The reasons for using most douching products are (a) to serve a therapeutic function by acidifying the vaginal tract and (b) to provide cleansing by removing material that may serve as a source of infection in the vagina.

Because of the brief time of contact with the vaginal mucosa douches can be of little value in changing the physiologic state of the vagina. From a medical point of view there is little indication for routine douching in the normal individual. In the case of vaginitis the primary use is acidification and cleansing. Most commercial products contain boric acid, acetic acid, or lactic acid. If acidification is recommended, 2 tablespoons of vinegar to 1 quart of water is much less expensive and serves the same purpose. Douching, however, probably has caused more problems than it has solved.

PREGNANCY TESTING

As was pointed out earlier, if pregnancy occurs, human chorionic gonadotropin (HCG) is released to maintain the high level of hormones needed during pregnancy. Immunoassay is currently the most widely used method of pregnancy testing. Two techniques are utilized. One is performed in a test tube and the other on a slide. These tests use an antigen antibody reaction to test for the presence of HCG in the urine. Sufficient quantities of gonadotropin for this test appear in the urine 4 weeks after conception, or 2 weeks after a missed menstrual period. The hemagglutination inhibition test performed in a test tube requires about 2 hours to perform and is the method used for the "do-it-yourself" OTC home pregnancy tests now marketed in the United States. When performed by consumers the accuracy is 97% for positive readings and 80% for negative readings.

The slide test is done in many office practices. This test is not extremely accurate, but can be done in a matter of minutes. Generally, the HCG value doubles every 2 days, starting from day 6 to 10, until approximately day 60 after the last menstrual period. This peak value, then, decreases slowly over the remaining 2 trimesters to approximately 10% of the peak value (70). By the third month of pregnancy, the corpus luteum ceases to produce enough HCG to be detected, and this method of pregnancy detection is no longer effective.

In addition to the immunoassay tests, a radioimmune assay has now been developed that can diagnose pregnancy 8 to 10 days after ovulation, or 2½ to 3 weeks earlier than the routine slide test. Recent technical advances have allowed measurements in 1 to 2 hours, permitting routine rapid diagnosis of ectopic pregnancy, a medical emergency.

THE MENOPAUSAL SYNDROME

The vasomotor disturbances which may occur in the early stages of menopause are part of the menopause syndrome. They are also called "hot flashes" because the effect is caused by a decrease in tone of the arterioles resulting in increased blood flow to the skin and a rise in temperature. The symptoms can cause considerable discomfort.

The conjugated estrogen preparations (Premarin) which consist primarily of sodium estrone sulfate, in doses of 0.3 to 1.25 mg daily, are very popular for the treatment of this syndrome. If therapy is to be initiated in menstruating women, cyclic administration is recommended. Beginning on day 5 the drug is usually given daily for 3 weeks then stopped for 1 week. In addition progesterone should be added to the estrogen for the last 7 to 10 days. The object is to avoid excessive proliferative changes in the endometrium. A cyclic administration is also recommended in nonmenstruating women but therapy is begun at once.

Estrogens should not be used to manage psychosomatic or anxiety and depression symptoms which may also be part of this syndrome. The long-term use of estrogens has most likely arisen from the belief that they promote a feeling of well-being and a youthful appearance as well as hoped for protection against coronary artery disease. These benefits have not been objectively documented.

In recent years, there has been increasing evidence that estrogen administration which is unopposed by progesterone may produce endometrial hyperplasia, which has been shown to advance to adenomatous hyperplasia, carcinoma in situ, or endometrial cancer. Some experts claim this increase is a result of better reporting technique and less liberal indications for hysterectomies. However, it is becoming obvious that the increase is indeed real and may in fact be related to the use of estrogens. In addition, it has been shown that progesterone competes with estrogen for binding sites in the endometrial cells and may reduce the stimulatory effect of estrogen (71).

The exposure of the normal estrogen-primed endometrium to progesterone converts the tissue to the secretory type seen in the secretory phase of the menstrual cycle. This effect of progesterone is thought to prevent the progression of endometrial hyperplasia. These findings may help to explain why no increase in endometrial carcinoma is noted in combined oral contraceptive users but has been reported with sequential oral contraceptives and with conjugated estrogens used alone. These findings have also led clinicians to include the administration of progesterone to the cyclic administration of estrogens in postmenopausal women. The use of norethindrone 2.5 mg, medroxyprogesterone 5 mg or ethynodiol diacetate 0.5 mg has been incorporated into the last 7 to 10 days of the usual 3-week estrogen therapy for women with intact uteri.

Estrogens may delay or prevent osteoporosis (72). Osteoporosis is a crippler of older women causing collapse of the vertebral column and broken hips in 25% of white women over 60 (73). More women die of secondary complications from broken hips after menopause than ever died of endometrial cancer from unopposed estrogens or other estrogen related side effects.

Intestinal absorption and dietary intake of calcium are decreased with age. Therefore, oral calcium, with or without a vitamin D supplement, should be recommended in conjunction with oral estrogens.

No cases of endometrial cancer have been attributed to postmenopausal use of estrogens since the addition of progestogin. Other risks associated with long-term use of estrogen continue to be studied. At this point there is no reason to withhold estrogen therapy from otherwise healthy postmenopausal women.

TERATOGENICITY

Many books and articles have now been written listing the harmful effects of particular drugs when taken during pregnancy. The discussion which follows will be concerned primarily with general principles involving the use of drugs during pregnancy.

"Terat" is a Greek root word referring to monster or monstrosity. A teratogen is an agent capable of producing a deformed fetus, i.e., congenital abnormalities. Gross abnormalities are present in 2% of all infants and are the third leading cause of infant mortality in the United States. Known teratogens cause one to two defects per 2000 births or about 5 to 10% of all birth defects. Genetic abnormalities cause 25% of congenital abnormalities which leaves the cause of 60 to 65% of congenital abnormalities unidentified (74). It is likely that a complicated interaction between genetic predisposition factors and subtle factors in the uterine environment account for the unidentified cases (75). Thus, only 5 to 10% of the birth defects could be eliminated by avoiding teratogens. As these figures show us, however, the prevention of one to two abnormalities in every 2000 births would be a significant accomplishment.

In order for a woman to avoid a potential teratogen, she must know she is pregnant. As was discussed under pregnancy testing earlier, it is probable that a woman will be pregnant approximately 1 month before her condition is recognized. Even if she suspects her pregnancy she cannot avoid potential teratogens unless she is aware which substances are harmful. In a study of drug consumption during pregnancy, including labor and delivery, each mother took an average of 10.3 drugs (3 to 29) while pregnant (76). Although some of these drugs were prescribed, many were taken without medical supervision. If aware of their potential harm, it is unlikely that these women would have consumed this many drugs.

The identification of teratogenic substances have been by three means: 1) case reports, 2) epidemiologic studies, and 3) animal studies. The shortcomings of these methods are obvious. However, it should also be obvious that it would be unethical to do cross over controlled double blind studies on potential teratogens in humans. In general, there is a gross lack of available knowledge on teratogenic effects of drugs. The ethical considerations of conducting controlled trial in humans, coupled with a high background rate of various defects in man makes a cause and effect relationship difficult to establish for any teratogen. Prescribers attempting to find information regarding the potential for harm of a given substance are confronted with this problem.

One of the common reference sources on drugs for physicians is the *Physicians' Desk Reference* (PDR). A standard statement in the PDR is "safety for use in pregnancy has not been established" and if not the statement then there is a confusing description of teratogenicity from animal studies which is difficult to interpret. In a recent survey, 65.9% of drugs listed in the PDR had no statement on use in pregnancy, another 14.3% had a statement that no data on use in pregnancy was available, and 8% gave animal data (77).

Human Embryology

To understand drug effects in pregnancy, it is first necessary to cover some concepts of human embryology. There are three basic periods in the development of fetus.

1. The *fertilization and implantation period* which extends from conception to about 15 days of gestation. This period is characterized by marked cell division. All cells are functionally equivalent in terms of their totipotential. During this period the developing organism is not highly susceptible to teratogenic agents. Toxic agents which interfere with all cells at this time would result in the death of the developing organism, hence pregnancy would be halted and products of conception would be expelled or absorbed.

2. The *embryonic period* which extends from approximately 16 to 55 days is the time of organogenesis. This is the period when developing fetus shows an extreme sensitivity to teratogenetic agents. In addition this period may well be before the mother to be is aware she is pregnant.

3. The *fetal period* ranges from about the 56th day to birth. It is the time of growth and development and although teratogenetic changes can occur, they are not as likely as during the embryonic period. The in utero exposure to noxious environmental influences at this time usually leads to a reduction in cell size and number (Table 4.6).

Placental Transfer

For a drug to be teratogenetic it must first cross from the maternal circulation to the fetal circulation via the placenta (Fig. 4.6). The so-called "placental barrier" is a myth. In general, the same considerations that apply to the passage of drug across any lipid membrane can be applied to the passage of drugs across the placenta.

Several mechanisms of drug transfer across the placenta have been identified:

1. Simple diffusion
2. Facilitated diffusion
3. Active transport

Table 4.6.
Teratogenicity during Embryogenesis

Days of Gestation	Cell Differentiation and Teratogenic Effects
<15	No differentiation of cells (germ layers formed). Embryo can be killed if enough cells are killed. Otherwise no teratogenic effects are seen
15–25	Central nervous system differentiation occurs
20–30	Precursors to axial skeleton and musculature occur and limb buds make appearance
24–40	Major differentiation of eyes, heart and lower limbs
60	Organ differentiation well under way and in many areas completed
90	Differentiation complete and maturation occurring
>90	Little susceptibility to the occurrence of congenital malformations

4. Metabolic conversion of transferred substrate
5. Physical disruption of the placental membrane

The major mechanism by which drugs cross the placenta is by passive diffusion. Estimating the rate of diffusion of a drug is complex, and the interrelationship of several factors can be described by the following equation:

Rate of diffusion = $K[A(C_m - C_f)/X]$

A = the surface area available for transfer
C_m = internal blood concentration
C_f = fetal blood concentration
X = thickness of the placental membrane
K = defusion constant of the drug

Many factors affect the rate of placenta drug transfer:

1. Surface area available for transfer
2. Maternal blood concentration
3. Fetal blood concentration
4. Thickness of placental membrane
5. Molecular weight
6. Degree of ionization (pK_a and pH)
7. Lipid solubility
8. Maternal placental blood flow
9. Protein binding

The thickness of the placental membrane becomes progressively thinner during pregnancy. In addition, there are thick and thin spots that create varying distances through which a drug must pass. Disease states such as diabetes or toxemia of pregnancy may also alter placental permeability. The diffusion constant of a drug appears to be primarily

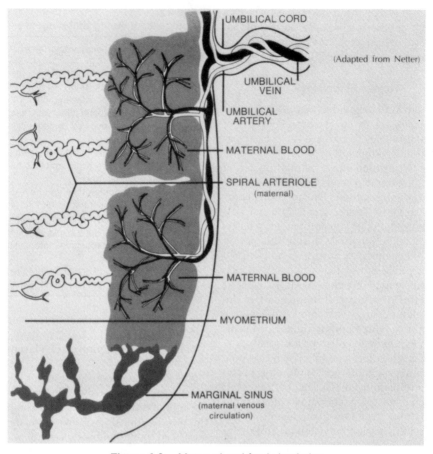

Figure 4.6.   Maternal and fetal circulation.

determined by its molecular weight, spacial configuration, degree of ionization, and lipid solubility. The majority of drugs have a molecular weight of 250 to 500 and cross the placenta quite easily depending on their state of ionization, lipid solubility and mechanism of transfer. It has often been stated, despite the absence of substantial data, compounds with molecular weight exceeding 1000 do not pass cross the placenta, whereas substances with molecular weights from 500 to 1000 cross with some difficulty. Drug molecules tend to penetrate biological membranes more quickly in an unionized state. This permeability seems relative rather than absolute. If sufficiently high maternal to fetal concentration gradients are achieved even polar compounds can cross the placenta and enter the fetal circulation.

In addition to the pK_a values for a drug, placental transfer is also influenced by the respective pH of the maternal and fetal circulations. The pH of umbilical vessel blood is normally 0.1 to 0.5 pH units lower than maternal blood. This partitioning may lead to a final drug concentration in the fetus which may be higher or lower than that of the mother at equilibrium.

More lipophilic compounds tend to defuse rapidly across the placenta into the fetal circulation. Another factor affecting drug transfer is maternal placental blood flow.

Protein binding may effect placental transfer. Protein binding does not appear to exert a significant affect on the placental transfer of drugs which are highly lipophilic and nonpolar, since the transfer of these drugs seems to be proportional to placental blood flow. However, compounds which move across the placenta more slowly because of high degrees of ionization or low lipid solubilities may be drastically altered by protein binding. Rate of diffusion of these drugs is limited by free drug concentration.

Teratogenetic Principles

Several teratogenetic principals have been developed through animal experimentation and epidemiologic study (74, 75, 78, 79).

1. The most sensitive period for teratogenesis is the phase of organ development (Table 4.6). This phase for developmental structural damage corresponds fairly well to the first trimester.

2. A variety of teratogens may produce the same malformation. Hundreds of agents have been shown to be teratogenic, among them are:
   a) Physical factors like x-rays
   b) Infection such as rubella toxoplasmosis and rickettsia
   c) Endotoxins
   d) A large variety of chemicals, e.g., drugs, poisons, industrial dyes, solvents, and pesticides.
   Any of these substances may cause decreases in organ formation and advancement. In addition, any of these agents may produce malformation similar to genetic abnormalities.

3. A variety of malformations may be produced by a single teratogen. As in the case of thalidomide, a great variety of congenital defects were traced to that drug. The type of defect was classified based on the specific number of days between conception and thalidomide ingestion.

4. The susceptibility to teratogenesis may differ by species and in different genetic strains of the same species. The implication for racial and familial differences within human studies are obvious. For example, a drug that is associated with the production of cleft palate produces its effect by slowing the rate of palate closure. Therefore the cleft would occur only in offsprings that had a genetically slow rate of palate closure, not in offspring with a normal or rapid rate of palate closure. This principle also explains why animal studies are frequently inconsistent among species and why extrapolation to humans is generally not valid.

5. Most malformations are due to an interaction between genetic and environmental factors.

6. Manifestations of teratogenicity are dose dependent. When drugs are used in pregnant women, dosage schedules and doses should be adjusted so that the lowest possible effective dose is used to prevent high fetal circulating levels.

7. A drug may have innocuous effects on an adult, but may be deleterious to the fetus. The use of thalidomide and subclinical maternal rubella infection are classic examples of this principle. Both of these agents are harmless to the mother, but can cause serious birth defects in the fetus.

As with all drug therapy, the therapeutic value of a drug must be weighed against possible adverse affects on the fetus before and after birth. Our knowledge of drug teratogenicity in humans is limited and characterized by suspected potential and theoretical risks. It is not practical to deny all drug therapy to pregnant women based upon some potential hazard, rather we must consider the risk benefit ratio using our present level of knowledge.

References

1. Hatcher RA, Stewart GK, Stewart FS, et al: *Contraceptive Technology, 1980–81*, ed 10. New York: Irvington Publishers, 1980.
2. Martinez-Manautou J, et al: Antiovulatory activity of several synthetic and natural estrogens. In Greenblatt RB: *Ovulation.* Philadelphia: J. B. Lippincott, 1966.
3. Delforge JP, Ferrin J: A histometric study of two estrogens: ethinyl-estradiol and its 3-methyl-ether derivative (mestranol); their comparative effect upon the growth of the human endometrium. *Contraception* 1:57, 1970.
4. Aufrere MB, Benson H: Progesterone: an overview and recent advances. *J Pharm Sci* 65:6, 1976.
5. McGee D: The Probability of Developing Certain Cardiovascular Disease in 8 years at Specified Values of Some Characteristics. Framingham Study 18 Years. DHEW Publ. No. (NIH) 74-618. Washington, D.C.: U.S. Government Printing Office, 1973.
6. Crane MG, Harris JJ, Winson W III: Hypertension, oral contraceptive agents and conjugated estrogens. *Ann Intern Med* 74:13, 1971.
7. Goodlin RC, Waechter V: Oral contraceptives and blood pressure. *Lancet* 1:1262, 1969.
8. Royal College of General Practitioners: *Oral Contraception Study. Oral Contraceptives and Health.* New York: Pitman & Sons, 1974.
9. Ramcharan S, Pellegran FA, Hoag E: The occurrence and cause of hypertensive disease in users and non-users of oral contraceptive drugs. In Fregley MJ, Fregley MS: *Oral Contraceptives and High Blood Pressure*, Gainesville, Fla.: Dolphin Press, 1974, p 1.
10. Fisch IR, Frank J: Oral contraceptives and blood pressure. *JAMA* 237:2499, 1977.
11. Kunin CM, McCormack RC, Abernathy JR: Oral contraceptives and blood pressure. *Arch Intern Med* 123:362, 1969.
12. Saruta T, Saade GA, Kaplan NM: A possible mechanism for hypertension induced by oral contraceptives. *Arch Intern Med* 126:621, 1970.
13. Laragh JH, Sealey JE, Ledingham JG, et al: Oral

contraceptives: renin, aldosterone, and high blood pressure. *JAMA* 201:918, 1967.

14. Effect on hypertension and benign breast disease of progestogen component in combined oral contraceptives: Royal College of General Practitioners Oral Contraception Study. *Lancet* 1:624, 1977.

15. Gershberg H, Hulse M, Janvier M: Hypertriglceridemia during treatment with estrogen and oral contraceptives. *Obstet Gynecol* 31:186, 1968.

16. Davidoff F, Tishler S, Rosoff C: Marked hyperlipidemia and pancreatitis associated with oral contraceptive therapy. *N Engl J Med* 289:552, 1973.

17. Glueck CJ, Scheel D, Fishbach J, et al: Progestogens, anabolic-androgenic compounds, estrogen: effects on triglycerides and post-heparin lipolytic enzymes. *Lipids* 7:110, 1971.

18. Bradley DB, Wingerd J, Petti DB, et al: Serum high-density lipoprotein cholesterol in women using oral contraceptive estrogens and progestins. *N Engl J Med* 299:17, 1978.

19. Briggs MH: Biochemical Basis for the selection of oral contraceptives. *Int J Gynaecol Obstet* 16:509, 1979.

20. Adams PW, Wynn V, Folkard J, et al: Influence of oral contraceptives, pridoxine (vitamin B_6) and tryptophan on carbohydrate metabolism. *Lancet* 1:759, 1976.

21. Mann JI, Doll R, Thorogood M, et al: Risk factors for myocardial infarction in young women. *Br J Prev Soc Med* 30:94, 1976.

22. Collaborative group for the Study of Stroke in Young Women: Oral contraceptives and stroke in young women; associated risk factors. *JAMA* 231:718, 1975.

23. Slone D, Shapiro S, Kaufman DW, et al: Risk of myocardial infarction in relation to current and discontinued use of oral contraceptives. *N Engl J Med* 305:420, 1981.

24. Sartwell PE, Masi AT, Arthes FG, et al: Thromboembolism and oral contraceptives: an epidemiologic case-control study. *Am J Epidemiol* 90:365, 1969.

25. Petitti DB, Wingerd J: Use of oral contraceptives, cigarette smoking, and risk of subarachnoid hemorrhage. *Lancet* 2:234, 1978.

26. Further analyses of mortality in oral contraceptive users: Royal College of General Practitioners' Oral Contraception Study. *Lancet* 1:541, 1981.

27. Inman WHW, Vessey MP, Westerholm B, et al: Thromboembolic disease and the steroidal content of oral contraceptives: a report to the Committee on Safety of Drugs. *Br Med J* 2:203, 1970.

28. Meade TW, Greenberg G, Thompson SG: Progestogens and cardiovascular reactions associated with oral contraceptives and a comparison of the safety of 50 and 30 mcg preparations. *Br Med J* 280:1157, 1980.

29. Stadel BV: Oral contraceptives and cardiovascular disease. *N Engl J Med* 305:672, 1981.

30. Oral contraceptives and venous thromboembolic disease, surgically confirmed gallbladder disease, and breast tumors: report from the Boston Collaborative Drug Surveillance Programe. *Lancet* 1:1399, 1973.

31. Oral contraceptives, venous thrombosis, and varicose veins: Royal College of General Practitioners' Oral Contraceptive Study. *J R Coll Gen Pract* 28:393, 1978.

32. Vessey MP, McPherson K, Yeates D: Mortality in oral contraceptive users. *Lancet* 1:549, 1981.

33. Irey NS, Manion WC, Taylor HB: Vascular lesions in women taking oral contraceptives. *Arch Pathol* 89:1, 1970.

34. Caspery EA, Peberdy M: Oral contraception and blood platelet adhesiveness. *Lancet* 1:1142, 1965.

35. Howie PW, Mallinson AC, Prentice CRM, et al: Effect of combined estrogen-progestogen oral contraceptives on antiplasmin and anti-thrombolic activity. *Lancet* 2:1329, 1970.

36. Peterson C, Kelly R, Minard B, et al: Antithrombin III: comparison of functional and immunologic assay. *Am J Clin Pathol* 69:500, 1978.

37. Conard J, Samama M, Salomon Y: Antithrombin III and the oestrogen content of combined oestrogen-progestagen contraceptives. *Lancet* 2:1148, 1972.

38. Fagerhol MK, Abilgaard U, Kornstad L: Antithrombin III concentration and ABO bloodgroups. *Lancet* 2:664, 1971.

39. Jick H, Slone D, Westerholm B, et al: Venous thromboembolic disease and ABO blood type: a cooperative study. *Lancet* 1:539, 1969.

40. Fechner RE: Benign hepatic lesions and orally administered contraceptives: a report of seven cases and a critical analysis of the literature. *Hum Pathol* 8:255, 1977.

41. Bennion LJ, Ginsberl RL, Garnich MB, et al: Effects of oral contraceptives on the gallbladder bile of normal women. *N Engl J Med* 294:189, 1976.

42. Adams PW, Wynn V, Rose DP, et al: Effect of pyridoxine hydrochloride (vitamin B_6) upon depression associated with oral contraception. *Lancet* 1:897, 1973.

43. Bolt HM, Bolt M, Kappus M: Interaction of rifampicin treatment with pharmacokineties and metabolism of ethinyloestradiol in man. *Acta Endocrinol* 85:189, 1977.

44. Breckenridge AM, Back DJ, Orme M: Interactions between oral contraceptives and other drugs. *Pharmacol Ther* 7:617, 1979.

45. Bacon JF, Shenfield GM: Pregnancy attributable to interaction between tetracycline and oral contraceptives. *Br Med J* 2:293, 1980.

46. Whitty CWM, Hockaday JM, Whitty MM: Effect of oral contraceptives on migraine. *Lancet* 1:856, 1966.

47. Kutt H, McDowell F: Management of epilepsy with diphenylhydantoin sodium. *JAMA* 203:969, 1968.

48. Smith MB: A quantitative estimate of ocular iatrogenic disease in humans. *J Am Optom Assoc* 45:751, 1974.

49. Wood JR: Ocular complications of oral contraceptives. *Ophthalmic Semin* 2:371, 1977.

50. Chapel TA, Burns RE: Oral contraceptives and exacerbation of lupus erythematous. *Am J Obstet Gynecol* 110:366, 1971.

51. Dickey RP: Initial pill section and managing the contraceptive pill patient. *Int J Gynaecol Obstet* 16:547, 1979.

52. Ostergard DR: DES-related vaginal lesions. *Clin Obstet Gynecol* 24:379, 1981.

53. Mishell DR: Intrauterine services: medicated and nonmedicated. *Int J Gynecol Obstet* 16:482, 1979.

54. Akerlund M: Pathophysiology of Dysmenorrhea. *Acta Obstet Gynecol Scand Supp* 87:27, 1979.

55. Todd J, Fishaut M, Kapral F, et al: Toxic-shock syndrome associated with phage-group I staphylococci. *Lancet* 2:1116, 1978.

56. Friedrich EG: Tampon effects on vaginal health. *Clin Obstet Gynecol* 24:395, 1981.

57. Kistner RW: *Gynecology—Principles and Practice*, ed 3. Chicago: Year Book, 1979, p 439.

58. Dmowski WP, Cohen MR: Antigonadotropin (danazol) in the treatment of endometriosis. *Am J Obstet Gynecol* 130:41, 1978.

59. Burmeister RE, Gardner HL: Vaginitis; diagnosis and treatment. *Postgrad Med* 54:159, 1970.

60. Diddle AW, Gardner WH, Williamson PJ, et al: Oral contraceptive medications and vulvovaginal candidiasis. *Obstet Gynecol* 34:3, 1969.

61. Pereyra AJ, Lansing JD: Urogenital trichomoniasis: treatment with metronidazole in 2002 incarcerated women. *Obstet Gynecol* 24:499, 1964.

62. Roe JRC: A critical appraisal of the toxicology of metronidazole. In Phillips I, Collier J: *Metronidazole*. London: Academic Press, 1979, pp 215–222.

63. Rustia M, Shubik P: Experimental induction of hepatomas, mammary tumors, and other tumors with metronidazole in non-inbred Sas: MRC (WI) BR rats. *JNCI* 63:863, 1979.

64. David JE, Frudenfeld JH, Goddard JL: Comparative evaluation of Monistat and Mycostatin in the treatment of vulvovaginal candidiasis. *Obstet Gynecol* 44:3, 1974.

65. Svendsen E, Lie S, Gunderson TH, et al: Comparative evaluation of miconazole, clotrimazole and nystatin in the treatment of candidal vulvovaginitis. *Curr Ther Res* 23:666, 1978.

66. Gardner HL, Dukes CD: *Haemophilus vaginalis* vaginitis. *Am J Obstet Gynecol* 69:962, 1955.

67. Vontver LA, Eschenbach DA: The role of gardnerella vaginalis in nonspecific vaginitis. *Clin Obstet Gynecol* 24:439, 1981.

68. Pheifer TA, Forsyth PS, Durfee MA, et al: Nonspecific vaginitis: role of *Haemophilus vaginalis* and treatment with metronidazole. *N Engl J Med* 298:1429, 1979.

69. Rigg LA, Hermann H, Yen SS: Absorption of estrogens from vaginal creams. *N Engl J Med* 4:195, 1978.

70. Goldstein DP, Aono T, Taymor ML, et al: Radioimmunoassay of serum chorionic gonadotrophin activity in normal pregnancy. *Am J Obstet Gynecol* 102:110, 1968.

71. Huggins GR: Neoplasia and hormonal contraceptions. *Clin Obstet Gynecol* 24:903, 1981.

72. Ryan KJ, Barrett-Connor E, Federman DD, et al: Estrogen use and postmenopausal women: a national institutes of health consensus development conference. *Ann Intern Med* 91:921, 1979.

73. Heaney RP: Estrogens and postmenopausal osteoporosis. *Clin Obstet Gynecol* 19:791, 1976.

74. Howard FM, Hill JM: Drugs in pregnancy. *Obstet Gynecol Surv* 34:643, 1979.

75. Pritchard JA, MacDonald PC: *Williams Obstetrics*, ed 15. New York: Appleton-Century-Crofts, 1976, p 825.

76. Hill RM: Drugs ingested by pregnant women. *Clin Pharmacol Ther* 14:654, 1973.

77. Hays DP: Teratogenesis: a review of the basic principles with a discussion of selected agents: part I. *Drug Intell Clin Pharm* 15:444, 1981.

78. Techmann-Duplessis H: *Drug Effects on the Fetus*. Acton, Mass.: Publishing Sciences Group, 1975.

79. Cohlan SQ: Fetal and neonatal hazards from drugs administered during pregnancy. *NY State J Med* 64:493, 1964.

CHAPTER 5

Alcoholism

THEODORE G. TONG, Pharm.D.
LINDA R. BERNSTEIN, Pharm.D.

Alcohol is the most misused drug in the United States today. According to knowledgeable estimates, the *incidence of* alcoholism in the United States ranges from 9 to 14 million, about 10% of the total number of adult Americans who use alcohol. It is a condition far more common than generally perceived, with only 3 to 5% of the country's alcoholic population classified as the "skid row" or public inebriate type. Alcoholics come from all levels of our society; the majority are found in the working and homemaking population. The largest percentage of American alcoholics are between the ages of 35 and 50 years. Alcoholics are primarily characterized socioeconomically as middle class men and women. Professionals and business people have high rates of alcoholism and alcohol consumption. The proportion of alcohol use in the younger school age population and "problem drinking" among women have increased alarmingly and appear to be continuing trends. Alcoholism represents one of the nation's most serious health concerns, and the problems related to alcohol abuse and alcoholism are increasing (1–5).

It has been shown that in half of all highway traffic fatalities an alcohol intoxicated driver is involved; it appears to be a leading causative factor in other accidents such as drownings, burns, trauma, suicides, and other violent crimes (6–8). Public intoxication alone accounts for nearly one third of all arrests reported annually (1).

The *economic costs* associated with the misuse of alcohol are conservatively estimated to be $40 billion a year. This estimate does not reflect the much greater costs of personal tragedy, disruption of family life, and the effects on the community in monetary terms. Health care costs attributable to alcohol overuse were estimated in 1971 at approximately 10% of the total health care costs. Of these expenses, most were allocated in direct hospital care (9, 10).

Alcoholism is an illness that can considerably shorten life span. Death rates from alcohol abuse in the major risk age groups are more than twice those for the general population (1). Alcoholism is a treatable illness when diagnosed in its early stages. Unfortunately, there is a serious deficit of accessible and high quality alcoholism treatment services. Moreover, the majority of the services available are designed to deal with only the late stages of alcoholism. Although much attention has been given to the problem of narcotic addiction and its economic and social costs to society, the more serious and widespread problem of alcoholism has been relatively ignored until recent years. In general, the prevailing attitude toward excessive alcohol consumption in the United States can be characterized as confused, ignorant, ambivalent, and often counterproductive.

Alcohol is an addicting drug, because those persons who abuse it generally experience physical and psychologic dependency and tolerance. What is addiction and how is it recognized? Addiction has three aspects: psychologic dependency, physical dependency, and tolerance. Psychologic dependency is perhaps the single most important factor and involves the compulsive use of and craving for a drug. Physical dependency is characterized by a series of physiologic events that occur when the drug is discontinued, including the withdrawal or abstinence syndrome. Tolerance develops when the continued use of a drug is required and increasing doses are needed to produce the same effect.

While the most important feature of addictive disorders is the psychologic dependency, it is the least understood of the three factors. A person can be made physically dependent on alcohol, but addiction or abuse may not be determined until behavioral effects secondary to psychologic dependence are present. Many persons consume alcoholic beverages but relatively few develop physical and psychologic dependency on the drug. The comparative risk of physical and psychological dependence and addiction are much greater with narcotics and other sedative-hypnotic drugs (barbiturates), than with alcohol. When the drug-dependent patients are detoxified, the physical symptoms of dependence (withdrawal syndrome and tolerance) are reversed, whereas this process will have little if any effect on the psychologic dependence.

The World Health Organization now recommends the use of the term drug-dependence in place of addiction and habituation.

PHARMACOLOGY

Alcohol is a psychoactive agent that can be characterized pharmacologically as a sedative-hypnotic drug. At low doses, the action of alcohol is an excitatory and stimulatory effect due to its depression of inhibitory centers in the brain. In a dose-response relationship, at sufficient doses, alcohol produces a depressant action. Although alcohol is able to provide anxiety relief and sedation at one dose level it produces sleep and depression of the central nervous system and respiratory system at higher levels.

Alcohol is present in a variety of popular beverages: beer and ale are products of the fermentation of cereals and contain 3 to 6% alcohol; wine is the result of the fermentation of yeast on sugars present in fruits and contains 11 to 20% alcohol; brandy is produced from the distillation of wine products and usually contains 40% alcohol; hard liquors are the distillates of fermented products such as grain, available as gin, rye, bourbon, scotch, and vodka, and contain approximately 40 to 50% alcohol by volume, commonly expressed by a proof number that is twice the alcohol concentration by volume.

METABOLISM

Alcohol is fully absorbed by the stomach and small intestine in 30 to 120 min after ingestion. Absorption is direct, by simple (passive) diffusion, and alcohol distributes freely in body tissues and fluids. The concentration of alcohol in the brain rapidly approaches that in the blood after completion of absorption. Factors that modify alcohol absorption are volume, dilution, rate of ingestion, and presence of food in the stomach. Interestingly, carbonation increases the absorption of alcohol. Alcohol crosses the placenta and may be found in the milk of lactating mothers.

The liver is the main site of the first step in the oxidation of ethyl alcohol. Ethanol is oxidized by alcohol dehydrogenase to acetaldehyde, which subsequently is oxidized by acetaldehyde dehydrogenase to acetate or acetyl coenzyme A. This enters the Krebs cycle to form carbon dioxide and water and also participates in protein and fat synthesis. Both oxidizing enzymes are responsible for converting nicotinamide adenine dinucleotide (NAD) to its reduced form, NADH, which contributes to the many metabolic abnormalities (e.g., hyperlipidemia, ketosis, hyperlactacidemia, hyperuricemia) associated with chronic alcohol ingestion. Acetaldehyde, the first metabolite of ethanol, may be more slowly metabolized in alcoholics and has been implicated in the pathogenesis of alcohol-induced tissue toxicity. A distinct microsomal ethanol-oxidizing system has also been characterized as having a major role in alcohol metabolism and may account for the observations that induction of microsomal enzyme activity can increase the clearance of alcohol and other drugs from the blood (11, 12).

Although most drugs are known to be metabolized or cleared from the body in a fixed percentage ("first order") of the dose taken, alcohol is unique in that it is eliminated from the blood in a fixed amount ("zero order") over time (13). Most of an ingested dose of alcohol is eliminated by liver metabolism. In a 70-kg (approximately 150-lb) person, the rate of alcohol metabolism approximates 7 g per hour. At this rate of metabolism, the blood alcohol level will decline at a rate of nearly 15 mg/100 ml/hour. An average "shot" of distilled spirit, 86 proof, contains about 15 g of ethyl alcohol; because body water approximates 65% of body weight in a 70-kg person, the blood ethyl alcohol content after one "shot" will be 15 g/50 liters, or 30 mg/100 ml, with 50 liters being the approximate volume of total body water calculated from the percentage of weight. If taken in one swallow, it will take approximately 2 hours for the blood ethyl alcohol level to return to zero. A 70-kg person would have a blood ethanol concentration of 100 mg/ml (the amount legally defined as intoxication in most states) after drinking, within 1 hour, any of the following: 5 12-oz cans of beer, 4 4-oz glasses of table wine, 5 1-oz glasses of liqueur, 5 1-oz shots of distilled spirits, or 3 3-oz martinis.

Exercise or administration of thyroid hormone, oxygen, glucose or multivitamins does not increase the rate of alcohol oxidation. Whether or not there are ethnic differences for developing tolerance to alcohol is unclear. There are no racial differences in the rate of alcohol metabolism to explain why there might be such an occurrence (14).

BLOOD ALCOHOL CONCENTRATIONS AND INTOXICATION

The relationship between blood ethyl alcohol concentration and clinical signs and symptoms of intoxication are variable and depend on rate of ingestion, amount consumed, alterations in absorption, metabolism, excretion, and chronicity of exposure (Table 5.1). The correlation of the blood alcohol concentration to behavioral effects has obvious significant medical and legal importance. As a consequence of tolerance, higher blood alcohol concentrations may be required to produce clinical effects in alcoholics than in occasional drinkers. The lethal blood alcohol level is variable but in the range of 400 to 700 mg/100 ml.

DIAGNOSIS OF ALCOHOLISM

The diagnosis of alcoholism is difficult because there is little agreement on the defini-

Table 5.1.
Blood Ethanol Concentrations and Clinical Effects in the Nontolerant Adult Drinker

Blood Ethanol Level (mg/100 ml)	Clinical Effects
20–99	Slight changes in mood and feelings progressing to muscular incoordination, impaired sensory function, personality and behavioral changes (talkative, noisy, morose)
100–199	Marked mental impairment, incoordination, clumsiness and unsteadiness in standing or walking, ataxia, prolonged reaction time, gross intoxication
200–299	Nausea, vomiting, diplopia, marked ataxia
300–399	Hypothermia, severe dysarthria, amnesia, stage 1 anesthesia
400–700	Coma, respiratory failure, and death

tion of alcoholism. The clinical signs and subtleties of the condition are varied, elusive, and without reliable parameters. Much depends on the experience and motivation of the observer in deciding whether a patient is suffering from alcoholism or not. Although not absolute, the criteria established by the National Council on Alcoholism (NCA) can serve as a convenient starting point for the diagnosis of alcohol dependence (15). These diagnostic criteria (Table 5.2) are of three kinds: (a) the classic criteria, considered definitive and obligatory, (b) a group of criteria frequently indicative of alcoholism, and (c) criteria indicating potential alcoholism or incidentally associated with alcoholism.

Early identification of an existing alcohol problem is important because the prognosis from treatment is much more promising when the difficulty is recognized early in its course (16). Clues that can provide early recognition can be found in demographic, social, familial, and cultural characteristics of alcohol consumers (Table 5.3). Awareness of the physical signs and symptoms of alcoholism at its earliest stages is also important.

The largest proportion of alcohol consumed in the United States is in the form of beer (46%) followed by distilled spirits (42%) and wine (12%). Comparison of consumption trends in the United States with 24 other countries where this information is available reveals that only 2 countries (West Germany and Italy) now outrank the United States in per capita consumption of distilled spirits (1).

ADVERSE EFFECTS FROM ALCOHOL

Alcoholics have an alarmingly high incidence of diseases and disorders. Alcohol effects almost every organ system in the body. The more important and known medical *complications* and pathologic consequences from excessive alcohol consumption are summarized in Table 5.4

ALCOHOLIC LIVER DISEASE

The risk of developing alcoholic liver disease is related to the quantity and duration of alcohol consumption. Factors such as genetics, nutritional state, and environment also predispose to the development of alcoholic liver disease (17–25, 54–56). Alcoholic fatty liver disease is the most common alcohol-induced he-

Table 5.2.
Summary of Diagnostic Criteria of Alcoholism (15)

A. Major criteria (definitive, obligatory: it is sufficient for the diagnosis of alcoholism that any of these criteria be fulfilled)

Physiologic conditions: (a) use of alcohol results in withdrawal symptoms upon cessation of drinking, e.g., gross tremor, hallucinations, seizures, delirium tremens; (b) use of alcohol results in tolerance, i.e., blood level of 150 mg/100 ml without apparent intoxication; a level of 300 mg/100 ml or more at any time, or a history of regular ingestion of 1 fifth of distilled spirits or 2 quarts of fortified wine or 3 quarts of table wine or 23 12-oz bottles of beer or equivalent in 1 day for a 70-kg (150-lb) person

Clinical conditions: use of alcohol results in diagnosable alcohol-related organ damage, e.g., alcoholic hepatitis or alcoholic cerebellar degeneration

Behavioral conditions: blatant and indiscriminate alcohol use continued in spite of medical and social contraindications, e.g., alcohol-related organ damage or social and psychologic disruption

B. Minor criteria (probable strong suspicion of alcoholism if several criteria are present

Physiologic and clinical conditions: use of alcohol results in amnesia ("blackout" periods), fatty liver in absence of other possible causes, pancreatitis with cholelithiasis, chronic gastritis, peripheral neuropathy, alcoholic myopathy, or cardiomyopathy

Behavioral conditions: constant and repetitive use of alcohol results in drinking alone; spouse complains about drinking; surreptitious use of alcohol; admits to drinking more than peers; outbursts of rage and suicidal gestures while drinking; loss of interest in activities not directly associated with drinking; repeated attempts at abstinence; "skid-row" social behavior

C. Minor criteria (possible manifestations are common in many persons but are not in themselves strong indicators of alcoholism; suspicion should be aroused and further evidence sought)

Physiologic and clinical conditions: patient presents with unexplained hypoglycemia, serum lactic acid and uric acid elevation, potassium and chloride depletion, SGOT elevation, EEG abnormalities, hyperreflexia or hyporeflexia, hematologic abnormalities (anemia), beriberi, scurvy, pellagra, decreased immune response, or increased incidence of infections

Behavioral conditions: patient presents with unexplained depression, paranoia, frequent accidents, major family disruptions, job loss, increasing interpersonal difficulties, employment choice that facilitates or encourages drinking, gulps drinks

Table 5.3.
Characteristics Associated with Alcohol-related Problems (1)

Most Likely to Have a Drinking Problem	Lower Risk
Male	Women*
Ages 18–20; 35–39	Farmers
Semiprofessional	< than 8th grade education
Middle socioeconomic level	Lower socioeconomic level
Separated, single, or divorced persons	Age greater than 50 years
Army, military	Married or widowed persons
Polydrug abuser	Residents of rural areas
Beer drinkers	Residents of the South
Residents of cities	Mostly drink wine
History of childhood disjunctions	

* Trend is toward increasing use.

patic abnormality, occurring in 90 to 100% of chronic alcoholics.

The postulated *mechanism* for fatty accumulation in the liver is that an increase in the NADH:NAD ratio during ethanol oxidation is responsible for accumulation of hepatic triglycerides (54). Uncomplicated fatty liver is usually asymptomatic, rarely presenting with usual signs of liver disease such as ascites, jaundice, or splenomegaly. Mild elevation of liver enzymes is the most frequent laboratory finding.

Alcoholic *hepatitis* is a much more serious disorder, 10 to 30% of alcoholics develop this syndrome, usually after years of excessive drinking or after an abrupt increase in alcohol intake. The clinical course of alcoholic hepatitis ranges from acute or chronic asymptomatic, mild, severe, and fulminant forms. It is often an incidental diagnosis when hepatomegaly and mild elevations in results of liver function studies are detected during a physical examination. Some patients who develop the fulminant course will rapidly progress to liver failure. The death rate in cases of severe alcoholic hepatitis is substantial. Approximately half of the survivors subsequently progress to development of cirrhosis of the liver.

The pathogenesis of alcoholic *cirrhosis* has

Table 5.4.
Complications of Alcoholism (Superior Numbers Are References)

Complication	Usual Onset	Comments
Increased morbidity and mortality[8]	Chronic	Most common causes cirrhosis, cancers of respiratory and gastrointestinal tracts, accidents, suicide, and ischemic heart disease
Fluid and electrolyte abnormalities[17–20]	Acute	Alcohol has diuretic action as blood alcohol concentration increases. Stable or decreasing blood alcohol concentrations result in antidiuresis. Hyperosmolarity, hypokalemia, hypophosphatemia, and hypomagnesemia are common. Mild lactic acidemia may contribute to asymptomatic elevation of uric acid due to interference with renal secretion of uric acid
Hypoglycemia[21, 22]	Acute or chronic	Alcohol depletes liver glycogen stores and decreases gluconeogenesis, blood sugar may drop precipitously. A dramatic but relatively uncommon complication.
Hyperglycemia	Acute	During early phases of alcohol withdrawal, blood sugar may be elevated because of increased release of catecholamines. Alcoholic pancreatitis and decreased peripheral glucose utilization are contributing factors
Hyperketonemia[23, 24]	Acute	Alcoholic patients frequently develop hyperketonemia and metabolic acidosis in the absence of hyperglycemia. Often the patient is hypoglycemic and without glycosuria. This is presumably due to alcohol-induced starvation ketosis. Insulin is not administered
Hypothermia	Acute	Occurs frequently as a result of prolonged exposure to cold (not uncommon in unconscious or stuporous state); pancreatitis and meningitis may also contribute
Liver disease[13, 25]		Best known sequela of chonic alcoholism and a leading cause of morbidity. Three common liver diseases often associated with alcoholism: acute fatty liver, alcoholic hepatitis, and alcoholic cirrhosis. Individual sensitivity is variable and degree of liver dysfunction does not appear to be related only to amount of alcohol ingested. Nutritional status, genetic composition, and immunologic factors appear to interact in development of alcoholic liver disease
a. Acute fatty liver	Acute	Develops in nearly all who ingest alcohol excessively (defined by some as an intake of at least 70 g ethyl alcohol daily) even for only a few days. Treatment: to stop drinking and give a diet with adequate vitamin and protein replacement
b. Alcoholic hepatitis	Acute or chronic	Apparently a toxic inflammatory response of liver in 10–30% of chronic or acute alcoholics. A high percentage who continue to drink with alcoholic hepatitis, develop cirrhosis within 5–10 yr. Most patients require 8–12 wk to show improvement from acute stage. Treatment is supportive, adequate diet, vitamin supplements, bed rest, and stop drinking. In severe cases, liver failure (hepatic coma), variceal bleeding, and hepatorenal syndrome often are present. Clinical features are similar to those of other forms of toxic or viral liver injury. Hepatomegaly, jaundice, splenomegaly, fever, and ascites are common. Corticosteroids may give benefit in fulminant cases, but their exact role in treatment of this disorder is still being investigated. Some studies have failed to show any benefit from their use
c. Alcoholic or Laennec's cirrhosis	Chronic	Symptoms frequently nonspecific in character, e.g., fatigue, weight loss, lethargy. Other physical signs include: slight hepatomegaly, splenomegaly, ascites, gy-

Table 5.4.—Continued

Complication	Usual Onset	Comments
		necomastia, spider angiomas, and palmar erythema. About 10–30% of alcoholics develop alcoholic cirrhosis, usually after drinking heavily for 10–15 yr. Three most common causes of death in alcoholic cirrhosis: bleeding esophageal varices, liver failure (encephalopathy and coma), and infection. Only treatment is to stop drinking
Portal hypertension	Acute or chronic	A sequela of hepatitis. Return of blood from abdominal viscera to heart is impaired as pressure rises, collateral blood vessels enlarge. All abdominal organs become congested; splenomegaly and ascites result
Ascites	Acute or chronic	Seen often in patients with portal hypertension and may be worsened by alcoholic liver disease and low serum albumin. Low sodium diet, spironolactone, and sometimes diuretics are helpful. As liver disease improves, ascites will often resolve. Careful monitoring of electrolytes must be done when diuretics and aldosterone antagonists are used
Esophageal varices	Acute	Thin-walled, collateral blood vessels of portal system are prone to hemorrhaging. Hemorrhage usually occurs when portal pressure rises because of expanded plasma volume, worsening liver involvement, or increased intraabdominal pressure. Thin walls and accompanying esophagitis are also contributing causes
Encephalopathy[26, 27]	Acute	Central nervous system is depressed by toxins, e.g., ammonia that reaches it through shunted blood that has bypassed liver. Patient usually is lethargic, has "flapping tremor," deterioration of fine movement, and unable to perform any purposeful activity before lapsing into coma. Central nervous system is more sensitive than usual to anoxia, sedative-hypnotics, opiates, or tranquilizers. Coma frequently precipitated by gastrointestinal hemorrhage, hypokalemia, infection or large amounts of nitrogen from dietary sources such as proteins
Gastrointestinal problems, e.g., pancreatitis, gastritis, peptic ulcer[28]	Acute or chronic	Acute pancreatitis occurs more commonly in alcoholics and is most often seen in persons who have been drinking heavily for 8–10 yr or more. Often no characteristic clinical picture except for abdominal pain is present. Nausea and vomiting are common. Is one of the more frequent causes for hospitalization of alcoholics following a drinking bout. Other manifestations of this condition include shock, hypocalcemia, hyperglycemia, marked fluid loss, or dehydration Acute gastritis, often hemorrhagic, is common in alcoholics. Made worse by chronic use of aspirin Incidence of peptic ulcer probably higher in alcoholics than nonalcoholics, but no definitive data support this impression. Tearing of gastroesophageal mucosa (Mallory-Weiss syndrome) with severe bleeding may occur as consequence of vomiting; this should be considered a medical and surgical emergency.
Malabsorption[28]	Chronic	Diarrhea after bout of drinking may cause temporary decreased absorption. Changes in gastrointestinal morphology and decreased enzyme activity in the intestinal tract have been observed in chronic alcoholic patients, even with adequate diet. Thiamine, vitamin B_{12}, folate, xylose, and fat malabsorption occur. Alcohol consump-

Table 5.4.—Continued

Complication	Usual Onset	Comments
		tion and poor diet are major contributors to malabsorption
Hyperlipidemia[29, 30]	Acute or chronic	Alcohol ingestion induces elevation of serum triglycerides in persons with Type IV hyperlipoproteinemia. Because alcoholic liver disease begins with fatty infiltrates, hypertriglyceridemia may be an early contributory factor to the hepatic and cardiac disorders from alcohol
Cardiomyopathies[31, 32]	Acute or chronic	Alcohol presumably affects the heart by depressing ventricular activity, reducing myocardial uptake or free fatty acids, enhancing uptake of triglycerides, or causing myocardial cell injury. Direct toxic effects of alcohol on myocardium, multiple vitamin deficiencies, inadequate protein intake, and electrolyte disturbances are all probably contributory
Myopathy[33–35]	Acute or chronic	Generalized and occasionally focal muscle weakness develops during or following heavy drinking bout. Muscle edema, pain, and cramps are common and may be accompanied by tenderness and edema. Elevated muscle enzymes may be accompanied by tenderness and edema. Elevated muscle enzymes (creatine phosphokinase and aldolase) may be present. In severe cases myoglobulinuria can occur. Mortality is significant (50%) when alcoholic myopathy occurs concomitantly with hyperkalemia and renal failure
Infection[36, 37]	Acute or chronic	Acute and chronic alcohol ingestion decreases resistance to bacterial infection especially in respiratory tract. Most pulmonary infection in alcoholics is due to *Pneumococcus*. Susceptibility to *Klebsiella* and *Haemophilus* organisms is also greater. Because they are debilitated, alcoholics are at higher risk of reactivated tuberculosis: has been claimed that 20% of patients with active tuberculosis are alcoholics. Aspiration pneumonia is also a major complication
Hematologic disorders, e.g., anemia, leukopenia, thrombocytopenia[38–42]	Chronic	Four major factors contribute to hematologic disorders: poor diet, blood loss, liver disease, and alcohol itself. Folate deficiency is probably the most important hematologic abnormality in alcoholics. Good diet alone cannot protect against bone marrow toxicity of alcohol if major portion of calories ingested is ethanol. Stopping of alcohol, nutritious diet including folic acid and multivitamins, and treatment of other medical complications nearly always will reverse hematologic abnormalities
Neurologic disorders, polyneuropathy[23, 43]	Chronic	A degenerative process of nerves secondary to nutritional deficiency is common with a long history of alcoholism. Clinical and pathologic features of polyneuropathy are almost identical with beriberi. Subjective sensory disturbances and loss of reflexes and motor activity occur. Recovery is slow and often incomplete, even with complete alcohol abstinence
Wernicke's disease	Acute or chronic	Clinical presentation includes ocular disturbances, e.g., nystagmus, muscle weakness or paralysis, diplopia, ataxia, disorientation, and confusion frequently accompanying signs of thiamine deficiency. Can be treated by giving thiamine.
Korsakoff's psychosis	Acute or chronic	Most apparent disturbance in this disorder is memory defect. Memory may be affected to exclusion of other components of mental function. Recent memory is affected most. Other clinical features often are confusion

Table 5.4.—Continued

Complication	Usual Onset	Comments
		and confabulation. Usually recovery is slow and incomplete, despite treatment with thiamine and other vitamins and cessation of drinking
Amblyopia	Chronic	Disorder of optic nerve occurring alone or in conjunction with other neuropathies; manifested by blurred vision
Skin disorders	Chronic	Skin disorders common (30–50%) in alcoholic patients can result from vitamin deficiency diseases such as scurvy or pellagra. Neglected skin disorders often result in secondary infections; seborrhea, lacerations, abrasions, acne, scabies and pediculosis are also frequent. When common skin conditions (e.g., psoriasis, eczema) are not responding to usual treatment measures, alcoholism may play a role
Teratogenesis[44–50]	Chronic	Multiple congenital defects, prenatal growth retardation, and delay in development are fetal abnormalities that result from heavy alcohol abuse during pregnancy
Neonatal intoxication and withdrawal[51–53]	Acute	Ethanol crosses the placental barrior freely. Clearance rate of alcohol is reduced in premature infants. Substantial impairment of motor activity, alertness, and respiration reported in neonates after ethanol infusion just before delivery
Cancer[1,8]	Chronic	Excessive use of alcohol combined with tobacco has been implicated in greater risks for cancers particularly of the mouth, pharynx, larynx, esophagus, and liver

not been determined completely. The liver is characterized as being finely nodular or grossly deformed, which may be smaller or larger than normal. Laboratory findings include hyperbilirubinemia, hypoalbuminemia, and prolonged prothrombin time. Complications from cirrhosis include encephalopathy, portal hypertension with bleeding at the esophageal varices, portal vein thrombosis, and hepatorenal syndrome.

Treatment of *hepatic encephalopathy* is to reverse the precipitating factors and lower serum ammonia levels. The immediate approach to bleeding esophageal varices is blood replacement, administration of vasopressin, and use of a Sengstaken-Blakemore tube if necessary. Surgery may be required to further decompress the varices by shunting the flow of hepatic portal circulation after the patient has stabilized. The development of the hepatorenal syndrome is a poor prognostic sign. This is characterized by sodium retention, progressively worsening oliguria, and eventually azotemia. There is no effective therapy.

ALCOHOL AND THE HEART

Recognition of alcoholic *cardiomyopathy* has been made difficult by its similarity to two other types of alcohol-related cardiomyopathies (57–59). Nutritional deficiency in thiamine can lead to an unusual type of cardiac disorder ("wet beriberi heart disease"), which is characterized by a state of high output failure, fluid retention, and cardiac dilatation. Another cause of cardiomyopathy is associated with excessive consumption of beers containing cobalt, an added foaming agent (60). There are patients with a history of alcoholism who have heart disease that is unrelated to either of these possible causes. There is increasing evidence that alcohol itself, acetaldehyde, or biogenic amines may produce chronic functional myocardial impairment.

ALCOHOL AND THE HEMATOPOIETIC SYSTEM

The association of *anemia*, *macrocytosis*, and alcoholism was long held to be attributable to nutritional deficiencies. Recent studies have shown that there is a direct role of alcohol on suppression of folate metabolism, depletion of folate from body stores, and malabsorption of folate (61–63). The direct toxicity of alcohol on erythropoiesis is demonstrated by vacuolation of erythroid and myeloid precursors. A sideroblastic or "iron-loading" anemia can result from alcohol's impairment of iron incorporation and metabolism in the red blood cell. Alcohol affects iron absorption by increasing jejunal absorption of iron, as reflected in hemochromatosis and a rise in serum iron levels. Iron deficiency anemia due to gastritis and to gastrointestinal bleeding can also occur. Alcoholic *thrombocytopenia* occurs in 25 to 30% of acutely ill alcoholics; platelets often have shorter than normal life spans and thrombopoiesis is ineffective because of marrow suppression and folate deficiency.

FETAL ALCOHOL SYNDROME

The relation between heavy alcohol consumption in pregnancy and fetal abnormalities has been suspected since antiquity. In 1973 Jones and Smith (47) described a unique clustering of fetal defects in offspring of mothers with chronic alcoholism as the fetal alcohol syndrome. Clarren and Smith (50) characterized this pattern of malformation as follows: 1) Prenatal and postnatal growth deficiency, 2) central nervous system dysfunction including physiologic depression, hypotonia, irritability and jitteriness, mental retardation, poor coordination and hyperactivity during childhood; 3) craniofacial abnormalities including short palpebral fissures, short upturned nose, hypoplastic philtrum, flat midface and thinned upper lip; and 4) other major organ system defects such as abnormalities of the eyes, ears and mouth, heart murmurs, septal defects, genitourinary abnormalities, hemangiomas and musculoskeletal problems such as hernias.

The reported incidence of fetal alcohol syndrome is rare, affecting 1 in 300 to 1 in 2000 infants (145). Approximately 450 cases have been documented in the world literature. Estimates of the proportion of women who drink heavily during pregnancy range from 2 to 13%, depending on the population studied and survey methodologies. There is evidence that the rate of heavy drinking among women is rapidly rising and approaching that seen in men. Heavy drinking by women may, in the future, exceed that in men. Furthermore, there may be a disproportionately large number of heavy users of alcohol among women of childbearing age relative to their proportion in the general population (146).

Many factors may influence the phenotypic outcome of pregnancy in the alcoholic mother including variable dose exposure at variable gestational periods, as well as the genetic background of the individual fetus. Alcohol, like other teratogens does not uniformly affect all those exposed to it. Rather there seems to be

a continuum of effects of alcohol on the fetus with increasingly severe outcomes generally associated with higher intakes of alcohol by the mother (147).

It should also be noted that alcohol readily enters breast milk, thereby providing alcohol to the nursing infant (148). There appears to be no established safe amount of alcohol or a safe time to drink it during pregnancy and *lactation*.

There have been numerous case reports and studies of alcohol use during pregnancy both in humans (149–152) and in animals (153–155). The limitations of these studies include variations in population characteristics, techniques for reporting alcohol consumption patterns and other outcome variables. Most of the studies lack adequate control groups and thus it is difficult to separate out direct effects of alcohol on the fetus from indirect effects by environmental, maternal and genetic factors. However, the numerous reports of fetal alcohol syndrome in these studies appear to be generally consistent in the findings that maternal alcohol abuse is related to adverse effects on fetal growth and development (156).

CLINICAL FEATURES OF ACUTE ALCOHOL ABSTINENCE (WITHDRAWAL) SYNDROME

An acute abstinence, or withdrawal, syndrome is a common problem experienced by the alcoholic when alcohol is discontinued abruptly; delirium tremens (DTs) is the most severe form (64–66). The severity of the withdrawal syndrome cannot always be predicted on the basis of the quantity or duration of alcohol ingestion. Although most patients experience only minor symptoms, described often as a "hangover," it is difficult to rule out the possibility that progressively more severe and even life-threatening withdrawal reactions may occur. The early physiologic and behavioral effects of acute alcohol abstinence experienced (8 to 36 hours after cessation of drinking) include tremors ("shakes"), increased blood pressure, pulse, respiration rate, and temperature, intermittent hallucinations, seizures ("rum fits"), sleep disturbance, and sweating. Late effects (1 to 6 days after cessation of drinking) may be severe tremors, marked agitation, profound disorientation and excitation, persistent hallucinations, marked sleep disturbance, fever, tachycardia, and other life-threatening complications.

Patients with delirium tremens are seriously ill. Although the mortality rate for this condition has decreased during the past 50 years, deaths from DTs still occur (variously estimated at 7 to 15%) particularly in patients with underlying or associated diseases such as pancreatitis, cirrhosis, gastrointestinal bleeding, pneumonia, or sepsis.

It should not be taken for granted that the intoxicated or bizarre behavior in alcoholics is an effect of alcohol; hyperosmolarity, hypomagnesemia, or hypoglycemia may be contributing to it.

The exact pathophysiologic mechanism for the acute alcohol withdrawal syndrome is uncertain. With hyperventilation and respiratory alkalosis, a corresponding rise in arterial pH and fall in serum magnesium takes place. Central nervous system excitability, altered sleep pattern, and other signs of withdrawal are experienced probably as a result of decreased cerebral blood flow and oxygen delivery to the brain and electrolyte imbalance.

MANAGEMENT OF ACUTE ALCOHOL ABSTINENCE SYNDROME

The object of *detoxification* is to remove alcohol from the body with as few withdrawal symptoms as possible. This process involves the substitution of a long-acting sedative-hypnotic drug for a shorter-acting one, alcohol (66). In the past 25 years, over 100 different drugs and drug combinations have been described in the medical literature on the treatment of acute alcohol withdrawal (65–72).

A recent review of studies that investigated the effectiveness of drugs in treating the withdrawal syndrome suggested that many such studies are poorly controlled and lack objective comparisons of effects (73). In carefully conducted studies drugs have not been shown to be necessarily or universally much more effective than placebos. The major benefit of the antianxiety agents may accrue to the nursing and medical staff as the patient is made more manageable.

Drug Therapy

BENZODIAZEPINES (DIAZEPAM, CHLORDIAZEPOXIDE, OXAZEPAM, CHLORAZEPATE)

The sedative-hypnotic drugs of this group when compared with others in this class of agents are longer-acting, safer, do not produce gastritis, and have antiseizure activity (74, 75). They are used also because of the convenient dose forms available. The usual therapeutic end point in the management of acute alcohol withdrawal symptoms is to produce a calmed but awake patient, using whatever doses are required to affect this end point.

The *pharmacokinetics* of these drugs in patients undergoing alcohol withdrawal or in patients with mild liver impairment have aroused a great deal of clinical and research interest (76, 77). In patients with alcoholic cirrhosis, the elimination of diazepam from the body is presumably decreased because of decreased clearance by the liver and increased tissue distribution. Because the major metabolites of all the benzodiazepines with the exception of oxazepam (Serax) are also psychoactive, accumulation of effects during chronic administration of this drug should be evaluated carefully in patients with cirrhosis. There is no evidence to suggest that any one of the benzodiazepines is better than another for use in acute detoxification. Most studies on use of benzodiazepines in this situation have been conducted with chlordiazepoxide (Librium). Oxazepam might be considered the drug of choice particularly in patients with liver disease who are likely to have impaired metabolism of these drugs, but it is available only in the oral form, which limits its usefulness in acute situations.

Dosage requirements of these drugs for detoxification are quite variable. The usual range for diazepam is 30 to 200 mg during the first 24 hours, but a few cases may require 1000 mg or more. It should be remembered that withdrawing alcoholics may require more sedative-hypnotic drug than other agitated patients, probably because of tolerance and decreased sensitivity. Some alcoholic patients are calmed by doses that would be severely depressive in nonalcoholic patients. Because dosage requirements are variable, no fixed dose schedule can be predicted for a given patient. In a patient undergoing a mild-to-moderate withdrawal syndrome, an initial oral dose of 20 mg diazepam can be administered orally, followed by 10 to 20 mg every 2 or 3 hours. However, elderly patients should receive only 10 mg initially, followed by doses every 4 to 6 hours if needed. The patient should be reevaluated and drug requirements reassessed every few hours until initial sedation is achieved and then at least daily during the maintenance phase. Standing orders for repetitive doses are not advisable. In cases of severe withdrawal, intravenous diazepam should be cautiously administered in a dose of 10 to 30 mg every 30 or more min until the patient is calm. Once calmed, a maintenance regimen of 10 to 20 mg can be given intravenously or orally as needed during the day and in the evening to enable sleep. Because of the risks of hypotension and respiratory depression the patient should be assessed before and periodically after every intravenous dose of a sedative-hypnotic drug. Intramuscular administration of the benzodiazepines should be avoided because of its slow and erratic absorption.

PHENOTHIAZINES

The major tranquilizers have not been shown to be any more effective than the sedative-hypnotic drugs and should not be used. They can result in increased incidence of seizures, extrapyramidal effects, and postural hypotention (68, 70). The syncope and arrhythmias that can result from these drugs can produce serious consequences in the acutely withdrawing alcoholic.

PHENYTOIN

Phenytoin has been advocated for routine use in acute alcohol withdrawal to prevent seizures, but there is no evidence that the drug actually prevents seizures associated with alcohol abstinence (78).

The seizures associated with acute alcohol withdrawal ("rum fits") are usually self-limiting and frequently do not require anticonvulsant medication (66, 79–81). The episode is brief, consisting usually (90%) of a single grand mal-like seizure, and only occasionally (10%) appears as a repeated flurry of seizures. This usually occurs in patients with a history of traumatic epilepsy or seizure onset in childhood or adolescence. In the postictal period following withdrawal seizures, only 9% show electroencephalographic abnormalities. In the acute situation during status epilepticus seizure activity, small doses (2 to 4 mg) of intravenous diazepam can be administered.

PARALDEHYDE

The difficulty in administering this drug, its variability in dose response, and current recommended use of safer drugs (e.g., benzodiaze-pines) should reduce the use of paraldehyde in treating alcoholic withdrawal (65). This traditional and once popular drug has been employed widely in the treatment of alcohol withdrawal. A major complication of this drug is metabolic acidosis, which can further complicate an already altered acid-base status. Intravenous administration has been associated with hypotension, pulmonary hemorrhage, depression of the respiratory center, and acute hepatic failure. Paraldehyde is primarily metabolized in the liver, and thus its potential for hepatotoxicity should be recognized when administered to a patient with an already significant degree of hepatic impairment. Oral or rectal administration causes local irritation of mucous membranes.

ETHANOL

The use of alcohol in the management of acute alcohol withdrawal symptoms in hazardous because of its short duration of action and the risk of continuing the metabolic, endocrine, and neurologic disturbances and pathologies.

ANTIHISTAMINES—HYDROXYZINE

These drugs have been recommended by some and are sometimes used, although clinical investigation suggests only equivocal therapeutic benefits. They are less effective in seizure control and their antianxiety effects have not been well established. Toxic doses of antihistamines may produce anticholinergic symptoms such as delirium that may be confused with acute alcohol withdrawal.

PROPRANOLOL

Theoretically a β-adrenergic blocking drug such as propranolol should be beneficial in preventing the adrenergic overactivity that occurs during alcohol withdrawal (71, 82). Carefully designed clinical investigations are still needed to assess the usefulness of this form of treatment for acute alcohol withdrawal, but some preliminary results are promising. Because propranolol can precipitate congestive heart failure, asthmatic attacks, and peripheral vascular insufficiency and mask the symptoms of hypoglycemia, benefits from its use should be weighed carefully against the risks before it can be considered in each case, as a possible therapeutic agent for acute alcohol withdrawal syndrome.

THIAMINE (VITAMIN B₁)

The most serious consequences of thiamine deficiency experienced by chronic alcoholics are neuromuscular effects (43). Wernicke's syndrome and Korsakoff's syndrome, characterized by ophthalmoplegia, ataxia, peripheral neuropathy, and progressive confusion, are manifestations of the deficiency. Thiamine is routinely administered intravenously (100 to 200 mg) to withdrawing alcoholics as a preventive measure. Furthermore, because glucose solutions are invariably administered to such patients, thiamine should be administered or deficient stores of thiamine may be further depleted as a result.

VITAMIN K

Vitamin K is used particularly in patients with alcoholic hepatitis or cirrhosis, because prothrombin production is frequently impaired.

FOLIC ACID

The moderate to severe anemia seen in alcoholics is usually of the megaloblastic type caused by folic acid deficiency (39, 40). A combined megaloblastic anemia and microcytic anemia indicating iron deficiency usually results from blood loss in addition to nutritional deficits (41).

FLUIDS, GLUCOSE, AND ELECTROLYTES

It is important to correct fluid and electrolyte, particularly sodium, potassium and magnesium, imbalances accompanying acute withdrawal (20, 83, 84). In some patients water is retained and renal resorption of sodium, potassium, and chloride is increased contrary to the notion that all acutely withdrawing alcoholics are dehydrated from the diuresis produced by alcohol.

FRUCTOSE

Several studies have demonstrated that intravenous administration of 10% and 40% fructose solutions, increases the rate of ethanol elimination and decreases the duration of acute intoxication (85, 86). However, side effects (e.g., lactic acidosis, hyperuricemia, fructose intolerance, gastrointestinal discomfort) make the use of fructose in the treatment of acute alcohol intoxication less than desirable

(87). Increasing the rate of clearance of alcohol from the body also leads to more rapid development of alcohol withdrawal symptoms.

Summary

The following considerations should be kept in mind when treating and caring for the alcoholic patient in the acute withdrawal phase. The acute alcohol wihdrawal syndrome and response to treatment both vary among alcoholic patients. Be suspicious of polydrug abuse in the chronic alcoholic because withdrawal from barbiturates or opiates is a further complication of therapy (88). Benzodiazepines are the drugs of choice for treating the acute alcohol withdrawal syndrome because they are distinctly safer than other medications. Consider the patient variables that influence the pharmacokinetics of benzodiazepines and assess the dose and route of administration accordingly. Taper the doses of the medication used to treat withdrawal symptoms to avoid delayed withdrawal symptoms. Avoid complete eradication of withdrawal symptoms since this may indicate overmedication. Search for medical and surgical illness that may worsen the acute withdrawal syndrome. Individualize all aspects of care and treatment. Nondrug factors such as staff attitude and ward environment can be effective in helping with the anxiety, insomnia, depression and other problems that often occur during acute detoxification. There is no evidence that drug therapy during acute alcohol detoxification modifies the outcome of long-term treatment of alcoholism. Detoxification is the first, not the final step in therapy for alcoholism. The most important factor in successful treatment of alcoholism is motivation of the patient to stop drinking.

ACUTE ALCOHOL INTOXICATION

The effects of acute alcohol intoxication and those from the alcohol abstinence syndrome should be distinguished and not treated as a single disorder. Intoxication from alcohol, like that of other sedative-hypnotics, is characterized by depressed tendon reflexes, slurred speech, staggering gait, stupor, and coma through a generalized depression of the central nervous system. Nystagmus and ataxia may also be present. Symptoms of acute intoxication are associated with elevated levels of alcohol in the blood, whereas the blood alcohol level during withdrawal is reduced.

The lethal dose of alcohol varies in adults: it ranges from 5 to 8 g per kg of body weight. In children this is lower, approximately 3 to 4 g per kg of body weight is considered at risk. The therapeutic index of alcohol is about 1:5, which is low in comparison with other sedative-hypnotic drugs. Diazepam (Valium) and chlordiazepoxide (Librium), for example, have a therapeutic index of approximately 1:7000. Occasionally alcohol substitutes such as methanol, or isopropyl alcohol are ingested. There are differences in the clinical manifestations following ingestion of these agents which distinguishes each (Table 5.5).

Diagnosis

The severity of the acute intoxication depends on the blood alcohol level and individual tolerance. Levels below 50 mg/100 ml or 0.05% rarely produce significant effects in adults. In children, signs of alcohol intoxication are often prominent at this level. The presence or absence of odor of alcohol on a patient's breath *cannot* be used to establish a diagnosis of alcohol intoxication. Unique odors should still be noted since they may offer a diagnostic clue as to the overall clinical condition of a toxic patient. The plasma osmolality

Table 5.5.
Toxicity of Alcohol and Alcohol Substitutes (Superior Numbers Are References)

Substance	Sources	Signs and Symptoms	Management
Ethanol (ethyl alcohol)	Found in solvents and beverages; toxic amounts usually ingested	Stupor, coma. A severe intoxication in children. Complicating concurrent problems: hypoglycemia, head injury, hepatic coma, pneumonia, pancreatitis	Treat coma and shock with volume replacement and vasopressors. In accidental overdose, activated charcoal useful only immediately after ingestion. Avoid analeptics. Support respiration, correct acid-base, electrolyte and temperature abnormalities. Dialysis may be useful
Methanol (methyl alcohol, "denatured alcohol")[89-91]	Found in solvents, denaturant and antifreeze; toxic amounts attained through inhalation and ingestion	Intractable metabolic acidosis and optic nerve injury can result in 12–24 hr after ingestion. Toxic metabolites are formic acid and formaldehyde. Find both metabolites in urine	Approximate lethal dose: 1–4 ml/kg in adult. Treat by administering intravenous ethanol to block the generation of toxic metabolites by alcohol dehydrogenase. Administer sodium bicarbonate. Peritoneal dialysis and hemodialysis can be useful
Isopropanol (isopropyl alcohol)[92-94]	Found in rubbing alcohol, solvents; toxic amounts attained through inhalation and ingestion	Severe hypoglycemia, acidosis, and coma; hypothermia and convulsions also occur. Infants and children at risk of hypoglycemia. Gastrointestinal irritant. Acetone in breath, urine, and serum in absence of hyperglycemia or glycosuria	Approximate lethal dose: 250 g for adult. Alkalinization to correct metabolic acidosis may be helpful. Manage primarily with support
Ethylene glycol[95-97]	Found in antifreeze	Clinical abnormalities of the central nervous and cardiopulmonary systems. Oxidation of ethylene glycol by alcohol dehydrogenase to oxalic acid and calcium oxalate, which precipitate in kidney. Oliguria and acute renal failure can occur	Approximate lethal dose: 100 mg for adult. Treatment by administration of intravenous ethanol. Alkalinization to correct metabolic acidosis and to solubilize calcium oxalate useful. Hemodialysis has been successful in removing ethylene glycol

can be a useful indicator since the relationship of osmolality with plasma alcohol is linear (125). A rise of approximately 22 milliosmoles/kg H_2O, reflects a 100 mg/100 ml or 0.1% increase in plasma alcohol. Concomitant conditions, such as trauma, infection, multiple drug use, will often complicate the recognition and assessment of an intoxicated patient; therefore the measurement or estimate of the blood alcohol level or comparable analysis of urine, saliva and expired air, is valuable for confirming alcohol intoxication and to establish an appropriate treatment plan in such cases.

Other toxicological tests, particularly for barbiturates and other sedative drugs, and also salicylates may be indicated to detect suspected commonly occurring poly drug toxicity. In addition, specific laboratory studies for liver function, renal function, serum electrolytes with particular attention to the potassium, magnesium, phosphate levels and the anion gap, arterial blood gases, blood ketone and glucose should be performed routinely. The urine should be examined for the appearance of any crystal-like material or myoglobin. An electrocardiogram should be taken and changes characteristic of abnormal calcium, magnesium and potassium levels or presence of hypoxia or hypothermia, should be recognized. An abnormal x-ray examination (kidney, ureter, and bladder) may offer useful clues to the identity of materials ingested in any possible multiple overdose involving an acutely alcohol-intoxicated patient. Some common drugs often taken in suicide attempts such as phenothiazines, tricyclic antidepressants, heavy metals including iron, arsenic and halides, iodides and bromides, chloral hydrate and enteric-coated tablets are radioopaque (126). X-rays of the skull and chest are also advisable at the time of initial examination.

Management

The basic treatment for acute alcohol intoxication is to maintain and support vital functions (i.e., maintain patent airway and adequate blood pressure, avoid aspiration) until no longer needed during the detoxification process, which takes from 7 to 10 days (13, 64–66). In the comatose patient, particularly if this involves accidental ingestion of alcohol by a child, acute alcoholic hypoglycemia and other possible causes of coma such as subdural hematoma should be ruled out. Central nervous stimulants should not be used. The major problems encountered in the management of acute alcohol intoxication are: (a) pneumonia; a leading cause of morbidity, (b) overhydration, and (c) complications from unnecessary therapeutic maneuvers.

The possible presence of alcohol should not be overlooked when evaluating a suspected acute case of drug intoxication. One study revealed that almost one of every five acute drug-overdosed patients in whom the presence of alcohol was unsuspected or thought to be insignificant were found to have significantly elevated blood levels of alcohol. The notion that acute alcohol intoxication is benign should be dispelled. Diagnosis of any drug intoxication should include a blood ethanol determination in addition to other laboratory tests.

Alcoholic coma is a life-threatening situation which usually responds well to supportive treatment. Establishment of a clear airway with assisted ventilation is essential in this condition. Oxygenation and volume replacement with intravenous fluids, generally improves the hypotension. In circumstances where recent ingestion of drugs is suspected, gastric lavage can be carefully performed in the unconscious patient with appropriate guarding of the airway to avoid the risk of aspiration. Emetics used to prevent the further absorption of drugs taken in an overdose should be employed with caution in any acutely intoxicated, but conscious alcoholic, since tearing of the gastroesophageal mucosa may occur as a life-threatening consequence of protracted vomiting.

A toxic psychosis associated with acute alcohol intoxication occasionally presents as an emergency situation. It is characterized by a markedly impaired sensorium with confusion, amnesia and disorientation. There is frequently a sudden onset of aggressive and hostile behavior with associated psychotic symptoms including hallucination and delusions. The treatment of this agitated phase can be accomplished with sedation to produce a calm, but still arousable condition. Benzodiazepines and haloperidol can be used judiciously in these circumstances.

ACUTE INTOXICATION FROM ALCOHOL SUBSTITUTES

Occasionally, alcohol substitutes such as methanol, ethylene glycol or isopropyl alcohol or paraldehyde are ingested. This is done perhaps for several reasons. Often the availability and low cost of products containing alcohol substitutes by comparison to alcoholic beverages, make it convenient for persons intent on drinking alcohol to seek out these products. Many are readily found around the home; they are sweet smelling and pleasant tasting, often colorless and appear innocuous enough to young children who might be attracted to them. Some are packaged in an attractive manner and not in childproof containers, thus contributing to risks of accidental ingestion. There are differences in the clinical manifestations following ingestion of these agents, which distinguishes each (see Table 5.5).

Methanol

Methanol is also referred to as methylalcohol, "wood" alcohol or "denatured" alcohol. It is used as a solvent and denaturant, and is found in canned heat, antifreeze, gasoline additives and paint removers. Toxic amounts of methanol can be attained systemically through either ingestion or inhalation of the vapors. Following ingestion, it is rapidly absorbed and distributed throughout the total body water, similar to ethanol. The toxic dose is extremely variable; as little as 4 ml has been reported to cause blindness, while no permanent impairment was demonstrated after an alleged 500 ml had been consumed. Methanol is metabolized by alcohol dehydrogenase enzymes in the liver to formaldehyde and formic acid. The rate of this process is independent of the dose and blood concentration and is approximately one-seventh the rate for ethanol metabolism. Formic acid accumulation is associated with the clinical symptoms experienced.

Methanol produces slight central nervous system depression; unlike ethanol, inebriation is not often observed (127). Intractable metabolic acidosis with significant anionic and osmolal gaps are experienced (128). Optic nerve and retinal injury from the toxic metabolites develop within 12 to 24 hours following acute exposure. An asymptomatic period of up to a day may follow an acute methanol poisoning before the onset of headache, nausea and vomiting. Severe abdominal pain, occasionally presumed mistakenly to be the result of ethanol-induced pancreatitis, is experienced. Central nervous system depression, coma and respiratory failure take place late in the course. Breath odor of alcohol or methanol is frequently not present. In the later stages of the intoxication, breath odor of formalin and Kussmaul respiration may be noticed. Visual disturbances will occur ranging in severity from mild diminished vision to total blindness, very often accompanied by photophobia, pain and conjunctival changes. Eye examination will show dilated, nonreactive pupils with optic disk hyperemia and retinal edema. The early recognition of the clinical presentation of acute methanol intoxication is commonly hampered by the effects from concomitant excessive ethanol ingestion.

Laboratory findings in acute methanol intoxication usually include significant metabolic acidosis, with a large anion gap and moderate ketonemia. Serum amylase is often markedly elevated. A significant leukocytosis is also part of this poisoning. Urine analysis will yield albuminuria with slight to moderate acetonuria. Differential diagnostic consideration would necessarily include: diabetic ketoacidosis, lactic acidosis, uremic acidosis, acute intoxication from ethylene glycol; paraldehyde, isoniazid, or salicylates. Detection of methanol and formic acid in the urine would be confirmatory evidence of methanol poisoning.

Early diagnosis and vigorous treatment of methanol poisoning can be sight-saving and life-saving. A methanol blood level determination can be obtained. It is estimated that for each 40 mg/100 ml of methanol in blood, there is an accompanying rise in plasma osmolality of 15 mOsm/kg H_2O. The plasma osmolality determination would therefore be a convenient and accessible means to determine presence of toxic levels of alcohols (128). Alkalinization to reverse the metabolic acidosis and administration of ethanol, either intravenously or by mouth, should be performed. Ethanol with its greater affinity for alcohol dehydrogenase, can competitively inhibit methanol's generation of its toxic metabolites. Blood ethanol levels of 100 mg/100 ml (or 100 mg%) or higher are required to saturate the liver enzyme alcohol dehydrogenase (129). The loading dose of intravenous or oral ethanol is 0.6 g/kg body weight, or about 40 g for a 70-kg person, to achieve this desired concentration of ethanol in the blood. This dose can be given conveniently by mouth with four 1-oz "shots" of 80-proof whiskey or intravenously as 500 ml of a 10% ethanol solution. In a comatose patient or a patient with variable ethanol absorption, as may be the case after activated charcoal administration, the intravenous route would be preferred. Maintenance doses of ethanol should average 7 to 10 g/hour or 109 mg/kg/hour. Hemodialysis is an effective method to treat methanol poisoning and should be initiated promptly where the blood methanol level is greater than 50 mg/ 100 ml (130, 131). The rapidity of blood methanol level reduction appears to be critical for a favorable outcome. Doses of ethanol required to maintain a blood level of 100 mg/100 ml should be increased to 237 mg/kg/hour. Therefore, a total of 17 g of ethanol must be given hourly during dialysis for a 70-kg person to satisfactorily maintain the desired ethanol blood level (128–133). Blood levels of ethanol should be monitored frequently until the methanol has been cleared from the blood.

If an acute ingestion of methanol has taken place within several minutes to hours from time of ingestion to treatment, such as in a child, methods should be employed to diminish further gastrointestinal absorption and removal by emesis or lavage. Respiratory and circulatory support should be established and maintained. Forced diuresis does not enhance elimination of either methanol or it metabolites. Experimental studies in animals recently suggest that folic acid deficiency can significantly enhance the systemic toxicity of formic acid (134). Since folic acid deficiency is not an uncommon disorder among chronic alcoholics, speculation that enhanced risks to the effects of methanol metabolites in this group has some basis for validity. Administration of folic acid may therefore be particularly helpful in some cases of acute methanol poisoning.

Ethylene Glycol

Ethylene glycol is a common ingredient of antifreeze solutions. It is rapidly absorbed when ingested. A potentially lethal quantity is often considered to be 100 ml. In children, much less has been associated with serious toxicity to the renal, cardiac, and central nervous system.

The initial symptoms of acute ethylene glycol poisoning are similar to those for acute ethanol intoxication except for differences in their onset and duration. The earliest signs of ethylene glycol intoxication is inebriation. Breath odor is conspicuously absent in persons who have ingested ethylene glycol alone. Central nervous system depression and gastrointestinal distress are experienced early in the course. During the first 12 hours, hypertension and leukocytosis are frequently encountered. Symptoms may progressively worsen until pulmonary edema, convulsions, respiratory failure and coma occur. Ethylene glycol itself is relatively non toxic, but its metabolic products are responsible for considerable toxicity. Severe metabolic acidosis, similar to that experienced with acute methanol poisoning is seen. Glyoxylic acid, oxalic acid and hippurate are the acid breakdown products of ethylene glycol which cause this profound acidosis (135). Contributing to this condition is also the overproduction and accumulation of lactate and other organic acids. Acute oliguric renal failure can occur. This is usually severe and believed to be irreversible, although survival from this condition has occurred (136). It is unclear whether the toxic damage to renal tubular epithelium is the direct result of ethylene glycol or the metabolites. There is marked renal pathology seen, including focal hemorrhagic necrosis, oxalate crystals in the convoluted renal tubules and epithelial cell destruction (136, 137). Calcium oxalate crystals, considered an important diagnostic marker for ethylene glycol poisoning, are frequently but not always encountered in the urine (136). Urinalysis normally will yield albumin, red blood cells and casts. The role of calcium oxalate crystals in the production of renal damage is probably a minor one. Myopathy is another common feature of ethylene glycol intoxication. Elevated muscle enzymes, such as creatine phosphokinase and a mild hypocalcemia are often seen. Searching for the signs of ethylene glycol toxicity usually described, is not often helpful for establishing early diagnosis. Blood ethylene glycol, if rapidly available, may be more useful. Serum osmolality can be used to provide an estimation of toxic ethylene glycol concentration. For every 50 mg/100 ml (50 mg%) of ethylene glycol, the plasma osmolality is exceeded by 10 mOsm/kg H_2O. A high anion and osmolal gap with metabolic acidosis is quite characteristic of this poisoning. Causes of death from ethylene glycol intoxication include central nervous depression, respiratory and cardiovascular failure. Treatment of acute ethylene glycol poisoning is focused on preventing its metabolism to the toxic metabolites and enhancing its elimination from the body (129, 138).

Ethanol inhibits the metabolism of ethylene glycol by competitively competing for alcohol dehydrogenase (139). A loading dose of ethanol to achieve a blood level of 100 to 150 mg/100 ml is initiated and then subsequent doses to maintain it for at least 24 hours, should be given. The monitoring and pharmacokinetic considerations of ethanol administration which has been described for methanol is applicable for ethylene glycol. The necessity for rapid treatment in ethylene glycol cannot be overstated. Since the half-life of ethylene glycol is approximately 3 hours, ethanol administration should be initiated promptly. Alkalinization should be attempted with cautious consideration for risks of volume overload and exacerbation of existing electrolyte imbalance (140).

Hemodialysis readily eliminates ethylene glycol and its metabolites from the body (140, 141). Blood ethylene glycol levels should be closely monitored since redistribution of the alcohol from tissue to the body water often occurs postdialysis. Repeated dialysis may be necessary to completely clear the ethylene glycol. If ethanol is concurrently administered, blood level determinations should also be routinely obtained in order to assess whether dosing adjustments are needed to maintain the desired level.

Support of vital functions such as ventilation, perfusion and volume are important as in all acute overdoses involving the alcohols. Emesis and lavage, whichever appropriate, should be attempted early in the course. Laboratory studies should include urinalysis for oxalates and myoglobin, arterial blood gases and electrolytes should also be determined. Urine output is measured, state of hydration, acid-base status and respiratory function need to be assessed frequently.

Isopropyl Alcohol

Isopropyl alcohol is commonly used as an antiseptic and solvent. Rubbing alcohol, which until recently was nearly always a 70% isopropyl alcohol solution, is an occasional source of childhood poisoning in the home. It is sometimes taken as a convenient substitute for ethanol by persons who are otherwise unable to obtain a suitable alcoholic drink. Lower concentrations of isopropyl alcohol can be found in various disinfectants, cosmetics, after-shave and skin lotions.

Isopropyl alcohol is rapidly absorbed following ingestion. Peak plasma levels with distribution throughout body fluids and tissues may be reached within an hour. With exception of children, skin absorption is insignificant. Inhalation of isopropyl alcohol vapors can produce considerable systemic absorption. Coma has been experienced by children who were bathed with excessive amounts of rubbing alcohol (142, 143). Isopropyl alcohol is metabolized by alcohol dehydrogenase enzymes in the liver to form acetone. Only 15% of this alcohol, when consumed, is eliminated as acetone via the saliva, lungs and kidneys. The remainder is further converted to acetate, formate and carbon dioxide. The rate of isopropyl alcohol metabolism to acetone is slower than that demonstrated for ethanol. Both isopropyl alcohol and acetone are central nervous system depressants. Tolerance to the toxic levels of both is experienced similar to the ethanol tolerance seen in chronic alcoholics. Toxic symptoms can occur with the ingestion of as little as 20 ml. Deaths from ingestion of 4 to 8 oz of 70% isopropyl alcohol, have been reported (142). The clinical effects of acute isopropyl alcohol intoxication are felt almost immediately after ingestion or significant exposure. The symptoms are similar to acute ethanol intoxication except for the absence of any early stimulatory phase. Dizziness, headache, confusion, flushing sensation, ataxia, stupor, hypothermia, and hypotension may be felt. Nausea, vomiting, diarrhea and severe gastritis occasionally accompanied with bleeding, are frequent. Children are often hypoglycemic. Concomitant ingestion of other sedative-hypnotic type drugs or ethanol, further complicates the neurologic and cardiovascular status of isopropyl alcohol intoxicated patients. Respiratory failure and death can occur within a few hours following a significant ingestion of isopropyl alcohol. Marked hypotension, renal and hepatic dysfunction are ominous predictors of a poor outcome on such occasions.

Volume for volume, the toxicity of isopropyl alcohol is considered twice that of ethanol. Toxic symptoms are noticed when blood isopropyl alcohol levels reach 50 mg/100 ml. In children, symptoms are likely to occur at even lower levels. Coma is associated with levels greater than 120 mg/100 ml. The range of blood levels between fatal and severe non-fatal intoxication is narrow. Acetonuria and acetonemia in the absence of glucosuria, hyperglycemia, or acidemia measured in an acutely intoxicated patient, should arouse suspicion of acute isopropyl alcohol poisoning. Blood level determinations and recovery of isopropyl alcohol in gastric contents should be considered diagnostically important and serve as a confirmation where poisoning is suspect. Unlike ethanol, there is no fixed relationship between the concentration of isopropyl alcohol in the blood and urine, therefore, blood level determination in such circumstances is necessary.

There is no specific treatment for acute isopropyl alcohol overdose. The usual methods for preventing further and continuous absorption, should be initiated, in addition to giving symptomatic and supportive treatment to maintain vital function. Forced diuresis is of little value. Hemodialysis has been shown to be life-saving in severe and unresponsive isopropyl alcohol poisoning (143). Repeated gastric lavage to prevent continued reabsorption of isopropyl alcohol has been reported to successfully reverse severe acute toxic symptoms. Use of serial activated charcoal may be effective in removing this alcohol. Many manufacturers of rubbing alcohol have recently begun to substitute ethanol for isopropyl alcohol, presumably because it is less toxic. Whenever dealing with a history of acute rubbing alcohol ingestion, determine which of these alcohols is in the product prior to treatment. A case of propylene glycol intoxication and lactic acidosis was recently reported (144). The patient, a 58-year-old man, with a history of chronic schizoprenia, was admitted to the hospital in stupor. Laboratory tests showed a metabolic acidosis with an anion gap of 28 mEq/liter and markedly elevated lactic acid. The patient's blood propylene glycol level was 70 mg/100 ml and 60 mg/100 ml in the urine. Propylene glycol is a chemical considered safe for use in food and cosmetics by the Food and Drug Administration. Previous cases have been described of children who became stuporous or experienced seizures after ingesting propylene glycol as a drug vehicle or cosolvent for vitamin therapy. The lactic acidosis produced is probably the result of excess propylene glycol metabolism. Bicarbonate therapy rapidly reversed the symptoms of intoxication and recovery was rapid and without sequela. Accumulation of propylene glycol, because of impaired renal clearance secondary to renal disease, was another explanation offered as the cause of this infrequent intoxication. A number of considerations should be kept in mind when treating and caring for the patient acutely intoxicated or overdosed with alcohol. The symptoms of acute alcohol intoxication and response to treatment vary among patients. Factors such as age, weight, tolerance and concomitant taking of other drugs, must be considered. Be suspicious of polydrug abuse in the adult with alcohol intoxication and be prepared for dealing with withdrawal from barbiturates or opiates as a further complication. In children, be aware of the toxicological effects of ingredients contained in alcoholic solutions, which are used for dealing with cough and colds, pain and allergic symptoms or for sleep. Search for medical and surgical illnesses that may contribute to the toxicological problems of acute alcohol poisoning. The basis of treatment should be to maintain and support vital functions. Individualize all aspects of care and treatment.

MANAGEMENT OF CHRONIC ALCOHOLISM

Although the period of detoxification is relatively short, it may take many months for the physiologic processes to return to normal. Treatment of the chronic alcoholic is enhanced by maintaining a prolonged alcohol-free period after detoxification. In managing the chronic alcoholic, the goal is to achieve and maintain sobriety or prolong the periods of sobriety to give the patient time to cope with the cause(s) of the excessive drinking (98, 99). It is commonly thought that alcoholism is primarily a manifestation of underlying psychiatric problems, and most methods of treatment and dealing with those problems will not succeed while the patient continues to drink. A variety of treatment approaches are available for management of chronic alcoholism including use of medications either alone or in combination with behavior-modification techniques.

Disulfiram

This drug is considered best used in the context of a close physician-patient or therapist-patient relationship with attempts at behavioral modification. Despite the fact that disulfiram has been available and used for more than 30 years, a consensus of its therapeutic utility has still not been developed. This is due in a significant way to methodologic problems inherent in studies in which there is a lack of accurate definitions for the stages of the disorder and an absence of a method to assess compliance.

MECHANISM OF ACTION

When administered alone, disulfiram is relatively nontoxic, but in the presence of alcohol it alters alcohol metabolism. Disulfiram causes an increase in the blood acetaldehyde levels by interfering with acetaldehyde dehydrogenase action, producing an acetaldehyde syndrome (100). It also inhibits dopamine-β-hydroxylase leading to the release and depletion of norepinephrine stores. The patient becomes flushed and develops a scarlet appearance; as the vasodilation continues, palpitations, hyperventilation, headache, tachycardia, and hypotension occur. Respiratory difficulty, nausea, vomiting, blurred vision, and vertigo may also occur. The reaction may be produced by as little as a few milliliters of alcohol and can last from 30 min to several hours (101).

TREATMENT OF THE DISULFIRAM-ALCOHOL REACTION

The intensity and duration of symptoms are related to the disulfiram dosage, the amount of alcohol consumed and individual sensitivity. Although the disulfiram-alcohol reaction is usually short-lived and without major sequelae, death can occur. In many fatal cases, the disulfiram dosage was excessive, but in others there was no apparent explanation. In these inexplicable cases, the causes of death were intracranial hemorrhage, acute myocardial infarction, cardiac arrhythmia, pulmonary edema, and cerebral edema (101, 102).

There are reports of antidotal treatment of the disulfiram-alcohol reaction with ascorbic acid, iron salts, or antihistamines, but the results are not definitive. Use of intravenous administration of ascorbic acid (0.5 to 2.0 g) is based on experimental evidence that ascorbic acid appears to reverse the disulfiram inhibition of cellular oxidation. However, nonspecific supportive measures, such as placing the patient in Trendelenburg posture, administration of oxygen, infusion of fluids and solutes, and (if needed) vasopressor agents, are more beneficial than the unproved use of these questionable antidotes (101). Table 5.6 summarizes the special factors to be considered in the use of disulfiram.

PHARMACOKINETICS

Disulfiram is rapidly absorbed from the gastrointestinal tract; it achieves full pharmacologic action in approximately 12 hours. Disul-

Table 5.6.
Considerations in the Use of Disulfiram

Assessment	Management	Evaluation
1. Assess for informed consent, motivation, social stability	1. Adequate blood level may take up to 4 days, although effect begins within 12 hr. The effect may last up to a week after discontinuation of disulfiram	1. Check for side effects (usually transient, lasting 2 weeks), drowsiness, fatigue, impotence, acneform eruption, metallic taste
2. Persons with moderate-to-severe hypertension, psychiatric problems, suicidal ideation should not receive this drug		2. Nausea and vomiting, dizziness, headache, hypotension, syncope, and flushed face in disulfiram-alcohol reaction
3. Interview patient	2. Metallic taste may cause anorexia; good oral hygiene may decrease taste	
	3. Tell patient to avoid alcohol; give list of OTC drugs and foods containing alcohol	3. Check for other medications being taken; i.e., phenytoin, barbiturates, isoniazid, metronidazole, or warfarin. Disulfiram can potentiate their therapeutic or toxic effects
	4. Paraldehyde may cause reaction, and should not be given	
	5. Give with caution concurrently with central nervous system depressants; may potentiate their effects	
	6. Patient should carry appropriate identification for this drug	

firam is eliminated slowly; approximately 20% still remains in the body after a week.

ADVERSE EFFECTS

Although disulfiram is relatively safe in most cases, it can cause acneform eruptions, fatigue, tremor, restlessness, impotence, and a garlicky or metallic taste in the mouth. With large doses, psychologic depression occurs probably as a result of interference in dopamine-β-hydroxylase activity in the brain. Disulfiram has also been shown to retard the metabolism of oral anticoagulants, isoniazid, and other drugs (103–106) (Table 5.6). Any patient receiving disulfiram should be warned to avoid medications that contain alcohol, particularly over-the-counter preparations such as some cough and cold medicines, tonics, antihistamines, body and shave lotions, colognes, after shave lotions, mouthwashes, and alcohol sponges (Table 5.7).

DOSAGE

The usual initial dosage of disulfiram is 250 to 500 mg/day for 5 to 7 days. The dosage may then be reduced to 125 to 250 mg/day (Table 5.6).

Sedative-Hypnotic Drugs

Anxiety, depression, and insomnia are common experiences for chronic alcoholics. Under most circumstances, these symptoms can be treated supportively, without psychotropic medications. The indiscriminate prescribing of antianxiety agents is all too frequent and has a high abuse potential in the alcoholic population. There is no evidence to support outpatient use of psychotropic drugs in the treatment of alcoholism. The use of placebos for relief of anxiety may be worthwhile when basic behavioral problems are dealt with concomitantly.

Tricyclic Antidepressants

Tricyclic antidepressants for patients in need of therapy for chronic and severe depression should be considered only after careful evaluation of the patient. Tricyclic antidepressant drugs are too frequently a convenient means of suicide in the depressed alcoholic patient. When antidepressants are prescribed for an alcoholic patient, the patient should be warned that the concomitant use of alcohol or other central nervous depressing agents with these drugs will produce severe impairment of motor and sensory function.

Lithium

It has been suggested that lithium, which is indicated for manic depressive disorders, may prevent the progress of primary alcoholism; however, further evidence in large populations is needed (72, 108). Lithium may also be an effective medication for the treatment of the acute alcohol withdrawal syndrome. Subjective symptoms of alcohol withdrawal appear to ameliorate when lithium is administered before discontinuation of the alcohol. The mechanism is unknown because patterns of catecholamine release, heart rate, blood pressure, and dopamine-β-hydroxylase are not affected.

Diet

Malnutrition is commonplace among alcoholics (109). Chronic alcohol consumption results in impaired digestion and absorption of essential nutrients. Nearly all alcoholics have diminished food intake while drinking because alcohol presumably suppresses appetite. *Nutritional problems* that alcoholics are most susceptible to are deficiencies of protein, water-soluble vitamins, and minerals. Many symptoms and signs of these deficiencies are readily recognized (110) (Table 5.8).

Accumulation of fluids with resultant ascites are frequent complications of alcohol cirrhosis. They are secondary to nutritional, endocrine, and metabolic disorders, resulting from alcoholism. The basis of management is to supply a normal or fortified diet with restricted sodium intake to replace only daily losses. "Hidden sources" of sodium such as intravenously administered fluids including plasma and drugs may be responsible for unexpected reaccumulation of fluids in these patients. Careful monitoring for problems that are related to nutritional balance of the hospitalized alcoholic patient is essential for successful management and care.

Nondrug Treatment Methods

Several techniques for behavioral modification are used with the chronic alcoholic. Individual psychotherapy is useful in those pa-

Table 5.7.
Alcohol Content of Nonprescription and Prescription Preparations Listed by Brand Name (Topical Agents Excluded) (107)

Brand Name	Alcohol Content (%)	Distribution Status[a]
Accurbron Liquid	7.5	Rx
Actol Expectorant	12.5	OTC
Acutuss Expectorant w/Codeine	5	C-V
Adatuss DC Expectorant	5	C-III
Airet G. G. Elixir	17	Rx
Alamine Expectorant	5	C-V
Alamine Liquid	5	OTC
Alamine-C Liquid	5	C-V
Almebex Plus B12 Syrup	10	OTC
Alurate Elixir	20	C-III
Alurate Elixir Verdum	20	C-III
Ambenyl-D Decongestant Cough Formula	9.5	OTC
Ambenyl Expectorant	5	C-V
Aminobrain PT Elixir	5	Rx
Amogel PG Suspension	5	CV
Amytal Elixir	34	C-II
Anatuss w/Codeine Syrup	12	C-V
Anatuss Syrup	12	Rx
A-Nil Expectorant	5	C-V
Antispasmodic Elixir	23	Rx
Anti-Tuss DM Expectorant	3.5	OTC
Anti-Tuss Syrup	3.5	OTC
Antrocol Elixir	20	Rx
Artane Elixir	5	Rx
Asbron G Elixir	15	Rx
Asma Syrup	10	Rx
Asmalix Elixir	20	Rx
Atarax Syrup	0.5	Rx
Atuss Syrup	3.5	C-III
Atuss-G Liquid	3.5	C-III
Atussin Expectorant	5	OTC
Bactalin Mouthwash	14	OTC
Barbidonna Elixir	15	Rx
Bayapap w/Codeine Elixir	7	C-V
Bayer Cough Syrup for Children	5	OTC
Benachlor (Improved) Cough Syrup	5	Rx
Benadryl Elixir	14	Rx
Bendylate Elixir	14	Rx
Bentyl w/Phenobarbital Syrup	19	Rx
Benylin Cough Syrup	5	Rx
Benylin DM Cough Syrup	5	OTC
Betalin Complex Elixir	17	OTC
Betalin S Elixir	10	OTC
Bewon Elixir	16	OTC
Black-Draught Syrup	5	OTC
Bowtussin Syrup	3.5	OTC
Breacol Liquid	10	OTC
Bromalix Elixir	2.3	Rx
Bromanyl Expectorant	5	C-V
Bromophen Elixir	2.3	Rx
Bromotuss Expectorant w/Codeine	5	C-V
Bromphen Elixir	3	OTC
Bromphen Expectorant	3.5	Rx

Table 5.7.—_Continued_

Brand Name	Alcohol Content (%)	Distribution Status[a]
Brompheniramine Compound Elixir	2.3	Rx
Brondecon Elixir	20	Rx
Brondelate Elixir	20	Rx
Bronkodyl Elixir	20	Rx
Bronkolixir Elixir	19	OTC
Brown Mixture	10	C-V
Butabarbitol Sodium Elixir	7	C-III
Butalan Elixir	7	C-III
Butazem Elixir	7	C-III
Butibel Elixir	7	Rx
Butisol Sodium Elixir	7	C-III
Calcidrine Syrup	6	C-V
Carbodec DM Syrup	<0.6	Rx
Caripeptic Liquid	18	OTC
Cenalene Elixir	15	Rx
Cepacol Mouthwash	14	OTC
Cerose DM Expectorant	2.5	OTC
Cetro-Cirose Liquid	1.5	C-V
Cheracol D Cough Syrup	4.75	OTC
Cheracol Syrup	3	C-V
Chlor-Mal Syrup	7	OTC
Chlor-Trimeton Expectorant	Not more than 1	OTC
Chlor-Trimeton Syrup	7	OTC
Choledyl Elixir	20	Rx
Citra Forte Syrup	2	C-III
Clistin Elixir	7	Rx
Coco-Quinine Suspension	4	OTC
Codehist DH Liquid	5	C-V
Codel AD Syrup	5	C-V
Codimal DM Syrup	4	OTC
Codistan No. 1 Liquid	1.4	OTC
Co-Histine DH Elixir	5	C-V
Co-Histine Expectorant	7.5	C-V
Colace Syrup	1	OTC
Cologel Liquid	5	OTC
Colrex Compound Elixir	9.5	C-V
Colrex Cough Syrup	4.5	OTC
Comtrex Liquid	20	OTC
Consotuss Antitussive Syrup	10	OTC
Contac Jr. Liquid	10	OTC
Coricidin Children's Cough Syrup	0.5	OTC
Coricidin Cough Syrup	<0.5	OTC
Corlin Infant Liquid Drops	<1	Rx
Corrective Mixture W/Paregoric Suspension	2	C-V
Corrective Mixture Suspension	1.5	OTC
Coryban-D Cough Syrup	7.5	OTC
Cosanyl Cough Syrup	6	C-V
Cosanyl-DM Syrup	6	OTC
Cotussis Cough Syrup	20	C-V
CoTylenol Cold Formula Liquid	7.5	OTC
CoTylenol Liquid for Children	8.5	OTC
Co-Xan (Improved) Syrup	10	C-V
C-Tussin Expectorant	7.5	C-V
Cytellin Suspension	.95	Rx

Table 5.7.—*Continued*

Brand Name	Alcohol Content (%)	Distribution Status[a]
DayCare Liquid	7.5	OTC
Decadron Elixir	5	Rx
Decohist Syrup	7.5	OTC
Deconamine Elixir	15	Rx
Dehist Elixir	5	OTC
Demazin Syrup	7.5	OTC
De-Tuss Liquid	7.5	Rx
Detussin Expectorant	12.5	C-III
Dexedrine Elixir	10	C-II
Dextro-Tuss GG Cough Syrup	1.4	OTC
Diahist Elixir	14	Rx
Dialixir Elixir	10	Rx
Dia-Quel Liquid	10	C-V
Dilantin-125 Oral Suspension	<0.6	Rx
Dilantin-30 Pediatric Oral Suspension	<0.6	Rx
Dilaudid Cough Syrup	5	C-II
Dilor Elixir	18	Rx
Dimacol Liquid	4.75	OTC
Dimetane Decongestant Elixir	2.3	OTC
Dimetane Elixir	3	OTC
Dimetane Expectorant	3.5	Rx
Dimetane Expectorant-DC	3.5	C-V
Dimetapp Elixir	2.3	Rx
Diphen Elixir	14	Rx
Diphenadril Syrup	5	Rx
Diphenallin Cough Syrup	5	Rx
Diphen-Ex Syrup	5	Rx
Diphenydramine Elixir	14	Rx
Diuril Oral Suspension	0.5	Rx
Dolanex Elixir	23	OTC
Donnagel-PG Suspension	5	CV
Donnagel Suspension	3.8	OTC
Donna-Phenal Elixir	23	Rx
Donna-Sed Elixir	23	Rx
Donnatal Elixir	23	Rx
Dorcol Pediatric Cough Syrup	5	OTC
Doxinate Solution	5	OTC
Dramamine Junior Syrup	5	OTC
Dri-Drip Liquid	3	OTC
Dristan Cough Formula Liquid	12	OTC
Duoprin-S Syrup	12	OTC
D-Vaso-S Elixir	18	Rx
Effacol Cough Formula	10	OTC
Eldadryl (Revised) Cough Syrup	7.6	Rx
ELdatapp Liquid	2.3	Rx
Eldertonic Liquid	13.5	Rx
Elixophyllin Elixir	20	Rx
Elixophyllin-KI Elixir	10	RX
Endotussin-NN Pediatric Syrup	4	OTC
Endotussin-NN Syrup	4	OTC
Enoxa Liquid	15	C-V
Entex Liquid	5	Rx
Ephedrol w/Codeine Liquid	3	C-V
Feosol Elixir	5	OTC
Fergon Elixir	6	OTC

Table 5.7.—Continued

Brand Name	Alcohol Content (%)	Distribution Status[a]
Ferrous-G Elixir	8	OTC
Fluorigard Rinse	6	OTC
Formula 3 Cough Mixture	10	OTC
Formula 44 Cough Mixture	10	OTC
Fumaral Elixir	5	OTC
Fynex Cough Syrup	5	Rx
2/G-DM Liquid	5	OTC
2/G Syrup	3.5	OTC
Ganatrex Elixir	15	OTC
Geravite Elixir	5	Rx
Genetuss Syrup	3.5	OTC
Geralix Liquid	15	OTC
Geriliquid Liquid	5	Rx
Gerilite Elixir	12	OTC
Geriplex-FS Liquid	18	OTC
Geritol Liquid	12	OTC
Geritonic Liquid	20	OTC
Gerix Elixir	20	OTC
Gerizyme Liquid	18	OTC
Geroniazol Elixir	12	Rx
Gevrabon Liquid	18	OTC
G G-CEN Syrup	10	OTC
g.g.i. Expectorant Liquid	5	Rx
G. G. Syrup	3.5	OTC
G-Tussin Syrup	3.5	OTC
GG-Tussin Syrup	3.5	OTC
Glybron Elixir	15	Rx
Glydeine Liquid	3.5	C-V
Glydm Liquid	1.4	OTC
Halenol Elixir	7	OTC
Halls Cough Syrup	22	OTC
Henotal Elixir	25	C-IV
Hexadrol Elixir	5	Rx
Histadyl E.C. Syrup	5	C-V
Histalet X Syrup	15	Rx
Histatapp Elixir	2.3	Rx
Hista-Vadrin Syrup	2	OTC
Histine Compound Expectorant	7.5	C-V
Histor-D Syrup	2	Rx
Histrey Syrup	7	Rx
Homicebrin Liquid	5	OTC
Hybephen Elixir	16.5	Rx
Hycotuss Expectorant	10	C-III
Hydergine Liquid	30	Rx
Hyonatol-B Elixir Improved	20	Rx
Hytinic Elixir	10	OTC
Iberet Liquid	1	OTC
I.L.X. B_{12} Elixir	8	OTC
Incremin with Iron Syrup	0.75	OTC
Infantol Pink Liquid	2	C-V
Isoclor Expectorant	5	C-V
Isogen Compound Elixir	19	Rx
Isolate Compound Elixir	19	Rx
Isuprel Compound Elixir	19	Rx

Table 5.7.—*Continued*

Brand Name	Alcohol Content (%)	Distribution Status[a]
Kaochlor 10% Liquid	5	Rx
Kaochlor S-F Liquid	5	Rx
Kaodonna PG Suspension	5	C-V
Kaomead w/Belladonna Suspension	3.8	OTC
Kaomead PG Suspension	5	C-V
Kaon-Cl 20% Liquid	5	Rx
Kaon Liquid	5	Rx
Kao-Nor Liquid	4.5	Rx
Kapectolin PG Suspension	5	C-V
Kay Ciel Liquid	4	Rx
Kaylixir Liquid	5	Rx
Kenpectin-P Suspension	6	C-V
KK-20 Liquid	5	Rx
Kloride Liquid	5	Rx
Klorvess 10% Liquid	1	Rx
K-Phen Expectorant w/Codeine	7	C-V
Lanophyllin Elixir	20	Rx
Lanoplex Elixir	11	OTC
Lanoxin Elixir, Pediatric	10	Rx
Lapav Elixir	10	Rx
Larylgan Throat Spray	1	OTC
Levsin Drops for Infants	5	Rx
Levsin Elixir	—[b]	Rx
Levsin w/Phenobarbital Elixvir	5	Rx
Liquitussin-AC Syrup	3.5	C-V
Liquitussin DM Syrup	1.4	OTC
Liquophylline Elixir	20	Rx
Lixaminol AT Liquid	20	Rx
Lixaminol Elixir	20	Rx
Lomanate Liquid	15	C-V
Lomoxate Liquid	15	C-V
Lonox Liquid	15	C-V
Lo-Trol Liquid	15	C-V
Lufyllin Elixir	20	Rx
Lufyllin-EPG Elixir	5.5	Rx
Lufyllin-GG Elixir	17	Rx
Mallergan Expectorant w/Codeine	7	C-V
Mallergan Expectorant, Plain	7	Rx
Mallergan-VC Expectorant w/Codeine	7	C-V
Marax DF Syrup	5	Rx
Mar-Tonic Liquid	5	OTC
Matropinal Elixir	15	Rx
Maxibolin Elixir	10	Rx
Mellaril Concentrate	4.2	Rx
Mentalert Elixir	5	Rx
Mercodol with Decapryn Syrup	5	C-V
Mestinon Bromide Syrup	5	Rx
Metrazol Liquidum Elixir	15	Rx
Midahist D.H. Liquid	5	C-V
Midahist Elixir	5	OTC
Midahist Expectorant	7.5	C-V
Midatane DC Expectorant	3.5	C-V
Midatane Elixir	3	Rx
Midatane Expectorant	3.5	Rx

Table 5.7.—*Continued*

Brand Name	Alcohol Content (%)	Distribution Status[a]
Midatap Elixir	2.3	Rx
Mini-Lix	20	Rx
Minocin Syrup	5	Rx
Mol-Iron Liquid	4.75	OTC
Morphine Sulfate Oral Solution	10	C-II
Mor-Tussin P.E. Syrup	1.4	OTC
Mor-Tussin Syrup	1.4	OTC
Motion-Aid Elixir	5	OTC
Mudrane GG Elixir	20	Rx
Mycostatin Oral Suspension	Not >1	Rx
Naldecon-Dx Syrup	5	OTC
Naldecon-Ex Pediatric Drops	0.6	OTC
Navane Concentration	7	Rx
Neothylline Elixir	18	Rx
Neothylline-GG Elixir	10	Rx
Neotrizine Suspension	2	Rx
Neozyl Liquid	5	C-V
Niapent Elixir	15	Rx
Nico-Metrazol Elixir	15	Rx
Nicotinex Elixir	14	OTC
Nicozol Elixir	5	Rx
Niferex Elixir	10	OTC
Nilcol Elixir	10	Rx
Nioric Elixir	15	Rx
N-N Cough Syrup	5	OTC
Noradryl Cough Syrup	5	Rx
Noradryl Elixir	14	Rx
Norisodrine w/Calcium Iodide Syrup	6	Rx
Normatane DC Expectorant w/Codeine	3.5	C-V
Normatane Elixir	2.3	Rx
Normatane Expectorant	3.5	Rx
Norophylline Elixir	20	Rx
Nortussin w/Codeine Liquid	3.5	C-V
Nortussin Syrup	3.5	OTC
Novafed A Liquid	5	OTC
Novafed Liquid	7.5	OTC
Novahistine Cough & Cold Formula Liquid	5	OTC
Novahistine Cough Formula Liquid	7.5	OTC
Novahistine DH Liquid	5	C-V
Novahistine DMX Liquid	10	OTC
Novahistine Elixir	5	OTC
Novahistine Expectorant	7.5	C-V
Novamor Elixir	5	OTC
Novamor Elixir DH	5	C-V
Novamor Expectorant	5	C-V
Novatuss Expectorant	7.5	C-V
Novrad Oral Suspension	1	Rx
Nucofed Syrup	12.5	C-III
Nu-Iron Elixir	10	OTC
Nyquil Liquid	25	OTC
Omnibel Liquid	15	Rx
Opium Tincture, Deoderized	19	C-II
Oralphyllin Elixir	20	Rx
Oraphen-PD Syrup	5	OTC

Table 5.7.—_Continued_

Brand Name	Alcohol Content (%)	Distribution Status[a]
Organidin Elixir	21.75	Rx
Ornacol Liquid	8	OTC
Ornade 2 Liquid for Children	5	OTC
Pabizol with Paregoric Suspension	9.6	C-V
Palbar Elixir	23	Rx
Pan-Kloride Liquid	5	Rx
Paradione Solution	65	Rx
Parelixir Liquid	18	C-V
Parepectolin Suspension	0.69	C-V
Pavadon Elixir	10	C-V
PBZ	12	Rx
Pediacof Cough Syrup	5	C-V
Pediaquil Liquid	5	OTC
Pedicran with Iron Liquid	1	OTC
Pedric Elixir	10	OTC
Penalate Elixir	15	Rx
Pentacresol 1:1000 Mouthwash	30	OTC
Pentazine Expectorant w/Codeine	7	C-V
Pentazine Expectorant, Plain	7	Rx
Pentazine VC Expectorant w/Codeine	7	C-V
Periactin Syrup	5	Rx
Peri-Colace Syrup	10	OTC
Pertussin Cough Syrup for Children	8.5	OTC
Pertussin 8 hour Cough Formula Syrup	9.5	OTC
Phen-Amin Elixir	14	Rx
Phenergan Expectorant w/Codeine	7	C-V
Phenergan Expectorant Pediatric w/Dextromethorphan	7	Rx
Phenergan Expectorant, Plain	7	Rx
Phenergan Syrup	1.5	Rx
Phenergan Syrup Fortis	1.5	Rx
Phenergan VC Expectorant w/Codeine	7	C-V
Phenergan VC Expectorant, Plain	7	Rx
Phenetron Syrup	7	Rx
Phenhist DH Liquid	5	C-V
Phenhist Elixir	5	OTC
Phenhist Expectorant	7.5	C-V
Point-Two Rinse	6	Rx
Polaramine Expectorant	7.2	Rx
Polaramine Syrup	6	Rx
Poly-Histine-D Elixir	4	Rx
Poly-Histine Elixir	4	Rx
Potasalan Liquid	4	Rx
Potassium Chloride Liquid (various)	4–5	Rx
Potassium Gluconate Liquid (various)	4–5	Rx
Proglycem Oral Suspension	7.25	Rx
Prolixin Elixir	14	Rx
Promethazine HCl Expectorant w/Codeine	7	C-V
Promethazine HCl Expectorant, Plain	7	Rx
Promethazine HCl VC Expectorant, w/Codeine	7	C-V
Promethazine HCl VC Expectorant, Plain	7	Rx
Propadrine Elixir	16	OTC
Prothazine w/Codeine Expectorant	7	C-V
Prothazine Expectorant	7	Rx
Prothazine Pediatric Liquid	7	Rx
Prunicodeine Liquid	25	C-V

Table 5.7.—*Continued*

Brand Name	Alcohol Content (%)	Distribution Status[a]
Pseudocodone Expectorant	12.5	C-III
Pseudo-Hist Expectorant	5	C-III
Puretane Expectorant	3.5	Rx
Puretane Expectorant DC	3.5	C-V
Puretapp Elixir	2.3	Rx
P-V-Tussin Syrup	5	C-III
Pyrralan Expectorant DM	6.5	OTC
Quad-Ramoid Suspension	5	Rx
Quelidrine Cough Syrup	2	OTC
Quibron Plus Elixir	15	Rx
Quiet-Nite Liquid	25	OTC
Quintess Suspension	0.9	OTC
Reletonic Liquid	15	OTC
Reletuss Pediatric Cough Syrup	8.2	OTC
Respinol-G Liquid	5	Rx
Rhinex DM Syrup	5	OTC
Rhinosyn-DM Syrup	1.4	OTC
Rhinosyn-PD Syrup	1.2	OTC
Rhinosyn Syrup	.45	OTC
Rhinosyn-X Syrup	7.5	OTC
Robitussin A-C Syrup	3.5	C-V
Robitussin-CF Liquid	4.75	OTC
Robitussin DAC Syrup	1.4	C-V
Robitussin DM Syrup	1.4	OTC
Robitussin-PE Syrup	1.4	OTC
Robitussin Syrup	3.5	OTC
Rohistine DH Liquid	5	C-V
Rohistine Elixir	5	OTC
Rohistine Expectorant	7.5	C-V
Romilar CF Syrup	20	OTC
Romilar 111 Decongestant Cough Syrup	20	OTC
Rondec DM Drops	<0.6	Rx
Rondec-DM Syrup	<0.6	Rx
Roniacol Elixir	—[b]	Rx
Rotane Expectorant	3.5	Rx
Rotane Expectorant DC	3.5	C-V
Rotapp Elixir	2.3	Rx
Ru-K-N Suspension	5	C-III
Ru-Tuss Expectorant	5	C-V
Ru-Tuss w/Hydrocodone Liquid	5	C-III
Rymed Liquid	5	Rx
Seconal Elixir	12	C-II
Secran/Fe Elixir	1	OTC
Secran Liquid	17	OTC
Sedacord Elixir	23	Rx
Senilezol Elixir	5	Rx
Senokot Syrup	7	OTC
Serentil Concentrate	0.61	Rx
Setamine Liquid	23	Rx
Sherry-Jen Tonic	9	OTC
SK-APAP Elixir	8	OTC
SK-Diphenhydramine Elixir	14.5	Rx
SK-Potassium Chloride Liquid	5	Rx

Table 5.7.—*Continued*

Brand Name	Alcohol Content (%)	Distribution Status[a]
SK Terpine Hydrate and Codeine Elixir	40	C-V
SK Tetracycline Syrup	1	Rx
Spalix Elixir	23	Rx
Spasaid Elixir	23	Rx
Spasmophen Elixir	23	Rx
Spasquid Elixir	23	Rx
Spendec DM Syrup	<0.6	Rx
Spen-Histine DH Liquid	5	C-V
Spen-Histine Elixir	5	OTC
Spen-Histine Expectorant	7.5	C-V
Spentane DC Expectorant	3.5	C-V
Spentane Expectorant	3.5	Rx
Spentapp Elixir	2.3	Rx
S/T Decongest Liquid	2.3	Rx
S-T Forte Liquid	5	C-III
Stopit Syrup	15	C-III
Sudafed Cough Syrup	2.4	OTC
Sulfonamides Duplex Suspension	3	Rx
Su-Ton Elixir	18	Rx
Su-Ton Liquid	18	Rx
Su-Zol Liquid	15	Rx
Symptom 3 Elixir	5	OTC
Symptom 1 Liquid	5	OTC
Symptom 2 Liquid	5	OTC
Synophylate Elixir	20	Rx
Synophylate GG Syrup	10	Rx
Tagatapp Elixir	2.3	Rx
Tamine Cough Syrup	2.3	Rx
Tamine Expectorant	3.5	Rx
Tamine Expectorant DC	3.5	C-V
Tedral Elixir	15	OTC
Tega-Atric w/Iron Elixir	15	Rx
Temaril Syrup	5.7	Rx
Tempra Drops	10	OTC
Tempra Syrup	10	OTC
Tenol Elixir	7	OTC
Terphan Elixir	40	OTC
Terpin Hydrate w/Codeine Elixir	40	C-V
Theofort Elixir	20	Rx
Theokin Elixir	9.5	Rx
Theolate Elixir	15	Rx
Theo-Lix Elixir	20	Rx
Theolixir Elixir	20	Rx
Theon Liquid	10	Rx
Theo-Organidin Elixir	15	Rx
Theophozine Liquid	5	Rx
Theophyl-225 Elixir	5	Rx
Theophylline Elixir	20	Rx
Theostat 80 Syrup	1	Rx
Tolu-Sed Cough Syrup	10	C-V
Tolu-Sed DM Cough Syrup	10	OTC
Trilafon Concentrate	<0.1	Rx
Triaminic Expectorant	5	OTC
Triaminic Expectorant w/Codeine	5	C-V
Triaminic Expectorant DH	5	C-III

Table 5.7.—*Continued*

Brand Name	Alcohol Content (%)	Distribution Status[a]
Trilafon Concentrate	<0.1	Rx
Tri-Medex Expectorant DH	5	Rx
Tri-Mine Expectorant	5	Rx
Trind DM Syrup	15	OTC
Trind Syrup	15	OTC
Tusquelin Syrup	5	Rx
Tuss-Ade Liquid	7.5	Rx
Tussafin Expectorant	12.5	C-III
Tussar-2 Cough Syrup	5	C-V
Tussar SF Cough Syrup	12	C-V
Tuss-Liquid	7.5	Rx
Tussend Expectorant	12.5	C-III
Tussend Liquid	5	C-III
Tussi-Organidin DM Expectorant	15	Rx
Tussi-Organidin Elixir	15	C-V
Tussi-Ornade Liquid	5	Rx
Tusstat Syrup	5	Rx
Tylenol w/Codeine Elixir	7	C-V
Tylenol Drops	7	OTC
Tylenol Elixir	7	OTC
Tylenol Extra Strength Liquid	8.5	OTC
Valadol Elixir	9	OTC
Valdrene Syrup	5	Rx
Veltap Elixir	2.3	Rx
Vicks Cough Syrup	5	OTC
Vi-Daylin Drops	<0.5	OTC
Vi-Daylin Liquid	<0.5	OTC
Viro-Med Liquid	16.63	OTC
Vita-Metrazol Elixir	15	Rx
Vitronic Liquid	12	OTC
Westapp Elixir	2.3	Rx
X-Prep Liquid	7	OTC
Zentron Liquid	2	OTC
Zymalixir Elixir	1.5	OTC
Zymasyrup	2	OTC

[a] Rx = prescription; OTC = over the counter; C-II to C-V are ratings from the schedules of the Drug Enforcement Administration. Drugs under the jurisdiction of the Controlled Substances Act are divided into five schedules based on their potential for abuse, physical and psychologic dependence. Schedule I (C-I): high abuse potential and no accepted medical use (heroin, marijuana, LSD). Schedule II (C-II): high abuse potential with severe dependence liability (narcotics, amphetamines, and barbiturates). Schedule III (C-III): less abuse potential than Schedule II drugs and moderate dependence liability (nonbarbiturate sedatives, nonamphetamine stimulants, limited amounts of certain narcotics). Schedule IV (C-IV): less abuse potential than Schedule III drugs and limited dependence liability (some sedatives and antianxiety agents and nonnarcotic analgesics). Schedule V (C-V): limited abuse potential. Primarily small amounts of narcotics (codeine) used as antitussives or antidiarrheals. Under federal law limited quantities of certain C-V drugs may be purchased without a prescription directly from a pharmacist. The purchaser must be at least 18 years of age and must furnish suitable identification. All such transactions must be recorded by the dispensing pharmacist.

[b] Elixirs contain ethyl alcohol by definition. However, the content varies greatly, from elixirs containing only a small percentage of alcohol, to those that contain a considerable portion as a necessary aid to solubility. Exact content of this product is unknown; contact manufacturer to ascertain.

Table 5.8.
Nutritional Problems Associated with Alcoholism

Source	Signs and Symptoms	Comments
Protein	Fatty liver and hypoalbuminemia may be result of deterioration of liver function or low protein intake. Others: hypocholesterolemia, edema, normocytic anemia	Association of alcohol with liver disease complicates the interpretation of many clinical signs or protein deficiency. Alcoholic liver disease is not prevented by eating well or limiting alcohol consumption only to certain types of beverages. Administration of protein to patients with severe active alcoholic cirrhosis can precipitate hepatic coma. Observation is important. When protein is poorly tolerated or the patient becomes progressively disoriented, showing asterixis or "flapping tremors," administration of protein should be discontinued
Water-soluble vitamins, vitamin B complexes, thiamine	The signs and symptoms are variable depending on severity of the deficiency Opthalmoplegia Sixth nerve palsy Nystagmus Ptosis Ataxia, peripheral neuropathies, Confusion Coma Death Wernicke's syndrome Heart failure "Beriberi" heart disease	Most common deficiency in alcoholics. Polyneuropathy is the mildest and most common form of thiamine deficiency Depressed tendon reflexes, muscle cramps, weakness, paresthesias and pain develop. The lower extremities are most often affected A grave prognosis and must be recognized early. Treatment is to give thiamine. Administration of glucose without thiamine may further deplete stores of thiamine. Coma can result Thiamine deficiency-induced heart failure does not respond well to digitalis or diuretics. Animal studies suggest that thiamine deficiency reduces myocardial oxygen consumption due to deficiency of the coenzyme thiamine pyrophosphate Average requirement for thiamine is 1.5 to 2 mg for adult per day. Alcoholics often will require 5–10 times more
Niacin	Weakness Photosensitive dermatitis Stomatitis Gastritis Diarrhea Peripheral neuropathy Dementia Encephalopathy	Alcoholic pellagra is the result of the lack of dietary nicotinic acid or its precursor, tryptopham. Niacin contributes to formation of specific coenzyme nucleotides (NAD) which participate in intracellular metabolism and cell respiration
Riboflavin	Weakness Photosensitive dermatitis Stomatitis Gastritis Diarrhea Peripheral neuropathy Dementia Encephalopathy	Sources include: animal proteins. Average daily amount is 250 mg for adults. Riboflavin deficiency usually accompanies alcoholic pellagra. Riboflavin is an essential constituent of coenzymes responsible for oxidative and electron transport processes
Pyridoxine	Irritability Insomnia Ataxia Skin lesions	Pyridoxine is responsible for a variety of enzymatic activities particularly related to nitrogen metabolism
Ascorbic acid	Anorexia Petechial ecchymoses Gingivitis and bleeding gums Dry mouth Loss of hair	Ascorbic acid is a coenzyme involved in the metabolism of amino acids. Usual amount recommended is 10 mg/day

Table 5.8.—Continued

Source	Signs and Symptoms	Comments
	Perifollicular hemorrhages	
	Purpuric lesions	
	Ecchymoses	
	Itchy dry skin	
	Weakness	
	Lethargy	
Folic acid	Macrocytic anemia	Deficiency of folic acid is the primary cause of macrocytic anemia in chronic alcoholics. Alcohol directly affects the hemotopoietic activity and interferes with utilization of folic acid. Must discontinue alcohol. Usual daily amount recommended is 50 μg/day
	Reticulocytosis	
Minerals		
Magnesium	Lethargy	Alcohol promotes the renal excretion of magnesium. Renal effect and inadequate diet cause significant depletion. Symptoms of acute alcohol withdrawal are often complicated by coexisting magnesium depletion. The total body magnesium deficits are not reflected by serum magnesium levels
	Muscle weakness	
	Coarse athetoid movements	
	Gross tremors of hands and tongue	
	Mental changes	
	Convulsions	
	Stupor	
	Coma	
Potassium	Weakness	Poor dietary intake of potassium and loss by diuresis, vomiting, and diarrhea can contribute to hypokalemia
	Lethargy	

tients who are intelligent, well-motivated, and financially secure. Group psychotherapy allows for interaction among alcoholics to deal with difficulties they have in common. "Halfway houses" or rehabilitation centers permit the recovering alcoholic to live with other recuperating alcoholics in an environment guided by trained staff. The group treatment approach of Alcoholics Anonymous (AA) takes a more structured and evangelistic attitude in dealing with alcoholism; it has returned many alcoholics to sobriety (111). Alcoholics Anonymous is a private organization whose members offer mutual support to each other to remain free of alcohol and has a current membership of 650,000 ex-alcoholics. Other similar groups such as the Salvation Army and Volunteers of America also have help groups for the rehabilitation of alcoholics.

ALCOHOL-DRUG INTERACTIONS

Because approximately 70 to 80% of adults consume alcoholic beverages, it is almost inevitable that medications either prescribed by a physician or bought over the counter (Table 5.7) will be taken concomitantly with alcohol or while alcohol is still in the body. Worsening of a patient's condition or failure to respond to drug therapy is almost always assumed to be due to exacerbation of the disease state; the concomitant use of alcohol is seldom considered as a contributing factor. Alcohol is not only found in alcoholic beverages, but also in many common prescription medications and readily available nonprescription preparations. Often these preparations are sources of the alcohol that interacts with prescribed medications to produce untoward effects in the unsuspecting patient (107) (Table 5.9).

The repeated administration of alcohol has been shown to increase the hepatic microsomal enzyme activity that metabolizes many drugs (115–117). This enzyme induction is nonspecific and may decrease the activity of some drugs (i.e., barbiturates) when alcohol is taken concurrently. This explains partially the "tolerance" to the action of sedatives observed in some chronic alcoholics. Warfarin, phenytoin, tolbutamide, and isoniazid are nonspychoactive drugs subject to hepatic microsomal enzyme activity (118, 119). The plasma half-lives of these drugs are markedly decreased in some chronic and heavy users of alcohol as a result of their increased rate of clearance. Clinical reports of significant problems from such interactions, however, are few (112, 114). Variable and unpredictable response to drugs in the alcoholic should arouse interest for the

Table 5.9.
Summary of Selected Alcohol-Drug Interactions (100, 112–114)

Drugs Interacting with Alcohol	Mechanism	Effect	Significance
Antabuse	Inhibits intermediate metabolism of alcohol	Abdominal cramps, flushing, vomiting, confusion, hypotension	Major
Anticoagulants (oral), warfarin	Metabolism enhanced with chronic alcohol abuse	Diminished anticoagulant effect	Moderate
	Metabolism reduced with acute alcohol intoxication	Increased anticoagulant effect	Moderate
Antihistamines	Additive	Increased central nervous system (CNS) depression	Moderate
Aspirin (and other salicylates)	Additive	Increased occult blood loss and damage to gastric mucosa	Moderate
Anticonvulsants: phenytoin (Dilantin) and others	Metabolism enhanced with chronic alcohol abuse	Diminished anticonvulsant effect	Moderate
	Metabolism reduced with acute alcohol intoxication	Increased anticonvulsant effect	Moderate
Antimicrobials Isoniazid	Metabolism enhanced in chronic alcohol abuse	Diminished isoniazid effect	Moderate
		Increased incidence of isoniazid hepatitis	Not established
Metronidazole, chloramphenicol, griseofulvin	Metabolism of alcohol reduced	Disulfiram-like reaction	Minor
Antidiabetic agents, Sulfonylureas, tolbutamide (Orinase)	Additive	Hypoglycemia effect increased	Moderate
Chlorpropamide (Diabinese)	Metabolism enhanced in chronic alcohol abuse	Decreased effect	Moderate in chronic alcoholic
Acetohexamide (Dymelor)	Accumulation of acetaldehyde	Disulfiram-like reaction	Moderate
Phenformin (DBI)	Alteration of biochemical pathway	Lactic acidosis	Major
Insulin	Interferes with hepatic gluconeogenesis	Increased hypoglycemic effects	Moderate but major if liver is damaged
Antihypertensive Methyldopa (Aldomet), reserpine	Additive	Sedation	Minor to moderate
Methyldopa (Aldomet), guanethidine (Ismelin), hydralazine (Apresoline), prazosin (Minipres)	Additive	Postural hypotensive effect increased	Minor to moderate
Monoamine oxidase inhibitor Pargyline	Alteration of tyramine metabolism	Increased CNS depression, hypertensive crisis	Moderate to major
Tranylcypromine Procarbazine	Additive		
Narcotic analgesics Meperidine (Demerol), morphine, methadone	Additive	Increased CNS depression	Major
Sedative-hypnotics Barbiturates (phenobarbital, pentobarbital, secobarbital)	Additive or metabolism enhanced with acute alcohol intoxication	Increased CNS depression	Major

Table 5.9.—Continued

Drugs Interacting with Alcohol	Mechanism	Effect	Significance
Nonbarbiturates (ethchlorvynol, glutethimide, meprobamate)	Tolerance with chronic alcohol use	Diminished CNS effect	Minor to moderate
Chloral hydrate	Additive with acute alcohol intoxication and competition for metabolic pathway	Increased CNS depression	Moderate
Tranquilizers Phenothiazines (Thorazine, etc.)	Additive	Impaired coordination and judgment, also increased CNS depression	Moderate
Chlordiazepoxide (Librium), diazepam (Valium), flurazepam (Dalmane)	Additive	Increased CNS depression	Major
Meprobamate	Additive with acute alcohol intoxication	Increased CNS depression	Major
Tricyclic antidepressants Amitriptyline (Elavil, Triavil) Imipramine (Tofranil) Nortriptyline	Additive	Possible increase in sedation, also additive to anticholinergic effects of tricyclics	Moderate
Vasodilators, Nitroglycerin	Additive	Hypotension potentiated may cause cardiovascular collapse	Major

possibility of some metabolic alteration of drug kinetics. It has become increasingly evident that toxicity to certain drugs and chemicals is enhanced in chronic alcoholics as a result of this mechanism (113).

The hepatotoxic manifestations of acetaminophen overdose or carbon tetrachloride ingestion are thought to be produced by the metabolites of these chemicals that are formed by the hepatic microsomal enzymes. Chronic consumption of alcohol enhances the activity of hepatic microsomal enzymes, which generates metabolites that result in further toxicity (120, 121).

Alcohol is primarily a central nervous system depressant. When combined with other drugs with similar depressing action on the central nervous system, an additive or synergistic effect occurs. This is perhaps the most important type of interaction between alcohol and other drugs (122).

Alcoholics taking tolbutamide and other antidiabetic drugs, chloramphenicol, griseofulvin, quinacrine, or metronidazole have reported a mild "disulfiram-like" reaction (Table 5.4). Recent experience suggests that moxalactam therapy may precipitate a disulfiram-like reaction (157). Some alcoholic beverages, such as chianti wines, contain appreciable amounts of tyramine that when taken by patients using monoamine oxidase (MAO)-inhibiting drugs (i.e., procarbazine, pargyline) will effect an acute hypertensive episode. Interference with tyramine metabolism by the MAO inhibitor results in the release of norepinephrine from the sympathetic nerve terminal.

ALCOHOL AS A THERAPEUTIC AGENT

There is a prevailing notion that alcohol may have some usefulness in the treatment of a variety of disorders and conditions. Clinical evidence, however, is not encouraging about alcohol's role in therapy, and it may actually worsen many conditions for which its use has been suggested (Table 5.10).

Intravenous administration of alcohol has been used with some success to delay premature labor. The efficacy of this method has not been sufficiently compared with other methods to delay premature labor. Blood alcohol levels of 100 to 150 mg/100 ml are required to inhibit uterine contractions. Studies of placenta cord blood alcohol levels following delivery were slightly less than that of the mother. In fact, neonatal depression of respiratory and circulatory activity after adminis-

Table 5.10.
"Therapeutic" Use of Alcohol

Proposed Use	Actual Effect
Relief of anxiety	Anxiety often worsens when blood alcohol level falls, as in withdrawal
Bedtime sedation	Sleeplessness is common as blood alcohol level declines
Improvement of nutrition	Blood sugar levels become more labile; although each gram of alcohol = 7.1 calories on oxidation, "empty" calories are gained. Overall nutrition not improved with alcohol because no vitamins, minerals or other essential dietary materials are in alcoholic beverages
Diuresis of edema	Diuretic response to alcohol occurs when blood alcohol level is on the rise; antidiuresis, hypersomality, and fluid retention occur as blood alcohol concentration falls
Anemia	Iron metabolism and bone marrow function are affected, and folate antagonism contributes to anemia in spite of frequent presence of iron in wines
Lowering of blood sugar in diabetics	Lowering of blood sugar is negligible. In fact, alcohol produces more labile blood sugar levels
Heart disease	The alcohol metabolite acetaldehyde is toxic to myocardium and not effective as a coronary vasodilator. Alcohol is a myocardial depressant. Although alcohol enhances coronary blood flow, myocardial oxygen consumption simultaneously increases
Anti-infective	Chronic alcoholism predisposes to systemic infections

tration of alcohol before delivery have been reported.

CONCLUSION

Much confusion has arisen in the midst of a widely publicized 1976 report by the Rand Corporation on alcoholism which seems to imply that some alcoholics can return to social drinking (123). The goal of alcohol abstinence by the alcoholic has been long advocated. For instance, Alcoholics Anonymous considers abstinence as the only goal for anyone with an alcohol problem. Careful evaluation of data from this report does not support the notion that alcoholics can safely return to drink. What it did point out was that after an 18-month period relatively few alcoholics were practicing long-term abstinence despite an impressive improvement rate (70%). Most had intermittent periods of abstinence interspersed with "controlled" drinking. Relapse to uncontrolled drinking by those who continued to drink in a "controlled" manner and those who continued abstinence were found to be no different. Major methodological problems are suggested by the large number (more than 80%) of subjects lost to follow-up at the end of the 18 month study period.

Abstinence from alcohol should not be a goal for treatment but rather a means to an end (124). The treatment of alcoholism for an alcoholic is best accomplished if conducted in a relationship of understanding and trust with others. This can be a concerned and interested friend or spouse, or a professional person such as a pharmacist, therapist, physician, or members of a therapeutic or rehabilitation group.

Admittedly, it is a rare circumstance that an alcoholic can fully achieve complete abstinence. Until it is possible to accurately select within the population of individuals with an alcohol problem who might be able to resume drinking in a "controlled" manner, total abstinence should continue to be the goal of treatment. Patients should be given emotional support and encouragement despite occasional relapses and even major hospitalizations as a result of resumption of drinking.

The recognition and management of the acute toxic effect or withdrawal reactions of alcohol is frequently complicated by the presence of complex physiologic and psychologic disturbances. The diagnosis and treatment of acute alcohol intoxication or withdrawal syndrome is often based simply on the clinical manifestations.

Dependence on alcohol is no different in any significant way from dependency on other addictive drugs such as opiates and barbiturates. Although there are differences in social attitudes toward drinking and drug abuse, many features of alcohol and "hard drugs" are remarkably similar. The similarities and differences should be appreciated and understood by those who are involved in the diagnosis, treatment, care, and rehabilitation of alcohol-dependent patients.

References

1. United States Department of Health, Education and Welfare: National Institute on Alcohol Abuse and Alcoholism: Second Special Report to the United States Congress on Alcohol and Health from the Secretary of Health, Education and Welfare, June 1974, Washington, D.C.
2. American Medical Association Council on Mental Health: The sick physician-impairment by psychiatric disorders, including alcoholism and drug dependence. JAMA 223:684, 1973.
3. Rising toll of alcoholism: new steps to combat it: U.S. News and World Report, (October 29) 1973.
4. Alcoholism: new victims, new treatment: Time 75. April 22, 1974.
5. American Academy of Pediatrics, Committee on Youth: Alcohol consumption–an adolescent problem. Pediatrics 55:557, 1975.
6. MacArthur JD, Moore FD: Epidemiology of burns: the burn-prone patient. JAMA 231:259, 1975.
7. Toll of traffic deaths mounts at last year's pace (Medical News). JAMA 236:2377,1976.
8. DeLint J, Levinson T: Mortality among patients treated for alcoholism. Can Med Assoc J 113:385, 1975.
9. Berry RE: Estimating the economic costs of alcohol abuse. N Engl J Med 295:620, 1976.
10. Girard DE, Carlton BE: Alcoholism—earlier diagnosis and definition of the problem. West J Med 129:1, 1978.
11. Mendelson JH: Biologic concomitants of alcoholism. Parts I and II. N Engl J Med 283:24 and 71, 1970.
12. Lieber CS: Hepatic and metabolic effects of alcohol. Gastroenterology 65:821, 1973.
13. Becker CE, Scott R: The treatment of alcoholism. Rational Drug Ther 6:1, 1972.
14. Bennion LJ, Li TK: Alcohol metabolism in American Indians and whites. Lack of racial differences in metabolic rate and liver alcohol dehydrogenase. N Engl J Med 294:9, 1976.
15. American Medical Association Criteria Committee and National Council on Alcoholism Criteria for the Diagnosis of Alcoholism: Ann Intern Med 77:249, 1972.
16. Davis CN: Early signs of alcoholism. JAMA 238:161, 1977.
17. Territo MC, Tanaka, KR: Hypophosphatemia in chronic alcoholism. Arch Intern Med 134:445, 1974.
18. Robinson AG, Loeb JN: Ethanol ingestion-commonest cause of elevated plasma osmolality. N Engl J Med 284:356, 1973.
19. Klock JC, Williams HE, Mentzer WC: Hemolytic anemia and somatic cell dysfunction in severe hypophosphatemia. Arch Intern Med 134:360, 1974.
20. Iseri LT, Freed J, Bures AR: Magnesium deficiency and cardiac disorders. Am J Med 58:837, 1975.
21. Kallas P, Sellers EM: Blood glucose in intoxicated chronic alcoholics. Can Med Assoc J 112:590, 1975.
22. Field JM, Williams HE, Mortimore GE: Studies on the mechanism of ethanol induced hypoglycemia. J Clin Invest 42:497, 1963.
23. Felig P: Alcoholic ketoacidosis. Prostgrad Med 59:153, 1976.
24. Levy LJ, Duga J, Girges M, et al: Ketoacidosis associated with alcoholism in non-diabetic subjects. Ann Intern Med 78:213, 1973.
25. Lieber CS: Hepatic and metabolic effects of alcohol. Gastroenterology 65:821, 1973.
26. Mendelson JH: Effects of alcohol on the central nervous system. N Engl J Med 284:104, 1971.
27. Freund G: Chronic central nervous system toxicity of alcohol. Ann Rev Pharmacol 13:217, 1973.
28. Mezey E, Jow E, Slavin RE, et al: Pancreatic function and intestinal absorption in chronic alcoholism. Gastroenterology 59:657, 1970.
29. Mendelson JH, Mello NK: Alcohol induced hyperlipidemia and betalipoproteins. Science 180:1372, 1973.
30. Ginsberg H, Olefsky J, Faruhar JW, Moderate ethanol ingestion and plasma triglyceride levels; a study in normal and hypertriglyceridemic persons. Ann Intern Med 80:143, 1974.
31. Factor SM: Intramyocardial small vessel disease in chronic alcoholism. Am Heart J 92:561, 1976.
32. Horwitz LD: Alcohol and heart disease. JAMA 239:959, 1975.
33. Hed R, Lundmark C, Fahlgren H, et al: Acute muscular syndrome in chronic alcoholism. Acta Med Scand 171:585, 1962.
34. Ekbom K, Hed R, Kirstein L, et al: Muscular affections in chronic alcoholism. Arch Neurol 10:449, 1964.
35. Schneider R: Acute alcoholic myopathy with myoglobinuria. South Med J 63:485, 1970.
36. Marr JJ, Spilber I: A mechanism for decreased resistance to infection by gram negative organisms during acute alcohol intoxication. J Lab Clin Med 86:253, 1975.
37. Brayton RG: Effect of alcohol and various diseases on leukocyte mobilization, phagocytosis and intracellular bacterial killing. N Engl J Med 282:123, 1978.
38. Sullivan IW, Herbert V: Mechanism of hematosuppression by ethanol. Am J Clin Nutr 14:238, 1964.
39. Herbert V, Zalusky R, Davidson CS: Correlation of folate deficiency with alcoholism and associated macrocytosis; anemia and liver disease. Ann Intern Med 58:977, 1963.
40. Eichner ER, Buchanan P, Smith J, et al: Variations in the hematologic and medical status of alcoholics. Am J Med Sci 263:35, 1972.
41. Eichner ER, Hillman RS: Evolution of anemia in alcoholic patients. Am J Med 50:218, 1971.
42. Cowan DH, Hines JD: Thrombocytopenia of severe alcoholism. Ann Intern Med 74:37, 1971.
43. Victor M, Adams RD: On the etiology of the alcoholic neurologic diseases with special reference in the role of nutrition. Am J Clin Nutr 9:379, 1961.

44. Palmer RH, Quellette EM, Warner L, et al: Congenital malformations in offspring of a chronic alcoholic mother. *Pediatrics* 53:490, 1974.

45. Jones KL, Smith DW, Ulleland CN, et al: Pattern of malformation in offspring of chronic alcoholic mothers. *Lancet* 1:1267, 1973.

46. Green HG: Infants of alcoholic mothers. *Am J Obstet Gynecol* 118:713, 1974.

47. Jones KL, Smith DW: Recognition of the fetal alcohol syndrome in early infancy. *Lancet* 2:999, 1973.

48. Tenbrinck MS, Buchin SY: Fetal alcohol syndrome; report of a case. *JAMA* 232:1144, 1975.

49. Hanson JW, Streissquth AP, Smith DW: The effects of moderate alcohol consumption during pregnancy on fetal growth and morphogenesis. *J Pediatr* 92:457, 1978.

50. Clarren SK, Smith DW: The fetal alcohol syndrome. *N Engl J Med* 298:1063, 1978.

51. Wagner L, Wagner G, and Guerrero J: Effect of alcohol on premature newborn infants. *Am J Obstet Gynecol* 108:308, 1970.

52. Nichols MM: Acute alcohol withdrawal syndrome in a newborn. *Am J Dis Child* 113:714, 1967.

53. Cook LN, Shott R, Andrew BF: Acute transplacental ethanol intoxication. *Am J Dis Child* 129:1075, 1973.

54. Rubin E, Lieber CS: Fatty liver, alcoholic hepatitis and cirrhosis produced by alcohol in primates. *N Engl J Med* 290:128, 1974.

55. Lieber CS: Alcohol and malnutrition in the pathogenesis of liver disease. *JAMA* 233:1077, 1975.

56. Patek AJ Jr, Toth IG, Sauders MG, et al: Alcohol and dietary factors in cirrhosis. *Arch Intern Med* 135:1053, 1975.

57. Burch GF, Giles TD: Alcoholic cardiomyopathy: concept of the disease and its treatment. *Am J Med* 50:141, 1971.

58. Demakis JG, Proskey A, Rahimtoola SH: The natural course of alcohol cardiomyopathy. *Ann Intern Med* 80:293, 1974.

59. Bashour TT, Fahdul H, Chong TO: Electrocardiographic abnormalities in alcoholic cardiomyopathy. *Chest* 61:24, 1975.

60. Marin YL, Foley AR, Martineau G, et al: Quebec beer-drinkers cardiomyopathy; forty-eight cases. *Can Med Assoc J* 97:881, 1967.

61. Lindenbaum J, Lieber CS: Hematologic effects of alcohol in man in absence of nutritional deficiency. *N Engl J Med* 281:333, 1969.

62. Eichner ER: The hematologic disorder of alcoholism. *Am J Med* 54:621, 1973.

63. Halsted CH, Robles EA, Mezey E: Intestinal malabsorption in folate-deficient alcoholics. *Gastroenterology* 64:526, 1973.

64. Sellers, EM, Kalant H: Alcohol intoxication and withdrawal. *N Engl J Med* 294:757, 1976.

65. Thompson WL, Johnson AD, Maddrey WC: Diazepam and paraldehyde for treatment of severe delirium tremens. *Ann Intern Med* 82:175, 1975.

66. Golbert TM, Sanz CJ, Rose HD, et al: Comparative evaluation of treatments of alcohol withdrawal syndrome. *JAMA* 201:99, 1967.

67. Klett CJ, Hollister LE, Caffey EM, et al: Evaluating changes in symptoms during acute alcohol withdrawal. *Arch Gen Psychiatry* 24:174, 1971.

68. Kaim SC, Klett CJ, Rothefeld B: Treatment of the acute alcohol withdrawal state; a comparison of four drugs. *Am J Psychiatry* 125:1640, 1969.

69. Kaim SC, Klett J: Treatment of delirium tremens. *Q J Stud Alcohol* 33:1065, 1972.

70. Sereny G, Kalant H: Comparative clinical evaluation of chlordiazepoxide and promazine in treatment of alcohol withdrawal syndrome. *Br Med J* 1:92, 1965.

71. Zilm DH, Sellers EM: Effect of propranolol on tremor of alcohol withdrawal (letter). *N Engl J Med* 294:785, 1976.

72. Sellers EM, Cooper SD, Zilm DH, et al: Lithium treatment of alcohol withdrawal. *Clin Pharmacol Ther* 20:199, 1976

73. Viamontes JA: Review of drug effectiveness in the treatment of alcoholism. *Am J Psychiatry* 128:120, 1972.

74. Greenblatt DJ, Greenblatt M: Which drug for alcohol withdrawal? *J Clin Pharmacol* 12:429, 1972.

75. Greenblatt DJ, Shader RJ: Drug therapy benzodiazepines; Parts I and II. *N Engl J Med* 291:1011, 1239, 1974.

76. Kloz UA, Avant GR, Hoyumpia A, et al: The effects of age and liver disease on the disposition and elimination of diazepam in adult man. *J Clin Invest* 55:347, 1975.

77. Boston Collaborative Drug Surveillance Program: Clinical depression of the central nervous system due to diazepam and chlordiazepoxide in relation to cigarette smoking and age. *N Engl J Med* 288:277, 1973.

78. Sampliner R, Iber FL: Diphenylhydantoin control of alcohol withdrawal seizures. *JAMA* 230:1430, 1974.

79. Victor M, Brausch C: The role of abstinence in the genesis of alcoholic epilepsy. *Epilepsia* 8:1, 1967.

80. Gessner PK: Is diphenylhydantoin effective in treatment of alcohol withdrawal? (letter) *JAMA* 219:1072, 1972.

81. MacDougall B: Treatment of alcohol withdrawal (letter). *N Engl J Med* 294:1240, 1976.

82. Mendelson JH: Propranolol and behavior of alcohol addicts after acute alcohol ingestion. *Clin Pharmacol Ther* 15:571, 1974.

83. Beard JD, Knott DH: Fluid and electrolyte balance during acute withdrawal in chronic alcoholic patients. *JAMA* 204:135, 1968.

84. Vetter WR, Cohn LH, Reichgott M: Hypokalemia and electrocardiographic abnormalities during acute alcohol withdrawal. *Arch Intern Med* 120:536, 1967.

85. Brown SS, Forest JA, Roscoe, PA: Controlled trial of fructose in the treatment of acute alcoholic intoxication. *Lancet* 2:892, 1972.

86. Coarse JF, Cardoni AA: Use of fructose in the treatment of acute alcoholic intoxication. *Am J Hosp Pharm* 32:518, 1975.

87. Rickett JW, Bowen DJ: Danger of intravenous fructose. *Lancet* 2:489, 1973.

88. Hirsch CS, Valentour JC, Adelson L, et al: Unexpected ethanol in drug-intoxicated persons. *Postgrad Med* 54:53, 1973.

89. Closs K, Solberg CO: Methanol poisoning. *JAMA* 211:497, 1970.

90. Cowen DL: Extracorporeal dialysis in methanol poisoning. *Ann Intern Med* 61:134, 1964.

91. Gonda A, Gault H, Churchill D, et al: Hemodialysis for methanol intoxication. *Am J Med* 64:749, 1978.

92. Adelson L: Fatal intoxication with isopropyl alcohol. *Am J Clin Pathol* 38:144, 1962.

93. Moss MH: Alcohol induced hypoglycemia and coma caused by alcohol sponging. *Pediatrics* 46:445, 1970.

94. Juncos L, Taguchi JT: Isopropyl alcohol intoxication. *JAMA* 204:186, 1968.

95. Underwood F, Bennett WM: Ethylene glycol intoxication. *JAMA* 226:1453, 1973.

96. Parry MF, Wallach R: Ethylene glycol poisoning. *Am J Med* 57:143, 1974.

97. Wacker WEC, Haynes H, Druyan R, et al: Treatment of ethylene glycol poisoning with ethyl alcohol. *JAMA* 194:1231, 1965.

98. Kissin B: The use of psychoactive drugs in the long term treatment of chronic alcoholics. *Ann N Y Acad Sci* 252:385, 1975.

99. Becker CE, Roe R, Scott R, et al: Rational drug therapy of alcoholism with sedative hypnotic drugs; is this possible? *Ann NY Acad Sci* 252:379, 1975.

100. Kitson TM: Disulfiram-ethanol reaction; a review. *J Stud Alcohol* 38:96, 1977.

101. Elenbaas RM: Drug therapy reviews; management of the disulfiram-alcohol reaction. *Am J Hosp Pharm* 34:827, 1977.

102. Amdor E, Gazdar A: Sudden death during disulfiram alcohol reaction. *O J Stud Alcohol* 28:649, 1967.

103. Whittington HG, Grey L: Possible interaction between disulfiram and isoniazid. *Am J Psychiatry* 125:1725, 1969.

104. O'Reilly RA: Interaction of sodium warfarin and disulfiram in man. *Ann Intern Med* 78:73, 1973.

105. Korboe E: Phenytoin intoxication during treatment with antabuse. *Epilepsia* 7:246, 1966.

106. Vessell ES, Passananti GT, Lee CH: Impairment of drug metabolism by disulfiram in man. *Clin Pharmacol Ther* 12:785, 1971.

107. Boyd JR: *Facts and Comparisons.* Facts and Comparisons Division, J. B. Lippincott Company, St. Louis, MO, 1982.

108. Kline NS, Wren JC, Cooper JB, et al: Evaluation of lithium therapy in chronic and periodic alcoholism. *Am J Med Sci* 268:15, 1974.

109. Leevy C, Baker H: Vitamins and alcoholism. *Am J Clin Nutr* 21:1325, 1968.

110. Davidson CS: Dietary treatment of hepatic diseases. *J Am Diet Assoc* 62:515, 1973.

111. OG: Alcoholic anonymous. *JAMA* 236:1505, 1976.

112. Parker WJ: Alcohol-drug interactions. *J Am Pharm Assoc (NS)* 10:664, 1970.

113. Seixas FA: Alcohol and its drug interactions. *Ann Intern Med* 83:86, 1975.

114. Adverse Interaction of Drugs: *Med Lett* 17:17, 1975.

115. Kater RM, Zieve P, Tobon F, et al: Accelerated metabolism of drugs in alcoholics. *Gastroenterology* 56:412, 1969.

116. Kater RM, Roggin G, Tobon F, et al: Increased rate of clearance of drugs from the circulation of alcoholics. *Am J Med Sci* 258:35, 1969.

117. Rubin E, Gang H, Misera PS, et al: Inhibition of drug metabolism by acute intoxication. *Am J Med* 49:801, 1970.

118. Kater RM, Tober F, Iber F: Increased rate of tolbutamide metabolism in alcoholic patients. *JAMA* 207:363, 1969.

119. Iber FL: Drug metabolism in heavy consumers of ethyl alcohol. *Clin Pharmacol Ther* 22:735, 1977.

120. Teschke R, Hasumura Y, Lieber CS: Increased carbon tetrachloride hepatotoxicity and its mechanism after chronic alcohol consumption. *Gastroenterology* 66:415, 1974.

121. Mitchell JR: Acetaminophen-induced hepatic injury; protective role of glutathione in man and rationale for therapy. *Clin Pharmacol Ther* 16:676, 1974.

122. Seppala T, Linnoila M, Elonen E, et al: Effects of tricyclic antidepressants and alcohol on psychomotor skills related to driving. *Clin Pharmacol Ther* 17:515, 1975.

123. Armor DJ, Polich JM, Stambul HB: Alcoholism and treatment R-1739-NIAA. The Rand Corporation. Santa Monica, Calif., 1976.

124. Nagy BR: Alcoholics returning to social drinking. *JAMA* 240:776, 1978.

125. Glasser L, Sternglanz PD, Combie J, et al: Serum osmolality and its applicability to drug overdose. *Am J Clin Pathol* 60:695–699, 1973.

126. Handy CA: Radiopacity of oral non-liquid medications. *Radiology* 98:525–534, 1971.

127. Closs K, Solberg CO: Methanol poisoning. *JAMA* 211:497–499, 1970.

128. Titinalli JE: Of anions, osmols and methanol poisoning. *JACEP* 6:417–421, 1977.

129. Peterson CD, Collins PJ, Himes JM, et al: Ethylene glycol poisoning pharmacokinetics during therapy with ethanol and hemodialysis. *N Engl J Med* 304:21–23, 1981.

130. Keyvan-Larijarni H, Tannenberg AM: Methanol intoxication. Comparison of peritoneal dialysis and hemodialysis treatment. *Arch Intern Med* 134:293–296, 1974.

131. Gonda A, Gault H, Churchill D, et al: Hemodialysis for methanol intoxication. *Am J Med* 64:749–758, 1978.

132. Tobin M, Lianos E: Hemodialysis for methanol intoxication. *J Dial* 3:97–106, 1979.

133. McCoy HG, Cipolle RJ, Ehlers SM, et al: Severe methanol poisoning. Application of a pharmacokinetic model for ethanol therapy and hemodialysis. *Am J Med* 67:804–807, 1979.

134. Norker PE, Lells JT, Tephly TR: Methanol toxicity: treatment with folic acid and 5-formyl tetrahydrofolic acid. *Alcoholism* 4:378–383, 1980.

135. Scully, RE, Galdabini JJ, McNeely BU: Case Records of the Massachusetts General Hospital

Case 38-1979 Ethylene glycol poisoning. *N Engl J Med* 301:650–657, 1979.

136. Collins JM, Hennes DM, Holzgang CR, et al: Recovery after prolonged oliguria due to ethylene glycol intoxication. *Arch Intern Med* 125:1059–1062, 1970.

137. Freed CR, Bobbitt WH, Williams RM, et al: Ethanol for ethylene glycol poisoning (letter). *N Engl J Med* 304:976–977, 1981.

138. Wacker WEC, Haynes H, Druyan R, et al: Treatment of ethylene glycol poisoning with ethyl alcohol. *JAMA* 194:1231–1233, 1965.

139. Underwood F, Bennett WM: Ethylene glycol intoxication. Prevention of renal failure by aggressive management. *JAMA* 226:1453–1454, 1973.

140. Stokes JB, Aueron F: Prevention of organ damage in massive ethylene glycol ingestion. *JAMA* 243:2065–2066, 1980.

141. Moss MH: Alcohol-induced hypoglycemia and coma caused by alcohol sponging. *Pediatrics* 46:445–447, 1970.

142. Lewin GA, Oppenheimer PR, Winger WA: Coma from alcohol sponging. *JACEP* 6:165–166, 1977.

143. Adelson L: Fatal intoxication with isopropyl alcohol (rubbing alcohol). *Am J Clin Pathol* 38:144–151, 1962.

144. Cate JC, Hedrick R: Propylene glycol intoxication and lactic acidosis (Letter). *N Engl J Med* 303:1237, 1979.

145. Sokol RJ: Alcohol and abnormal outcomes of pregnancy. *Can Med Assoc J* 125:143–148, 1981.

146. Abel EL: Fetal alcohol Syndrome: behavioral teratology. *Psychol Bull* 87:29–30, 1980.

147. Little RE, Streissguth AP: Effects of alcohol on the fetus: impact and prevention. *Can Med Assoc J* 125:159–164, 1981.

148. Binkiewicz A, Robinson MJ, Senior B: Pseudo-Cushing's Syndrome caused by alcohol in breast milk. *J Pediatr* 93:965, 1978.

149. Dehaene P, Samaille-Villette C, Samaille P, et al: Le syndrome d'alcoolisome foetal dans le nord de la France. *Rev Alcoholism* 23:145–148, 1977.

150. Olegard R, Sabel KG, Arronsson M, et al: Effects on the child of alcohol abuse during pregnancy. *Acta Paediatr Scand [Suppl]* 275:112–121, 1979.

151. Ouellette EM, Rosett HL, Rosman NP, et al: Adverse effects on offspring of maternal alcohol abuse during pregnancy. *N Engl J Med* 297:528–530, 1977.

152. Sokol RJ, Miller SI, Debanne S, et al: The Cleveland NIAAA Prospective Alcohol in Pregnancy Study: The First Year. Paper presented at the NIAAA Fetal Alcohol Syndrome Workshop, Seattle, 1980.

153. Chernoff GF: The fetal alcohol syndrome in mice: an animal model. *Teratology* 15:223–230, 1977.

154. Randall CL, Taylor WJ: Prenatal ethanol exposure in mice: teratogenic effect. *Teratology* 19:305–311, 1979.

155. Randall CL, Taylor WJ, Walker DW: Ethanol-induced malformations in mice. *Alcohol Clin Exp Res* 1:219–224, 1977.

156. Secretary of Health and Human Services: Fourth Special Report to the U.S. Congress on Alcohol and Health, Ch. 3. Biomedical Consequences of Alcohol Use and Abuse. Jan. 1981.

157. Elenbaas RM, Ryan JL, Robinson WA, et al: On the disulfiram-like activity of moxalactam. *Clin Pharmacol Ther* 32:347–355, 1982.

SECTION 2
Infectious Disease

CHAPTER 6

Respiratory Infections

ROBERT H. LEVIN, Pharm.D.

UPPER RESPIRATORY TRACT

An upper respiratory tract infection (URI) is defined as one that involves the head and neck above the vocal cords or larynx. Any infection below the larynx in the trachea or bronchial tree is considered a lower respiratory infection, such as bronchitis or pneumonia. Upper respiratory infections are a major societal health and economic problem, constituting more than half of all illnesses reported in the United States. From 1957 to 1962 there were 1,000,000,000 acute respiratory illnesses or about 227,000,000 per year (1). This figure has been steadily rising proportionally to increases in population, so that more recently there are approximately 1,000,000,000 cases of respiratory disease each year of which a majority are URIs (2). About 52% of the time the patient is required to spend at least 1 day at home in bed. This corresponds to a loss of productivity of 2 days per person per year.

The incidence of acute URI in childhood has been reported to be 7 or more episodes per year per child (3, 4). The incidence is age-dependent with very little difference in sexes. Most cases occur between birth and 2 years of age and thereafter the incidence decreases with age to about 4 to 6 episodes of acute URI per year for adolescents and adults. The frequency of per capita infections in the last 40 years has remained relatively unchanged (5).

Etiology

VIRAL

Krugman and Ward (1) stated that greater than 90% of all acute respiratory infections are probably viral in origin. There are more than 100 different viruses that can cause URIs (Table 6.1). The major viral groupings are the orthomyxoviruses, picornaviruses, adenoviruses, herpesvirus, poxvirus and paramyxoviruses (6). Hable et al. (7) found that viruses causes 19% of URIs in children from birth to 16 years of age. The viruses responsible were

influenza A$_2$/Hong Kong (5.5%), adenovirus (4.9%), parainfluenza (4.7%), rhinoviruses (1.2%), and herpes simplex (1.8%). Respiratory syncytial virus (RSV), coxsackie B, cytomegalovirus (CMV) and polio account for less than 1% each. Mufson et al. (8) identified specific viruses 34% of the time in a group of adults with URIs. The most predominant were rhinoviruses, found in 18% of the cases. Influenza A virus, parainfluenza virus type 1 or 3 and herpesvirus each occurred in 2 to 5% of patients. Coxsackie virus, adenovirus and RSV accounted for less than 1% each in Mufson's study.

General Characteristics of Viruses

Viruses are characterized by a lack of metabolism and only proliferate in living host cells, in tissue culture medium or in the developing chick embryo. The size of viruses is quite variable. For example, the picornavirus is extremely small and can be seen only with an electron microscope, whereas more complex viruses such as the poxvirus can be visualized with a light microscope. The nucleus of a virus has either a core of ribonucleic acid (RNA) or deoxyribonucleic acid (DNA). DNA and RNA are nucleic acids that govern viral replication since they carry the genetic codes which determine all hereditary characteristics.

There are three hypothesis to help explain the origin of viruses (9).

1. Viruses originated as parasites of the first cellular organisms. These first viruses gradually developed into present viruses as new organisms and animals evolved.

2. Viruses are not individual organisms but only components of normal cells which occasionally and inexplicably get out of hand. In this sense, viruses may be likened to uncontrolled genes which continue to replicate as long as there is building material available. A corollary to this hypothesis is that viruses are

Table 6.1.
Infectious Agents in Acute Respiratory Disease[a]

Group	Nucleic Acid	Size (nm)	Subgroups	Total No.	Clinical Syndromes
VIRAL					
Adenovirus	DNA	70–90	Adenoviruses, human	31	URI, pneumonia, bronchitis, croup, influenza-like illness
Herpesvirus	DNA	120–180	Herpes simplex 1, 2	2	Acute tonsillopharyngitis with vesicles or ulcers
			Varicella-zoster virus	1	Pneumonia
			Cytomegalovirus (CMV)	1	Pneumonia
			Mononucleosis (EBV)	1	URI
Poxvirus	DNA	230–300	Variola (smallpox)	1	Severe URI
Picornavirus	RNA	15–30	Rhinoviruses	>90	URI mainly in adults; bronchitis
			Enteroviruses:		
			Coxsackie virus A	24	URI, tonsillopharyngitis, influenza-like illness
			Coxsackie virus B	6	URI, influenza-like illness, bronchitis, pneumonia
			Echovirus	33	URI, croup
			Poliovirus 1, 2, 3	3	URI
Togavirus	RNA	20–70	Rubella	1	URI
Orthomyxovirus	RNA	80–120	Influenza A, B, C,	3	Influenza, croup, URI
Paramyxovirus	RNA	100–200	Rubeola	1	Measles, laryngitis, bronchitis pneumonia
		100–300	Parainfluenza 1, 2, 3, 4	4	URI, croup, bronchitis
		120–300	Respiratory syncytial	2+?	URI, croup, bronchitis, pneumonia
NONVIRAL AGENTS					
Mycoplasma (PPLO)		125–150	*M. pneumoniae*	1	URI, pneumonia
			Other mycloplasmas	7	
Chlamydia					Conjunctivitis, pneumonia
Pneumocystis carinii					Pneumonia
Kawasaki's organism					Pharyngitis
Bacterial					
Streptococci group A, β-hemolytic					URI, "strep throat," otitis media
Streptococcus pneumoniae					Otitis media, pneumonia
Haemophilus influenzae					Epiglottitis, otitis media, pneumonia
Diphtheria					Pharyngitis
Pseudomonas aerugenosa					Pneumonia
Staphylococcus aureus					Pneumonia
Fungi					
Candida					Stomatitis, pneumonia

[a] Others causing disease are reoviruses, psittacosis-ornithosis virus, lymphocytic choriomeningitis virus.

derivatives of normal cellular genes (nucleic acids) which centuries ago developed the capability of reproducing by themselves and forming a protective envelope to stabilize the structure as it passed from cell to cell.

3. Viruses have evolved from pathogenic bacteria through a retrograde evolutionary process. There is no evidence to support this theory. However, it remains viable because there are bacteria which have developed a parasitic existence and grow only with great difficulty outside host cells.

Most viruses, such as measles, mumps, rubella and polio, have remarkably stable immunological characteristics, so that after countless replication cycles, they have little or no genetic change. In contrast, a few are unstable and change continuously, such as the influenza viruses, rhinoviruses and adenoviruses. This instability creates difficulty in developing effective immunizations against the latter groups (see immunizations in Chapter 3, "Pediatrics"). The protective envelope of the virus and the other structured proteins serve several important functions; protection from enzymatic (nuclease) inactivation; participation in attachment to susceptible cells; and provision of structural symmetry. The proteins in the viral envelope are also responsible for the antigenicity of the virus; an important consideration in vaccine production.

BACTERIAL

Nonviral causes of URI and its complications are *Mycoplasma pneumoniae*, other bacteria, such as streptococci, *Haemophilus influenzae*, some fungi and some rickettsia. However, these nonviral agents are much more commonly associated with lower respiratory tract infections and other manifestations or complications of URIs. Group A β-hemolytic streptococci commonly cause sore throat (38%) and otitis media (5%). *Streptococcus pneumoniae* is the most common organism in infectious otitis media (40%) and a very common cause of pneumonia. *H. influenzae* is the second most common cause of bacterial pneumonia and otitis media in children from 6 months to 6 years old and the predominant cause of epiglottitis.

Pathogenesis

The viruses causing URI gain entrance to the human host through the respiratory or gastrointestinal (GI) tract. Discharges from the mouth and nose of infected persons are transmitted to susceptible people by direct contact or droplet infection or by recently contaminated articles. Those viruses causing colds, flu or croup have a short incubation period of approximately 1 to 3 days. Those causing lower tract disease such as measles and mumps, where viral replication occurs in the lymph nodes rather than in the respiratory tract, have a long incubation period which may be as long as 3 weeks.

As the virus replicates and disseminates, the human body responds to the foreign invader, producing an inflammatory condition in affected areas to increase blood perfusion. Increased perfusion brings lymphocytes to fight the infection and allows circulating antibodies, if present, to come in contact with the virus and inactivate it. Other local physiologic changes which aid the body in combating infection are pyrexia, lowered cellular pH, and hypoxia. A cell-mediated immunity, which is not clearly understood, is also present (10–12) and involves sensitized lymphocytes, activated macrophages and interferon, a nonspecific antiviral protein. Most viruses are potent stimulators of interferon production.

Viral infection generally results in antibody production that aids in preventing reinfection. Viral infections induce both local and systemic antibody production. Viruses which invade the respiratory tract and proliferate in the superficial respiratory epithelium induce a local antibody response. Secretory immunoglobulin A (IgA) is produced in the mucous cells and is secreted into the mucous blanket to locally inhibit viruses (10, 13). The IgA is very specific and only protects against that specific virus. Unfortunately, these resistant epithelial cells rapidly turn over and are replaced by susceptible cells. Furthermore, only secretory IgA is of any benefit in fighting local infection, since serum gamma globulins provide only partial local protection.

Serum IgA, serum immunoglobulin G (IgG), and immunoglobulin M (IgM) afford complete protection only when systemic viremia occurs. These γ-globulins are produced after systemic viral infection, and afford excellent protection against those diseases with long incubation periods, such as measles, rubella and smallpox.

SUSCEPTIBILITY TO COLDS

There are some interesting observations that can be made about colds. Cold weather per se does not increase the probability of getting colds, nor does chilling of the body and wet feet induce colds; however, a chilly body will result in a decrease in body temperature. The nose, which is especially sensitive to cold, becomes irritated when chilled, and sneezing and a serous discharge follow. This ensuing rhinitis is frequently confused with actual viral infections. Susceptibility to infection does not appear to be affected by the general state of a person's health but a poor state of nutrition is a large factor for increasing the severity of colds or developing complications. Fatigue or emotional disturbances may temporarily lower one's resistance to infection. Allergic people develop colds more easily after exposure than nonallergic people, 45% and 30% incidence, respectively (14). Finally, women who are chilled or exposed to cold in the middle third of their menstrual cycle (10 to 20 days after menstruation) are more susceptible to colds than at any other time in their cycles (14).

DIAGNOSIS

The etiological agents of colds can be divided into groups of viruses which cause similar symptoms. Picornaviruses, adenoviruses, orthomyxoviruses and paramyxoviruses, with few exceptions, cause nearly identical disease states (15, 16). Viral cultures to ascertain the etiological agent are seldom done because of the time and difficulty in culturing viruses. Two weeks are required to report the results of a culture so that standard cultures are done only with epidemics. New techniques are being developed which are capable of determining the identity of viral agents in 24 hours. The use of immunofluorescent staining is one very promising method (17). In this procedure, a patient's nasal secretion is mixed with conjugated horse antiparainfluenza antibody. If there is parainfluenza virus in the nasal secretions, this antibody attaches to the virus and fluoresces in 24 hours giving a positive identification.

In patients, especially children, with repeated colds, it is important to differentiate an infectious process from an allergic one. The symptoms of both a cold and allergic rhinitis are clinically indistinguishable. Fortunately, a patient with allergic rhinitis does have some characteristic symptoms, such as constant watery rhinorrhea, frequent sneezing, nasal itching, wheezing and night cough. The allergic child also has a greater incidence of skin rashes.

Clinical Findings and Symptoms

Many of the viruses can cause similar symptoms of URI, and the same virus may cause various forms of illness in different individuals (18). The common cold in children and adults and croup in children are the most common forms of URIs and can be caused by most of the viruses discussed. The common cold encompasses a number of entities; coryza, rhinitis, rhinopharyngitis, acute catarrh and tonsillopharyngitis with or without exudate, vesicles or ulcers. The incubation period is short, being from 1 to 6 days with an average of 2 days. Colds are spread by direct person-to-person contact through contaminated droplets in the air or by touching contaminated personal items.

The common cold causes a wide range of symptoms which are all too familiar to each of us. Varying degrees of nasal congestion and discharge will occur. Initially, this discharge is clear and watery but, with progression of the disease, it becomes thicker and opaque. It may also become purulent if secondarily infected with bacteria. Conjunctivitis and watering eyes, a sore throat and unproductive cough are also rather common manifestations of the cold. If a lower respiratory infection complicates a cold, the increased pulmonary secretions will lead to a productive cough. Redness of the pharynx and tonsils without an exudate commonly occurs and is usually accompanied by a sore throat. If an exudate is present on the tonsils, bacterial agents such as streptococci or diphtheria are suspected, although some forms of adenoviruses and herpesvirus can also cause exudates. Herpesvirus is the probable causative agent when vesicles or ulcers are seen. Body temperature usually is not elevated to more than 38°C (101°F). Chilly sensations are common, as are sneezing and headache. Infection with influenza virus also causes marked prostration, muscular aches and a high incidence of lower respiratory symptoms.

The common cold is usually a short-lived benign disease. Although the symptoms can be very discomforting, they seldom cause serious complications. The usual complications, which are more common in children are otitis media and croup and secondary bacterial infection, chiefly in the pulmonary tree because of mucus plugging of the bronchioles. Bacterial agents and some viral agents will cause bronchitis, bronchiolitis, pneumonia and other lower respiratory tract infections.

Medicinal Treatment

The treatment of colds is carried out on a completely symptomatic basis. With the plethora of medications on the market (19, 20), it seems more of an art than a science to select the proper treatment. The sheer number of combination products "boggles the mind." This large number of products plus the reported high placebo response to cold medications leads one to believe that effective treatment is difficult to quantify. The inclusion of many pharmacological agents in one "shotgun" preparation, some of which negate the action of others, makes it difficult to understand the rationality of the formulation. The combination "shotgun" preparations containing antihistamines, decongestants, expectorants and antitussives seem to temporarily alleviate some symptoms of colds. Some may be useful, some not, and this enigma exists because people desire one pill or liquid to cure all symptoms and the manufacturers claim to have produced such entities. Cold formulas should be kept simple with the judicious use of a few drugs to treat a limited number of specific symptoms because combination products do not allow dosing of individual agents and produce complicated toxicological problems with overdoses.

ANALGESICS

Analgesics, such as aspirin and acetaminophen, are commonly used for the minor aches, pains and fever associated with colds. Aspirin is the drug of choice for adults and older children but not for children under 2 years old. This young age group is particularly sensitive to the toxic effects of aspirin and small overdoses can cause serious acid-base and fluid electrolyte problems. Acetaminophen is an excellent substitute for aspirin in this age group. It is equivalent to aspirin as an analgesic and antipyretic and is much less toxic (19). An overdose of acetaminophen, however, can be extremely toxic and lead to hepatic damage or hepatic failure (21).

Caution should be observed when using salicylates to treat fever or pain in children less than 16 years old who have chicken pox, influenza or possibly viral URIs (22–25). The Secretary of the U.S. Health and Human Services Department has proposed new labeling for salicylates to warn against the possible link between salicylate use and Reye's syndrome (22). Reye's syndrome consists of encephalopathy associated with hepatic failure and occurs in children between 5 and 16 years old, is a rare disease, accounts for about 600 to 1200 cases/year, has a 20 to 30% fatality rate and may cause permanent brain damage in survivors. Pharmacists can order patient brochures on Reyes syndrome as part of an established awareness program (26, 27).

ANTIBIOTICS

Antibiotics should not be used prophylactically for colds but only for proven or highly suspected bacterial infections (28, 29). The indiscriminate use of antibiotics has not changed the incidence of respiratory infections (5) and may lead to the development of resistant strains of microorganisms, which may be a major problem. The proper antibiotic should be used for suspected bacterial otitis media or pneumonia and will be covered later.

NOSE DROPS AND SPRAYS

Nose drops and sprays containing decongestants sometimes provide impressive and immediate relief of congestion. They are useful for local decongestant effect for short periods of time. The drops and spray are equally effective, but the spray is easier to use and has a better distribution in the nasal mucosa. Unfortunately, this relief does not last unless the drops or sprays are used repeatedly every 6 to 12 hours. Tolerance to these preparations is common. Upon withdrawal of the drops, a rebound congestion as severe as the original congestion may occur. For this reason patients may abuse nose drops and develop a nose drop habit. In short, nose drops or sprays should be used judiciously, as infrequently as possible and not for periods of over a week at a time.

Nose drops in oily vehicles should not be used because aspiration of the drops may result in lipoid pneumonia, especially in infants. Those containing antibiotics and antiseptics are not effective and should not be used. Antiseptics like eucalyptus and thymol can paralyze the cilia and prevent the clearing of mucus, which may cause more problems than the disease (1). Hypotonic or very hypertonic solutions may also paralyze the cilia. If a physician requests a mother to use normal saline drops for her infant, she should obtain the solution prepared by a pharmacist, which would be isotonic and relatively sterile. Because infants less than 6 months of age breathe only through their nose, drops may be helpful just prior to meals in congested infants who are having difficulty feeding. The two most common drops used for infants are phenylephrine and xylometazoline, both now available over the counter (OTC) (19). Phenylephrine causes more rebound congestion that xylometazoline, but the latter is more toxic causing profound sedation when absorbed systemically.

ORAL DECONGESTANTS

The most frequently used oral decongestants are ephedrine, pseudoephedrine, phenylpropanolamine and phenylephrine (Table 6.2). Most are now available OTC, individually or in combination with other ingredients including antihistamines. Because these agents may increase blood sugar and raise blood pressure, people with diabetes mellitus, heart disease, hypertension, hyperthyroidism or cardiovascular disease and elderly patients or infants should be appropriately cautioned regarding these products. The elderly patient is much more sensitive to the effects of these agents. Nasal secretions in infants less than 6 months of age can become so viscous after oral decongestant use that nasal passage obstruction and extreme difficulty in breathing may occur.

Oral decongestants have certain advantages over the nasal decongestants.

1. They reach all the respiratory membranes via the blood and are not dependent on absorption through the thick mucous layer in the nose as are the drops.

2. They generally have a longer duration of effect.

3. They cause no rebound nasal congestion.

4. Nose drop habit does not ocurr.

5. They are easily administered in an accurate dosage which is not easily achieved with drops.

6. They cause no pathological changes in the cilia or nasal mucosa.

The oral decongestants also have disadvantages:

1. Systemic side effects are common, such as nervousness, increased heart rate and in-

Table 6.2.
Common Decongestants

Drug	Equivalent Adult Dose[a]	Pediatric Dose	CNS Stimulation
	mg	*mg/kg/24 hr*	
Ephedrine	50	3	+++
Phenylephrine	10–25	4	–
Phenylpropanolamine	50	3	+
Pseudoephedrine	60	1–2	++

[a] Frequency of dosage (all drugs) is t.i.d.–q.i.d.

somnia. Such side effects are unusual with normal doses of the nasal decongestants.

2. Tolerance develops so that increasing doses must be given.

3. They have not been conclusively proven to be efficacious in the treatment of nasal congestion (30). They are used traditionally and empricially as a rational way to treat rhinorrhea.

Ephredrine is probably the best orally absorbed of these agents. Phenylephrine is the most poorly absorbed since it is readily destroyed in the stomach by the enzyme monoamine oxidase (31). It is so readily inactivated that an adequate oral dose is very difficult to achieve, making its use in oral preparations at best questionable. Ephedrine causes the most central nervous system (CNS) stimulation and phenylephrine the least (Table 6.2). Phenylpropanolamine has a greater vasopressor effect than ephedrine or pseudoephedrine but less than phenylephrine. Antihistamines are sometimes combined with these agents in an effort to counteract their central stimulating effect.

COMBINATION PRODUCTS

Because of their sedative properties, the antihistamines do counteract some of the stimulant effects of the oral decongestants. This theorectical balancing of effects does not always achieve the anticipated results. Some people are more sensitive to the effects of either the antihistamines or the decongestants and react accordingly. Not surprisingly, parents seek those products which produce sedation in children. The combination products are more attractive to parents because they want to give as few different doses of medications as possible to their sick, cranky and obstinate children. Successful combinations for each individual are usually found only after considerable trial and error using many products. This combination also has an additive effect in decreasing rhinorrhea—the decongestant due to vasoconstriction thereby decreasing edema and the antihistamine due to its anticholinergic effect of mucous drying (32). The combination products, however, reduce flexibility in dosing. It is not possible to recommend one combination oral decongestant and antihistamine preparation over another. Minimal side effects, symptomatic relief and palatability will determine the product used by each individual. Children or adults with asthma, acute otitis media or sensitivity to antihistamines are probably better served with decongestants alone.

Furthermore, the usual practice is to put numerous drugs in cold preparations to treat all URI symptoms. Analgesics, antitussives, expectorants, decongestants, anticholinergics, vitamins and antihistamines are commonly found together in the same preparation. This combination of ingredients increases the incidence of adverse effects. These products also pose a major treatment problem when accidentally ingested in toxic quantities. Some ingredients in combination products are in suboptimal doses, requiring doses above the recommended ones to achieve therapeutic results. This can result in serious side effects or toxicity. Lack of flexibility in dosing is an obvious drawback to the use of combinations. Finally, there is no convicing evidence that combination products are any better than placebos in treating the common cold.

When recommending products and doses, a pharmacist must carefully check the quantity of each ingredient in the product against its recommended dose. Most combination products, especially those sold OTC are labeled with directions that usually result in underdosing. An OTC product should be initially given at the recommended dose level to ascertain whether the patient will react adversely. If no adverse effects ensue, the recommended dose generally must be increased before any therapeutic effect becomes evident. In general, the dose should be increased until a therapeutic effect is achieved or until side effects become evident.

ANTIHISTAMINES

The antihistamines are most effective for allergic reactions, such as allergic rhinitis, chronic allergic otitis media, angioneurotic edema and other conditions in which histamine blockade is required (33, 34). They have equivocal effects in the treatment of asthma and may exacerbate wheezing because of their mucus drying effect. There is little difference between the antihistamines based on their efficacy as histamine blockers. Finally, the antihistamines are most effective as drying agents only in the initial stages of a cold.

The preference of one product over another rests purely on the side effects each produces (Table 6.3). The prominent side effects are anticholinergic in nature, sedation, tachycardia, mucus drying and decreased GI motility. Since the differences in products are based on side effects and somewhat on cost, the antihistamine chosen should be inexpensive and cause only desired side effects. For example, if a daytime dose is needed, a product with a low incidence of sedation, e.g., chlorpheniramine, should be chosen so as not to interfere with one's routine. If a nightime medication is needed, the reverse would be true—use the antihistamine with the greatest incidence of sedation, e.g., diphenhydramine. If one antihistamine does not achieve the desired effects after being given in doses large enough to elicit side effects, another product, preferably in a different chemical class, should be tried.

Table 6.3.
Common Antihistamines

Drug	Equivalent Adult Dose[a]	Pediatric Dose[a]	CNS Sedation
	mg	*mg/kg/24 hr*	
Ethanolamines			
Bromodiphenhydramine	25	2.5	+++
Carbinoxamine	4	0.4	+
Diphenhydramine	50	5.0	+++
Doxylamine	12–25	2.0	+++
Ethylenediamines			
Methapyrilene	50–100	5.0	+
Pyrilamine	50	2.5	++
Tripelennamine	50	5.0	++
Alkylamines			
Brompheniramine	4	0.5	+
chlorpheniramine	4	0.35	+
Triprolidine	2.5[b]	0.2[b]	+
Phenothiazines			
Promethazine	25	1.5[b]	+++

[a] All taken t.i.d.-q.i.d., except as noted.
[b] Taken b.i.d.-t.i.d.

COUGH PREPARATIONS

The cough associated with URI is usually brief, self-limiting and does not require an arsenal of medication to treat. If the cough is nonproductive and is caused by irritation of the respiratory tract from inflammation or postnasal drip, the treatment objective is to ameliorate the cough. A rational approach would dictate the use of demulcents for the irritation with or without an antitussive. If a postnasal drip complicates the picture, a decongestant with or without an antihistamine could be separately added and individually titrated. If the patient has a lower respiratory infection and has a nonproductive cough, the aim of treatment should be to induce a productive cough to facilitate the removal of pulmonary secretions. Dehydration, a common problem in infections with high fever and patients with poor appetites, causes mucus to become viscous and tenacious. This is not reversed with medications until the patient is rehydrated. Expectorants are available and utilized to decrease mucus viscosity and facilitate its removal. Cool mist and steam vaporizers are also effective in loosening mucus, providing they are capable of increasing the relative humidity of the air in the room to 100%.

EXPECTORANTS

There are a number of expectorants utilized in cough medications which are of little or no value, e.g., ammonium citrate and other ammonium compounds, terpin hydrate, creosote, chloroform and squill (35). There are three commonly used expectorants which in proper doses do seem to have some value although this is unproven (35): guafenisin, syrup of ipecac and iodide salts.

Blanchard and Ford (36) reported in 1954 that guafenisin with desoxyephedrine is an effective antitussive-demulcent-expectorant. The definition of an antitussive used by Blanchard is a drug which reduces cough by facilitating the removal of mucus. The addition of desoxyephedrine, however, is of doubtful efficacy in this preparation. Also, the subjectivity of this study makes the results difficult to interpret. Other studies done during the 1950s could be cited, but all suffer from being subjectively done with few or no controls. If guafenisin is to be effective at all, it must be given

in therapeutic doses. Chodosh (37) stated that only at doses of 300 to 600 mg 4 times daily is there a definite decrease in sputum viscosity. Thus, the commonly recommended dose of 100 mg (usually 1 teaspoonful) 4 times daily is a substantial underdose. A therapeutic dose of guafenisin cough syrup for adults is 15 to 30 ml 4 times daily, and for children there should also be a proportional increase of dose. Generally, hydration alone is sufficient for children with URI.

Syrup of ipecac can be utilized as an expectorant in doses that are lower than the 15-ml emetic dose. Traditionally, 1 to 2 teaspoonfuls were given to children with croup to induce emesis and force up tenacious sputum (36) (see "Croup," p. 179). This proved to be effective but was usually only temporary and was unpleasant for the patient and family. The doses recommended now, 5 drops for a 1-year-old plus a drop for each year, is an underdose. Furthermore, most commercial preparations contain less than 10% of the therapeutic dose.

Potassium and sodium iodide are the most commonly used iodides. They are effective in adults when given in therapeutic doses of at least 300 mg (0.3 ml saturated solution of potassium iodide) every 2 to 4 hours and in children at doses of 100 mg per year of age per 24 hours. Most preparations containing iodides have considerably less than these therapeutic doses. More important, long-term use of iodides has caused goiters and symptoms of hypothyroidism, thus only short-term use should be considered.

ANTITUSSIVES

The antitussives are drugs which depress the cough reflex either centrally in the medulla or locally in the respiratory tree. The narcotics used (codeine, hydrocodone and ethylmorphine) work centrally as do the nonnarcotics, dextromethorphan, noscapine and levopropoxyphene. Other non-narcotics, such as chlophedianol HCL, dimenthoxanate HCl, benzonate HCl, or pipazethate, act as local anesthetics in the respiratory tree to produce their antitussive effect. The high cost and dubious value of the non-narcotic drugs other than dextromethorphan make their use questionable.

Codeine is by far the most commonly employed antitussive in adults. The recommended dose of 10 mg every 3 to 4 hours can usually be safely increased to 20 to 40 mg every 3 to 4 hours to achieve effects (38, 39). Occasionally 60 mg every 4 hours may be needed (35, 40). The usual dose range for children is 5 to 15 mg (35). Dextromethorphan, however, is the drug of choice for children.

Dextromethorphan is recommended especially for children, but it is also popular with adults because it does not have the sedative, analgesic, gastric irritating, constipating or habituating properties of codeine. It is as effective as codeine when used in adequate doses. The recommended dose in children of 1 mg per kg every 24 hours has been exceeded 4-fold without causing any apparent ill effects (38). Adult doses of 20 mg every 4 hours are minimal doses but 45 to 60 mg every 4 hours is a good therapeutic dose (39, 40). A prudent policy a pharmacist should follow when recommending doses would be to start with the recommended dose. If no cough suppression is noted, a careful increase in dose is warranted until the cough or side effects occur.

General Treatment

Bed rest and sufficient fluids, especially with fever, are very important for treating colds. Hydration is extremely important and must be achieved either through oral or respiratory intake. The steam vaporizers are somewhat effective in increasing room humidity and, therefore, fluid intake occurs via the lungs; however, they must be used in a small closed room to achieve this effect. They have the disadvantage of causing serious burns when tipped over—a decided problem where small ambulatory children are being treated. The cool mist vaporizers do not have this disadvantage but they also must be used in a small closed room to be effective. Generally, the most effective humidifier is the steam from a hot shower. A croupy child may be put to sleep in the bathroom near the shower, in a portable bed, with the hot water slowly running (see "Croup," p. 179). Heat lamps have also been used to treat colds. The warmth they produce feels good but has a dubious value in ameliorating the symptoms of a cold.

Prevention of Colds

Numerous panaceas have been proposed in the hopes of preventing the incidence of colds. Combined bacterial catarrhal vaccines (36), antihistamines, ultraviolet radiation and vitamins have all been tried and have been proven worthless. Vitamin C received a wide press coverage for its proposed effects on colds. Linus Pauling claimed large doses (1 to 5 g per day) can prevent colds and 15 g a day can cure colds (41). The *Medical Letter* (42, 43) carefully reviewed his book and concluded, "In the absence of convincing evidence of its effectiveness and safety, the *Medical Letter* does not recommend the use of large doses of vitamin C for the prevention or treatment of the common cold." Studies done by Hornick (44) and Charleston and Clegg (45) shed little new light on this subject.

Hornick used only 21 patients, ½ of which were controls, and found no difference between the test group and controls in preventing experimental rhinovirus infection in adults. The test subjects received 1 g of ascorbic acid 3 times a day starting 2 weeks before the infection and continued for 1 week past the infection. A placebo was given to the control group. He found no difference between groups in onset of illness, in the peak illness, virus excretion, antibody levels or nasal mucus flow. He did find that the test group on day 4 of the illness had less severe rhinitis and rhinorrhea than did the control group. Because of the small number of patients, this study is not very meaningful. Charleston with 47 patients and 43 controls and using 250 mg of ascorbic acid 4 times daily for 15 weeks did find a reduction in the incidence of colds in the test group. The average number of colds per person in the test group was 0.94 compared to 1.86 in the control group. He also found a significant reduction in the average duration of cold symptoms (3.5 days compared with 4.2 days). This study was reported to the editor so very little information about control procedures is known. This study is also difficult to interpret but does indicate additional research needs to be done to elucidate the role of vitamin C in the prevention of colds. Prevention of colds is important to preclude the development of other sequalae such as otitis media, pharyngitis, croup, etc.

Sequelae of Colds

Lower respiratory infection (LRI) is one of the sequelae of URI and it is usually caused by bacteria or *M. pneumoniae*. *M. pneumoniae* was thought to be a virus and to be the cause of "atypical pneumonia." In 1962, it was reclassified to pleuropneumonia-like organism, a bacterium. It may account for as much as 30 to 50% of lower respiratory disease of young adults (1, 46). In epidemics, as many as 10% of children with URI will be afflicted. Its incidence in younger children is about 1%. Other bacteria causing both LRI and URI symptoms are streptococci, staphylococci, pneumococci, diptheria and *H. influenzae*. All of these are treated primarily with appropriate antibiotics and also symptomatically. Fungal agents producing coccidiodomycosis or histoplasmosis and rickettsial agents, such as *Rickettsia burnetii*, the cause of Q fever, can also cause URI symptoms and are treated with appropriate antibiotics.

OTITIS MEDIA

Incidence and Etiology

Disease of the middle ear is among the most common illnesses of early childhood, and may account for as many as 40% of a pediatricians office visits (47). The highest incidence of otitis media occurs in children 6 months to 6 years of age. The infecting bacterial organisms generally responsible are: *S. pneumoniae* (40%), *H.influenzae* (24%), group A β-hemolytic streptococci (4%), *Staphylococcus aureus* (2%) and with the balance being aseptic or viruses (30%). In neonates, *Escherichia coli*, group B streptococci, *S. aureus*, *Listeria* and *Klebsiella pneumoniae* are the common infecting organisms (48, 49). In children over 6 years of age and adults, *S. pneumonia*, group A β-hemolytic streptococci and viruses are the etiologic agents. It is important to remember these differences because cultures of the middle ear are rarely done, due to the difficulty in performing tympanocentesis in young children.

Diagnosis and Symptoms

The child with otitis media is frequently irritable and may be lethargic. Over 50% have pain and fever greater than 100°F. Many have symptoms of an URI, some have a cough and a few may present with a draining ear secondary to a perforated tympanic membrane. Ear pulling by the child, commonly thought to be indicative of otitis media, occurs in less than 4% of children with otitis media. The physician makes the definitive diagnosis by observing the ear through an otoscope. The tympanic membrane in acute suppurative otitis media is red, bulging and the middle-ear bony landmarks cannot be observed. Newer methods of

evaluating middle ear function using acoustic impedance measurement through tympanometry are very accurate and useful (50).

Complications

Treated otitis media is associated with a conductive hearing loss. This loss may progress and lead to permanent loss and deafness in untreated cases. Rupture of the tympanic membrane may occur, and if left untreated, the continual drainage of pus may cause a permanent hole in the eardrum. Recurrent untreated cases may disseminate and lead to serious cases of mastoiditis or meningitis.

Pathogenesis

Acute otitis media, middle ear infection, is almost always associated with an URI. Infectious agents enter the middle ear through the eustachian tube, and normally are also excreted via the eustachian tube. However, children less than 6 years of age have short, horizontal eustachian tubes which are prone to obstruction from inflamed tonsils, adenoids or mucus plugging. If a tube is obstructed, the infectious agents will propagate in the middle ear and cause suppurative otitis media. To prevent damage to the ear and a possible loss of hearing, it is important to treat probable bacterial otitis media with medications.

Treatment

ANTIBIOTICS

The treatment of choice is a 10-day course of antibiotics. This is routinely done by outpatient management with an oral antibiotic preparation (51). Neonatal or complicated otitis media may have to be managed in a hospital with IV medications (49). The choice of antibiotics in a child less than 6 years old should be dictated by the most likely infecting organisms, i.e., *S. pneumoniae* and *H. influenzae*. The antibiotic of choice should be chosen on the basis of efficacy, incidence of side effects, cost and patient acceptance.

There has been an increasing resistance of lactamase-producing *H. influenzae* to ampicillin and amoxicillin. This may necessitate therapy with lactamase-resistant drugs in areas where the resistance level is 50% or more. Penicillin or erythromycin alone have little if any efficacy against *H. influenzae*. Of the oral cephalosporins used for otitis media, cefaclor

Table 6.4.
Common Antibiotics in Respiratory Disease[a]

Drug	Route[b]	Pediatric Dose[c]	Adult Dose[d]
Amikacin	IV, IM	15–25 mg/kg/24 h q 8–12 h	15 mg/kg/24 h q 8–12 h
Amoxicillin	PO	<20 kg 20–40 mg/kg/24 h q 8 h >20 kg 40–100 mg/kg/24 h q 8 h	250–500 mg q 8 h
Ampicillin	PO	50–100 mg/kg/24 h q 6 h	250–500 mg q 6 h
	IV, IM	<40 kg 100–300 mg/kg/24 h q 6 h >40 kg 1–14 g/24 h q 6 h	8–14 g/24 h q 6 h
Azlocillin	IV	50–150 mg/kg/24 h q 8 h	2–5 g q 8 h
Carbenicillin sodium	IV, IM	50–500 mg/kg/24 h q 4–6 h	15–30 g/24 h q 4–6 h
Cefaclor	PO	20–40 mg/kg/24 h q 8 h	250–500 mg q 8 h
Cefamandole	IV, IM	50–100 mg/kg/24 h q 4–8 h	0.5–2 g q 4–6 h
Cefazolin	IV, IM	25–100 mg/kg/24 h q 6–8 h	0.5–3 g q 6–8 h
Cefoperazone	IV, IM	50–100 mg/kg/24 h q 12 h	2–12 g/24 h q 12 h
Cefotaxime	IV, IM	50–180 mg/kg/24 h q 4–6 h	1–2 g q 4–8 h maximum 12 g/24 h
Cephalexin	PO	25–100 mg/kg/24 h q 6 h	250–500 mg q 6 h
Cephradine	PO	25–100 mg/kg/24 h q 6–12 h	250–500 mg q 6–12 h
	IV	>9 months old 50–100 mg/kg/24 h q 6–12 h	2–4 g/24 q 6 h
Chloramphenical	PO, IV	50–100 mg/kg/24 h q 6 h	250–500 mg q 6 h
Cloxacillin	PO	50–200 mg/kg/24 h q 6 h maximum 8 g/24 h	250–500 mg q 6 h
Co-trimoxazole	PO	48–120 mg/kg/24 h q 6–12 h (trimethoprim 8–20 mg + sulfamethoxazole 40–100 mg)	960 mg q 6–12 h (trimethoprim 160 mg + sulfamethoxazole 800 mg)
Dicloxacillin	PO	12.5–100 mg/kg/24 h q 6 h	125–500 mg q 6 h
Doxycycline	PO	>8 years and <45 kg: 2.2 mg/kg/24 h q 12–24 h; >45 kg: 100 mg/24 h q 12–24 h	100–200 mg q 12–24 h
Erythromycin	PO	30–50 mg/kg/24 h q 6 h	250–500 mg q 6 h
	IV, IM	10 mg/kg/24 h q 8–12 h	200 mg q 8–12 h
Gentamicin	IV, IM	3–7.5 mg/kg/24 h q 8 h	40–80 mg q 8–12 h
Methicillin	IV, IM	100–400 mg/kg/24 h q 4–6 h	1–4 g q 4–6 h
Mezlocillin	IV, IM	150–300 mg/kg/24 h q 4 h	1.5–4 g q 4–6 h maximum 24 g/24 h
Moxalactam	IV, IM	50–200 mg/kg/24 h q 6–8 h	0.5–4 g q 8 h maximum 12 g/24 h
Nafcillin	IV, IM	50–200 mg/kg/24 h q 4–8 h	4–12 g/24 h q 4–6 h
Penicillin G			
Aqueous	PO	25,000–50,000 units/kg/24 h q 4–6 h	400,000–800,000 units q 4–6 h
	IV	50,000–400,000 units/kg/24 h q 4–6 h	4–30 million units/24 h q 4–6 h
Procaine and benzathine	IM	0.6–1.2 million units q 12 h	1.2–2.4 million units q 12 h
Penicillin V	PO	25,000–100,000 units/kg/24 h q 6–8 h	400,000–800,000 units q 6–8 h
Pipiracillin	IV, IM	>12 years old: 100–300 mg/kg/24 h q 4–6 h	2–4 g q 4–6 h maximum 24 g/24 h
Sulfisoxazole	PO	150 mg/kg/24 h q 6 h	1 g q 6 h
	IV	100 mg/kg/24 h q 6–8 h	0.5–1 g q 6–8 h
Tetracycline	PO	>8 years: 25–50 mg/kg/24 h q 4–6 h maximum 500 mg/dose	250–500 mg q 4–6 h
	IV	>8 years: 10–15 mg/kg/24 h q 12 h maximum 2 g	500 mg q 12 h

Table 6.4.—*Continued*

Drug	Route[b]	Pediatric Dose[c]	Adult Dose[d]
	IM	>8 years: 10–25 mg/kg/24 h q 8–12 h maximum 250 mg/ dose	250 mg q 8–12 h
Ticarcillin	IV, IM	200–300 mg/kg/24 h q 4–6 h	200–300 mg/kg hr q 4–6 h
Tobramycin	IV, IM	3–5 mg/kg/24 h q 8 h	1 mg/kg q 8 h

[a] Modified from A. M. Rudolph: *Pediatrics*, Ed. 17. Norwalk, Conn.: Appleton-Century-Crofts, 1982, pp. 787–813.

[b] The oral doses are for mild to moderate infections like strep throat and otitis media. The IV, IM doses are for moderate to severe infections like pneumonia and epiglottitis.

[c] These doses are for infants greater than 1 month of age and children, and when used should not exceed adult dose. Doses are expressed as 24-h doses and should be divided as indicated for each drug.

[d] These doses are for adolescents and adults.

is clearly more active against *H. influenzae* than either cephalexin or cephradine. Tetracycline and chloramphenical, historically used for otitis media, have no place in contemporary therapy, because of their respective side effects of tooth staining and skeletal growth suppression; and aplastic anemia and bone marrow suppression. In comparison, penicillins and cephalosporins produce the fewest side effects. Ampicillin, amoxicillin, penicillin, erythromycin and sulfasoxazole are the least expensive agents. Co-trimoxazole, cephalexin and cephradine are more expensive and cefaclor is the most expensive product.

Patient acceptance is also important. Children prefer the good taste of chewing-gum flavored Keflex (cephalexin) and grape-flavored Ceclor (cefaclor). Taking into consideration all of the preceding factors the currently recommended antibiotics for children less than 6 years old in order of preference are: ampicillin, amoxicillin, penicillin or erythromycin with sulfasoxazole; co-trimoxazole, cephalexin, cephradine and cefaclor. (See doses in Table 6.4.) Decongestants, antihistamines and ear drops have also been used for otitis media.

DECONGESTANTS AND ANTIHISTAMINES

No convincing evidence exists showing that decongestants or antihistamines are of any benefit in treating or preventing otitis media (52–54). Topical nasal decongestants have been used prophylactally with questionable results to keep the eustachian tube open and prevent otitis media (55). Oral decongestants, however, along with antihistamines have been used mainly to treat otitis media. The antihistamines are most effective if there is an allergic component (52) but probably only act as sedatives. Sulfasoxazole, co-trimoxazole, and ampilcillin have been helpful in some patients as prophalaxis (56).

EAR DROPS

Ear drops containing local anesthetics have been used to reduce the pain of otitis media by anesthetizing the tympanic membrane. Most pediatricians, however, prefer to use systemic acetaminophen or aspirin for pain relief. The use of ear drops containing antibiotics and/or corticosteroids for otitis media is irrational. These agents do not penetrate the tympanic membrane. However, a perforated ear drum secondary to a case of otitis media can discharge purulent material into the external canal. This discharge can lead to an otitis externa which is amenable to local therapy with an antibiotic otic solution. One consideration that has not been studied with otic solutions is the problem of local absorption through the perforated ear drum of neomycin, an ototoxic drug and a common constituent of otic solutions. If the perforated drum allows a significant absorption of neomycin, ear damage might occur.

Prognosis

The prognosis is generally excellent. Complete resolution without loss of hearing or sequalae is expected with adequate antibiotic treatment. In cases of recurrent serous otitis media, polyethylene tubes may have to be surgically implanted in the tympanic membrane to prevent suppurative otitis media (57). Otitis media is a very easily treated entity, however, there is a considerable lack of compliance with prescribed medications. It is therefore incumbent on the pharmacist to counsel the patient to improve therapy through proper compliance.

PHARYNGITIS

Sore throat is one of the common results of upper airway infections. Continuous coughing and dryness irritates the pharynx, and causes inflammation and painful swallowing. Sore throat may also be the first sign of infection for an immunosuppressed host. It is very important for the pharmacist to be aware of this and carefully monitor patients receiving cancer chemotherapeutic agents, steroids, phenylbutazone, etc.

Etiology

The usual cause of pharyngitis in children and adults is a viral infection. Adenovirus, rhinoviruses, influenza or parainfluenza are the most common etiologic agents and usually cause a mild to moderately severe case. More severe cases are caused by enteroviruses, echovirus, respiratory syncytial, and rubella and the most severe by herpes simplex, Epstein Barr virus (EBV) (mononucleosis) and smallpox virus. Bacteria are the next most frequent agent and may cause secondary or primary infections. β-Hemolytic streptococci, S. pneumoniae, and H. influenzae are the most common bacterial culprits. Diphtheria and pertussis are rare causes of pharyngitis and should be ruled out. An immunocompromised person, or a patient on antibiotics or beclomethasone may have a monilial pharyngitis. Other cases of sore throat are chronic smoking or other ingested irritants, i.e., irritating gases, caustics, corrosives, etc.

Diagnosis and Symptoms

The presenting symptoms of pharyngitis are usually sore throat, painful swallowing and mild fever. The pharynx is usually inflamed, swollen and sore and may have pustules or blisters. The patient may also have concomitant laryngitis with loss of voice. The tonsils may be inflamed and swollen. In the most severe infections, the tonsils may be so swollen and painful as to prevent the patient from swallowing and cause difficulty in breathing. Pharyngitis caused by streptococci ("strep throat") is an important disease to differentiate from a viral sore throat because it can cause numerous serious sequelae, such as rheumatic fever, kidney damage and scarlet fever. If a bacterial infection is suspected a throat culture should be done. It usually takes about 2 days for the definitive results.

Complications

The infecting agent may invade adjacent tissues in the pharynx. A cellulitis or abscess may develop in the tonsils. This process can lead to airway obstruction and require surgery to relieve it.

Treatment

For a viral pharyngitis systemic analgesics and topical agents are usually employed. The patient should be adequately hydrated and the pharynx moistened by breathing in humidified air. Topical preparations such as demulcents, sprays and gargles may be utilized.

DEMULCENTS

A demulcent is any product that will coat the throat and soothe the irritated mucous membrane, e.g., compound tincture of benzoin, elm bark or linseed. These products can be in the form of liquids, pastilles or lozenges. The liquids are thick and act as a protective blanket. Normal oral secretions act as the diluting liquid when pastilles or lozenges are used. In order to properly employ these agents to relieve sore throats, they must be able to coat the inflamed area in the back of the throat. The most effective way to achieve this with lozenges is for the patient to lie on his back and allow the lozenge to dissolve and slowly coat the back of the throat. This procedure can be utilized with liquids but care must be taken in order not to aspirate them.

GARGLES AND SPRAYS

Most gargles and sprays are combinations of antiseptics and/or local anesthetics. Neither of these is effective for fighting viral or bacterial infections. The gargles, in addition, do not reach the pharynx, the painful area of a sore throat. Some local pain relief can be achieved from the local anesthetics in the sprays, but it is transient in nature.

SYSTEMIC MEDICATIONS

Importantly, a sore throat that lasts longer than 3 days should be treated because it may be a streptococcal infection. If streptococci are suspected, a 10-day course of oral penicillin V is the treatment of choice. Ampicillin, amoxicillin, erythromycin or an oral cephalosporin are also appropriate. Penicillin is also effective for diphtheria and pertussis (see Chapter 3, "Pediatrics"). Nystatin suspension applied directly to lesions can be used to treat oral moniliasis.

For severe disseminated cases of infectious mononucleosis and herpes infections additional medications may be needed. Systemic steroids have been used in infectious mononucleosis and cytarabine and acyclovir are employed IV to treat herpes.

Prognosis/Conclusion

The prognosis is excellent if there are no complications or sequelae. The signs and symptoms of uncomplicated viral pharyngitis usually are over in 3 days. Strep throat symptoms may persist for a week or more. Adequate antibiotic treatment for bacterial and fungal infections will prevent complications. Rheumatic heart disease can be prevented if strep throat is completely treated. Pertussis and diphtheria can be prevented by adequate prophylactic immunizations.

CROUP

Croup is a clinical syndrome having multiple etiologies and characterized by upper airway obstruction. Patients have inspiratory stridor, a seal-like barking cough and hoarseness. The etiologies of this syndrome are spasmodic, viral, or bacterial and the symptoms can be mild in nature to life-threatening respiratory failure.

Spasmodic croup (acute spasmodic laryngitis) is characterized by sudden attacks of acute inspiratory stridor and cough in children ages 1 to 3 years old. The child has no fever and the posterior pharynx has minimal if any inflammation. The child may have severe breathing difficulties so that hospitalization may be necessary. Home treatment consists of putting the child in a bathroom and having him breathe steam from a hot running shower. Epinephrine, if needed, can be administered either parenterally or by aerosal nebulization as racemic epinephrine (58).

Viral croup (acute laryngotracheobronchitis) is the most common croup syndrome. The most common virus implicated in this syndrome is parainfluenza, but influenza A, respiratory syncytial and adenovirus can also cause similiar symptoms (59). It affects children 6 months to 3 years of age in the winter months which is viral season. It is usually preceded by 2 to 3 days of a URI which spreads to the larynx and trachea causing inspiratory stridor and a seal-like barking cough. The child usually has a low grade fever and does not appear to be very ill. This is to be contrasted with the symptoms of epiglottitis.

The treatment is with inhaled mist either from a cool mist humidifier, steam vaporizer or steam from a shower. The child should have bed rest and adequate hydration. Syrup of ipecac has been used historically but is now rarely employed. In severe obstruction hospitalization may be necessary. The hospitalized child may need oxygen and aerosolized epinephrine. The use of corticosteroids is controversial, and they should probably be used only in the hospitalized child who does not respond to routine therapy and who gets progressively worse. Hydrocortisone in doses of 5 to 10 mg/kg/24 hours should be used with maximum doses of 500 mg every 6 hours, and should be continued until acute symptoms are alleviated. In rare cases, the child may have to be intubated or have a tracheostomy performed to prevent death by respiratory obstruction.

EPIGLOTTITIS

Epiglottitis is the most serious form of croup and is characterized by an inflamed and swollen epiglottis. It is a bacterial infection and the etiologic organism is almost always *H. influenzae* type B. Diphtheria can also produce a similar picture and must be ruled out. The child is typically over 3 years old and suddenly becomes ill with acute inspiratory stridor. There usually is no antecedent URI. The disease progresses over 4 to 12 hours leading to almost total upper airway obstruction. The child typically arrives at the physician's office febrile and looking very sick. Saliva is drooling from the mouth due to dysphagia and the neck and chin are pushed forward in order to open the airway.

These children are always hospitalized and commonly intubated, however tracheostomy is rarely performed. They are given aerosolized mist and oxygen as with other forms of croup. Immediate treatment is begun with suitable IV antibiotics. The American Academy of Pediatrics current recommended treatment is to utilize IV ampicillin plus IV chloramphenical (Table 6.4). When the culture and sensitivity report is back in 48 hours, if the *H. fluenzae* is sensitive to ampicillin the chloramphenical is stopped. If the *H. influenzae* is resistant to ampicillin, usually because it produces lactamase, the ampicillin is stopped. Either the chloramphenical or ampicillin is continued for 7 to 10 days until the child is better. Recently the third generation cephalosporins, moxalactam, cefoperazone and cefotaxime have been used in place of the chloramphenical with the most experience being with moxalactam. They seem to offer the same efficacy for *H. influenzae* without the risk of chloramphenical-induced aplastic anemia. The use of steroids for epiglottitis is controversial (60). If the child is not improving after 24 to 48 hours on antibiotics, then steroids can be added. Hydrocortisone 5 to 10 mg/kg/24 hours given every 6 hours, or an equivalent steroid, should be employed.

LOWER RESPIRATORY TRACT: PNEUMONIA

Introduction

Lower airway infections are usually the complications of the spread of upper airway disease. The lungs are affected several days after the onset of the URI. Pneumonias are the chief cause of death from infectious diseases. There is a particularly high mortality in infants, elderly patients, and those with debilitating underlying disease (61).

Etiology

The primary infecting agent is viral with secondary infections involving bacteria. The most common viruses are rhinovirus, adenovirus, respiratory syncytial, parainfluenza and influenza viruses. In children, varicella and rubeola virus can also cause pneumonia. Of the secondary bacterial invaders, *S. pneumoniae* and group A β-hemolytic streptococci are the most common in adults and children. Infants may have chlamydia and children may have *S. aureus* or *H. influenzae*, uncommon causes of adult pneumonia. Both immunocompromised children and adults may develop pneumonia from opportunistic organisms, i.e., *Pseudomonas*, or *Pneumocystis carinii*. Myco-

plasma may also cause pneumonia in both children and adults.

Diagnosis/Clinical Findings

The viral pneumonias usually begin with the onset of rapid breathing, a nonproductive cough, a low grade fever and malaise. The pharynx is usually red and there is nasopharyngeal discharge. There is usually no physical signs of lung disease even though there is local lung infiltration. The patients are usually sick, remain home, and occasionally are hospitalized for complications. On the contrary, bacterial pneumonias are characterized by severe symptoms, necessitating hospitalization for their treatment. There is a rapid onset of symptoms including fever, chills, chest pain, difficulty in breathing, sore throat and hoarseness. The patient appears very sick and may cough up blood-tinged sputum. When opportunistic organisms invade immunosuppressed hosts severe sequelae may ensue with very little in the way of symptoms due to the patient's diminished response to infection.

Complications

Viral infections may lead to airway obstruction that may necessitate the administration of oxygen, but rarely intubation. Bacterial and opportunistic organisms may lead to pleurisy, emphysema, sterile pleural effusions, abscesses, and less common pericarditis, peritonitis, and purpura fulminans.

Pathogenesis

The initial viral infection of the lungs tends to produce an inflammation of the interstitial spaces. In severe cases, the inflammation may extend to and involve the alveolar sacs. The inflammation can damage the lung surface and allow secondary invaders an opportunity to invade the tissues. Bacteria, fungi and parasites can then proliferate in the susceptible tissue, extend the infectious process and lead to bronchial or lobar pneumonia.

Treatment

Viral pneumonia has no specific drug therapy. General symptomatic care is indicated, i.e., rest, adequate fluids, good nutritional intake and analgesics for pain and fever. In children under 16 years of age, acetaminophen should be used in place of salicylates due to the possible development of Reyes syndrome. If airway obstruction develops and causes hypoxia, oxygen and bronchodilators should be used, such as intravenous theophylline, in therapeutic doses depending on age, and inhaled metaproterenol. Appropriate antibiotic therapy is indicated for bacterial and opportunistic organisms.

Streptococcus pneumonia and group A-β-hemolytic streptococci can both be treated with IV or IM penicillin (Table 6.4). For those with nonanaphylactic allergy to penicillin, a first generation cephalosporin (cefazolin) or erythromycin should be used. For serious infections treatment may last as long as 3 to 4 weeks.

Staphylococcal pneumonia should be treated quickly and adequately to prevent complications. Because of the high incidence of resistant lactamase-producing strains, penicillin can no longer be recommended for treatment. Intravenous nafcillin or methicillin are the preferred drugs. For nonanaphylactic penicillin-allergic patients cefazolin or other 1st generation cephalosporin can be used. For resistant strains of staphylococcus, clindamycin, vancomycin or chloramphenicol are alternate drugs of choice for pneumonia.

H. influenzae encapsulated type B is also a common cause of pneumonia. In spite of the increasing incidence of lactamase positive ampicillin-resistant strains, ampicillin is still the drug of choice. Cephamandol, moxalactam, cefoperazone, cefotaxime, co-trimoxazole, or chloramphenicol are also very effective treatments.

Opportunistic organisms will usually first involve the lungs of immunosuppressed patients. *Pseudomonas aerugenosa* infections can be very severe and difficult to cure. Combination antibiotics, a penicillin plus an aminoglycoside, are used routinely. Pipericillin, mezlocillin, azlocillin, ticarcillin, or carbenicillin are the appropriate penicillins in order of preference. This should be combined with either tobramycin, gentamicin or amikacin. A penicillin should never be used alone because of the rapid development of resistant pseudomonas strains. Tobramycin is probably the preferred drug because it seems to have a lower incidence of renal and ototoxicity. The other common opportunistic pathogen is *Pneumocystis carinii*, which is a protozoa. Co-trimoxazole is the preferred agent because of a low incidence of adverse effects. Pentamidine isothianate, an investigational drug from the

Centers for Disease Control, is also used. Symptoms of *M. pneumoniae* infection closely resemble those of viral infections. Oral erythromycin can be used in all ages and tetracycline in persons over 8 years old.

Prognosis/Conclusions

The rapid utilization of antibiotics has decreased the complications and hospitalizations needed for pneumonias. Children and adults usually recover without sequelae. However, infants, immunosuppressed patients, and debilitated or elderly patients may develop severe complications and take years to recover.

Prevention of Lower Respiratory Viral Infections

A number of killed viral vaccines have been utilized and have been somewhat effective. Influenza vaccines are efficacious if the patient receives the immunization 1 month before exposure occurs. Unfortunately, the Hong Kong flu and the London flu were epidemics in the United States 6 months after the virus was initially isolated. It takes approximately 1 year to produce a new vaccine. This lag time severely diminishes the prophylactic effect of the vaccine. Additionally, the rapid mutation of influenza virus makes production of an effective immunization for all influenza strains all but impossible. The influenza A_2/Hong Kong vaccine was used for the London flu and proved to be about 50% effective because of the mutation of the virus. The lay press has reported a possible major breakthrough in developing a somewhat permanent influenza vaccine. Professor Claude Hannoun of the Pasteur Institute in Paris (62) reported the development of an influenza vaccine to protect people from the present strain plus all its proposed mutant forms (produced experimentally in his laboratory) for the next 5 years. They reported their new vaccine is ready for use and is 84% effective against the London flu. Unfortunately, not all mutant strains were tested or accounted for in laboratory experiments so that this promising vaccine probably will never be developed. Killed parainfluenza vaccine has also been produced and has proven somewhat efficacious when used intranasally (63).

The effect of immunity on preventing epidemics has been challenged by Fox et al. (64). Fox and his associates carried out a mathematical analysis of herd immunity and concluded "the important determinants of an epidemic were the number of susceptibles plus the number of opportunities for their exposure to the disease, and that if these two variables remained constant, the total number of immune persons in the population had no influence on the epidemic."

In addition to vaccines, one medication has been produced to be used specifically for prophylaxis and treatment against influenza A_2 (65). Amantadine given for 10 days after an exposure has been somewhat effective in preventing infection and is recommended only for high risk influenza patients—those with chronic debilitating disease or the elderly.

Chemotherapeutic agents can attack the virus in a number of different ways (2). Drugs may be effective in attacking the virus extracellularly during its attachment to host cells, during penetration of the cells by the virus, during the uncoating of the virus in the cells, during the synthesis of certain critical enzymes by other virus, by inactivating certain viral components, during assembly of virus particles by the host cell or during the release of virus particles from the cell. As can now be appreciated, drugs can interfere and destroy viruses in a variety of ways. Additionally, chemotherapeutic agents do not always destroy virus but may only suppress symptoms of a viral infection. They may only stimulate natural defenses such as interferon production or antibody production, or they may only act to slow down the infectious process and allow the body's own defenses to work. Each agent, however, is rather specific for only certain viruses; e.g., amantadine works only on the RNA-coating influenza A_2 virus by preventing the virus from penetrating the host cell (2).

Research on treatment for cancer has produced many chemotherapeutic agents. Recently, some cancers have been shown to be caused by viruses, spurring on the use of many chemotherapeutic agents to treat various viral infections. In addition to amantadine, cytarabine (ARA-C), vidarabine (ARA-A), acyclovir, methisazone and idoxuridine (IDU), have been employed and there seems to be little doubt that many other drugs will shortly be utilized to treat other viral infections.

A great deal of research is being done in the area of interferon and its inducers (2, 66). Interferon is a protein made by white cells in the spleen, liver, thymus and lymph nodes in response to viral infection (2, 67–69). It is a nonspecific entity so that it is active against virtually all viruses, some bacteria and some protozoa (67–69). There are five known human varieties of interferon which probably are produced by at least two specific genes in white blood cells. Interferon has a rapid onset and is produced shortly after the onset of illness. It is effective both before and during an infection. In addition to viruses (67–71) activating these genes, at least 30 synthetic chemical inducers (67–70) of interferon have been produced. Because of cost, induction of endogenous interferon is preferable to isolation, purification and administration of exogenous interferon. It has been estimated that it would require $5000 worth of parenteral interferon to treat one case of the common cold (66).

CONCLUSIONS

The causes of respiratory disease are many, but the symptoms are largely similar. The treatment of choice is generally symptomatic with specific therapy for only a few indicated infections. Diseases that have been largely eliminated by the use of immunizations can only remain so if vaccinations are routinely done. Work on interferon, new vaccines and chemotherapeutic agents will continue with further research being done with lymphocyte transfusions, lymphocyte mediator substances and other immunological preparations. The next few years should herald major breakthroughs in the treatment of many viral-induced illnesses.

References

1. Krugman S, Ward R: *Infectious Diseases of Children*, ed. 5. St. Louis: C. V. Mosby, 1972, p 221.
2. Stevens DA, Merigan TC: Approaches to the control of viral infections in man. *Ration Drug Ther* 5:1, 1971.
3. Loda RA, Glezen PE, Clyde WA: Respiratory disease in group day care. *Pediatrics* 19:428, 1972.
4. Hope-Simpson EE, Higgins PG: A respiratory virus study in Great Britain: review and evaluation. *Prog Med Virol* 11:354, 1969.
5. McCammon RW: Natural history of respiratory tract infection patterns in basically healthy individuals. *Am J Dis Child* 122:232, 1971.
6. Melnick JL: Classification and nomenclature of animal viruses. *Prog Med Virol* 13:462, 1971.
7. Hable KA, Washington JA, Herrmann EC: Bacterial and viral throat flora, comparison of findings in children with acute upper respiratory tract disease and in healthy controls during winter. *Clin Pediatr* 10:199, 1971.
8. Mufson MA, Webb PA, Kennedy H, et al: Etiol-

ogy of upper-respiratory-tract illnesses among civilian adults. *JAMA* 195:91, 1965.

9. Jawetz E, Melnick JL, Adelberg EA: *Review of Medical Microbiology*, ed 10. Los Altos, Calif.: Lange Medical Publications, 1972, p 279.

10. Chang TW: Recurrent viral infection (reinfection). *N Engl J Med*, 284:765, 1971.

11. Craddock CG, Longmire R, McMillan R: Lymphocytes and the immune response, Part I. *N Engl J Med* 285:324, 1971.

12. Craddock CG, Longmire R, McMillan R: Lymphocytes and the immune response, Part II. *N Engl J Med* 285:378, 1971.

13. Tomasi TB: Secretory immunoglobins. *N Engl J Med* 287:500, 1972.

14. Dowling HF, Jackson GG, Inouye T: Transmission of the experimental common cold in volunteers. *J Lab Clin Med* 50:516, 1957.

15. Moffet H, Siegel AC, Doyle HK: Nonstreptococcal pharyngitis. *J Pediatr* 73:51, 1968.

16. Jacobs JW, Peacock DB, Corner BD, et al: Respiratory synctyial and other viruses associated with respiratory disease in infants. *Lancet* 1:871, 1971.

17. Marks MT, Nagahama H, Eller JJ: Parainfluenza virus immunofluorescence in vitro and clinical application of the direct method. *Pediatrics* 48:73, 1971.

18. Kempe H: *Current Pediatric Diagnosis and Treatment*, ed 7. Los Altos, Calif.: Lange Medical Publications, 1982.

19. APHA Project Staff: *Handbook of Non-prescription Drugs*, ed 7. Washington, D.C.: American Pharmaceutical Association, 1982, p 123.

20. Kastrup E, Boyd JR: In Schwach GM: *Facts and Comparisons*, St. Louis: Facts and Comparisons, Inc., 1983, p 184.

21. Anon: Aspirin or paracetamol. *Lancet* 2:287, 1981.

22. Salicylate labeling may change because of Reye's syndrome. *FDA Drug Bull* 12:9, 1982.

23. Waldman RJ, et al: Aspirin as a risk factor in Reye's syndrome. *JAMA* 247:3089, 1982.

24. Halpin TJ, Holtzhauer FJ, Campbell RJ, et al: Reye's syndrome and medication use. *JAMA* 248:687, 1982.

25. Starko KM, Ray CG, Dominguez LB, et al: Reye's syndrome and salicylate use. *Pediatrics* 66:859, 1980.

26. National Surveillance for Reye's Syndrome, 1981; Update, Reye's Syndrome and Salicylate usage. *MMWR* 31:55, 1982.

27. Anon: Reye's syndrome. HHS publication No. (FDA) 82-3126.

28. Lexomboon Y, Duangmani C, Kusalassai V, et al: Evaluation of orally administered antibiotics for treatment of upper respiratory infections in Thai children. *J Pediatr* 78:772, 1971.

29. Anon: Antimicrobial cold remedies. *Med Lett Drugs Ther* 9:30, 1967.

30. Lampert RP, Robinson DS, Soyka LF: A critical look at oral decongestants. *Pediatrics* 55:550, 1975.

31. Elis J, Laurence DR, Mattie H, et al: Modification by monoamine oxidase inhibitors of the effect of some sympathomimetics on blood pressure. *Br Med J* 1:75,1967.

32. Callagahan RP, Cox AJ, Boulder RVM, et al: Combination therapy in hay fever and allergic rhinitis. *Practitioner* 198:713, 1967.

33. Hartman MM: Capabilities and limitations of major drug groups in allergy: Their role within current theories. *Ann Allergy* 27:164, 1969.

34. Feinberg SM: The antihistamines: pharmacologic principles in their use. *Pharmacol Physicians* 1:1, 1967.

35. Anon: Cough remedies. *Med Lett Drugs Ther* 13:9, 1971.

36. Blanchard K, Ford RA: Effective antitussive agent in the treatment of cough in childhood. *Lancet* 74:443, 1954.

37. Chodosh S: Newer drugs in treatment of chronic bronchitis. *Med Clin North Am* 51:1177, 1967.

38. Carter CH: Evaluation of the effectiveness of Novrad and acetysalicylic acid in children with cough. *Am J Med Sci* 245:713, 1963.

39. Calesnick B, Christensen JA: Latency of cough response as a measure of antitussive agents. *Clin Pharmacol Ther* 8:374, 1967.

40. Committee on Drugs, American Academy of Pediatrics: Use of codeine- and dextromethorpham-containing cough syrups in pediatrics. *Pediatrics* 62:118, 1978.

41. Pauling L: *Vitamin C and the Common Cold*. San Francisco: W. H. Freeman, 1970.

42. Anon: Vitamin C: were the trials well controlled and are large doses safe? *Med Lett Drugs Ther* 13:46, 1971.

43. Anon: Vitamin C and the common cold. *Med Lett Drugs Ther* 12:105, 1970.

44. Hornick RB: Does ascorbic acid have value in combating the common cold? *Med Counterpoint* 4:50, 1972.

45. Charleston SS, Clegg KM: Ascorbic acid and the common cold (letter). *Lancet* 1:1401, 1972.

46. Steigman AJ: *Report of the Committee on Infectious Disease*, ed 19. Evanston, Ill.: American Academy of Pediatrics, 1982.

47. Teele DW, Klein JO, Rosner B, et al: Middle ear disease and the practice of pediatrics. *JAMA* 249:1026, 1983.

48. Shurin PA, Howie VM, Pelton SI, et al: Bacterial etiology of otitis media during the first six weeks of life. *J Pediatr* 92:893, 1978.

49. Berman SA, Balkany TJ, Simmons MA: Otitis media in the neonatal intensive care unit. *Pediatrics* 62:198, 1978.

50. Northern SL: Advanced techniques for measuring middle ear function. *Pediatrics* 61:761, 1978.

51. Rowe DS: Acute suppurative otitis media. *Pediatrics* 56:285, 1975.

52. Bluestone CD: Eustachian tube function and allergy in otitis media. *Pediatrics* 61:753, 1978.

53. Olson AL, et al: Prevention and therapy of serous otitis media by oral decongestant: a double-blind study in pediatric practice. *Pediatrics* 61:679, 1978.

54. Cantekin EF, Mandel EM, Bluestone CD, et al: Lack of efficacy of a decongestant-antihistamine combination for otitis media with effusion ("secretory" otitis media) in children. *N Engl J Med* 308:297, 1983.

55. Bierman CW, Furukawa CT: Medical manage-

ment of serous otitis in children. *Pediatrics* 61:768, 1978.

56. Perrin JM, et al: Sulfasoxazole as chemoprophylaxis for recurrent otitis media. *N Engl J Med* 291:664, 1974.

57. Donaldson JA: Surgical management of eustachian tube dysfunction and its importance in middle ear effusion. *Pediatrics* 61:774, 1978.

58. Fogel JM, Berg JI, Gerber MA, et al: Racemic epinephrine in the treatment of croup: nebulization alone versus nebulization with intermittent positive pressure breathing. *J Pediatr* 101:1028, 1982.

59. Denny FW, Murphy TF, Clyde WA, et al: Croup: an 11-year study in a pediatric practice. *Pediatrics* 71:871, 1983.

60. Rudolph AM: *Pediatrics,* ed 7. Norwalk, Conn.: Appleton-Century-Crofts, 1982.

61. Kannangora DW, LeFrock JL: Targeting pneumonia therapy. *Drug Therapy Hospital,* p. 49, 1982.

62. Anon: Anticipating the flu virus. *Time* 101:68, 1973.

63. Wigley FM, Fruchtman MH, Waldman RH: Aerosol immunization of humans with inactivated parainfluenza type 2 vaccine. *N Engl J Med* 283:1250, 1970.

64. Fox JP, Elveback L, Scott W, et al: Herd immunity: basic concept and relevance to public health immunization practices. *Am J Epidemiol* 94:179, 1971.

65. Anon: Amantadine for high risk influenza. *Med Lett Drugs Ther* 20:25, 1978.

66. Meyer HM: The control of viral disease: problems and prospects viewed in perspective. *J Pediatr* 73:653, 1968.

67. Grossberg SE: The interferons and their inducers: molecular and therapeputic considerations, Part I. *N Engl J Med* 287:79, 1972.

68. Grossberg SE: The interferons and their inducers: Molecular and therapeutic considerations, Part II. *N Engl J Med* 287:79, 1972.

69. Grossberg SE: the interferons and their inducers: molecular and therapeutic considerations, Part III. *N Engl J Med* 287:122, 1972.

70. Ho M: Interferon and herpes zoster (editorial). *N Engl J Med* 283:1222, 1970.

71. Armstrong RW, Gurwith MJ, Waddell D, et al: Cutaneous interferon production in patients with Hodgkins disease and other cancers infected with varicella or vaccinia. *N Engl J Med* 283:1182, 1970.

CHAPTER 7

Urinary Tract Infections

DONALD T. KISHI, Pharm.D.

Infections of the urinary tract are the most common form of urologic disease encountered in the hospitalized and ambulatory patient population. It represents an area in which pharmacists can provide potentially significant contributions to the rational prescribing of antiinfectives, therapy monitoring, and patient education and compliance. While considerable clinical research has been done in the treatment of the urinary tract infection, many issues remain to be resolved and, consequently, this area remains invitingly open to pharmacist participation.

DEFINITIONS

The urinary tract consists of the urethra, prostate gland (in males), the urinary bladder, the ureters and the kidneys. The term urinary tract infection (UTI) describes a variety of conditions relating the components of the tract in which the common basis is the presence of microorganisms in significant quantities.

A UTI may be evidenced solely by the presence of bacteria in the urine (bacteriuria) and/or signs and symptoms of bacterial invasion of one or more components of the tract. It should be recognized that however localized the infection initially, once any component of the tract is invaded, the entire tract is at risk for infection.

A UTI can be designated as asymptomatic or symptomatic, complicated or uncomplicated and/or acute, chronic or recurrent. The terms asymptomatic, symptomatic, chronic and acute are self-explanatory and will not be defined. An uncomplicated UTI is defined as an infection in which there is no structural or neurologic abnormality of the urinary tract which interferes with the normal flow of urine or the voiding mechanism. A complicated UTI is the result of the presence of a congenital abnormality or distortion of the tract, stone, indwelling catheter, enlarged prostate gland, or neurological deficit which will interfere with the basic urinary tract defense of washing

bacteria out of the system. The term recurrent refers to the reoccurrence of a UTI in a given patient. The recurrent infection is subcategorized into relapse or reinfection. If a UTI is recurrent, it can be the result of invasion by the same, specific serotype of microorganism, as was present in the previous infection, in which case it is termed a relapse; or it can be the result of a completely different microorganism or same microorganism but of a different serotype, in which case the recurrence is termed a reinfection.

INCIDENCE

In general UTIs are predominantly found in women and girls. It is only during the first year and after the fifth decade of life that the incidence of UTIs in males is high or begins to increase. These latter findings are attributable to the higher incidence of congenital abnormalities in the males, in the former instance, and the development of prostatic hypertrophy and interference with urinary flow in the latter instance. In adult males less than 50 years of age, the incidence of UTIs is 0%; 50 to 59 years—0.6%; 60 to 69 years—1.5%; and greater than 70 years—3.6% (1).

In school girls the prevalence rate of UTIs approximates 1.2% and by age 18 approximately 5% will have had at least one UTI (2). During the childbearing age women appear to have a particular predisposition to UTIs. This is evidenced by the syndromes of "honeymoon" cystitis and the pyelonephritis of pregnancy. Sexual intercourse has been documented to increase bacterial counts on clean catch postcoital specimens (3). Urethral milking of anesthetized women has been demonstrated to increase bacterial counts in specimens obtained by suprapubic bladder aspiration (4). The incidence of UTIs and pyelonephritis in women who were bacteriuric during pregnancy is 27 to 38% and 20 to 30%, respectively (5–8). The significance of sexual intercourse and pregnancy and their relationship to UTIs is emphasized by the incidence of UTIs of less than 2% in nuns between 15 and 54 years of age (9). When all women are considered, the incidence of UTIs increases at an estimated 1 to 2% per decade of life. By age 70, 10% of women have UTIs. It is also estimated that during their lifetime 20% of women will have experienced a UTI (10).

Concomitant disease states, such as diabetes or hypertension, are associated with an increased incidence of UTIs. In a diabetic clinic population, for example, a 19% incidence of UTIs in women and a 2% incidence in males has been reported. In this patient population upper tract and recurrent infections were common. The propensity for diabetics to develop UTIs is not correlated with age, degree of glucosuria or urinary tract instrumentation. The predisposing cause remains to be defined (11).

Urologic manipulation—catheterization, cystoscopy, etc.—account for over 400,000 UTIs annually. This figure represents approximately 75% of the nosocomial UTIs (16).

PATHOGENESIS

Microorganisms invade the urinary tract by two routes—through the urethra and by hematogenous spread. The hematogenous route is much less common and results from seeding the kidney from a primary site of infection-carbuncle, osteomyelitis, endocarditis, or empyema (12). The UTI thus becomes a secondary infection.

The most common route of invasion of microorganisms into the urinary tract is via the urethral route. The source of these organisms is the fecal reservoir of enteric bacteria as is evidenced by the 75 to 80% correlation of the etiologic microorganisms of bacteriuria and those cultured from rectal swab (13, 14). In women these bacteria colonize the vaginal vestibule and through urethral milking and trauma of sexual intercourse, as previously noted, are introduced via the short female urethra into the bladder (15). Vaginal and urethral contamination may occur simply as a result of poor personal hygiene of the anal-perineal areas.

Urologic manipulation can introduce bacteria into the bladder by contamination at the time of instrument insertion, by bacterial migration, and by breaks in the sterility of the catheter system. Normally bacteria inhabit the distal third of the urethra. Thus, the introduction of an instrument through the urethra can

contaminate the bladder. In the instance of the indwelling urinary catheter, microorganisms can migrate from the periurethral area into the bladder via the fluid which separates the urethral mucosa and the catheter (17). Loss of sterility of the catheter system can contribute to catheter-associated UTIs. This can occur if the closed collecting system is broken or disconnected at any time, if retrograde urine flow occurs from bag to bladder, or if cross-contamination of patients in close proximity occurs due to improper hand cleansing of hospital personnel caring for the patients (16). Other factors which increase the rate of catheter-associated UTIs include age, sex, duration of the catheterization, catheter care techniques, training of the health care personnel inserting the catheter, and clustering of catheterized patients. The elderly, debilitated women appear to be at highest risk for developing this form of infection.

A major intrinsic defense mechanism against the UTI is the washing out of bacteria which occurs with each urinary void (44). This defense mechanism is compromised if urinary flow is slowed or obstructed or if a post-void residual urine develops. Since the urine is a good culture medium, urinary stasis provides an ideal situation for bacterial growth. Obstructed or slowed urine flow can occur with urologic tumors, strictures, stones or prostatic hypertrophy. Post-void residual urine can occur with neurologic lesions affecting the bladder or sphincter musculature—bladder spasticity or flaccidity; drugs—anticholinergic, anesthetic medications; or poor micturition habits.

Vesicoureteral reflux provides a mechanism for bacteria to ascend from the bladder to the kidney. This reflux occurs when the anatomic valve at the vesicoureteral junction is incompetent. This lesion may result from a congenital abnormality or a distortion of the bladder such as that which occurs during pregnancy.

Etiologic Agent

The enteric bacteria—*Escherichia coli*, proteus, klebsiella, enterobacter, enterococcus, pseudomonas—are responsible for the vast majority of UTIs (Table 7.1). The predominant infecting agent is *E. coli*, accounting for over 90% of initial infections and approximately 50% of recurrent infections. When a UTI is hospital acquired or if the urinary tract is complicated by obstruction, stone, catheter, or

Table 7.1.
Etiologic Organisms of Urinary Tract Infections (UTIs) (65)

Organism	% of Total UTI	% of Inpatient UTIs	% of Outpatient UTIs
GRAM-NEGATIVE			
Escherichia coli	55.4	47	64
Proteus mirabilis	18.8	21	15
Klebsiella aerogenes	8.8	7	4
Pseudomonas aeruginosa	2.9	2.9	0
Other coliforms	6.1	14.1	9
GRAM-POSITIVE			
Streptococcus faecalis	4.1	8	8
Others	3.9		
	100	100	100

other urologic manipulation, the predictability of the causative microorganism is pure speculation. The use of repeated courses of antiinfectives and the presence of these complicating factors tends to select out organisms other than E. coli and also results in an increased incidence of mixed infections. Occasionally staphylococcal UTIs occur. This can be the result of contamination during urologic manipulation or the hematogenous spread of the microorganism from a primary site of infection.

CLINICAL PRESENTATION

The clinical presentation of a UTI can be divided into those findings associated with lower tract and upper tract infections. Classically the signs and symptoms of lower tract infection—cystitis, urethritis—include dysuria, frequency, urgency and a vague lower abdominal discomfort. Grossly the urine is turbid, dark and foul smelling. A urinalysis reveals pyuria (more than 5 to 10 white blood cells per high power field), bacteria, and occasionally hematuria. Leukocytosis in a peripheral blood smear is absent unless the upper tract or prostate is involved.

The presentation of prostatitis is primarily that of a lower UTI; however, fever, perineal pain, and urethral discharge are also present. A rectal examination reveals an enlarged, tender, firm prostate gland. In the acute prostatic infection leukocytosis is present, while in the chronic infection the patient will typically also complain of a lumbosacral backache.

The classical presentation of an upper UTI includes nonspecific complaints of headache, malaise, and nausea and vomiting. In association with these nonspecific findings, the patient may complain of abdominal pain, costovertebral angle (CVA) tenderness, and fever and chills. Pyuria, WBC casts, bacteria, and proteinuria are found in the urinalysis. Examination of the blood reveals a leukocytosis with a predominance of polymorphonucleocytes and band forms on the differential count. Blood cultures are positive for the infecting organism. In addition to these upper tract findings, lower tract symptomatology can also be present.

Unfortunately not all UTIs present with classical findings. For example, both upper and lower tract UTIs can be asymptomatic. Asymptomatic UTIs occur in 1% of newborns (18), 2 to 2.7% of infants (19, 20), 1.1 to 1.2% of school girls (20–22), 0.03% of school boys (20) and in 5% of pregnant women (23). Conversely, about 50% of women with symptoms have sterile urine (24). Pyuria occurs in only 50% of asymptomatic women with significant bacteriuria (25). Conversely, pyuria can occur without bacteriuria (25). In this latter instance vaginal contamination of the specimen or tuberculous infection, tumor, foreign body or medications could cause inflammation of the tract (26). Similarly, dysuria can be caused by irritation of the bladder or urethra by medications e.g., methenamine, cyclophosphamide.

DIAGNOSIS

The diagnosis of a UTI should be based on the demonstration of a significant quantity of bacteria in the urine. Symptomatology, as was alluded to in the previous section, is unreliable. The presence or absence of pyuria on urinalysis can be misleading and should not be relied upon as the sole screening or diagnostic test. Gram stain examination of the urine may provide information as to whether the microorganism is Gram-positive or Gram-negative, but it does not specifically identify the organism nor does it provide quantitative information. Gram staining can be also misleading as is evidenced by a 20% error rate (25). Consequently, the most reliable method of diagnosing the UTI is the properly performed urine culture and sensitivity. The presence of symptoms and pyuria while unreliable alone, are suggestive and supportive evidence for the diagnosis of UTI.

Collection of the Specimen

Collection of urine for culture and sensitivity testing has been performed using four different methods: the suprapubic needle aspirate, single catheterization, the whole void collection, and the midstream void collection. Each method has a different accuracy potential and a different level of bacteriuria indicative of the presence or absence of a UTI.

The suprapubic aspirate is performed by inserting a needle in the midline, 2 cm above symphysis pubis and aspirating the urine. The sample is then cultured. A colony count of 5 $\times$ 10^3/ml or greater of the same organism is diagnostic of a UTI. A single culture using this technique is 99% accurate in detecting infection (26).

The single or in and out catheterization method is advocated to alleviate the problem of contamination of the specimen which occurs, primarily in women, with voiding. The patient's periurethral area is cleansed and a catheter is aseptically inserted, the urine is drained, the catheter removed, and an aliquot of urine is cultured. The bacterial colony count diagnostic of a UTI is 1 $\times$ 10^5/ml or greater of the same microorganism. This method is 95% accurate in detecting UTIs (27).

The whole void collection method is performed by cleansing the periurethral area and collecting the entire voided specimen. An aliquot of urine is then cultured. A bacterial colony count of 1 $\times$ 10^5/ml or greater of the same microorganism is diagnostic of a UTI. This method is 80% accurate if the results are based on a single void, 91% accurate if two separate voids are cultured, and 95% accurate if three separate voids are cultured (27).

The most common technique for obtaining urine for culture is midstream void method. The patients periurethral area is cleansed with soap. The female patient is asked to separate her labia to avoid contamination. During the midpoint of the void, an aliquot of urine is collected and cultured. If the patient is asymptomatic, midstream samples from two separate voids should be obtained; if symptomatic, a single specimen is sufficient. A bacterial colony count of 1 $\times$ 10^5/ml or greater of the same microorganism is diagnostic of the UTI. This method is 95% accurate in detecting UTIs (27).

Collection of a urine specimen from a patient with an indwelling catheter can be obtained with relative ease. The catheter is clamped closed a short distance from the meatus for an hour. After this interval the clamp is released and a few milliliters of urine are allowed to drain before the clamp is reapplied. An alcohol swab is used to wipe clean the area on the catheter between the meatus and clamp. Finally, a needle and syringe are used to aspirate the urine from the catheter just distal to the meatus. The sample is then cultured (16).

Culture and Sensitivity Testing

The standard method of identifying, quantitating and determining the sensitivity and resistance pattern to antiinfectives of the invading microorganism is the culture and sensitivity test. The most popular of these tests is the Kirby-Bauer method. In this test the urine sample is plated onto the culture medium and a disc containing the various antiinfectives utilized to treat UTIs is placed on the plated medium. After 24 hours of incubation the organism and colony count can be delineated, after 48 hours the sensitivities of the microorganism can be defined. Since the sensitivity and resistance pattern of the microorganism is based on the size of zone of growth inhibition surrounding a particular antiinfective, the concentration of antiinfective in the disc is of importance.

The antiinfective concentration in the disc varies with the agent and may reflect either the concentration achievable in the urine or serum. Which concentration is utilized by a laboratory should be investigated by the practitioner in order to gain the proper perspective of the sensitivity and resistance pattern of the microorganism. This paradox of using serum concentrations is, in part, based on the controversy of whether urine or serum levels of antiinfective is of importance in treating pyelonephritis. Since many antiinfectives are excreted and concentrated in their active form in the urine, a disc sensitivity which uses the antiinfective concentration achievable in the serum will not reflect the effective resistance/sensitivity pattern of the microorganism infecting the urine (28).

Methods other than the standard culture and sensitivity test for urinary infections are available. These methods are designed primarily to circumvent the cost and time factors required by the culture and sensitivity test. These other methods are summarized in Table

7.2. Their major drawbacks include their non-specific results with respect to microorganism identification and no sensitivity testing. Their place in the diagnosis and treatment should be limited to screening for and post-therapy follow-up of UTIs.

Localization Studies

A positive culture and sensitivity only confirms that bacteria are present in the bladder. It provides no information regarding the presence or absence of infection in the kidney. Various tests, including renal concentrating ability and antibody titers, have been devised in an attempt to determine if pyelonephritis is present. Since in pyelonephritis the kidney often loses its ability to concentrate urine, a

test of this function following overnight dehydration has been devised. This test unfortunately requires ureteral catheterization and can be influenced by other noninfectious renal conditions, e.g. analgesic nephropathy.

The use of serum antibody titers to the microorganism is based on patients with classic upper UTIs having high titers and those with classic cystitis having low titers. However, since there is considerable overlap, the test is not definitive (27).

Another promising test for differentiating upper from lower tract UTIs is the presence or absence of antibody-coated bacteria in urinary sediment. In upper tract infections the bacteria are coated with antibody and in UTIs confined to lower tract the bacteria are unaffected (40, 41). This method has been tried clinically and

Table 7.2.
Urine Screening Tests

Test	Principle	Type of Result Obtained	Reference
Low glucose indicator (Uriglox)	Bacterial consumption of urinary glucose to less than 2 mg/100 ml. Urine glucose concentration measured by color reaction to reagent Time required for test: 6–10 min	Indicates presence of bacteria	29, 30
Agar cup quantitative culture (Speci-Test)	Culture with comparison to photographic standard for colony count Time required for test: 10–24 hr	Estimate of bacterial colony count	31
Dip-slide method (Uricult)	Culture with two media. Nutrient agar and McConkey agar. Nutrient agar supports Gram-negative and Gram-positive bacteria. McConkey agar supports Gram-negative bacteria only. Standard method for bacterial colony count Time required for test: 12 hr	Estimate of bacterial colony count. Differentiates Gram-positive and Gram-negative organism	32
Greiss or nitrite indicator (Stat-Test) (Bac-U-Dip)	Bacterial reduction of urinary nitrates to nitrite. Color reaction of Greiss reagent in the presence of nitrite concentration associated with bacterial colony count in excess of 10^5 Time required for test: 1 min	Positive test in presence of bacterial colony count of 10^5	33–36
Tetrazolium test (Uroscreen)	Bacterial reduction of triphenyl tetrazolium Cl to triphenylformazan. Color reaction occurs only if bacterial colony count exceeds 10^5 Time required for test: 4 hr	Positive test in presence of bacterial colony count of 10^5	37–39
Combination test (Microstix)	Greiss or nitrite indicator. Dip-slide method tetrazolium test Time required for test: 12–18 hr	Estimate of bacterial colony count. Differentiates Gram-positive and Gram-negative organism	31

appears to be an accurate, noninvasive method for detecting upper UTIs (42).

The intravenous pyelogram (IVP) is another study which can provide evidence of pyelonephritis. Classically in the early stages, localized scarring and calyceal distortion are present. In advanced cases of pyelonephritis the above findings plus cortical scarring are found (27).

The indications for using localization studies in males revolves around the infrequent occurrence of UTIs. The presence of an infection, especially in boys and men less than 50 years of age, usually indicates a structural deformity within the tract. Consequently localization studies should be done with the first infection.

Since incidence of UTIs in women is quite high due to their anatomic predisposition, localization studies are usually not performed until the third UTI recurrence. The need for localization studies in women with recurrent infections is based on the statistic that approximately 50% will have upper tract involvement (43).

THERAPY

The therapeutic approaches available for the patient with a urinary tract infection can be broadly classified as preventive, eradicative, suppressive or prophylactic. The approach or approaches utilized are dependent on the extent of the current illness, the patient's past history of UTIs, the patient's urologic status—complicated or uncomplicated, and the presence or absence of other diseases which will predispose or affect the severity of the current and future UTIs.

Preventive

Preventive measures are those which are directed toward minimizing the chance of a UTI developing. These measures are directed toward patient populations which are at particular risk of infection. Included in this group are females, patients who are or are about to be catheterized or have some form of urologic manipulation, diabetics, hypertensive patients, debilitated or otherwise compromised patients.

As was alluded to previously, females are prone to UTIs due to the anatomical proximity of the anal and urethral orifices. The perineal-anal toilet and micturition habits of these patients should be assessed prior to or with the first infection. Should the habits be improper—wiping from back to front after defecation or incomplete micturition—the patient should be instructed in the proper techniques and why they predispose to UTIs. These preventive, educative measures are particularly applicable for pregnant women and women who, due to advancing age or concurrent chronic diseases, are particularly susceptible to infection.

Since urologic manipulation is such a well-known risk factor for UTIs, the need for performing the procedure should be weighed against the potential risks. Should the necessity be compelling, proper preparation of both the patient and the practitioner in order to minimize the risk of infection should be made and the procedure should be performed using aseptic techniques.

The urinary catheter poses a special predisposing problem and has been studied extensively. The incidence of catheter associated UTIs is related to a variety of factors including the method and duration of catheterization, the health care personnel inserting the catheter, the catheter system and catheter care. The Center for Disease Control (CDC) has developed recommendations for the use of the indwelling catheter. While the complete recommendations are too extensive for discussion in this text, a summary is presented (16):

1. Indwelling catheters should be used only when indicated and for as short a time as is possible.
2. Insertion should be done by adequately trained personnel.
3. Insertion should be done aseptically.
4. Perineal and meatal catheter junction should be cleansed once or twice daily with an antiseptic soap. The use of an antimicrobial ointment is optimal.
5. A sterile closed drainage system should always be used.
6. At no time should the collecting bag be above the level of the patient's bladder. The urine flow should be "downhill" and unobstructed.
7. Any closed collecting system which is contaminated by inappropriate technique, accidental disconnection, etc., should be replaced.
8. If a patient is catheterized for 2 weeks or less, a routine catheter change is not required except when obstruction, contam-

ination or other malfunction of the system occurs.

9. In patients who are chronically catheterized, replacement is not necessary until a malfunction or obstruction occurs.

10. Patients who are catheterized should be in separate rooms and not in adjacent beds to avoid cross contamination.

11. Daily bacteriologic monitoring of the urine of catheterized patients may be useful; however, the cost-effectiveness requires evaluation.

12. The use of systemic antibiotics as prophylaxis in catheterized patients when combined with aseptic care and a closed drainage system reduces the rate of infection for the first four days and delays bacteriuria in patients catheterized for longer periods. The cost effectiveness and the cost benefit, however, remain to be evaluated.

13. The effectiveness of continuous antiinfective irrigations in reducing the incidence and delaying the onset of UTIs in open indwelling catheter drainage systems has been demonstrated. However, their value, when used in patients with a closed system, has not been demonstrated. Prophylactic irrigations may be useful if the closed system is difficult to maintain (Table 7.3).

Patients with other concurrent conditions, which predispose to UTIs, should be routinely screened for infection. This preventive measure is particularly applicable to debilitated, immunosuppressed or pregnant patients.

Maintenance of the patient in a well-hydrated state is a simple and worthwhile preventive measure which inhibits or minimizes the risk of developing pyelonephritis. The value of maintaining hydration is based on its effect on the activity of phagocytes in the renal medulla. Dehydration and resultant hypertonicity of urine in the renal medulla inhibit leukocyte mobilization and phagocytic activity (59, 60).

Eradicative Therapy

The goal of eradicative therapy is the sterilization of the tract. This approach is used when there is bacterial colonization occurring in any part of the tract. It is indicated prior to the institution of prophylactic or suppressive therapy and prior to insertion of an indwelling catheter or other urologic manipulation should an infection be present.

The efficacy of eradicative therapy is usually more dependent on the host environment than on the choice of drug. In the patient with a complicated infection, the structural abnormality whether it be a stone, renal disease prostatic hypertrophy, vesicoureteral or urethrovesical reflux can negatively affect the outcome of therapy by preventing adequate antimicrobial-organism contact. Similarly, should the patient have a disease such as diabetes mellitus which predisposes or otherwise modifies the patient's response to infection the outcome of therapy can be adversely affected. Control or correction of the underlying predisposing factors is essential to effective eradicative therapy (Table 7.4).

The drug which is selected should reflect variables encountered in the individual patient. In this regard, the patient's immunologic

Table 7.3.
Bladder Irrigants

Irrigant	Infusion Rate	Comments
PROPHYLACTIC AGENT[a]		
Acetic acid ¼%	1 ml/min	Locally irritating. Check for hematuria—if present, reduce to ⅛%
Neomycin-polymixin (Neosporin GU)	1 amp in 1 L normal saline over 24 hr	Resistant organisms can develop
Chlorhexidine digluconate, 0.02% solution	1 L over 24 hr or 60 ml with single catheterization	Locally irritating at greater than 0.02% concentration
ERADICATION AGENT		
Amphotericin B 25–50 mg/L of sterile water	1 L over 24 hr	No systemic absorption; effective in treating candiduria

[a] No prophylactic irrigation should be used until the urine has been cleared of active infection.

Table 7.4.
Eradictive Agents for Urinary Tract Infections (UTIs)

Medication	Adult Dose	$t_{1/2}$ (hr)	$t_{1/2}$ (hr) Anuric	Relatively Common Toxicity	Comments
Amikacin	7.5 mg/kg q12h IM or IV	2	>48	Renal; ototoxicity, auditory (high frequency hearing loss); vestibular	Can potentiate a neuro-muscular blockade
Amoxicillin	250 mg q6–8h PO	0.5	16	Rashes, gastrointestinal	Absorption is not greatly influenced by food. Rashes less common than with ampicillin
Ampicillin	250–500 mg q6h PO; 500–1000 mg q6h IM or IV	0.5	10	Rashes, gastrointestinal	Rashes in 10% of patients treated; usually morbilliform or macular-papular; higher incidence with mononucleosis. Cross-hypersensitivity with penicillin allergy. Avoid giving with meals
Carbenicillin indanyl sodium	1.0 g (2 tabs) q6h PO	?	14	Rashes, gastrointestinal	Reserve for pseudomonas, other organisms resistant to other agents. In patients with severely impaired renal function seizures and coagulapathies noted. Do not use if creatinine clearance (C_{cr}) <10 ml/min. Cross-hypersensitivity with penicillin allergy
Cefachlor	250 mg q6–8h PO	0.5	24	Gastrointestinal, moniliasis	Cross-hypersensitivity with penicillin allergy. Coombs (+). False (+) urine glucose (copper reduction method)
Cefaman-dole	500 mg q6h IM or IV	1	16	As above plus phlebitis	As above
Cefoxitin	250 mg q6–8h PO	0.5	24	Gastrointestinal, moniliasis	Cross-hypersensitivity with penicillin allergy. Coombs (+). False (+) urine glucose (copper reduction method)
Cephalexin	250–500 mg q6h PO	0.5	24	As above	As above
Cephalothin	0.5–1.0 g q6h IV	0.5	3	As above plus phlebitis	As above
Cephazolin	1.0 g q12h IM or IV	4	35	As above plus pain at injection site	As above
Cephapirin	500 mg q6h IM or IV				
Erythro-mycin	500 mg q6h PO	1.5	4.5	Gastrointestinal, ? hepatotoxic	Effective in alkaline urine only. Penetrates prostate gland

Table 7.4.—Continued

Medication	Adult Dose	$t_{1/2}$ (hr)	$t_{1/2}$ (hr) Anuric	Relatively Common Toxicity	Comments
Flucytosine	50–75 mg/kg/ day PO	3.4	70	Gastrointestinal, dose-related bone marrow suppression	Converted to 5FU
Gentamycin	1 mg/kg q8h IM or IV	2	30–76	Renal, ototoxicity: vestibular, auditory	Can potentiate neuromuscular blockade. Reserve for pseudomonas or organisms resistant to other agents
Kanamycin	7.5 mg/kg q12h IM	3	85	Ototoxicity: auditory, vestibular, renal; neuromuscular	Effective against most common urinary tract pathogens. Reserve for organisms resistant to less toxic drugs
Nalidixic acid	1.0 g q6h PO	1.5	?	Gastrointestinal, headache, visual disturbance, drowsiness, G6PD hemolysis	Resistance develops rapidly
Nitrofurantoin	100 mg q6–8h PO	0.5	?	Gastrointestinal, eosinophilic pulmonary infiltrate G6PD hemolysis, peripheral neuropathy if renal dysfunction	Contraindicated with C_{cr} of <40 ml/min. Give with food or milk. Good for prophylaxis or suppression
Sulfamethoxazole	1.0 g q12h PO	9	23	Rash, G6PD hemolysis, crystalluria, hematologic	Available alone or in combination with trimethoprim. Maintain adequate fluid intake. An intermediate acting sulfonamide. Caution in patients with asthma or liver dysfunction
Sulfisoxazole	1.0–2.0 g q6h PO; 2.0–3.0 g q6h IV	3.5	10	Rash, G6PD hemolysis, hematologic	Short-acting sulfonamide. Dilute parenteral form with sterile water for injection only. Caution in patients with asthma or liver dysfunction
Tetracycline	250–500 mg q6h PO	6	80	Rash, gastrointestinal, superinfection, dental staining	Do not use in children less than 8 years old or in last half of pregnancy
Tobramycin	1.5 mg/kg q8–12h IM or IV	2	48	Renal; ototoxicity: vestibular auditory	Reputedly less nephrotoxic than gentamycin
Trimethoprim	160 mg q12h PO or 100 mg q12–24h PO	10.5	23	Folate deficiency	Not approved for use during pregnancy, in breast feeding women or children less than 12 years old. Available in combination with sulfamethoxazole

status, age, allergy history, race, renal and hepatic function, previous history of UTIs and sex can influence the choice of antimicrobial used. Aside from these patient variables, the sensitivity of the organism to the available agents is a factor which must be considered. Finally, the relative differences of the agents themselves—kinetics, cost, dosage form availability, toxicity—are practical considerations which will influence the choice of agents.

Once an agent is selected, the currently recommended duration of eradicative therapy for an episode of acute, uncomplicated bacterial cystitis or pyelonephritis ranges from 10 to 14 days. This standard of therapy is effective in clearing an infection; however, compliance may be decreased when the patient becomes asymptomatic or if diarrhea or other side effects develop. On this basis, in addition to the obvious drug cost factor, there have been attempts to shorten the required duration of therapy. Ronald et al. (45) reported that a single 500-mg intramuscular injection with kanamycin cleared 92% of infections in adult patients. Fang et al. (42) found that a single 3.0-g oral dose of amoxicillin was as effective as conventional therapy—250 mg q.i.d. orally for 10 days—in clearing lower tract infections. The efficacy rate for both dosing regimens was 92%. However, a similar study by Brumfitt et al. (46) reported a success rate of only 44% following a single intramuscular dose of 2 g of cephaloridine. While the issue of duration of therapy for uncomplicated lower tract UTIs is unclear, based on the first two studies cited above, the single dose regimen deserves further evaluation especially in view of its potential impact on cost and compliance (Table 7.5).

While the duration of therapy of 10 to 14 days appears adequate for lower tract infections, the efficaciousness of this regimen for upper tract infection is questionable in view of the high relapse and failure rate. Fang et al. (42) reported a 50% failure rate in patients with upper tract infections treated with amoxicillin 250 mg q.i.d. for 10 days. Turck et al. (47, 48) noted that in upper tract infections treated for additional 6 weeks, the relapse rate was reduced by 50%.

The site of infection will influence the selection of an agent. In bacterial prostatitis the efficacy of eradicative therapy is dependent on the ability of the medication to penetrate into the prostate gland and its activity against the usual urinary tract pathogens. Both erythromycin and trimethoprim are able to achieve high prostatic concentrations; however, the antibacterial spectrum of erythromycin is primarily against gram positive microorganism. Trimethoprim, on the other hand, is quite effective against Gram-negative bacteria. Erythromycin's activity is further compromised due to the acidic environment of the prostate gland. Currently, trimethoprim is the drug of choice in prostatic infections. It is available, in this country, alone or in combination with sulfamethoxazole which does not penetrate the prostate gland well (49).

In the treatment of bacterial pyelonephritis the selection of an agent has been complicated by the controversy based on importance of serum versus urinary levels of the agent in treating pyelonephritis. McCabe and Jackson (28) clarified the issue in their study of 252 patients with pyelonephritis. In this study serum antiinfective levels could not be correlated with the cure or failure rates of the therapy; however, urinary levels of the agents did correlate with cure rate. While higher urinary levels are of importance, of equal significance is the ability of the antiinfective to diffuse into the kidney tissue. The diffusion characteristics are determined by the degree of protein binding of the agent and its ionic state in the urinary pH range (50). Drugs with a lower degree of protein binding are cleared primarily by glomerular filtration of the unbound fraction. In the tubular fluid, the drug in the nonionized state can passively diffuse into renal tissue along a concentration gradient. Since the nonionized ionized ratio is dependent on the pK_a of the drug and the urinary pH, the fraction of nonionized drug can be increased by adjusting the urinary pH in the appropriate direction. The significance of this pH adjustment on the outcome of therapy was demonstrated by Brumfitt and Percival (51). In patients in whom the urinary pH was appropriately adjusted for the antiinfective used, a cure rate approximating 87% was achieved. This is in marked contrast to the 67% cure rate when urinary pH was not altered (Table 7.6).

Patient variables such as pregnancy, renal and hepatic function and previous medication allergies should be considered prior to selecting an agent. Since women who are pregnant are particularly prone to UTIs, the selection of an agent should be viewed also from the perspective of potential teratogenic or neonatal

Table 7.5.
Singe Dose and Short Course Urinary Tract Infection (UTI) Therapy (42, 45)

Drug/Regimen	Patients[a]	Cured Initial Infection	Relapse	Reinfection	Reference
Amoxicillin 3.0 g PO	38 women, 18–55 yr old, uncomplicated ACB negative	34	4 (in 4 wk)	1 (in 4 wk)	66
	15 women, 18–55 yr old, ACB positive	5	10 (in 72 hr)		
	22 women, 18–54 yr old, uncomplicated ACB negative	20	0	2 (in 4 wk)	42
50 mg/kg (max 2.5 g) PO	18 girls, 12–18 yr old, with dysuria, frequency, urgency	14			
Cefaloridine, 2.0 g IM	25 women with bacteriuria in pregnancy	13	4 (in 3 mo)		70
	23 women with dysuria/frequency	8	12 (in 4–6 wk)		46
			15 (in 4–6 wk)		
	23 women with ACB negative	15	?	?	
	16 women with ACB positive	2	?	?	
Cefamandole, 1.0 g IM	44 women and 2 men with 53 infections	37	16 (in 1 wk)	1	67
	27 with abnormal IVP	16	11		
	23 with normal IVP	18	5		
Kanamycin, 0.5 g IM	104 women 15–64 yr old 39 with cystitis	36	3 (in 1 wk)	5 (in 4 wk)	45
	65 with upper tract infection	18	47 (in 2 wk)		
Nitrofurantoin ≤20 kg:25 mg/day × 3 days >20 kg:1.25 mg/kg/day × 3 days	26 girls 2–18 yr old	24	2 (in 1 wk)	12 (in 6 mo)	68
Trimethoprim-Sulfamethoxazole 0.48 g TMP PO 2.4 g SMX PO Based on age	20 women 17–55 yr old with cystitis or asymptomatic UTI	17		3 (in 1 wk)	69
	10 children 14 mo to 11 yr old with cystitis or asymptomatic UTI	7	1	2	

[a] ACB = antibody-coated bacteria test; IVP = intravenous pyelogram.

toxicity; for example, tetracyclines and tooth discoloration, sulfonamides and kernicterus. Renal and hepatic dysfunction can predispose the patient to accumulation of the agent and unnecessary toxicity. The use of aminoglycosides with renal dysfunction and the use of ammonium chloride as an acidifying agent in patients with hepatic dysfunction are examples of potential iatrogenically aggravated situations.

The use of antibiotic irrigations to treat bacterial infections of the lower tract have not been effective and have the added disadvantage of causing superinfections. However, fungal cystitis has been effectively treated with amphotericin irrigations (71).

Suppression

Long-term suppressive therapy is used primarily to reduce the incidence of recurrence and acute exacerbations of chronic infections.

Table 7.6.
Parameters Influencing the Renal Clearance of Eradicative Agents

Agent	% Protein Bound	% Excreted Unchanged	Effect of Urinary pH
Amikacin	Very low	90	?
Amoxicillin	17	73	?
Ampicillin	25	45	—
Carbenicillin (oral)	50	85	—
Cefachlor	Very low	90	?
Cefamandole	70	90	?
Cefoxitin	70	80	?
Cephalexin	15	90	↑ in alkaline
Cephalothin	60	60	↑ in alkaline
Cefazolin	74	90	↑ in alkaline
Erythromycin	20	10	↑ in alkaline
Flucytosine	10	95	?
Gentamycin	25	90	↑ in alkaline
Kanamycin	Very low	90	↑ in alkaline
Nalidixic acid	90	10	↑ in alkaline
Nitrofurantoin	25	35	↑ in alkaline
Sulfisoxazole	85	65	↑ in acidic
Sulfamethoxazole	65	30	↑ in acidic
Tetracycline	30	55	↑ in acidic
Tobramycin	Very low	90	?
Trimethoprim	45	55	↑ in alkaline

This form of therapy is indicated in patients who have a persistent focus of infection from which the microorganism cannot be eradicated. Examples of this type of infection include men with chronic bacterial prostatitis, patients with urinary calculi or other structural defect in the urinary tract system and/or the presence of a chronic indwelling catheter.

Methenamine appears to be the most suitable agent for suppressive therapy because of its action as a urinary antiseptic and resulting obviation of the problem of bacterial resistance. It has a low order of toxicity (dysuria and diarrhea) and can be used for prolonged periods. Other agents such as nitrofurantoin, sulfamethazole, trimethoprim-sulfamethoxazole and ampicillin have been used for suppression and are less than satisfactory when the problems of bacterial resistance, superinfection and toxicity are considered, especially when compared to methenamine. Consequently, the therapy of choice for protracted or long term suppression of UTIs is methenamine mandelate 1.0 g q.i.d. in conjunction with a urinary acidifier—ammonium chloride or ascorbic acid—to maintain the urine pH at 5.5 or less (52) (Table 7.7). Prior to instituting suppressive therapy, an attempt to clear the urine of any active infection should be made.

Prophylaxis

Prophylactic therapy is used to prevent infections in patients who have uncomplicated urinary tracts and a history of closely spaced, recurrent UTIs. Since recurrent, uncomplicated UTIs are primarily a problem of women and are usually reinfections, a prophylactic agent should continue to be effective with extended use. The agent used should be effective in low doses to minimize side effects (Table 7.8).

Three antiinfectives appear to be effective as prophylactic agents: methenamine, nitrofurantoin and trimethoprim-sulfamethoxazole. Since uncomplicated reinfections are the result of periurethral contamination by colonic flora, the prophylactic agent should not alter the sensitivity-resistance pattern of these bacteria. Both methenamine and nitrofurantoin do not affect the sensitivity of these organisms and thus remain effective with continued use (54). Trimethoprim's effectiveness is based on its ability to achieve bacteriocidal concentrations in vaginal fluid and thus inhibit periurethral colonization of enteric flora (55).

The dosage and regimens for nitrofurantoin or trimethoprim-sulfamethoxazole as prophy-

Table 7.7.
Urinary Acidifying and Alkalinizing Agents

Agent	Dose	Comments
Acidifiers		
Ascorbic acid	>6 g/day in divided doses	Titrate dose and urine pH; caution with patients who are receiving other medications whose clearance will be affected by acidic pH
Ammonium chloride	2–3 g q6h	As above; caution in patients with decreased hepatic or renal function; effectiveness limited by renal compensation; can cause systemic acidosis
Alkalinizers:		
NaHCO₃	4 g initially, 1–2 g q4h PO	Caution in patients with congestive heart failure, hypertension; titrate urine pH; can cause systemic alkalosis
Sodium citrate	1 g q4h PO	As above

Table 7.8.
Prophylactic and Suppressive Agents for UTIs

Drug	Dose	Comments
Methenamine mandelate	1.0 g q.i.d.	Requires urine pH <5.5; contraindicated in renal insufficiency, dehydration; can cause dysuria, GI irritation; avoid concurrent use with sulfonamides
Methenamine hippurate	1.0 g b.i.d.	As above
Nitrofurantoin	50–100 mg q.h.s.	See Table 7.4
Trimethoprim-sulfamethoxazole	½–1 tab q.h.s.	See Table 7.4

lactic agents are significantly less than those required for eradicative therapy. Nitrofurantoin in a dose of 50 or 100 mg at bedtime or one-half tablet of trimethoprim-sulfamethoxazole (80 mg-400 mg/tablet) at bedtime have been demonstrated to be effective prophylactic measures (56, 57).

Methenamine has been tried in a single bedtime dose of 1.0 g; however, this has been shown to be less effective than the other agents (58). Consequently, full doses of 0.5 to 1.0 g q.i.d. of methenamine in addition to urinary acidification to a pH of 5.5 or lower should be used if this agent is used for prophylaxis.

As with suppressive therapy, prophylactic therapy should not be instituted until an existent infection is cleared using eradicative therapy.

Follow-up

One of the most important yet most frequently omitted components in the total treatment of UTIs is adequate follow-up. A culture after the first 48 to 72 hours of therapy to check for antiinfective failure is indicated. Since pyuria can persist during this initial phase of treatment, a urinalysis is a poor screening test for ineffective therapy.

Reculturing the urine following any course of therapy, whether it is eradicative, prophylactic or suppressive, is a mandatory check for recurrent infection. Since relapses occur shortly after discontinuation of the antiinfective agent, a culture 7 to 10 days after completion of therapy should be done. Reinfections can occur at any time following treatment. Follow-up cultures should be performed periodically during the first 2 years in uncomplicated infections, initially at monthly intervals during the first 3 months, then every 3 to 6 months during the remainder of the 2-year period. In patients with a history of recurrent infections, periodic cultures should be done routinely and indefinitely.

Since cultures and office visits are relatively expensive, the use of a test which a patient can perform at home has been advocated. The Microstix (see Table 7.1) has been tested and is 93% accurate in detecting significant bacteriuria (61). This test offers a viable, inexpensive alternative method for follow-up of UTIs.

PROGNOSIS

The prognosis for UTIs is highly variable, even with adequate therapy. Urologic structural abnormalities, presence of an indwelling catheter, sexual activity, and pregnancy favor the potential for recurrent infections. Concurrent predisposing conditions such as sex, age, debility and urologic manipulation favor the spread of infection beyond the urinary tract.

In young girls with UTIs which were treated, only a 20% cure rate was achieved; within two years following the initial infection 80% had a recurrence (22). Following an episode of bacteriuria during pregnancy, the possibility of recurrence is markedly enhanced when compared to patients who were nonbacteriuric during pregnancy (54% vs. 5%) (8). Of note is the increased incidence of urologic abnormalities on radiologic exam on follow-up examination in the patients who were bacteriuric during pregnancy as compared to the control population (54% vs. 22%) (8).

Metastatic infections secondary to UTIs can occur. Men appear to be more prone to developing metastases from lower UTIs and women more prone to the developing metastases from upper tract infections. In general predisposing factors to developing these ectopic infections include a complicated urinary tract, urologic manipulation and impaired host defenses—diabetes, malignancy, cirrhosis, uremia, malnutrition, anemia and collagen disease. The sites of metastases reported include skeletal (59%), endocarditis (29%), chest (4%), eye (2%) and miscellaneous (3%). Of note is that within the skeletal metastatic lesions, 83% were to the vertebrae (62).

The uncomplicated UTI has the most favorable prognosis. In women this type of infection has been reported to clear spontaneously in 40 to 50% of patients (63). With a single course of therapy up to 94% of uncomplicated infections can be eradicated (64).

CONCLUSION

The rational management of UTIs requires knowledge of the pathogenesis, methods of detection and their interpretations, approaches to therapy, and follow-up care. In spite of the voluminous literature in these areas, the UTI is still considered to be a minor problem and is often taken lightly. This unfortunate circumstance can and has led to unnecessary morbidity and an increased expense to the patient and health care system. The pharmacist through his routine monitoring activities is in a position to promote the detection, the rational therapy, and follow-up for UTIs. The universal nature of UTIs requires that all pharmacists be well versed in this disease. It also offers the pharmacist interested in clinical and/or patient care research the opportunity to impact on a health care problem which tends to be minimized at the community and nonresearch oriented institutional level.

With respect to the patient, the pharmacist is in a position to provide education and counseling regarding the disease, methods of prevention and therapy. An emphasis on the patient's responsibility to participate in his own health care by complying with the entire course of therapy and follow-up should be part of this educational process.

References

1. Friedman LR, Phair JP, Seki M: The epidemiology of urinary tract infections in Hiroshima. *Yale J Biol Med* 37:262, 1965.
2. Kunin CM: Emergence of bacteriuria, proteinuria, and symptomatic urinary tract infections among a population of school girls followed for 7 years. *Pediatrics* 41:968, 1968.
3. Buckley RM Jr, McGuckin M, Mac Gregor RR: Urine bacterial counts after sexual intercourse. *N Engl J Med* 298:321, 1978.
4. Bran JL, Levison ME, Kaye D: Entrance of bacteria into the female urinary bladder. *N Engl J Med* 286:626, 1972.
5. Whalley PJ, Martin FG, Peters PC: Significance of asymptomatic bacteriuria detected during pregnancy. *JAMA* 193:879, 1965.
6. Gower PE, Haswell B, Sidaway ME, et al: Follow up of 164 patients with bacteriuria of pregnancy. *Lancet* 1:990, 1968.
7. Leigh DA, Grueneberg RN, Brumfitt W: Long term follow-up of bacteriuria of pregnancy. *Lancet* 1:603, 1968.
8. Zinner SH, Kass EH: Long term (10 to 14 years) follow up of bacteriuria of pregnancy. *N Engl J Med* 285:820, 1971.
9. Kunin CM, McCormack RC: An epidemiologic study of bacteriuria and blood pressure among nuns and working women. *N Engl J Med* 278:635, 1968.
10. Kass EH, Savage WD, Santamarina BAG: The significance of bacteriuria in preventive medicine. In Kass EH: *Progress in Pyelonephritis.* Philadelphia: F. A. Davis, 1965, p 3.
11. Forland M, Thomas V, Shelokov A: Urinary tract infections in patients with diabetes mellitus. *JAMA* 238:1924, 1977.
12. McCabe W: Pyelonephritis. In Hoeprich PD: *Infectious Diseases,* New York: Harper & Row, 1973, p 507.

13. Turck M, Petersdorf RG: The epidemiology of nonenteric E. coli infections: prevalence of serologic groups. J Clin Invest 41:1760, 1962.
14. Vosti KL, Goldberg LM, Monto AS, et al: Host-parasite interaction in patients with infections due to Esch. coli; 1. Serogrouping of Esch. coli from intestinal and extra-intestinal sources. J Clin Invest 43:2377, 1964.
15. Stamey TA, Timothy M, Millar M, et al: Recurrent urinary infections in adult women. The role of introital enterobacteria. Calif Med 115:1, 1971.
16. Stamm WE: Guidelines for prevention of catheter-associated urinary tract infections. Ann Int Med 82:386, 1975.
17. Kass EH, Schneiderman LJ: Entry of bacteria into the urinary tracts of patients with inlying catheters. N Engl J Med 256:556, 1957.
18. McCarthy JM, Pryles CV: Clean voided and catheter neonatal urine specimens: bacteriology in the male and female neonate. Am J Dis Child 106:473, 1968.
19. Randolph MF, Greenfield M: The incidence of asymptomatic bacteriuria and pyuria in infancy. J Pediatr 65:57, 1964.
20. Siegel SR, Sokoloff B, Siegel B: Asymptomatic and symptomatic urinary tract infections in infancy. Am J Dis Child 125:45, 1973.
21. Scheinman JI, Hester DJ, Integlia SS, et al: Antibiotic treatment of asymptomatic baceriuria. Am J Dis Child 125:349, 1973.
22. Kunin CM, Deutscher R, Pacquin A, Jr: Urinary tract infection in school children: an epidemiologic, clinical and laboratory study. Medicine 43:91, 1964.
23. Whalley P: Bacteriuria of pregnancy. Am J Obstet Gynecol 97:723, 1967.
24. Gallagher DJA, Montgomerie JZ, North SDK: Acute infections of the urinary tract and the urethral syndrome in general practice. Br Med J 1:622, 1965.
25. Kass EH: Asymptomatic infections of the urinary tract. Trans Am Assoc Physicians 69:56, 1956.
26. Marple CD: The frequency and character of urinary tract infections in an unselected group of women. Ann Intern Med 14:2220, 1941.
27. Stamey TA, Pfau A: Urinary infections: a selective review and some observations. Calif Med 113:6, 1970.
28. McCabe WR, Jackson GG: Treatment of pyelonephritis: bacterial, drug and host factors in success or failure among 252 patients. N Engl J Med 272:1037, 1965.
29. Matsoniotis N, Danelatou-Athanassiadou C, Katerelos C, et al: Low urinary glucose concentration: a reliable index of urinary tract infection. J Pediatr 78:851, 1971.
30. Scherstein B, Dahlquist A, Fritz H, et al: Screening for bacteriuria with a test paper for glucose. JAMA 204:205, 1968.
31. Craig WA, Kunin CM, DeGroot J: Evaluation of new urinary tract infection screening devices. Appl Microbiol 26:196, 1973.
32. Cohen SN, Kass EH: A simple method for quantitative urine culture. N Engl J Med 277:176, 1967.
33. Smith I, Schmidt J: Evaluation of three screening tests for patients with significant bacteriuria. JAMA 181:159, 1962.
34. Schaus R: Greiss' nitrate test in the diagnosis of urinary infection. JAMA 161:528, 1956.
35. Smith LG, Thayer WR, Malta EM, et al: Relationship of the Greiss nitrite test to bacterial culture in the diagnosis of urinary tract infection. Ann Intern Med 54:66, 1961.
36. Randolph MF, Morris K: Instant screening for bacteriuria in children: analysis of a dipstick. J Pediatr 84:246, 1974.
37. Neter E: Evaluation of the tetrazolium blue test for the diagnosis of significant bacteriuria. JAMA 192:769, 1965.
38. Eliot CR, Pryles CV: Observations on the use of triphenyltetrazolium for the detection of bacteriuria. Pediatrics 34:421, 1964.
39. Bulger RJ, Kirby WM: Simple tests for significant bacteriuria. Arch Intern Med 112:742, 1963.
40. Thomas V, Shelokov A, Forland M: Antibody-coated bacteria in the urine and the site of the urinary tract infection. N Engl J Med 290:588, 1974.
41. Jones SR, Smith JW, Sanford JP: Localization of urinary tract infections by detection of antibody coated bacteria in urine sediment. N Engl J Med 290:591, 1974.
42. Fang LST, Tolkoff-Rubin NE, Rubin RH: Efficacy of single-dose and conventional amoxicillin therapy in urinary tract infection localized by the antibody-coated bacteria technic. N Engl J Med 298:413, 1978.
43. Stamey TA, Govan DE, Palmer SM: The localization and treatment cf urinary tract infections. The role of bactericidal urine levels as opposed to serum levels. Medicine 44:1, 1965.
44. Fass RJ, Klainer AS, Perkins RL: Urinary tract infection: practical aspects of diagnosis and treatment. JAMA 225:1509, 1973.
45. Ronald AR, Boutros P, Mourtada H: Bacteriuria localization and response to single-dose therapy in women. JAMA 235:1854, 1976.
46. Brumfitt W, Faiers MC, Franklin INS: The treatment of urinary infection by means of a single dose of cephaloridine. Postgrad Med J 46 (Suppl):65, 1970.
47. Turck M, Anderson KN, Petersdorf RG: Relapse and reinfection in chronic bacteriuria. N Engl J Med 275:70, 1966.
48. Turck M, Anderson KN, Petersdorf RG: Relapse and reinfection in chronic bacteriuria (Part II). N Engl J Med 278:422, 1968.
49. Stamey TA, Meares EM, Winningham DG: Chronic bacterial prostatitis and the diffusion of drugs into prostatic fluid. J Urol 103:187, 1970.
50. Romankiewicz JA: Factors influencing renal distribution of antibiotics: a key to therapy of pyelonephritis. Drug Intell Clin Pharm 8:512, 1974.
51. Brumfitt W, Percival A: Adjustment of urine pH in the chemotherapy of urinary tract infections. Lancet 1:186, 1962.
52. Freeman RB, Smith WM, Richardson JA, et al: Long term therapy for chronic bacteriuria in men. Ann Intern Med 83:133, 1975.
53. Gleckman RA: Trimethoprim-sulfamethoxazole vs. ampicillin in chronic urinary tract infections. JAMA 233:427, 1975.
54. Winberg J, Bergström T, Lincoln K, et al: Treatment trials in urinary tract infection with special deference to the effect of antimicrobials on the

fecal and periurethral flora. *Clin Nephrol* 1:142, 1973.

55. Stamey TA, Condy M: The diffusion and concentration of trimethoprim in human vaginal fluid. *J Infect Dis* 131:261, 1975.
56. Stamey TA, Condy M, Mihara G: Prophylactic efficacy of nitrofurantoin macrocrystals and trimethoprim-sulfamethoxazole in urinary infection: biologic effects on vaginal flora. *N Engl J Med* 296:780, 1977.
57. Harding GKM, Ronald AR: A controlled study of antimicrobial prophylaxis of recurrent urinary infections in women. *N Engl J Med* 291:597, 1974.
58. Kincaid-Smith P, Kalowski S, Nanra RS: Cotrimoxazole in urinary tract infection. *Med J Aust* 1(Suppl):49, 1973.
59. Andriole VT, Epstein FH: Prevention of pyelonephritis by water diuresis: evidence for the role of medullary hypertonicity in promoting renal function. *J Clin Invest* 44:73, 1965.
60. Andriole VT: Acceleration of the inflammatory response of the renal medulla by water diuresis. *J Clin Invest* 45:847, 1966.
61. Kunin CM, DeGroot JE: Self-screening for significant bacteriuria: evaluation of a dip-strip combination nitrite/culture test. *JAMA* 231:1349, 1975.
62. Siroky MB, Moylan RA, Austin G, Jr, et al: Metastatic infection secondary to genitourinary tract sepsis. *Am J Med* 61:351, 1976.
63. Kass EH: Prevention of apparently non-infectious disease by detection and treatment of infections of the urinary tract. *J Chronic Dis* 15:665, 1962.
64. Bailey RR: Urinary tract infection—some recent concepts. *Can Med Assn J* 107:316, 1972.
65. McAllister TA, Percival A, Alexander JG, et al: The sensitivities of urinary pathogenesis—a survey: multicentric study of sensitivities of urinary tract pathogens. *Postgrad Med J* 47(Suppl):7, 1971.
66. Rubin RH, Fang LST, Jones SR, et al: Single-dose amoxicillin therapy for urinary tract infections. Multicenter trial using antibody coated bacteria localization technique. *JAMA* 244:561, 1980.
67. Shaw PG, Fairley KF, Whitworth JA: Treatment of urinary tract infection with a single dose intramuscular administration of cephamandole. *Med J Aust* 1:489, 1980.
68. Lohr JA, Hayden GF, Kesler RW, et al: Three day therapy of lower urinary tract infections with nitrofurantoin macrocrystals: a randomized clinical trial. *J Pediatr* 99:980, 1981.
69. Bailey RR, Abbott GD: Treatment of urinary tract infection with a single dose of trimethoprim-sulfamethoxazole. *J Can Med Assn* 118:551, 1978.
70. Shapiro ED, Wald ER: Simple dose amoxicillin treatment of urinary tract infections. *J Pediatr* 99:989, 1981.
71. Wise GJ, Weinstein S, Goldberg P, et al: Candidal cystitis—management by continuous bladder irrigation with amphotericin B. *JAMA* 174:359, 1960.

CHAPTER 8

Enteric Infections

ELAINE OBSTARCZYK REALE, Pharm.D.

Infectious gastroenteritis (GE) is a cause of significant morbidity and mortality throughout the world. Acute diarrheal disease in developing countries is a major contributor to mortality in infants and morbidity in all age groups. An estimated 3 to 5 billion cases of diarrhea occurred during the year 1977 to 1978 resulting in 5 to 10 million deaths in Asia, Africa and Latin America (1). In contrast, in the United States, GE is rarely fatal, although it is a common cause of morbidity and decreased productivity. Elderly and debilitated persons and infants are often hospitalized because of the severe diarrhea.

The most common symptom of acute infectious GE is diarrhea which is often self-medicated. Thus, the pharmacist will have frequent opportunities to educate patients regarding diarrheal illness and to advise them on appropriate use of over-the-counter medications. Knowledge of the disease and treatment will assist the pharmacist in screening patients and referring them to physicians, choosing medications, and educating patients and other health care personnel.

ETIOLOGY AND EPIDEMIOLOGY

Viruses are the most common etiology of infectious diarrhea in the United States. Only recently have researchers shown that the Norwalk virus and rotavirus are responsible for the majority of cases (2). Bacterial GE is less frequent. Staphylococci, salmonella and shigella have been recognized as causes of acute diarrheal illness for decades, but recently other bacteria were isolated and identified as etiologic agents, important examples being campylobacter and yersinia. Likewise, the role of *Escherichia coli* as a diarrheal pathogen has been elucidated of late. An increasingly important parasite causing diarrheal illness is giardia which will be discussed with other intestinal parasites in Chapter 13 (*Parasitic and Mycotic Diseases*).

The discussion will be limited to agents which are common or of increasing epidemiologic importance, or agents that merit special treatment considerations. Information regarding other viral infections, overgrowth of normal flora, antibiotic-induced *Clostridium difficile* colitis, and agents that cause diarrhea mainly through food poisoning, may be found elsewhere (3, 4).

Viruses

GE due to a parvovirus, the Norwalk agent, is usually epidemic because secondary spread is very rapid. Outbreaks occur in schools, institutions and communities. Infection is acquired by the fecal-oral route, through contaminated water and improperly cooked seafood, and possibly through airborne transmission. In the United States, infection with Norwalk virus is uncommon during infancy, but occurs in all other age groups and at any time of the year. The virus is excreted in the stool for 3 days after onset of the illness (2).

Rotavirus infection is usually sporadic and occasionally epidemic, commonly affecting young children and infants over 4 months of age. The virus has spread among hospital patients and employees, as well as within families of infected children who attend day-care centers. Adult contacts of infected children occasionally are symptomatic but frequently may have subclinical infection. Transmission is mainly by the fecal-oral route. The incubation period is 1 to 3 days and the virus is excreted in the feces for up to 8 days or more (2). Rotavirus has also been implicated as a cause of traveler's diarrhea (5).

Bacteria

Shigellae are Gram-negative bacilli which reside in the gastrointestinal tract of higher primates. Four types of shigella are human pathogens. *Shigella sonnei* is the most prevalent, followed by *Shigella flexneri*. Both *Shigella dysenteriae*, the most virulent, and *Shi-*

gella boydii are rare. In developed countries shigellosis primarily affects children less than 10 years of age. The small inoculum size required to cause clinical illness facilitates spread, particularly in closed populations such as day-care and resident-care centers. Community epidemics of shigellosis have occurred as a result of secondary spread to families of children attending day-care centers (6) and as a result of large scale food and water contamination. It may also be acquired during travel to foreign countries. Transmission is primarily by the fecal-oral route, with man as the sole reservoir. Fourteen thousand cases of shigella infection were reported to the Center for Disease Control in the United States in 1980 (7).

Salmonellae are also Gram-negative bacilli. The most common serotype associated with disease in the United States is *Salmonella typhimurium* (30%). Other types, including *Salmonella typhi* which is associated with typhoid fever, are reported in less than 10% of cases. Salmonella organisms have been isolated from almost all types of animals. The ingestion of contaminated poultry, poultry products, beef or pork, dairy products, or water is usually responsible for human acquisition of salmonella. Home, community or institutional outbreaks almost always occur in this manner. Closed-population epidemics may also occur secondary to spread from an environmental reservoir or a convalescent carrier. The chronic carrier state occurs most frequently with *S. typhi* (2 to 4%) and is associated with biliary tract disease. The 25 to 30 thousand cases of salmonellosis reported in the United States each year may be only a small percentage of the true incidence (8).

Campylobacter is a gram-negative bacillus. The human pathogenic species are *Campylobacter jejuni* and *Campylobacter fetus* ssp. *fetus*. Of the two, *C. jejuni* is the most frequent cause of acute diarrheal disease. Person-to-person or animal-to-person spread is by the fecal-oral route as occurred in cases of secondary intrafamilial infection, vertical transmission from mother to newborn, and infection from sick animals, particularly puppies and kittens. Infection has also been contracted from contaminated water or food, as in recent raw milkborne epidemics (9). Proper preparation of foods, especially fowl, will help prevent infection. Campylobacter may also cause traveler's diarrhea (4). Since the refinement of isolation methods for *Campylobacter* species,

this organism has been noted to cause as much or more GE in the United States as salmonella or shigella (10, 11).

Escherichia coli, a Gram-negative bacillus, is the most common normal inhabitant of the human intestinal tract. Its role in acute GE has only recently been clarified. *E. coli* is now categorized into three groups, enteropathogenic (EPEC), enterotoxogenic (ETEC) and enteroinvasive (EIEC). EPEC has caused nursery outbreaks of diarrhea since the late 1800s although this type of epidemic has mysteriously disappeared in developing countries. ETEC and EIEC can affect persons of all ages. Along with rotavirus, they are the major causes of diarrheal morbidity and mortality in young children of developing countries. GE due to ETEC or EIEC is uncommon in developed countries including the United States (12). Most cases of *E. coli* GE are associated with ingestion of contaminated food or water. In several studies, 30 to 70% of the cases of traveler's diarrhea were due to ETEC (12).

Yersinia enterocolitica is another Gram-negative organism recently recognized as a cause of GE in both children and adults (13). Most cases in the United States have been associated with contaminated milk, although sporadic cases may occur. Person-to-person spread is strongly suggested by outbreaks in hospitals and within families. Yersinia seems to be transmissible from animals to man because pigs, dogs, and cats carry the organism and simultaneous infection of animals and children in the same household has been noted. Recent refinement of isolation methods will facilitate further epidemiologic characterization of this agent in the United States.

PATHOGENESIS
Host Defenses

Among the host factors which act against pathogenic organisms, four have been well established as defense mechanisms: colon gastric acidity, peristalsis, immune response and resident microflora. Most enteric pathogens are sensitive to gastric acidity. The peristaltic action of the small intestine, aided by mucus secretion, also minimizes colonization and assists in eliminating pathogenic organisms. Enteric immunity consists of intraluminal phagocytic cells, cell-mediated immune processes and secretory IgA production. Finally, resident microflora provide competition for pathogenic

colonization by attaching to intestinal epithelium and acting synergistically with other enteric immunity. Interference with these factors
may increase host susceptibility to infection.

Patients with achlorhydria or gastric resection are more susceptible to enteric infection.
Antacid therapy can dramatically reduce the
inoculum required to produce GE from certain
organisms. Delay in intestinal motility, such
as occurs with opiate antidiarrheals, may encourage colonization and increase the contact
time of organisms with the mucosa, leading to
mucosal invasion. Compromise or immaturity
of immune status predisposes to infection, as
in cancer patients or during infancy. Antibiotics may decrease normal flora of the intestinal
tract and create an environment more condu-
cive to infection. These will be discussed further under treatment.

Viral and Bacterial Virulence

Norwalk and rotavirus both cause lesions of
the small intestine mucosal cells, whereas colonic mucosa remains normal. The exact
mechanism of diarrhea production is uncertain although the clinical features most closely
resemble enterotoxin-mediated diarrhea. Alteration of duodenal mucosal function usually
accompanies these infections, as indicated by
decreased xylose absorption and/or reduced
fat absorption.

Among the many bacterial properties that
promote infection three of the most important
are the abilities to produce enterotoxin, adhere
to mucosa, and invade the mucosa. Organisms
which cause disease mainly by enterotoxin
production primarily colonize the upper small
intestine and produce secretory diarrhea (isotonic fluid loss in excess of 10 ml/kg/24 hours)
(14). Salmonella, shigella, ETEC and Y. enterocolitica produce enterotoxins, also called ex-
otoxins (15). These proteins are secreted by the
organisms and bind to receptors located on the
brush border of the villus epithelial cell. The
bound exotoxin then stimulates adenyl cyclase or guanyl cyclase to dramatically increase intestinal secretion of water and electrolytes. When the volume of fluid over-
whelms the reabsorptive capacity of the colon,
diarrhea results. The importance of enterotoxin in the pathogenesis of salmonella, shigella and yersinia diarrhea is unknown.

Cytotoxin, a type of exotoxin which alters
mucosal cell histology, causes diarrhea by an
unkown mechanism. S. dysenteriae, some
strains of E. coli, and possibly C. fetus ssp. jejuni
produce cytotoxins (15).

Evidence exists indicating the importance of
bacterial adherence to intestinal mucosa for
salmonella, shigella, and E. coli. Bacteria possess structures called fimbriae, fine protein
filaments protruding from their surfaces.
These attach to specific receptor sites on the
intestinal cell. The presence or absence of the
specific receptor sites is inherited; thus susceptibility or resistance to infection is partly genetically determined (15).

S. enteritidis, shigella, C. fetus ssp. jejuni and
enteroinvasive strains of E. coli must invade
the colonic mucosa and multiply there causing
inflammation. Spread to other epithelial cells
(shigella) or to the lamina propria with systemic dissemination (salmonella) may occur.
Inflammation and gross or minute ulceration,
as in shigella or salmonella infections, respectively, are followed by diarrhea. The mechanism of fluid secretion is not due to increased
mucosal permeability, but is probably a mul-
tifactorial process involving inflammatory
processes and enterotoxin production (15). S.
typhi, yersinia and C. fetus ssp. intestinalis
usually penetrate the intact mucosa of the
distal small bowel and multiply in the lymphatic or reticuloendothelial system (3). These
organisms often cause systemic illness with or
without diarrhea. The exact mechanism of
diarrhea in these cases is unclear.

Prostaglandins may be involved in the production of diarrhea. There is some preliminary
evidence that bacteria stimulate production of
prostaglandins which increase adenyl cyclase
activity, thereby causing fluid and electrolyte
loss (16).

Electrolyte Depletion

In addition to increased fluid secretion
caused by the pathogenic mechanisms discussed above, these processes are responsible
for electrolyte loss. Sodium and bicarbonate
regulation occur, in part, in the intestinal epithelial cell (Fig. 8.1). Within the cell H_2CO_3
dissociates into hydrogen and bicarbonate.
The bicarbonate is secreted into the intestine
along with sodium and the hydrogen is reabsorbed into the blood. In the diarrheal process
increased sodium loss increases the bicarbonate loss into the intestine, and therefore more
hydrogen is reabsorbed resulting in systemic

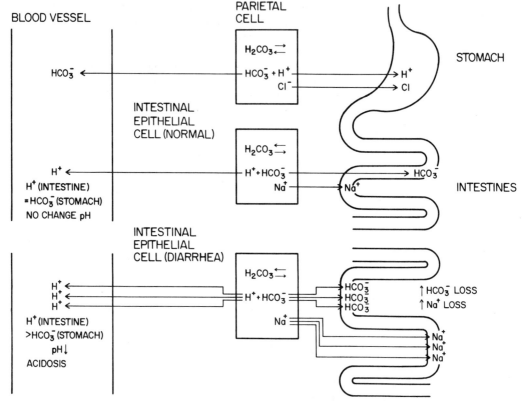

Figure 8.1. Bicarbonate secretion in diarrhea (43).

metabolic acidosis. Potassium loss may also be greater secondary to interference with reabsorption. Activation of aldosterone by hyponatremia and/or hypovolemia may increase renal potassium excretion as well.

Clinical Features

In patients with enterotoxin-mediated diarrhea (ETEC and possibly salmonella), there is abrupt onset of nausea, vomiting, cramps, and large volume, watery stools. Mild constitutional symptoms and low grade fever may be present. Fluid and electrolyte loss may result in hypovolemic shock. Blood, mucus and leukocytes are absent from the stool since the mucosal surface is not damaged. The clinical picture of viral enteritis most closely resembles that of the enterotoxin-mediated diarrheas. These infections are usually self-limited (Table 8.1). Various other noninfectious processes can cause similar symptoms. Among them are solute loads, tropical sprue, excessive bile salts or fatty acids, lactase or other enzyme deficiencies, or neoplasms associated with in-

creased serum prostaglandins or vasoactive polypeptides.

Enteroinvasive organisms (EIEC), S. enteritidis and C. jejuni can produce a more severe clinical picture with higher fever, moderate to severe constitutional symptoms, and stools containing blood, mucus and leukocytes. The latter results from inflammation and other colonic mucosal damage. Ulcerative colitis and pseudomembranous colitis cause similar symptoms.

Organisms which penetrate the mucosa and multiply in lymphatic or reticuloendothelial systems also tend to produce systemic symptoms more frequently. Campylobacter diarrheal illness has been associated with fever and bacteremia (9). Extraintestinal manifestations of yersinia are common, including various vasculitic rashes, and arthritis which may occur during or after the diarrheal symptoms. Yersinia may also cause a chronic colitis resembling Crohn's disease (13). Additional clinical features due to each infectious agent are given in Table 8.1.

Since many of these bacteria cause symp-

Table 8.1.
Features of Gastroenteritis

	Norwalk Virus	Rotavirus	Shigella sonnei	Shigella flexneri and Shigella dysenteriae	Salmonella	Escherichia coli EI	E. coli ET	Campylobacter	Yersinia
Stool	Clear	Clear, brown	Clear	Bloody	Green, brown	Bloody	Clear	Bloody	Pale, green
WBCs[a]	−	−	−	++	−	++	−	++	+
Volume[b]	var	lg	lg	sml	mod	sml	lg	mod-lg	sml-mod
>39°C	−	−	++	+	−	++	−	++	
Incubation period (days)	1–2	1–3	1.5–3	1.5–3	1–2	?	1–3	1–7	4–10
Duration (days)	1–2	5–8	2–3	7–14	3–7	?	5–10	2–3	7–14
Carrier state	−	−	+	+	+	−	−	−	?
Age	Any	<2 yr	2 yr	Any	Any	Any	Any	Any	Any

[a] −, Unlikely; +, likely; and ++, very likely.
[b] var, variable; sml, small; mod, moderate; lg, large.

toms which resemble other noninfectious diarrheal illnesses, an appropriate diagnostic approach is important.

A careful history including recent travel, antibiotic use, illnesses in contacts, weight loss, underlying diseases, and appearance of stool, can provide clues to the etiology. Actual examination of a stool specimen for blood, mucus and leukocytes is preferable to a description of the stool by the patient. A stool culture can be very valuable in diagnosis, although a laboratory may not always be available. Culture technique is critical in the isolation of many enteric bacteria since some require special media and procedures. Physical assessment of the patient for signs of dehydration and other abnormalities will help to determine the therapeutic approach. Radiologic and endoscopic evaluation may be necessary if routine diagnostic procedures fail. Information on differential diagnosis of infectious vs. noninfectious diarrhea can be found elsewhere (3).

TREATMENT

Fluid and Electrolyte Therapy

The mainstay of treatment for any type of infectious diarrhea is fluid and electrolyte replacement. Fluids may be given by the oral or intravenous route, depending on the severity of losses and the patient's ability to maintain oral intake. If the patient's intake is less than output, intravenous therapy is recommended. Severe dehydration, manifest as oliguria or anuria, thirst, dry mucous membranes, irritability, lethargy, hypotension, sunken fontanel (infants) and lack of tears (infants), often requires intravenous therapy, in whole or part. Infants become dehydrated more rapidly than children or adults. Thus, infants most often require hospitalization and intravenous rehydration.

The volume of fluid administered is dependent on the size of the individual, stool losses, degree of dehydration and the presence of fever. Severely dehydrated patients may require a 10 to 20 ml/kg bolus of normal saline initially.

A commonly used method for calculating fluid requirement is shown in Table 8.2. According to this method, a 56-kg person with a fever of 10°C and 2-kg weight loss would require 2530 ml maintenance, plus 2000 ml replacement, plus the appropriate volume for

Table 8.2.
Fluid Requirements in Diarrheal Disease

Fluid requirements = deficit + maintenance + ongoing losses

I. Deficit = % body wt lost (kg) × 1000 ml/kg

II. Maintenance = $X + Y + Z$ + Stool losses

   X = 1st 10 kg body wt × 100 ml/kg
   Y = 2nd 10 kg body wt × 50 ml/kg
   Z = remaining body wt × 20 ml/kg

   Increase maintenance for increased respiratory rate or increased temperature (12% per °C)

III. Ongoing losses = diarrhea and emesis, replace ml for ml

---

stool losses in the first 24 hours. The calculations are shown below.

Maintenance:
   10 kg × 100 ml/kg = 1000 ml
   10 kg × 50 ml/kg = 500 ml
   38 kg × 20 ml/kg = 760 ml
   ———————
                        2260 ml

Maintenance increase for fever: 12/100 × 2260 ml = 271.2 ml

Replacement: 2 kg × 1000 ml/kg = 2000 ml

Total 24-hour requirement (first 24 hours): 4530 ml plus stool losses

Maintenance fluids for the next 24 hours would be 2260 ml adjusted for fever and stool losses.

The type of fluid administered is determined by the electrolyte loss and the need for caloric support. Fluids should routinely contain carbohydrate as an energy source to prevent hypoglycemia, particularly in the infant. The electrolyte content of diarrheal stool varies greatly depending on age, food intake, type of infectious organism, and stool volume. Stool and/or serum electrolyte content may assist in determining replacement needs.

The interpretation of serum concentrations and the treatment of electrolyte imbalances are discussed in Chapter 29. An intravenous solution of dextrose 5% with 0.25 or 0.5 N saline will meet the needs of most patients with mild to moderate diarrheal losses if their serum sodium is in the range of 130 to 150 mEq/liter.

Potassium supplementation should be withheld until urination is present to avoid hyperkalemia. An intravenous solution of 20 to 40 mEq/liter should maintain serum potassium once replacement of deficits is complete. Correction of metabolic acidosis with sodium bicarbonate is usually unnecessary unless the bicarbonate deficit is severe (less than 15 mEq/liter).

Oral fluid and electrolyte therapy has been used extensively in countries where diarrhea is endemic. In these countries and in the United States, oral rehydration and electrolyte replacement have been accomplished even in severely dehydrated infants and children (17–19). Oral rehydration is not yet the standard of treatment for severe dehydration in the United States. However, oral therapy may prevent the need for hospitalization for mild to moderately dehydrated patients and is a helpful adjunct to intravenous therapy. Commercial products made specifically for oral hydration are available, although many household products are suitable and are less expensive (Table 8.3). Household products high in one electrolyte may be alternated with those high in others to provide balanced supplementation. An example of this would be alternating half-strength apple juice with Gatorade to provide adequate quantities of potassium and sodium, respectively. Commercial electrolyte solutions may be tolerated better than household products. They do not contain flavorful food substances which may be undesirable to a nauseated patient and are isoosmolar.

The carbohydrates present in the oral solutions are glucose, sucrose or fructose. In addition to providing an energy substrate, glucose facilitates the transport of water and sodium across the cell membrane during its absorption, reducing stool losses (20). Sucrose must be hydrolyzed by intestinal mucosal disaccharidases to glucose and fructose, which are then absorbed. During enterotoxigenic and viral enteric infections, intestinal disaccharidases are decreased, leading to the hypothesis that glucose is the preferred carbohydrate for oral replacement. Although glucose may be slightly more efficient in rehydration and restoration of electrolytes, sucrose has been demonstrated to be an acceptable alternative (17, 18). Fructose alone has not been evaluated.

The sodium content of the commercially available oral replacement solutions listed is 30 to 60 mEq/liter. This is less than the 90 mEq/liter of sodium present in the standard rehydration formula recommended by the World Health Organization (WHO). The WHO formula was designed for patients suffering

Table 8.3.
Products for Oral Hydration

	Carbohydrate	Electrolyte (mEq/liter)			
		Na+	K+	Cl−	Base
Pedialyte	Glucose	30	20	30	28
Pedialyte RS[a]	Glucose	60	20	50	28
Infalyte	Glucose	50	20	40	30
Gatorade	Glucose Sucrose	23	3	17	3
Orange juice[b]	Glucose	0.4	50	—	50
Apple juice[b]	Glucose	0.4	30	—	—
Grape juice[b]	Glucose	0.5	30	—	32

[a] Pedialyte RS contains 25 g/liter of glucose vs. 50 g/liter in Pedialyte, in order to reduce the chance of carbohydrate overload of the intestinal tract in enteritis accompanied by carbohydrate malabsorption.

[b] Also contain fructose.

from choleragenic diarrhea in which diarrheal losses of electrolytes are usually greater than in patients with noncholera diarrhea. Free water is usually administered along with the WHO rehydration formula to avoid occasional hypernatremia which results with the standard formula alone. A solution of 50 mEq/liter of sodium has been used successfully for rehydration of severely dehydrated children without free water supplementation (18). Others have stated that 30 to 40 mEq/liter is adequate for a majority of patients, i.e. those with mild to moderate noncholeragenic diarrhea who can be orally rehydrated and maintained (19). For home rehydration and maintenance when losses are mild, solutions of lower sodium content (30 to 60 mEq/liter) are adequate and safe, if not supplemented with free water. Patients who have acute, large volume losses may require higher sodium concentrations. Free water alone should always be avoided since this may result in hyponatremia. Although the standard practice is to withhold food until diarrhea begins to resolve, Santosham et al. (18) found that early food intake along with the rehydration solution had no effect on duration or severity of diarrheal illness. A more conservative approach is to administer soft foods (banana, rice cereal, applesauce, toast), breast milk, or half strength formula once resolution of diarrhea begins. Food or formula should then be advanced as tolerated.

Other Supportive Therapy

The value of antidiarrheal agents in treatment of infectious GE depends on the partic-

ular product, the infectious agent, and the age of the patient. Antidiarrheals such as tincture of opium, Immodium and diphenoxylate-atropine are considered to be safe and may reduce the frequency of stool in some types of acute, self-limited GE in adults and older children. However, some studies in children have challenged the effectiveness of diphenoxylate-atropine (21, 22). Diphenoxylate-atropine increased the duration of illness in patients with shigella GE in one study (23) and increased mortality in guinea pigs having salmonella intestinal infections in another (24). Based on this evidence, agents which slow gastrointestinal motility are not recommended for treatment of bacterial enteritis, in general. Decreasing peristaltic activity may be especially adverse if the pathogenesis of an infection is mucosal invasion, since this is probably dependent on bacterial contact time with the mucosa.

Diphenoxylate-atropine should be avoided in young children, particularly those less than 2 years of age (25). This age group may be more sensitive to the toxic effects of atropine in combination with diphenoxylate, and may experience atropinism with normal doses. There is concern that antispasmodics may actually mask fluid losses in young children by reducing peristalsis without decreasing fluid and electrolyte loss into the bowel (26). Documentation of these problems at normal doses is scanty. However, a conservative approach is recommended.

Kaolin-pectin suspension aids in the production of firmer stools, but does not reduce water loss (21). Thus, use of this preparation may lead to false sense of security. Various other nonprescription antidiarrheal agents are available, but have not been proven effective. Any expected benefits of such agents should be weighed against the risks.

There is some evidence, in vivo and in vitro, that the prostaglandin inhibitors, indomethacin and aspirin, reduce the sodium and fluid loss induced by enterotoxigenic microorganisms. In one clinical study, aspirin reduced fluid losses in children suffering from GE of unspecified infectious etiology (27). The appropriate place of prostaglandin inhibitors in the treatment of infectious GE requires further study, with special consideration given to potential adverse effects.

Bismuth subsalicylate has been shown to inhibit fluid secretion caused by E. coli and cholera toxin (28). The incidence of traveler's diarrhea can be reduced by prophylactic bismuth subsalicylate in the form of Pepto-Bismol, 60 ml 4 times per day. This regimen reduces the incidence of gastrointestinal symptoms and the excretion of infectious organisms in stool of persons who do become ill (29).

The use of Lactobacillus to recolonize the intestinal tract was not effective in preventing or altering diarrheal illness in experimentally induced ETEC diarrhea (30).

Antimicrobial Therapy

There is no effective cure available for viral GE. The use of antibiotics to treat bacterial GE depends on the infecting organism, the severity and chronicity of infection, and the effectiveness of antibiotics in reducing the severity of the illness as well as the carrier state. Since most of the bacterial enteritides are self-limiting, antibiotic therapy is usually not recommended unless the infection is severe, systemic or chronically symptomatic and debilitating.

Antimicrobial Resistance

An important factor in the prevalence of multiresistant strains is the indiscriminate use of antibiotics in humans and animals. The use of antibiotics is clearly related to development of plasmid-mediated resistance in microorganisms. Recently, multiple drug-resistant salmonella and shigella have been associated with epidemics in developing countries. One multiresistant strain of salmonella was associated with an epidemic which spread from Af-

rica to Europe and the Middle East (31). Multiple drug resistance has been found in developed countries as well. This could easily occur with any of the organisms known to cause GE. Thus, patients who receive antibiotic therapy for GE must be selected carefully. This precaution is necessary to help ensure the usefulness of presently available antibiotics in cases of true need. If a patient requires treatment, antibiotic susceptibilities of the isolated organism should be determined to assist in choosing the appropriate drug.

Antibiotics of Choice

Antibiotic treatment of shigellosis may reduce severity, duration of symptoms and carrier state to a slight extent (32). The disease is self-limited in otherwise normal patients, and routine treatment is controversial. However, the slight edge treatment provides may be of benefit to compromised patients, and to the very young and elderly, in whom dehydration occurs more rapidly. The shigella carrier state is rarely more than 3 to 4 weeks and hygienic measures can be as effective as antibiotic therapy in reducing the spread.

Ampicillin is considered to be the drug of choice for treatment of shigella, unless the organism is resistant. In one study, oral ampicillin was shown to be superior to amoxicillin in achieving a bacteriologic and clinical cure (33). The increased absorption of amoxicillin is not likely to be the explanation for the difference in effectiveness since parenteral therapy of shigella GE alone is effective. Greater susceptibilities of shigella to ampicillin in this study may explain the difference.

Many reports of ampicillin-resistant shigella exist. Trimethoprim-sulfamethoxazole (TMP-SMX) is usually an appropriate alternative for ampicillin-resistant organisms. In some institutions, it is considered the drug of choice since there are fewer resistant strains to this combination than to ampicillin. Due to widespread resistance, sulfonamides alone are unsuitable for treatment of shigella. Pickering et al. (34) have demonstrated the effectiveness of a single 2.5-g dose of tetracycline in adults with acute shigellosis. The trial was not placebo controlled and the results require confirmation before this can be routinely recommended. In addition, resistance to tetracycline is common. Tetracyclines should be avoided in children less than 12 years of age and in pregnant women during the second and third trimesters due to the potential staining of teeth which results from deposition of these drugs in teeth. There is also evidence that nalidixic acid 55 mg/kg/day, up to 1 g q6h for 5 days is effective for sensitive shigella (35). Chloramphenicol may be used if the situation precludes the use of ampicillin and TMP-SMX. Resistance to both TMP-SMX and chloramphenicol has been reported, although it is uncommon. Duration of therapy is 5 days. Dosage guidelines are provided in Table 8.4.

Table 8.4.
Antibiotics

Drug	Dose	Side Effects	Monitoring Parameters
Ampicillin	*Adults:* 500 mg q6h or 50–100 mg/kg/day *Children:* 50–200 mg/kg/day	*7.7% incidence* of rashes including a benign (nonhypersensitivity) macular, measles-like rash and a urticarial, hypersensitivity related rash *Diarrhea*, nausea, SGOT elevations reported after IM injection *1.6–8% incidence* of rashes, most probably due to SMX	*Skin changes:* macular rashes often; onset: 4–5 days into therapy *GI complaints:* difficult to establish drug-induced because of disease-related GI symptoms, but can monitor for changes in GI complaints or continued symptoms despite infection cure *Skin changes:* urticarial rashes
Trimethoprim (TMP)-Sulfamethoxazole (SMX); (cotrimoxazole)	*Adults:* TMP/SMX 160 mg/800 mg q12h *Children:* (>6 wks) TMP/SMX 5/25 mg/kg q12h Renal failure (severe): decrease by ½ to ⅔	*Megaloblastic* anemia rare but more common in pregnancy or in patients on anticonvulsants; reversible with folinic acid *Bone marrow* toxicity (leukopenia, anemia, thrombocytopenia) more common with high doses, if there are preexisting marrow abnormalities or in renal failure *Nausea* and diarrhea uncommon with recommended doses *SMX-induced* Stevens-Johnson syndrome and toxic epidermal necrolysis rarely *TMP safety* in pregnancy not established	*Megaloblastic anemia:* peripheral smear and/or RBC indices, periodically during long-term therapy, reversible with 60 μg folinic acid/day for 1–2 wk *Bone marrow toxicity:* CBC with platelets periodically
Chloramphenicol	*Adults:* 500 mg-1 g q.i.d.; doses above 4 g rarely needed *Children:* 6.25–25 mg/kg q.i.d.	*Nausea*, vomiting, diarrhea *Aplastic* anemia (hypersensitivity) *Bone marrow* depression (dose-related) *Gray syndrome*, unusual if serum levels 20 μg/ml or less *Optic neuritis* with prolonged courses, only partially reversible *Hypersensitivity* skin reactions are rare *Inhibits* metabolism of tolbutamide, phenytoin, dicumarol	*Bone marrow depression:* reticulocyte count, RBC count, hematocrit, platelets, leukocyte count *Gray syndrome:* vomiting, cyanosis, symptoms of circulatory failure; blood level data could help prevent *Aplastic anemia:* cannot be monitored for occurrence, consider when leukopenia or thrombocytopenia are present

The most common complications of ampicillin therapy are diarrhea and rashes (7 to 10% incidence). Drug-induced diarrhea may make assessment of response difficult and an alternative medication may be warranted in these cases. Rashes due to ampicillin may be of two types. The urticarial-type (hivelike) which is allergic in nature and requires discontinuing the drug. The maculopapular type (measles-like) is not allergic in nature and ampicillin may be continued without life-threatening sequelae. The maculopapular rash occurs in up to 90% of patients who have mononucleosis while taking ampicillin (36).

TMS is contraindicated in patients allergic to sulfonamides. Gastrointestinal upset may occur and the incidence of rashes is approximately 1%. Effects on the bone marrow are manifested as megaloblastic anemia, neutropenia and/or thrombocytopenia. These effects are uncommon, usually mild and reversible when the drug is discontinued (36). Red cell indices and white blood cell and platelet counts are useful monitoring parameters. Use of sulfonamides should be avoided in newborns, breast-feeding mothers, and pregnant women near term because of possible hyperbilirubinemia in the child due to displacement of bilirubin from protein (37). SMX may induce hemolysis in patients with G6PD deficiency. If intravenous therapy is required, TMP-SMX must be appropriately diluted to ensure stability. A concentration of 80 mg TMP/400 mg SMX per 75 ml may be used in a volume-restricted patient.

Chloramphenical may cause gastrointestinal upset. Rash or drug fever are uncommon. A dose-related bone marrow suppression commonly occurs if serum levels are greater than 25 μg/ml repeatedly or for prolonged periods. However, this can occur at lower levels as well. The first indication of dose-related bone marrow suppression is an increase in serum iron due to decreased iron utilization. A decrease in reticulocyte count follows as a result of vacuolation of erythroblasts. There is probably interference with the production and maturation of erythroid cells. Leukopenia and thrombocytopenia may also occur. Reticulocyte, hematocrit, red and white cell counts, and platelets are practical monitoring parameters. There is no information regarding the risk of dose-related bone marrow suppression leading to bone marrow aplasia (see below). Therefore, the practitioner must decide when to discontinue chloramphenicol based on treatment alternatives, the severity of the illness and the severity of the bone marrow suppression. If chloramphenical must be continued, one should consider dosage reduction. Dose-related bone marrow suppression is distinguished from aplastic anemia with pancytopenia, which is thought to be a hypersensitivity reaction. Although rare, it is often irreversible and difficult to monitor for occurrence. It may appear after 1 to 2 weeks of therapy, but there are many reports of the onset weeks to months after the end of treatment (36). In patients with severe liver disease and in infants less than 2 months of age who may have impaired clearance, chloramphenicol serum levels should be monitored.

Antibiotic treatment of salmonella GE has been shown to be of no benefit in reducing severity or duration of diarrhea, may increase the incidence of carriers as well as the relapse rate (38) and does not decrease the duration of the carrier state (39). However, chemotherapy is indicated for salmonella bacteremia, salmonellosis and chronic biliary carriers. Because reports of resistance of salmonella to ampicillin and chloramphenicol have been increasing, sensitivity testing should be done if possible. Chloramphenicol is preferable to ampicillin if sensitivities are unavailable since there is more resistance to ampicillin.

More controlled studies are needed to evaluate the role of antibiotics in the treatment of acute enteric infections with E. coli. Many strains of ETEC are resistant to ampicillin and tetracycline (40). TMP-SMX and TMP alone decreased the severity and duration of illness significantly more than placebo in one study. However, more resistant strains developed in patients treated with TMP alone and relapse occurred in two of these cases (40). Chronic E. coli GE causing malnutrition and failure to thrive may be treated with a nonabsorbable antibiotic such as kanamycin (50 mg/kg/day divided q6h up to 8 g/day). Since kanamycin is poorly absorbed from the gastrointestinal tract, side effects are minimal. In patients who have renal impairment and receive the drug for a prolonged period, an occasional serum level may be warranted to determine serum accumulation.

Propylaxis of traveler's diarrhea with antimicrobial agents has been shown to be effective (29, 41, 42) and may be more convenient than transporting the necessary volume of

Pepto-Bismol (see "Other Supportive Therapy"). Doxycycline (100 mg daily) and TMP-SMX are effective and practical prophylactic regimens (41, 42). Dosage of TMP-SMX is listed in Table 8.4. These regimens have been tested only during the first 3 weeks of residence in foreign countries. Prolonged efficacy and the potential for development of resistance after this time have not been studied. It is important to inform the patient that continued protection requires continued antibiotic therapy. TMP-SMX may be preferable to doxycycline because susceptibility of organisms to doxycycline is variable in different parts of the world. For example, salmonella and shigella may be resistant to doxycycline, whereas TMP-SMX is active against most isolates. The same precautions and side effects as for tetracycline apply to doxycycline. Photosensitization, leading to sunburn is probably the most significant for travelers. Although rashes can occur with TMP-SMX, photosensitization is not a problem. The most effective way of preventing traveler's diarrhea is to avoid food and water which may be contaminated.

Anecdotal reports have suggested that antibiotic treatment of campylobacter resulted in rapid resolution of symptoms and fewer relapses. However, one unpublished double-blind, controlled clinical trial failed to show an advantage of treatment with erythromycin over placebo (9). Until further information is available, routine antibiotic therapy is not recommended for campylobacter GE.

Yersinia GE is usually mild and self-limiting, requiring no treatment. Prospective studies in patients with chronic or systemic infection have not been reported.

References

1. Walsh JA, Warren KS: Selective primary health care: an interim strategy for disease control in developing countries. *N Engl J Med* 301:967–974, 1979.
2. Wolf JL, Schreiber DS: Viral gastroenteritis. *Med Clin North Am* 66:575–595, 1982.
3. Mandell GL, Douglas RG, Bennett JE: *Principles and Practice of Infectious Diseases.* New York: John Wiley & Sons, 1979, vol I, ch 70–74.
4. Tedesco FJ: Pseudomembranous colitis: pathogenesis and therapy. *Med Clin North Am* 66:655–664, 1982.
5. Nye FJ: Traveler's diarrhea. *Clin Gastroenterol* 8:767–781, 1979.
6. Pickering LK, Evans DG, DuPont HL, et al: Diarrhea caused by Shigella, rotavirus and Giardia in day-care centers: prospective study. *J Pediatr* 99:51–56, 1981.
7. Anon: Shgellosis—United States 1980. *MMWR* 30:462–463, 1981.
8. Bauer H: The growing problem of salmonellosis in modern society. *Medicine (Balt)* 52:323–330, 1973.
9. Blaser MJ, Reller LB: Campylobacter enteritis. *N Engl J Med* 305:1444–1452, 1981.
10. Lopez CE, Jackson D: Campylobacter enteritis. *J Med Assoc Ga* 69:597–600, 1980.
11. Mosenthal AC, Mones RL, Bokkenheuser VD: *Campylobacter fetus jejuni* enteritis. *NY S J Med* 321–323, 1981.
12. Rowe B: The role of *Escherichia coli* in gastroenteritis. *Clin Gastroenterol* 8:625–644, 1979.
13. Vantrappen G, Geboes K, Ponette E: Yersinia enteritis. *Med Clin North Am* 66:639–653, 1982.
14. Carpenter, CCJ: Pathogenesis of secretory diarrheas. *Med Clin North Am* 66:597–610, 1982.
15. Giannella RA: Pathogenesis of acute bacterial diarrheal disorders. *Ann Rev Med* 32:341–357, 1981.
16. Rachmilewitz D: Prostaglandins and diarrhea. *Dig Dis Sci* 25:897–898, 1980.
17. Black RE, Merson MH, Taylor PR, et al: Glucose vs sucrose in oral rehydration solutions for infants and young children with rotavirus-associated diarrhea. *Pediatrics* 67:79–83, 1981.
18. Santosham M, Daum R, Dillman L, et al: Oral rehydration therapy of infantile diarrhea. *N Engl J Med* 306:1070–1076, 1982.
19. Nichols BL, Soriano HA: A critique of oral therapy of dehydration due to diarrheal syndromes. *Am J Clin Nutr* 30:1457–1472, 1977.
20. Hirschhorn N, Kinzie J, Sachar D, et al: Decrease in net stool output in cholera during intestinal perfusion with glucose-containing solutions. *N Engl J Med* 279:176–181, 1968.
21. Portnog BL, DuPont HL, Pruitt D, et al: Antidiarrheal agents in the treatment of acute diarrhea in children. *JAMA* 236:844–846, 1976.
22. Harris MJ, Beveridge J: Diphenoxylate in the treatment of acute gastroenteritis in children. *Med J Aust* 921–922, 1965.
23. DuPont HL, Hornick RB: Adverse effect of lomotil therapy in shigellosis. *JAMA* 226:1525–1528, 1973.
24. Kent TH, Formal SB, LaBree EH: Acute enteritis due to *Salmonella typhimurium* in opium treated guinea pigs. *Arch Pathol* 81:50, 1966.
25. Rosenstein G, Freeman M, Standard AL, et al: Warning: the use of Lomotil in children. *Pediatrics* 51:132–133, 1973.
26. Anon: Lomotil. *Med Lett* 11:46, 1969.
27. Suharyono VB, Sunato MG: Reduction by aspirin of intestinal fluid loss in acute childhood gastroenteritis. *Lancet* 1:1329–1330, 1980.
28. Ericsson DC, Evans DG, DuPont HL, et al: Bismuth subsalicylate inhibits activity of crude toxins of *Escherichia coli* and *Vibrio cholerae*. *J Infect Dis* 136:693–696, 1977.
29. DuPont HL, Sullivan P, Evans DG: Prevention of traveler's diarrhea (emporiatic enteritis). *JAMA* 243:237–241, 1980.
30. Clements ML, Levine MM, Black RE, et al: *Lactobacillus* prophylaxis for diarrhea due to enterotoxigenic *E. coli*. *Antimicrob Agents Chemother* 2:104–108, 1981.

31. WHO Scientific Working Group: Enteric infections due to campylobacter, yersinia, salmonella and shigella. *Bull WHO* 58:519–537, 1980.

32. Haltalin KC, Nelson JD, Ring R III, et al: Double-blind treatment study of shigellosis comparing ampicillin, sulfadiazine and placebo. *J Pediatr* 70:970–981, 1967.

33. Nelson JD, Haltalin KC: Amoxicillin less effective than ampicillin against shigella *in vitro* and *in vivo*: relationship of efficacy to activity in serum. *J Infect Dis* 129:5222–5227, 1974.

34. Pickering LK, DuPont HL, Olarte J: Single dose tetracycline therapy for shigellosis in adults. *JAMA* 239:853–854, 1978.

35. Haltalin KC, Nelson JD, Kusmiesz HT: Comparative efficacy of nalidixic acid and ampicillin for severe shigellosis. *Arch Dis Child* 48:305–312, 1973.

36. Kucers A, Bennet NM: *The Use of Antibiotics*, ed 3. Philadelphia: J. B. Lippincott, 1979.

37. Pagliaro LA, Levin RH: *Problems in Pediatric Drug Therapy.* Hamilton, Ill.: Drug Intelligence Publications, 1979.

38. Nelson JD, Kusmiesz H, Jackson LH, et al: Treatment of salmonella gastroenteritis with ampicillin, amoxicillin or placebo. *Pediatrics* 65:1125–1130, 1980.

39. Smith ER, Badley BWD: Treatment of salmonella enteritis and its effect on carrier state. *Can Med Assoc J* 104:1004, 1971.

40. Black RE, Levine MM, Clements ML, et al: Treatment of experimentally induced enterotoxigenic *Escherichia coli* diarrhea with trimethoprim, trimethoprim-sulfamethoxazole and placebo. *Rev Infect Dis* 4:540–545, 1982.

41. Sack DA, Kaminsky DC, Sack RB: Prophylactic doxycycline for traveler's diarrhea. *N Engl J Med* 298:758–763, 1978.

42. DuPont HL, Evands DG, Rios N: Prevention of traveler's diarrhea with trimethoprim-sulfamethoxazole. *Rev Infect Dis* 4:33–39, 1982.

43. Clibon U, Enteric infections. In Herfindal ET, Hirschman JL: *Clinical Pharmacy and Therapeutics*, ed 2. Baltimore, Williams & Wilkins, 1979, p 163.

CHAPTER 9

Central Nervous System Infections

DONALD P. ALEXANDER, Pharm.D.
STEVEN L. BARRIERE, Pharm.D.

Meningitis is generally defined as an inflammation of the membranes of the brain or spinal cord (meninges). This is distinguished from encephalitis, which is inflammation of the brain tissue itself. This discussion will be limited to inflammation caused by infectious agents (bacteria, fungi and viruses). In addition, the pathogenesis and management of brain abscess will be discussed. Cerebrospinal fluid (CSF) shunt infection and subdural empyema will not considered. For an excellent discussion of these topics, the reader is referred to two recent reviews (1, 2). Further general reviews on meningitis and brain abscess are available and should also be consulted (3–7).

ETIOLOGY

The most commonly encountered organisms producing meningitis and brain abscess are listed in Table 9.1. It should be noted that they are listed in an approximate order of frequency of occurrence, and that the categories are divided into age-related and history-related incidence. Neonatal meningitis is most commonly caused by group B streptococci, *Escherichia coli* and *Listeria monocytogenes* (8–10). Other Gram-negative organisms known to cause neonatal meningitis include *Proteus* species, *Klebsiella-Enterobacter*, and *Pseudomonas*. Staphylococci and *Streptococcus pneumoniae* together account for about 10% of the cases. Infection with *Mycobacterium tuberculosis* is dealt with in Chapter 11, "Tuberculosis."

Haemophilus influenzae type B, *Neisseria meningitidis*, and S. *pneumoniae* are the organisms responsible for 95% of cases of meningitis in children over 2 months of age (6). *H. influenzae* is usually the most significant pathogen between the ages of 2 months and 4 to 5 years of age. After 4 to 5 years of age the incidence of *H. influenzae* meningitis decreases and *N. meningitidis* (meningococcus),

and S. *pneumoniae* (pneumococcus), become the significant pathogens which cause meningitis (8).

In adults, *N. meningitidis* and S. *pneumoniae* are the major pathogens which cause meningitis (4, 8). In adults under 40 years of age and without a prior history of trauma, the meningococcus is more frequently reported than the pneumococcus as a cause of meningitis. After 40 years of age, the pneumococcus is the most frequent cause of meningitis. Staphylococci are infrequent causes of acute spontaneous meningitis in this age group.

In adults greater than 60 years of age the incidence of meningitis caused by Gram-negative bacilli and *Listeria* again begins to increase, but the pneumococcus remains a significant pathogen (4, 8, 11).

Meningitis following trauma is caused by a variety of bacteria. Most commonly the pneumococcus in closed skull fracture and Enterobacteriaceae or staphylococci in penetrating injuries (12, 13). Postsurgical meningitis nearly always follows procedures performed directly on the CNS. The most commonly encountered bacteria in this setting are Gram-negative bacilli: *Klebsiella*, *Enterobacter*, *E. coli*, *Serratia*, and *Pseudomonas*. Staphylococci are occasionally causative agents (14).

Fungal meningitis may be roughly divided into two groups for etiologic purposes: (a) disease in a "normal" (nonimmunocompromised) host and, (b) infection in the immunocompromised patient. Fungal CNS infection in otherwise normal patients is most often seen in disseminated coccidioidomycosis, and in infection with *Cryptococcus neoformans*. Fungal meningitis in the compromised host is primarily due to *C. neoformans*, *Candida* sp., and *Aspergillus* sp. However, there is a good deal of overlap between these two groups.

Viral infections of the central nervous system are quite common. Most cases are self-limited and mild to moderate in severity. We

Table 9.1.
Common Pathogens in CNS Infections[a]

Bacterial Meningitis	
Premature infants and neonates (up to 2 mo)	*Escherichia coli* Group B streptococci Other Enterobacteriaceae *Listeria monocytogenes* *Streptococcus pneumoniae* *Streptococcus faecalis*
Infants and children (2 mo to 10 yr)	*Haemophilus influenzae* *Neisseria meningitidis* *S. pneumoniae*
Adults	*N. meningitidis* *S. pneumoniae* Staphylococci
Associated with trauma or surgery	*Staphylococcus aureus* *S. pneumoniae* Enterobacteriaceae

Fungal Meningitis	
"Normal" host	*Coccidioides immitis* *Cryptococcus neoformans*
Immunocompromised host	*C. neoformans* *Candida albicans* *Aspergillus* sp.

Viral Meningoencephalitis[b]	
Neonates Immunocompromised host	Herpes simplex Herpes zoster

Brain Abscess	
General	Streptococci Mixed anaerobes Enterobacteriaceae
Associated with trauma or surgery	*S. aureus* Mixed anaerobes Enterobacteriaceae
Immunocompromised host	*Nocardia asteroides*

[a] In approximate order of frequency.
[b] Many viruses can produce "aseptic" meningitis, but herpesvirus is listed here as the only *treatable cause.*

shall limit our discussion to severe viral meningoencephalitis, caused by herpes simplex virus, in the neonate and the immunocompromised host (15).

The causative agents of brain abscess are many and varied, and most individual abscesses are polymicrobial. Aerobic and anaerobic streptococci, and anaerobic Gram-negative bacilli are the most common causes of abscess in patients without a history of trauma or surgery. The latter history predisposes to infection with staphylococci, aerobic Gram-negative bacilli, and streptococci. *Nocardia as-*

teroides may produce brain abscess as a manifestation of disseminated infection.

INCIDENCE

The overall incidence of bacterial meningitis has remained approximately the same for decades, affecting approximately 2.7 persons per 100,000 population (8). This figure does not reflect the age-related disparity in incidence: 0.04% of cases occur in neonates (1 case per 2500 live births), 15% occur under 1 to 2 months of age, 20 to 25% between ages 2 to 12 months, and 40% in children and adolescents 1 to 15 years of age. This disease is, therefore, mostly a pediatric problem. There is no racial predilection and only a slightly greater prevalence of males over females.

Recently, it has been estimated that between 6 and 9% of all cases of acute bacterial meningitis are acquired in the hospital (13).

PATHOGENESIS

Meningitis is most common in the very very young and elderly population. In the neonate the host defenses against infection are not well developed and deficiencies exist in leukocyte and complement system functions. Immunoglobulin deficiency of IgA and IgM may also be present at birth and result from the lack of placental transfer from the mother (6). Lower levels of immunoglobulins and slightly depressed leukocyte function in the elderly contributes to a decreased resistance to infection. Splenectomy, diabetes mellitus, and alcoholism also increase the risk of infection because of defective leukocyte function. Individuals with altered cellular immunity from severe underlying disease or immunosuppressive therapy are also at higher risk for developing meningitis.

Most cases of meningitis in children, less than 4 years of age, are caused by encapsulated microorganisms. The presence of this capsule protects the bacteria from neutrophil phagocytosis and may enhance the bacteria's penetration into the CSF. The role of bacterial endotoxin, produced by many Gram-negative organisms, is uncertain but may result in damage to the CSF barrier thus allowing entry of bacteria into the CSF.

Bacteria may reach the CSF by the hematogenous route, spread from contiguous tissues or by direct implantation. Bacteremia, resulting from a distant site of infection appears to be an important predisposing factor for the establishment of infection. Bacteria may also reach the CSF by spread from contiguous tissues. Otitis media, sinusitis, dental infections and mastoiditis are known to be predisposing conditions in meningitis. It is probably the combination of these two processes that result in bacterial entry into the CSF. Direct implantation of bacteria by trauma or neurosurgical procedures represents only a small percentage of the cases of meningitis.

Brain abscess, not induced by trauma or surgery, is usually the result of hematogenous seeding.

DIAGNOSIS AND CLINICAL FEATURES

The clinical course of meningitis may be acute or subacute depending on whether the signs and symptoms have been present for less than or greater than 24 hours. In the acute presentation (approximately 10% of cases) the signs and symptoms are usually present for less than 24 hours and are rapidly progressive. The etiology is usually bacterial in nature; S. pneumoniae or N. meningitidis are most common (prognosis is inversely related to the length of time from the onset of symptoms until presentation for medical care). In the subacute presentation (approximately 75% of cases) the signs and symptoms are present for 1 to 7 days before evaluation and may be caused by a number of different agents (viruses, fungi, bacteria).

Signs and symptoms are usually nonspecific and may vary in different age groups. In neonates and infants the symptoms are often absent or very nonspecific. The most common clinical findings are lethargy, irritability, poor feeding, respiratory distress, cyanosis or hypothermia. Because these findings are nonspecific the infection may go unrecognized until irreversible brain damage has occurred. It is therefore important to identify recognized risk factors to the development of meningitis in

this age group; prolonged labor, premature rupture of fetal membranes, peripartum maternal infection, or any neonatal or infant infection.

In infants greater than 1 year of age, older children and adults symptoms are more indicative of meningitis inflammation. Fever and altered mental status are the most common findings. Other symptoms include nausea, vomiting, headache, and photophobia and may reflect increased intracranial pressure or cerebral inflammation. Neurologic signs may vary and convulsions or coma occur in approximately one third of patients. Nuchal rigidity is a classical finding which results from meningeal inflammation. Helpful clues include Brudzinski's sign (neck flexion producing knee and hip flexion) or Kernig's sign (pain and difficulty in raising the extended leg).

The clinical presentation of patients with brain abscess is usually headache and an altered state of consciousness which may vary from lethargy, irritability and confusion to coma. Focal neurologic signs maybe due to an expanding intracranial mass and, depending on the location in the brain, the presentation may vary from indolent to rapidly progressive.

The clinical presentation does not permit the etiologic agent causing meningeal inflammation to be determined. A careful history and physical examination should be performed. If a mass lesion is not a concern, a lumbar puncture should be performed to obtain information which includes: CSF pressure and appearance, cell count and differential, sugar, protein, CSF Gram stain and culture. Table 9.2 lists the common parameters of the CSF that are altered in various forms of meningitis. It must be emphasized that these are only general principles and the use of the numbers in this table can not be absolute (for example, the CSF white blood cell count may be less than 500 in bacterial meningitis, or may not be predominantly polymorphonu-

Table 9.2.
Cerebrospinal Fluid (CSF) Findings in Meningitis

	Appearance	WBC	Type[a]	Protein	Glucose Ratio CSF/Serum
Bacterial	Turbid	>500	PMN	Elevated	<50%
Fungal	Clear	10–500	MN	Elevated	Variable
Viral	Clear	10–500	MN	Normal or elevated	>50%

[a] PMN, polymorphonuclear; MN, mononuclear.

clear (PMN), or the glucose CSF/serum ratio may be normal).

A repeat lumbar puncture within 12 to 72 hours may be helpful in circumstances where patients with symptoms of meningeal inflammation have normal CSF parameters, or to distinguish bacterial from aseptic (viral) meningitis. Early viral infection may show a predominantly neutrophilic white blood cell count that will soon change to mononuclear cells (16).

The clinical presentation and CSF findings may be consistent with meningitis but the diagnosis is confirmed by laboratory culture of the causative agent. However, the CSF culture may not always be positive. One explanation for this finding in bacterial meningitis is the use of antibiotics prior to the lumbar puncture. It has been estimated that approximately 50% of all children with bacterial meningitis under the age of 5 years receive some form of antibiotic therapy prior to the lumbar puncture (17). This practice does not significantly alter the CSF findings in Table 9.2, but will frequently lead to negative Gram stain and culture results.

Standard laboratory analysis of the CSF does not always provide definitive information regarding the presence or absence of meningitis or nature of the causative agent. A few additional laboratory tests may be helpful in the differentiation of bacterial meningitis, especially when the CSF culture and Gram stain are negative. These include: (a) CSF lactate concentration may be of value to differentiate bacterial from viral meningitis, (b) limulus lysate assay may detect the presence of Gram-negative endotoxin, (c) counterimmunoelectrophoresis (CIE), latex agglutination, and enzyme-linked immunosorbent assay (ELISA) may detect minute quantities of bacterial antigen (18).

Fungi are occasionally cultured from the CSF. The detection of fungal antigen (e.g. cryptococcal) or antibody (e.g. coccidiodomycosis) in the CSF is often essential to the diagnosis of these causative agents.

Herpesvirus encephalitis usually presents with diffuse neurologic findings and nonspecific CSF findings which usually requires brain biopsy for diagnosis.

The diagnosis of brain abscess is complicated by a number of factors. Routine laboratory tests are usually not helpful (e.g. 20 to 40% of patients have normal white blood cell counts).

A lumbar puncture is occasionally mildly abnormal and nonspecific. Gram stain and culture of the CSF are usually negative unless the abscess has ruptured into the subarachnoid space or ventricles. Lumbar puncture is contraindicated in the presence of increased intracranial pressure or if a mass lesion is suspected. Computerized axial tomography (CAT scan), brain scan, arteriogram or pneumoencephalogram are diagnostic aids used to detect brain abscesses.

COMPLICATIONS

The complications of bacterial meningitis include brain abscess, lateral sinus thrombosis, cerebral thrombophlebitis, and subdural empyema. Generalized or focal convulsions may occur as well as septic shock, and disseminated intravascular coagulation, especially in meningococcemia. Cerebral edema results from leukocytic and toxic factors, blood vessel thrombosis and encephalitis. This may lead to an elevated CSF pressure resulting in cortical necrosis and brain infarction progressing to herniation and eventually death.

Neurological sequelae such as mental retardation, hydrocephalus, permanent seizure disorders, paresis, ataxia, deafness, psychosis, and blindness occur frequently as a result of neonatal and childhood meningitis. Generally infections with H. influenza and the pneumococcus carry the poorest prognosis with respect to neurological sequelae (approximately 25 to 50%) (6, 19). It is felt that the degree of neurological sequelae may be related to the size of the bacterial inoculum or antigen load in the CSF which causes the intense inflammatory response.

The results of treatment of herpes simplex encephalitis with adenine arabinoside have shown that neurological sequelae will be present in approximately 50% of survivors (20).

Approximately one third of patients with brain abscess will have some residual neurologic disability.

TREATMENT

The effective treatment of central nervous system (CNS) infections is largely dependent upon: (a) attaining and maintaining adequate antibiotic concentrations in the CSF or brain extracellular fluid (ECF), (b) the microbiological activity of the antibiotic while in the CNS, and (c) effective management of the complications resulting from the infection.

The blood, CSF and brain comprise three different compartments which intercommunicate and maintain the homeostasis of the CNS (21). These three compartments are separated functionally and anatomically by three barriers; the blood-brain extracellular fluid barrier the blood-CSF barrier and the CSF-brain extracellular fluid barrier. Traditionally what is recognized as the blood-brain barrier (BBB) can be functionally and anatomically explained as two separate barriers (the blood-brain ECF barrier and the blood-CSF barrier). Physiologically both of these barriers contain capillaries whose cellular wall structure is different from capillaries elsewhere in the body in that the junctions between the cells are "tight." Functionally these barriers require substances to pass through the cellular wall rather than between the cells. Because of this requirement, the physical properties of each antibiotic determine how well it passess from the blood into the brain extracellular fluid or CSF. Once the antibiotic has gained access to the brain ECF or CSF, equilibration between these compartments occurs relatively quickly.

The physical properties of a drug will govern its penetration into the CNS and include: (a) the relative affinity to lipid or water (degree of ionization and the relative lipid solubility of the unionized form), (b) the relative affinity for serum plasma proteins (only the free fraction would be expected to penetrate the CNS barrier), and (c) carrier mediated transport (usually insignificant for antibiotics). The degree of ionization of a drug is dependent upon its characteristics at plasma pH. The ionized form of the drug has increased affinity to plasma water and it is the unionized form which is available to cross cellular membranes. The lipid solubility of the unionized form of the drug is determined by the relative affinity of that drug to lipid or water. Therefore, for a drug to readily penetrate into the CNS, three properties are important: low ionization at plasma pH, higher affinity for lipid than water, and low protein binding (22) (Table 9.3).

The failure of many drugs to reach detectable levels in the CSF, despite their ability to penetrate the barriers, is due to the rapid clearance of the drug from the CSF. Most drugs are removed by bulk flow through the arachnoid villi. The high turnover rate of the CSF prevents accumulation of these drugs in the CNS. Active transport of various organic acids and

Table 9.3.

Cerebrospinal Fluid (CSF) Penetration of Various Antibiotics during Meningitis

Adequate CSF Penetration with Systemic Therapy Alone	
Penicillin G	Ticarcillin
Ampicillin/Amoxicillin	Chloramphenicol
Methicillin/Nafcillin	Cefoxitin[a]
Mezlocillin/Piperacillin	Sulfonamides
Cefotaxime/Moxalactam	Trimethoprim
Isoniazid	Flucytosine
Rifampin	Metronidazole

Limited CSF Penetration and/or Requiring CSF Instillation	
Carbenicillin (40 mg)[b]	Polymixin B[d] (2.5–5
Vancomycin (20 mg)	mg)
Amphotericin B (0.25–0.5	Ketoconazole[d]
mg)[c]	(oral)
Miconazole (20 mg)	Clindamycin[d]
Streptomycin (20–40 mg)	Cephalothin/Ceph-
Gentamicin/Tobramycin	aloridine[d]
(4–8 mg)	Cefazolin/Cefa-
Kanamycin/Amikacin	mandole[d]
(10–20 mg)	Tetracyclines[d]
	Erythromycin[d] (3–
	10 mg)

[a] Usually administered with probenicid 500 mg every 6 to 8 hours.
[b] Usual daily intrathecal or intraventricular dose.
[c] Diluted with CSF and given intrathecally (lumbar or intraventricular) or use in a hyperbaric solution of 10% dextrose given intralumbar.
[d] Limited use because of poor penetration or lack of bactericidal activity.

bases has also been demonstrated. This mechanism is felt to be similar to the secretory action which occurs in the kidney. Many penicillins and cephalosporins have been shown to have some degree of tubular secretion which contributes to their elimination. Probenicid has been shown to decrease the renal excretion of these antibiotics as well as the elimination of these antibiotics from the CSF resulting in higher measured levels.

There are conditions (infection, tumors, chemicals, etc.) which impair these normal physiologic mechanisms and increase the BBB permeability. Many drugs do not penetrate into the CSF with normal intact meninges, but do readily cross when the meninges are inflamed. This is true for most antibiotics. For example, penicillin is not detectable in the CSF of animals or humans with normal meninges. It is important to note that in meningitis both the CSF barrier and clearance mechanisms are usually altered. As the meningitis resolves, the permeability to drugs is reduced and the clearance mechanisms begin to work more efficiently.

Once the antibiotic penetrates into the CSF it must be microbiologically active. A better understanding of the CSF environment and in vitro susceptibility testing should provide information to make a more rational selection of an antibiotic.

Infections of the CSF occur in an area of impaired host resistance. Normal CSF contains only low concentrations of immunoglobulins. Low levels of CSF complement has been found in patients with meningitis together with reduced bactericidal and opsonic activity (23). Additionally, an intact BBB impedes the entrance of peripheral white blood cells to the site of infection. Therefore, antibiotics which actually kill the organism (bactericidal) rather than just inhibit their growth (bacteriostatic) are required.

Treatment of meningitis with antibiotics which achieve CSF concentrations that are similar to or just exceed the minimum inhibitory concentration (MIC) of the organism often result in bacteriologic failures (24, 25). It is suggested that the peak drug concentrations in the CSF should exceed the minimum bactericidal concentrations (MBC) by several fold to produce bacterial killing. However, the size of the bacterial inoculum, the use of broth instead of CSF as the growth media for susceptibility testing and the altered pH of the CSF may markedly influence the in vitro activity of these antibiotics. The aminoglycosides are an excellent example. The bactericidal activity of the aminoglycosides decreases when the pH decreases. The MBC of E. coli for gentamicin at a pH of 7.35 is 1 μg/ml and increases to 8 μg/ml when the pH is changed to 7.0 (as may occur in meningitis). Recent experience suggests that concentrations 10 to 30 times the MBC are necessary to achieve bacterial killing in vivo (31). This may be impossible with aminoglycosides because of the narrow therapeutic-toxic ratio. Also, the use of antibiotic concentrations far above what may be attained in the CSF, to determine the microorganism's in vitro susceptibility, may be misleading.

The need for prompt antimicrobial therapy is emphasized by the high incidence of mortality within hours in patients with an acute presentation of meningitis. In this situation, it is not appropriate to wait for culture results to initiate therapy. After the patient history, physical examination and specimens for the appropriate laboratory tests are collected, the patient should be started on intravenous antibiotics. The choice of empiric therapy should be based upon the patient's age, history and any specific underlying disease; and tailored further by the results of the CSF Gram stain. Once the culture results are known and the antimicrobial sensitivities have been performed, more specific antibiotic therapy can be initiated (Table 9.4). It is important that full doses of antibiotics be administered for the entire course of therapy. As the patient responds, meningeal inflammation will decrease and result in decreased antibiotic penetration into the CSF. Reduction in antibiotic dose as the patient responds has been correlated with relapse of the infection.

A repeat lumbar puncture is usually performed at 24 to 48 hours after beginning therapy to monitor the clinical and bacteriologic response of the patient. CSF Gram stain and culture should be negative for bacteria. Occasionally Gram stains and cultures remain positive. If so, a parameningeal focus should be investigated. In enteric Gram-negative bacillary meningitis, Gram stain and culture may remain positive for several days. Persistence of Gram-negative bacteria in the CSF is often associated with ventriculitis.

The optimal duration of therapy for meningitis is not known, but should be a minimum of 2 weeks of systemic antibiotics. More serious cases and Gram-negative bacillary meningitis may require 3 or more weeks of therapy. Treatment of fungal meningitis may require long-term therapy (3 to 6 months or longer). The duration of treatment for brain abscess is usually 4 to 6 weeks of systemic antibiotic therapy after surgical drainage of the abscess.

Neonatal Meningitis

The antibiotics of choice for E. coli meningitis have traditionally been ampicillin plus an aminoglycoside in the doses listed in Table 9.4 for a minimum of 14 days. The use of intraventricular aminoglycoside is controversial. The newer cephalosporins, cefotaxime and moxalactam, have been very effective in treating this form of meningitis. Both drugs penetrate into the CNS and have exceptional activity against this organism. The use of these newer agents could provide effective therapy

Table 9.4.
Empiric Antibiotic Therapy in CNS Infection

Neonates (up to 2 mo old)	Ampicillin plus	100–200 mg/kg/day (every 8–12 hr)	Intravenous
	Aminoglycoside[a,b] or	5–7 mg/kg/day 1 mg/day (intraventricular preferred)	Intravenous Intrathecal
	Moxalactam or Cefotaxime	100–150 mg/kg/day (max. q8h) (q4–6h)	Intravenous
Infants and children (2 mo to 10 yr)	Ampicillin and Chloramphenicol[c] or	200–300 mg/kg/day 50–100 mg/kg/day	Intravenous
	Moxalactam[d] or Cefotaxime	150–200 mg/kg/day	Intravenous
Adolescents and adults (≥10 yr)	Penicillin G	200–300,000 units/kg/day every 2–4 hr	Intravenous
Associated with trauma or surgery (any age)	Penicillin G plus	200–300,000 units/kg/day (every 2–4 hr)	Intravenous
	Nafcillin plus	150 mg/kg/day (every 4 hr) Neonates (up to 14 days)	Intravenous
	Aminoglycoside[a]	20 mg/kg/day (every 8–12 hr) 5–6 mg/kg/day	Intravenous
	or	plus 4–8 mg (intraventricular preferred)	Intrathecal
	Moxalactam or Cefotaxime	150–200 mg/kg/day	Intravenous
	Penicillin allergy: Vancomycin	20–30 mg/kg/day (2 g max./day) 20 mg intrathecal (intraventricular preferred)	Intravenous

[a] Gentamicin/tobramycin/amikacin (amikacin: 15 mg/kg/day every 12 hours for infants <7 days, 22.5 mg/kg/day for older children).
[b] If enterococci are cultured use gentamicin.
[c] Intravenous or oral.
[d] If found susceptible.

without requiring multiple intrathecal or intraventricular injections of aminoglycoside. The doses most commonly used are listed in Table 9.4.

Group B streptococci are usually less sensitive to penicillin than other streptococci, therefore penicillin G must be given in doses of 200,000 to 250,000 units/kg/day in divided doses every 8 to 12 hours for 14 days. Ampicillin may be substituted for penicillin G even though the organism is slightly less susceptible. Of the newer agents, only cefotaxime possesses good activity against group B streptococci. Moxalactam is not very active against most Gram-positive organisms, including group B streptococci, and should not be considered for the treatment of this form of men-

ingitis. Empiric therapy with a combination of penicillin or ampicillin plus cefotaxime or moxalactam would provide adequate coverage for meningitis caused by these two organisms. In the penicillin-allergic patient with documented group B streptococcal meningitis, chloramphenicol may be used as an alternative antibiotic.

Meningitis caused by other Enterobacteriaceae such as *Proteus* species and the *Klebsiella-Enterobacter-Serratia* group have usually required the use of an aminoglycoside both systemically and intrathecally. If these organisms are sensitive to the newer cephalosporins, these antibiotics may be the best alternative to treat this serious form of meningitis. For more resistant organisms, such as *Serratia mar-*

cescens and *Pseudomonas aeruginosa*, an aminoglycoside alone or in combination with a penicillin (ticarcillin, piperacillin, or mezlocillin) or a newer cephalosporin should be used depending upon the sensitivities of the pathogen. Amikacin may be required and should be dosed at 15 mg/kg/day for infants less than 7 days of age, and 22.5 mg/kg/day for older infants. If intrathecal or intraventricular administration of aminoglycosides is required, doses are listed in Table 9.4. Therapy should continue for a minimum of 2 weeks, preferably 3 weeks or longer.

Appropriate therapy for *Listeria* meningitis is ampicillin or penicillin intravenously for 14 days. The addition of an aminoglycoside to the regimen depends upon the clinical response of the patient. In the penicillin-allergic patient, trimethoprim/sulfamethoxazole should be used. A dose of 10 mg/kg/day of trimethoprim in the fixed combination should be effective.

Childhood and Adult Meningitis

H. influenzae is the most common cause of childhood meningitis. Because of the incidence of ampicillin-resistant organisms, both ampicillin and chloramphenicol should be initiated pending sensitivites of the organism. Once these sensitivities are known, definitive therapy can be continued and one of the antibiotics discontinued. Therapy should be continued for a minimum of 14 days. Chloramphenicol should never be given by intramuscular injection because of poor absorption. Oral absorption produces excellent serum concentrations and may be considered after the initial few days of intravenous therapy. Ampicillin is well absorbed from intramuscular injection sites and satisfactory clinical results have been demonstrated (26). In the penicillin-allergic patient, chloramphenicol is generally the accepted alternative agent. Another effective alternative would be the combination of intravenous sulfisoxazole with intramuscular or intravenous streptomycin plus intrathecal streptomycin for 14 days (27). The newer cephalosporins have excellent activity against *H. influenzae* and may also be considered as an alternative.

Meningitis due to *S. pneumoniae* or *N. meningitidis* should be treated with intravenous penicillin G. Doses are listed in Table 9.4. Treatment should be given for 10 to 14 days. In the penicillin-allergic patient, chloramphenicol is a useful alternative. Neither of the newer cephalosporins offer any advantage over penicillin. Because of the poor Gram-positive activity of moxalactam, it should not be considered for therapy of pneumococcal meningitis.

Staphylococcal meningitis is nearly always caused by *S. aureus*; and, therefore, seldom responds to penicillin G, as most strains are resistant. The therapy of choice is a penicillinase-resistant penicillin. Our choice is nafcillin, over methicillin, as it is significantly less nephrotoxic. Oxacillin would be an acceptable alternative. Appropriate dosages are 150 to 200 mg/kg/day intravenously for 14 days. These doses have been demonstrated to achieve therapeutic concentrations in the CSF of patients with staphylococcal meningitis. Vancomycin would be the drug of choice for meningeal infections due to methicillin-resistant staphylococci and may be used as an alternative therapy for patients allergic to penicillin. Older cephalosporins should not be used because of poor CSF penetration and chloramphenicol should not be used because of poor bactericidal activity against staphylococci.

Enterococcal (*Streptococcus faecalis*) meningitis is uncommon, but the causative organism is difficult to kill due to its relative insensitivity to penicillins. A combination of a penicillin (penicillin G or ampicillin) plus an aminoglycoside (gentamicin or streptomycin) is the therapy of choice. It may be that intrathecal aminoglycoside is not always necessary to treat this infection but careful clinical monitoring during the first 48 to 72 hours must dictate this decision. Doses may be found in Table 9.3 and 9.4. In patients allergic to penicillin, vancomycin may be used alone or in combination with an aminoglycoside and intrathecal vancomycin may be required. Doses are listed in Tables 9.3 and 9.4. The cephalosporins do not have activity against the enterococcus and should not be used to treat this form of meningitis.

The most common fungi causing meningitis are *Cryptococcus*, *Coccidioides*, and *Candida*. Each of these causative agents are treated in approximately the same manner. Cryptococcal meningitis is treated with intravenous amphotericin B in doses up to 0.5 mg/kg/day with or without flucytosine. Intrathecal therapy with amphotericin B is usually unncessary, and is given only when there has not been an adequate clinical response with intravenous therapy. The use of flucytosine in this infection has been studied, and those patients who received both drugs did slightly better clinically but they also suffered more frequent and severe adverse reactions due to flucytosine (28). Thus, flucytosine should be reserved for those situations where the patients do not improve adequately on amphotericin B alone. The patients should be treated until CSF cryptococcal antigen titers are negative.

Coccidioidomycosis is more difficult to treat since the causative organisms are less sensitive to amphotericin B and are completely resistant to flucytosine (29). The systemic dose of amphotericin B must be increased to 0.75 to 1.0 mg/kg/day; and daily to every other day intrathecal or, preferably, intracisternal or intraventricular injection of 0.25 to 0.5 mg is necessary. As with cryptococcosis, the course of this disease tends to be relapsing, so that amphotericin B must be given until the coccidioides antibody in the CSF is significantly reduced (equal to or more than 4-fold decrease in titers). This may require 3 to 6 months of therapy. Outpatient amphotericin B therapy, given 3 times a week, is preferred in many situations.

Intravenous miconazole has been shown to be effective in some cases; dosage is 25 to 30 mg/kg/day intravenously, with or without 20 mg/day intrathecally. There have been several reports of failure of miconazole and it should be used only as an alternative. Ketoconazole, a newly marketed imidazole antibiotic, is active against various fungal infections including coccidiodomycosis. Only limited data concerning its penetration into the CNS and its use in fungal meningitis are available.

Candidal meningitis is unusual and many reported cases have resolved spontaneously (30). Nevertheless, appropriate treatment seems to be the same as for cryptococcal meningitis.

The treatment of herpesvirus meningitis has been unsuccessful until recently. Previous attempts have used cytosine arabinoside (ara-C) and idoxuridine which only produced severe toxicity. Clinical trials have demonstrated the efficacy of adenine arabinoside (vidarabine) in the treatment of neonatal and adult herpes simplex encephalitis and disseminated herpes zoster infection in the immunosuppressed (20). Unfortunately, although survival was definitely increased in those patients given the drug, severe morbidity was common. Therapy must be instituted early in the course of the disease (within the first 48 to 72 hours) to be of any benefit. The dose of vidarabine is 15 mg/kg/day in a single daily infusion for 5 days;

if there seems to be clinical response, therapy is continued for 10 to 14 days.

CONTROVERSIES IN ANTIBIOTIC THERAPY
Chloramphenicol

Chloramphenicol penetrates well into the CSF in concentrations ranging from 35 to 45% of serum concentrations and is frequently used in the treatment of meningitis. As has been mentioned before, bactericidal activity is required for effective treatment of meningitis. Chloramphenicol has been shown to be bactericidal against H. influenzae, S. pneumoniae, and N. meningitidis. Treatment of meningitis caused by these organisms with chloramphenicol usually results in eradication of the organisms from the CSF. Treatment of Gram-negative meningitis with chloramphenicol is controversial. Most gram-negative organisms are only inhibited by chloramphenicol and are not killed until very large concentrations are used. Reports of treatment failures with the development of bacterial resistance during therapy are common (11). There is also evidence that the combination of chloramphenicol and an aminoglycoside may be less effective than an aminoglycoside alone (31). This information would suggest that the use of chloramphenicol in meningitis should be reserved for cases where the antibiotic is known to be bactericidal. Chloramphenicol may be used in gram-negative meningitis but only if the susceptibility (MBC) of the organism to chloramphenicol is known.

Aminoglycosides

The aminoglycosides do not diffuse readily from the blood into the CSF. Little antibiotic passes the uninflamed meninges but during periods of inflammation up to 30% of serum concentrations can be found in the CSF. However, the amount of antibiotic which is present does not result in a consistently bactericidal effect due to the acid pH of infected CSF. Because of variable penetration and inconsistent bactericidal effect, direct instillation into the subarachnoid space (SAS) is required.

The CSF is formed in the third and fourth ventricles and is circulated from the ventricles into two directions: (a) ascending to the lateral SAS and bathes the cerebral hemispheres and (b) descending through the SAS to the spinal cord. If an antibiotic is placed into the SAS by lumbar injection, the normal physiology of CSF flow would preclude its entrance into the ventricles. Direct instillation into the ventricles does provide drug concentrations throughout the entire SAS.

There is considerable controversy regarding the benefit of intrathecal use of aminoglycosides in treating neonatal Gram-negative meningitis (32). In 1976, the Neonatal Meningitis Cooperative Study Group investigated the treatment of neonatal meningitis with and without the intralumbar instillation of gentamicin added to intravenous therapy. Their results showed no benefit in the use of intralumbar gentamicin over systemic therapy alone. A large percentage of the neonates were found to have ventriculitis which was thought to have contributed to the lack of effect.

In 1980, a second Neonatal Meningitis Cooperative Study Group investigated the intraventricular use of gentamicin in the treatment of Gram-negative meningitis. In this study there was a higher death rate in the group receiving intraventricular gentamicin plus systemic therapy vs. those receiving systemic therapy alone. The increased mortality experienced in this group may have been caused by repeated percutaneous intraventricular injections. Recently, a controlled clinical trial of the intraventricular use of amikacin instilled into a Rickman reservoir did not substantiate the second Neonatal Meningitis Cooperative Study Group's findings. In fact, all of the neonatal deaths occurred in the group which received systemic antibiotics alone. From these data, the role of intraventricular aminoglycoside therapy for treatment of neonatal Gram-negative meningitis and ventriculitis remains unclear. In adults, the use of intraventricular aminoglycoside has been shown to reduce the mortality of Gram-negative meningitis.

When using aminoglycosides to treat meningitis the following points should be remembered: (a) these agents penetrate variably into the CSF, (b) the amount of antibiotic which passes into the CSF may not be consistently bactericidal, (c) direct instillation into the CSF is usually required to reach bactericidal concentrations, (d) intralumbar instillation provides drug levels to all areas except the ventricles, (e) ventriculitis is common in Gram-negative meningitis, and (f) repeated direct drug administration into the ventricles should be done through a reservoir.

Cephalosporins

Cephalothin and cephaloridine should not be used to treat patients with meningitis (24).

Poor penetration, minimal antibacterial activity and toxicity of these agents has led to the previous widespread avoidance of cephalosporin antibiotics in the treatment of meningitis. Cefamandole demonstrates moderate CSF penetration and greater antibacterial activity than earlier cephalosporins. Treatment failures and the development of resistance during therapy has discouraged its use for treating meningitis. Cefoxitin, a cephamycin, penetrates moderately into the CSF and also has greater antibacterial activity than earlier cephalosporins. Probenecid is frequently given with cefoxitin to increase the CSF levels. However, cefoxitin has limited utility and should only be used in cases of meningitis caused by highly susceptible organisms. Both cefotaxime and moxalactam penetrate moderately into the CSF during meningitis. Because these drugs have excellent antibacterial activity against most Enterobacteriaceae, their use in Gram-negative meningitis may be of great importance in the management of this serious infection. Although these antibiotics have increased Gram-negative activity, their activity against most Gram-positive organisms is markedly decreased. This is especially important in meningitis caused by group B streptococci, *S. pneumoniae*, *S. aureus*, and *Listeria*. Moxalactam should not be used to treat Gram-positive meningitis. In addition, the activity of these antibiotics against most *Pseudomonas* is limited, as many strains have minimum bactericidal concentrations that are not readily attainable in the CSF.

Successful single drug therapy has been documented in meningitis caused by susceptible organisms. However, these new agents will not totally replace the use of the aminoglycosides in the treatment of Gram-negative meningitis. Also because of the poor Gram-positive activity of moxalactam, this agent should not be used alone for empiric therapy. Further clinical experience will be needed to establish a place for these agents in the treatment of meningitis.

BRAIN ABSCESS

Unlike meningitis, the key to the successful treatment of brain abscess is surgery. Drainage of the abscess not only allows clinical cure, but provides accurate identification of the infecting organism(s) since CSF laboratory findings are often normal in patients with brain abscess. The importance of surgery is underlined by the study of Black et al. (34) who found adequate concentrations of antibiotics in excised abscesses, but viable organisms could still be cultured.

Since the abscesses are often polymicrobial, a combination of antibiotics, especially penicillin G plus chloramphenicol, is usually employed (Table 9.5): If the culture results reveal aerobic Gram-negative bacilli or staphylococci, therapy should include an aminoglycoside or a penicillinase-resistant penicillin, respectively (7). These agents should be given in doses similar to those employed in the treatment of meningitis. Therapy should be prolonged (at least 4 weeks) following surgical removal or evacuation of the abscess. *Nocardia asteroides* produces brain abscess primarily in the immunocompromised patient and should be treated with a sulfonamide (preferably sulfadiazine) in a dosage of 100 to 150 mg/kg/day for extended periods of time (a minimum of 3 to 6 months in usually required) (35). Trimethoprim/sulfamethoxazole in a dose of 10/50 mg/kg/day has also been effective. Other possible alternatives are a combination of erythromycin and ampicillin in high dosage or perhaps minocycline. These alternatives are inferior to the sulfonamides, however, and there is little experience with them in the treatment of brain abscess.

NONANTIBIOTIC THERAPY

Supportive therapy should be used only as an adjuvant to use of appropriate antibiotic therapy. Shock should be managed with fluids, vasopressors and possibly high dose corticosteroids. Cerebral edema and hydrocephalus should be quickly managed with mannitol or a ventricular shunt. The use of corticosteroids to reduce cerebral edema from meningitis remains controversial. A recent review of steroid usage in meningitis suggests that steroids are neither helpful nor harmful when administered to patients less than 16 years of age but several case reports have cited treatment failures attributed to the prolonged use of corticosteroids (36, 37). The proposed mechanism for this detrimental effect was that the steroid therapy alters the immunological status of the patient and decreases the BBB inflammation resulting in reduced antibiotic penetration. The controversy regarding their use is not resolved at the present time.

PREVENTION

The use of antibiotics (sulfonamides, minocycline and rifampin) and meningococcal vaccines have been shown to be effective in the prevention of meningococcal disease (38). The most common types of meningococci known to cause disease are serogroups A, B, C, and Y. The current commercially produced vaccines are: monovalent A, monovalent C and bivalent A–C. Serogroup B is not sufficiently immunogenic to produce a reliable antibody response. The increased incidence of serogroup Y in the last few years has stimulated interest in evaluating the group Y capsular polysaccharide as a vaccine material. Confirmation of the effec-

Table 9.5.
Empiric Antibiotic Therapy in Brain Abscess

Unassociated with trauma or surgery	Penicillin G plus	200–300,000 units/kg/day (every 2–4 hr)	Intravenous
	Chloramphenicol[a] or	40–60 mg/kg/day	Intravenous/oral
	Metronidazole[a]	30–40 mg/kg/day (every 6–8 hr)	Intravenous
Associated with trauma or surgery	Nafcillin Penicillin allergy:	150–200 mg/kg/day	Intravenous Intravenous
	Vancomycin plus	30–40 mg/kg/day	
	Chloramphenicol[a] or	As above	Intravenous
	Penicillin plus	As above	Intravenous
	Metronidazole[a] plus	As above	Intravenous
	Aminoglycoside[b]	As above	Intravenous

[a] Oral therapy may be given subsequent to initial intravenous therapy.
[b] Enterococcus—use gentamicin.

tiveness of serogroup A vaccine has been found in children ages 3 months of age and older but the serogroup C vaccines does not appear to be effective in children less than 2 years of age.

Serogroup B strains currently cause the majority of infections in the United States, most frequently in infants. Serogroup C strains account for about one third of the cases and approximately 70% of these cases occur in persons over 2 years of age. Secondary cases of infection occur more frequently in household contacts, of the person with the primary infection than in the general population. Since most secondary cases occur within 2 weeks after the primary case, protection should be provided promptly. The Center for Disease Control (CDC) has provided an algorithm for meningococcal prophylaxis (Fig. 9.1) (39).

Sulfonamides have been classically used in prophylaxis and treatment of meningococcal infection. Their use has declined because of the changing patterns of resistance of the serogroups. It has been found that 25% of strains submitted to the CDC are sulfonamide resistant. Because of the lack of oropharyngeal pen-

etration of penicillins, these drugs are unsuitable for prophylaxis. Minocycline and rifampin have been shown effective in eradicating the carrier state and reducing the secondary attack rate of meningococcal infection. Minocycline is associated with an unacceptably high incidence of vestibular toxicity, therefore, rifampin is the drug of choice for prophylaxis.

The pneumococcal vaccine was developed to prevent infection caused by the 14 pneumococcal serotypes most commonly encountered. The vaccine is recommended for individuals who are at increased risk of developing pneumococcal infections only if they are capable of producing an antibody response to the vaccine (40). There have been few studies investigating the effectiveness of the pneumococcal vaccine in children. The vaccine is poorly immunogenic in children less than 2 years of age (41). Since secondary cases of pneumococcal meningitis have not been reported, antimicrobial prophylaxis of family and household contacts have not been required. The exact role for the use of pneumococcal vaccine is still not well defined.

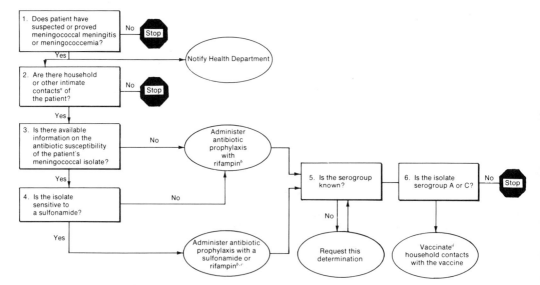

[a] Intimate contact is defined as direct exposure to oral secretions of patients (such as through mouth-to-mouth resuscitation or kissing).

[b] Dosage regimen is 2 days of 600 mg twice daily for adults; 10 mg/kg twice daily for children 1 to 12 years of age; and 5 mg/kg twice daily for children less than 1 year.

[c] Dosage regimen is 2 days of sulfisoxazole or sulfadiazine 1 g twice daily for adults; 500 mg twice daily for children 1 to 12 years of age; and 500 mg once daily for children less than 1 year.

[d] Group A and C vaccines are administered as a single 50-μg injection.

Figure 9.1. Algorithm for administration of meningococcal prophylaxis. (Copyright 1976 American Medical Association.)

Young children, less than 6 years old, with known exposure to children who have documented invasive *H. influenzae* infections, are at increased risk for developing serious infections caused by this organism. The exposure may occur in individual households or in other closed settings such as nursery schools or day-care centers. Nasopharyngeal colonization is felt to result from personal exposure to droplets of respiratory secretions from infected or colonized individuals. Antibiotic prophylaxis is believed to interrupt transmission of the organism by eradicating the carrier state. The use of ampicillin, cefaclor, erythromycin-sulfisoxazole and trimethoprim-sulfamethoxazole has not been successful in eradicating the *H. influenzae* carrier state. Rifampin has been used with success in some closed populations (42). Therefore, the current recommendations for prophylaxis are: (a) rifampin prophylaxis should be given to all contacts of the index case (adults and children) in households where there are other children less than 4 years of age. The dose of rifampin is 20 mg/kg/day (maximum of 600 mg/day) given once daily for 4 days; (b) other closed communities such as nursery schools and day-care centers should be considered a "household." Rifampin prophylaxis is recommended for children attending these centers and for the adult personnel. The use of prophylaxis in this group is controversial. Some experts advise against prophylaxis unless at least 2 cases occur among attendees; and (c) children recovering from serious *H. influenzae* infections have often been found to carry the organism in their nasopharynx despite appropriate systemic antibiotic therapy. Thus prior to discharge, all children with invasive diseases who have young siblings at home should receive rifampin prophylaxis to avoid introduction of the organism into their households (43).

It is possible that prophylaxis may fail to reduce the incidence of secondary disease. This may result because some carriers within the "household" group remain untreated because of poor medication compliance or contraindications to the use of rifampin.

PROGNOSIS

The overall mortality rate for treated bacterial meningitis is about 10 to 20%. This incidence may vary depending upon the organism; meningococcal meningitis (without sepsis) and meningitis due to *H. influenzae* carry a better prognosis than pneumococcal or Gram-negative bacillary meningitis, where as many as 15 to 30% of patients may die as a result of the infection. Fungal meningitis due to *C. immitis* is ultimately a fatal disease in 100% of patients despite treatment but the use of amphotericin B may prolong survival for months to years. Mortality of neonatal meningitis is between 60 to 75% of cases.

Statistical analysis of clinical parameters demonstrates a significant risk of death or morbidity in those patients younger than one year of age or older than 40 years, those with predisposing illness, in patients presenting with neurological deficits or in patients in shock with positive blood cultures. Other findings such as low CSF leukocyte counts, markedly elevated CSF protein, very low CSF glucose concentration, and a delay in diagnosis may or may not predict significant morbidity or mortality (44).

CONCLUSION

Because meningitis produces a great deal of concern and anxiety in the lay public, the pharmacist is in a key position to be able to allay many of these fears and to refer patients who do need medical attention or prophylactic antibiotics.

When treating bacterial meningitis, it should be remembered that early diagnosis and the prompt institution of appropriate antibiotic therapy may be lifesaving in many instances. The pharmacist should clearly understand the mechanism of action, pharmacology, dosage and side effects of antibiotics useful in treating meningitis.

References

1. Yogev R, Davis AT: Neurosurgical shunt infections: a review. *Childs Brain* 6:74, 1980.
2. Kaufman DM, Miller MH, Steigbigel NH: Subdural empyema; analysis of 17 recent cases and review of the literature. *Medicine* 54:485, 1975.
3. McGee ZA, Kaiser AB: Acute meningitis. In Mandell GL, Douglas Jr, RD, Bennett JE: *Principles and Practice of Infectious Diseases.* New York: John Wiley & Sons, 1979, p 738.
4. Underman AE, Overturf GD, Leedom JM: Bacterial meningitis: 1978. *DM* 24:1, 1978.
5. Crane LR, Lerner AM: Non-traumatic gram-negative bacillary meningitis in the Detroit Medical Center 1964–1974 (with special mention of cases due to *Escherichia coli*). *Medicine* 57:197, 1978.
6. Feigin RD, Dodge PR: Bacterial meningitis: newer concepts of pathophysiology and neurologic sequelae. *Pediatr Clin North Am* 23:541, 1976.
7. de Louvois J: The bacteriology and chemother-

apy of brain abscess. *J Antimicrob Chemother* 4:395, 1978.

8. Anon: Bacterial meningitis and meningococcemia-United States, 1978. *MMWR* 28:277, 1979.

9. Heckmatt JZ: Coliform meningitis in the newborn. *Arch Dis Child* 51:569, 1976.

10. McSwiggan DA: Neonatal and perinatal infection: routes of transmission and prevention. *J Antimicrob Chemother* 5 (Suppl A):1, 1979.

11. Cherubin CE, Marr JS, Sierra MF, et al: Listeria and gram-negative bacillary meningitis in New York City, 1972–1979. *Am J Med* 71:199, 1981.

12. Geiseler PJ, Nelson KE, Levin S, et al: Community-acquired purulent meningitis: a review of 1,316 cases during the antibiotic era, 1954–1976. *Rev Infect Dis* 2:725, 1980.

13. Hodges GR, Perkins RL: Hospital-associated bacterial meningitis. *Am J Med Sci* 271:335, 1976.

14. Buckwold FJ, Hand R, Hansebout RR: Hospital acquired bacterial meningitis in neurosurgical patients. *J Neurosurg* 46:494, 1977.

15. Nahmias AJ, Roizman B: Infection with herpes simplex viruses 1 and 2. *N Engl J Med* 289:667, 719, 781, 1973.

16. Feigin RD, Shackelford PG: Value of repeat lumbar puncture in the differential diagnosis of meningitis. *N Engl J Med* 289:571, 1973.

17. Lewin EB: Partially treated meningitis. *Am J Dis Child* 128:145, 1974.

18. Lauwers S, Clumeck N: Rapid diagnosis of bacterial meningitis. *J Infection* 3 (Suppl):27, 1981.

19. Alon U, Naveh Y, Gardos M, et al: Neurological sequelae of septic meningitis. A follow-up study of 65 children. *Isr J Med Sci* 15:512, 1979.

20. Whitley RJ, Soong S-J, Hirsch MS, et al, and the NIAD Collaborative Antiviral Study Group: Herpes simplex encephalitis: vidarabine therapy and diagnostic problems. *N Engl J Med* 304:313, 1981.

21. Pollay M, Roberts PA: Blood-brain barrier: a definition of normal and altered function. *Neurosurgery* 6:675, 1980.

22. Allinson RR, Stach PE: Intrathecal drug therapy. *Drug Intell Clin Pharm* 12:347, 1978.

23. Simberkoff MS, Moldover NH, Rahal Jr JJ: Absence of detectable bactericidal and opsonic activities in normal and infected human cerebrospinal fluids. *J Lab Clin Med* 95:362, 1980.

24. Landesman SH, Corrado ML, Shah PM, et al: Past and current roles for cephalosporin antibiotics in treatment of meningitis: emphasis on use in gram-negative bacillary meningitis. *Am J Med* 71:693, 1981.

25. Sande MA: Antibiotic therapy of bacterial meningitis: lessons we've learned. *Am J Med* 71:507, 1981.

26. Wilson HD, Haltalin KC: Ampicillin in *Haemophilus influenzae* meningitis. Clinicopharmacoloic evaluation of intramuscular vs. intravenous administration. *Am J Dis Child* 129:208, 1975.

27. Meade III RH: Streptomycin and sulfisoxazole for treatment of *Haemophilus influenzae* meningitis. *JAMA* 239:324, 1978.

28. Bennett JE, Dismukes WE, Duma RJ, et al: A comparison of amphotericin B alone and combined with flucytosine in the treatment of cryptococcal meningitis. *N Engl J Med* 301:126, 1979.

29. Bouza E, Dreyer JS, Hewitt WL, et al: Coccidioidal meningitis: an analysis of thirty-one cases and review of the literature. *Medicine* 60:139, 1981.

30. Bayer AS, Edwards JE, Seidel JS, et al: Candida meningitis. Report of seven cases and review of the literature. *Medicine* 55:477, 1976.

31. Strausbaugh LJ, Sande MA: Factors influencing the therapy of experimental *Proteus mirabilis* meningitis in rabbits. *J Infect Dis* 137:251, 1978.

32. Swartz MN: Intraventricular use of aminoglycosides in the treatment of gram-negative bacillary meningitis: conflicting views. *J Infect Dis* 143:293, 1981.

33. Dacey RG, Sande MA: Effect of probenecid on cerebrospinal fluid concentrations of penicillin and cephalosporin derivatives. *Antimicrob Agents Chemother* 6:437, 1974.

34. Black P, Graybill JR, Charache P: Penetration of brain abscess by systemically administered antibiotics. *J Neurosurg* 38:705, 1973.

35. Palmer DL, Harvey RL, Wheeler JK: Diagnostic and therapeutic considerations in *Nocardia asteroides* infection. *Medicine* 53:391, 1974.

36. Harbin GL, Hodges GR: Corticosteroids as adjunctive therapy for acute bacterial meningitis. *South Med J* 72:977, 1979.

37. Brady MT, Kaplan SL, Taber LH: Association between persistence of pneumococcal meningitis and dexamethasone administration. *J Pediatr* 99:924, 1981.

38. Public Health Service Advisory Committee on Immunization Practices: Meningococcal polysaccharide vaccines. *Ann Intern Med* 89:949, 1978.

39. Jacobson JA, Fraser DW: A simplified approach to meningococcal disease prophylaxis. *JAMA* 236:1053, 1976.

40. Public Health Service Advisory Committee on Immunization Practices: Pneumococcal polysaccharide vaccine. *Ann Intern Med* 96:203, 1982.

41. Schwartz JS: Pneumococcal vaccine: clinical efficacy and effectiveness. *Ann Intern Med* 96:208, 1982.

42. Daum RS, Glode MP, Goldmann DA, et al: Rifampin chemoprophylaxis for household contacts of patients with invasive infections due to *Haemophilus influenzae* type B. *J Pediatr* 98:485, 1981.

43. Committee on Infectious Diseases American Academy of Pediatrics: In Klein JO: *Haemophilus influenzae Infections*. Evanston, Ill.: American Academy of Pediatrics, 1982, pp 105–107.

44. Hodges GR, Perkins RL: Acute bacterial meningitis: an analysis of factors influencing prognosis. *Am J Med Sci* 270:427, 1975.

CHAPTER 10

Infective Endocarditis

STEVEN L. BARRIERE, Pharm.D.
DONALD P. ALEXANDER, Pharm.D.

Endocarditis is, by strict definition, an infection of the inner lining of the heart and the mucosa which underlies it. The term, however, refers most commonly to an infection of a heart valve. The heart wall, papillary muscles, and chordae tendineae can be involved in the infection, but the complications and clinical manifestations arise from the involvement of the tricuspid, mitral, or aortic valves.

Subacute disease is an indolent infection that may produce signs and symptoms over periods as long as several months before a diagnosis is made. Acute infection is of rapid onset, with fulminant symptomatology. Classically, patients with subacute disease had all of the "typical" manifestations of the disease (see below); however, the diagnosis is now suspected in any febrile illness of unclear etiology, so that progression to chronicity is becoming less common.

ANATOMY

As mentioned above the tissues involved in endocarditis are primarily the tricuspid, mitral and aortic valves; the valve of the pulmonary artery is only rarely infected. The tricuspid valve is a common site of infection in intravenous drug users. The mitral and aortic valves are also involved in this group of patients, and damage to these valves leads to more severe hemodynamic alterations than tricuspid disease.

The sites of the lesions are the atrial surfaces of the mitral and tricuspid valves and the ventricular surfaces of the aortic and pulmonic valves. Lesions of the chordae, atrial or ventricular walls and the pulmonary artery or aorta are all considered satellite infections to the primary valvular involvement (1).

PATHOPHYSIOLOGY

Four factors are necessary in the pathogenesis of the infection: (a) a previously damaged cardiac valve or a hemodynamic situation in which a so-called jet effect is produced by blood flowing from an area of high pressure to one of relatively low pressure, as in mitral insufficiency; (b) a platelet-fibrin thrombus; (c) bacteremia; and (d) bacterial adherence (1, 2). In patients with endocarditis the mitral valve is involved in 66 to 86%, the aortic vlave in 45 to 55%, tricuspid valve in 5 to 20% and pulmonic valve in only 1% (3, 4). Correlating the pressure gradient across these valves with the relative frequency of infection makes a strong argument for mechanical stress as an important factor in the pathogenesis of endocarditis. Similarly, the hemodynamic alterations that occur across an incompetent valve result in abnormal "jets" of blood that may damage the endocardium and provide a locus for infection. This change in hemodynamics also creates a low pressure "sink" which sets up an additional site for infection as illustrated by the Venturi model (Fig. 10.1). A bacterial aerosol (bacteremia) flows from the high pressure source (left ventricle) through the narrowed orifice (incompetent mitral valve) into the low pressure area (left atrium). The development of vegetations, just distal to the orifice, has been demonstrated with this model. Vegetations in endocarditis are indeed most commonly found on the low pressure side of the valve (1).

Once the endothelial surface of the valve is traumatized by the aforementioned jet effects, collagen is exposed and a platelet-fibrin thrombus is formed which is sterile.

The next critical factor in the pathogenesis of the infection is bacteremia. The microorganism is delivered to the valve surface by the bloodstream. Finally, the ability of the organisms to stick to fibrin and platelets correlates directly with their ability to produce endocarditis (2).

ETIOLOGY

Infection due to viridans streptococci has declined over the last 2 decades. Half or more of all cases of endocarditis were due to these

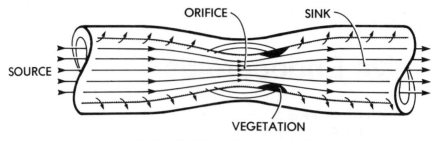

Figure 10.1. The Venturi model. (Modified from S. Rodbard: Blood Velocity and Endocarditis. *Circulation,* 27:18, 1963, by permission of the American Heart Association, Inc.)

organisms 10 years ago. Now approximately one third are caused by these streptococci (3, 4). Enterococci are the causative pathogens in approximately 6% of cases, and other streptococci account for 7 to 14% of cases. Staphylococci account for 25% of all cases, particularly in intravenous drug users (5). Gram-negative bacteria such as *Serratia marcescens* and *Pseudomonas aeruginosa* have been reported to be responsible for as many as 11% of cases (6, 7); again, frequently occurring in habitual intravenous drug users. Fungi, particularly *Candida albicans* are seen in 5% or less of cases (3–6).

Intravenous drug users develop endocarditis more frequently than the general population, probably due to frequent nonsterile intravenous injections. The bacteriology of endocarditis in this population is comprised of staphylococcus (50 to 60%), and Gram-negative bacilli and fungi (30 to 35%). Anaerobes and other organisms produce only a few cases of disease in this population.

The other group of patients who are at special risk to developing endocarditis are those who have prosthetic cardiac valves. Prosthetic valve endocarditis (PVE) occurring within the first 2 months after surgery (early PVE) is caused by organisms introduced during surgery. The most frequently cultured organisms are staphylococci, especially *Staphylococcus epidermidis*. Infection occurring beyond 2 months (late PVE) are caused by the same organisms which produce disease on native valves (i.e., primarily streptococci). Fungi are also a concern in these patients. Endocarditis is especially devastating in these patients since fatal complications can occur quickly (8, 9).

BACTEREMIA

Infecting organisms must reach the cardiac tissues by means of the general circulation.

Bacteremias and fungemia are the initiating events in the genesis of the actual infection as noted above.

The viridans streptococci, nonenterococcal group D streptococci, and other facultative organisms are normal flora of the nasopharynx. *Streptococcus faecalis* (enterococcus) and Gram-negative bacilli usually arise from the urinary tract. Staphylococci are quite often found on the skin. Fungi may arise from the bowel, as can certain Gram-negative and anaerobic organisms. Fungi may also colonize certain areas of skin, and thus gain entrance to the circulation via intravenous catheters.

Staphylococcal bacteremia and its management is enmeshed in a good deal of controversy. Iannini and Crossley (10) reported on 29 patients with no previous evidence of endocarditis who developed *Staphylococcus aureus* bacteremia associated with a removable focus of infection—usually an intravenous catheter. The patients were treated for only 10 to 21 days with appropriate antibiotics and none developed endocarditis. This suggests that early recognition of the problem and prompt therapy for a short duration prevents the development of endocarditis. Watanakunakorn and Baird (11) reviewed 21 similar patients in whom bacteremia with *S. aureus* developed secondary to an intravenous device. They found that without therapy endocarditis developed in 8 patients (38%) and they felt that endocarditis had been established by the time bacteremia was detected. It seems reasonable then, based upon the limited information available, to treat staphylococcal bacteremia, due to a removable focus for 2 to 3 weeks with appropriate therapy, while monitoring for signs of endocarditis. This has not been demonstrated for bacteremias caused by other microorganisms, in the absence of previous cardiac disease.

Endocarditis has been described following bacteremias arising from gentiourinary infection and the use of an oral irrigation device. In addition, transient bacteremias, with the potential for producing endocarditis, have been described following tooth extraction, periodontal surgery, liver biopsy, endoscopy or sigmoidoscopy, and manipulations of the gentiourinary tract (Table 10.1).

DIAGNOSIS AND CLINICAL FEATURES

The classical signs and symptoms of endocarditis such as Osler's nodes, Janeway lesions, clubbing of the fingers, splinter hemorrhages, and retinal lesions, are all infrequently seen in modern clinical medicine (3, 4). The primary reason for this is the high index of suspicion for the disease in a patient with fever of unknown etiology, leading to early diagnosis. The most common presenting signs and symptoms are the following: presence of a heart murmur or a change in a previously noted murmur, fever, embolic episodes, splenomegaly, skin manifestations (primarily petechiae), weakness, dyspnea, sweats, anorexia, weight loss, malaise, and cough (3). The aforementioned are not present in 100% of cases, but the most crucial criterion for the diagnosis of the disease is positive blood cultures.

The bacteremia of endocarditis is qualitatively continuous, but quantitatively variable. Negative blood cultures may be due to uremia, poor bacteriologic technique, fastidious organisms (e.g., *Cardiobacterium hominis*, *Eikenella corrodens*) nonbacterial disease (e.g., Q fever, fungi, viruses), or prior antibiotic therapy (12, 13). The number of blood cultures necessary to establish or exclude the diagnosis has been determined to be at least three and perhaps as many as five. In practice, three cultures taken over a 24 hour period, in a patient who is not critically ill, should produce a very high yield. In acutely ill patients, 2 to 3 samples of blood should be taken from different sites in rapid fashion prior to instituting antibiotic therapy.

Most of the classic signs and symptoms are due either to emboli from the infected endocardium, or local vasculitis. Subacute disease is characterized by one or more of the "classic" signs or symptoms, but acute disease may often present as hemorrhage, embolus, or metastatic

Table 10.1.
Incidence and Types of Bacteremia

Procedure	Incidence of Bacteremia (%)	Organisms
Dental extraction	30–80	Streptococci Diphtheroids *Staphylococcus epidermidis*
Periodontal surgery	80–90	As above Anaerobes
Tooth brushing, oral irrigation	25–50	Streptococci Staphylococci
Tonsillectomy	30–40	Streptococci
Upper GI endoscopy	10	Streptococci Staphylococci Diphtheroids
Lower GI endoscopy (sigmoidoscopy)	5–10	Enterococci Gram-negative bacilli *Bacteroides*
Liver biopsy	3–13	Streptococci Staphylococci Gram-negative bacilli
Cystoscopy, urethral dilation, etc.	20–80	Gram-negative bacilli Enterococci

infection (meninges, eye, kidneys). Echocardiography is sometimes useful in detecting vegetations on valve leaflets, especially in those patients with symptoms suggestive of endocarditis but negative blood cultures. This procedure is more useful in assessing valvular competence in candidates for valve replacement.

The laboratory parameters (other than cultures) used to establish the diagnosis of endocarditis are elevated titers of rheumatoid factor; increased erythrocyte sedimentation rate; normochromic, normocytic anemia, and a decline in renal function with hematuria.

All of the above, in conjunction with a history compatible with the disease, put endocarditis at the top of the differential diagnosis list. Compatible histories would include: intravenous drug abuse, underlying heart disease or presence of an indwelling prosthetic device.

Endocarditis in intravenous drug users is frequently heralded by neurologic dysfunction or pulmonary emboli (6). This may misdirect the efforts toward a diagnosis, and again points to the importance of obtaining sufficient blood cultures in the febrile patient with a history of symptoms compatible with endocarditis.

TREATMENT

The cure of infective endocarditis requires the *sustained* application of antimicrobial agents that are capable of *killing* the organisms causing the infection.

As mentioned previously, the sequestration of the infecting organisms within valvular vegetation protects the organisms from antibodies and macrophages and, in addition, results in slowed microbial metabolism. This slowed replication leads to relative insusceptibility to many antibiotics, and requires that the organisms be killed by the antibiotics used (14). This has been proven clinically by the failure of bacteriostatic antibiotics such as the tetracyclines, erythromycin, and chloramphenicol to cure endocarditis. This relative impermeability of antibiotics and slowed microbial replication also require prolonged therapy with antibiotics.

The bactericidal or fungicidal activity of the patient's serum during therapy should be assessed in infections due to more resistant organisms (enterococci, Gram-negative bacilli, fungi and, in some cases, staphylococci) or if treatment with oral antibiotics is to be employed after a shortened course of parenteral therapy. It is generally accepted that bactericidal activity should be present at no less than 1:8 dilutions of serum (Fig. 10.2). This has been found to correlate with good results in the therapy of other infectious diseases (15), and in the therapy of endocarditis (16). These results in Gram-negative bacillary infection often do not correlate with the clinical outcome, however.

Empiric therapy is often instituted prior to the results of culture and sensitivity tests, especially in patients who are acutely ill. The choice of empiric therapy is based upon the facts of history, the physical examination and the course of the disease. For example, an elderly man with evidence of chronic disease and a history of urinary tract infections due to the enterococcus should be treated for enterococcal endocarditis. Likewise, an IV drug user with acute disease should be treated for staphylococcal, enterococcal, and Gram-negative endocarditis until culture results are obtained.

Table 10.2 lists drugs of first choice and alternative drugs for the treatment of the most common causes of endocarditis.

Most streptococci (except enterococci) are highly susceptible to penicillin G or ampicillin, and therapy with either of these drugs alone is adequate in nearly all cases (15–18).

Therapy for 2 weeks, rather than the usual 4, has been evaluated and been found to be effective as long as the combination of procaine penicillin plus streptomycin is employed (19). This regimen is most beneficial but may be more toxic because of the necessity of the aminoglycoside. This regimen should not be used in the elderly, patients in shock, with PVE or extracardiac foci of infection, or for patients infected with less susceptible streptococci (17). Nonenterococcal streptococci may be less sensitive to penicillin G (minimal inhibitory concentration (MIC) equal to or more than 0.1 μg/ml) and should be treated with penicillin G or ampicillin plus an aminoglycoside (streptomycin or gentamicin) (17, 20). Group D streptococci include S. faecalis (enterococcus) and *Streptococcus bovis*. The latter organism is usually highly susceptible to penicillin G. The enterococcus, however, is only moderately susceptible (MIC = 1 to 2 μg/ml) and therapy with a penicillin alone has resulted in a high failure rate. The addition of an aminoglycoside results in synergistic killing of the organism in vitro, and clinically produces improved cure rates (20). In vitro, approximately 20% of enterococci are highly re-

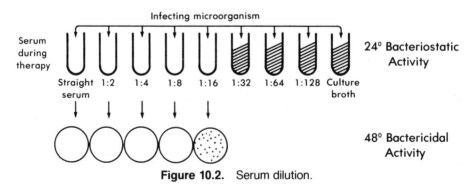

Figure 10.2. Serum dilution.

sistant to streptomycin (MIC equal to or more than 1000 μg/ml). These organisms are not killed in vitro by the penicillin-streptomycin combination and frequently not by penicillin-tobramycin, but the combination of penicillin and gentamicin is routinely bactericidal (20). Combinations of penicillinase-resistant penicillins or cephalosporins plus an aminoglycoside, although sometimes shown to provide in vitro killing of enterococci, have not demonstrated this effect in vivo. Gentamicin is recommended as the preferred aminoglycoside over streptomycin in combination with a penicillin only when high level resistance is found.

In penicillin-allergic patients, vancomycin or a cephalosporin (except in enterococcal infection) are acceptable alternatives. The addition of an aminoglycoside to vancomycin in the management of enterococcal infection is often necessary. A cephalosporin should never be given to a patient with a history of an immediate or accelerated reaction to penicillin.

In the authors' experience, doses of vancomycin 25 to 50% lower than those generally recommended have been shown to be adequate in providing bactericidal activity of serum (Table 10.2). If inadequate levels are demonstrated, increased activity can be obtained by the addition of an aminoglycoside; but caution must be taken as their respective toxicities may be additive.

S. aureus is nearly always resistant to penicillin G necessitating the use of a β-lactamase resistant antibiotic (e.g., isoxazolyl penicillins or cephalosporins).

Staphylococcal endocarditis is best treated with a penicillinase-resistant penicillin. Our choice is nafcillin since it appears to be essentially devoid of the renal toxicity of methicillin (21). Oxacillin would be an acceptable alternative. There is controversy over the relative susceptibility to β-lactamase of the various cephalosporins. A few reports of failure of cefazolin have been attributed to a lack of resistance to β-lactamase. However, successful therapy with cefazolin is reported, and experimental models of endocarditis support the use of this drug.

Another therapeutic attempt to improve in vivo effectiveness of the therapy of S. aureus endocarditis has been the addition of gentamicin to a penicillinase-resistant penicillin. This has been shown to be effective in an animal model and in scattered case reports. However, a large multicenter study was performed to assess the benefit of adding gentamicin to nafcillin compared to nafcillin alone. The results indicated that although the duration of bacteremia was shorter with the combination therapy the overall cure rate was no different in the two groups (20). However, these patients were predominantly young intravenous drug abusers, in whom endocarditis appears to be easier to treat. An additional smaller study reported similar results (22). Each case must be evaluated by determination of clinical response and bactericidal activity to determine if the addition of aminoglycoside is necessary (23). The mortality rate of this infection in patients over 50 years of age is very high and these patients should be treated aggressively with large doses of nafcillin or vancomycin. The addition of an aminoglycoside should be weighed against the potential toxicity in an older patient.

Rifampin also has excellent in vitro activity against staphylococci and may be considered for addition to β-lactam or vancomycin regimens to enhance bactericidal activity (24). Despite reports of successful treatment of staphylococcal endocarditis with clindamycin, it is imperative that bactericidal activity be demonstrated before embarking on therapy with this agent since several reports of failure and the development of resistance during therapy have been published.

S. epidermidis is often resistant to the semisynthetic penicillins. Infections due to these organisms should be treated with vancomycin plus either an aminoglycoside or rifampin (20).

The treatment of other forms of endocarditis is less well established. Infections due to Gram-negative bacilli, fungi, and anaerobes are extremely difficult to cure with antimicrobial therapy alone (20): and often require surgical intervention to repair the valve, or replace the infected valve with a prosthesis. The prime indications for surgery are the development of emboli, impending heart failure, persistent bacteremia, fungal infection, pericarditis, or relapse following "adequate" therapy (25).

Should a prosthetic valve become infected, as is often the case when surgery is performed on intravenous drug users who continue to inject drugs intravenously, the mortality rate is very high. Sterilization of the prosthesis is difficult, and prolonged combination therapy

Table 10.2.
Antimicrobial Therapy for Endocarditis

Organism	Regimen(s) of Choice	Daily Dosage	Alternatives	Daily Dosage	Comments
Streptococci (penicillin MIC <0.2 unit/ml)	1. Penicillin G, aqueous × 4wk or	200–300,000 units/kg IV	Cephalosporin[b]	CZ:75 mg/kg IV CP:150–200 mg/kg IV	Choice of regimen should be dictated by severity of disease and patient's predisposition to aminoglycoside toxicity (i.e., elderly, renal dysfunction, underlying 8th nerve impairment). Preferred regimen is No. 2. Infection caused by organisms that are less susceptible or which are not killed by penicillin alone (tolerant) should be treated with combination therapy
	2. Penicillin G, aqueous × 4 wk plus Aminoglycoside[a] × 2 wk	As above S:15 mg/kg (max 1 g/day IM) T/G:3–4 mg/kg IM/IV	Vancomycin	25–30 mg/kg IV	
	3. Procaine Pen G × 2 wk plus Streptomycin × 2wk	1.2 million units q6h IM As above			
Enterococci (Streptococcus faecalis and others)	Penicillin G, aqueous × 4–6 wk plus Aminoglycoside × 4–6 wk	300,000 units/kg IV S:15 mg/kg (max:1g/d IM) G:3–4 mg/kg IV/IM	Vancomycin with or without Aminoglycoside	25–30 mg/kg IV Same	Many isolates are not killed by vancomycin alone and require addition of aminoglycoside. Cephalosporins are not effective in the treatment of enterococcal infection, even in combination with aminoglycoside
Staphylococcus aureus	Nafcillin or Oxacillin × 4–6 wk	150–200 mg/kg IV	Cephalosporin[b] Vancomycin	As above As above	"Tolerant" strains require addition of aminoglycoside or rifampin for bactericidal effect. However, clinical significance of tolerance remains unknown

Organism	Drug	Dose	Alternative	Alternative dose	Comments
Staphylococcus epidermidis	Native valve: Same as for S. aureus Prosthetic valve: Vancomycin plus Aminoglycoside × 6 wk or Rifampin	25–30 mg/kg/IV As above 600 mg/day	None		Most cases of S. epidermidis infections are on prosthetic valves
Gram-negative bacilli (Serratia, Pseudomonas, Enterobacter)	Aminoglycoside plus Cephalosporin[c] × 4–6 weeks or Penicillin[d]	G/T:5–6 mg/kg IV/IM A:15 mg/kg IV/IM MX: CP: 100–150 mg/kg CT: IV TIC: MEZ: 300 mg/kg IV PIP:	Cephalosporin[c] Cotrimoxazole	Same 10 mg/kg (as TMP) IV	Surgery is often required for cure. Combination therapy is preferred since there is little experience with newer agents alone in the treatment of endocarditis. Duration of therapy is probably at least 4 weeks
Anaerobes (Bacteroides fragilis)	Metronidazole × 6 wk or Penicillin[d]	30 mg/kg IV 300–400 mg/kg IV	Cefoxitin or Moxalactam	150–200 mg/kg IV	Traditional agents for anaerobic infection (clindamycin, chloramphenicol) are bacteriostatic. Newer penicillins (piperacillin, mezlocillin) may be bactericidal
Fungi (Candida, Aspergillus)	Amphotericin B	0.5–1.0 mg/kg IV	None		Some candida sp. are killed synergistically by addition of flucytosine or rifampin to amphotericin B. Newer agents such as miconazole and ketoconazole have not been tested

[a] Streptomycin (S), gentamicin (G) or tobramycin (T).
[b] Cephalothin/cephapirin (CP) or cefazolin (CZ).
[c] Cefotaxime (CT), moxalactam (MX) or cefoperazone (CP).
[d] Mezlocillin (MEZ), piperacillin (PIP), or ticarcillin (TIC).

is indicated (8, 9, 20). Failure of the valve may lead to rapid heart failure and death.

Gram-negative bacillary endocarditis should be treated with bactericidal antibiotics to which the infecting organisms are sensitive. Unfortunately, the most common organisms found in this category are not the relatively antibiotic-sensitive E. coli or Proteus mirabilis, but rather S. marcescens and P. aeruginosa. Both of these organisms are relatively insensitive to most antibiotics and many Serratia have become resistant to all antibiotics except amikacin and trimethoprim-sulfamethoxazole.

The empiric treatment of Gram-negative endocarditis should include an aminoglycoside in maximum dosage probably in combination with a β-lactam compound (20).

Newer cephalosporins (cefotaxime, moxalactam) and new penicillins (piperacillin, mezlocillin) may provide bactericidal therapy for endocarditis due to S. marcescens and P. aeruginosa. To date, little clinical experience has been gained with these agents in the management of endocarditis. Additionally, many isolates of P. aeruginosa are not highly susceptible to these agents and combination therapy with an aminoglycoside plus an antipseudomonal penicillin is probably necessary.

Trimethoprim-sulfamethoxazole (TMP/SMX) is becoming a valuable antimicrobial for the treatment of many extraurinary infections including endocarditis. We have treated Gram-negative bacillary endocarditis with large doses of TMP/SMX resulting in negative blood cultures. Bactericidal activity of the patients' serum must be assured, however. Endocarditis caused by Pseudomonas cepacia has also been effectively treated with TMP/SMX, sometimes in combination with polymyxin B. In an area with a high percentage of Gram-negative bacilli resistant to gentamicin, amikacin may be the empiric aminoglycoside of choice, since most Gram-negative bacilli retain sensitivity to it, unlike tobramycin.

Anaerobic Gram-negative organisms present a special problem, since the two antibiotics most frequently used to treat the infections caused by these organisms, clindamycin and chloramphenicol, are bacteriostatic.

Carbenicillin, in doses of 400 to 500 mg per kg daily has been shown to be effective in the treatment of Bacteroides fragilis endocarditis. Most other anaerobic organisms are highly susceptible to penicillin G. Metronidazole has also been shown in vitro to be highly bactericidal against B. fragilis, and isolated reports have shown it to be effective in treating anaerobic infections other than endocarditis (26). Experience in the treatment of endocarditis is needed to verify this efficacy. Cefoxitin and moxalactam are also active in vitro against B. fragilis and should be considered (27).

Fungal endocarditis is virtually impossible to cure without surgery and, even with optimal therapy, the mortality rate is very high. This is probably due to the invasiveness of the organisms, the large vegetations produced in the valve, the lack of fungicidal activity often found with amphotericin B, and the negligible penetration of the antifungal agent into the vegetation. The mainstay of therapy is amphotericin B given for prolonged periods of time. Therapy 2 to 3 times a week on an outpatient basis has been recommended to suppress the infection and possibly achieve a cure with long-term treatment. Dosage should be tailored to the patient's tolerance. The addition of 5-fluorocytosine for the treatment of candidal infection should be based upon in vitro sensitivity and the assessment of fungicidal activity of the patient's serum. Flucytosine is toxic, however, and this is manifested primarily in the presence of renal failure, which is often a result of amphotericin B therapy. The toxicities include agranulocytosis and hepatic necrosis.

Coxiella burnetii, the agent of Q fever, can produce endocarditis. The treatment is long-term tetracycline therapy, 2.0 g per day orally. This disease, however, is nearly always fatal.

Prosthetic valve replacement is becoming more widespread due to advances in surgical and life support techniques. Along with this has come an increase in the infections involving these valves (PVE). The mortality rate as a result of this infection has been reported to be as high as 90%, depending upon the onset and types of organisms, with an overall mortality figure approaching 70%.

The greatest mortality in PVE is associated with an onset within the first few months after surgery, with Gram-negative bacillary, fungal, and S. aureus infections, with aortic valve involvement, and the presence of congestive heart failure (8, 9). As mentioned previously, the most common infecting organisms are staphylococci (40 to 50%) and streptococci (30 to 40%).

Therapy with antibiotics alone has resulted in a cure rate of approximately 40%, but many patients have required replacement of the infected prosthesis to achieve cure. Antibiotics

Table 10.3.
Antibiotic Regimens for Dental Procedures and Surgery of the Upper Respiratory Tract

Regimen A—Penicillin	Regimen B—Penicillin-Streptomycin
1. Parenteral-oral combined:	*Adults:* Aqueous crystalline penicillin G (1,000,000 units intramuscularly) *mixed with* procaine penicillin G (600,000 units intramuscularly) *plus* streptomycin (1 g intramuscularly). Give 30 min to 1 hr prior to the procedure; then penicillin V 500 mg orally every 6 hr for 8 doses[a]
Adults: Aqueous crystalline penicillin G (1,000,000 units intramuscularly) *mixed with* procaine penicillin G (600,000 units intramuscularly). Give 30 min to 1 hr prior to procedure and then give penicillin V (formerly called phenoxymethyl penicillin) 500 mg orally every 6 hr for 8 doses[a]	
Children[b]: Aqueous crystalline penicillin G (30,000 units/kg intramuscularly. Timing of doses for children is the same as for adults. For children less than 60 lb (27 kg) the dose of penicillin V is 250 mg orally every 6 hr for 8 doses[a]	*Children[b]:* Aqueous crystalline penicillin (30,000 units/kg intramuscularly) *mixed with* procaine penicillin G (600,000 units intramuscularly) *plus* streptomycin (20 mg/kg intramuscularly). Timing of doses for children is the same as for adults. For children less than 60 lb (27 kg) the recommended oral dose of penicillin V is 250 mg every 6 hr for 8 doses[a]
2. Oral[c]:	*For Patients Allergic to Penicillin:*
Adults: Penicillin V (2.0 g orally 30 min to 1 hr prior to the procedure and then 500 mg orally every 6 hr for 8 doses)[a]	*Adults:* Vancomycin (1 g intravenously over 30 min to 1 hr). Start initial vancomycin infusion ½ to 1 hr prior to procedure; then erythromycin 500 mg orally every 6 hr for 8 doses[a]
Children[b]: Penicillin V (2.0 g orally 30 min to 1 hr prior to procedure and then 500 mg orally every 6 hr for 8 doses. For children less than 60 lb use 1.0 g orally 30 min to 1 hr prior to the procedure and then 250 mg orally every 6 hr for 8 doses)[a]	*Children[b]:* Vancomycin (20 mg/kg intravenously over 30 min to 1 hr).[d] Timing of doses for children is the same as for adults. Erythromycin dose is 10 mg/kg every 6 hr for 8 doses[a]
Children[b]: Erythromycin (20 mg/kg orally 1½– 2 hr prior to the procedure and then 10 mg/kg every 6 hr for 8 doses)[a]	

[a] In unusual circumstances or in the case of delayed healing, it may be prudent to provide additional doses of antibiotics even though available data suggest that bacteremia rarely persists longer than 15 min after the procedure. The physician or dentist may also choose to use the parenteral route of administration for all of the doses in selected situations.

[b] Doses for children should not exceed recommendations for adults for a single dose or for a 24-hr period.

[c] For those patients receiving continuous oral penicillin for secondary prevention of rheumatic fever, α-hemolytic streptococci which are relatively resistant to penicillin are occasionally found in the oral cavity. While it is likely that the doses of penicillin recommended in Regimen A are sufficient to control these organisms, the physician or dentist may choose one of the suggestions in Regimen B or may choose oral erythromycin.

[d] For vancomycin the total dose for children should not exceed 40 mg/kg/24 hr.

should be used as in endocarditis occurring on natural valves and should be continued for a minimum of 6 weeks of parenteral therapy. Early replacement of infected prostheses should be considered in all patients except those with uncomplicated streptococcal or mitral valve PVE (8, 25).

COMPLICATIONS

Complications in infective endocarditis are due to the disease, the antibiotics used or both. The overall mortality for *all* forms of infective endocarditis is approximately 25 to 30%. However, the mortality ranges from 10 to 15% in penicillin-sensitive streptococcal endocarditis to 90% or more in fungal infection.

A poor prognosis is associated with old age, serious underlying cardiac or other disease, aortic or mitral valve involvement, infection of a prosthetic valve, presence of emboli, and infection with Gram-negative bacilli or fungi.

Patients with subacute disease may develop renal insufficiency. This may be due to one or more of several factors: nephrotoxicity of antimicrobials, metastatic abscess within the kidney from infected emboli (predominantly staphylococcal infection), infarction of the kidney due to compromised blood flow caused by aseptic emboli, or, immune complex nephritis due to deposition of immunoglobulins and complement on the glomerular basement membrane.

Involvement of the central nervous system occurs in nearly one third of all patients with endocarditis. The predominant manifestations are stroke and hemorrhage. Less common are meningitis, toxic encephalopathy, mononeuritis, convulsions and visual impairment. The visual impairment is usually due to emboli or infarction, but may be caused by secondary endophthalmitis which may rapidly progress to loss of the eye.

The most common complications of endocarditis involve the lung, in the form of pulmonary emboli, and congestive heart failure due to valvular insufficiency.

PREVENTION OF ENDOCARDITIS

Bacteremia from most sources is usually transient and nearly always inconsequential in the normal individual. However, in the patient with congenital or acquired heart disease or a prosthetic valve, any bacteremia may lead to endocarditis. In assessing the risk of a bacteremia to an individual patient, important considerations are the incidence of bacteremia with a given procedure (Table 10.2). The most likely organisms, the type of cardiac abnormality, and perhaps, the concentration of the bacteria in the bloodstream are important, although data are lacking on this latter point. In general, Gram-positive cocci infect congenital defects or acquired valvular diseases, while Gram-negative aerobic bacilli and fungi are not uncommon pathogens in prosthetic valve infection. It has been estimated that as much as 15% of all cases of endocarditis are related to dental surgical procedures (28).

General measures to reduce the risk of bacteremia are to avoid manipulation or instrumentation of infected areas, avoid procedures which may traumatize mucous membranes usually colonized with a normal flora (e.g., mouth), and avoidance of intravenous catheterization with plastic devices. Topical antisepsis does not decrease the incidence of bacteremia during dental procedures.

Only indirect evidence from animal studies exists to demonstrate the effect of prophylactic antibiotics in bacteremia-producing procedures. No controlled trials are available and the recommended regimens are derived from

Table 10.4.
Prophylaxis for Dental Procedures and Surgical Procedures of the Upper Respiratory Tract

	Most congenital heart disease[c]; rheumatic or other acquired valvular heart disease; idiopathic hypertrophic subaortic stenosis; mitral valve[d] prolapse syndrome with mitral insufficiency	Prosthetic heart valves[e]
All dental procedures that are likely to result in gingival bleeding[a,b]	Regimen A or B[g]	Regimen B
Surgery or instrumentation of the respiratory tract[f]	Regimen A or B	Regimen B

[a] Does not include shedding of deciduous teeth.

[b] Does not include simple adjustment of orthodontic appliances.

[c] For example, ventricular septal defect, tetralogy of Fallot, aortic stenosis, pulmonic stenosis, complex cyanotic heart disease, patent ductus arteriosus or systemic to pulmonary artery shunts. Does not include uncomplicated secundum atrial septal defect.

[d] Although cases of infective endocarditis in patients with mitral valve prolapse syndrome have been documented, the incidence appears to be relatively low and the necessity for prophylaxis in all of these patients has not yet been established.

[e] Some patients with a prosthetic heart valve in whom a high level of oral health is being maintained may be offered oral antibiotic prophylaxis for routine dental procedures except the following: parenteral antibiotics are recommended for patients with prosthetic valves who require extensive dental procedures, especially extractions, or oral or gingival surgical procedures.

[f] Tonsillectomy, adenoidectomy, bronchoscopy, and other surgical procedures of the upper respiratory tract involving disruption of the respiratory mucosa.

[g] See Table 10.3.

Table 10.5.
Antibiotic Regimen for Gastrointestinal and Genitourinary Tract Surgery and Instrumentation[a]

Adults: Aqueous crystalline penicillin G (2,000,000 units intramuscularly or intravenously or ampicillin (1.0 g intramuscularly or intravenously) *plus* gentamicin [1.5 mg/kg (not to exceed 80 mg) intramuscularly or intravenously] *or* streptomycin (1.0 g, intramuscularly)

Give initial doses 30 min to 1 hr prior to procedure. If gentamicin is used then give a similar dose of gentamicin and penicillin (or ampicillin) every 8 hr for 2 additional doses.[b] If streptomycin is used then give a similar dose of streptomycin and penicillin (or ampicillin) every 12 hr for two additional doses[b]

Children[c]: Aqueous crystalline penicillin G (30,000 units/kg) intramuscularly or intravenously *or* ampicillin (50 mg/kg intramuscularly or intravenously) *plus* gentamicin (2.0 mg/kg intramuscularly). Timing of doses for children is the same as for adults[a]

For Those Patients Who Are Allergic To Penicillin[b]

Adults: Vancomycin (1.0 g intravenously given over 30 min to 1 hr) *plus* streptomycin (1.0 g intramuscularly). A single dose of these antibiotics begun 30 min to 1 hr prior to the procedure is probably sufficient, but the same dose may be repeated in 12 hr[b]

Children[d]: Vancomycin (20 mg/kg given intravenously over 30 min to 1 hr) *plus* streptomycin (20 mg/kg intramuscularly). Timing of doses for children is the same as for adults[a]

---

[a] In patients with significantly compromised renal function, it may be necessary to modify the dose of antibiotics used. Some of these doses may exceed manufacturer's recommendations for a 24-hr period. However, since they are only recommended for a 24-hr period in most cases it is unlikely that toxicity will occur.
[b] During prolonged procedures, or in the case of delayed healing, it may be necessary to provide doses of antibiotics. For brief outpatient procedures such as uncomplicated catheterization of the bladder 1 dose may be sufficient.
[c] Doses for children should not exceed recommendations for adults for a single dose or for a 24-hr period.
[d] For vancomycin the total dose for children should not exceed 40 mg/kg/24 hr.

---

experiments in the rabbit model. Nevertheless, the American Heart Association (AHA) recommends the use of prophylactic antimicrobials prior to, during and after a procedure likely to produce a bacteremia (29). The AHA guidelines for prophylaxis are given in Tables 10.3 to 10.5.

No specific recommendations are made for cardiac surgery other than to direct short-term (3 days or less) prophylaxis against staphylococci, with a penicillinase-resistant penicillin or a cephalosporin.

Prophylaxis is not indicated for "clean" surgeries such as thyroidectomies; however, it is indicated for surgery or manipulation of infected or contaminated tissues.

Alternatively, Petersdorf (30) has outlined a less aggressive set of regimens than the AHA which may be more reasonable and practical considering cost factors and patient compliance.

References

1. Weinstein L, Schlesinger JJ: Pathoanatomic, pathophysiologic, and clinical correlations in endocarditis. *N Engl J Med* 291:832, 1974.
2. Sande MA, Scheld WM: Bacterial adherance in endocarditis: interaction of bacterial dextran, platelets, fibrin, and antibody. *Scand J Infect Dis Suppl* 24:100, 1980.
3. Von Reyn CF, Levy BS, Arbeit Rd, et al: Infective endocarditis: analysis based on strict case definitions. *Ann Intern Med* 94:505, 1981.
4. Kaplan EL, Rich H, Gersony W, et al: A collaborative study of infective endocarditis in the 1970's: emphasis on infections in patients who have undergone cardiovascular surgery. *Circulation* 59:327, 1979.
5. Hubbell G, Cheitlin MD, Rapaport E: Presentation, management, and followup evaluation of infective endocarditis in drug addicts. *Am Heart J* 102:85, 1981.
6. Lange M, Salaki JS, Middleton JR, et al: Infective endocarditis in heroin addicts: epidemiologic observations and some unusual cases. *Am Heart J* 96:144, 1978.
7. Geraci JE, Wilson WR: Endocarditis due to gram-negative bacteria: report of 56 cases. *Mayo Clinic Proc* 57:145, 1982.
8. Masur H, Johnson WD: Prosthetic valve endocarditis. *J. Thorac Cardiovasc Surg* 80:31, 1980.
9. Wilson WR, Danielson GK, Giuliani ER, et al: Prosthetic valve endocarditis. *Mayo Clinic Proc* 57:155, 1982.
10. Iannini PB, Crossley K: Therapy of S. aureus bacteremia associated with a removable focus of infection. *Ann Intern Med* 38:281, 1976.
11. Watanakunakorn C, Baird IM: *Staphylococcus aureus* bacteremia and endocarditis associated

with a removable infected intravenous device. *Am J Med* 63:253, 1977.

12. Van Scoy RE: Culture-negative endocarditis. *Mayo Clin Proc* 57:149, 1982.

13. Pazin GJ, Saul S, Thompson ME: Blood culture positivity: suppression by outpatient antibiotic therapy in patients with bacterial endocarditis. *Arch Intern Med* 142:263, 1982.

14. Wilson WR, Nichols DR, Thompson RL, et al: Infective endocarditis: therapeutic considerations. *Am Heart J* 100:689, 1980.

15. Jordan GW, Kawachi MM: Analysis of serum bactericidal activity in endocarditis, osteomyelitis and other bacterial infections. *Medicine* 60:49,1981.

16. Karchmer AW, Moellering RC, Maki DG, et al: Single-antibiotic therapy for streptococcal endocarditis. *JAMA* 241:1801, 1979.

17. Bisno AL, Dismukes WE, Durack DT, et al: Treatment of infective endocarditis due to viridans streptococci. *Circulation* 63:730A, 1981.

18. Malacoff RF, Frank E, Andriole VT: Streptococcal endocarditis (nonenterococcal, non group A); single vs combination therapy. *JAMA* 241:1807, 1979.

19. Wilson WR, Thompson RL, Wilkowske CJ, et al: Short term therapy for streptococcal infective endocarditis-combined intramuscular administration of penicillin and streptomycin. *JAMA* 245:360, 1981.

20. Sande MA, Schild WM: Combination antibiotic therapy of bacterial endocarditis. *Ann Intern Med* 92:390, 1980.

21. Barriere SL, Conte JE Jr: Absence of nafcillin associated nephritis: a prospective analysis of 210 consecutive patients. *West J Med* 133:472, 1980.

22. Abrams B, Sklaver A, Hoffman T, et al: Single or combination therapy of staphylococcal endocarditis in intravenous drug abusers. *Ann Intern Med* 90:789, 1979.

23. Kaye D: The clinical significance of tolerance of *Staphylococcus aureus*. *Ann Intern Med* 93:924, 1980.

24. Massanari RM, Donta ST: The efficacy of rifampin as adjunctive therapy in selected cases of staphylococcal endocarditis. *Chest* 73:371, 1978.

25. Dinubile MJ: Surgery in active endocarditis. *Ann Intern Med* 96:650, 1982.

26. Brogden RN, Heel RC, Speight TM, et al: Metronidazole in anaerobic infections: a review of its activity, pharmacokinetics, and therapeutic use. *Drugs* 16:387, 1978.

27. Rolfe RD, Finegold SM: Comparative in vitro activity of new β-lactam antibiotics against anaerobic bacteria. *Antimicrob Agents Chemother* 20:60, 1981.

28. Conte JE Jr: Prophylaxis of endocarditis during surgical and dental procedures. *West J Med* 133:141, 1980.

29. Kaplan EL: Prevention of bacterial endocarditis—AHA committee report. *Circulation* 56:139A, 1977.

30. Petersdorf RG: Antimicrobial prophylaxis of bacterial endocarditis. Prudent caution of bacterial overkill. *Am J Med* 65:220, 1978.

General Reference

Scheld WM, Sande MA: Endocarditis and intravascular infection. In Mandell GA, Douglas RG, Bennett JE: *Principles and Practice of Infectious Diseases.* New York: John Wiley & Sons, 1981, ch 51.

CHAPTER 11

Tuberculosis

DAVID S. TATRO, Pharm.D

Chemotherapy is central to the diagnosis, treatment and prevention of tuberculosis. Since drugs play such an important role in the treatment of tuberculosis, it is essential that the practicing pharmacist have a thorough knowledge of the disease as well as its treatment. The pharmacist is in an ideal position to monitor drug usage and may be the first to learn of an adverse reaction that a patient is experiencing as a result of drug therapy. In addition, there is a move away from long hospitalization in the management of patients with tuberculosis toward more prolonged outpatient treatment. Along with this shift, there is a decrease in the number of physicians specializing in this area and an increase in the need for other members of the health profession to become more familiar with the management and treatment of tuberculosis.

Tuberculosis is an infection caused by *Mycobacterium tuberculosis*. The disease derives its name from the characteristic lesion that is formed—the tubercle. When infection occurs, the host response leads to the formation of cells around the bacilli in an attempt to keep the reaction localized. In most instances, infection stops at this point, leaving its characteristic scar. If the host response is unable to halt the infection, growth continues and an active case of infectious tuberculosis develops.

ETIOLOGY AND PATHOGENESIS

Any infection caused by *M. tuberculosis* is referred to as tuberculosis. Three types of tubercle bacilli are pathogenic to man—human, bovine, and avian. Avian tuberculosis is extremely rare in the United States, and, with the advent of pasteurization of milk and testing of cows, the human type has become the more significant. The most prevalent means of spreading tuberculosis between individuals is by coughing and sneezing. The sputum of actively infected patients is contaminated with many bacilli. These droplets are airborne and may be inhaled by unsuspecting persons. If the organisms in the inhaled droplets reach the bronchioles or alveoli, these people may develop tuberculous infection; however, if the bacilli only contact the upper bronchi, they will be eliminated without subsequent infection (1).

Since the tuberculous bacillus is an aerobe, the high oxygen tension in the apices of the lungs offers an ideal environment for harboring the organism; however, even though pulmonary infection is most common, tuberculosis may affect any organ in the body. With few exceptions, the infecting organism gains entry into the body via the lungs. It is here that primary tuberculosis is established. From the lungs, infection spreads to other organs by way of the lymphatic system and the bloodstream.

At this stage, the infection usually becomes dormant, and immunity, on the part of the host, prevents further spread. The lesions may become walled off by the production of fibrous tissue and calcification. The time during which tuberculosis remains dormant varies greatly. Organisms may remain inactive for the life of the host or, following a breakdown in the host's defenses, they may become reactivated at any time. Three to 10% of the patients infected will develop the disease within the first year, and the incidence decreases with subsequent years (2).

Following the period of dormancy, reactivation of a latent infection may take one of two courses—chronic tuberculosis or miliary tuberculosis. The factors allowing recurrence of infection are not completely understood; however, a breakdown in the host's immune mechanism is an important factor. Thus, reactivation is more common in patients suffering from or recovering from another illness. Reactivation may also occur in a patient receiving immunosuppressive drugs or steroid therapy.

CHRONIC TUBERCULOSIS

Although chronic tuberculosis may develop in any organ of the body, the most frequently encountered sites are those with the greatest oxygen tension. Therefore, the kidneys and brain provide a suitable environment in which M. tuberculosis may grow. When the primary infection occurs during childhood, the epiphysis of the long bones (wrist, elbow, knee) and spine is undergoing rapid growth. The oxygen tension at these sites is high and may harbor the tubercle bacilli. Tuberculosis may remain dormant in these areas for many decades only to manifest itself in the elderly patient.

Other organs involved in tuberculosis include lymph nodes, meninges, skin, peritoneum, eyes, larynx, pericardium, adrenal glands and gastrointestinal tract. The infection of these sites by the invading organism results from the spread of small quantities of tubercle bacilli by hematogenous dissemination.

MILIARY TUBERCULOSIS

It is also possible for large numbers of bacilli to be released from a primary focus, spreading throughout the body. The occurrence of this is referred to as miliary tuberculosis.

Like chronic tuberculosis, miliary tuberculosis may develop any time after primary infection. However, the occurrence of this form of tuberculosis is seen most frequently in children under 4 years of age. It is most feared by clinicians since death may rapidly ensue.

INCIDENCE

Presently, the incidence of tuberculosis is steadily declining. Although many adults still demonstrate a positive tuberculin test, the prevalence of these adult reactors is much less than it was in 1900. In many instances, adults showing positive reactions to the tuberculin skin test acquired their primary infection as children. It has been estimated by the Center for Disease Control that approximately 15,000,000 Americans are infected with tuberculosis and that 70% of these individuals are over 35 years old (3). Ninety-eight percent of the people under 20 years of age show negative tuberculin skin tests (4). Each year, over 20,000 people in the United States become newly infected with tuberculosis.

Many factors are responsible for the declining rate of tuberculosis in today's society. Some of these considerations are listed in Table 11.1. Tuberculosis now tends to occur within a family, rather than in the epidemic proportions of the past. Thus, several children living under the same roof may become infected owing to a common contact with an infectious adult (parent, grandparent). The decreasing incidence of tuberculin-positive skin tests in 16-year-olds in the 40 years from 1928 to 1968 may well reflect the decreasing threat of tuberculosis in young patients (Table 11.2).

DIAGNOSIS AND CLINICAL FINDINGS

Signs and symptoms that may be present in tuberculosis include malaise, fever, anorexia, fatigue, nausea, night sweats and weight loss. However, it should be noted that, in either primary or chronic tuberculosis, patients may be asymptomatic. Indeed, symptoms may be absent even in the presence of extensive infection. Most cases of asymptomatic childhood infections are uncovered during routine physical examinations.

Skin Tests

Tuberculin and its purified protein derivative (PPD) are used for the diagnosis of tuberculosis. Intradermal injection of tuberculin or PPD in individuals infected with M. tuberculosis will elicit a positive response (5). This reaction represents a cutaneous hypersensitivity to bacterial protein from the culture media. Multiple puncture techniques such as the Tine or Heaf tests are difficult to interpret because inoculations contain an unstandardized amount of tuberculin. Therefore, to ensure uniformity in testing in tuberculosis control

Table 11.1.
Factors Contributing to the Decreasing Incidence of Tuberculosis

1. Effective antitubercular drugs
2. Rapid identification of disease
3. Adequate nutrition
4. Less crowded living conditions
5. Declining rate of infection in adults
6. Vaccination
7. Isolation of infectious cases

Table 11.2.
Tuberculin-Positive Tests in 16-Year-Old Patients

Year	Incidence of Positive Test Results (%)
1928	53
1948	16.4
1968	1.4

programs and private practice, a stabilized form of PPD is recommended.

Test materials are isolated from a broth in which human strains of *M. tuberculosis* are cultured. The tubercle bacilli are grown in the synthetic medium and later precipitated in ammonium sulfate. The PPD is then obtained from the filtrates of the heat-killed cultures. Since tuberculoprotein is adsorbed onto glass and plastic, Tween 80 is added as a stabilizing agent to minimize the loss of material to the container, ensuring greater consistency in the strength of the administered dose, and resulting in less false-negative skin tests (4, 6). Tuberculin should be stored in its original container and injected immediately after transfer into a syringe. Following the intracutaneous injection of the appropriate dilution of test materials, one waits 48 to 72 hours before interpreting the results. For the initial intradermal tuberculin test it is customary to use 5 tuberculin units (TU), PPD intermediate, per test dose. The 1 TU (first strength PPD) per dose is used for individuals suspected of being highly sensitive since larger initial doses may result in severe skin reactions. The 250 TU (second strength PPD) per test dose should be used exclusively for testing individuals who fail to react to a previous injection of either 1 TU and/or 5 TU. It should never be used for the initial injection.

In keeping with the criteria established by the U.S. Public Health Service for interpreting tuberculin reactions, a positive response is indicated by an induration of 10 mm or more. For patients with reactions of 5 to 9 mm, it is considered doubtful that they have tuberculosis; while a test less than 5 mm is taken to be negative. Since considering the results of a test to be "doubtful" (5 to 9 mm) would not aid in the diagnosis of the disease, it would be in the patient's best interest to accept a palpable induration of greater than 5 mm as a positive reaction. A positive reaction to very low concentrations (e.g., PPD first strength, 1 TU) of material supports a diagnosis of active tuberculosis. A slight reaction (induration of 5 to 9 mm to a skin test with PPD intermediate) or no reaction to a low concentration of test substance is an indication for retesting with the next highest concentration (e.g., PPD second strength). Severe local reactions to PPD skin testing can be treated with topical steroids (4). Positive test results on either test dosage are an indication for further diagnostic testing.

Common diagnostic errors which would lead one to interpret the results of a skin test for *M. tuberculosis* as positive in the absence of infection are listed in Table 11.3.

The greatest value of tuberculin testing probably can be attributed to a negative test. With very few exceptions, the lack of a response to either the 5 TU or 250 TU solutions rules out active tuberculosis. It should be noted, however, that as many as 20% of the patients with active *M. tuberculosis* may fail to respond to the stabilized intermediate strength PPD. Nearly all of these nonreactive patients will respond to additional testing with the second strength (6). A negative test may be seen in severe tuberculosis (i.e., miliary tuberculosis) where the body's defense mechanisms are overwhelmed. Patients receiving corticosteroids or immunosuppressive therapy may also show false-negative skin tests. The most frequent reasons for false-negative results to tuberculin skin testing are listed in Table 11.3 (4, 7).

Bacterial Infection

Isolation of *M. tuberculosis* from an infected site provides positive proof of tuberculosis in the patient. The most frequent source of the bacillus is sputum and tracheal or gastric washings. Material from washings or biopsy

Table 11.3.
Diagnostic Errors when Interpreting Skin Tests for *Mycobacterium tuberculosis*

Factors resulting in a positive interpretation:
1. Previous BCG vaccination
2. Mycobacterial infection other than *M. tuberculosis* (e.g., *Mycobacterium kansasii*)

Factors leading to inhibition of tuberculin reactions:
1. Overwhelming tuberculosis infection (immunologic blockade)
2. Administration of corticosteroids, immunosuppressive therapy, or cytotoxic agents
3. Vaccinations with live virus
4. Early infection with tuberculosis where hypersensitivity has not yet developed
5. Presence of a concurrent disease that depresses cell-mediated immunity (e.g., chronic renal failure)
6. Incorrect reading of skin test results
7. Administering an insufficient amount of tuberculin
8. Anergy

should be cultured for identification of the acid-fast bacillus.

Mycobacterial infections by organisms other than M. tuberculosis are also possible. These have been categorized as "unclassified," "anonymous," "opportunistic," or "atypical" mycobacterium infections. Examples of Mycobacterium other than M. tuberculosis include Mycobacterium kansasii, Mycobacterium scrofulaceum, Mycobacterium batteyi (Battey bacillus) and Mycobacterium fortuitum. Infections by these organisms are not known to be communicable, and, it is, therefore, not necessary to isolate patients. Although some of the infections are very similar to M. tuberculosis on clinical and radiographic appearances (8), response to drug therapy is frequently unpredictable, and surgical excision is necessary. Infections by "opportunistic" mycobacteria may result in pulmonary disease (e.g., M. kansasii) or lymphadenitis (e.g., M. scrofulaceum) or both pulmonary disease and lymphadenitis (M. batteyi) (8). These other mycobacterial infections may result in a positive skin test for tuberculosis (9).

X-rays

Chest x-rays are valuable in the identification of pulmonary tuberculosis. Repeated films are usually necessary to establish the presence of the disease. X-rays are essential in evaluating the progress of therapy.

COMPLICATIONS

The complications associated with tuberculosis are dependent on the organ involved. A complete discussion covering every conceivable complication in conjunction with each vulnerable organ is beyond the scope of this chapter. However, the most frequent and serious complications will be considered.

In active pulmonary tuberculosis, necrosis with liquefaction develops. As this fluid empties, cavities remain. Arteries to the resulting cavities may burst, causing frank pulmonary hemorrhage. Atelectasis is a further complication associated with respiratory lesions.

A similar process occurs with renal involvement. When lesions are in the kidney, cavitation may also occur. Ruptured blood vessels in this area lead to hematuria.

When tuberculosis strikes the lining of organs in the body, such as the peritoneum, pleura and pericardium, several types of complications may result. Tuberculous peritonitis may take two forms—wet or dry. In the wet form, serous fluid is present in the abdominal cavity and numerous white tubercles are spread over the peritoneal surface. The dry form of peritonitis is characterized by little effusion of fluid. However, numerous adhesions may form between peritoneal surfaces or fibrous membranes which will lead to constriction and impairment of intestinal motility. In infants and children, if the abdominal lymph nodes are infected with tuberculosis, the consequence may be life-threatening. When the lining of the heart is involved, its function can be seriously impeded by the formation of inelastic fibrous tissue. However, once again, the course of infection is variable and may instead result in large amounts of fluid accumulating in the pericardium.

Two very serious complications are miliary tuberculosis and tuberculosis meningitis. Miliary tuberculosis (discussed earlier) is a hematogenous disease, allowing widespread infection throughout the body. In tuberculosis meningitis, fluid collects around the base of the brain causing adhesion. Since these lesions are in the area of the hypothalamus, fatal brain damage may occur.

There is a high incidence of tuberculosis in patients with Addison's disease. Infection leads to progressive destruction of the gland with resulting adrenal cortical insufficiency. Patients with Addison's disease must be routinely tested for tuberculosis.

TREATMENT

Drug therapy is indicated for all forms of tuberculosis. Patients will receive antitubercular therapy for extended periods of time, usually in excess of 1 year. Because of the long duration of treatment, special attention must be directed to dose-related side effects (Table 11.4).

In many instances, the selection of drugs to be used in tuberculosis is based on their toxicity. Medication with the most serious and frequent side effects is generally reserved for treatment of resistant organisms.

Aminosalicylic Acid

In combination with isoniazid and streptomycin, p-aminosalicylic acid (PAS) delays the emergence of resistant strains of tuberculosis. However, there is little need for this drug in

Table 11.4.
Drugs Used in the Treatment of Tuberculosis

Drug	Dosage	Duration	Special Considerations
Aminosalicylic acid, K^+ = 25%, Ca^{2+} = 30%	*Adult:* 4 g t.i.d. PO (25% higher if salts are used) *Child:* 200 mg/kg/24 hr PO	24 mo	Gastrointestinal side effects are frequent
Capreomycin	*Adult:* 15 mg/kg/24 hr IM (1 g maximum) *Child:* 15 mg/kg/24 hr IM (1 g maximum)	24 mo	Monitoring of renal and eighth nerve function is indicated
Cycloserine	*Adult:* 250 mg 2–4 times daily PO (1 g maximum) *Child:* 10–20 mg/kg/24 hr PO (500 mg maximum)	18–24 mo	Reduce dosage in renal impairment
Ethambutol	*Adult:* 25 mg/kg/24 hr PO, then 15 mg/kg/24 hr PO (may give as a single dose) *Child:* 20 mg/kg/24 hr PO, then 15 mg/kg/24 hr PO	For up to 2 mo then for remainder of therapy Up to 2 mo then for remainder of therapy	Frequent tests for ocular changes are indicated
Ethionamide	*Adult:* 250 mg t.i.d. or q.i.d. PO or rectal (may give as single dose) *Child:* 15–30 mg/kg/24 hr PO or rectal	24 mo	Perform liver function tests frequently
Isoniazid (INH)	*Adult:* 300 mg daily PO (may give as single dose) *Child:* 10–20 mg/kg/24 hr PO (300 mg maximum)	12–24 mo; 24 mo for miliary tuberculosis or meningitis	Administer with pyridoxine 10 mg/100 mg isoniazid
Kanamycin	*Adult:* 7.5–15 mg/kg/24 hr IM (usually give 1 g 3–5 times/wk) *Child:* 7.5–15 mg/kg/24 hr IM	18–24 mo	Audiometric tests should be performed
Pyrazinamide	*Adult:* 2 g/24 hr PO (maximum 35 mg/kg/24 hr, but not more than 3 g) *Child:* 20–30 mg/kg/24 hr PO (2 g maximum)	18–24 mo	Fatal hepatic reactions may occur; liver function should be monitored
Rifampin	*Adult:* 600 mg/24 hr PO *Child:* 10–20 mg/kg/24 hr PO (600 mg maximum)	12–24 mo	Complete blood counts should be performed
Streptomycin	*Adult:* 1 g/24 hr IM then 1 g 2–3 times/wk *Child:* 20–40 mg/kg/24 hr IM	Until 1 mo after negative culture then for remainder of therapy	Audiometric tests and tests for vestibular function are important

current therapy. Although PAS is widely distributed in body fluids following oral administration, drug levels within cells are low and therapeutic concentrations are not achieved. Like isoniazid, PAS is metabolized by acetylation. Therefore, concurrent administration of the two drugs will increase the plasma levels of isoniazid. However, at this point, clinical data are lacking as to whether this elevation is of any benefit. The most frequently encountered adverse reactions are nausea, vomiting, diarrhea and anorexia. These untoward effects may be circumvented by careful adjustments of dosages. In some instances, where gastrointestinal reactions persist, it may be necessary to discontinue therapy. Aminosalicylic acid-induced hepatitis and blood dyscrasias may also occur. One may observe acute tubulointerstitial toxicity as a rare hypersensitivity re-action (10–13). Potassium loss and other elec-trolyte disturbances have also been seen with administration of PAS. Since these complica-tions are dependent upon the manner in which PAS is excreted in the urine when given as the acid per se, the drug is usually given as the sodium salt which will minimize these reactions. However, patients with cardiovas-cular disease cannot tolerate the increased so-dium load. Thus, other salts or drugs should be selected for these patients.

Capreomycin

The antitubercular drug capreomycin is poorly absorbed following oral administration and is, therefore, given by intramuscular in-jection. Tubercle bacilli resistant to capreo-mycin are also resistant to kanamycin. Like streptomycin, this antitubercular drug may cause vestibular damage. Since capreomycin is excreted by the kidneys, the dose must be reduced in renal impairment to prevent loss of hearing. Tubular toxicity, as a direct nephro-toxic reaction, has been infrequently reported (10, 13).

Cycloserine

Absorption occurs readily following oral ad-ministration. This drug is well distributed throughout body fluids and tissue, including the cerebrospinal fluid. However, in the treat-ment of tuberculosis, cycloserine appears to be less effective than streptomycin (14). Serious side effects include neurological manifesta-tions, such as anxiety, depression, convulsions and psychoses. Additional adverse reactions include dizziness, headache, insomnia, slurred speech and tremor. Since cycloserine decom-poses in the presence of moisture, it must be dispensed and stored under dry conditions.

Ethambutol

Ethambutol is a frequently used oral agent in tuberculosis chemotherapy. Previously, ocular side effects limited the widespread use of this compound. However, in the dosages currently administered (15 to 25 mg/kg/day) ocular toxicity has not been a problem. When considering the ocular side effects, two types of retrobulbar neuritis are manifest. In one instance, there is a constriction in peripheral vision while in the other, there is a loss of visual acuity. In the latter type, central sco-toma and green color-blindness may also oc-cur. Monthly eye examinations should accom-pany therapy. Acute tubulointerstitial toxicity has been reported with ethambutol therapy. The mechanism is not known (10, 13, 15, 16).

Therapeutic doses of ethambutol have been shown to cause mild elevations in serum uric acid levels (17). In one study the majority of significant increases occurred between the first day and third week of therapy. Fifty per-cent of the patients studied were classified as hyperuricemic—none demonstrated symp-toms of gout. Elevated serum uric acid levels were seen in patients receiving ethambutol alone and in combination with isoniazid and pyridoxine. Drug regimens containing etham-butol should be suspected when hyperuri-cemia occurs.

Ethionamide

The greatest incidence and variety of side effects occur with this drug. The most fre-quently encountered untoward reactions are those affecting the gastrointestinal tract. These include nausea, vomiting, and diarrhea, as well as increased salivation and metallic taste. In addition, loss of appetite and cramps may be experienced. These adversities appear to be mediated through the central nervous system and occur even with parenteral administration of ethionamide. Other adverse reactions in-clude convulsions, diplopia, deafness, hypo-tension, gynecomastia, peripheral neuritis, im-potence and hepatitis. Dermatological reac-tions consist of photosensitivity, alopecia and acneform eruptions. Although ethionamide is absorbed orally and is distributed to all body tissues and fluids, its use should be limited to that of a second-line drug when no preferable alternative is available.

Isoniazid

To date, isoniazid (INH) is still the most effective drug for the treatment of tuberculo-sis. It may be administered as either a 100-mg dosage 3 times daily, or a 300-mg dosage once daily. Neither regimen alters the efficacy of the drug. However, a single daily dose offers greater convenience to the patient and possi-bly results in better compliance.

Rapid absorption occurs after oral adminis-tration of the drug. Isoniazid is widely distrib-uted in the body, with therapeutic levels achieved in all tissues and fluid including skin, feces, urine and saliva. Although patients vary in the rate at which they metabolize (acetylate) this drug, this does not appear to be of therapeutic significance. However, it is noteworthy that slow metabolizers appear to develop pyridoxine deficiency anemia with a greater frequency than normal acetylators. Peripheral neuritis resembling pyridoxine deficiency is also encountered with high doses of this antitubercular agent. In those patients considered to be at risk of developing peripheral neuritis, concomitant administration of pyridoxine, 10 mg/100 mg of isoniazid daily, will prevent the reaction. Other side effects which have been encountered are nausea, anorexia, cutaneous reactions, optic neuritis, systemic lupus erythematosus, drug fever, methemoglobinemia, agranulocytosis, acute tubulointerstitial toxicity, and liver damage.

Both retrospective and prospective studies indicate that isoniazid can cause liver damage (18, 19). The mechanism of isoniazid-induced hepatitis remains ill-defined (20). In patients receiving isoniazid significant elevations in serum glutamic oxaloacetic transaminase (SGOT) levels may occur in up to 20%. In most instances SGOT levels will return to normal or remain slightly elevated with continued therapy. Elevated SGOT, in the absence of any signs or symptoms, is not necessarily an indication for withdrawal of the antitubercular drug; however, concomitant symptoms, such as markedly abnormal liver function tests, liver enlargement with tenderness, jaundice, dark urine, tiredness, fever, chills, nausea, vomiting, or loss of appetite, are indications for discontinuing isoniazid (18, 19, 21). Cessation of therapy with the first signs of isoniazid-induced hepatitis will usually result in reversal of the adversity; continuation of the drug may be fatal. Most reactions resemble viral hepatitis and occur in the first 3 months of therapy. Patients should be monitored and questioned most closely for signs and symptoms of hepatitis during this period (18, 19, 21). Isoniazid hepatitis is seen with the greatest frequency in persons older than 35 years (22). Approximately 1% of patients receiving isoniazid may develop liver damage (23).

An interesting interaction may occur when phenytoin and isoniazid are administered concurrently. The incidence of phenytoin toxicity is increased 10-fold when usual dosages of the two drugs are given simultaneously (24, 25). A possible mechanism for this reaction is the inhibition of phenytoin metabolism, allowing plasma concentrations to increase to toxic levels. Monitoring the patient and reduction of anticonvulsant dosage will result in adequate drug therapy.

Kanamycin

This antitubercular drug is administered parenterally. The long-term use of kanamycin is limited by the various side effects that include vestibular damage, ototoxicity and nephrotoxicity. Ethacrynic acid and furosemide can also produce ototoxicity. Thus, patients receiving concurrent therapy with kanamycin and ethacrynic acid or furosemide should be monitored closely to avoid deafness (26). Respiratory paralysis may result when kanamycin and curareform skeletal muscle relaxants are administered jointly (27). These drugs should be used with particular caution in surgical patients. Since kanamycin is excreted by the kidney, dosage must be carefully adjusted to avoid toxic reactions in patients with renal insufficiency.

Pyrazinamide

This drug can be administered orally. However, since fatal hepatic reactions have occurred, its use in the treatment of tuberculosis has been limited. Elevated plasma uric acid levels and gout may also result from the administration of pyrazinamide. Other reported reactions include cutaneous hypersensitivity, photosensitivity, flushing, nausea, vomiting, anorexia and arthralgia.

Presently, pyrazinamide is available for distribution only from the manufacturer directly to hospitals. Therapy is to be initiated in hospitalized patients and frequent tests of liver function are to be performed.

Rifampin

Rifampin is one of the more important of the newer antitubercular agents. Clinical findings indicate that this drug may have an efficacy similar to isoniazid. Rifampin is readily absorbed following oral administration. As a pediatric dosage form, pharmacists may prepare capsules, the contents of which can be mixed with applesauce or jelly. Also, a suspension containing 10 mg/ml of rifampin can be prepared by emptying the contents of 4 rifampin

300-mg capsules into a 4-oz amber bottle; adding 20 ml of simple syrup and shaking vigorously, followed by an additional 100 ml of simple syrup, once again shaking. The suspension should be stored at 2 to 8°C (36 to 46°F) for no more than 6 weeks. The suspension should be shaken vigorously before withdrawal of each dose (28). It has a wide distribution in the body reaching most organs, body fluids and cerebrospinal fluid. The incidence of side effects with daily administration of rifampin is apparently low. Reported adverse reactions include cutaneous reactions and gastrointestinal disturbances, such as nausea, vomiting, diarrhea, "heartburn" and loss of appetite. These reactions are seldom severe enough to require discontinuation of treatment. More serious side effects include blood dyscrasias, hearing defects, and hepatic damage. The possibility that rifampin may contribute to isoniazid hepatotoxicity has been raised (29, 30) and further clinical study of this potential additive toxicity is needed (31). In addition to liver toxicity, rifampin may also cause a false elevation in the bromsulfophthalein excretion test since the antitubercular drug competes with bilirubin and bromsulfophthalein for excretion via the liver (32). Patients should be warned that rifampin causes an orange discoloration of the urine, tears and perspiration. Soft contact lenses may become stained. The high cost of rifampin has led to the investigation of alternative dosing schedules (33). Intermittent regimens consisting of rifampin once or twice weekly have resulted in lower total weekly doses of rifampin but have also been associated with a higher incidence of hypersensitivity reactions (33). Adversities consist of a flu-like syndrome, cutaneous eruptions, renal toxicity (including tubular necrosis or interstitial nephritis), and blood dyscrasias (thrombocytopenia and hemolytic anemia) (33, 34). Rifampin-dependent antibodies have been demonstrated by an indirect antiglobulin test in a patient experiencing prolonged, acute renal failure (35). Similarly, immunoglobulin (IgG and IgM) antibodies capable of fixing complement in the presence of the patient's red blood cells and platelets have been found in patients with rifampin-induced hemolytic anemia and thrombocytopenia (36). Because of the increased incidence in immune reactions associated with intermittent administration of rifampin, it is felt, at this time, that this type of dosing schedule should not be used.

Streptomycin

Like kanamycin and capreomycin, streptomycin is poorly absorbed from the gastrointestinal tract. It is, therefore, administered by intramuscular injection. Streptomycin will not cross the blood-brain barrier unless the meninges are inflamed. Its use, for this reason, is limited in tuberculosis involving the central nervous system. The most serious side effect encountered with streptomycin therapy is eighth nerve damage leading to loss of vestibular function. Deafness may also be encountered, although less frequently than with kanamycin. Streptomycin-induced nephrotoxicity has been reported; observations demonstrate the presence of proximal tubular necrosis (13, 37, 38).

As with kanamycin therapy, ethacrynic acid and furosemide should be administered with caution to patients receiving streptomycin since loss of hearing may result. Neuromuscular blockage leading to respiratory paralysis can occur when curareform skeletal muscle relaxants are given concurrently with streptomycin therapy. Thorough drug histories are essential in patients about to receive preoperative relaxants. Neuromuscular blockade occurring with the aminoglycoside antibiotics may be reversed by neostigmine and atropine administration.

Dosage adjustments are necessary in patients with impaired renal function since streptomycin is excreted via the kidneys. Vestibular damage and deafness occur more frequently in patients with renal insufficiency, unless the dose is reduced.

Resistant strains of *M. tuberculosis* develop rapidly if streptomycin is used alone. It should, therefore, always be administered in combination with another antitubercular drug.

Corticosteroids

In the treatment of certain life-threatening and severe infections, steroids are administered. Prednisone is the most frequently used oral agent, although therapeutically equivalent dosages of other corticosteroids may be substituted with the same clinical response. When used, these medications are given for their anti-inflammatory action.

Treatment Regimens

Once the diagnosis of tuberculosis is established, prompt treatment with antituberculosis agents is instituted (Table 11.4). These drugs are bacteriostatic. As such, they exert their action by arresting the growth of M. tuberculosis, while relying on host response to eradicate the infection and repair tissue. Because this process is slow, medication is administered on a long-term basis. It will be necessary for patients to continue drug therapy for 12 months to 2 years. Clinical trials utilizing short-term treatment regimens with two or three drugs for time periods of as little as 6 months are still under investigation. Although initial results are encouraging, more study is needed before any recommendations can be made for short-course chemotherapy using drugs other than isoniazid, ethambutol, and rifampin (see Table 11.4). If treatment failures occur, they tend to be seen soon after completion of the regimen; therefore, patients should be monitored for one year after the completion of therapy (39–42).

As in choosing any anti-infective agent, drugs should be selected on the basis of culture and sensitivity testing in order to insure optimal therapeutic response. Tuberculosis is no exception. However, M. tuberculosis grows slowly and up to 6 weeks may elapse before results of these cultures are available. In patients with either the appropriate clinical findings or a positive acid-fast smear, therapy should be initiated prior to receiving results of culture and sensitivity tests. Appropriate adjustments in the drug regimen can be made when these data become known. Drugs to which the bacilli are resistant should be discontinued and effective drugs substituted.

Of the agents discussed in the preceding section, two have been widely used in treating tuberculosis for nearly three decades. Over the years, isoniazid and streptomycin have proven to be very efficacious. The high rate of clinical success and relatively low incidence of toxicity have led to their use in the treatment of this disease. Isoniazid is the single most effective drug, and when possible, all treatment regimens should include this medication. Ethambutol and rifampin are two antitubercular drugs that have been in use for a considerably shorter amount of time, but have shown great promise in the treatment of tuberculosis and must join isoniazid and streptomycin as first-line drugs. Ethambutol has been shown to be quite effective and somewhat less toxic than rifampin. The ocular toxicity associated with ethambutol does not appear to be as much of a concern with the lower doses (15 to 25 mg/kg/day) administered now, compared to the doses administered several years ago (50 mg/kg/day). Since rifampin inhibits RNA synthesis and is widely distributed in the body tissues and cells, clinical trials should focus on the incidence of gastrointestinal and hematological side effects that may occur. These adversities have yet to be evaluated fully.

The remaining antituberculosis agents are viewed as back-up drugs or second-line therapy by clinicians. Their use is limited to the treatment of patients with M. tuberculosis resistant to isoniazid, streptomycin, ethambutol and/or rifampin. Generally, the second-line drugs are less effective and more toxic. These drugs are acceptable companion drugs, minimizing the emergence of drug resistance. Resistance may be evidenced by culture and sensitivity tests as well as failure of the infection to respond during the treatment period. These drugs are also indicated when toxicity or hypersensitivity makes it impossible to continue with one or more of the first-line drugs.

Resistance develops rapidly to treatment with any single drug, although less frequently with isoniazid. For this reason, therapy of active disease should always be instituted with at least two drugs. This will minimize the emergence of resistance. However, there are situations, such as the prophylactic use of isoniazid, where a single agent may be used efficaciously.

Varying drug regimens consisting of one to three or more drugs may be indicated, depending on the nature and severity of infection (Table 11.5).

When a single drug is to be utilized, isoniazid is the drug of choice. Ethambutol, rifampin, or streptomycin should never be used as sole agents to treat tuberculosis since resistance develops rapidly. For the two-drug regimen, isoniazid with ethambutol or isoniazid with rifampin is the combination of choice. If an alternative drug is required, kanamycin, capreomycin, ethionamide, pyrazinamide or cycloserine should be considered. Severe infections necessitating administration of three drugs should include one of the following combinations (listed in order of decreasing preference):

> Isoniazid-ethambutol-rifampin
> Isoniazid-streptomycin-rifampin
> Isoniazid-ethambutol-streptomycin

When possible, each drug regimen should include isoniazid. Few populations of tuber-

Table 11.5.
Drug Regimen Indicated in Tuberculosis

One Drug	Two Drugs	Three Drugs
Asymptomatic primary	Skin	Miliary
Children with positive skin test	Joints and bones	Meningitis
Prophylaxis	Lymph nodes	Renal
	Chronic pulmonary	Pleural effusion
		Severe pulmonary

culosis are totally resistant to this drug (43, 44). If drug toxicity or bacterial resistance prevents use of isoniazid, either rifampin or ethambutol should be considered as an alternative to be used in combination with streptomycin. If a third drug is essential, pyrazinamide should be used.

In certain instances, it is necessary to add corticosteroids to the treatment protocol. An inflammatory response is part of the host's normal defense against tuberculosis infection. Since corticosteroids have an antiinflammatory action which may allow rapid progression of the disease if the organism is resistant to the drug being administered, they have no role in the chronic treatment of tuberculosis. However, in certain acute situations where the loss of either life or permanent function of an organ may result, steroid therapy is indicated (45). Clinical situations for which steroids may be administered are listed in Table 11.6. When necessary, corticosteroids are given concurrently with antituberculosis therapy and are administered only for short-term use until beneficial effects are achieved. At this point, steroid therapy is discontinued by tapering the dosage to circumvent serious adverse reactions that may occur from sudden drug withdrawal.

The patient's reliability in taking medication must be taken into consideration. A serious factor leading to drug-resistant tuberculosis is failure on the part of the patient to follow a prescribed drug regimen. Side effects, long duration of treatment and frequency of dosage are all factors that may contribute toward the patient's poor compliance in following the drug regimen.

The pharmacist, being physically involved in the distribution of the medication, is in an ideal position to advise the patient of the importance of following directions as prescribed. The contribution in this area is invaluable. Further, access to drug records allows determination of whether or not the time proximity for prescription renewals is consistent with the

Table 11.6.
Indications for Administration of Corticosteroids

1. Treatment of allergic reactions to antitubercular agents
2. Prevention of permanent loss of function in an organ, e.g., ocular tuberculosis
3. Life-threatening tuberculous infections:
   A. Miliary
   B. Meningitis
   C. Pleurisy with effusion
   D. Severe pulmonary

dosing regimen. Something is obviously amiss when the patient receiving 100 tablets to be taken 3 times a day returns for a renewal after a 6-month period. The patient-oriented pharmacist should not hesitate to discuss any findings of concern with both the patient and physician.

PROPHYLAXIS

The most common prophylactic measure used worldwide to prevent tuberculosis is the administration of bacillus Calmette-Guérin (BCG) vaccine. However, for a number of reasons, this vaccine has not gained wide acceptance in the United States. The vaccine is used more frequently in underdeveloped countries where there is a high rate of primary infection as well as inadequate facilities for diagnostic screening of patients with tuberculosis (45–48). BCG vaccine is a suspension of living cells of the BCG strain of bovine M. tuberculosis, maintained so as to preserve its power of sensitizing man to tuberculin while maintaining a relative nonpathogenicity to man.

Vaccination with BCG, at best, provides 80% protection against tuberculosis (49). Its routine use is not advocated. However, administration is offered to high risk patients. These individuals are in an environment where contact with tuberculosis is unavoidable. Circumstances under which this arises include children of parents with tuberculosis, family and friends of a tuberculosis patient and hospital and rest home employees where contact is likely to occur. Vaccination converts tuberculin-negative reactors to positive reactors. This is a disadvantage because skin testing of vaccinated individuals becomes meaningless. Therefore, before a patient is skin tested for tuberculosis, the patient must be questioned to determine if there is a previous history of BCG vaccination. If patients who have had a BCG vaccination have annual or intermittent tuberculin skin tests, the results of the skin test will remain positive indefinitely; however, in the absence of skin testing, 75% of patients will be tuberculin negative 10 years after BCG vaccination (7).

Since BCG is a live vaccine, the material should be boiled or sterilized prior to disposal. This will destroy any remaining live vaccine and prevent unsuspected contamination (50).

In addition to the use of BCG vaccine, the administration of isoniazid to household contacts of tuberculosis patients and positive skin test reactors in endemic areas and, of course, the isolation of patients with infectious tuberculosis have also proved to be effective preventive measures against tuberculosis. The prophylactic dose of isoniazid is 5 mg per kg per day (maximum of 300 mg/day) for up to 1 year. At this dosage level, good protection is afforded those individuals exposed to active tuberculosis. Since the incidence of isoniazid hepatotoxicity is higher in patients 35 years old or older, isoniazid prophylaxis should not be administered in this age group unless other factors are indicative of a high risk of developing tuberculosis. Currently, opinions as to whether or not the benefits of isoniazid prophylaxis outweigh the risk of isoniazid-induced hepatitis are equivocal (51, 52).

CLINICAL DILEMMAS

Pregnancy

There is a striking paucity of information regarding the safe clinical use of antitubercular drugs in pregnancy. This is in part due to the following: the populations studied are too small to allow adequate statistical handling, certain defects may not manifest for many years, fetal abnormalities occur with some frequency even in the absence of drugs, and tuberculosis itself may have adverse effects on the fetus.

The incidence of malformations associated with the use of PAS, isoniazid and streptomycin in pregnancy has been reported to be 2 to 3 times higher than normally occurs (53). However, the possibility that tuberculosis or some other undefined variable may have caused the abnormalities was not ruled out. A review of side effects of drugs on the fetus, as well as a recent case history, indicate eighth nerve damage and impaired psychomotor activity may be present in the newborn when streptomycin and isoniazid, respectively, are administered during pregnancy (54, 55). In a review of nearly 2000 reported births to mothers receiving isoniazid, ethambutol, rifampin, and streptomycin alone or in combination, it was shown that there was no significant increase in birth defects with the first three drugs (56). Streptomycin, however, was associated with mild auditory and vestibular defects. Therefore, the use of streptomycin in pregnant patients should be avoided.

In order to prevent progressive tissue damage and to minimize dissemination of the disease in the mother, as well as to reduce the likelihood of infecting the fetus and neonate, it is important to treat pregnant patients. Based upon currently available information, those drugs which appear to be safest to use during pregnancy include isoniazid, ethambutol and rifampin (57–63). However, there is evidence of teratogenicity to laboratory animals with the latter two agents. The risk of teratogenicity is reduced if treatment can be initiated after the first trimester of pregnancy and if minimally effective doses are administered (57–63). With respect to all other antitubercular drugs, their safety has not been established. Physicians must weigh the benefits to the mother against the potential harm to the unborn child in making a decision.

Renal Function

The dosages of the antitubercular drugs listed in Table 11.4 are for patients with normal kidney function. There is ample evidence indicating that the occurrence of adverse reactions to drugs increases in patients with renal impairment. Unless appropriate alteration in dosages is made, certain of the drugs used to treat tuberculosis may accumulate in the body and lead to more frequent or serious side effects. This cumulative effect of drug administration can often be circumvented by reduction in dosage, an increase in the dosing interval or a combination of these. Dosage adjustments which should be made in patients with abnormal renal function are listed in Table 11.7. Although patients with impaired renal function may be receiving lower dosages of drugs, they must still be closely observed for signs of toxicity.

Tuberculosis Meningitis

Not all drugs will pass the blood-brain barrier. Ionized and lipid-insoluble drugs do not readily transfer into the cerebrospinal fluid (CSF), whereas therapeutic concentrations of lipid-soluble compounds may be achieved. In addition, the rate of penetration is inversely related to the size of the molecule; i.e., small molecules enter more freely than do large (64). The picture is further complicated in that, although some drugs may not gain access into the CSF of healthy individuals, they do enter in patients with inflamed meninges (tuberculosis meningitis). The agents used in treating tuberculosis differ in the degree with which they cross into the CSF (Table 11.8).

Although PAS does not enter the CSF, it is

Table 11.7.
Dosing of Antitubercular Drugs in Patients with Abnormal Renal Function

Drug	Dosage
Aminosalicylic acid	The drug accumulates in patients with impaired renal function and dosage adjustments should be based upon drug serum levels (65), 2 g of aminosalicylic acid following each dialysis in a patient with renal failure has resulted in satisfactory treatment
Capreomycin	This drug is renal toxic; more data are needed before recommending doses in patients with poor kidney function
Cycloserine	Since most of this drug (60%) is excreted unchanged in the urine, the dose should be reduced in patients with renal insufficiency (66). Guidelines for dosage adjustments have not been established
Ethambutol	As much as 80% of ethambutol is eliminated unchanged in the urine; dosage adjustments are needed in patients with renal impairment (64–66). The following guidelines have been recommended:

Creatinine Clearance	Dose
25–50 ml/min	15–20 mg/kg/day
10–25 ml/min	7.5–15 mg/kg/day
<10 ml/min	5 mg/kg/day

Drug	Dosage
Isoniazid	In patients who are both slow acetylators and have serum creatinines greater than 1.2 mg%, the dose of isoniazid should be slightly reduced (67). In almost all other instances, it is not necessary to reduce the dose (64)
Kanamycin	Following a normal loading dose of kanamycin, clinically therapeutic levels may be maintained by administering 7 mg/kg every third half-life (68). The serum half-life, in hours, may be estimated by multiplying the serum creatinine concentration, in mg/100 ml, times 3
Pyrazinamide	Not enough clinical data are available to allow a recommendation
Rifampin	Only about 13% of a dose is eliminated unchanged in the urine; the major route of elimination is biliary; therefore, problems would not be expected in patients with decreased renal function (66)
Streptomycin	Doses of 500 mg twice weekly should be adequate for patients with a creatinine clearance below 50 ml/min (64, 69)

still used in combination with isoniazid to treat tuberculosis meningitis because simultaneous administration results in higher and prolonged blood levels of isoniazid. Cycloserine, ethionamide, isoniazid and rifampin enter the CSF of healthy patients and those with tuberculosis meningitis (70, 71). However, therapeutic concentrations of ethambutol and streptomycin are attained only in meningitis (70, 72, 73). Only low levels of kanamycin can be achieved (64).

When treating tuberculous meningitis, a three-drug regimen should be utilized. The dose and duration of treatment are listed in Table 11.4, except isoniazid, which should be given as 600 mg daily (14). The distribution of drugs into the CSF must also be considered (Table 11.8).

Drug Interactions

Whenever a patient receives more than one medication, the possibility of a drug-drug interaction exists. Management of tuberculosis is no exception. Since therapy is to be continued for 12 to 24 months, patients will often have numerous opportunities to receive multiple agents which can result in drug interactions. Table 11.9 summarizes the data reported for antitubercular agents. Emphasis is placed on clinical studies substantiating these interactions and on the possible mechanisms involved. Suggestions for circumventing or minimizing the effects of each potential interaction are included in the table. Several well-documented texts on drug interactions are available for those individuals desiring more detailed information (88, 89). For those drug interactions listed in Table 11.9 only clinical references which have appeared in the medical literature during the past few years are cited. In addition, several of the aminosalicylic acid interactions presented in the table are based on studies that involved acetylsalicylic acid and not aminosalicylic acid. Because of the close structural similarity between these drugs, the extrapolation of the results of aspirin studies to aminosalicylic acid seems warranted.

PROGNOSIS

The prognosis for patients with tuberculosis is variable and dependent on several factors. Drug therapy is the single most important con-

Table 11.8.
Passage of Antitubercular Drugs into the Cerebrospinal Fluid

	Healthy and Tuberculosis Meningitis	Tuberculosis Meningitis	Low Levels	Not at All
Aminosalicylic acid				×
Cycloserine	×			
Ethambutol		×		
Ethionamide	×			
Isoniazid	×			
Kanamycin			×	
Rifampin	×			
Streptomycin		×		

sideration in the outcome of the disease. Prior to the advent of chemotherapy for tuberculosis, mortality figures were high. However, today few people die from this disease. Early identification and prompt treatment with the correct drug regimen are usually sufficient to render patients free of active infection. After 2 weeks of chemotherapy it is unlikely that patients with pulmonary tuberculosis will be infectious to their contacts. Patients should be able to return to work as soon as sputum cultures are negative. At the completion of therapy, it is not necessary to have routine periodic examinations since reactivation has been shown to occur only in a small percentage of cases (90). However, patients should be instructed to report for an examination if symptoms of reactivation are noted. The most serious danger exists in miliary tuberculosis where the infecting organisms are spread rapidly in the blood. Even in this instance, therapy usually results in striking clinical improvement within 2 months.

CONCLUSION

There is no simple cure for tuberculosis. In its present stage, therapy is complicated and treatment involves long-term administration of multiple medications. Drug selection must often be made despite potential serious adverse reactions. A comprehensive understanding of the disease and its treatment places the pharmacist in a situation where therapy can be effectively discussed with both physician and patient. With this understanding, the pharmacist can make a valuable contribution to rational drug usage.

Table 11.9.
Antitubercular Drug-Drug Interactions

Drug Combination	Mechanism	Suggestions
Aminosalicylic acid-amino-benzoic acid	Both decreased metabolism and excretion of the salicylate	Monitor serum salicylate level and decrease dose accordingly
Aminosalicylic acid-cortico-steroids	Corticosteroid therapy may increase aminosalicylic acid excretion	Adjust the dose of aminosalicylic acid based on salicylate blood level
Aminosalicylic acid-folic acid	Decreased gastrointestinal absorption of folic acid	If folic acid is required, it should be administered parenterally
Aminosalicylic acid-probenecid	Aminosalicylic acid may impair the uricosuric effect of probenecid	Avoid concurrent use of the two drugs
Aminosalicylic acid-rifampin (74)	Decreased gastrointestinal absorption of rifampin, possibly due to the bentonite excipient	Do not administer the two drugs orally within 8 hr of each other
Aminosalicylic acid-spironolactone	Decreased renal excretion of a spironolactone metabolite	Monitor therapeutic response and increase the dose of the diuretic if necessary
Aminosalicylic acid-sulfinpyrazone	Impairment of the uricosuric effect of sulfinpyrazone	Avoid concurrent administration of the two drugs
Aminosalicylic acid-sulfonylureas	Displacement from plasma protein binding sites; both drugs have hypoglycemic activity	Make the appropriate adjustments in the oral hypoglycemic agent based upon the blood glucose level
Aminosalicylic acid-vitamin B_{12}	Decreased gastrointestinal absorption of the vitamin	If vitamin B_{12} administration is needed while a patient is receiving aminosalicylic acid, the former drug should be given parenterally
Aminosalicylic acid-warfarin	Probably additive hypoprothrombinemic effects	Monitor the patient's prothrombin time and decrease anticoagulant dosage if indicated
Capreomycin-curare	Both drugs have neuromuscular blocking activity	May require a lower dose of curare
Isoniazid-diazepam (74)	Inhibition of hepatic microsomal enzymes by isoniazid	May require a reduction in diazepam dosage
Isoniazid-phenytoin	Inhibition of hepatic microsomal enzymes	May require a lower dose of phenytoin
Kanamycin-curare	See Capreomycin	
Kanamycin-ethacrynic acid	Both drugs may be ototoxic	Monitor eighth nerve function
Kanamycin-ether	Both drugs may have neuromuscular blocking activity	If possible, avoid this drug combination; may require a lower dose of ether
Kanamycin-furosemide	Both drugs may be ototoxic	Monitor eighth nerve function
Kanamycin-gallamine	Both drugs may have neuromuscular blocking activity	If possible, avoid this drug combination; may require lower dose of gallamine
Kanamycin-succinylcholine	Both drugs may have neuromuscular blocking activity	If possible, avoid this drug combination; may require lower dose of succinylcholine
Rifampin-barbiturates (75)	Induction of hepatic microsomal enzymes	May require higher dose of barbiturates
Rifampin-corticosteroids (76)	Induction of hepatic microsomal enzymes	May require higher dose of corticosteroids
Rifampin-diazepam (75)	Induction of hepatic microsomal enzymes by diazepam	May require higher doses of diazepam

Table 11.9—*Continued*

Drug Combination	Mechanism	Suggestions
Rifampin-digoxin (77)	Possible induction of microsomal enzymes by rifampin	May require higher doses of digoxin
Rifampin-oral contraceptives (78–81)	Probably induction of hepatic microsomal enzymes	Select an alternate method of birth control
Rifampin-quinidine (82)	Induction of hepatic microsomal enzymes by rifampin	May require higher doses of quinidine
Rifampin-sulfonylurea hypoglycemics (83, 84)	Induction of hepatic microsomal enzymes	May require a higher dose of hypoglycemic agent; monitor blood glucose
Rifampin-warfarin (85–87)	Induction of hepatic microsomal enzymes	Monitor prothrombin times and adjust warfarin dose accordingly
Streptomycin interactions	*See* Kanamycin	

References

1. Glassroth J, Robins AG, Snider DE: Tuberculosis the 1980's. *N Engl J Med* 302:1442, 1980.
2. Sbarbaro JA: Tuberculosis. *Med Clin North Am* 64:417, 1980.
3. Stein SC: Tuberculosis infection in a metropolitan city; an epidemiologic review. *Am Rev Respir Dis* 99:298, 1969.
4. Mayock RL, MacGregor RR: Diagnosis, prevention and early therapy of tuberculosis. *DM* 22:3, 1976.
5. Comstock GW, Daniel TM, Snider DE, et al: The tuberculin skin test. *Am Rev Respir Dis* 124:356, 1981.
6. Holden M, Dubin MR, Diamond PH: Frequency of negative intermediate-strength tuberculin sensitivity in patients with active tuberculosis. *N Engl J Med* 285:1506, 1971.
7. Comstock GW, Edwards LB, Nabangxang M: Tuberculin sensitivity eight to fifteen years after BCG vaccination. *Am Rev Respir Dis* 103:572, 1971.
8. Selkon JB: "Atypical" mycobacteria; a review. *Tubercle* 50 (Suppl):70, 1969.
9. Pitchenik AE: PPD-Tuberculin and PPD-Battey dual skin testing of hospital employees and medical students. *South Med J* 71:917, 1978.
10. Appel GB: The nephrotoxicity of antimicrobial agents. *N Engl J Med* 296:784, 1977.
11. Owen D: Renal failure due to para-aminosalicylic acid. *Br Med J* 2:483, 1958.
12. Silverman JD: Simultaneous hypersensitivity to streptomycin and para-aminosalicylic acid. *Dis Chest* 30:103, 1956.
13. Mangini RJ, Gambertoglio JG: Adverse effects of drugs on the kidney. In Koda-Kimble MA, Katcher BS, Young LY: *Applied Therapeutics for Clinical Pharmacists*, ed 2. San Francisco: Applied Therapeutics Inc., 1978.
14. Kendig EL Jr: Tuberculosis. *Pediatr Clin North Am* 15:213, 1968.
15. Collier J, Joekes AM, Philalithis PE, et al: Two cases of ethambutol nephrotoxicity. *Br Med J* 2:1105, 1976.
16. Stone WJ: Acute diffuse interstitial nephritis related to chemotherapy of tuberculosis. *Antimicrob Agents Chemother* 10:164, 1976.
17. Postlethwaite AE, Bartel AG, Kelley WN: Hyperuricemia due to ethambutol. *N Engl J Med* 286:761, 1972.
18. Garibaldi RA, Drusin RE, Ferebee SH, et al: Isoniazid-associated hepatitis; report of an outbreak. *Am Rev Respir Dis* 106:357, 1972.
19. Byrd RB, Nelson R, Elliott RC: Isoniazid toxicity; a prospective study in secondary chemoprophylaxis. *JAMA* 220:1471, 1972.
20. Alexander MR, Louie SG, Guernsey BG: Isoniazid-associated hepatitis. *Clin Pharm* 1:148, 1982.
21. Martin CW, Arthaud JB: Hepatitis after isoniazid administration. *N Engl J Med* 282:433, 1970.
22. Mitchell JR, Zimmerman HJ, Ishak KG, et al: Isoniazid liver injury; clinical spectrum, pathology, and probable pathogenesis. *Ann Intern Med* 84:181, 1976.
23. Maddrey WC, Boitnott JK: Isoniazid hepatitis. *Ann Intern Med* 79:1, 1973.
24. Kutt H, Brennan R, Dehejia H, et al: Diphenylhydantoin intoxication: a complication of isoniazid therapy. *Am Rev Respir Dis* 101: 377, 1970.
25. Brennan R, Dehejia J, Kutt H, et al: Diphenylhydantoin intoxication attendant to slow-inactivation of isoniazid. *Neurology* 20:687, 1970.
26. Mathog RH, Klein WJ: Ototoxicity of ethacrynic acid and aminoglycoside antibiotics in uremia. *N Engl J Med* 280:1223, 1969.
27. Pittinger CB, Eryasa Y, Adamson R: Antibiotic-induced paralysis. *Anesth Analg* 49:487, 1970.
28. Anon: The preparation of rifampin suspension for pediatric use. *Calif Morbid* Nov. 27, 1981.
29. Johnston RF, Wildrick KH: The impact of chemotherapy on the case of patients with tuberculosis. *Am Rev Respir Dis* 109:636, 1974.
30. Pessayre D, Bentata M, Degott C, et al: Isoniazid-rifampin fulminant hepatitis. *Gastroenterology* 72:284, 1977.
31. Girling DJ: Adverse effects of antituberculosis drugs. *Drugs* 23:56, 1982.
32. Capelle P, Dhumeaux D, Mora M, et al: Effect of rifampin on liver function in man. *Gut* 13:366, 1972.
33. Aquinas M, Allan W, Horsfal P, et al: Adverse

reactions to daily and intermittent rifampin regimens for pulmonary tuberculosis in Hong Kong. *Br Med J* 1:765, 1972.

34. Blajchman MA, Lowry RC, Pettit JE, et al: Rifampin-induced immune thrombocytopenia. *Br Med J* 3:24, 1970.

35. Kleinknecht D, Homberg JC, Decroix G: Acute renal failure after rifampin (letter). *Lancet* 1:1238, 1972.

36. Lakshminarayan S, Sahn SA, Hudson LD: Massive haemolysis caused by rifampin. *Br Med J* 2:282, 1973.

37. Apple GB, Neu HC: The nephrotoxicity of antimicrobial agents. *N Engl J Med* 296:722, 1977.

38. Falco FG: Nephrotoxicity of aminoglycosides and gentamicin. *J Infect Dis* 119:406, 1969.

39. Spagnolo SV, Raver JM: Nine-month chemotherapy for pulmonary tuberculosis. *South Med J* 75:134, 1982.

40. Iseman MD, Albert R, Locks M, et al: Guidelines for short-course tuberculosis chemotherapy. *Am Rev Respir Dis* 121:611, 1980.

41. Grossett J: Studies in short-course chemotherapy for tuberculosis. *Chest* 80:719, 1981.

42. Dutt AK, Stead WW: Short-course therapy for patients with tuberculosis. *Arch Intern Med* 140:827, 1980.

43. Mitchell RS: Control of tuberculosis. *N Engl J Med* 276:842, 1967.

44. Mitchell RS: Control of tuberculosis. *N Engl J Med* 276:905, 1967.

45. Horne NW: Advances in the treatment of tuberculosis. *Practitioner* 199:465, 1967.

46. Anon: Chemoprophylaxis for tuberculosis. *Tubercle* 61:69, 1981.

47. Crispen RG: BCG vaccine in perspective. *Semin Oncol* 1:311, 1974.

48. Eickhoff TC: The current status of BCG immunization against tuberculosis. *Ann Rev Med* 28:411, 1977.

49. Miller FJ: The prevention and treatment of tuberculosis in childhood. *Practitioner* 204:117, 1970.

50. Mitchell JF: Disposal of BCG vaccine. *Am J Hosp Pharm* 34:575, 1977.

51. Taylor WC, Aronson MD, Belbanco TL: Should young adults with a positive tuberculin test take isoniazid? *Ann Intern Med* 94:808, 1981.

52. Editorial: Evaluating isoniazid preventive therapy; the need for more data. *Ann Intern Med* 94:817, 1981.

53. Varpela E: On the effect exerted by first-line tuberculosis medicines on the foetus. *Acta Tuberc Scand* 35:53, 1964.

54. Nishimura H, Tanimura T: *Clinical Aspects of the Teratogenicity of Drugs.* Amsterdam: Exerpta Medica, 1976, pp 129–131.

55. Donald PR, Sellars SL: Streptomycin ototoxicity in the unborn child. *S Afr Med J* 60:316, 1981.

56. Scheinhorn DJ, Angelillo VA: Antituberculosis therapy in pregnancy. *West J Med* 127:195, 1977.

57. Good JT, Iseman MD, Davidson PT, et al: Tuberculosis associated with pregnancy. *Am J Obstet Gynecol* 140:492, 1981.

58. Warkany J: Teratogen update-antituberculosis drugs. *Teratology* 20:133, 1979.

59. Snider DE, Layde PM, Johnon MW, et al: Treatment of tuberculosis during pregnancy. *Am Rev Respir Dis* 122:65, 1980.

60. Schaefer G, Zervoudakis IA, Fuchs FF, et al: Pregnancy and pulmonary tuberculosis. *Obstet Gynecol* 46:706, 1975.

61. Bobrowitz ID: Ethambutol in pregnancy. *Chest* 66:20, 1974.

62. Potworowska M, Sianozeka E, Szufladowicz R: Ethionamide treatment and pregnancy. *Pol Med J* 5:1152, 1966.

63. O'Brien TE: Excretion of drugs in human milk. *Am J Hosp Pharm* 31:844, 1974.

64. Finegold SM, Davis A, Zimmet I, et al: Medical progress; chemotherapy guide. *Calif Med* 111:362, 1969.

65. Anderson RJ, Gambertoglio JG, Schrier RW: *Clinical Uses of Drugs in Renal Failure.* Springfield, Ill: Charles C Thomas, 1976, pp 90–108.

66. Reidenberg MM: *Renal Function and Drug Action.* Philadelphia: W. B. Saunders, 1971, p 73.

67. Bowersox DW, Winterbauer RH, Steward GS, et al: Isoniazid dosage in patients with renal failure. *N Engl J Med* 289:84, 1973.

68. Cutler RE, Orme BM: Correlations of serum creatinine concentration and kanamycin half-life, therapeutic implications. *JAMA* 209:539, 1969.

69. Bennett WM, Muther RS, Parker RA, et al: Drug therapy in renal failure: dosing guidelines for adults. *Ann Intern Med* 93:286, 1980.

70. Gilman AG, Goodman LS, Gilman A: *The Pharmacological Basis of Therapeutics,* ed 6. New York: Macmillan, 1980.

71. Doliveira JJG: Cerebrospinal fluid concentrations of rifampin in meningeal tuberculosis. *Am Rev Respir Dis* 106:432, 1972.

72. Piheu JA, Maglio R, Centrangolo R, et al: Concentrations of ethambutol in the cerebrospinal fluid after oral administration. *Tubercle* 52:117, 1971.

73. Bobrowitz ID: Ethambutol in tuberculosis meningitis. *Chest* 61:629, 1972.

74. Boman G, Lundgren P, Stjernstrom G: Mechanism of the inhibitory effect of PAS granules on the absorption of rifampin; adsorption of rifampin by an excipient, bentonite. *Eur J Clin Pharmacol* 8:293, 1975.

75. Ochs HR, Greenblatt DJ, Roberts GM, et al: Diazepam interaction with antituberculosis drugs. *Clin Pharmacol Ther* 29:671, 1981.

76. Buffington GA, Dominguez JH, Piering WF, et al: Interaction of rifampin and glucocorticoids; effect on renal allograft function. *JAMA* 236:1958, 1976.

77. Novi C, Bissoli F, Simonati V, et al: Rifampin and digoxin: possible drug interaction in a dialysis patient. *JAMA* 244:2521, 1980.

78. Altschuler SL, Valenteen J: Amenorrhea following rifampin administration during oral contraceptive use.*Obstet Gynecol* 44:771, 1974.

79. Skolnick JL, Stoler BS, Katz DB, et al: Rifampin, oral contraceptives, and pregnancy. *JAMA* 236:1382, 1976.

80. Joshi JV, Joshi UM, Sankolli GM, et al: A study of introduction of a low-dose combination oral contraceptive with anti-tubercular drugs. *Contraception* 21:617, 1980.

81. Back DJ, Breckenridge AM, Crawford FE, et al:

The effect of rifampicin on the pharmacokinetics of ethynylestradiol in women. *Contraception* 21:135, 1980.

82. Twum-Barima Y, Carruthers SG: Quinidine-rifampin interactions. *N Engl J Med* 304:1466, 1981.

83. Self TH, Morris T: Interaction of rifampin and chlorpropamide. *Chest* 77:800, 1980.

84. Syvalanti E, Pihlajamaki KK, Iisalo EI: Half-life of tolbutamide in patients receiving tuberculostatic agents. *Scand J Respir Dis* 88 (Suppl):17, 1974.

85. O'Reilly RA: Interaction of sodium warfarin and rifampin; studies in man. *Ann Intern Med* 81:337, 1974.

86. O'Reilly RA: Interaction of chronic daily warfarin therapy on rifampin. *Ann Intern Med* 83:506, 1975.

87. Romankiewicz JA, Ehrman M: Rifampin and warfarin; a drug interaction. *Ann Intern Med* 82:224, 1975.

88. Hansten PD: *Drug Interactions*, ed 4. Philadelphia: Lea & Febiger, 1979.

89. *Evaluations of Drug Interactions*, ed 2: Washington, D.C.: American Pharmaceutical Association, 1976.

90. Albert RK, Iseman M, Sbarbaro JA, et al: Monitoring patients with tuberculosis for failure during and after treatment. *Am Rev Respir Dis* 114:1051, 1976.

CHAPTER 12

Sexually Transmitted Diseases

MICHAEL L. RYAN, Pharm.D.
MICHAEL N. DUDLEY, Pharm.D.
RICHARD F. DE LEON, Pharm.D.

The two most common sexually transmitted diseases in the United States today are non-gonococcal urethritis (NGU) and gonorrhea. NGU, which is not a reportable disease in the United States, is a more recently recognized venereal disease that has been reported with a frequency twice that of gonorrhea in several European countries. NGU, unlike gonorrhea, is a disease primarily of sexually inexperienced, well-educated, heterosexual whites of higher socioeconomic standing.

Gonococcal infections, the incidence of which has not increased since 1975, continues to be a major health problem in the United States today. Gonorrhea is characteristically seen in patients between the ages of 20 and 24, with 70% of all gonorrhea being reported in persons under 24 years of age. Complications of *Neisseria gonorrhoeae* infection continue to plague these patients, with 10% of female patients developing gonococcal pelvic inflammatory disease and 1 to 3% of patients developing gonococcal arthritis or other signs of gonococcal bacteremia. However, it is the continued influx of penicillin-resistant strains of *N. gonorrhoeae* into the United States, the incidence of which has grown more than 2-fold in the past year, that most alarms health care practitioners today.

The incidence of syphilis in the United States has increased 26.3% since 1974; the majority of this increase is due to an astonishing 187% rise in the frequency of homosexually acquired male syphilis. Syphilis is seen most frequently in patients between the ages of 15 to 25. Unlike gonorrhea, the resistance patterns of *Treponema pallidum* have not changed over the past 2 decades. Thus, the treatment regimens for syphilis have remained relatively constant.

Lymphogranuloma venereum (LGV) has a worldwide distribution, but tends to be more common in tropical and subtropical areas. In the past, LGV was usually described in travelers, seamen, prostitutes, and in people of lower socioeconomic status in the southeastern United States, but recent reports have described outbreaks in affluent college students and Vietnam veterans (1). In 1980, fewer than 200 cases of LGV were reported to the Centers for Disease Control (2).

Herpes genitalis is not a reportable disease in the United States. Recent data suggest that an epidemic of genital herpes has occurred in the United States during the past decade. One recent survey showed an almost 9-fold increase in the number of office-based physician consultations for genital herpes infection from 1966 to 1979 (3). Genital herpes is now thought to be the third most common sexually transmitted disease in the United States, accounting for well over 40% of all diagnosed genital ulcers. In Britain, reports now show that genital herpes is more common than primary syphilis (4).

NGU AND GONORRHEA

NGU, which was formerly referred to as nonspecific urethritis, has a complex microbiological etiology. Several organisms, as well as urethral stricture, chronic prostatitis and mechanical or chemical trauma, have been suggested as possible causes of NGU.

Of a multitude of organisms isolated from the genitourinary (GU) tract, only *Chlamydia trachomatis* has been firmly established as having a causal relationship. *C. trachomatis* is an intracellular obligate parasite which is responsible for 40 to 50% of all NGU. Other serotypes of *C. trachomatis* are known to cause hyperendemic blinding trachoma, lymphogranuloma venereum, proctitis, epididymitis, cervicitis, and salpingitis. *C. trachomatis* infections at term have been associated with a higher frequency of stillbirths or neonatal death as well as chlamydial pneumonia and inclusion conjunctivitis in the newborn. Other possible, but certainly rarer, infectious causes of NGU include *Trichomonas vaginalis*, herpes simplex virus, and *Candida albicans*.

Neisseria gonorrhoeae, a gram-negative diplococcus, is the causal organism for all forms of gonorrhea. Unlike syphilis, both the relative and absolute resistance patterns of *N. gonorrhoeae* have changed significantly over the past decade. Substantially higher doses of penicillin are required to treat gonorrhea today than were used 20 years ago. In addition, the first strains of *penicillinase-producing N. gonorrhoeae (PPNG)*, which are resistant to penicillin and often tetracyclines as well, were introduced in the United States in 1976. Since that time, the frequency of PPNG infections, which are most prevalent in Southeast Asia, the Far East and West Africa, in the United States has remained low (approximately 0.6% of all gonococcal infections). However, the rate of occurrence of PPNG within the United States continues to rise, having increased 167% from 1980 to 1981.

Pathogenesis

Most cases of NGU are limited to the genitourinary tract. Untreated chlamydial NGU may progress to urethral strictures, epididymitis, salpingitis, venereally acquired Reiter's syndrome, and proctitis in individuals who engage in rectal intercourse. In addition, infants exposed to *Chlamydia* infected birth canals are at risk for acquiring inclusion conjunctivitis and chlamydial pneumonia. Approximately 50% of exposed infants will develop *inclusion conjunctivitis*, which is usually seen during the second and third weeks of life; with 10–20% of infants acquiring *chlamydial pneumonia*, which is first seen during the second and third months of life.

The symptomatology of gonococcal urethritis and NGU is very similar. However, the dysuria associated with NGU usually appears later (8 to 20 days after exposure) in the course of the infection and is milder in nature than gonococcal urethritis. Another difference between gonococcal urethritis and NGU is the consistency of the discharge, which is usually mucoid (65%) with NGU and purulent (80%) with gonococcal urethritis.

A gonorrheal infection is first manifested in males 4 to 10 days after the initial contact with an infected source. The first signs are usually a milky urethral discharge associated with meatal pain, especially on voiding, and frequency of urination. As the disease progresses, the discharge becomes more profuse, purulent, and may be blood-tinged. The discharge is caused by the irritating endotoxin released by the gonococcus when it dies. The infection may extend into the seminal vesicles, epididymis and prostate, resulting in inflammation, pain, and sometimes fever. Urethral stricture after repeated attacks and sterility after epididymitis are complications of gonococcal infection.

In women, the disease may often remain asymptomatic (about 75% of infected women are asymptomatic); however, a purulent urethral discharge may be reported. Dysuria, frequency and urgency occur, as does involvement of the cervix and Bartholin's and Skene's glands. Symptoms of lower genital tract involvement may last for only a month; however, the patient may remain an asymptomatic carrier of gonorrhea. Spread of the infection to the upper genital tract can cause salpingitis. *Salpingitis* may lead to fibrosis and scarring of the fallopian tubes resulting in sterility. *Pelvic inflammatory disease* (PID) is manifested by acute onset of fever and lower abdominal pain and is a result of the extension of infection with abscess formation in the peritoneal cavity. PID tends to be a recurrent problem.

The most common manifestation of gonorrhea in infants is a destructive conjunctivitis that frequently caused blindness before antibiotics were introduced. Infection with N. gonorrhoeae takes place during birth as the neonate passes through the birth canal or makes contact with the hands of infected persons with poor personal hygiene. Acute purulent conjunctivitis develops 3 to 4 days after infection. If untreated, the disease causes corneal ulceration, perforation, scarring and may lead to blindness.

Gonococcal arthritis occurs in about 1% of patients with genital infections and is manifested by fever, arthralgia and painful arthritis. The arthritis involves more than one joint in about 80% of the cases; the knee is the most frequently involved joint. Following the knee in order of frequency of involvement are the wrists, ankles, hands, elbows, hips and shoulders. Before antibiotics became available, permanent joint damage was a common occurrence because of the muscle wasting around the joint.

Gonococcal bacteremia, endocarditis and perihepatitis are rare complications of gonorrhea.

Diagnosis

One cannot accurately distinguish between nongonococcal and gonococcal urethritis on the basis of clinical history and presentation alone. Since the two major causes of NGU (*C. trachomatis* and *Ureaplasma urealyticum*) cannot be cultured by routine laboratory procedures, NGU is currently diagnosed by exclusion. The diagnosis of NGU is made by confirming the absence of typical intracellular Gram-negative diplococci on a Gram stain of the patient's urethral discharge which is positive for urethritis (four or more polymorphonuclear leukocytes).

Gonorrhea is more easily diagnosed in male than in female patients. The history of recent sexual contact combined with positive clinical findings and the microscopic demonstration of Gram-negative diplococci in urethral exudate smears constitutes a positive diagnosis of gonorrheal infection. Subtherapeutic doses of antibiotics such as penicillin, tetracycline or erythromycin, 3 to 4 hours before the urethral smear will prevent the identification of characteristic gonococci and cultures will be required. If the history and clinical picture are suggestive of gonorrhea, but no diplococci can be seen on microscopic examination, a culture specimen from the anterior urethra should be obtained. The diagnosis of gonorrhea in the female is difficult and presents major obstacles to control programs. Direct smears taken during the acute phase of the disease are fairly reliable, however, they become unreliable as the disease progresses or if the patient is asymptomatic. Specimens from the cervix and anal canal can be inoculated on Thayer-Martin (TM) medium for diagnosis. The culture procedure must be repeated after treatment as a test-for-cure. Gram staining with microscopic examination is recommended only as an adjunct to TM culture because of the likelihood of obtaining false-negative and false-positive reactions. Gonococcal infections in women must be differentiated from leukorrhea due to trichomoniasis vaginitis, monilia, or physical or chemical irritants.

Treatment

C. trachomatis, like the two other major causes of NGU, *U. urelyticum* and *Corynebacterium genitalium* type 1, is sensitive to both tetracycline and erythromycin but unresponsive to penicillin, cephalosporins, aminoglycosides and metronidazole. Either oral tetracycline or erythromycin at 250 mg, 4 times a day, for 7 to 14 days can be used to effectively treat NGU. However, since NGU often occurs or is confused with gonococcal urethritis, many practitioners elect to use higher dosages of tetracycline or erythromycin (500 mg orally, 4 times a day, for 7 to 14 days) which will effectively eradicate both infections (5). Contact tracing and concurrent treatment of all sexual partners, up to 70% of whom may be asymptomatic, is essential for preventing reinfection. The major problem with the treatment of NGU is the high rate of recurrent infections. Patients with recurrent infections, who did not comply with this treatment regimen or whose sexual partners were not adequately treated, should be retreated with the same antibiotic regimen. If therapy has been completed appropriately, alternative causes of NGU such as tetracycline-resistant *U. urealyticum*, *T. vaginalis*, herpes simplex virus, urethral stricture or prostatitis should be ruled out.

At present, there are four drug regimens recommended for the *treatment of uncomplicated gonorrhea* (see Table 12.1). The pharmacokinetic determinants for penicillin cure of gonococcal urethritis have recently been published by Jaffe et al. (6). Their studies of experimentally induced gonococcal urethritis in prisoner-volunteer men demonstrated that penicillin cure was best predicted by dosage regimens that produced serum penicillin concentrations that remained 3 to 4 times the minimum inhibitory concentration of *N. gonorrhoeae* to penicillin for 7 to 10 hours (6). This study confirmed clinical observations of the ineffectiveness of regimens producing low concentrations of penicillin (i.e., benzathine penicillin for syphilis) in gonococcal urethritis and confirmed the pharmacokinetic rationale for other single high dose therapies.

The treatment failure rate in uncomplicated genital gonorrhea for all four regimens is similar, and ranges from 3 to 7%. However, the regimens differ in their microbiological spectra, restrictions, and dosing frequency (7). Therefore, the final decision as to the most appropriate therapy is patient specific.

Aqueous procaine penicillin G (APPG) plus probenecid therapy is effective against incubating syphilis, genital, pharyngeal, and anorectal gonorrhea, and is the therapy of choice in patients with multiple foci of infection. Either ampicillin or amoxicillin, each with probenecid, are effective single dose, one time

Table 12.1.
Drug Regimens for the Treatment of Gonorrhea, Nongonococcal Urethritis and Chlamydial Infections[a]

Condition	Drug	Dose	Route	Regimen	Total Dose
Uncompli-cated gon-orrhea	APPG and	4.8 million units	IM	Single dose; probenecid given prior to injec-tion; APPG given in 2 sites	4.8 million units
	Probenecid	1.0 g	PO		1.0 g
	or				
	Amoxicillin and	3.0 g	PO	Single dose; both drugs given simultaneously	3.0 g
	probenecid	1.0 g	PO		1.0 g
	or				
	Tetracycline hydrochlo-ride	500 mg	PO	500 mg every 6 hr for 5 days	10.0 g
	or				
	Ampicillin and	3.5 g	PO	Single dose; both drugs given simultaneously	3.5 g
	probenecid	1.0 g	PO		1.0 g
				Alternative Drugs	
PPNG	Spectinomycin hydrochlo-ride	2.0 g	IM	Single dose	2.0 g
	Cefoxitin and	2 g	IM	Single dose; probenecid given prior to injection	2.0 g
	probenecid	1 g	PO		1.0 g
PID: outpa-tient	Tetracycline hydrochlo-ride	500 mg	PO	500 mg every 6 hr for 10 days	20.0 g
	APPG and pro-benicid fol-lowed by ampicillin	4.8 million units	PO	Single dose divided into 2 injections with pro-benecid given before injection and followed with ampicillin in 500 mg every 6 hr for 10 days	4.8 million units
		1.0 g	PO		1.0 g
		500 mg	PO		20.0 g
	Ampicillin and	3.5 g/500 mg	PO	Loading dose of ampicil-lin given with proben-ecid and followed by 500 mg of ampicillin every 6 hr for 10 days	23.5 g
	probenecid	1.0 g	PO		1.0 g
PID: Inpatient	Aqueous crys-talline peni-cillin G fol-lowed by ampicillin	20 million units	IV	Given daily until clinicial improvement	—
		500 mg	PO	Given every 6 hr daily to complete 10 days of therapy	—
	Tetracycline hydrochlo-ride followed by tetracy-cline hydro-chloride	250 mg	IV	Every 6 hr until clinical improvement	—
		500 mg	PO	Given every 6 hr to complete 10 days of therapy	—
Disseminated gonorrhea	Aqueous crys-talline peni-cillin G fol-lowed by Ampicillin	10 million units	IV	Daily until clinical im-provement	—
		500 mg	PO	Every 6 hr to complete 7 days of therapy	

Table 12.1.—*Continued*

Condition	Drug	Dose	Route	Regimen	Total Dose
				Alternative Drugs	
Disseminated gonorrhea—*continued*	Ampicillin and probenecid	3.5 g/500 mg 1.0 g	PO PO	3.5 g ampicillin loading dose given with probenecid and followed by 500 mg ampicillin every 6 hr for 7 days	—
	Tetracycline	500 mg	PO	500 mg every 6 hr for at least 7 days	—
	Erythromycin, amoxicillin, and probenecid	500 mg 3.0 g/500 mg 1.0 g	PO PO PO	Every 6 hr for 7 days 3.0 g amoxicillin loading dose given with probenecid and followed by amoxicillin, 500 mg, every 6 hr for 7 days	— —
	Spectinomycin	2.0 g	IM	Twice daily for 3 days for disseminated infections due to penicillinase-producing *N. gonorrhoeae*	—
NGU	Tetracycline or	500 mg	PO	Every 6 hr for 7–14 days	—
	Erythromycin	500 mg	PO	Every 6 hr for 7–14 days	—
Chlamydial pneumonia	Erythromycin	10 mg/kg	PO or IV	Every 6 hr for 14 days	—
Chlamydial ophthalmia	Erythromycin	10 mg/kg	PO or IV	Every 6 hr for 14 days	—

[a] Abbreviations are: APPG, aqueous procaine penicillin G; PPNG, penicillinase-producing *Neisseria gonorrhoeae*; PID, pelvic inflammatory disease; NGU, nongonococcal urethritis. (Adapted from: Treatment of sexually transmitted disease. *The Medical Letter*, 24:29, 1982.)

oral therapies for the treatment of uncomplicated gonorrhea. However, both ampicillin and amoxicillin, each with probenecid, have been demonstrated to have a 15% failure rate in patients with *anorectal* and/or *pharyngeal gonorrhea*, and should not be used in these patients. In addition to incubating syphilis, uncomplicated genital and pharyngeal gonorrhea, tetracycline, unlike the previous penicillin therapies, is effective against *C. trachomatis* and is the therapy of choice for patients with a documented or suspected concomitant nongonococcal infection. Tetracycline is associated with a 15% failure rate in patients with anorectal gonorrhea and is contraindicated in pregnant patients and children who are 8 years of age or younger. Noncompliant patients in whom qid tetracycline is a problem should receive a single dose, one-time penicillin regimen.

Benzathine penicillin G should not be used to treat gonorrhea since adequate serum levels cannot be attained. Oral penicillin preparations, such as Pen-VK, are also ineffective in the treatment of gonorrhea.

Spectinomycin (2 gm IM in a single injection), unlike APPG, is not effective against syphilis or pharyngeal gonorrhea. In addition, spectinomycin is ineffective in the treatment of chlamydial NGU. However, spectinomycin, which is not a first line drug in the treatment of uncomplicated gonococcal urethritis, is the drug of choice for the treatment of penicillin allergic patients who are unable to tolerate or comply with tetracycline. Spectinomycin is also the drug of choice for the treatment of PPNG as well.

Some newer β-lactam antibiotics have been useful in the treatment of gonorrhea. The newer, cephalosporin-type antibiotics, such as cefoxitin, cefotaxime, and moxalactam, are attractive agents because of potent activity against N. gonorrhoeae and their stability to β-lactamases. A single IM injection of 2 g of cefoxitin with a 1-g oral dose of probenecid is effective in gonococcal urethritis caused by PPNG. This regimen is currently recommended by the Center for Disease Control (CDC) for the treamtent of uncomplicated infections due to PPNG in patients allergic to spectinomycin, or for isolates of PPNG resistant to spectinomycin. A single intramuscular injection of 500 mg or 1 g of cefotaxime has been effective in urethral, endocervical, rectal, and pharyngeal infections due to N. gonorrhoeae, including penicillinase-producing strains. A single 1-g intramuscular injection of moxalactam has also been effective in urethral and endocervical gonorrhea. The newer penicillin derivatives, azlocillin, mezlocillin, and piperacillin are also active against N. gonorrhoeae but offer no advantages in the treatment of uncomplicated gonorrhea.

Test-of-cure procedures should be done 5 to 7 days after therapy. Retreatment of the male patient is indicated if a Gram-stained smear from the anterior urethra is positive. If the smear is negative, a TM culture specimen should be taken and the decision to retreat the patient based upon culture results. Culture specimens should be taken from the endocervical and anal sites in female patients to determine the need for retreatment. Two successive negative cultures should be obtained before the patient is declared free of gonorrhea.

Disseminated gonococcal infections may be treated with aqueous crystalline penicillin G, 10 million units given intravenously each day for at least 3 days or until the patient has improved significantly. Ampicillin (500 mg, 4 times daily) should then be given orally to complete 7 days of antibiotic treatment. Alternatively, oral ampicillin 3.5 g and probenecid 1.0 g may be used followed by at least 7 days of ampicillin 500 mg taken orally 4 times per day to complete the therapy. Patients allergic to penicillin or probenecid may receive tetracycline 500 mg orally 4 times a day for 7 days. Oral erythromycin 500 mg may also be given for 7 days at 6-hour intervals. Amoxicillin, 3.0 g, orally with probenecid, 1.0 g, followed by amoxicillin, 500 mg, 4 times daily for 7 days is also recommended for treatment of disseminated gonorrhea. Intramuscular spectinomycin 2.0 g, twice daily for 3 days, should be used to treat disseminated infections due to penicillinase-producing N. gonorrhoeae.

Pelvic inflammatory disease is a severe complication of gonococcal infections. The patient may be treated on an outpatient or inpatient basis, depending upon the severity of symptoms. Outpatients who cannot tolerate penicillin or ampicillin can be treated with tetracycline 500 mg, 4 times a day, for 10 days. APPG may be used if 4,800,00 units is administered intramuscularly in two doses in two sites and is preceded by the oral administration of 1 g of probenecid. The parenteral dose of APPG should be followed up with oral ampicillin 500 mg taken four times daily for 10 days. Another effective regimen utilizes oral ampicillin 3.5 g and probenecid 1.0 followed by 500 mg of oral ampicillin taken 4 times daily for 10 days. Amoxicillin, 3.0 g, and probenecid, 1.0 g, given orally and followed by 500 mg of amoxicillin 4 times daily for 10 days is also effective.

Hospitalized patients should receive 20 million units of aqueous crystalline penicillin G IV until there is significant clinical improvement. Oral ampicillin 500 mg should then be given 4 times daily to complete 10 days of therapy. Intravenous tetracycline 250 mg may be used instead of penicillin. It should be given 4 times daily until improvement occurs, then changed to oral tetracycline 500 mg 4 times daily to complete 10 days of therapy. The use of tetracycline in patients with compromised renal function or who are pregnant should be avoided.

Due to the high mortality and rapid progression of *gonococcal ophthalmia neonatorum* infections as well as the possibility of a secondary infection, prophylactic therapy is recommended for all infants, whether delivered vaginally or by cesarean section. The instillation of 1% *silver nitrate* drops has been the standard of prophylactic therapy for the past 100 years. However, due to the high frequency of chemical conjunctivitis associated with silver nitrate prophylaxis and the growing prevalence of neonatal chlamydial conjunctivitis, many practitioners now elect to use either 1% tetracycline or 0.5% erythromycin ophthalmic ointments for the routine prevention of gonococcal ophthalmia neonatorum (8). Both the silver nitrate and ophthalmic antibiotic regimens are associated with a 2% failure rate. Therefore, infants born to mothers with a documented gonococcal infection at term should receive, in addition to local prophylactic therapy, 50,000 units of aqueous crystalline penicillin G IV or IM for a full term infant and 20,000 units for low birth weight infants. Documented gonococcal ophthalmia neonatorum infections should be treated with 50,000 units/kg/day of aqueous crystalline penicillin G given in two intravenous doses per day for several days. Topical antibiotic therapy of an active infection is not required when appropriate systemic therapy is administered.

SYPHILIS

Treponema pallidum, a spirochete, is the causative organism of syphilis. *T. pallidum* can invade any tissue or organ of the body causing acute, chronic or contagious syphilis. Infection usually occurs through sexual activity, but a fetus may become infected during birth if the mother has syphilis (congenital syphilis) or a patient may become infected if donated blood contaminated with *T. pallidum* is received. The organism cannot survive outside of body tissues or fluids and infection by means other than personal contact is rare.

Pathogenesis

Syphilis is transmitted by direct contact with an active lesion. *T. pallidum* invades the body by directly penetrating the epithelium. The site of penetration is usually on the genitals but may occur in the rectum, mouth or any other cutaneous tissue. After penetration, the organism spreads through the lymphatics, resulting in regional lymph node tenderness. The spirochete also travels to the lungs by way of the venous circulation and through the arteries. During this sojourn, *T. pallidum* leaves the small vessels and establishes numerous metastatic foci along the way. This dissemination of the disease occurs within a few days after the initial implantation of *T. pallidum*. During the incubation period, which lasts from 10 to 90 days, the patient is asymptomatic and not infectious. However, fetal infections have been known to result from an incubating maternal infection.

The first clinical expression of syphilis is seen with the onset of the primary stage of syphilis about 3 weeks after the initial exposure. *Primary syphilis* is characterized by the development of a primary chancre at the original site of invasion. The chancre, which resolves spontaneously in 2 to 6 weeks, is indurated, painless, filled with numerous spirochetes, and may be single or multiple in number. Primary chancres are frequently missed by the patient since they are painless and may occur in obscure sites. Primary syphilis is the most infectious stage and lasts 6 to 8 weeks.

The *secondary stage of syphilis* commences about 6 weeks to 6 months after the appearance of the primary chancre. This stage is characterized by a generalized involvement of the skin and mucous membranes. The maculopapular skin rash that develops may be confused with many other rashes, resulting in an incorrect diagnosis. The rash is usually widespread and frequently involves the palms of the hands and the soles of the feet in addition to the trunk and extremities. The mucous membranes may be involved simultaneously or independently of the skin. The lesions that develop in the mucous membranes of the mouth and genitalia are usually superficial and painless and may be covered with a gray exudate. During the secondary stage the patient may complain of fatigue, malaise, headache and fever. A generalized lymphadenopathy, hair loss, and iritis may also occur. Patients with secondary syphilis are infectious to others.

If untreated, the lesions of the secondary stage of syphilis heal in about 4 to 12 weeks, heralding the beginning of the *latent stage* of the syphilitic process. The latent stage is characterized by the absence of clinical lesions, a negative darkfield examination, a normal cerebrospinal fluid (CSF) examination and positive serological tests. The early latent phase, which is defined to be less than 4 year's duration of disease, is considered to be potentially infectious following relapse to the secondary stage. However, the late latent phase, which is greater than 4 year's duration, is considered to be noninfectious.

Latent syphilis may remain dormant for the patient's life or may spontaneously erupt and affect virtually every organ system and tissue. The skeletal system is affected in about 5% of patients with late syphilis. The skull and tibia are most frequently involved; however, the clavicle, humerus and ribs may also be affected. Pain, tenderness and inflammation over the affected area are common complaints.

Syphilitic involvement of the cardiovascular system and CNS is the most serious complication of the disease and accounts for 90% of the deaths due to syphilis. Cardiovascular manifestations usually appear 20 to 30 years after the original infection. The fundamental lesion is in inflammation of the ascending aorta. *T. pallidum* invades the media of the aorta causing a destruction of the tissues and a loss of elasticity which may lead to aneurysm formation. The aneurysm can subsequently enlarge and rupture, causing death.

The clinical symptoms of neurosyphilis may range from a reversible meningitis to irreversible paralysis and insanity. The mildest symptoms, such as headache, vomiting and malaise, are manifestations of a meningitis that is usually reversible upon institution of appropriate therapy. However, invasion of the nervous system tissues by T. pallidum may lead to general paresis, tabes dorsalis or optic atrophy. General paresis, or dementia paralytica, usually occurs 10 to 25 years after the primary lesion and is first evidenced by loss of memory, confusion and impaired judgment. The disease rapidly progresses to the point where the patient is physically, mentally and socially disabled. General paresis is fatal, usually within 3 years. Tabes dorsalis, or locomotor ataxia, may become evident 10 to 20 years after the primary lesion. Destruction of portions of the nervous system affects the patient's sense of joint position and causes stumbling while walking. A characteristic gait is developed as the disease progresses. Sharp jabs of pain may appear anywhere in the body; these "lightning pains" are experienced by most patients with tabes dorsalis. Optic atrophy occurs in 1% of untreated syphilitics and eventually leads to blindness.

Syphilis may be transmitted to a fetus through the placenta by the infected mother after the fifth month of pregnancy. As a result of infection, the pregnancy may result in spontaneous abortion, a stillborn infant or a premature or full term infant with syphilis. A serological examination for syphilis should be a routine test taken at the first prenatal visit of every pregnant women.

Congenital syphilis is often a severe disease manifested by dehydration and malnutrition. The infants also display skin lesions, persistent rhinitis, tenderness over the long bones and pseudoparalysis. Roentgenograms of the long bones may demonstrate areas of bone destruction and osteochondritis. Late congenital syphilis is often manifested 20 years after birth with signs of central nervous system (CNS) involvement. Eighth nerve deafness, optic atrophy and juvenile paresis occur. Hutchinson's teeth are an unusual manifestation of late congenital syphilis; the peglike teeth are widely spaced, smooth and notched. Congenital neurosyphilis

poses a serious prognosis due to a lack of response to therapy.

Diagnosis

Darkfield microscopic examination is the method of choice for the diagnosis of early lesion syphilis. In darkfield examination, serous material from a suspected syphilitic lesion is viewed through a compound microscope fitted with a darkfield condenser. The identification of organisms with the characteristic morphology and motility of T. pallidium with darkfield microscopy is a positive diagnosis of infectious syphilis. Since Treponema microdentium, a nonpathogen that is part of the normal flora of the mouth, is morphologically indistinguishable from T. pallidum, darkfield examination of oral lesions is not reliable.

The serological tests used for the diagnosis of syphilis are divided into treponemal and nontreponemal types. Both serological tests have a high rate of false negative results (15 to 25%) during the primary stage of syphilis when the patient's immune response may not yet be sufficiently developed. The treponemal tests utilize antigens from T. pallidum to detect antibodies to the pathogen. The treponemal test of choice is the *FTA-Abs* (fluorescent treponemal antibody absorption) test. The FTA-Abs test is more specific than nontreponemal tests, and has a much lower rate of false-positive reactions. However, unlike the treponemal tests, the FTA-Abs test cannot be quantified and, therefore, is not of value in judging the effectiveness of therapy. In fact, the FTA-Abs test may remain positive for the patient's life, even after the patient has been effectively treated. The FTA-Abs is most commonly used to distinguish between a biological false-positive treponemal test result and a true positive diagnosis of syphilis.

Nontreponemal tests for syphilis measure serum reagin titers. Therefore, unlike treponemal tests, nontreponemal test results can be quantified and used to determine the effectiveness of antisyphilitic therapy. The Venereal Disease Research Laboratory (VDRL) test is the most commonly used treponemal test. The VDRL reports the most dilute serum concentration having a positive reaction. Since reagin levels are nonspecific antibodies and may result from conditions other than syphilis, such as autoimmune diseases, there is a high rate (3 to 10%) of false-positive VDRL results.

Treatment of syphilis is considered to be

adequate if the VDRL reagin titer decreases 4-fold. Patients who receive adequate intramuscular or intravenous therapy return to a state of seronegativity within 6 to 12 months with primary syphilis and 12 to 24 months with secondary syphilis. However, patients treated with oral antibiotic therapies, or who have latent syphilis, may never become seronegative.

Treatment

The drug of choice for the treatment of all stages of syphilis is parenteral penicillin G (Table 12.2). Patients with primary, secondary, and latent syphilis (with a negative CSF) of less than 1 year's duration are treated with either a single intramuscular dose of 2.4 million units of benzathine penicillin given in two

Table 12.2.
Drug Regimens for the Treatment of Syphilis[a]

Condition	Drug	Dose	Route	Regimen	Total Dose
Early syphilis (primary, secondary, and latent syphilis of <1 year duration)	Benzathine penicillin G or	2.4 million units	IM	Single dose	2.4 million units
	Aqueous procaine penicillin G (APPG)	600,000 units	IM	Daily for 8 days	4.8 million units
Late syphilis (latent syphilis of >1 yr duration or cardiovascular syphilis)	Benzathine penicillin G	2.4 million units	IM	Three doses given 7 days apart	7.2 million units
	APPG	600,000 units	IM	Daily for 15 days	9.0 million units
Neurosyphilis with positive CNS findings	Aqueous crystalline penicillin G	2 to 4 million units	IV	Every 4 hr for 10 days	—
Alternative Drugs					
Early syphilis	Tetracycline hydrochloride and	500 mg	PO	Every 6 hr for 15 days	30.0 g
	Erythromycin	500 mg	PO	Every 6 hr for 15 days	30.0 g
	Cephalexin	500 mg	PO	Every 6 hr for 15 days	30.0 g
Late syphilis	Tetracycline hydrochloride[b], Erythromycin stearate[b], ethylsuccinate, or base	500 mg	PO	Every 6 hr for 30 days	60.0 g
		500 mg	PO	Every 6 hr for 30 days	60.0 g
	Cephalexin	500 mg	PO	Every 6 hr for 30 days	60.0 g
Congenital with abnormal CSF	Aqueous crystalline penicillin G	50,000 units/kg	IM or IV	Two divided doses for at least 10 days	—
	APPG	50,000 units/kg	IM	Daily for at least 10 days	—
Congenital with normal CSF	Benzathine penicillin G	50,000 units/kg	IM	Single dose	—

[a] Adapted from: Syphilis—CDC recommended treatment schedules, 1976. *Morbidity and Mortality Weekly Report*, 28:13, 1979.
[b] Avoid use in pregnant women.

sites or 600,000 units of aqueous procaine penicillin G (APPG) given intramuscularly daily for 8 days. Patients with latent syphilis and those with cardiovascular involvement should be treated with 2.4 million units of benzathine penicillin G given intramuscularly weekly for 3 weeks or 600,000 units of APPG given intramuscularly each day for 15 days.

Tetracycline, erythromycin, and cephalexin are oral alternatives to penicillin for the treatment of syphilis. Either tetracycline or erythromycin may be substituted for penicillin in patients who are allergic to penicillin. However, tetracycline should be avoided in pregnant patients because of the potential for adverse effects on the teeth and bones of the developing fetus. For the same reasons, tetracycline should not be given to children under 8 years of age. Penicillin, in the same dosage regimen as that used in other infected individuals, is the treatment of choice for pregnant women. Since erythromycin achieves only 6 to 20% of the maternal blood levels in the fetus and its use in pregnant women has been associated with aborted and stillborn infants, documentation of penicillin allergy is especially important before resorting to erythromycin.

The current CDC recommendations for the treatment of neurosyphilis are the same as for any other form of syphilis of greater than 1 year's duration: either 2.4 million units of benzathine penicillin IM weekly for 3 successive weeks, or 600,000 units of APPG IM daily for 15 days. However, due to the lack of well-controlled studies documenting the efficacy of benzathine or procaine penicillin in the treatment of neurosyphilis, and the numerous recent reports of treatment failures with both of these CDC recommended treatment regimens, the therapy of choice for neurosyphilis remains controversial.

Penicillin penetrates the blood brain barrier poorly in the presence of uninflamed meninges, resulting in CSF concentrations which are less than 10% of the corresponding serum concentrations. Meningeal inflammation increases the penetration of penicillin into the CSF. However, therapy with CDC recommended dosages of benzathine penicillin has frequently been associated with subtherapeutic or negligible CSF levels of penicillin in patients with neurosyphilis. Therefore, the use of benzathine penicillin should be reserved for asymptomatic patients with positive serum FTA-Abs and no evidence of CNS involvement. Patients who are symptomatic and have CSF findings consistent with neurosyphilis (a positive CSF FTA-Abs or CSF-VDRL, or documented *T. pallidum* within the CSF) should be treated with 2 to 4 million units of aqueous crystalline penicillin G intravenously every 4 hours for 10 days.

The Jarisch-Herxheimer reaction is usually a benign complication of anti-treponemal therapy with an antibiotic, usually penicillin. This reaction is seen in 50% of patients with primary syphilis and 75% of patients with secondary syphilis. Six to 10 hours after an injection of penicillin, syphilitic skin lesions may become intensified and the patient may complain of fever and malaise. The exacerbation of lesions is thought to be due to the sudden release of antigenic substances from lysed treponemes and is not an allergic reaction to the penicillin. Symptoms of the reaction subside spontaneously in 18 to 24 hours and may be controlled with antipyretics or corticosteroids.

The treatment of infants over 2 months of age with *congenital syphilis* is best accomplished with APPG. The use of aqueous crystalline penicillin G in patients who are less than 2 months of age will avoid abscess formation. Infants with congenital syphilis and an abnormal CSF should receive either 50,000 units per kg of aqueous crystalline penicillin G or 50,000 units per kg of APPG each day for at least 10 days. Infants with a normal CSF should receive 50,000 units per kg of benzathine penicillin G in a single IM dose.

LYMPHOGRANULOMA VENEREUM

Lymphogranuloma venereum (LGV) is caused by *C. trachomatis*, the same organism responsible for the majority of cases of nongonococcal urethritis. Only *Chlamydia* serotypes L_1, L_2, and L_3 produce LGV; these serotypes have been shown to be more invasive in animal models than in humans. Infection is usually acquired by sexual exposure, but laboratory or fomite spread is possible.

Pathogenesis

LGV resembles syphilis in that infection may manifest itself in three stages. Three days to 3 weeks postexposure, a 2- to 3-millimeter evanescent vesicle appears at the site of inoculation. In men, the primary lesion is usually found on the penis. The primary lesion may be found in the vagina, cervix or labia of women. This lesion is painless and usually resolves within 2 to 3 days. The transient, nonthreatening nature of the lesion rarely results in patients seeking medical assistance; in fact this lesion is noted in only 24 to 40% of cases, the majority of which are males. The secondary stage of LGV usually presents 2 to 6 weeks postexposure. From the site of initial inoculation, organisms spread to the regional lymphatic nodes through lymphatic channels. Penile infection results in the development of enlarged, painful inguinal lymph nodes (bubo). Unilateral bubo formation is usually seen, but up to one third of patients may have bilateral disease. Lymphadenopathy is usually painful, resulting in the patient seeking medical assistance. The location of lymphadenopathy in women depends on whether the primary lesion is drained by lymphatics to the inguinal, obturator, iliac, or deep iliac lymph nodes. Patients may be systematically ill with fevers, chills, myalgias, arthralgias, and gastrointestinal complaints. Laboratory studies show an elevated or normal white blood cell count, elevated erythrocyte sedimentation rate (ESR), and occasionally elevated liver function tests. When left untreated, infection may progress to involve the entire chain of lymph nodes. These nodes may eventually coalesce to form large, fluctuant, suppurative masses. The areas may enlarge and rupture spontaneously, forming multiple fistulous tracts.

Late complications of untreated LGV include progressive, infiltrative, and ulcerative lesions of the genitalia. Fibrosis and scarring may occlude lymph draining resulting in formation of "lymphorkhoids" or genital elephantiasis.

Up to 25% of patients with LGV may present with anorectal complaints, particularly women and homosexual men. These patients complain of a rectal discharge of blood, mucus, and pus; rectal pain may be present or absent initially. Rectal strictures with accompanying constipation or tenesmus develop in many patients.

Diagnosis

LGV must be differentiated from genital herpes, syphilis, and chancroid. The diagnosis of LGV in men is usually based upon the clinical presentation of inguinal adenopathy. LGV is less easily diagnosed in women. Isolation of Chlamydia from aspirated bubo pus is possible in approximately 30% of cases when there is clinical and serologic evidence of LGV. Culturing the organism requires special techniques not routinely available in most laboratories.

A skin test (Frei test) containing crude antigens from LGV producing Chlamydia has been utilized in the diagnosis of LGV in patients with suggestive clinical symptoms. Unfortunately, this test is negative in approximately one third of patients with LGV and is frequently positive in patients with infections due to non-LGV strains of C. trachomatis and Chlamydia psittaci. In view of the insensitivity and nonspecificity of the test, its usefulness in confirming the clinical diagnosis is limited, and a commercial preparation of the Frei test is no longer available. Tests for complement fixation (CF) may be useful in diagnosing LGV, but like the Frei test, it may be positive in other chlamydial infections. Patients with LGV usually have CF titers of 1:64 or greater, while other infections due to Chlamydia cause CF titers of 1:16 or less (9). Detection of antichlamydial antibody by microimmunofluorescence (MIF) or enzyme-linked immunosorbent assay (ELISA) appear to be sensitive tests that are more specific than the CF test.

Treatment

There have been no significant advances in the treatment of LGV during the past 2 decades. Management of LGV includes antimicrobial therapy, and when indicated, surgery for drainage of bubos or complications due to chronic infections. Fluctuant bubos should be aspirated to prevent spontaneous rupture and fistula formation. Incision and drainage are unnecessary and are discouraged because of the possible formation of sinus tracts.

C. trachomatis is usually sensitive in vitro to tetracyclines, sulfonamides, erythromycin, and chloramphenicol. Susceptibility testing has shown penicillin to have an inhibitory but not lethal effect on C. trachomatis. Rifampin is often active in vitro, but resistance develops rapidly. Relative resistance to erythromycin and sulfonamides in tissue culture susceptibility testing has been reported, but the clinical significance of these isolates is not known (10).

The impact of antimicrobial chemotherapy on the course of LGV is poorly studied. Most authors claim that all patients "get better" with whatever drug they use. Since the growth cycle of Chlamydia is approximately 48 hours, prolonged antimicrobial therapy would be expected to be necessary for clinical response. Response to antimicrobial therapy in the early inguinal phase appears to be better than the response in chronic infections (11). Antimicrobial therapy probably has the greatest effect on the relief of constitutional symptoms. In the only controlled evaluation of the treatment of bubonic LGV, Greaves et al. (11) compared chloramphenicol, oxytetracycline, chlortetracycline, and sulfadiazine to symptomatic aspirin therapy. Resolution of bubos was more rapid in the group receiving antimicrobial therapy, but bubos in a few patients persisted for as long as 181 days following completion of therapy. It was concluded that clinical response to antimicrobial therapy (measured by duration of bubos after therapy) was not significantly superior to symptomatic therapy alone. The incidence of complications (bubonic relapse, sinus tract formation, and skin lesions) in the antimicrobial therapy group was less than that observed in the symptomatic therapy group (11% vs. 53%).

Most authorities recommend a course of either oral tetracycline 500 mg, 4 times daily, or sulfisoxazole 1 g, 4 times daily, in uncomplicated cases of LGV. Multiple courses may be necessary in chronic or complicated cases. The development of bubos at another site or increase in size of existing undrained bubos shortly after initiating antimicrobial therapy does not connote antibiotic failure. Response to therapy is usually evaluated by the patient's clinical response. Serial CF titers are not reliable as a monitoring parameter, as some studies have failed to show a fall in CF titers in patients showing a good clinical response. Furthermore, antibody titers may fall spontaneously in patients not receiving antimicrobial therapy (11, 12).

HERPES GENITALIS

Herpes simplex virus (HSV, Herpesvirus hominus) is a double-stranded DNA virus belonging to the Herpetoviridae family of viruses. In the past, herpesviruses have been separated based on clinical and epidemiologic patterns, although certain biochemical differences exist. Herpes simplex type 1 (*HSV-1*) is usually associated with infection "above the waist" (i.e., labialis, keratitis, and encephalitis in adults), while herpes simplex type 2 (*HSV-2*) is usually associated with infections "below the waist" acquired through genital contact. However, changing sexual mores and increasing oral-genital contact have likely contributed to the increasing incidence of oral HSV-2 and genital HSV-1 infections; one recent study reported that 37% of genital herpes infections in college women were due to HSV-1.

Pathogenesis

Genital herpes infections are usually acquired through contact with an infected symptomatic lesion, although the virus can be excreted by asymptomatic patients. After inoculation, the virus replicates locally in epithelial cells, resulting in cell lysis and an inflammatory response. When the virus is acquired via genital contact, it ascends through peripheral nerves to sacral ganglia where it becomes latent, undisturbed by host defenses. Recurrence happens when the virus becomes reactivated and replicates within the ganglia. Newly formed virus then migrates through an intra-axonal pathway to nerve endings to form new lesions.

After exposure to the virus, an incubation period of 2 to 20 days (mean approximately 6 days) precedes the onset of symptoms (13). The first occurrence of genital herpes infection may be described as primary or nonprimary. A patient has a *primary genital infection* when there is no previous history of *any* infection due to HSV. *Nonprimary herpes genital infection* occurs when a patient has no previous history of *genital* HSV infection, but has had a prior HSV infection at another site (i.e., labialis, keratitis). The distinction between primary and nonprimary infection is important in that recent data suggest that prior HSV-1 exposure (i.e., labialis) may prevent the acquisition of symptomatic genital HSV-1 infection (14).

Prior to the appearance of herpetic lesions, patients may experience local prodromal syndromes of mild aching, itching, paresthesia or burning at the affected site. Following these symptoms, erythema (without induration) ensues with development of papules, and ultimately, 1- to 2-mm vesicles. These vesicles may number as many as 20 in primary infections. In men, these lesions are usually found on the penile shaft or glans of the penis. Women may have lesions on the lower legs, thighs, vulva, perineum, buttocks, cervix or vagina. These vesicles eventually rupture, forming erosions which crust over and heal. The duration of these primary lesions is usually 2 to 3 weeks, but they may persist for up to 6 weeks. Other symptoms may include urethral or vaginal discharge, perianal pain, or dysuria. These symptoms tend to be of shorter duration (10 to 14 days). Primary perianal and anal infection with HSV-2 has been reported, particularly in homosexual men. Symptoms include rectal pain, tenesmus, itching and rectal discharge.

Recent studies have shown that initial genital herpes infection in patients with previous HSV infection (usually due to HSV-1) are milder with more rapid resolution of symptoms and lesions than that observed in patients with no history of prior HSV infection. Following the initial genital infection, the duration of virus shedding is approximately 10 days; however, the duration of viral shedding has been shown to vary from 3 to 33 days depending on the frequency of follow-up cultures.

One of the most intriguing yet frustrating aspects of genital HSV infection is the tendency for recurrence in the majority of patients. In men, greater than two thirds of all cases will recur within the first year after initial presentation (14). One study reported that recurrence in women was less than that in men; however, some recurrences may occur on the cervix and are asymptomatic, thereby going undetected. Recurrence is more likely in patients with genital infections due to HSV-2, especially in those patients developing high titers of neutralizing antibody to HSV-2 (14). Various factors have been implicated as causes for recurrence, including fever, emotional or physical stress, trauma, increased sexual activity, and menstruation. However, controlled studies have shown only menstruation to have a relationship with the appearance of recurrent lesions. Fortunately, the frequency of recurrence tends to decline with time.

Recurrent genital herpes lesions tend to develop in the vicinity of the initial infections. Patients will experience a prodrome similar to that of the first infection. The important difference between initial and recurrent infection is that the course of recurrent HSV infection is milder and of shorter duration. In most patients, pain appears to subside after the fourth day. Herpetic lesions tend to be less numerous and most heal in approximately 8 days (13, 15). The virus is shed from recurrent lesions for only 4 days; it has been suggested that all recurrent lesions are culture-negative after 10 days (15).

There is considerable controversy about the association of genital HSV infection and neoplasms of the female genital tract. Although many studies are fraught with methodological problems, several available retrospective studies have suggested that genital HSV infection may be involved in the later development of *cervical cancer.* One study has demonstrated the presence of HSV-2 DNA binding proteins within the cells of lesions diagnosed as squamous-cell carcinoma in situ of the vulva. Clearly, prospective study of the role of genital HSV infection and development of neoplastic disease in women is necessary.

Maternal genital herpes infection has been associated with spontaneous abortion, premature delivery and occasionally with congenital malformations. HSV infection in the neonate is associated with a 60% fatality rate, with greater than 50% of survivors having neurologic sequelae. Disseminated infection in the mother leading to hepatitis, pancreatitis, and death has been reported. Neonatal infection presumably occurs during either vaginal delivery in mothers with active lesions or ascending infection from the maternal genital tract after fetal membranes have ruptured. Neonatal infection may also be acquired by contact with nongenital sources (e.g., nosocomial infection from nursery personnel). Early institution of intravenous *vidarabine* (15 to 30 mg/kg/day) appears to decrease the morbidity and mortality associated with HSV infection in the neonate. Prophylactic cesarean section is recommended when there is symptomatic or cytological or virological evidence of maternal infection at term (16).

Diagnosis

HSV infection must be differentiated from other sexually transmitted diseases, including syphilis, LGV and chancroid. Isolation of HSV by tissue culture of vesicles (ideally only 24 to 48 hours old) remains the most definitive form of diagnosis. Microscopic examination of scrapings from lesions using Giemsa, Tzanck or Papanicolaou techniques may be used to show the characteristic cellular morphology of HSV infection. However, these tests are frequently associated with false-negative results. Serologic tests for detecting antibodies to HSV are helpful only in primary infections, since antibody titers remain relatively unchanged during recurrent disease. In addition, antibodies may cross-react with both HSV-1 and HSV-2 because of antigenic similarities. In view of the limited availability and reliability of laboratory methods of diagnosis, genital

HSV infections are usually diagnosed based on the history and clinical presentation.

Treatment

Therapy of genital HSV infection remains controversial, although some promising regimens have recently emerged. The goals of therapy are to: 1) decrease the severity and duration of the symptoms of active infection, 2) decrease the frequency of recurrence, and 3) decrease the duration of viral shedding from herpetic lesions. The clinical and virologic course of untreated primary and recurrent genital HSV infection and identified variables that must be controlled or analyzed to determine the effects of antiviral therapy has been carefully documented. Table 12.3 summarizes some of the considerations that should be applied when evaluating or designing studies dealing with the treatment of genital HSV infection.

Over a dozen treatment regimens with photodynamic inactivators, immunostimulants, vaccines, topical surfactants, or nucleoside derivatives have been studied. Many of these evaluations have been conducted in uncontrolled or poorly controlled clinical trials. The efficacy of specific agents based on controlled trials is described below. Unfortunately, the results from many studies are now inconclusive in view of the recent literature describing the natural course of untreated genital HSV infection.

PHOTODYNAMIC INACTIVATION

When early work showed that certain heterotricyclic dyes bound to HSV and briefly exposed to ordinary fluorescent or incandescent light inactivated HSV, a number of clinical trials were initiated to determine the in vivo efficacy of this therapy. Herpetic lesions were painted with methylene blue, proflavine, or neutral-red dyes and exposed to visible light for up to 15 min with multiple exposures during the first 24 hours after application. While early experience with this therapy suggested a decrease in healing time and recurrence rate, subsequent placebo-controlled studies failed to show any benefit (17). In addition, photodynamic inactivation of mammalian cells containing HSV has been demonstrated to enhance the oncogenic potential of HSV. In view of these observations and the lack of demonstrable benefit, photodynamic inactivation therapy has been largely abandoned.

Table 12.3.
Aspects of the Natural History of Genital Herpes Simplex Virus (HSV) Infection to Consider for Proper Evaluation of Therapeutic Regimens (14, 15, 20, 21, 28)

Considerations for Evaluating the Effect of Therapy on Severity and Duration of Symptoms of Active Infection:

1. Difficulty in determining if formation of new lesions on therapy represent additional viral replication in ganglia or skin
2. Difference in clinical course between "wet" skin lesions and "dry" skin lesions
3. Necessity for rapid institution of therapy to evaluate the effects on symptoms, especially in recurrent infections
4. Difficulty in defining "healing" especially in women with intravaginal or cervical infection
5. Pronounced interpatient and inter-sex variability in clinical course on recurrent infection

Considerations for Evaluating the Effect of Therapy on Recurrence Rates:

1. Differences between the propensity of HSV-1 and HSV-2 to cause recurrent infection
2. Difference beween men and women in the frequency of recurrence

Considerations for Evaluating the Effect of Therapy on Virus Shedding from Lesions:

1. Necessity for rapid institution of therapy in recurrent disease to determine effect since period of virus shedding in untreated infections is brief
2. Pronounced interpatient variability in virologic course of recurrent disease

IMMUNOSTIMULANTS AND VACCINES

There is considerable evidence that there is an association between decreased host immunity and recurrence of HSV infection. *Levamisole* has been shown to have immunostimulating properties and was shown in early studies to enhance the immune response to HSV. However, double-blind placebo controlled trials have demonstrated that oral levamisole (50 mg, 3 times daily, for 3 days) had no effect on the duration of lesions, degree of pain, or the number of days between attacks (18). Another immunostimulant, Isoprinosine, has been shown in preliminary studies to have some benefits in primary genital HSV infection (13).

Immunostimulation through the use of *BCG* and *smallpox vaccination* has also been studied. While initial reports suggested that BCG decreased the frequency of recurrence of genital HSV infection, subsequent controlled studies failed to demonstrate any benefit (13). The use of frequent smallpox vaccinations prophylactically to decrease the rate of recurrent infections has been shown to be ineffective and to carry a significant risk of morbidity.

Vaccines for HSV have been developed and undergone limited evaluation. A preparation containing formalin-inactivated HSV-1 was studied briefly in the United States by Eli Lilly Company, but further study was abandoned when studies demonstrated that protection was only transient and production problems arose. Heat-inactivated HSV-1 and HSV-2 vaccines are available in Europe. These vaccines have been recommended by the manufacturer for the prevention of recurrent HSV infection, but controlled studies to support this contention are not available.

TOPICAL SURFACTANTS

Various lipid solvents and nonionic surfactants have been shown to have activity against HSV in vitro. Controlled evaluation in patients with primary or secondary episodes of HSV infection of topical *ethyl ether* applied 4 times daily for 7 days have failed to show any significant beneficial effect on the duration of symptoms or the rate of recurrent infections. The application of ether is extremely painful; in fact, several patients felt that the pain was "worse than the disease" (19). Topical application of the nonionic surfactant *nonoxynol-9* (5 times daily for up to 7 days) in initial or recurrent disease, has been shown to have no effect on the duration of symptoms, lesions, viral shedding, or the recurrence rate (20).

NUCLEOSIDE DERIVATIVES

Topical *vidarabine (adenosine arabinoside, Ara-A)* in a 3% petrolatum base has been shown in two double-blind controlled trials to have no effect on the duration of healing time, pain, viral shedding or formation of new lesions (21).

Topical application of 0.19% 2-deoxy-D-glucose in 2% *miconazole* cream 4 times daily was found to decrease the duration of lesions, positive viral cultures, and also decreased the frequency of recurrence. However, the control (miconazole alone) group appeared to have prolonged clinical and virologic courses which were markedly different from observations of untreated patients reported by other groups

(22). No other clinical studies of this agent have since been reported.

Idoxuridine (IDU) in a 0.5% ointment applied 3 times daily for 5 days has been shown to be no more effective than normal saline or proflavine photodynamic inactivation therapy in reducing the duration of lesions or viral shedding (23). Five and 20% IDU in *DMSO* (dimethyl sulfoxide) was shown to heal lesions of recurrent infections more rapidly than those treated with DMSO alone. The duration of viral shedding from lesions was also shorter in the IDU group. IDU appeared to have no effect on recurrent rate, although only a small number of patients was evaluated (24).

Acyclovir (Zovirax) is a prodrug which is converted to its active form, acyclovir triphosphate, by a viral-coded thymidine kinase. Acyclovir triphosphate then interferes with viral DNA polymerase activity and inhibits viral DNA replication.

Acyclovir is the only antiviral agent currently approved for the topical therapy of HSV infections. Topical acyclovir (5% ointment) is indicated in the management of initial herpes genitalis and in limited non-life-threatening mucocutaneous herpes simplex virus infections in immunocompromised patients. Topical acyclovir has been shown to be of limited value (small decreases in the duration of viral shedding only) in the treatment of recurrent herpes genitalis and of herpes labialis in patients who are not immunocompromised. A well-controlled, double-blind study by Corey et al. (25) has shown topical acyclovir to be effective in decreasing the duration of local pain (5.2 vs. 7.0 days), itching (3.6 vs. 8.0 days), viral shedding (2.3 vs. 5.6 days) and the time of healing (11.4 vs. 15.8 days) when compared to a placebo in the treatment of primary genital herpes (25). However, topical acyclovir has not been shown to either prevent the transmission of infection nor to decrease the rate of recurrent infections. These two facts, plus the potential for acquired resistance (via the rapid selection of mutant HSV which is deficient in viral thymidine kinase activity) with prolonged exposure, preclude the use of topical acyclovir prophylactically for recurrent herpes. Topical therapy with 5% acyclovir in PEG ointment should be initiated as early as possible to attain maximal benefit. It is recommended that it be applied 6 times daily, although preliminary results suggest that four daily applications are sufficient. To prevent autoinoculation of other body sites and transmission of the infection to other persons, a finger cot or rubber glove should be used to apply acyclovir topically. The necessity and safety of intravaginal administration has not been established. Preliminary data on intravenous acyclovir (5 mg/kg every 8 hours for 5 days) in patients with primary genital HSV infection has demonstrated it to be effective in decreasing the duration of lesions, local symptoms, and viral shedding. Studies of the effect of IV acyclovir on the recurrence rate of herpetic infections are in progress (26). Oral acyclovir in doses of 200 mg 5 times a day was recently tested in a double-blind placebo controlled trial (27). Virus shedding, new lesion formation after 48 hours and duration of genital lesions were significantly reduced in both men and women. The duration and severity of symptoms were reduced by the third day for males and the fourth day for females. Oral acyclovir did not prevent virus latency or recurrent episodes.

Other therapies that have been suggested but have not been evaluated in controlled clinical trials include topical zinc sulfate, tannic acid and urea in HEB cream with ultrasound, influenza vaccine, carbon dioxide laser therapy, povidone-iodine, lysine, and thymol.

SUPPORTIVE MEASURES

Symptomatic therapy attempts to reduce the discomfort associated with active herpetic lesions. Analgesics (narcotic and non-narcotic) may be useful in reducing neuralgic pain and dysuria. Sitz or colloidal oatmeal baths may provide some relief. Topical lidocaine and use of warm air from hair dryers may also decrease the pain. Topical steroids should be avoided since they appear to be of no therapeutic benefit and could lead to secondary bacterial infections of the herpetic lesions.

The greatest concerns in the management of patients with genital HSV are overcoming the social problems and stigma concerning the disease. Many patients are unable to continue or initiate interpersonal relationships because of the fear of having a chronic, transmissible infectious disease. Supportive services are available, through HELP (Herpetics Engaged in Living Productively) by writing to P.O. Box 100, Palo Alto, CA 94032, USA. The patient should be educated regarding the chronicity of the disease and must understand that sexual abstinence is necessary when active lesions are present. Women should be advised of the possible link between genital HSV infection and cervical cancer; it is recommended that women with genital HSV infections have a yearly Papanicolaou (Pap) smear.

SEXUALLY TRANSMITTED DISEASES IN HOMOSEXUAL MEN

The study of sexually transmitted diseases in homosexual patients has increased in importance over the past few years. As in heterosexual couples, intimate contact between homosexual men frequently includes oral, oral-genital, and genital contact. These practices have resulted in new presentations of the classic sexually transmitted diseases, as well as the frequent observation of certain infectious diseases that are not usually associated with venereal transmission. Transmission of any of these diseases may occur between heterosexual couples; however, certain factors in the life-style of some homosexual men as well as closer surveillance of sexually transmitted diseases in this population have resulted in more complete documentation of these apparently "newer" syndromes. A number of social factors among homosexual men have also been cited as possible reasons for the apparently higher prevalance of certain transmitted diseases in this population than that observed among heterosexual men or lesbians (29).

The necessity for unimpeded communication between the health care practitioner and the homosexual patient cannot be overemphasized. Many practitioners may have difficulty interacting with homosexual patients for various social or moral reasons. Homosexual patients may be reluctant to disclose pertinent information regarding the type of sexual contact, particularly if they do not understand the possible relationship between their complaints and sexual activity.

Sexually transmitted diseases in the homosexual patient may present in the colorectal or pharyngeal area as well as in the genital region. Colorectal complaints in homosexual men are often referred to as the "gay bowel syndrome," but this term has been discouraged because of its lack of specificity. Enteric infections may present with complaints of proctitis, enteritis, or both. Table 12.4 lists the organisms associated with proctitis, enteritis, and pharyngitis in homosexual men.

Table 12.4.
Clinical Presentation and Possible Etiology of Complaints Due to Sexually Transmitted Diseases in Homosexual Men

Presentation	Possible Etiologies
Proctitis (anal discharge, rectal pain, perianal lesions, pruritis, change in bowel habit, abdominal pain)	Herpes simplex virus *Neisseria gonorrhoeae* *Treponema pallidum* *Giardia lamblia* *Entamoeba histolytica* *Chlamydia trachomatis* *Shigella* *Campylobacter* Trauma Allergy
Enteritis (diarrhea, abdominal pain)	*E. histolytica* *Giardia lamblia* *Shigella* *Salmonella* *Campylobacter* Nonpathogenic organisms and amoeba (i.e., *Escherichia coli*, *Entamoeba hartmanii*, *Chilomastix mesnili*, *Iodamoeba bütschlii*, *Dientamoeba fragilis*)
Pharyngitis	*N. gonorrhoeae* Group A streptococcus Herpes simplex virus *Chlamydia*

PROCTITIS

Homosexual men with proctitis may present with a variety of symptoms. It is important to note that these symptoms are not specific for any infectious etiology and may be described by patients without infection. Proctitis and other constitutional symptoms may be due to rectal trauma from a penis, foreign object (vibrators, bottles, enema nozzles), fist or even a forearm. Many topical preparations applied to the anorectal region may be sensitizing and exacerbate the problem through local allergic reactions. Lubricants used during sexual practices (e.g., soaps, shampoos, cooking oil and even K-Y jelly) may also be sensitizing, especially when applied to abraded skin or mucosa.

The clinical presentation alone is insufficient to determine the etiology of infection; in fact, 21 to 66% of all homosexual men with positive rectal cultures for gonorrhea will be asymptomatic (29, 30). Visualization of lesions through direct examination or sigmoidoscopy may not be helpful, as some lesions may be difficult to distinguish from Crohn's disease or even carcinoma; therefore, rectal culture is necessary to determine the specific infectious etiologies.

ENTERITIS

Bacterial and parasitic causes of gastroenteritis in homosexual men are listed in Table 12.4. Outbreaks of *Shigella* dysentery in homosexual men have been reported in San Francisco, New York, Seattle and London. Only two cases of *Salmonella* gastroenteritis in homosexual contacts have been reported. *Campylobacter* has recently been recognized as a frequent cause of acute gastroenteritis in the general population. Venereal transmission of the organism among homosexual men is suspected, but has not been adequately documented. The high prevalence of *Entamoeba histolytica* infection among homosexual men has been well documented in New York City and San Francisco. Infection with *E. histolytica* may be asymptomatic with only cyst passage for many years, with later development of symptomatic disease. Infection with *Giardia lamblia* frequently causes diarrhea of variable duration or may only cause a mild case of flatus, bloating, and cramping. Generally accepted "nonpathogenic" parasites have been implicated as causes of gastrointestinal complaints in homosexual patients when symptoms resolved following the eradication of these organisms through chemotherapy; however, treatment of these pathogens may simply eliminate undetected *E. histolytica* or *G. lamblia* which are responsible for clinical disease.

PHARYNGITIS

Symptomatic pharyngeal gonococcal infection may present as an acute exudative tonsillitis or pharyngeal pain and fever. Remarkably, up to 89% of pharyngeal gonococcal infections in gay men are asymptomatic (29). Group A streptococci is often carried in the rectum and, therefore, may be a source for pharyngitis. An outbreak of scarlet fever in homosexual men due to a rare group A β-hemolytic streptococcus occurred in San Francisco in 1976. *C. trachomatis* has been isolated from the throats of homosexual men but production of symptomatic disease has not been reported. Development of pharyngitis due to herpes simplex virus following orogenital contact has been reported.

Hepatitis

Both hepatitis A and B appear to be prevalent among homosexual men. The risk of acquiring hepatitis A is greatest in homosexual men having frequent oro-anal contact with different partners. Hepatitis B appears to be transmitted by contact of abraded rectal mucosa with saliva or semen infected with hepatitis B virus. It is not known whether non-A non-B hepatitis is transmitted sexually, although infection in homosexual men has been reported (see Chapter 16, "Hepatitis").

Cytomegalovirus

Cytomegalovirus (CMV) may be a cause of hepatitis in homosexual men. CMV is also one of the causes of a mononucleosis like syndrome. CMV infection appears to be prevalent among homosexual men; one study showed that 93% of homosexual men between 18 and 29 years of age had serologic evidence of prior infection while 47% of heterosexual men in the same age group had evidence of past CMV infection.

Acquired Immunodeficiency Syndrome

Recently a number of reports have described the occurrence of certain opportunistic infections in homosexual men (31). Some of these patients also had an uncommon neoplasm known as *Kaposi's sarcoma*. Opportunistic infections have included *Pneumocystis carinii* pneumonia, esophageal candidiasis, cryptococcosis, chronic herpes simplex lesions, and CMV infections. The mortality of this syndrome has been high; approximately 40% of patients with *P. carinii* pneumonia have died. Immunologic studies in some of these patients have demonstrated alterations in T-lymphocyte populations, generalized lymphopenia, or skin-test anergy. Concurrent or prior CMV infection appears to have been present in many of these patients. This finding is significant because of the ability of CMV to induce abnormalities in cellular immune response in vitro and in vivo in mice. Other studies have suggested that CMV is involved in the pathogenesis of Kaposi's sarcoma. Further studies are currently in progress to define the etiology, spectrum, and proper management of this emerging syndrome.

Treatment and Prevention

In view of the epidemiology of sexually transmitted diseases in homosexual men, asymptomatic as well as symptomatic infections should be treated. Follow-up cultures and examinations are necessary to determine cure, treatment failure or possible reinfection. Patients should be informed of the relationship between sexual practices and the etiology of their ailments. Sexual abstinence is necessary (and often curative) during episodes of active infection. Use of condoms may prevent acquisition and transmission of infections, but this remains speculative. A recent field trial of a hepatitis B vaccine in homosexual men significantly reduced the incidence of hepatitis B infection. Since prophylaxis of other infections is not feasible, it may be necessary for promiscuous patients to undergo periodic screening for detection of asymptomatic infection. Table 12.5 lists the treatment of some sexually transmitted diseases in homosexual men.

THE ROLE OF THE PHARMACIST

The prevention of sexually transmitted diseases requires the active participation of pharmacists. Pharmacists can act as information sources and ensure the dissemination of accurate, factual information, thereby dispelling many of the myths related to the transmission of venereal diseases. For example, a common belief among the lay public is that spermicidal gels and creams can prevent the transmission of an infection. However, numerous studies have shown this not be true for gonorrhea, NGU or genital herpes infections. Condoms have been available for many years, yet there is concern and confusion about their effectiveness as a device for prevention of venereal disease. Evidence gathered during World War I and World War II have shown condoms to be effective mechanical barriers to the transmission of gonorrhea and syphilis, however, they have not been shown to effectively prevent the transmission of genital herpes.

Pharmacists can also play an important role in advising practitioners on the most appropriate therapeutic regimen. Even the present CDC recommendations for the treatment of gonorrhea and syphilis are not clear cut. For example, the CDC recommendations for the treatment of gonorrhea provides the practi-

Table 12.5.
Antimicrobial Therapy of Common Sexually Transmitted Diseases in Homosexual Men

Etiology	Site	Regimen(s)	Penicillin Allergic Patients
Neisseria gonorrhoeae	Proctitis	Aqueous procaine penicillin G (APPG) 4.8 million units IM *plus* probenecid 1 g PO	Spectinomycin 2 g IM × 1
		or	
		Ampicillin 3.5 g PO *plus* probenecid 1 g PO repeat dose 8–14 hr later[a]	Tetracycline 500 mg QID for 5 days
	Pharyngitis	APPG, 4.8 MU IM *plus* probenecid 1 g PO	Tetracycline 500 mg QID for 15 days
Treponema pallidum (syphilis)	Pharyngitis or anorectal infection	Benzathine penicillin 2.4 million units/IM × 1	Tetracycline 500 mg QID for 15 days
Chlamydia trachomatis	Proctitis	Tetracycline 250–500 mg PO QID for 2–6 wk	—
		or	
		Trimethoprim 160 mg/sulfamethoxazole 800 mg PO BID for 2–6 wk	—
		or	
		Erythromycin 250–500 mg PO QID for 3 wk	—
Shigella sp.	Enteritis	Ampicillin 500 mg PO QID for 7 days	
		or	
		Trimethoprim 160/sulfamethoxazole 800 mg BID for 7 days	—
Giardia lamblia (giardiasis)	Enteritis	Quinacrine 100 mg PO TID for 5 days	—
		or	
		Metronidazole 250 mg PO TID for 5 days	—
Entamoeba histolytica (amebiasis)	Asymptomatic carriage	Diiodohydroxyquin 650 mg PO TID for 20 days	—
		or	
		Paromomycin 25–30 mg/kg/d in 3 divided doses for 7 days	
	Enteritis	Metronidazole 750 mg PO TID for 5–10 days *plus* diiodohydroxyquin 650 mg PO TID for 20 days	—

[a] Intramuscular penicillin (with probenecid) and spectinomycin appear to be the most effective agents in anorectal infection. Oral tetracycline and the single dose ampicillin regimens are also effective, but are associated with higher failure rates; however, the efficacy of the ampicillin regimen is greatly enhanced when the dose is repeated 8–14 hours later.

tioner with several possible therapeutic regimens from which to chose, and their recommendations for the treatment of neurosyphilis are inadequate. The pharmacist can enhance the appropriateness of therapy by assessing the advantages and disadvantages of each therapeutic regimen as it pertains to the individual patient and by remaining abreast of current therapeutic breakthroughs and changing microbiological susceptibilities.

The ultimate answers to the VD problem are education and therapeutics. The therapeutic aspect will see the development of vaccines for mass inoculation and, thus, the mass prevention of gonorrhea and herpes. Unfortunately, these vaccines are still not available. Standard education, however, is available. Pharmacists can and must participate in the dissemination of factual information about standards. More and more pharmacists have correctly identified that they have a serious and significant obligation to educate the public in matters of personal health. But there is a long way to go, and the antivenereal disease effort can use all the help it can get. A cooperative effort by pharmacist, public health workers, and physicians can help control venereal disease. This challenge of cooperation and participation is, therefore, extended to all pharmacy practitioners.

References

1. McLellard BA, Anderson PC: Lymphogranuloma venereum outbreak in a university community. *JAMA* 235:56, 1976.
2. Annual Summary of 1980: *MMWR* 29 (Suppl): 1981.
3. Anon: *MMWR* 31:127, 1982.
4. Editorial: Genital herpes. *Br Med J* 1:1335, 1980.
5. Felman YM, MPhil MA, Nikitas JA: Nongonococcal urethritis: a clinical review. *JAMA* 245:381, 1981.
6. Jaffe HW, Schroeter AL, Reynolds GM, et al: Pharmacokinetic determinants of penicillin cure of gonococcal urethritis. *Antimicrob Agents Chemother* 15:587, 1979.
7. McCormack WM: Treatment of gonorrhea. *Ann Intern Med* 90:845, 1979.
8. Anon: Prophylaxis and treatment of neonatal gonococcal infections. *Pediatrics* 65:1047, 1980.
9. Schacter J: Chlamydial infections. *N Engl J Med* 298:428, 490, 540, 1978.
10. Movrad A, Sweet RL, Sugg N, et al: Relative resistance of erythromycin in *Chlamydia trachomatis*. *Antimicrob Agents Chemother* 18:696, 1980.
11. Greaves AB, Hillman MR, Taggart SR, et al: Chemotherapy in bubonic lymphogranuloma venereum: a clinical and serological evaluation. *Bull WHO* 16:277, 1957.
12. Schacter J, Dawson H: *Human Chlamydial Infections*. Littleton Mass.: PSG Publishing, 1978.
13. Davis LG, Keeney RE: Genital herpes simplex virus infection; clinical course and attempted therapy. *Am J Hosp Pharm* 38:825, 1981.
14. Reeves WC, Corey L, Adams HG: The risk of recurrence after first episodes of genital herpes. *N Engl J Med* 305:315, 1981.
15. Guinan ME, MacCalman J, Kern ER, et al: The course of untreated recurrent genital herpes simplex infection in 27 women. *N Engl J Med* 304:759, 1981.
16. Committees on Fetus and Newborn and Infectious Diseases: Perinatal herpes simplex virus infections. *Pediatrics* 66:147, 1980.
17. Kaufman RM, Adam E, Mirkovic RR, et al: Treatment of genital herpes simplex virus infection with photodynamic inactivation. *Am J Obstet Gynecol* 132:861, 1978.
18. Chang TW, Fiumara N: Treatment with levamisole of recurrent herpes genitalis. *Antimicrob Agents Chemother* 13:809, 1978.
19. Corey L, Reeves WC, Chiag WT et al: Ineffectiveness of topical ether for the treatment of genital herpes simplex virus infection. *N Engl J Med* 199:237, 1978.
20. Vontver LA, Reeves WC, Rattray M et al: Clinical course and diagnosis of genital herpes simplex virus infection and evaluation of topical surfactant therapy. *Am J Obstet Gynecol* 133:548, 1979.
21. Adams HG, Benson EA, Alexander ER, et al: Genital herpetic infection in men and women: clinical course and effect of topical application of adenine arabinoside. *J Infect Dis* 133 (Suppl):A151, 1976.
22. Blough HA, Gluntoli RL: Successful treatment of human genital infections with 2-deoxy-D-glucose. *JAMA* 241:2798, 1979.
23. Taylor PK, Doherty NR: Comparison of the treatment of herpes genitalis in men with proflavine photoinactivation idoxuridine ointment, and normal saline. *Br J Vener Dis* 51:125, 1975.
24. Parker JD: A double-blind trial of idoxuridine in recurrent genital herpes. *J Antimicrob Chemother* 3 (Suppl A):131, 1977.
25. Corey L, Benedetti J, Critchlow C, et al: Topical therapy of genital HSV infection with acyclovir: the Seattle experience. Proceedings of the Interscience Conference on Antimicrobial Agents and Chemotherapy, Chicago, Abst 31, 1981.
26. Fife KH, Corey L, Keeney RE, et al: Double-blind placebo controlled trial of intravenous acyclovir for severe primary genital herpes. Proceedings of the 21st Interscience Conference Antimicrobial Agents and Chemotherapy, Chicago, Abstr 31, 1981.
27. Bryson YJ, Dillon M, Lovett M, et al: Treatment of first episodes of genital herpes simplex virus infection with oral acyclovir. *N Engl J Med* 308:916, 1983.
28. Brown ZA, Kerner, Spruance SL, et al: Clinical and virologic course of herpes simplex genitalis. *West J Med* 130:414, 1979.
29. Owen WF: Sexually transmitted diseases and traumatic problems in homosexual men. *Ann Intern Med* 92:805, 1980.
30. Quinn TC, Corey L, Chaffee RG, et al: Etiology of anorectal infections in homosexual men. *Am J Med* 7:395, 1981.
31. Durack DT: Opportunistic infections and Kaposi's sarcoma in homosexual men. *N Engl J Med* 305:1465, 1981.

CHAPTER 13

Mycotic and Parasitic Infections

PETER J. S. KOO, Pharm.D.

MYCOTIC INFECTIONS

Mycotic infections can be classified into two major categories, superficial and systemic. Infections caused by these fungi in man are usually accidental and it is not necessary for the propagation of the species, with the exception of only a few dermatophytes. These dermatophytes do not invade the living tissue, but they survive on the dead tissue structures of the stratum corneum of the skin, the hair and the nails. They are dependent on man to man or object to man transmission. These dermatophytes exist in the saprophytic form and can be found anywhere in the world, not being restricted to any particular geographic or temperate area.

Fungi causing systemic infections are almost always soil saprophytes with the ability to adapt to a host and therefore cause disease. These fungi are usually dimorphic, they can either grow in soil as the mycelial forms that are responsible for the spore production or as the budding yeast while in a host. Infection is acquired by inhaling the airborne spores. These dimorphic fungi are generally restricted to particular geographic environments. Infections of the population in these endemic areas are common, but rarely manifest clinical disease.

Another important category of fungal infection is caused by the opportunistic fungi. These organisms are generally not infective to the normal host. However, they produce disease in the host who is compromised due to diabetes, neoplastic disease or immunosuppression from drugs. Tissue response varies greatly from no response to pyogenic or granulomatous reactions. These fungi are committed mycelial forms and are not restricted to any particular geographic area.

Subcutaneous mycoses usually occur through trauma to the host. They have some ability to adapt to dimorphism. Clinically, they cause diseases known as chromomycosis and mycetoma, and are caused by a diverse varieties of soil organisms. In the tissue these organism form grains, granules, and sclerotic bodies. Infections develop slowly and so is recovery. Most of these subcutaneous mycotic organisms are restricted geographically, but some occur throughout the hemisphere.

SYSTEMIC MYCOSES
Aspergillosis

Aspergillosis is a group of diseases caused by a mycotic organism from the genus *Aspergillus*. *Aspergillus fumigatus* is a primary offending organism in animals and birds and it is often associated with opportunistic infections in the human. Other aspergillus species such as *Aspergillus terreus* and *Aspergillus flavus*, have also being associated with opportunistic infections. Aspergillus usually infect the pulmonary system of the human host, but systemic infection can also occur. On rare occasion aspergillus also may cause mycetoma, subcutaneous granuloma, and other superficial mycotic infections.

Aspergillus species are ubiquitous in nature and are therefore a constant threat as an infective organism in debilitated individuals. They grow in moist environments like other "molds" and their spores are readily available for infection.

CLINICAL FEATURES

Aspergillus bronchitis or pneumonia can mimic infections caused by other organisms. Often bronchitis develops into a chronic state, secondary to ineffective antibiotic therapy. Allergic bronchopulmonary reaction can occur from aspergillus growing in the bronchioles and the mucus plugs. Eosinophilia and asthmatic attacks are also commonly precipitated when aspergillus is present in the bronchiole lumen. Invasive aspergillosis can occur in debilitated patients and can present as a generalized systemic infection, which can be rapidly fatal.

DIAGNOSIS

The diagnosis of aspergillosis is based on the isolation of the aspergillus from the sputum and mucus plugs from a patient who has clinical symptoms of pulmonary infection. The isolation of aspergillus from a known lesion of tuberculosis, bronchiectasis, or cancer presents a serious complication. Eosinophilia, and concomitant allergic bronchitis with the isolation of aspergillus from the mucus plug should make a definitive diagnosis. Serum precipitin test is an useful aid in the diagnosis, but is not absolute.

TREATMENT

Aspergillus endobronchial infection need only be treated with measures to improve bronchopulmonary toilet (Table 13.1). Aspergillomas, however, can lead to exsanguinating hemoptysis, and therefore require surgical intervention. Systemic aspergillus infection will require appropriate antifungal therapy, and, if applicable, reduction or discontinuation of immunosuppressive therapy may also become necessary.

Amphotericin B is the primary agent used for the treatment of systemic aspergillosis. However, flucytosine has also been used in the treatment of aspergillus pneumonia and meningitis (102), but flucytosine alone is not the best regimen for those infections. Combinations of flucytosine and amphotericin B as well as amphotericin B and rifampin have been used to treat aspergillus infections as well (103, 118).

Meningeal aspergillus infection may require intraventricular or intrathecal administrations of amphotericin B.

Blastomycosis

Blastomycosis is a mycotic disease caused by the organism *Blastomyces dermatitidis* which frequently involves the lungs and can disseminate to the skin and other internal organs. The lesions caused by this organism resemble that of tuberculosis due to its granulomatous nature. Blastomycosis was first thought to occur only on the American continent, however recent information seems to

indicate that it can also occur on the other continents as well. Unlike histoplasmosis or coccidioidomycosis, the blastomyces organism is rare in nature.

CLINICAL FEATURES

The clinical presentation of blastomycosis can closely emulate that of tuberculosis. Systemic dissemination is usually a result of primary pulmonary infection. The lesions produced by the blastomyces is granulomatous-pyogenic in nature, with multiple abscesses containing polymorphonuclear leukocytic infiltrations. The cutaneous involvement first appears as a papule or pustule, but then extends to form the chronic nonpainful ulcers. Usually these ulcers do not produce any local reaction or lymphadenopathy. The systemic and the cutaneous lesions are almost always the result of dissemination from the primary pulmonary infection.

DIAGNOSIS

The diagnosis of blastomycosis is based upon finding the characteristic budding mycoses within the cells from the lesion or the sputum of the infected individual. Serological tests, skin tests and compliment fixation tests are of limited value, because the serological tests cross react with histoplasmosis, and the skin and complement fixation tests are often negative with active disease.

TREATMENT

The treatment of choice for blastomycosis is amphotericin B; it is the most active antifungal agent (Table 13.1). Other agents such as miconazole and hydroxystilbamidine have also been reported to have activity against this infection (105, 106), but the toxicity of hydroxystilbamidine and the high incidence of relapse has limited its usefulness.

Meningeal infection may require intrathecal or intraventricular administration of amphotericin B or miconazole.

Candidiasis

Candidiasis is an infection of the host by the organism *Candida albicans*. *C. albicans* is found in the gastrointestinal tract and vagina of normal healthy individuals. Candida infec-

Table 13.1.
Treatment of Mycotic Infections

AMPHOTERICIN B (119–124)

Indications (see text);
  Aspergillosis, blastomycosis, candidiasis, coccidioidomycosis, cryptococcosis, histoplasmosis
Dose:
Adult and child:
  Intravenous:
    0.6 mg/kg to 1.0 mg/kg per day given intravenously for disseminating systemic mycosis
  Intrathecal or intraventricular:
    0.5–1.0 mg in 10 ml of spinal fluid every other day
Side effects:
  Immediate side effects include nausea, vomiting, anorexia, headache, myalgias, and arthralgia occur in 20–90% of amphotericin B recipients. Many measures have been formulated to combat these common side effects, but only hydrocortisone 25 mg iv at the beginning of the amphotericin B infusion has been shown to be effective in a controlled trial. Thrombophlebitis at the infusion site will develop in 70% of patients with prolonged therapy. The severity of thrombophlebitis might be reduced by the addition of 500–1000 units of heparin to 500 to 1000 ml of the amphotericin B infusion solution. However, controlled studies are lacking to support this procedure. Renal toxicity is a serious complication of amphotericin B therapy. Hypokalemia, renal tubular acidosis, and decrease in glomerular filtration rate (GFR) have been described. These toxicities are usually reversible, unless the total amphotericin B dose is in excess of 4–5 g. Side effects from intrathecal administration of amphotericin B may include headache, vomiting, paresthesias, arachnoiditis and nerve palsies. Intrathecal corticosteroids may be effective in reducing inflammatory reactions, although their efficacy has not been proven

FLUCYTOSINE (107, 124–126)

Indications (see text):
  Aspergillosis, candidiasis, cryptococcosis
Dose:
Adult and child:
  100–200 mg/kg/day given orally in 4 divided doses
Side effects:
  Frequent side effects include nausea, vomiting, diarrhea, and headaches. Less frequent side effects may include vertigo, sedation, hallucination, confusion, and on rare occasion flucytosine may also cause bone marrow supression, and hepatotoxicity. Most of these reported hematological adverse reactions are associated with patients with renal failure, although many renal failure patients have received flucytosine without complications

MICONAZOLE (124, 127–130)

Indications (see text):
  Blastomycosis, coccidioidomycosis, cryptococcosis, histoplasmosis, nonsystemic candidiasis
Dose:
Adult and child older than 1 year of age:
  Intravenous:
    30–60 mg/kg/day iv in 3 divided doses. Manufacturer recommends not to exceed 15 mg/kg per infusion dose. In children, the total daily of 20–40 mg/kg is usually sufficient
  Intrathecal or intraventricular:
    20 mg/day in 5% dextrose is used for intrathecal instillation in adults
Side effects:
  Peripheral vein thrombophlebitis has been reported to occur in 29–38% of patients receiving miconazole. Occasional pruritus, nausea, fever, chills, vomiting, hyperlipidemia, hyponatremia, and skin eruptions have also been reported. Rare side effects such as anemia and thrombocytosis, and anaphylaxis have been described as well. Arachnoiditis has been reported after intrathecal miconazole instillation

tions are generally opportunistic infections due to the weakening of the host's defense by some other causes such as diabetes, neoplastic diseases, immunosupressive therapy, broad- spectrum antiobiotics, or surgical stress. Prolonged indwelling catheter use can also predispose the individual to opportunistic candida infection (110).

CLINICAL FEATURES

C. albicans is frequently present in the gastrointestinal tract of both the normal healthy individual as well as patients with candidiasis. Therefore, it is sometimes difficult to diagnose candidiasis based on candida isolates alone. It is well known that candida infection can be systemic as well as cutaneous (110). The most common cutaneous infection being candida dermatitis involving the moist skin area such the axilla, gluteal folds, perineal folds and the folds beneath the breast. Systemic infections can often involve the bladder, the lungs, and the meninges.

TREATMENT

Candida dermatitis and mucocutaneous infections can be effectively treated with nystatin, clotrimazole, and miconazole (Table 13.1). However, systemic infection will require treatment with more active agents such as amphotericin B and flucytosine. Flucytosine is generally not used alone for systemic candidiasis, except in cases of nonfulminating sensitive candida systemic infection, but more commonly in combination with amphotericin B (107, 111). Meningeal candidal infection may require administration of amphotericin B intraventricularly or intrathecally.

Coccidioidomycosis

Coccidioidomycosis is also known as San Joaquin Valley fever, valley fever, and Posada-Wernicke disease. It is an infection caused by the organism *Coccidioides immitis*, a dimorphic fungus which grows in soil and in culture media as a mold that reproduces by arthrospores, and in tissues and under special conditions of culture it grows spherical cells which reproduce by endospore formation. This disease is endemic in the arid areas of United States, Mexico, Honduras, Guatemala, Venezuela, Bolivia, Paraguay and Argentina, but dusty fomites from endemic areas can also transmit infections elsewhere. This infection can present as acute, self-limiting primary pulmonary infection or as malignant disseminating systemic infection after inhalation of the infective dust borne *C. immitis* arthrospores. *C. immitis* has been isolated from the soil as well as from pulmonary lesions in various animals in endemic areas. There is no evidence of direct animal to man or man to man transmission. The incidence of primary infection appears to have a cyclical seasonal nature, the highest incidence occurring during the arid summer and autumn months.

CLINICAL FEATURES

Primary infection may be entirely asymptomatic or resemble an acute influenzal illness with fever, chill, cough, and pleural pain with effusion. In the majority of the cases recovery occurs within 2 to 3 weeks without sequelae leaving only fibrosis or calcification of pulmonary lesions, or a persistent thin-walled cavity. However, about 5% of the cases develop sensitivity to the organism and may be manifest as erythema nodosum, a complication most frequent in white females and rarest in black males. It is this form of the disease that is known as San Joaquin Valley fever or valley fever. These infections are accompanied by an initial leukocytosis with a normal differential count and later, lymphocytosis, monocytosis and eosinophilia.

The rare secondary or progressive coccidioidal granulomatous disease is characterized by lung lesions and single or aggregated abscesses throughout the body, especially in subcutaneous tissues, skin, bone, peritoneum, testes, thyroid and central nervous system. Coccidioidal meningitis resembles tuberculous meningitis. These disseminative complications occur 10 times more frequently in blacks and Filipinos than in Caucasians.

DIAGNOSIS

Diagnosis is based upon demonstration of the organism by microscopic examination of the sputum or by culture. Reactivity to skin test with coccidioidin appears usually within 2 to 3 days after onset of symptoms but may not develop for up to 3 weeks. Precipitin and complement-fixation tests are usually positive within the first 3 months of clinical disease. Serial skin and serological tests may be necessary to confirm a recent infection. There is an increase in titer of the complement-fixation test with disseminating disease.

TREATMENT

Primary pulmonary coccidiodal infection usually does not require treatment, healing occurs spontaneously without complications. Systemic infections, however, will require antifungal therapy (Table 13.1). The most active antifungal agent is amphotericin B, but other less active agents such as miconazole and amphotericin methyl ester have also been used with some success (115, 116). More recently ketoconazole has also been reported to produce promising results (108, 109). The later agents have lower incidence of toxicity as compared to amphotericin B. Coccidioidomycosis of the meninges may also require intrathecal or intraventricular administration of amphotericin B or miconazole. Although high dose oral ketoconazole produces significant CSF levels, experience with its use is very limited (108).

Cryptococcosis

Cryptococcosis is also known as torulosis, European blastomycosis, or Busse-Buschke's disease. It is usually presented as a subacute or chronic meningoencephalitis. Infection of lung, kidney, prostate, bone or liver occurs, often without local symptoms. Skin may show acneform lesions, ulcers or subcutaneous tumor-like masses filled with gelatinous material. In the central nervous system, cryptococcus may produce a variety of pathologic changes which includes meningitis, granulomas in the meninges, endarteritis, infarcts, and areas of softening and destruction of nerve tissue. Cryptococcosis is caused by the fungus *Cryptococcus neoformans*, which is widely distributed in nature in all parts of the world. This infectious agent has been isolated from the soil, and from old pigeon nests and pigeon droppings. It is presumably transmitted by inhalation of the infectious fungi.

CLINICAL FEATURES

The clinical presentation of cryptococcosis resembles that of tuberculosis. It is a systemic disease with cutaneous manifestations. Lung infections are usually accompanied by cough and signs of chronic bronchitis with peribronchial involvement, which may be confused with pulmonary tuberculosis. A low grade fever is also frequently present. The onset of central nervous system involvement is insidious, although occasionally sudden, with fever, headache and vomiting, and associated increase in cerebral spinal fluid pressure and monocytosis.

DIAGNOSIS

The diagnosis is based on the microscopic isolation of the cryptococcal fungi in the infected tissue, spinal fluid, sputum or the gelatinous content of the subcutaneous mass. The fungi are characteristically in an encapsulated budding form. Diagnosis can also be based on culture or histopathology.

TREATMENT

Amphotericin B therapy (Table 13.1) is usually required, and treatment failures can occur. Flucytosine alone is not recommended, due to it high failure rate. However, the combination of amphotericin B and flucytosine is reported to be superior to either of those two agents alone (117).

Miconazole has also been reported to have varied success in treating cryptococcal infection, although experience with this therapeutic application is still limited (112). Most recently, ketoconazole has also been shown to produce significant success in treating nonmeningeal cryptococcosis (109).

Cryptococcal meningitis may necessitate the use of intraventricular or intrathecal administration of amphotericin B or miconazole in addition to the intravenous regimen (113, 114).

Histoplasmosis

Histoplasmosis, also known as reticuloendothelial cytomycosis, cave disease and Darling's disease is caused by the fungus *Histoplasma capsulatum*. Foci of infection are common over wide areas of the Americas, Europe, eastern Asia, and Australia. *H. capsulatum* has been isolated from the soil and from numerous animals. Infection of man occurs by inhalation of the infectious soilborne spores and there is no evidence for man or animal to man transmission. Clinical disease is infrequent. Histoplasmin hypersensitivity, sometimes in as much as 80% of a population and indicating antecedent infection, is prevalent in parts of eastern and central United States. Prevalence increases from childhood to 30 years of age.

CLINICAL FEATURES

Primary pulmonary infection may be asymptomatic, detectable only by acquired hypersensitivity to histoplasmin, or simulate a mild respiratory illness with general malaise, weakness, fever, chest pains, and cough. Erythema multiforme and erythema nodosum may occur. Recovery is usually spontaneous, with residual multiple scattered lung calcifications, which can be detected by x-ray. Secondary disseminated disease often resemble miliary tuberculosis, and symptoms may vary from unexplained fever, anemia, patchy pneumonia, hepatitis, endocarditis, meningitis, or mucosal ulcerations. Adrenal infection is common in secondary disseminated infections, but are usually asymptomatic. Dissemination occurs more frequently in the generally debilitated individual who is receiving cytotoxic or immunosupressive therapy, and in individual who is greater than 54 years of age (98).

DIAGNOSIS

Clinical diagnosis can be made based on finding the fungus in Giemsa's or Wright's stained smears of the ulcer exudate, bone marrow, sputum or blood. Final identification is based on cultures which demonstrate the typical *H. capsulatum* colonies and spores. Antihistoplasma antibody serum titer tests are available, but recent positive skin tests with histoplasmin can induce false-positive results and additionally the serological tests can cross-react with other mycoses. Cultures for histoplasma are disappointing, because, in noncavitary infections, cultures are rarely positive, and requires 2 to 4 weeks for identification. The compliment fixation test may prove to be of value in detecting histoplasma infections (99).

TREATMENT

Amphotericin B is the antifungal drug of choice (Table 13.1). It is very effective against acute disseminated histoplasma infection, however, with chronic disease the organism may persist in the cavitary lesions. Miconazole has also been used with limited success (100, 101). Recently, ketoconazole has reported to be effective in treating disseminated histoplasmosis, but numbers of reported cases are limited (104, 108).

PARASITIC INFECTIONS

Parasites infect humans in all regions of the world, but there is a particular prevalence of them in the areas where climates are mild, and sanitation is poor. In those underdeveloped regions there is an abundance of both species and infected individuals. Many of these parasites require special environmental conditions for both reproduction and survival. There are other parasites that require an intermediary host for the complement of their life cycle. These intermediary hosts gain access to humans, because of the absence of preventive measures in these underdeveloped countries. In contrast to the more developed countries in the temperature zones where the degenerative diseases, cardiovascular diseases, and malignant diseases are major causes of disability and death, the underdeveloped countries have to deal with diseases that afflict the younger age groups. Infections and malnutrition are sometimes so severe that 40 to 50% of the population may die before reaching the age of 50. Eating habits can also determine the incidence of parasitic infection. The practice of eating raw or partially cooked foods increases the risk of getting a parasitic infection.

Parasitic infections are not limited to the endemic areas. Infections are frequently observed in the migrant population or in travelers who acquire their infection in endemic areas. Thus, health care practitioners outside the tropics must also have adequate knowledge in the diagnosis and treatment of parasitic diseases.

Enterobiasis (1, 2, 20)

Enterobiasis (pinworm, threadworm, or seatworm) infection is an infection of the human gastrointestinal tract caused by *Enterobius vermicularis*. It is one of the most common parasitic infection in the world today. It has been estimated that 5 to 15% of the general population of the United States harbor this helminth, the most prevalent being in school age children, followed by children of preschool age and mothers of infected children. The infection rate is lowest among adults. Infection can be transmitted directly by oral fecal contact or indirectly through clothing, bedding, food, or dust contaminated with viable eggs.

CLINICAL FEATURES (1, 3–8)

Pinworm infection may be asymptomatic, but the most frequent symptom is intense pruritus ani produced by the migrating female helminth and the presence of eggs. This intense pruritus ani may cause secondary dermatitis, eczema, and bacterial infection from the host's constant scratching. A parasitic vulvovaginits and urinary tract infection may also occur in young girls due to enterobiasis. Behavior changes including inattention, irritability, and lack of cooperation can also occur in children infected with pinworm.

DIAGNOSIS

Stool examination for pinworm infection is of little value since adult worms are only occasionally found in heavy infections but the enterobius eggs are almost always present in the perianal areas. The most satisfactory method of diagnosing pinworm infection is by the use of a perianal swab made of a wooden tongue blade and transparent tape. The resulting tape is then placed on a glass slide and examined under a microscope for enterobius ovums. The swabs should be employed in the morning prior to bathing and defecation. Eosinophil count is usually normal in enterobiasis.

TREATMENT (4, 10, 17)

There are numerous anthelmintics available for the treatment of enterobius infection, among them are mebendazole, piperazine citrate, pyrantel pamoate, pyrvinium pamoate, and thiabendazole (Table 13.2). Besides medical management of pinworm infection with pharmacological agents, the treatment should also include prevention of reinfection and screening of the other family members. Personal hygiene and adequate sanitary facilities are paramount in the prevention of pinworm infection. The therapeutic agent of choice for the management of enterobiasis is mebendazole, because it is easy to give and has minimal side effects.

Ascariasis (19, 20)

Ascariasis (roundworm) infection is an infection of the human gastrointestinal tract by *Ascaris lumbricoides*. Ascaris infection occurs worldwide, with the highest incidence in the tropics. In the United States the disease in most prevalent in the southern states among the preschool and early school-aged children. There have been estimates made that approximately 4 million people in the United States are infected by this parasite (20). Ascariasis is transmitted via ingestion of soil contaminated with human feces and viable ascaris eggs. Direct man to man transmission does not occur because the eggs require a minimum soil incubation of 2 weeks.

CLINICAL FEATURES (21–25)

Symptoms caused by ascariasis are often vague and variable or absent. However, children with a heavy parasitic burden may present with symptoms of abdominal pain, vomiting, sleep disturbance, intestinal obstructions, and malnutrition. Individuals who ingest large numbers of ascaris eggs may develop fever, cough, ascaris pneumonitis, and prominent eosinophilia secondary to the large number of migrating larvae. Other rare but more serious complications include obstructions of the pancreatic duct, bile duct, intestinal perforation, and appendicitis.

DIAGNOSIS (26)

Diagnosis is made based upon the demonstration of ascaris ova in the stool or the recovery of a passed adult worm. On occasion diagnosis is made upon visualizing the adult worm in the intestine by x-ray with or without contrasting material. Administrating barium can increase the x-ray visualization of the adult worm after the barium is passed, because the barium is adsorbed onto the surface of the ascaris as well as sometimes stored in their alimentary canal.

TREATMENT

Treatment of ascariasis involves treatment of the disease and prophylaxis (Table 13.2). There are several drugs available for the treatment of ascariasis, among them are mebendazole, piperazine citrate, and pyrantel pamoate. These agents have replaced some of the older and more toxic agents. Prophylaxis against ascariasis should include good hygiene habits especially with respect to proper disposal of human feces, and prevention of ingestion of contaminated soil. The time honored method of fasting before treatment and purgation post treatment has proved to be unnecessary. Unless the patient has total intestinal ascaris obstruction, these pharmacological agents are effective in eradicating the worm and symptoms. It is also common to see an increase in abdominal complaints prior to the expulsion of the ascaris.

Trichuriasis (20)

Trichuriasis (whipworm or trichocephaliasis) is an infection of the large intestinal tract of the human by the parasite *Trichurus trichiura*. Trichuriasis has a similar geographic distribution to ascariasis. The prevalence of trichuriasis is highest among young children in the tropics. In the United States approxi-

Table 13.2.
Treatment of Helminthic Infections

Enterobiasis

MEBENDAZOLE (VERMOX) (8, 9, 14, 17, 74)

Dose:
Adult and child greater than 2 years of age:
  A single dose of 100 mg and repeat in 2 wk
Side effects:
  Occasional abdominal cramps and diarrhea has been reported. Rarely can cause leukopenia

PIPERAZINE CITRATE (ANTEPAR) (12, 13, 74)

Dose:
Adult and child:
  65 mg/kg not to exceed 2.5 g daily for 7 days and repeat in 2 wk
Side effects:
  Occasionally can cause nausea, vomiting, diarrhea, abdominal cramps, and headaches. On rare occasions it can cause transient vertigo, incoordination, muscle weakness, lethargy, erythema multiforme, urticaria, and visual disturbance. It can also exacerbate underlying seizure disorders and cause other CNS toxicity especially in patients with renal dysfunction (14–16)

PYRANTEL PAMOATE (ANTIMINTH) (8, 9, 14, 74)

Dose:
Adult and child:
  A single dose of 11 mg/kg not to exceed 1 g and repeat in 2 wk
Side effects:
  Occasional abdominal cramps, diarrhea, dizziness, headaches, rash, and fever. Transient rise in SGOT has been reported

PYRVINIUM PAMOATE (Povan)

Dose:
Adult and child:
  A single dose of 5 mg/kg not to exceed 250 mg and repeat in 2 wk
Side effects:
  The pyrvinium pamoate will turn stool red and it can stain clothing. Occasionally it can cause nausea, vomiting, and diarrhea. Pyrvinium pamoate can also cause photosensitivity on rare instances

THIABENDAZOLE (MINTEZOL) (18, 27, 74)

Dose:
Adult and child:
  25 mg/kg twice daily not to exceed 3.0 g per day for 1 day only and repeat in 2 wk
Side effects:
  Side effects of thiabendazole include anorexia, headache, nausea, vomiting, and dizziness. On rare occasion it can also cause fever, chills, urticaria, and pruritus

Ascariasis:

MEBENDAZOLE (VERMOX) (8, 13, 17, 32, 74)

Dose:
Adult and child:
  100 mg orally twice daily for 3 days
Side effects:
  Abdominal cramps and diarrhea, and occasionally can cause leukopenia

PIPERAZINE CITRATE (ANTEPAR) (8, 13, 15, 30, 31, 74)

Dose:
Adult and child:
  75 mg/kg orally once daily not to exceed 3.5 g per day for 2 consecutive days
Side effects:
  Adverse reactions can include nausea, vomiting, diarrhea, abdominal cramps, and headaches. Muscle weakness, vertigo, incoordination, lethargy, urticaria, erythema multiforme, and visual disturbance do also rarely occur. In patients with renal dysfunction, CNS toxicities can occur as well

Table 13.2.—*Continued*

PYRANTEL PAMOATE (ANTIMINTH) (8, 13, 18, 28, 29, 74)
Dose:
Adult and child:
   A single dose of 11 mg/kg not to exceed 1 g is effective against ascaris.
Side effects:
   Abdominal cramps, diarrhea, headache, dizziness, rash and fever can occasionally occur. Transient increase in SGOT has also been reported

THIABENDAZOLE (MINTEZOL) (18, 27, 74)
Dose:
Adult and child:
   25 mg/kg orally twice daily not to exceed 3.0 g per day for 1 day and repeat in 2 wk
Side effects:
   Occasional side effects include anorexia, headache, nausea, vomiting, and dizziness. In rare instances pruritus, fever, chills, and urticaria can also occur

Trichuriasis

MEBENDAZOLE (VERMOX) (13, 17, 37, 39, 40, 74)
Dose:
Adult and child over 2 years of age:
   100 mg orally twice daily for 3 days. This is the treatment of choice
Side effects:
   Generally well tolerated, but occasional abdominal cramps and diarrhea can occur. On rare instances leukopenia can also occur

---

mately 2.2 million individuals have been estimated to have trichuriasis. Trichuriasis is transmitted via ingestion of soil contaminated with feces containing viable eggs. Direct man to man transmission does not occur because the eggs require a minimum of 10 days in the soil to mature.

CLINICAL FEATURES (13, 33–35)

Trichurus infections usually produce no clinical symptoms unless a large worm burden is present. Severe infestation of trichurus can produce symptoms including dysentary, mucoid stools, abdominal cramps, weight loss, prolapsed rectum, and malnutrition. Moderate blood eosinophilia and stool Charcot-Leyden crystals may also be found.

DIAGNOSIS (36)

Diagnosis depends on recovery of the trichurus eggs in the stool or upon visualizing the adult worms through sigmoidoscopy or colonoscopy. Three stool samples should be collected on alternate days, and preserved in PVA (polyvinyl alcohol fixative) for shipment or laboratory analysis. (This method of stool sampling will allow one to screen for other concurrent parasitic infection as well.)

TREATMENT (10, 38)

Mebendazole is the drug of choice for the treatment of trichuriasis, although other less active agents like thiabendazole can be used (Table 13.2). Thiabendazole is not recommended for use during pregnancy. Light infection of trichuriasis is usually self-limiting and requires no treatment; however, this may be a source of infection for other family members and contacts.

Treatment of trichuriasis should also include screening of all family members and playmates when children are involved.

Amebiasis (41–43, 56–60)

Amebiasis (amebic dysentery, amebic colitis, or amebic enteritis) specifically refers to an infection of the human host by the protozoa *Entameba histolytica*. Amebiasis occurs in temperate areas worldwide. The *E. histolytica* cysts passed in the stool are immediately infective, and therefore man to man transmission can occur. Unlike the cysts, however, the motile trophozoites are not infective because they can easily be destroyed by stomach acid after ingestion. The most common mode of transmission of amebiasis is from person to person. The asymptomatic cyst passer is an important source of infection, especially if the individual is involved in food preparation. Other modes of transmission may involve contaminated water source, houseflies, cockroaches, and as a venereal disease. The exact incidence of amebiasis is not known, but the prevalence is highest in areas of questionable water source and sanitation. Amebiasis also has a relatively high incidence among the homosexual population.

CLINICAL FEATURES (44–46, 63)

The clinical manifestations of amebiasis varies greatly depending upon the site of infection. The most common amebic infection is that of the intestine. Infected individuals may present with mild diarrhea to bloody dysentary, or without any symptoms at all. Thus, amebiasis is known as the great imitator. Amebiasis can also disseminate to any organ of the body. The most common extraintestinal organ involved is the liver. Liver abscesses may occur many years after the primary intestinal infestation; therefore, one is obligated to treat possible liver involvement at the time of treating the intestinal amebiasis. The factors which determine the virulence of amebiasis are poorly understood, but there is some evidence to indicate that the pathogenesis of disease due to amebae requires the presence of symbiotic bacteria.

DIAGNOSIS (47–54, 61, 62, 70)

The stool from a patient with suspected amebiasis should be examined over a period of 7 to 10 days. If direct on location examination of stool is not possible, the stool specimens should be preserved in PVA fixative for transport and future use. The stool should be passed into the container directly or onto paper and then transferred to container with wooden sticks. The specimens collected during sigmoidoscopy examination may also be examined. The most difficult part of making a correct diagnosis comes from laboratory interpretation errors. A positive stool finding is the only indisputable evidence for diagnosing intraluminal amebiasis. However, the indirect hemagglutination (IHA) test for amebiasis is a valuable diagnostic test for extraluminal amebiasis. The usefulness of this test is limited by its inability to differentiate currently active extraluminal amebiasis from old dormant extraluminal amebic infection. A IHA titer of greater than 1:512 is a reasonably good indicator for recent extraluminal infection. Less then 50% of the patients with hepatic amebiasis will yield a positive stool examination while 95 to 100% of them will have a positive IHA titer of greater than 1:128. Liver function tests are generally not very helpful in detecting hepatic amebiasis because 75% of these patients will have a normal liver function tests. However, radioisotope scan is of value if amebic abscess is present. When stool examinations are performed correctly, 90% of the intestinal amebiasis cases can accurately be diagnosed by three formed and one purged samples, and a 95% accuracy level can be achieved from six samples taken from patients with diarrhea. Diarrhea can be achieved by giving patient magnesium sulfate.

TREATMENT (55, 64, 69, 70)

The chemotherapy of amebiasis is not as clearly defined as that of the other parasitic infections (Table 13.3). The opinions on the drug of choice among the experts are divergent, and this confusion is compounded by the toxicities of the most active drugs. Because there are increasing numbers of reports of treatment failures after using a single agent for amebic dysentary, the therapeutic regimen usually requires two active agents, one for the intestinal amebiasis and the other for the extraluminal infection. It is necessary to repeat the stool examination at least at 6 months after the treatment to confirm total eradication of the infective organism.

Since no single drug is adequate in curing both types of amebiasis, a luminal and extraluminal amebicide must be employed for patients with only intestinal or hepatic amebic infection. The combination of metronidazole followed by diiodohydroxyquin is generally well tolerated and adequate for this purpose, but other drug combinations can also be used. This regimen is not recommended during pregnancy, however, because of the possible teratogenicity and deafness. Other agents used for treating amebiasis include chloroquin phosphate, diloxanide furoate, and paromomycin. Although emetine and emetine hydrochloride have been used very effectively for treatment of extraluminal amebic infections in the past, their use has now been limited by, cardiotoxicity.

Table 13.3.
Treatment of Protozoal Infections (Amebiasis)

I. Intestinal Amebiasis:

DIIODOHYDROXYQUIN (VARIOUS) (67, 68, 74)

Dose:
Adult:
  650 mg orally 3 times daily for 20 days
Child:
  40 mg/kg orally in 3 divided doses daily, not to exceed 2 g per day, for 20 days
Side effects:
  Occasional abdominal cramps, diarrhea, weakness, rash, acne, pruritus ani, optic atrophy, and blindness in children with prolonged exposure (65, 66, 74). Diiodohydroxyquin may cause deafness in children from prenatal exposure, and therefore this drug should be avoided during pregnancy (65)

DILOXANIDE FUROATE (FURAMIDE)

Dose:
Adult:
  500 mg taken orally 3 times daily for 10 days
Child:
  20 mg/kg/day given in 3 divided doses daily, not to exceed 1.5 g per day, for 10 days
Side effects:
  Frequently causes flatulence, and other gastrointestinal symptoms such as cramps, diarrhea, vomiting, and nausea. Occasional urticaria has also been reported

METRONIDAZOLE (FLAGYL) (67, 74)

Dose:
Adult:
  750 mg taken orally 3 times daily for 10 days
Child:
  50 mg/kg/day given in 3 divided doses daily, not to exceed 2250 mg per day, for 10 days
Side effects (67, 74):
  Metronidazole at amebicidal doses may exhibit disulfiram-like side effects when alcohol is taken. Other side effects may include occasional anorexia, nausea, vomiting, diarrhea, flatulence, blurred vision, headaches, confusion, disorientation, depression, and metallic taste in mouth. Leukopenia may also be observed in some patients. Recently, metronidazole has been reported to be carcinogenic in rodents and mutagenic in bacteria. Therefore, this drug is relatively contraindicated for at least during the first trimester of pregnancy (71)

PAROMOMYCIN (HUMATIN) (74)

Dose:
Adult and child:
  25–30 mg/kg/day in 3 divided doses, not to exceed 2.0 g per day, for 10 days
Side effects:
  Gastrointestinal disturbances including nausea, vomiting, diarrhea, and abdominal cramps are most common. These side effects are frequently associated with giving doses in excess of the 2.0 g total daily dose. On rare occasions, eighth nerve damage and nephrotoxicity can also occur, since paromomycin is an aminoglycoside

II. Extraintestinal Amebiasis:

CHLOROQUIN (ARALEN) (67, 72–74)

Dose:
Adult:
  600 mg of base (1 g of chloroquin phosphate) taken orally once daily, for 2 to 3 wk
Child:
  10 mg base (16.67 mg of chloroquin phosphate) per kg per day, not to exceed 300 mg base (500 mg of chloroquin phosphate) given orally once daily, for 2 to 3 wk
Side effects:
  Nausea, vomiting, skin rashes, corneal opacity, alopecia, muscle weakness, and exfoliative dermatitus have been occasionally observed. Rare blood dyscrasias and deafness can also occur

Table 13.3.—*Continued*

METRONIDAZOLE (FLAGYL) (73, 74)
Dose:
Adult:
   750 mg taken orally 3 times daily for 10 days, or 2.0 g taken orally once daily for 3 days. These two regimens are equally effective
Child:
   50 mg/kg/day given in 3 divided doses, not to exceed 2250 mg per day, for 10 days
Side effects:
   Metronidazole may have effects similar to disulfiram when taken with alcohol. Other side effects include nausea, vomiting, diarrhea, anorexia, flatulence, blurred vision, headaches, confusion, disorientation, and depression. Leukopenia has also been observed in some patients. Metronidazole is relatively contraindicated during the first trimester of pregnancy due to recent reports of mutagenicity and carcinogenicity in bacteria and rodents, respectively (71)

Scabies (75, 76)

Scabies (itch mite, or 7-year itch) belong to the family of Sarcoptidae itch mites. Scabies infection occurs most frequently when overcrowding and poor sanitation situations exist. It also appears to be cyclic in nature. Scabies mites are most readily spread through close bodily contact for prolonged periods of time. Only the female mite is implicated in transmission and can survive apart from the host for 2 to 3 days. She is activated by warmth and perspiration of the skin and burrows into the stratum corneum. The mite will live for approximately 2 months in the host and lay a total of several hundred eggs during its lifespan. The incubation period for the eggs is 3 to 4 days, and the larval stage, 10 to 12 days. Fortunately for the human host only 1% of all the eggs will successfully hatch.

CLINICAL FEATURES (77)

Most of the clinical symptoms are caused by the female mite moving through the burrows. She leaves secretions and excreta which elicit erythema, edema and severe itching. The part of the body most commonly infested by scabies mite include the arms, hands, feet, and especially in the skin folds, but other areas such as the belt line, scrotum, the penis, and in women the skin around the nipples can be infected.

DIAGNOSIS (75)

Diagnosis of scabies is made based on clinical presentation of intense pruritus with associated burrow lesions measuring 1 to 10 mm in length caused by the female mite while laying her eggs. Distribution of excoriation marks can help with the diagnosis, but is not conclusive. Skin scrapings of suspicious areas may contain mite or eggs when examined under microscope, and a positive finding is diagnostic of scabies.

TREATMENT

Good personal hygiene is paramount in the treatment of scabies infection, for reinfection is common when infested clothing or bedding are used. Treatment should include laundering of all clothing, especially bedclothes, treating all household contacts, and application of scabicides after a thorough bath (Table 13.4). The scabicides used include γ-benzene hexachloride, crotamiton, benzyl benzoate, and sulfur ointment. Even after adequate treatment, the itching may persist for days and should not be construed as a sign of reinfection, superinfection, or treatment failure. Overtreatment is common and can lead to toxicity especially with γ-benzene hexachloride. In less than 5% of the cases a second course of treatment will be necessary 7 to 10 days after the initial course.

Pediculosis

Pediculosis (human lice) belongs to the family of Pediculidae and there are three species that infest man. These species are 1) *Pediculus humanus corporis*, body lice; 2) *Pediculus humanus capitis*, head lice; and 3) *Phthirus pubis*, crab or pubic lice.

1) *Pediculus humanus corporis* (78–81)

Like the other ectoparasites, the body louse is cosmoplitan in distribution. It is this species that has been implicated in the transmission of diseases such as relapsing fever, trench fe-

Table 13.4.
Treatment of Human Lice and Scabies

Scabies:

1% γ-BENZENE HEXACHLORIDE (GBH) (86–90, 96) CREAM OR LOTION

Directions:
1. Warm bath at night
2. Apply lotion or cream with soft brush from neck down
3. Allow application to dry
4. Repeat application of lotion or cream in the morning
5. Second warm bath in the evening
6. This 24-hr procedure may be repeated in 4–7 days

Cautions:
1. Avoid over treatment
2. Symptoms may persist for 1 month post adequate treatment
3. Avoid use of GBH on face or urethral meatus

CROTAMITON 10% (92–96) CREAM OR LOTION

Directions:
1. Warm bath at night
2. Apply lotion or cream from neck down thoroughly in a massage motion
3. Reapply lotion or cream in 24 hr
4. Second warm bath in 48 hr after the second application

Cautions:
1. Avoid the head, grossly inflamed areas, or excoriated areas

SULFUR OINTMENT (92, 93, 96) 2.5%, 5%, 10% IN PETROLATUM

This is the preferred treatment in children

Directions:
1. Warm bath at night
2. Apply ointment over entire body from neck down nightly for 3 consecutive nights
3. Final bath 24 hr after final application

Cautions:
1. Avoid the head
2. The ointment will stain clothing

BENZYL BENZOATE 25% (91–94) SOLUTION

Directions:
1. Warm bath at night
2. Apply solution by hand or spray over body from neck down for 3 consecutive nights
3. Final bath 24 hr after last application

Cautions:
1. Avoid the head

Body Lice:

1% γ-BENZENE HEXACHLORIDE (93–96) SHAMPOO

Directions:
1. Sterilize clothing, bedding by laundering and hot drying, dry cleaning, or ironing
2. Use 1 oz of shampoo for adult and less for child and lather trunk and extremities for at least 4 min, then rinse thoroughly
3. Repeat procedure in 7 days

Cautions:
Same as in the treatment for scabies

1% MALATHION OR 0.2% PYRETHRINS OR 0.3% ALLETHRIN WITH 1:10 PIPERONYL BUTOXIDE IN AN INERT DUST

Directions:
This procedure is used in cases of heavy infestation or where cleaning facility is not available
1. Dust body and clothing with duster or a sifter can
2. Pay special attention to seams and insides of the clothing

Table 13.4.—*Continued*

Cautions:
1. Avoid excessive use of the dust
2. Avoid inhalation of dust or contamination of foods

Head and Crab Lice (93–95):

1% γ-BENZENE HEXACHLORIDE SHAMPOO

Directions:
1. Clean and wash affected areas well
2. Apply one ounce of shampoo for adult and proportionally less for children and work into hair for at least 4 minutes
3. Thoroughly rinse out shampoo and remove nits with a fine tooth comb
4. Procedure may be repeated in 7–10 days
5. Sterilization of bedding and clothing used within the past 7 days
Cautions:
Same as in the treatment of scabies

PYRETHRINS 0.16%, PIPERONYL BUTOXIDE 2.0%, AND DEODORIZED KEROSENE 5.0%, LIQUID OR GEL

Directions:
1. Clean and wash affected area
2. Massage liberal quantities of solution into hair for at least 1 min
3. Rinse area thoroughly and comb out nits and dead lice with a fine tooth comb within 10 min after application
4. May repeat procedure in 24 hr
Cautions:
1. Avoid face and excessive contact with solution

PHYSOSTIGMINE 2.0% OR AMMONIATED MERCURY 2.0% OINTMENT

Used primarily for treatment of eyelash infestations

Directions:
1. For infestation involving eyelashes one of these ointments may be applied twice daily for 7–10 days
Cautions:
1. Avoid excessive use

---

ver, and epidemic typhus. Body lice are most commonly found in the seams of clothing where tight contact with the body occurs, especially in areas of the axilla, perineum, belt line, neck, and shoulders. The female has a lifespan of 3 to 4 weeks and can lay up to 300 eggs during that lifespan. The eggs hatch in 11 to 13 days depending on conditions and mature to adults in 10 to 20 days. The adult parasite feeds 2 to 3 times daily. The adult and the eggs can survive without the host for up to a month. Body lice are transmitted through direct contact with a louse-infested individual or his/her clothing.

CLINICAL FEATURES

Most of the clinical symptoms are caused by the adult louse feeding on the host daily by digging through the skin with its claws and sucking the blood. It is the saliva and the excretion which produces the intense itching and irritation. Together, they produce the classic clinical presentation.

DIAGNOSIS

Diagnosis is made based on the intense itching, excoriation and infection from scratching and upon finding of the adult louse or the eggs in the seams of the clothing from the suspected infested individual.

TREATMENT

Since concurrent infections are common, treatment must include all members of the family or group, and sterilization of all articles that are possible vehicles of transmission such as clothing, bedding, and cosmetic objects. The agents used to treat body lice include γ-benzene hexachloride and malathion (Table 13.4).

Malathion is used as a 1% dusting powder in endemic areas with good results for quite a number of years, but now there are reports of strains of pediculi that are resistant to malathion. In those resistant strain areas, World Health Organization (WHO) has recommended the use of the insecticide ABATE as a 2% dusting powder.

Often secondary bacterial infections accompany body lice infestation as a result of poor hygiene and excoriation, and these secondary infections may require appropriate antibiotic therapy.

2) *Pediculus humanus capitis* (82, 83)

These pediculi are similar to the body lice in geographic distribution. They are typically found on the hair located around the occiput and ears. The adult female has a lifespan of 33 to 40 days, and can lay 50 to 100 eggs which she attaches individually to the hair shaft with a cement substance. The eggs hatch in 1 to 3 weeks, and reach maturity in 10 to 20 days. The adults can survive without a host for up to 10 days. The infestation is communicated by shared hats, combs, brushes, towels and direct contact.

CLINICAL FEATURES

Pruritus is a cardinal clinical symptom, and excoriation frequently lead to impetigo and pyoderma.

DIAGNOSIS

The itching and the sequelae of scratching usually brings the patient to seek medical help. The diagnosis of head lice is made when the adult louse or the nits of the head lice are found.

TREATMENT

Treatment of head lice involves cleaning and washing of affected areas of the scalp, and applying the pediculocide such as γ-benzene hexachloride, or pyrethrins (Table 13.4). The nits must be physically removed with a fine tooth comb, because they are attached to the hair shaft by a cement-like substance. A second application may be necessary if the infestation is severe.

Secondary impetigo and pyoderma may also require appropriate antibiotic therapy.

3) *Phthirus pubis* (84–86)

The pubic louse is also distributed worldwide. These organisms infest primarily the pubic hairs, but not to the exclusion of others areas. Infestation of the eyelashes can also occur. The lifespan of the female louse is about 20 to 30 days, and she can produce approximately 50 eggs during this time period. The eggs will hatch in about 1 week, and develop into mature adults in 15 to 17 days. The adult crab louse can live for a maximum of 42 hours without feeding and the eggs can stay viable for up to a month under ideal conditions. Transmission almost always occurs during sexual contacts, but in rare circumstances transmission can occur by sharing bedding, underwear, or other objects.

CLINICAL FEATURES

Pruritus and the host's inflammatory response to the crab lice saliva and excreta at the site of feeding accounts for most of the clinical symptoms. Secondary infection can also occur as a result of scratching and excoriation. On rare occasions, infestation of the eyelashes can also occur, resulting in irritation and inflammation of the eyelids.

DIAGNOSIS

Diagnosis of crab lice infestation is made based on the clinical symptoms, distribution of the feeding sites of the pubic lice, and upon the isolation of either the adult louse or the eggs that are cemented to the hair shaft.

TREATMENT (97)

Treatment of crab lice infestation is very similar to the treatment of head lice (Table 13.4). It requires the cleaning and washing of the affected areas, and the application of a delousing agent. Since crab lice infestation is sexually transmitted, the treatment must also include sexual partners. The delousing agents used include γ-benzene hexachloride, pyrethrin, and physostigmine or ammoniated mercury for eyelash involvement.

References

1. Beneson AS: *Control of Communicable Diseases in Man*, ed 12. Washington, D.C.: American Public Health Association, 1975.
2. Cram EB: Studies on oxyuriasis; XXVII. Sum-

mary and conclusion. *Am J Dis Child* 65:46–59, 1943.

3. Simon RD: Pinworm infestation and urinary tract infection in young girls. *Am J Dis Child* 128:21–22, 1974.

4. Royer A, et al: Pinworm infestation in children; the problem and its treatment. *Can Med Assoc J* 86:60–5, 1962.

5. McDonald GSA, et al: Ectopic *Enterobius vermicularis*. Gut 13:621–6, 1972.

6. Sachdev YV, et al: *Enterobius vermicularis* infestation and secondary enuresis. *J Urol* 113:143–144, 1975.

7. Brook STJ Jr, et al: Pelvic granuloma due to *Enterobius vermicularis*. *JAMA* 179:492–494, 1962.

8. Blumenthal DS: Current concept: intestinal nematodes in the United States. *N Engl J Med* 297:1437–1439, 1978.

9. Bambalo TS, et al: Treatment of enterobiasis with pyrantel pamoate. *Am J Trop Med Hyg* 18:50–52, 1969.

10. Miller MJ, et al: Mebendazole, an effective anthelmitic for trichuriasis and enterobiasis. *JAMA* 230:1412–1414, 1974.

11. Beck NJ: Treatment of pinworm infections with reduced single dose of pyrvinium pamoate. *JAMA* 189:511, 1964.

12. Brown HW, et al: Treatment of enterobiasis and ascariasis with piperazine. *JAMA* 161:515, 1956.

13. Johnston TS: Diagnosis and treatment of five parasites. *Drug Intell Clin Pharm* 15:103–110, 1981.

14. Belloni C, et al: Neurotoxic side-effects of piperazine. *Lancet* 2:369, 1967.

15. Nickey LN: Possible prescription of petit mal seizure with piperazine citrate. *JAMA* 195:1069, 1966.

16. Miller CG, et al: Neurotoxic side-effects of piperazine. *Lancet* 1:895, 1967.

17. Keystone JS, Murdoch JK: Mebendazole. *Ann Int Med* 91:582–586, 1979.

18. Most H: Office management of common intestinal parasites. *Drug Ther* 3:39–45, 1973.

19. Schultz MG: The surveillance of parasitic diseases in the United States. *Am J Trop Med Hyg* 23:744–751, 1974.

20. Warren KS: Helminthic disease endemic in the United States. *Am J Trop Med Hyg* 23:723–30, 1974.

21. Tripathy K, et al: Effects of ascaris infection on human nutrition. *Am J Trop Med Hyg* 20:212–218, 1971.

22. Tripathy K, et al: Malabsorption syndrome in ascarians. *Am J Clin Nutr* 25:1276–1281, 1972.

23. Blumenthal DS, et al: Effects of ascaris infection on nutritional status in children. *Am J Trop Med Hyg* 25:682–690, 1976.

24. Jenkins MQ, et al: Intestinal obstruction due to ascariasis: report of thirty-one cases. *Pediatrics* 13:419–425, 1954.

25. Waller CE, et al: Ascariasis: surgical complications in children. *Am J Surg* 120:50–54, 1970.

26. Middlemiss H: *Tropical Radiology*. Bath, England: Intercontinental Medical Book Corporation and Pittman Press, 1961.

27. Shirkey HC: *Pediatric Dosage Handbook, 1971.* Washington, D.C.: American Pharmaceutical Association, 1971.

28. Desowitz RS, et al: Anthelmintic activity of pyrantel pamoate. *Am J Trop Med Hyg* 19:775–778, 1970.

29. Vallarejos VM, et al: Experience with the anthelmintic pyrantel pamoate. *Am J Trop Med Hyg* 20:842–845, 1971.

30. Mathias AW Jr: *Enterobius vermicularis* infection: certain effects of host-parasite relationships. *Am J Dis Child* 101:174, 1961.

31. Swartzwelder JC, et al: The use of piperazine for the treatment of human helminthiases. *Gastroenterology* 33:87–96, 1957.

32. Pena C, et al: Mebendazole, an effective broad-spectrum anthelmintic. *Am J Trop Hyg* 22:592–595, 1973.

33. Jung RC, et al: Clinical observations on *Trichocephalus trichiuras* (whipworm) infestation in children. *Pediatrics* 8:548–557, 1952.

34. Layrisse M, et al: Blood loss due to infections with *Trichuris trichiura*. *Am J Trop Med Hyg* 16:613–9, 1967.

35. Lotero H, et al: Gastrointestinal blood loss in trichuris infection. *Am J Trop Med Hyg* 23:1203–1204, 1974.

36. Melvin DM, et al: Laboratory Procedure for the Diagnosis of Intestinal Parasites (DHEW Publication No. [CDC] 75-8282). Atlanta Center for Disease Control, 1974.

37. Mebendazole—a new anthelminthic: *Med Lett Drugs Ther* 17:37–38, 1975.

38. Sargent RG, et al: A clinical evaluation of mebendazole in the treatment of trichuriasis. *Am J Trop Med Hyg* 23:375–377, 1974.

39. Wagner ED, et al: Morphologically altered eggs of *Trichuris trichiura* following treatment with mebendazole. *Am J Trop Med Hyg* 23:154–157, 1974.

40. Wagner ED, et al: In vivo effects of a new anthelmintic mebendazole (R-17,635) on the eggs of *Trichuris trichiura* and hookworm. *Am J Trop Med Hyg* 23:151–153, 1974.

41. Kean BH: Venereal amebiasis. *NY State J Med* 76:930–931, 1976.

42. Mildvan D, et al: Venereal transmission of enteric pathogens in male homosexuals. *JAMA* 238:1387, 1977.

43. Schmerin MD, et al: Amebiasis. An increasing problem among homosexuals in New York City. *JAMA* 238:1387, 1977.

44. Jones RW: Amoebic liver abscess presenting thirty-two years after acute amoebic dysentary. *Proc R Soc Med* 68:593–594, 1975.

45. Phillips BP, et al: Studies on the ameba-bacteria relationship in amebiasis: comparative results of the intracecal inoculation of germ-free monocontaminated and conventional guinea pigs with *E. histolytica*. *Am J Trop Med Hyg* 4:675–692, 1955.

46. Powell SJ: Latest development in the treatment of amebiasis. *Adv Pharmacol Chemother* 10:91–103, 1972.

47. Krogstad DJ, et al: Amebiasis: epidemiologic studies in the United States, 1971–1974. *Ann Intern Med* 88:89–97, 1978.

48. Juniper K Jr, et al: Serologic diagnosis of amebiasis. *Am J Trop Med Hyg* 21:157–168, 1972.
49. Krupp IM: Antibody response in intestinal and extraintestinal amebiasis. *Am J Trop Med Hyg* 19:57–62, 1970.
50. Krupp IM, et al: Comparative study of the antibody response in amebiasis: persistence after successful treatment. *Am J Trop Med Hyg* 20:421–424, 1971.
51. Healy GR, et al: Use of indirect hemagglutination test in some studies of seroepidemiology of amebiasis in the western hemisphere. *Health Lab Sci* 7:109–116, 1970.
52. Healy GR: The use and limitations to the indirect hemagglutination test in the diagnosis of intestinal amebiasis. *Health Lab Sci* 5:174–179, 1968.
53. Kim CW: The diagnosis of parasitic diseases. *Prog Clin Pathol* 6:267–288, 1975.
54. Kagan IG: Serologic diagnosis of parasitic diseases. *N Engl J Med* 282:685–86, 1970.
55. Barrett-Connor E: Amebiasis, today, in the United States. *West J Med* 114:1–6, 1971.
56. Sexton DJ, et al: Amebiasis in a mental institution: serologic and epidemiologic studies. *Am J Epidemiol* 100:414–423, 1974.
57. Brooke MM: Epidemiology of amebiasis. *Am J Gastroenterol* 41:371–375, 1964.
58. Hardy AV, et al: The occurrence of infestations with *E. histolytica* associated with waterborne epidemic diseases. *Public Health Rep* 50:232–234, 1935.
59. McCoy GW, et al: Epidemic amebic dysentery. The Chicago outbreak of 1933. *Natl Inst Health Bull*, No. 166, Washington, D.C., 1936.
60. Spencer HC, et al: Endemic amebiasis in an extended family. *Am J Trop Med Hyg* 26:623–635, 1977.
61. Kessel JG, et al: Indirect hemagglutination and compliment fixation tests in amebiasis. *Am J Trop Med Hyg* 14:540–555, 1951.
62. Debakey ME, et al: Hepatic amebiasis: a 20-year experience and analysis of 263 cases. *Surg Gynecol Obstet* 92:209–231, 1951.
63. Wittner MR: Role of bacteria in modifying virulence of *Entamoeba histolytica*: studies of amebae from axenic cultures. *Am J Trop Med Hyg* 19:755–761, 1970.
64. Powell SJ: Therapy of amebiasis. *Bull NY Acad Med* 47 (Ser 2):469–477, 1971.
65. Oakley GP: The neurotoxicity of the halogenated hydroxyquinolines. *JAMA* 225:395–397, 1973.
66. Behrens MM: Optic atrophy in children after diiodohydroxyquin therapy. *JAMA* 228:693, 1974.
67. Krogstad DJ, et al: Amebiasis. *N Engl J Med* 298:262–265, 1978.
68. Most H: Treatment of common parasitic infections of man encountered in the United States. *N Engl J Med* 287:698–702, 1972.
69. Tsar SH: Experience in the therapy of amebic liver abscesses on Taiwan. *Am J Trop Med Hyg* 22:24–29, 1973.
70. Gregory PB: A refractory case of hepatic amoebiasis. *Gastroenterology* 70:585–587, 1976.
71. Is Flagyl Dangerous? *Med Lett Drug Ther* 17:53–54, 1975.
72. Coher HG, et al: Comparison of metronidazole and chloroquin for the treatment of amebic liver abscess. *Gastroenterology* 69:35–41, 1975.
73. Hunter GW, et al: Amebiasis and related infections. In Hunter GW, et al: *Tropical Medicine*, ed 5. Philadelphia: W. B. Saunders, 1976.
74. Drugs for parasitic infections. *Med Lett* 24:601, 1982.
75. Mellanby K: The development of symptoms; parasitic infection and immunity in human scabies. *Parasitology* 35:197, 1944.
76. Orkin M: Resurgence of scabies. *JAMA* 217:593, 1971.
77. Parlette HL: Scabietic infestations of man. *Cutis* 16:47, 1975.
78. Snyder JC: Typhius fever rickettsia. In Hoosfall FL Jr, Tamm I: *Viral and Rickettsial Infections of Man*, ed 4. Philadelphia: J. B. Lippincott, 1965, pp 1059–1094.
79. Zolrodovskii PF, Golinevich EH: Wolhynian on five-day fever. In *The Rickettsial Diseases*, ed 2. London: Pergamon Press, 1960, p 630.
80. Geigy R: Relapsing fevers: In Wienman D, Ristie M: *Infectious Blood Diseases of Man and Animals*. New York: Academic Press, 1968, vol 2, pp 175–216.
81. NuHall G: The biology of *Pediculus humanus*. *Parasitology* 10:80, 1917.
82. Gratz NG: The current status of louse infestations throughout the world. The control of lice and louse-borne diseases. In *Proceedings of the International Symposium on Control of Lice and Louse-Borne Diseases*. Washington, D.C.: Pan American Health Organization, 1973, p 23.
83. Grothaus RH, et al: Class Insecta (Hexapoda). In Hunter GW, et al: *Tropical Medicine*, ed 5. Philadelphia: W. B. Saunders, 1976.
84. Nuttall G: The biology of *Phthirus pubis*. *Parasitology* 10:383, 1918.
85. Koehn GG: Current trends in scabies. *Rocky Mt Med J* 526, 1975.
86. Nuhal G: The pathological effects of *Phthirus pubis*. *Parasitology* 10:375, 1918.
87. Feldman RJ: Percutaneous penetration of some pesticides and herbicides in man. *Toxicol Appl Pharmacol* 28:126, 1974.
88. Council on Pharmacy and Chemistry. Toxic effects of technical benzene hexachloride and its isomers. *JAMA* 147:571, 1951.
89. Joslin EF: Fatal case of lindane poisoning. National Association of Coroners, Proceedings of 1958 Symposium.
90. Nicholls RW: A case of acute poisoning by benzene hexachloride. *Med J Aust* 42: Jan. 11, 1958.
91. Rajan U: Treatment of head lice infestation with benzyl benzoate and pyrethrum. *Singapore Med J* 16:297, 1975.
92. Kawaaheh MA: Eradication of a large scabies outbreak using community-wide health education. *Am J Public Health* 66:564, 1976.
93. Orkin M: Treatment of today's scabies and pediculosis. *JAMA* 236:1136, 1976.
94. Nierhuis M: Pediculosis and scabies. *U.S. Pharmacist* 35, Oct. 1976.
95. Maibach HI: Therapeutic agents for human skin infestations. *JAMA* 230:759, 1974.

96. Kwell and other drugs for treatment of lice and scabies. *Med Lett* 19:473, 1977.

97. Cogan DG: Treatment of pediculosis ciliaris with anticholinesterase agents. *Arch Opthalmol* 41:627, 1949.

98. Wheat LJ, et al: Risk factors for disseminated or fatal histoplasmosis. *Ann Intern Med* 96:159–163, 1982.

99. Wheat J, et al: The diagnostic laboratory tests of histoplasmosis analyses of experience in a large urban outbreak. *Ann Intern Med* 97:680–685, 1982.

100. Goodwin RA Jr, et al: Disseminated histoplasmosis: clinical and pathological correlations. *Medicine (Baltimore)* 59:1–33, 1980.

101. Reddy P, et al: Progressive disseminated histoplasmosis as seen in adults. *Am J Med* 48:629–636, 1970.

102. Atkinson GW, Israel HL: 5-Flurocytosine treatment of meningeal and pulmonary aspergillosis. *Am J Med* 55:496–504, 1973.

103. Ribner B, Keusch GT, Hana BA, et al: Combination amphotericin B-rifampin therapy for pulmonary aspergillosis in a leukemic patient. *Chest* 70:681–683, 1976.

104. Hawkins SS, Gragory DW, Alford RH: Progressive disseminated histoplasmosis: favorable response to ketoconazole. *Ann Intern Med* 95:446–449, 1981.

105. Wade TR, Jones HE, Chanda JS: Intravenous miconazole therapy of mycotic infections. *Arch Intern Med* 139:784–786, 1979.

106. Rose HD, Varkey B: Miconazole treatment of relapsed pulmonary blastomycosis. *Am Rev Resp Dis* 118:403–408, 1978.

107. Bennett JE: Flucytosine. *Ann Intern Med* 86:319–322, 1977.

108. Craven PC, Graybill JR, Jorgensen JH, et al: High-dose ketoconazole for treatment of fungal infection of the central nervous system. *Ann Intern Med* 98:160–167, 1983.

109. Dismukes WE, Stamm AM, Graybill JR, et al: Treatment of systemic mycoses with ketoconazole: emphasis on toxicity and clinical response in 52 patients. *Ann Intern Med* 98:13–20, 1983.

110. Torres-Rojas JR, Stratton CW, Sanders CV, et al: Candidal suppurative peripheral thrombophlebitis. *Ann Intern Med* 96:431–435, 1982.

111. Edwards JE Jr, Lehrer PI, Stiehm ER, et al. Severe candidal infections: clinical perspective, immune defense mechanisms, and current concepts of therapy. *Ann Intern Med* 89:91–106, 1978.

112. Young RC, Bennett JE, Geelhoed GW, et al: Fungemia in patients with compromised host resistance: a study of 70 cases. *Ann Intern Med* 80:605–612, 1974.

113. Weinstein L, Jacoby I: Successful treatment of cerebral cryptococcoma and meningitis with miconazole. *Ann Intern Med* 93:569–571, 1980.

114. Graybill JR, Levine MB: Successful treatment of cryptococcas meningitis with ventricular miconazole. *Arch Intern Med* 138:814–816, 1978.

115. Hoeprich PD, Heath LK, Lawrence RM: The methyl ester of amphotericin B: evolution to therapy in man. Proceedings and Abstracts of the 16th Interscience Conference on Antimicrobial Agents and Chemotherapy, Chicago, 1976, Abstr 306.

116. Stranz MH: Micronazole. *Drug Intell Clin Pharm* 14:86–95, 1980.

117. Bennett JE, Dismukes WE, Duma RJ, et al: A comparison of amphotericin B alone and combined with flucytosine in the treatment of cryptococcal meningitis. *N Engl J Med* 301:126–131, 1979.

118. Kitahara M, Seth VK, Medoff G, et al: Activity of amphotericin B, 5-fluorocytosine, and rifampin against six clinical isolates of aspergillus. *Antibicrob Agents Chemother* 9:915–919, 1976.

119. Utz JP, Bennett JE, Brandriss MW, et al: Amphotericin B toxicity. *Ann Intern Med* 61:334–354, 1964.

120. Douglas J, Healy J: Nephrotoxic effects of amphotericin B, including renal tubular acidosis. *Am J Med* 46:154–162, 1969.

121. Takacs F, Tomkiewicz Z, Merrill J: Amphotericin B nephrotoxicity with irreversible renal failure. *Ann Intern Med* 59:716–724, 1963.

122. Miller H, Bates J: Amphotericin-B toxicity: a follow-up report of 53 patients. *Ann Intern Med* 71:1089–1095, 1969.

123. Maddux MS, Barriere SL: A review of complications of amphotericin-B therapy: recommendations for prevention and management. *Drug Intell Clin Pharm* 14:177–181, 1980.

124. Meade RH III: Drug therapy review: clinical pharmacology and therapeutic use of antimycotic drugs. *Am J Hosp Pharm* 36:1326–1334, 1979.

125. Steer PL, Marks MI, Klite PD, et al: 5-Fluorocytosine: oral antifungal compound. *Ann Intern Med* 76:15–22, 1972.

126. Meyer R, Axelrod JL: Fatal aplastic anemia resulting from flucytosine. *JAMA* 224:1573, 1974.

127. Bagnarello AG, Lewis LA, McHenry MC, et al: Unusual serum lipoprotein abnormality induced by the vehicle of miconazole. *N Engl J Med* 296:497–479, 1977.

128. Sawyer PR, Brodgen RN, Pinder RM, et al: Miconazole: a review of its antifungal activity and therapeutic efficacy. *Drugs* 9:406–423, 1975.

129. Sung JP, Campbell GD, Grendahl JG: Miconazole therapy for fungal meningitis. *Arch Neurol* 35:443–447, 1978.

130. Stranz MH: Miconazole. *Drug Intell Clin Pharm* 14:86–95, 1980.

SECTION 3
Gastrointestinal Diseases

CHAPTER 14

Peptic Ulcer Disease

JOHN K. SIEPLER, Pharm.D.
WALTER L. TRUDEAU, B.M., B.Ch.

Most estimates suggest that between 5 and 10% of the general population will develop a peptic ulcer during their lifetime. Duodenal ulcers are 4 times more common than gastric ulcers, and males are 3 times as likely as females to develop an ulcer. Peptic ulcer is a recurrent disease and most clinical studies have shown that approximately 50% of patients will have a recurrence within 1 year of diagnosis. Duodenal ulcers are almost never malignant, but 5% of gastric ulcers are cancerous. For this reason evaluation of the patient and follow-up is extremely important in patients with gastric ulcer disease.

Peptic ulcer disease includes ulceration anywhere in the gastrointestinal tract where gastric mucosal (parietal) cells secrete hydrochloric acid. The Barrett ulcer of the esophagus, ulcers in the stomach (gastric ulcer), duodenal ulcer in the first part of the duodenum, postbulbar ulcer, some cases of Meckel's diverticulum, and stomal or jejunal ulcers following surgery for peptic ulcer are all classified as peptic ulcer disease. The Zollinger-Ellison syndrome is rare but of major importance in its implications with regard to the hormone gastrin (1).

GASTRIC SECRETION

The physiology of gastric secretions has been the subject of many studies since Prout demonstrated hydrochloric acid in the human stomach in 1824 and since Beaumont published his classic studies on Alexis St. Martin in 1833. The secretion of gastric hydrochloric acid is intimately related to peptic ulcer disease. A peptic ulcer does not develop when there is no acid secretion. Although measurement of gastric HCl (gastric analysis) is a time-honored procedure, improved knowledge of the physiology of gastric secretion, has allowed a more clear-cut definition of its indications and recognition of its limitations.

Gastric secretion occurs continuously, and is termed "basal" when no stimuli are applied. Stimulated gastric secretion can be divided into three phases: cephalic, gastric and intestinal.

Basal acid secretion in humans ranges between 0 and 5 mEq/hour. A circadian rhythm of acid secretion occurs, with the lowest output between 5 A.M. and 11 A.M. and the highest rate in the evening between 6 P.M. and 1 A.M. The factors responsible for basal acid secretion are unknown. Tonic vagal stimulation and a steady release of small amounts of gastrin probably play a role. Basal acid secretion is decreased by vagotomy or by antrectomy (2).

The major physiologic stimulant to acid secretion in man is the ingestion of meals (Table 14.1). The work of Pavlov in the last century led to clinically important understanding of the cephalic stimulation of secretion resulting from sight, taste, smell and chewing of food. Two mechanisms are responsible for the cephalic phase (a) vagal stimuli acting directly on the parietal cell through release of acetylcholine, and (b) vagal stimuli that cause release of gastrin from the antrum. The peak acid response to slow feeding, a measure of the cephalic phase, is about 50% of the maximal acid response to a potent stimulant such as pentagastrin. Vagotomy and atropine abolish the cephalic phase.

Like the cephalic phase, the gastric phase of acid secretion is mediated both by gastrin and by cholinergic nerves. The stimulus to secretion arises from mechanical and chemical stimuli acting in the stomach, but in this phase distention of the stomach is the only form of mechanical stimulation that is known to be effective in stimulating acid secretion. It is assumed to be mediated by cholinergic reflexes through long and short vagal nerves in the gastric wall. The chemicals in food known to stimulate acid secretion are amino acids and peptides. The principal mechanism by which they stimulate acid secretion is through the release of gastrin, which in turn stimulates the

Table 14.1.
Phases of Acid Secretion

Phase	Mediator

Cephalic	1. Vagus nerve
	  (a) Direct innervation of parietal cell
	  (b) Gastrin release

Gastric	1. Distention of stomach
	  (a) Vagus nerve
	2. Amino acids
	  (b) Direct release of gastrin
	  (c) pH dependent

Intestinal	1. Food in jejunum
	  (a) Entero-oxyntin (?)
	  (b) Gastrin (?)

Table 14.2.
Stimulants of Acid Secretion

Stimulant	Action	Blocker
Acetylcholine	Direct receptor on parietal cell	Anticholinergics
Gastrin	Direct receptor	Anti-gastrin antibody (experimental)
Histamine	Direct receptor or parietal cell (final common mediator (?))	H_2 receptor antagonists (cimetidine, ranitidine)

parietal cells to secrete acid. The acid response provides a negative feedback on the further secretion of gastrin. Lowering of the gastric pH from 5.5 to 2.5 completely suppresses gastrin output in response to amino acids.

The intestinal phase is less well understood. Food in the upper small intestine stimulates gastric acid secretion, which is thought to be mediated in part by the release of intestinal gastrin. An as yet unidentified hormone, called entero-oxyntin to distinguish it from gastrin, may be the principal mediator of the intestinal phase of acid secretion. In addition, fats and hypertonic solutions instilled into the duodenum inhibit acid secretion through the release of cholecystokinin (CCK) and gastric inhibitory peptide (GIP) (1).

Histologic studies have shown that patients with duodenal ulcer have a greater number of parietal cells than do normal patients. Each cell is capable, with maximal stimulation, of secreting maximally. Increases and decreases in total gastric hydrochloric acid secretion are thus a function of the number of cells present and functioning. The total parietal cell population is termed the "parietal cell mass." Following maximal stimulation, the amount of acid output correlates well, both in dogs and man, with parietal cell mass.

NEUROHUMORAL STIMULANTS OF ACID SECRETION

Three substances, acetylcholine, gastrin and histamine, are capable of stimulating the parietal cells to produce hydrochloric acid (Table 14.2). For many years the physiologic role of histamine in gastric secretion has been controversial. With the discovery by Black and co-workers of a new class of antihistaminic drugs, the H_2 receptor antagonists, histamine is now considered to have an important physiologic role in gastric acid secretion. H_2 receptor antagonists both block the receptor for histamine on the parietal cell and inhibit acid secretion stimulated by gastrin and acetylcholine.

Acetylcholine

Acetylcholine is released at the parietal cell by local nerves, stimulation of the vagus and by distention of the stomach that is mediated through receptors in the gastric wall. These cholinergic reflexes can be blocked by atropine. Acetylcholine also sensitizes the parietal cell to other stimuli, such as gastrin and histamine, and plays a role in the cholinergic release of gastrin from the antral G-cell in man.

Gastrin

Almost 70 years ago Edkins discovered a hormone in the gastric antrum, which he named "gastrin," that stimulates gastric secretion. Like many fundamental discoveries, it was almost forgotten until Gregory and Tracy isolated, determined the chemical structure and synthesized pure gastrin in 1964. There are two gastrins, gastrin I and gastrin II, each being a polypeptide of 17 amino acids. Their physiologic properties stem from the terminal residues of the molecule, the smallest being the tetrapeptide. Its congener, pentagastrin, is a synthetic preparation that is now commercially available and that eventually should supplant histamine as the standard stimulant of gastric secretion in performing a gastric analysis. It is as effective as maximal histamine stimulation and is without side effects.

The known actions of gastrin are as follows: (a) potent stimulation of gastric acid; (b) moderate stimulation of pepsinogen secretion; (c) moderate stimulation of hepatic bile flow, insulin release from pancreas and pancreatic secretion; (d) stimulation of gastric and intestinal motility; and (e) increases lower esophageal sphincter pressure; i.e. promotes closure of the sphincter mechanism.

The three gastrointestinal hormones, gastrin, cholecystokinin (now known to be the same as pancreozymin) and secretin, that have been isolated and whose chemical structure is known, have important interrelationships. Other hormones exist, but they are less well defined.

Gastrin may now be accurately determined in the blood by radioimmunoassay. Gastrin assays are now obtainable from many commercial laboratories and in most medical centers. The normal gastrin level is less than 200 pg/ml. The gastrin assay is imperative for the diagnosis of the gastrin-producing pancreatic adenoma (Zollinger-Ellison syndrome) in which fasting blood levels are extremely high. Gastrin levels are not elevated in chronic peptic ulcer. In pernicious anemia with its achlorhydria, serum gastrin levels are significantly elevated because the stimulus to the "turning off" of gastric, i.e. acid production, is absent.

Histamine

Histamine is present in many of the tissues of the body, including the gastric mucosa. Recent studies with the histamine H_2 antagonists suggests that histamine is the "final common mediator" of acid secretion. The H_2 receptor antagonist cimetidine has been shown to inhibit acid secretion stimulated not only by histamine, but also by other agents such as gastrin, insulin and caffeine, implying that histamine is involved in all forms of acid secretion.

DUODENAL ULCER

A duodenal ulcer is a benign ulcer in the wall of the duodenum, passing into the muscularis mucosae. Most duodenal lesions that are discovered by endoscope, or by upper GI x-rays, fall into this category.

This true cause of duodenal ulcer is unknown, although it has been assumed for years that it is related to excessive secretion of hydrochloric acid by the parietal cells of the stomach. One third to one half of patients with duodenal ulcer exhibit basal hypersecretion, and show evidence of an increased parietal cell mass by a markedly increased peak acid secretion on gastric analysis testing. Part of the evidence for acid hypersecretion as the cause of duodenal ulcer is indirect: Dragstedt and Owens (2), in 1943, demonstrated that truncal vagotomy caused healing of peptic ulcers. It has been assumed that this is due to interruption of the vagal innervation of the parietal cell with a resulting 70% reduction in acid secretion.

Duodenal ulcer disease is both chronic and remittent. Upper GI endoscopy has demonstrated that it is unlikely that an individual will suffer from a single ulcer for any great length of time. Duodenal ulcers probably represent a stage in a disease process which begins with acute inflammation of the duodenal mucosa, and progresses through more severe stages of duodenitis until a frank ulcer develops.

The ulcer usually persists for 4 to 6 weeks, but may on occasion heal rapidly. The whole process then repeats itself at some later stage, depending upon as yet unknown stimuli. Psychosomatic factors probably do not play an important role in the development of the ulcer, and a relationship to a variety of stress situations seems at best only vaguely associated with the development of new ulcers. A recurrent ulcer may or may not develop in the same location as previously. There is a no site predilection in the duodenal bulb, except that 95% occur in close association with the pyloric ring, the mucosal junction between stomach and duodenum (1).

BENIGN GASTRIC ULCER

In the United States, gastric ulcer occurs about one fourth as frequently as duodenal ulcer. Like duodenal ulcer, it is more common in men than in women. It is unusual in the younger age population, the incidence increasing after age 50 years.

Unlike duodenal ulcer which is thought to be a disorder of gastric acid hypersecretion, gastric ulcers tend to be associated with lower rates of secretion when compared to normal subjects. As do other ulcers, it tends to occur at areas where two different types of epithelium join; i.e. junctional epithelial areas. It is most common at the junction between the antrum and the fundus of the stomach on the lesser curvature. It may, however, occur high on the lesser curvature. Oi et al. (3) found that 96% of all gastric ulcers occur within 2 cm of the transitional zone between the body and the antrum or the stomach, containing both fundic and pyloric glands.

Within the last 10 years, various authors have shown that gastric ulcer, although an acid peptic disease like other ulcers, may be due primarily to breakage of the mucosal barrier by back-diffusion of acid secreted by the fundic parietal cells. Normally, less than one tenth of the gastric hydrochloric acid secreted by the parietal cells is reabsorbed into the gastric mucosa by back-diffusion. In patients with gastric ulcer, the figure tends to be much higher. The question then becomes: What is responsible for the breakage of the mucosal barrier?

It has repeatedly been demonstrated that healing of a gastric ulcer does not result in restitution of the gastric mucosal barrier to back-diffusion. Back-diffusion remains high, even if the ulcer has disappeared. Furthermore, a gastric ulcer does not necessarily recur at the site of the previous ulcer, suggesting that the defect in the mucosal barrier is generalized, rather than localized. Davenport (5) defined the gastric mucosal barrier as that property of the gastric mucosa which impedes diffusion of acid from the lumen into the mucosa and impedes diffusion of sodium ion from mucosal interstitial space into the lumen.

The mucosal barrier consists of the plasma membrane of the surface epithelial cells which, because of their high phospholipid content, and because of tight junctions between cells, renders it impermeable to ionized materials. A number of agents are capable of damaging the mucosal barrier. It has been shown that salicylates, fatty acids, ethanol, lysolecithin and bile salts all disrupt the normal mucosal barrier. This allows rapid back-diffusion of hydrogen ion from the lumen into the mucosa, causing cellular destruction and increased capillary permeability within the damaged mucosa. This in turn results in extravasation of plasma proteins producing mucosal edema. The rapid cell turnover of the gastric mucosa is also disrupted, leading to desquamation and loss of gastric epithelial cells in the area. Capper (7), who demonstrated a high incidence of bile reflux in patients with gastric ulcer, suggested that these changes are caused by regurgitation of duodenal content into the stomach. He suggests that bile reflux

produces a gastritis, which may predispose to ulcer in some patients. The mucosal damage which follows bile reflux appears to be closely related to the back-diffusion of hydrogen ion from gastric contents into the mucosa. This concept is of importance in view of the development of compounds which strengthen the mucosa against bile damage and reduce the back-diffusion of hydrogen ion.

Other theories for the cause of gastric ulcer have also been proposed. The Dragstedt theory (8) of antral stasis, with resultant hypersecretion of gastrin, was popular for a time, but has largely been disproven. Other authors have suggested that gastric ulcer may be caused by a deficiency of gastric mucous secretion or an alteration of gastric mucous composition. It has been well demonstrated that normal gastric mucus does not provide an adequate barrier to acid diffusion, diffusion occurring freely both ways through gastric mucus. The currently prevailing theory for the etiology of gastric ulcer is the back-diffusion theory of Davenport (5).

SYMPTOM COMPLEX

The symptoms of peptic ulcer disease are quite varied. The slight differences that may appear between duodenal ulcer and gastric ulcer are so subtle that the differentiation between these two entities cannot be made on symptoms alone. Burning pain in the epigastric area is most common. Less commonly, it radiates to other areas, such as the back or lower abdomen. It most often occurs when the stomach is empty, and is relieved by meals.

Zollinger-Ellison (Gastrinoma) Syndrome

The Zollinger-Ellison syndrome is caused by a gastrin-producing adenoma of the pancreas and, sometimes, other endocrine glands. Gastrin isolated from the tumor is usually identical to antral gastrin. It has been suggested that this syndrome should be redesignated "gastrinoma," a more exact term (Table 14.3).

The syndrome, first described in 1955, is moderately rare but important in leading to a better understanding of gastric secretion—especially the role of gastrin. Characteristically there are severe, often unremitting and numerous recurrences of peptic ulcers. These may be either gastric or duodenal and are often multiple, occurring in unusual locations such as the third part of the duodenum or even the jejunum. It occurs in adults of both sexes with equal frequency and rarely in children, 11 pediatric cases having been reported up to 1967. In a large general hospital two or three cases probably will be found each year, especially if the syndrome is kept in mind as a possible cause of severe peptic ulcer disease. Because the disease is caused by a gastrin-secreting adenoma that may be in multiple location in the pancreas and in other endocrine glands, there is a continuous stimulation of HCl secretion that cannot be turned off as in the normal physiologic mechanism. This is the explanation for the very high basal acid secretion and for the fact that histamine or pentagastrin stimulation does not increase this significantly.

To properly identify this disease, further studies are necessary, including a measurement of serum gastrin. Serum gastrin measurements by radioimmunoassay are done in most large hospital nuclear medicine departments. The range of basal gastrin concentration in patients with duodenal ulcer disease without gastrinoma is usually from 0 to 120 pg/ml, depending on the sensitivity of the assay being utilized. A serum gastrin concentration above 500 pg/ml strongly supports the diagnosis of Zollinger-Ellison syndrome.

The most valuable tests in identifying patients with the Zollinger-Ellison syndrome are the presence of striking hypergastrinemia in patients with acid hypersecretion and consistent clinical features. The combination of hypersecretion of acid and marked hypergastrinemia is virtually diagnostic, even in the absence of demonstrable tumor. In those patients with less prominent hypergastrinemia, performance of provocative tests of gastrin release have made the detection of Zollinger-Ellison syndrome easier and more precise (1).

DIAGNOSTIC TECHNIQUES
Gastric Analysis

Although it is now generally agreed that duodenal ulcer is caused primarily by hypersecretion of hydrochloric acid by the parietal cells, there is still a place for gastric analysis. More correctly, we should refer to it as analysis of the magnitude of gastric acid secretion. The wide individual variations and overlapping are indicative of the lack of pronounced value in assessment of findings on a quantitative basis for a given patient. However, the data do support the concept that duodenal ulcer tends to

be associated with acid secretion that is almost twice normal, that gastric ulcer patients secrete less acid then normal persons, and that gastric cancer patients secrete much less. Women secrete less acid than men in all categories. In the majority of patients with demonstrable duodenal ulcer, a gastric analysis adds little, if anything, to the clinical evaluation of the problem and need not be done. Only when the ulcer is intractable or when complications requiring surgery occur may quantitative assessment of gastric secretion be helpful—especially if Zollinger-Ellison syndrome is a possible diagnostic consideration. If the same techniques are closely observed, constant and reliable results may be obtained.

Most experienced gastric surgeons and gastroenterologists now rely upon the 1-hour calculated basal secretion, and the 1-hour maximally stimulated secretion (Table 14.4). This test requires four 15-min, carefully aspirated samples, obtained from the patient in as close to a basal condition as possible.

Radiology and Endoscopy

The current literature is replete with comparative studies assessing the relative accuracy of endoscopy and radiology in GI diagnosis. The time-honored central role that radiology has played in this field has been challenged by the development of fiberoptic endoscopes. Endoscopes permit the direct examination of the esophagus, stomach and first and second portions of the duodenum. Thus,

Table 14.3.
Zollinger-Ellison Syndrome

1. Severe recurrent ulcers frequently in distal duodenum or jejunum
2. Very high basal acid secretion rates (see Table 14.4)
3. Elevated fasting gastrin (200 pg/ml—frequently 7500)
4. Diarrhea and steatorrhea

Table 14.4.
Acid Secretion—Condition

HCl (mEq/hr)		Consistent with
Basal	Stimulated	
0–5	4–10	Normal, gastric cancer
5–10	6–15	Normal, gastric ulcer
10–20	15–25	Duodenal ulcer
15–45	20–60	Zollinger-Ellison syndrome

most areas in which upper GI disease occur are readily accessible to direct visualization and biopsy. Equivocal lesions can be biopsied with relative ease, and one can obtain adequate visualization of superficial erosions not readily visible radiographically. Endoscopy has become the primary modality in the diagnosis of sources of upper GI bleeding. Additionally, endoscopy should be the preferred procedure in evaluating upper GI problems in pregnant women, where radiation is to be avoided.

Several important considerations must be kept in mind when comparing endoscopy with radiography in the diagnosis of upper GI tract disorders. Technique and experience are very important factors. The diagnostic accuracy of endoscopy is no better than the specialist performing the procedure. Experienced endoscopists have a very high diagnostic accuracy rate. In contrast, it is estimated that in using a standard upper GI x-ray series 20 to 40% of all lesions will be missed. The air contrast x-ray examination consists of the use of a thick barium suspension and effervescent pellets or powder to release gas within the stomach and distend it. After rotating the patient to ensure uniform barium coating, air contrast views of the stomach and duodenum can be obtained. This procedure may be followed by the ingestion of standard barium for completing the examination with the standard technique. The combined approach offers the advantage of both an air contrast and a standard upper GI examination in the same study.

An upper GI series should be the initial examination in evaluating the patient with ulcer pain or dyspepsia. Fifteen to 30% of lesions will be missed in the standard upper GI series, many of these lesions being superficial and nonpenetrating erosions. The diagnostic accuracy rate of endoscopy in ulcer disease is in the 95% range. Using the air contrast technique, diagnostic accuracy of 90 to 95% can be obtained with radiographic techniques. If duodenal ulcer is demonstrated on performance of the air contrast upper GI series, no further diagnostic procedure is required, provided that the stomach is normal. In such a situation, a patient can be treated medically, since duodenal ulcer lesions are usually benign and the radiographic picture has a high diagnostic accuracy. Endoscopy is required only if the response to treatment is inadequate or the symptoms are atypical. If the patient responds symptomatically to treatment, there is no need to follow a duodenal ulcer to endoscopic healing. Since the finding of a gastric ulcer radiographically raises the question of a possible gastric carcinoma, endoscopy is indicated for biopsy and brush cytology of the ulcer. Certainly no patient with a gastric ulcer should undergo surgery without endoscopic confirmation of the presence of the ulcer and exclusion of other lesions not seen on x-ray. If the initial x-ray examination discloses a completely normal stomach and duodenum despite the presence of upper GI symptomatology, the patient should then be endoscoped in order to identify a possible gastric or duodenal ulcer that may have been missed radiographically.

MEDICAL THERAPY

One may classify the medical treatment of peptic ulcer disease (PUD) into three phases. In the early part of this century, treatment consisted primarily of dietary manipulation, which remained popular until the early 1950s, when "alkalis" were used with increasing frequency. Early "alkalis" were proprietary products, made in local pharmacies. They contained magnesium oxide, calcium carbonate, aluminum oxide and other antacids. Hourly dosing was common, and studies attempting to document effectiveness usually measured disappearance of symptoms, or long-term radiologic evidence of healing.

Commercial availability of antacids put peptic ulcer therapy into a second and transitional phase. Studies began to document and compare the in vitro and in vivo efficacy of these products in their capacity to buffer gastric acid. The flexible fiberoptic endoscope was used with increasing frequency during this period. This development, more than any other, allowed the clinician to actually document the healing of gastric and duodenal ulcers. Widespread use of this instrument for investigation of efficacy of medical treatment and the development of new antisecretory drugs, such as cimetidine, bring us into the latest and present phase of therapy.

Despite the abundance of well-controlled studies that document ulcer healing endoscopically, traditional clinical goals remain unchanged. Relief of pain, prevention of recurrence, and prevention of complications are just as important today as they were 80 years ago. Elimination of gastric acid either by neutralization, or by preventing its secretion, is the central concept around which all current therapy revolves (1, 2). Indeed, in the past, "dietary programs" and "alkalis" provided substantial buffering capacity. The real advance in recent years is in the documentation of efficacy of the various medical regimens, using fiberoptic endoscopy. Attempts at documentation have produced many well-controlled studies which will be discussed under separate headings of duodenal and gastric ulcers.

DUODENAL ULCER THERAPY

There is no shortage of controlled studies evaluating therapy for duodenal ulcers. Various therapeutic modalities have been studied, mostly within the last 5 years. Three things appear to have spawned this new interest in studying duodenal ulcers. First is the realization that rather large amounts of antacid may be required to neutralize acid and heal ulcers (3). Second is the development and extensive use of flexible fiberoptic endoscopes, capable of entering the duodenum, and viewing the ulcer closely. Third is the development of new drugs, such as the H_2 receptor blockers and ulcer coating agents and prostaglandin. In this section, we will review the therapy of duodenal ulcers, including commonly used drugs and pertinent experimental drugs.

Antacids

Antacids have been used in treatment of duodenal ulcer for many years. Before World War I, "alkalis" were commonly used in patients with ulcer disease. After 1950, proprietary antacids came into common use, and were the subject of many studies in the 1950s through 1970s (4, 5, 9).

Antacids heal duodenal ulcers through elimination of gastric acid by neutralization. In order to buffer the acid that the stomach constantly produces, the antacid must be present in the stomach. Gastric emptying limits the amounts of antacid present in the stomach. The fasting stomach empties its contents into the duodenum as often as every 20 to 30 min (1). Frequent administration of antacid to buffer the constant secretion of acid is therefore necessary. This has led to the use of continuous antacid administration via nasogastric tube. A more practical regimen, however, is hourly administration or every other hour. A regimen that administers antacids several times between meals to take advantage of the meals' buffering ability is the most frequently used dosage schedule today (10). Fortran showed that administration of 30 ml of a high

potency antacid 1 hour after a meal caused neutralization of the acid secreted in response to the meal for 3 hours. The *Fortran regimen* is to give the antacid 1 hour and 3 hours after a meal and again at bedtime for a total of seven administrations of antacid per day. This is the regimen most commonly used now in the treatment of duodenal ulcer. The efficacy has been repeatedly shown in numerous studies (11).

In order to evaluate different dosage regimens, a measurement of success must be made. Until the development of the flexible fiberoptic endoscope which allowed direct visualization of ulcer healing, that measurement was usually based on relief of symptoms alone. Recently, studies evaluating actual ulcer healing have appeared with some frequency. This section will note the important earlier studies, and concentrate on the more recent ones.

In vitro evaluation has revealed that antacids vary in ability to neutralize acid, depending on their composition (Table 14.5) (12). Most magnesium- and aluminum-containing antacids are of sufficient potency to provide 80 to

Table 14.5.

A. Antacid Comparison Chart

Product	Acid Neutralizing Capacity (mEq/30 ml)	Sodium Content (mg/30 ml)	Ingredients[a]
Delcid	172	9.0	Mg/Al
Maalox TC	170	4.9	Mg/Al
Mylanta II	152	6.6	Mg/Al, S
Gelusil II	141	7.8	Mg/Al, S
Maalox	80	7.8	Mg/Al
Maalox plus	80	7.8	Mg/Al, S
Mylanta	76	4.5	Mg/Al, S
Alternagel	72	12.0	—Al—
Gelusil	69	4.2	Mg/Al, S
Riopan	66	1.5	Magaldrate
Amphogel	42	46.0	—Al—

B. Antacid Tablet Neutralizing Capacity

	Acid Neutralizing Capacity (mEq/tablet)	Dose Containing (140 mEq/tablet)
Camalox	16.7	8
Mylanta II	11.0	13
Tums	10.5	13
Rolaids	6.9	20
DiGel	4.7	30
Amphogel	2.0	70

[a] Mg, magnesium hydroxide; Al, aluminum hydroxide; S, simethicone.

140 mEq of neutralizing ability with one 30-ml dose.

Studies that evaluate antacid effect on patients have generally had two goals: clinical improvement and endoscopic evidence of ulcer healing. It is clear, however, that pain relief from antacids is a poor indicator of healing of duodenal ulcers. Pain relief has been compared between antacids and placebo with little difference (11). Subsequent studies have also clearly supported this finding. The lack of correlation between pain relief and healing becomes important when attempting to ensure compliance for a patient.

Trials that use endoscopy to evaluate success of antacid treatment have all had a similar double-blind design. They compare antacid with placebo for a trial of 4, 6, or 8 weeks, with confirmation of healing at the end of the trial. Most studies include an additional antacid for patients to take if they have pain. (The studies are summarized in Table 14.6.)

Petersen and associates (11) gave the equivalent of 30 ml of Mylanta II (without simethicone) 7 times daily, 1 and 3 hours after meals, and at bedtime (the Fortran regimen). Patients were randomized between this regimen and a placebo. Both groups were instructed to take 30 ml of an antacid if they had pain. If diarrhea developed, an equivalent dose of an aluminum-containing antacid or placebo was given. The total daily acid neutralizing ability of this regimen exceeds 1000 mEq. Pain relief, antacid usage, and ulcer healing, as demonstrated by endoscopy, were all measured. Ulcers healed in 78% of the patients receiving antacids and 45% of those receiving placebo. Besides being a significant difference, there was no correlation between ulcer healing and pain relief. Two thirds of the antacid group developed diarrhea requiring addition of an aluminum containing antacid.

Marks (14) used a lower dose of antacid (15 ml t.i.d., plus 5 chewed tablets daily), and found similar rates of ulcer healing, 86%. Their study design did not allow the inclusion of a true placebo group.

Lam (15) assessed the success of 800 mg of Mg/Al tablets, given 1 and 3 hours after meals, and at bedtime. He found that over 90% of patients treated with this regimen demonstrated a healed ulcer in 4 weeks. The control group healed the ulcers at a 46% rate. These studies, while not as complete or large as Petersen's, appear to confirm the assumption that antacids do indeed speed the healing of duodenal ulcers. There also appears to be confirmation of a high placebo healing rate and a lack of correlation between ulcer healing and pain relief. The high placebo healing rate is effectively demonstrated by a study conducted in Germany, where patients were given placebo or only 5 ml of antacid to be taken 3 times daily. In 3 weeks, 36% of the patient's ulcers had healed, and 80% healed in 6 weeks (16).

While many have demonstrated efficacy, the lowest effective antacid dose required for healing is still unknown. A treatment period of 4 to 6 weeks appears to be the standard. There is little evidence that prolonging therapy beyond 6 weeks further will heal a larger percentage of patients.

The safest recommendation is 30 ml of a highly potent antacid suspension, 1 and 3 hours after meals and at bedtime. If diarrhea develops, an aluminum antacid may be added

Table 14.6.
Duodenal Ulcer Treatment with Antacids

Reference	Regimen[a]	H$^+$ Neutralized (mEq/day)	Study Length (weeks)	% of Patients Healed-Placebo[b]	% Patients Healed-Treatment Group
11 (77)	30 ml t.i.d., 1 and 3 hr p.c. and h.s.	1008	4	45	78
13 (79)	15 ml t.i.d. and h.s. and Mg/Al tablets[c] 5 times a day	175	6	0	69
			12	0	85
12 (79)	Mg/Al tablets[c] t.i.d., 1 and 3 hr p.c. and h.s.	175	4	36	92
15 (77)	15 ml t.i.d. and h.s.	125	3	0	36
			6	0	80

[a] All magnesium/aluminum suspensions unless noted.
[b] 0 = no true placebo group.
[c] Magnesium/aluminum tablets (chewable), 800 mg.

to the regimen. Less aggressive regimens may be successful, but are less conclusively proven.

Antacid tablets provide a convenient alternative to using the suspension. They are, however, much less potent (Table 14.5). It can be seen that 10 to 15 of even the most potent antacid tablets would be required per dose to achieve a similar buffering capacity to the suspension.

Cimetidine (Tagamet)

The development of cimetidine has changed forever the way that patients with peptic ulcer disease are treated. Since it was released in the United States in August 1977, it has become the most popular prescription medicine in the world (17).

Black (18), in 1972, demonstrated the concept of prevention of acid secretion through histamine-mediated receptors when he synthesized certain compounds he called histamine H_2 receptor antagonists. The first compound, burimimide, was not orally absorbed. The second, metiamide, was associated with certain blood dyscrasias (19) causing Smith, Kline and French to withdraw the drug from investigation in November 1975. Cimetidine was found to be more potent on a milligram for milligram basis. It was also found to be effective at suppressing acid secretion following all known physiologic and pharmacologic stimuli. A 300-mg oral dose will reduce 70% of acid secretion for 4 to 5 hours (20). About 70% of the drug is absorbed and about 70 to 80% is excreted unchanged in the urine. It has a half-life of 2 hours in patients with normal renal function (20).

Cimetidine's promise became clear when several uncontrolled trials showed that over 90% of duodenal ulcers healed within 6 weeks (21). Controlled trials in the United Kingdom (using 1.0 gm daily: 200 mg t.i.d. and 400 mg h.s.) and the United States (using 1.2 g daily: 300 mg q.i.d., with meals and at bedtime) have consistently shown significant duodenal ulcer healing at 4 and 6 weeks (22–38) (Table 14.7). Ulcer healing was assessed endoscopically in all trials and weak antacids were used for occasional pain. The initial U.S. trial found a nonsignificant difference between the treatment and placebo groups because of a very high placebo healing rate (22). The "p.r.n." antacid used in these patients was very potent compared to the antacid used in the British

Table 14.7.
Cimetidine Duodenal Ulcer Treatment

Daily Dose (g)	Length of Study (weeks)	No. of Patients		% Healed	
		Placebo	Drug	Placebo	Drug
1.0	4	360	402	37.8	73.8
1.2	2–6	283	232	44.8	81.4
1.6–2.0	4–12	94	113	25.5	72.5

studies and may have played a role in the high placebo healing rate.

The accepted dose in patients with normal renal function is 300 mg, 4 times daily (taken with meals and at bedtime). Patients with impaired renal function should be given lower doses (39). Raising the dose to 1.6 g per day has not been shown to improve healing rate (Table 14.7).

Clinical response of patients is dramatic, with pain relief being seen early in the course of therapy for most patients.

Like many drugs, cimetidine carries a long list of side effects. Side effects ranging from CNS toxicity to bone marrow suppression have been reported but are really relatively low in frequency (3 to 7% of patients (40). Alteration in bowel habits, usually diarrhea, but occasionally constipation, may occur. Headache has been reported with a frequency of less than 2 to 3% and mental status alteration (ranging from mild to severe) probably occurs less than 1% of the time. Mental status alteration (confusion, agitation and somnolence) appears to occur more frequently in acutely ill patients in hospital intensive care units and has been very rare in outpatients (36). Severe side effects such as bone marrow suppression, liver toxicity and renal failure occur much less frequently.

Drug interactions occur with some frequency since cimetidine inhibits the cytochrome P-450 enzyme systems that metabolize drugs in the liver (12). Diazepam, chlordiazepoxide, theophylline, phenytoin, warfarin, lidocaine and propranolol have all been shown to have decreased clearance with concurrent cimetidine use (16). Oxazepam and lorazepam appear unaffected by cimetidine. Cimetidine does not decrease the absorption of tetracyclines as antacids do. The clinical significance of these drug interactions is questioned; however, cases of theophylline toxicity have been reported so care in concurrent use of these drugs is advised.

There is little question that cimetidine has an important place in the treatment of duodenal ulcers. A dose of 300 mg, 4 times daily (with meals and at bedtime), will heal 70 to 80% of patients within 4 to 6 weeks. Treatment longer than 6 to 8 weeks provides minimal increased benefit in ulcer healing in most patients.

Ranitidine (Zantac)

Ranitidine is an H_2 receptor antagonist that has recently been approved for the short-term treatment of duodenal ulcer. Ranitidine differs from cimetidine in that it has a furan ring instead of an imidazole ring like cimetidine. This structural alteration makes ranitidine 8 to 10 times more potent than cimetidine and decreases its inhibition of the cytochrome P-450 system. It has a half-life of 2 hours with absorption and elimination characteristics similar to cimetidine (Table 14.8).

Ranitidine in a dose of 150 mg twice daily heals patients at about the same rate as cimetidine [41]. Relief of symptoms of duodenal ulcer is similar to cimetidine. In most patients, duodenal ulcer symptoms are relieved early in the therapeutic course.

As expected, ranitidine does not appear to inhibit the metabolism of drugs oxidized by the cytochrome P-450 system. Early reports appeared to suggest that ranitidine causes mental status alteration less frequently than cimetidine but careful post marketing surveillance is necessary before any broad statements can be made.

Ranitidine is an important addition to the medications available for treatment of duodenal ulcer. Its twice daily dosing (because of its potency, not pharmacokinetics) and equal efficacy are sure to make it a popular alternative to other available drugs used to treat duodenal ulcer. It is too soon to make an assessment about its frequency of side effects.

Sucralfate (Carafate)

Sucralfate was approved by the FDA late in 1981 for the short-term treatment of duodenal ulcer.

It is a complex of sulfated sucrose and aluminum hydroxide. It has a unique mechanism of action since it neither buffers nor inhibits acid production. Sucralfate does have significant antipeptic activity which is strongest at the acid pH values expected to occur in the stomach. Sucralfate also binds to free proteins which suggest that the concentration of sucralfate at the ulcer site was higher than in noninvolved areas [42]. Sucralfate also effectively binds bile salts. This binding is greater at acid pH values [43].

In several studies, sucralfate 1 g given 30 to 60 min before meals and at bedtime (4 times daily) has been found to heal duodenal ulcers about 80% of the time (in 4 to 6 weeks). Placebo healing rate in studies ranges from 40 to 50% [44–46]. Studies comparing cimetidine with sucralfate for duodenal ulcer healing show similar healing rates for both drugs [47, 48]. Relapse rates in duodenal ulcer patients treated with sucralfate appear to be similar to other drugs (about 70% in 1 year) [47].

Side effects are minimal since the drug is very poorly absorbed. Drug-associated laboratory abnormalities have yet to be observed. The most frequent side effect appears to be constipation, however other minor complaints have also been noted. Among them are: diarrhea, nausea, indigestion, dry mouth and dizziness. As with many drugs, it is often difficult to distinguish side effects of drugs from complaints associated with the condition to be treated.

In summary, sucralfate appears to be an effective addition to a growing number of drugs that treat peptic ulcer disease. Its somewhat cumbersome administration schedule (30 to 60 min before meals) is offset by its infrequent side effects. It appears neither more nor less effective than other agents in healing ulcers.

Table 14.8.
Cimetidine Treatment of Gastric Ulcer (Controlled Trials)

Reference	Cimetidine		Placebo	
	No.	% Healed	No.	% Healed
50	26	69[a]	27	37
51	23	78	22	27
52	30	60	29	41
53	68	59[b]	62	31
54	60	70[a]		
All	207	67[c]	140	43[c]

[a] Cimetidine plus antacid.
[b] Cimetidine alone.
[c] Overall healing rate (all studies combined).

Anticholinergics

This class of drugs is decreasing in importance in the treatment of duodenal ulcer. Although they are effective antagonists of acid secretion, the magnitude of their acid secretory reduction is in the order of 30 to 35%, rather than the 85 to 90% reduction achieved with cimetidine (20). There are no good studies using endoscopy that document the effectiveness of anticholinergics alone in the treatment of duodenal ulcer. This class of drugs, therefore, is relegated to an adjunctive role, to be used with antacids to help prevent stomach emptying, and to prolong the buffering activity of antacids. They may also be used at bedtime to prolong the effect of the night time dose.

In certain cases, anticholinergics have been used to increase the antisecretory effect of cimetidine in patients who continue to secrete acid despite "normal" doses of the H_2 receptor antagonist (49).

Summary

Antacids, anticholinergics, cimetidine, ranitidine and sucralfate are all available as treatment modalities for duodenal ulcer. Of these, antacids and anticholinergics probably offer the least benefit to the patient in terms of efficacy and ease of administration and frequency of side effects. It is possible, therefore, that the two older treatment modalities will be used less and less frequently as cimetidine, ranitidine and sucralfate are used more. We recommend, therefore, using appropriate doses of cimetidine, ranitidine, or sucralfate. Ranitidine may offer an advantage in elderly patients, patients receiving drugs concurrently that interact with cimetidine, or patients that fail to heal on cimetidine.

GASTRIC ULCER

Medical treatment of patients with gastric ulcer is not easy. Due to the similarity in symptoms, one is tempted to treat them as we treat duodenal ulcers. The two diseases are, however, different. First, the gastric ulcer is characterized by a chronic course. It also has a much higher chance of being malignant than does the duodenal ulcer, and this possibility must be recognized in the diagnostic work-up. Gastric ulcers are not associated with gastric hypersecretion as duodenal ulcers so often are (Table 14.5). Also, there are many theories regarding the cause of gastric ulcers that do not involve acid production.

Despite all of the above statements, elimination of acid remains the cornerstone of gastric ulcer treatment. We will review the current place of medical treatment for gastric ulcer.

Antacid Therapy

Antacid therapy for gastric ulcers has been in wide use for over 75 years. Older texts suggest "alkali" therapy will give good results, without defining how frequently these good results occur. More recent studies exist, but are not nearly as common as those for duodenal ulcer.

The classic study is by Hollander and Harlan (49). They gave patients either calcium carbonate or placebo, and followed their results with rigid endoscopy. They found that 45% of their treated patients, and 27% of their placebo patients healed in 6 weeks. This study clearly shows that benign gastric ulcers will heal with medical therapy, but follow-up studies are lacking.

Cimetidine

With the success cimetidine has had in the treatment of duodenal ulcer, it seems natural that it should be tried in gastric ulcer. Despite much work by many respected investigators, however, there remain a question of effectiveness.

Early uncontrolled trials showed some promise. Controlled trials using cimetidine in gastric ulcer are less numerous than for duodenal ulcer (50–54). All trials used a design that allowed *all* patients, even those receiving a placebo, free access to antacids for pain relief. Treatment was 1.0 to 1.2 g per day in 4 divided doses for 4 to 6 weeks (Table 14.8). The most interesting trial is the one conducted by Englert in the United States. There were two treatment groups: cimetidine alone, and cimetidine plus high doses of antacids. Each was compared with the standard placebo plus occasional antacids, used only for pain. The three groups had very similar healing rates. In fact, the high placebo healing rate has lead at least one respected gastroenterologist to suggest that the p.r.n. antacid consumption in the placebo group in the U.S. trials was large enough to serve as "treatment" for gastric ulcers (55). Most cimetidine trials report an average gastric ulcer healing rate of 67% at 6 weeks.

Ranitidine

Several studies have shown that ranitidine has promise in the treatment of benign gastric ulcer. Healing rates are similar to cimetidine (41). While only cimetidine is FDA approved for this condition, most feel that their efficacy in benign gastric ulcers renders these H_2 receptor agents the treatment of choice.

Sucralfate

Sucralfate appears to be effective in healing gastric ulcers as well. About 80% of the patients treated for 6 to 8 weeks appear to heal compared with 40% of patients receiving placebo (46).

Other Treatment Modalities

Anticholinergics have no place in the treatment of patients with gastric ulcers. The minor antisecretory activity of this class of drugs is offset by its ability to reduce the motility of the GI tract. This causes significant retention of acid and pepsin in the stomach where it can do the most damage.

Carbenoxolone has been in use for nearly 20 years. Geismar et al. (56) reported effectiveness in gastric ulcer healing in 1973. Over the next 10 years, the results were confirmed by many studies (57). This drug has also been compared to cimetidine, resulting in similar healing rates (58, 59). Its primary side effect, sodium retention, is its chief drawback. Adding spironolactone to the regimen can reverse the sodium retention, but it also reverses the effectiveness. Carbenoloxone is available in Mexico and the United Kingdom, but is still investigational in the United States. Despite its apparent promise, its eventual release in this country is doubtful.

Summary of Treatment of Gastric Ulcer

The effectiveness of medical treatment of gastric ulcers remains somewhat controversial. The use of antisecretory drugs in a disease where the patients do not produce more acid than normal will probably remain controversial and unproven until more answers are found that uncover the actual cause of ulceration. Until then, despite the lack of proof, we recommend using either antacids, cimetidine, ranitidine or sucralfate in doses recommended for duodenal ulcer. After treatment for 6 to 8 weeks, the patient's response should be assessed. Further treatment may often be necessary.

Anticholinergics have no place in the treatment of gastric ulcer. Carbenoxolone appears promising, but its sodium retaining properties are bothersome.

MAINTENANCE THERAPY

About 50 to 75% of the patients with a healed duodenal ulcer will suffer a recurrence within 1 year. The agent used to heal the patient initially does not appear to affect the recurrence rate. About ¼ to ⅓ of these recurrences will be asymptomatic.

Maintenance treatment with cimetidine (400 mg h.s.) (16), ranitidine (150 mg h.s.) (40) or sucralfate (1 g b.i.d.) (55) will prevent recurrence, with only 20% of the patients treated experiencing a relapse in the first year following initial healing. While maintenance treatment appears to prevent recurrence in most patients, may clinicians are reluctant to recommend life-long treatment for patients with duodenal ulcer. Surgery is, therefore, an alternative that the patient who is intractable (difficult to heal and difficult to prevent recurrence) may derive most benefit.

ZOLLINGER-ELLISON SYNDROME

The medical treatment of patients who have developed ulceration from a gastrin-secreting tumor has been frustrating until recently. Total gastrectomy to remove all the acid-secreting cells of the GI tract was (and still is) an effective treatment modality. The development of H_2 receptor antagonists which can effectively inhibit the large amounts of acid produced in these patients has allowed patients the option of effective medical therapy that was not available before.

Both Stadil (60) and McCarthy (61) have large series of patients on chronic treatment. Doses are usually higher than the 1.2 g per day daily dose recommended for duodenal ulcer. Chronic treatment (lifetime) is necessary unless the patient has a total gastrectomy or the tumor is surgically removed.

The incidence of side effects on the chronic high dose therapy required for this condition is still low. Gynecomastia and impotence appear to pose a problem in as many as 50% of patients (62). In a recent series of 22 men who were being treated with cimetidine in high doses for Zollinger-Ellison syndrome, 11 developed gynecomastia, impotence or both. All 11 patients were switched to ranitidine with resolution of their side effects. Ranitidine, therefore, may be the drug of choice for medical therapy of Zollinger-Ellison syndrome.

SUMMARY

The medical treatment of peptic ulcer disease has been revolutionized in the last 10 years by the development of the fiberoptic endoscope and effective antisecretory drugs. Effective treatment can be obtained with antacids, cimetidine, sucralfate, or ranitidine. Careful evaluation of efficacy of treatment on an individual basis is necessary since recurrence rates following healing are high.

References

1. Sleisenger MH, Fordtran JS: *Gastrointestinal Diseases*, ed 2. Philadelphia: W.B. Saunders, 1978.
2. Dragstedt LR, Owens FM: Supra diaphragmatic section of the vagus nerve in the treatment of duodenal ulcer. *Proc Soc Exp Biol Med* 53:152, 1943.
3. Oi M, Oshida K, Sugimara S: The location of gastric ulcer. *Gastroenterology* 39:45, 1959.
4. Capper WM, Laidlow CBA, Buckler K, et al: The pH fields of the gastric mucosa. *Lancet* 2:1200, 1962.
5. Davenport HW: The gastric mucosal barrier. *Digestion* 5:162, 1972.
6. Capper WM: Factors in the pathogenesis of gastric ulcer. *Ann R Coll Surg Engl* 40:21, 1967.
7. Capper WM, Airth GR, Kolby JO: A test for pyloric regurgittion. *Lancet* 2:621, 1966.
8. Dragstedt LR: A concept of the etiology of gastric and duodenal ulcers. *Gastroenterology* 30:208, 1956.
9. Rovelstad RA, Owen CA, et al: Factors influencing the stomach contents. *Gastroenterology* 20:609, 1952.
10. Piper DW, Fentar BM: Antacid therapy of peptic ulcer; I. The mathematical determination of an adequate dose. *Gut* 5:581, 1964.
11. Petersen WL, Sturdevant R, Fordtran J: Healing of duodenal ulcer with an antacid regimen. *N Engl J Med* 297:341–344, 1977.
12. Dutro MP, Ammerson AT: Comparison of liquid antacids. *N Engl J Med* 302:967, 1980.
13. Fordtran JS, Morawski S, Richardson C: In vitro and in vivo evaluation of antacids. *N Engl J Med* 288:923, 1973.
14. Marks IN: Healing of peptic ulcers on antacids. *S Afr Med J* 55:331, 1979.
15. Lam I: Treatment of duodenal ulcer with sulpiride. *Gastroenterology* 76:315, 1979.
16. Schuerer U: Gastric and duodenal ulcer healing with or without butriptyline? *Gastroenterology* 72:838, 1977.
17. Freston JW: Cimetidine: developments, pharmacology and efficacy. *Ann Intern Med* 97:573–580, 1982.
18. Black JW, Duncan WA, Durant CJ, et al: Definition and antagonism of histamine H_2 receptors. *Nature* 236:385–390, 1972.
19. Feldman EJ, Isenberg JI: Effects of metiamide and gastric acid hypersecretion, steatorrhea, and bone marrow function in a patient with systemic mastocytosis. *N Engl J Med* 295:1178–1179, 1976.
20. Griffiths R, Lee RM, Taylor DC: Kinetics of cimetidine and man and experimental animals. In Burland WL, Simkins MA: *Cimetidine, Proceedings of the Second International Symposium on Histamine H_2 Receptor Antagonists*. New York: Excerpta Medica, 1977, pp 38–53.
21. Blackwood WS, MacDougaal DP: Cimetidine in duodenal ulcer. *Lancet* 2:174–176, 1976.
22. Bardhan KD, Blum A: Long term treatment with cimetidine for duodenal ulceration. *Lancet* 1:900–901, 1977.
23. Albano O, Barara L: Trattamento ra breve termine con cimetidine nell ulcera duodenale. In Lucchelli P: *Cimetidina, Farmacologica e Clinica*. Philadelphia: Smith Kline & French, 1978.
24. Bank S, Barbezat GO: Histamine H_2 receptor antagonist in the treatment of duodenal ulcer. *S Afr Med J* 50:1781–1784, 1976.
25. Bianchi P: Cimetidine in duodenal ulcer. Presented at the Round Table Meeting, Sixth World Congress of Gastroenterology, Madrid, June 7, 1978.
26. Binder HJ, Cocco A, Crossley RJ, et al: Cimetidine in the treatment of duodenal ulcer. *Gastroenterology* 74:380–388, 1978.
27. Blackwood WS, Mandgal DP, Pickard RG, et al: Cimetidine in duodenal ulcer. *Lancet* 2:174–176, 1976.
28. Bodemar G, Walan A: Cimetidine in the treatment of active duodenal ulceration and prepyloric ulcers. *Lancet* 2:161–164, 1976.
29. Crenner M, Dermuier J: Traitment des ulceres gastriques et duodenaux par la cimetidine. Presented at the Sixth World Congress of Gastroenterology, Madrid, May 8, 1978.
30. Gray GR, McKenzie I, Smith IS, et al: Oral cimetidine in severe duodenal ulceration. *Lancet* 1:4–7, 1977.
31. Hentschel E, Schultze J: Treatment of duodenal and prepyloric ulcer by cimetidine. Presented at the Sixth World Congress of Gastroenterology, Madrid, May 8, 1978.
32. Hetzel DJ, Taggert GJ, Sherman DJC, et al: Cimetidine in the treatment of duodenal ulcer. *Med J Aust* 1:317–319, 1977.
33. Lambert R, Bader JP: Treatment of gastric and duodenal ulcers with cimetidine. *Gastroenterol Clin Biol* 1:855–860, 1977.
34. Malchow H, Sewing KF: In-patient treatment of peptic ulcer with cimetidine. *Dtsch Med Wochenschr* 103:149–152, 1978.
35. Moshal MG, Spitaels JD, Booha R: Treatment of duodenal ulcers with cimetidine. *S Afr Med J* 52:760–763, 1977.
36. Northfield TC, Blackwood WS: Controlled clinical trial of cimetidine for duodenal ulcer. In Burland WL, Simkins MA: *Cimetidine: Proceedings of Second International Symposium on H_2 Receptor Antagonists*. New York: Excerpta Medica, 1977.
37. Petrillo M, Proda A, et al: Traitmento con cimetidina del ulcera duodenale. *Recenti Prog Med* 12:362–365, 1978.
38. Lamb LS, Berstad A: A double blind center comparative study of cimetidine and placebo. In Burland WL, Simkins MA: *Proceedings of the Second International Symposium on H_2 Receptor Antagonists*. New York: Exerpta Medica, 1977, pp 248–253.

39. Norlander B, Bodemar G, Carsson R, et al: Therapeutic plasma concentrations of cimetidine in normal renal function and dosage requirements in renal failure. *Ther Drug Monit* 2:147–148, 1980.

40. Sawyer D, Conner C, Scalley R: Cimetidine: adverse reactions and acute toxicity. *Am J Hosp Pharm* 38:188–197, 1981.

41. Berner BD, Conner CS, Sawyer DR, et al: Ranitidine: a new H_2 receptor antagonist. *Clin Pharm* 1:499–508, 1981.

42. Nagashima R: Development and characteristics of sucralfate. *J Clin Gastroenterol* 3 (Suppl 2):103–110, 1981.

43. Nagazawa S, Nagashima R, Samloff IM: Selective binding of sucralfate to gastric ulcer in man. *Dig Dis Sci* 26:297–300, 1981.

44. Hollander D: Efficacy of sucralfate for duodenal ulcers: a multicenter, double-blind trial. *J Clin Gastroenterol* 3 (Suppl 2):153–157, 1981.

45. Moshal MG, Spaetels JM, Kahn F: Sucralfate in the treatment of duodenal ulcers. *S Afr Med J* 57:742–744, 1980.

46. Marks IN, Lucke W, Wright JP, et al: Ulcer healing and relapse rates after initial treatment with cimetidine or sucralfate. *J Clin Gastroenterol* 3 (Suppl 2):163–165, 1981.

47. Marks IN, Wright JP, Denyerm J, et al: Comparison of sucralfate with cimetidine in the short term treatment of chronic peptic ulcers. *S Afr Med J* 57:567–573, 1980.

48. McCarthy DM, Peikin SR, Lopatkin RN, et al: H_2 receptor antagonists in the treatment of gastric hypersecretory states. In Creutzfeld W: *Cimetidine: Proceeding of an International Symposium.* New York: Excerpta Medica, 1978, pp 137.

49. Hollander D, Harlan J: Antacids vs placebo in peptic ulcer disease treatment. *JAMA* 266:1181, 1973.

50. Isenberg J, Elashof J, Sandersfeld M, et al: Double blind comparison of cimetidine and low dose antacid in the healing of benign gastric ulcer. *Gastroenterology* 82:1090, 1982.

51. Akamar K, Dyck W, Englert E, et al: Cimetidine vs placebo in the treatment of benign gastric ulcer. *Gastroenterology* 80:1098, 1981.

52. Dyck W, Belsito A, et al: Cimetidine and placebo in the treatment of benign gastric ulcer. *Gastroenterology* 74:410–415, 1978.

53. Englert E, Freston JW, et al: Cimetidine, antacid and hospitalization in the treatment of benign gastric ulcer. *Gastroenterology* 74:416–425, 1978.

54. Semb L, et al: Cimetidine in the treatment of gastric ulcer. *Scand J Gastroenterol* 12:115–117, 1977.

55. Ashton MG, Holdswert CD, Ryan FP, et al: Healing of gastric ulcers after 1, 2, and 3 months of ranitidine. *Br Med J* 284:467–468, 1982.

56. Geismar P, Mosbech J, Myren J: A double-blind study of the effect of carbenoxolone sodium in gastric ulcer. *Scand J Gastroenterol* 8:251–256, 1973.

57. Oselladere D, Chierichetti SM, Norbetto L, et al: Pirenzapine in severe duodenal acid gastric ulcer. *Scand J Gastroenterol Suppl* 57:33–39, 1979.

58. La Brooy S, Taylor R, Hunt R, et al: Controlled comparison of cimetidine and carbonoxolone sodium in gastric ulcer. *Br Med J* 1308–1309, 1971.

59. Levis JH: Treatment of gastric ulcer. *Arch Intern Med* 143:264–274, 1983.

60. Stadil F, Stage JG: Cimetidine and the Zollinger-Ellison syndrome. In Wastell C, Lance P: *Cimetidine: The Westminster Hospital Symposium.* Edinburgh: Churchill-Livingstone, 1978, p 91.

61. McCarthy DM: Report on the U.S. experience with cimetidine in Zollinger-Ellison syndrome. *Gastroenterology* 74:453–456, 1978.

62. Jensen RT, et al: Cimetidine induced impotence and gynecomastia in patients with gastric hypersecretory states. *N Engl J Med* 308:883–887, 1983.

CHAPTER 15

Ulcerative Colitis

GARY H. SMITH, Pharm.D.

Ulcerative colitis is a disease of the bowel which can be characterized by the presence of diffuse inflammation and necrosis of the colonic and rectal mucosa. The clinical course of the disease is complex and unpredictable, and it can be expressed either continuously or intermittently. The duration is almost always prolonged with a wide variety of systemic and local manifestations of varying intensity. Although considered to be the most common of the "idiopathic" inflammatory bowel diseases, ulcerative colitis constitutes only a small proportion of the disorders the pharmacist encounters in his practice. However, the opportunity for a pharmacist to contribute significantly to patient care can be most rewarding since few diseases require more skill, consideration and understanding than ulcerative colitis for successful rehabilitation of those afflicted. As a consequence of pathological changes, ulcerative colitis is associated with many complex, sometime life-threatening, problems. Prognosis for survival can never be assured of the basis of symptom remission or absence of disease activity alone. Complex problems associated with this disease and its treatment represent a formidable therapeutic challenge for its successful management.

ETIOLOGY

Little is definitely known about the etiology of ulcerative colitis, although investigations into its pathogenesis have been extensive in number and scope. There appear to be multiple pathogenic factors involved, but their relationship to the clinical course, symptoms and response to therapy is still unclear (1). It has been suggested that the etiological agent, possibly a mucolytic enzyme, within the lumen of the bowel, attacks the mucosal surface. This has not been demonstrated by the proponents of this postulate. Neither have bacteria, parasites, fungi, virus or their destructive toxins been successfully demonstrated to be etiological factors. However coexisting infections with ulcerative colitis have been observed with the bacteria *Clostridium difficle, Campylobacter fetus* and *Yersinia enterocolitica* (2). Antibodies reacting with certain fecal anerobic bacteria have been recovered in the rectocolonic mucosa of patients with ulcerative colitis; it remains, however, to be resolved whether this is a reflection of an altered immunological status or an underlying etiological factor. A great deal of emphasis and study recently has been placed on the immunological process as the cause of ulcerative colitis. The pathological changes seen in colitis are compatible with an autoimmune response and frequently are associated with concurrent diseases thought to be autoimmune in nature. Antibodies to colonic epithelial antigens also have been demonstrated (1). There appears to be increasing support for a cell-mediated response in the gut wall evidenced by lymphocyte hyporesponsiveness to mitogen stimulation, depressed T-lymphocyte counts and cutaneous anergy (3). People who develop inflammatory bowel disease may be predisposed to this response. The immunological component may, however, be a secondary phenomenon since removal of the target organ is followed by a disappearance of immune suppression. (3). Further evidence to support that the immunologic etiological theory is insufficient in that immunosuppressive drugs have failed to improve significantly the treatment outcomes for patients with ulcerative colitis (4, 5). Allergy and sensitivity to certain foods also have been suggested as possible causative factors in this disorder (1).

It is widely held that ulcerative colitis patients are of a particular personality type. They are thought to be compulsive, hostile, immature, depressed, and they frequently have difficulties expressing their aggression and sexual identity. The behavior of young patients has been described as obsessive, passive, neurotic and emotionally dependent on a parent. The mother of the child with colitis has often been characterized as being overly strict, punitive and domineering. The impression that the frequency of personality disorders among ulcerative colitis patients is greater than for patients with other medical problems has not been confirmed. Controlled studies have failed to demonstrate any relationship of personality type or psychological factors to the pathogenesis of ulcerative colitis. There is greater acceptance of the association of exacerbations and remissions of colitis with changes in the emotional state once the disease has been established. It appears that the most appropriate approach for the moment is to consider ulcerative colitis as a manifestation of many underlying factors and to monitor its clinical course for complications and empirically provide symptomatic treatment. In the majority of cases, medical therapy does not offer a permanent cure.

INCIDENCE

The incidence of ulcerative colitis varies from country to country. In the United States the incidence of the population at risk has been estimated to be from 6 to 8 per 100,000 per year (1). On a worldwide basis the occurrence of the disease is increasing, and the available figures represent perhaps a fraction of the true incidence. Caucasians comprise a significant majority of all cases, and the condition is relatively rare among blacks. The greater frequency among the Jewish population, nearly 4 times more common, suggests that genetic or ethnic predisposition plays an important etiological role in ulcerative colitis. Observations that the incidence of inflammatory bowel disease is higher among Israeli Jews of occidental rather than oriental extraction and the equal occurrence of the disorder in American Jews from rural or urban backgrounds support impressions that the occurrence of colitis is significantly influenced by genetics. About 10 to 15% of patients with ulcerative colitis also have a family history of inflammatory bowel disorders. Environment does not, however, appear to be a significant factor since nonfamilial individuals living with families which have a predilection for ulcerative colitis have not demonstrated a greater tendency to develop this disease. The disease appears to be evenly distributed between the sexes although a number of studies indicate a 3 to 2 preponderance of male children to female children with colitis. Although

it affects all ages, ulcerative colitis is considered to be a disease of adolescents and young adults. The majority of cases occur initially between the 1st and 4th decade of life, with peak rate of occurrence in the 3rd decade. The relationship between age and the incidence of the disease remains unclear (1).

PATHOPHYSIOLOGY

Ulcerative colitis is an inflammatory and suppurative process which involves the mucosa and submucosa of the colon. Involvement at its onset is usually most active in the rectum and distal colon, progressing proximally to other portions of the colon in a continuous manner. The extent of colonic disruption varies considerably, with about one-third of the patients developing "universal" colitis with involvement of the entire length of the colon. The intensity of colitis varies throughout the clinical course. It may be acutely fulminant and severe or gradual with chronic recurrences of exacerbations and remissions. The morbidity and mortality risks are greatest during severe attacks where extensive total or near total colonic involvement is present. Relapses are quite common with more than half of them experienced within a year following the acute episode. About 25 to 30% of patients during their initial attack will unexpectedly present with the pathology of universal colitis similar to that encountered in patients with a history of long-term colitis. A small proportion (less than 10%) of patients have ulcerative proctitis where the disease is confined to the rectum and distal sigmoid colon only. Patients with extensive colonic involvement and severe symptoms must be vigorously and rationally managed medically. Surgery must be considered where hemorrhage is acute, perforation is imminent, sepsis a complication or medical means have been unsuccessful in alleviating the acute attack.

DIAGNOSIS AND CLINICAL FINDINGS

The clinical history of patients with ulcerative colitis usually reveals the presence of bloody purulent diarrhea often of long duration. Many patients initially experience only mild rectal bleeding with either normal bowel function or mild constipation. As the bleeding gradually increases, bowel movements become greater in frequency, a characteristic of colitis. Abdominal cramping and pain are common, particularly during the early stages of the disease. The patient with advanced colitis may have as many as 30 to 40 watery purulent and bloody bowel movements throughout the day and night. Incontinence may develop during severe episodes. When the disease is in remission or inactive, the bowel may appear to be functioning normally. Constipation is occasionally experienced by patients with colitis limited to the rectum. In some patients, usually those with disease of greater severity and extensive colonic involvement, the symptoms are acute and occur abruptly with intense diarrhea, severe abdominal cramping, pain and rectal bleeding. Malaise, weakness, easy fatigability, mild fever, pallor, dehydration and abdominal tenderness are usually observed on physical examination in the patients with acute colitis. Local and systemic manifestations involving the skin and joints are sometimes encountered. Weight loss and deficiency anemias are not uncommon since anorexia and malabsorption are frequently experienced during acute and chronic periods of the disease. Hematological evaluation may reveal a hypochromic anemia which parallels the course of the disease. During active periods of colitis, slight to moderate leukocytosis and elevated erythrocyte sedimentation rates can be seen. The clinical impression of ulcerative colitis cannot be firmly established without sigmoidoscopic examination and rectal biopsy. Edema and hyperemia of the colonic mucosa are early sigmoidoscopic findings. As the disease becomes more active, ulcerations and infiltration by inflammatory cells are seen in the mucosa of the rectum and the sigmoid colon. Uniform and continuous enlargement and coalescence of ulcerations spreading to the submucosa occur as the extent and activity of the colitis progress. The bowel becomes thickened, scarred and inflexible with narrowing of the lumen as a result of continuous disease activity or episodes of exacerbation. Abdominal pain often diminishes during the later stages of the clinical course and is responsible for the erroneous impression that the disease has become less active or extensive. As a result, therapeutic management is often abated or even discontinued. Unfortunately the symptoms often recur as a consequence. The clinical course most frequently consists of spontaneous remissions and relapses varying in severity and duration. The unpredictable and remitting pattern of this disorder may continue for years. For some patients permanent remis-

sion may be possible while for others symptoms evolve gradually into a chronic continuous course. Radiological examination establishes the extent of colonic involvement in ulcerative colitis. It can reveal significant information with respect to the degree of mucosal and luminal changes and the presence of localized complications. The differentiation of ulcerative colitis from a number of conditions with a similar clinical course and symptoms must always be considered during the diagnostic workup. Serum electrolytes, proteins, liver function and other changes which diagnostically reflect the sequelae of ulcerative colitis or complications arising from its treatment must be monitored. Selection of appropriate treatment and assessment of therapeutic responsiveness must be done using the results of such tests while concurrently considering the clinical symptoms of the disease.

COMPLICATIONS

A variety of systemic and extracolonic complications can occur as a consequence of ulcerative colitis. Anemia due to occult blood loss and depletion of body iron stores is a frequent problem, especially where disease involvement is extensive. Hemoglobin levels lower than 10 g/100 ml, hypochromic microcytic red cells on peripheral blood smear, low serum iron and elevated total serum iron-binding capacity characteristically are seen. Factors other than blood loss appear to be of minor significance as a source of anemia. Hemolysis is rarely a primary cause of anemia in ulcerative colitis. Few cases of acquired secondary autoimmune hemolytic anemia in ulcerative colitis have been reported. These patients present with fever, slight jaundice, tachycardia, hemoglobin of less than 7 g/100 ml, thrombocytopenia and marked reticulocytosis. A situation which merits special attention is the occurrence of hemolytic anemia following sulfasalazine therapy in erythrocyte glucose-6-phosphate dehydrogenase (G6PD)-deficient individuals. Several cases have been reported in which several black patients with ulcerative colitis have developed hemolytic anemia following sulfasalazine. Appropriate laboratory studies should be monitored when sulfasalazine or any other sulfonamide is used in high risk individuals such as black males or Caucasians of Sardinian descent. A rare condition known as Heinz-Ehrlich body anemia has been reported to occur following sulfasalazine administration but reversed subsequent to its withdrawal (1).

Deficiencies in vitamin K and erythropoietic factors such as vitamin B_{12} and folic acid can occur after longer periods of malnutrition. Thrombophlebitis, platelet deficiency, and cardiac and thyroid abnormalities have been associated extracolonic complications of ulcerative colitis. Severe electrolyte abnormalities, particularly with hypokalemia and acid-base imbalances, frequently complicate the severe form of the disease.

Toxic megacolon is the most severe and acute consequence of ulcerative colitis (6, 7). Toxic megacolon occurs in about 2 to 6% of all cases and 10 to 20% of severe attacks of ulcerative colitis and may be fatal if surgical intervention is not timely (6, 7). Perforation and peritonitis are the most feared consequences of toxic megacolon. Development of this comlication is usually preceded by a rapidly deteriorating and fulminating clinical course with symptoms of severe toxicity. Patients who develop toxic megacolon most frequently have involvement of the entire colon. The development of this extremely severe complication is influenced by the severity of the colitis rather than its duration; therefore, it may even occur during the initial episode of colitis, or during an exacerbation of the remitting type (6, 7). Symptoms may suggest infarction, perforation, septicemia or partial obstruction. Appearing quite ill, the patient will have fever, leukocytosis, abdominal distention and bloody, purulent diarrhea. A decrease in the number of bowel movements without clinical improvement is not an uncommon experience. Many factors have been alleged to precipitate toxic megacolon including the use of opiate antidiarrheal agents, hypokalemia, anticholinergic drugs, barium enemas and others (6, 8). However, evidence of association between its occurrence and most of these factors remains equivocal and circumstantial. The use of corticosteroids in acute colitis is not related to the development of colonic distention or perforation (1, 6). Barium enemas should, however, be postponed until the disease is less active since the further distention of an overly dilated colon could have disastrous consequences. Table 15.1 summarizes the drugs which could complicate the diagnosis, course or treatment of ulcerative colitis.

Hepatobiliary abnormalities in the form of inflammatory liver changes are experienced by patients with ulcerative colitis. In 3 to 4% of the patients, generally those with longstanding and extensive disease involvement, cirrhosis will develop. The other most serious hepatic complication associated with ulcerative colitis is sclerosing cholangitis with inflammatory destruction of the large and small biliary ducts. Fatty hepatic infiltrations are a frequent consequence of nutritional disturbances in the colitis patient. Resolution of relatively minor and nonspecific type hepatic changes usually occurs as the clinical course improves. However, the prognosis for cirrhosis and pericholangitis is not related as clearly to the clinical course.

Ulcerative colitis patients may experience a rheumatoid type of arthritis. Unlike the classical presentation of rheumatoid disease, the rheumatoid factor is absent from the circulation. The arthritis is usually a disorder affecting the joints of the lower limbs. Nodules are absent. The severity of symptoms will often parallel the clinical course of the colitis, although ankylosing spondylitis and sacroiliitis may progressively worsen in spite of remission of the colitis.

Skin abnormalities such as erythema nodosum, erythema multiforme and purpura are associated with ulcerative colitis in some patients. Lesions tend to necrose and form chronic ulcers on the lower limbs. The severity of these dermatological disorders are greatest during periods of exacerbation of the colitis. Pyoderma gangrenosum is a rare dermatological disorder which can be associated with ulcerative colitis patients. Appearing usually on the limbs, these bullae-like lesions resembling "bedsores" produce chronic and severe ulcerations. The onset, duration or severity of this condition, however, does not correlate well with either the extent or severity of the ulcerative colitis. Aphthous ulcers of the mouth are also common. Conjunctivitis, iritis, uveitis, blepharitis and corneal ulcerations are inflammatory eye disorders which often accompany active colitis. They tend to be recurrent and have been experienced during all stages of the systemic disease. The association of ulcerative colitis with many of the extracolonic disorders remains unclear; however, the suggestion that the etiology of the disease is an underlying autoimmune or hyperimmune response receives much support from their apparent relationship.

Table 15.1.
Untoward Effects of Drugs on Ulcerative Colitis[a]

Drug	Comments
A. *Drugs associated with "ulcerative colitis-like" syndrome*[b]	
1. Antibiotics:	
Chloramphenicol	Pseudomenbranous enterocolitis; a necrotizing inflamma-
Neomycin	tory process affecting the mucosa of the ileum and
Penicillin	colon; symptoms of fever, abdominal pain, oliguria, ful-
Tetracycline	minating diarrhea, hypotension and collapse are experi-
Chlortetracycline	enced and appear abruptly 4–6 days following intes-
Sulfonamides	tinal surgery, injury, or antibiotic therapy; broad-spec-
Ampicillin	trum antibiotics are most frequently implicated and the
Cephalosporins	onset may be delayed up to 10–14 days after stopping
Erythromycin (17)	therapy; increased risk also associated with use of
Carbenicillin (16)	postoperative systemic antibiotics after preoperative
	courses of antibiotics; suspect resistant *Clostridium*
	difficle postantibiotic enteritis but not always a consist-
	ent find; combination antibiotic therapy and even peni-
	cillin alone have been associated with occurrence
Lincomycin	Patients receiving oral lincomycin or its congener subse-
Clindamycin	quently may develop fulminant diarrhea; sigmoido-
	scopy reveals hyperemic and friable colonic mucosa
	without ulcerations; barium enema often will show mu-
	cosal changes consistent with inflammatory bowel dis-
	ease; diarrhea is not uncommon following oral lincomy-
	cin; however, in cases developing protracted ulcerative
	colitis-like symptoms, pseudomembranous enterocolitis
	should be ruled out
2. Oral contraceptives	Ulcerative colitis-like symptoms and sigmoidoscopic ex-
	amination following oral contraceptives suggest vascu-
	lar occlusion of the distal ileum and colon in several
	case reports; remission of symptoms following discon-
	tinuation of drug suggests causal relationship
3. Chlorpropamide	Edema and multiple small ulcerations of rectal and sig-
	moid mucosa following 500 mg for 5 days for mild
	hyperglycemia; concurrent exfoliative dermatitis sug-
	gests allergic disorder
4. 5-Fluorouracil	Colonic mucosal ulceration and necrosis very similar to
	findings of chronic ulcerative colitis have appeared in
	patients receiving this drug; gastrointestinal effects are
	commonly experienced by patients taking this drug;
	most of the difficulties and symptoms stop following
	discontinuation of drug administration
5. Cyclophosphamide	Gastrointestinal symptoms are commonly experienced
	particularly with higher doses; acute hemorrhagic coli-
	tis has been reported following long-term and short-
	term cyclophosphamide administration with return to
	normal soon
6. 6-Mercaptopurine	Reports suggest intestinal ulceration is an often over-
	looked complication from this chemotherapeutic agent
7. Soap suds	Colon became edematous and inflamed without ulcera-
	tion following use as an enema during labor
8. Phenylbutazone	Inflammatory infiltrate and ulcer of sigmoid colon follow-
	ing long-term use reported in one patient; remission of
	symptoms on discontinuation and subsequent return
	when drug was reintroduced suggests a common etiol-
	ogy

Table 15.1.—*Continued*

Drug	Comments
9. Gold	Clinical and radiographic evidence of colitis, esophagitis, gastritis or enteritis following gold therapy should arouse suspicion of toxicity
10. Lithium carbonate	Underlying gastrointestinal disorder may be exacerbated; one manic depressive patient reportedly developed "acute abdomen" soon after lithium therapy was begun; diagnosed as regional enteritis; diarrhea continued for several months until lithium was discontinued
11. Laxatives, cathartics	Radiographic appearance of chronic inflammatory bowel has been seen in patients following excessive and chronic use of laxatives and cathartics
12. Digitalis	Cases of enterocolitis with acute hemorrhagic necrosis of the bowel have been described in patients with congestive failure and receiving high doses of digitalis; some of these patients had definite symptoms of digitalis toxicity; whether this is a causal relationship between colitis and therapy for congestive failure remains to be established
13. Ergot	Ischemic colitis and mesenteric-vascular occlusions, probably related to ingestion of a large dose of ergotamine tartrate has been described
B. *Drugs associated with production of paralytic ileus*	
1. Anticholinergics; atropine	Therapeutic doses have been demonstrated to have an inhibitory effect on colonic motility and tone; the use of anticholinergic antispasmodics for the control of diarrhea in fulminant colitis contributes little therapeutically in moderate to severe colitis since colonic tonus is already diminished; diarrhea is symptomatic of the inflammatory activity, not of hypermotility
2. Antidepressants Nortriptyline Imipramine Amitriptyline	Anticholinergic side effects have been associated with paralytic ileus in several reported cases; concomitant use of drugs with anticholinergic side effects, i.e., phenothiazines, tricyclic antidepressants, antiparkinsonian drugs, should be closely monitored, particularly in the older schizophrenic or severely depressed patient or any with a concomitant disorder such as hypothyroidism
3. Anticoagulants Dicumarol	Intestinal obstruction occurs secondary to intraperitoneal or intraabdominal hemorrhage; partial or complete mechanical obstruction by an adynamic condition may be produced by intestinal hematomas; presence of echymoses, epitaxis, bloody stools with symptoms indicative of obstruction should arouse suspicion; associated with long-term anticoagulant use before onset of acute abdomen
Phenidione	Severe hemorrhagic colitis occurring several days after administration of drug reported in 2 patients
4. Antihypertensives Mecamylamine Hexamethonium Pentolinium tartrate Reserpine Hydralazine	Paralytic ileus due to parasympatholytic effects of sympatholytic antihypertensives; cases reported often involve combinations of these agents used in attempts to enhance antihypertensive effects; abdominal pain is prominent feature of ileus induced by ganglionic blockade unlike "classical" paralytic ileus or acute abdomen

Table 15.1.—Continued

Drug	Comments

5. Narcotics
   Meperidine
   Tincture of opium
   Tincture of paregoric
   Diphenoxylate
   Loperamide
	In usual therapeutic doses are potent inhibitors of gastrointestinal motility; toxic dilation of the colon has occurred in patients with mild to moderate severe ulcerative colitis; colonic motility in fulminant colitis is already impaired; diarrhea is a reflection of the generalized inflammatory activity, and treatment must be directed at managing the underlying causes; there is no therapeutic rationale for using narcotics in such situations since they can contribute to further problems such as paralytic ileus and the development of toxic dilation of the colon

6. Phenothiazines
   Chlorpromazine
   Mepazine
	Cases have been reported; paralytic ileus probably secondary to anticholinergic side effects; in one report, the patient had myxedema concurrently

7. Barium enema	Rapid distention of the acutely inflamed colon can induce toxic dilation and perforation

8. Others
   Methocarbamol
   Antacids
	—

[a] For specific references (except those specifically noted) for each agent, see those listed in Ref. 1.

[b] A patient who experiences "colitis-like" symptoms during or soon after therapy with a drug of which diarrhea is a known or suspected side effect or complication should always be evaluated for gastrointestinal disease; the reaction should not simply be considered an idiopathic or unique "sensitivity" to the agent.

Patients with inflammatory bowel disease may have elevated concentrations of serum calcium and uric acid and appear to be predisposed to formation of renal stones. However, the pathogenesis of nephrolithiasis in patients with colitis is poorly understood.

Children often experience a more fulminant clinical course and respond more poorly to medical management than adults (9, 10). Physical growth often is severely impaired by the disease in children. The risk of mortality from ulcerative colitis is greatest where the onset of symptoms is rapid, colonic involvement is extensive and severe and the patient is very young or old. Carcinoma of the colon occurs more frequently among colitis patients than in the general population. This risk of malignancy increases proportionately with the duration of disease and is greatest for those patients whose disease began in childhood. It has been estimated that mortality from carcinoma increases by 20% during each decade of the disease beginning after the 1st decade. Premalignant mucosal changes may be seen in colonic biopsies of patients with longstanding ulcerative colitis (11). This fact supports the suggestion for yearly colonoscopy in patients with ulcerative colitis of greater than 10 years' duration. The survival rate of colitis patients with colonic carcinoma is significantly lower than in patients with colonic carcinoma only (11). It is quite likely that the manifestation of neoplasms in colitis patients is frequently erroneously associated with the underlying disorder, thus delaying surgery and other means for eradicating the neoplasm and quite possibly contributing to the higher mortality. An awareness of the extracolonic and systemic manifestations of the disease is necessary for the early recognition and management of complications secondary to ulcerative colitis since their amelioration may significantly influence the prognosis of the high risk patients (1).

DRUG-ASSOCIATED PSEUDOMEMBRANEOUS COLITIS

The association between a variety of drugs, e.g., antimicrobials, oral contraceptives, phenylbutazone, etc., and the occurrence of "ulcerative colitis-like" syndrome is well recognized. See Table 15.1 for a summary of drugs associated with this syndrome. Clindamycin and lincomycin have been incriminated most often but cases have been associated with a number of other antimicrobials, e.g., ampicillin, chloramphenicol, cephalosporins, sulfonamides, neomycin, tetracycline, erythromycin and carbenicillin. A prospective study of 200 hospitalized patients who were given either oral or parenteral clindamycin reported a 20% of diarrhea and 10% incidence of pseudomembraneous colitis. Since all symptoms disappeared upon withdrawl of clindamycin, the cases were presumed to be drug related. Other reports indicate the incidence to be less. There have been at least 50 cases including several fatalities of clindamycin-associated pseudomembranous colitis in the literature. In recent reports indicate that the cephalosporins and ampicillin may produce pseudomembranous colitis with equal frequency (12). The clinical course is characterized by the acute onset of profuse, watery or mucoserous diarrhea which occurs following a week or more of antibiotic administration. In some cases, symptoms did not develop until several days to weeks following the discontinuation of the antibiotic. Low grade fever, elevated white blood cell counts, abdominal pain and ileus often accompany the diarrhea. Occasionally these physical findings can be mistaken for symptoms of an acute surgical condition of the abdomen. The stools are not grossly bloodied and often are guaiac negative. It appears that older patients are at higher risk for this disorder. There is a preponderance of women involved and the reason for this is unclear. The oral route of antibiotic administration had been thought to be important in the etiology of the antibiotic-induced colitis. Colitis has, however, occurred following intravenous administration. The course of this illness varies from a week to several months. Complications include toxic megacolon and perforation of the sigmoid colon. Diagnosis of antibiotic-associated pseudomembranous colitis can best be established by the presence of pseudomembranes on sigmoidoscopic examination. Biopsy of the colonic mucosa for the presence of typical discrete plaque-like lesions is useful and probably justified in light of the high fatality risk of cases of undetected colitis. Radiographic findings of large bowel dilatation with mucosal thickening may be seen. Barium enema is generally not useful for diagnosis and may exacerbate symptoms.

Recent investigations into the pathogenesis of antibiotic colitis suggest that a toxin produced by *C. difficle*, a normal inhabitant of the intestinal flora, may be responsible. In most all patients evaluated following antibiotic associated colitis *C. difficle* has been present in significant amounts (12, 13).

Management of antibiotic associated colitis is directed at providing symptomatic relief and support and removing the toxic bacteria. Current recommendations include the use of cholestyramine or colestipol, anion exchange resins, for mild cases. These resins act to bind the *C. difficle* toxin. In more severe forms of the colitis oral vancomycin 0.5 to 2 g per day in divided doses for 7 to 14 days is usually effective (14). *C. difficle* is very sensitive to vancomycin but relapses have been reported. Bacitracin in doses of 25,000 units (500 mg) 4 times daily has also been shown to be effective and provides a significant cost advantage (14, 15). Metronidazole has also been proposed as effective therapy but more evidence is needed at this time (14).

Antibiotic-induced colitis will continue to be a problem with the newer antibiotics on the horizon having broader spectrum of activity. The newer agents as well as those already shown to cause pseudomembranous colitis should be constantly monitored for this severe complication.

TREATMENT

The goal of treatment in ulcerative colitis is to provide relief from symptoms and complications, correct deficiency states and attempt to arrest or reverse the disease process. Tailoring treatment for a disorder which is expressed by a variety of manifestations, complications and obscure etiology is a formidable task. The unpredictable clinical course, with its spontaneous remissions and exacerbations and the subjectivity by which therapeutic effectiveness is assessed, intensifies the dilemma of selecting the most appropriate and rational therapy for ulcerative colitis. Drug therapy for ulcerative colitis is nonspecific and directed against factors which have been suspected to play a role in the etiology of the disease. Agents used in the treatment of inflammatory bowel disease may be divided conveniently into those that have been found to influence the clinical course and those that correct deficiency states. Therapeutic failure with medical management and the presence of life-threatening complications are important indications for surgery.

Antimicrobials

Clinical experience with the use of antimicrobials for the treatment of ulcerative colitis has been confined primarily to the sulfonamides. Sulfasalazine, a diazo-linked combination of salicyclic acid and sulfapyridine, has been the mainstay of therapy of most clinicians (18). The choice of sulfasalazine is based on the widely held impression that it has been found more effective than any other sulfonamide for controlling ulcerative colitis. Recent evidence strongly indicates that the 5-aminosalicylic acid portion of sulfasalazine is the active component and that sulfapyridine serves as a carrier molecule to ensure 5-aminosalicylic acid being released in the colon (19, 20). Reliable studies have demonstrated that sulfonamides reduce the severity of colitis and the occurrence of relapses (21, 22). The basis for the successful use of sulfonamides in ulcerative colitis is unclear. Alteration of intestinal bacterial flora does not appear to be the mode of action. It has been thought that sulfasalazine, having been demonstrated to possess an affinity for connective tissue, exerts a nonspecific anti-inflammatory effect on the surface of the colonic wall. Evidence for the anti-inflammatory effect of sulfasalazine has recently been demonstrated by its effectiveness when given by rectal enema (20, 23). Furthermore the 5-aminosalicylic acid component of sulfasalazine, which is anti-inflammatory, produced a greater effect than sulfapyridine (20).

The usual dosage of sulfasalazine recommended for maintenance therapy is 2 g daily in divided doses for several weeks to months until symptoms are completely resolved. Higher doses of 4 to 8 g have been employed by some clinicians for the treatment of active and acute disease. Recently it has been shown that 2 g per day produces a significant reduction in relapses over 1 g and that 4 g is better than 2 g (24). However symptomatic side effects occurred much more frequently at the higher dose and is therefore not recommended for routine therapy (24). Concomitant administration of corticosteroids with sulfasalazine has been successful in controlling moderate to severe symptoms. Whether therapy with sulfonamides is to be continued intermittently or indefinitely should be determined by the frequency of relapses and the success of the regimen in maintaining the patient in a relatively asymptomatic state. In a few patients with mild disease and limited colonic involvement, sulfonamides may eventually be discontinued when remission of the active disease has been present for a year or more (21, 22). During acute episodes of fulminating colitis, i.e., toxic megacolon, the use of oral sulfonamides including sulfasalazine appears to serve little purpose. Administration of rationally selected antibiotics parenterally is certainly an appropriate and worthwhile consideration in severe toxic dilation of the colon, threatened perforation or suspected secondary infection.

The incidence of severe untoward effects of sulfasalazine is relatively low especially at doses of 2 g per day or less, although minor reactions range from occasional to frequent. It can be expected that 20 to 30% of the patients receiving sulfasalazine on short-term therapy will experience unpleasant side effects, usually gastrointestinal in nature. In a recent large cooperative controlled study the side effects experienced from sulfasalazine although ranging up to 46% of patients complaining of nausea and vomiting with higher doses, none of the side effects were significantly different from placebo (25). Intolerance to the gastrointestinal effects can possibly be overcome by taking the medication during meals or by gradually increasing the dose as tolerated to reach optimal therapeutic levels. Enteric-coated sulfasalazine tablets are available; however, there is no clinical evidence available to demonstrate their comparative effectiveness or toxicities with the plain tablets in ulcerative colitis patients. A recently controlled study demonstrated a relationship between sulfasalazine and the incidence of folate deficiency in ulcerative colitis patients (26). Dietary intake of folic acid should therefore be increased in patients on sulfasalazine therapy.

Table 15.2 summarizes the untoward effects from sulfasalazine. Investigation into the absorption, metabolism and excretion of sulfasalazine and its metabolites following single dose and repeated dosage administration in man was recently reported. The investigators concluded that the serum concentration of sulfasalazine is determined by highly individualized rates of absorption. About one third of the dose absorbed is unchanged sulfasalazine while the remaining portion is reduced by the

Table 15.2.
Untoward Effects from Sulfasalazine (1, 24)[a]

Complaints	Comments
A. *Minor*	
1. Headache, nausea, gastrointestinal distress, arthralgia	These complaints comprise the majority of side effects experienced from this drug; apparently dose-related, these complaints have been minimized by reducing the dosage; increasing the frequency of administration with smaller dose might be a worthwhile attempt
2. Dermatological reactions	Sulfonamides produce a spectrum of cutaneous reactions ranging from minor pruritus to life-threatening and even fatal toxic epidermal necrosis; dermatological reactions are not uncommon with the class of drugs having sulfasalazine as a member
3. Urine discoloration	Orange discoloration of alkaline urine; no color change in acid urine; should inform patient to avoid undue alarm
B. *Major[b]*	
1. Agranulocytosis	The most serious of untoward effects induced by sulfasalazine appears to be an allergic reaction, cutaneous reactions often precede the detection of agranulocytosis; complaints of sore throat, chills, fever or appearance of rash should arouse suspicion of this life-threatening reaction
2. Hemolytic anemia	Particularly important in glucose-6-phosphate dehydrogenase-deficient individuals
3. Heinz body anemia	Heinz bodies occurred following sulfasalazine administration; immediate return to normal following discontinuation of drug
4. Cholestatic hepatitis	Bilirubin levels increased following sulfasalazine in several patients who also had cholestatic jaundice; sulfonamides have been implicated in drug-induced cholestatic hepatitis
5. Pancreatitis	Epigastric distress and marked elevation of serum amylase occurred following administration of sulfasalazine; the association of sulfonamide derivatives with the occurrence of pancreatitis is known; pancreatitis may be overlooked since gastrointestinal side effects most frequently encountered are considered benign; in colitis, patients symptoms may be erroneously construed as originating from underlying inflammatory disorder rather than drug-induced
6. Serum sickness-like syndrome	A patient reported to have experienced serum sickness, skin rash, hemolytic anemia, plasmacytosis, lymphocytosis and elevation of immunoglobulins; a hypersensitivity reaction most likely cause; a patient with the allergic history of sulfonamide or salicylate sensitivity should not receive sulfasalazine
7. Systemic lupus erythematosus	Several patients with chronic ulcerative colitis experienced onset of exacerbation of symptoms compatible with systemic lupus erythematosus when given sulfonamides; sulfonamides have been documented to elicit clinical manifestations of systemic lupus erythematosus in susceptible individuals
8. Impaired folic acid absorption	Recent study demonstrated folic acid malabsorption in patients on sulfasalazine therapy; dietary intake of folic acid should be increased
9. Sinus tachycardia	A patient reported to have experienced sinus tachycardia of up to 126 beats/min after large initial doses of sulfasalazine (5–6 g/day)

Table 15.2.—_Continued_

[a] Adverse reactions to drugs of the sulfonamide class have been reported to involve all major organ systems, and the severity can range from mild discomfort to severe life-threatening reactions. The use of such agents is always accompanied by risk of complications; and an awareness of their clinical manifestations and significance and factors which contribute to their occurrence must always be exercised. Also beware of clinical significant drug-drug interactions associated with sulfonamides such as potentiation of hypoglycemic effects of sulfonylureas or increasing the anticoagulant activity of coumarin and its derivatives, etc.

[b] Incidence reported relatively infrequent to date.

gut flora in the cecum and colon to sulfasalazine and 5-aminosalicylic acid. Further absorption then occurs in the large intestine. Only a small portion of sulfasalazine is recovered unchanged in the urine and feces (1).

It has been suggested recently that the capacity to metabolize sulfasalazine by acetylation may influence the onset and severity of its adverse effects. In experimental studies with healthy individuals as well as patients who were given 2 to 8 g daily, up to 86% of subjects studied experiencing side effects were of the slow acetylator phenotype. This phenomenon is not unique in therapeutics but rather reminiscent of the higher incidence of polyneuropathy in patients receiving isoniazid who were considered to be slow acetylators (1).

Corticosteroids

Corticosteroids are therapeutically effective in producing remission of active ulcerative colitis. Their mode of action is considered to be primarily by suppression of inflammatory activity, and their effectiveness supports the impression than an abnormally responsive immune system may be a significant etiological factor in ulcerative colitis.

Corticosteroids rapidly reduce the severity of acute colitis but they cannot alter the basic disease process. Their use during periods of remission or in chronic continuous type colitis is controversial. Although relapses have been experienced following the discontinuation of corticosteroids, there is no evidence to justify their use as a prophylactic measure against recurrence. The risk from their long-term use has to be considered greater than any benefit which may be achieved by such use in ulcerative colitis.

Systemic corticosteroids should be given by the intravenous route in cases of acute, severe colitis. The usual dose during acute episodes is 60 to 80 mg of prednisone or equivalent doses of hydrocortisone per day. Steroid dosage may be increased to as high as 160 mg prednisone per day in acute, severe colitis with 40 to 50% chance of improvement when 80 mg failed to achieve a remission (27). Although hydrocortisone is recommended most frequently for intravenous use, it has salt- and water-retaining activity which may be undesirable where large doses are to be used and for prolonged periods. The dose of corticosteroid required to achieve the therapeutic response must be determined for every patient individually, based on the severity of symptoms and clinical course. In moderately severe active colitis oral prednisone in doses of 40 mg daily is recommended as the optimum starting dose (18). Although incidence of adverse effects from corticosteroids varies considerably, these effects are related to the amount and type administered and duration of therapy. The smallest possible dose needed to produce rapid and sustained improvement should be used. This dosage is then maintained until the patient has improved sufficiently enough to have the corticosteroids decreased or withdrawn which is usually 1 to 2 weeks. Up to 75% of patients with acute, severe colitis will respond to high dose steroids within 5 to 6 days and if a response is not seen within that time frame emergency surgery may be indicated (26).

Oral corticosteroids can be given to the patient whose condition has improved sufficiently to allow the discontinuation of intravenous administration or who is able to tolerate oral intake. Although the goal of therapy is to improve the condition to where corticosteroids are no longer required, too rapid or premature withdrawal can result in undesirable consequences. The dosage regimen must be gradually reduced following long-term use, minimizing the risk of recurrence of disease activity or adrenal-hypothalmic-pituitary insufficiency. Many of the undesirable side effects experienced following chronic therapy can be avoided if large doses of corticosteroids are given systemically over a short interval of several days to a week. Adrenal insufficiency is not seen following parenteral corticosteroids when the duration of therapy does not exceed 3 or 4 days. However, coincident diseases such as diabetes, psychological and cardiovascular disease can be exacerbated even following short-term corticosteroid therapy.

When prolonged corticosteroid therapy is necessary for control of chronic severe colitis unresponsive to medical management, an alternate day single dose regimen has been suggested as a desirable method of treatment. The risk of significant complications, especially adrenal insufficiency, is minimized by the intermittent administration of a cumulative single 48-hour dose every other day. The dose is given in the early morning in order to simulate the normal diurnal pattern of endogenous steroid secretion. Comparisons of the effect of giving corticosteroids in divided daily doses with alternate day therapy in ulcerative colitis patients have demonstrated less adrenal suppression during intermittent therapy; however, whether clinical effectiveness is equivalent to the daily continuous regimen of therapy is equivocal. Adrenal insufficiency and growth suppression following the long-term use of corticosteroids must always be considered serious complications. Children with ulcerative colitis preferably should be treated with high doses of corticosteroids on a short-term basis to induce remission, and long-term therapy with these agents should be avoided if at all possible. Alternate day corticosteroid therapy has reportedly been successful in remitting symptoms without adrenal suppression in several children. More studies of the long-term effects of intermittent therapy on the clinical course of the disease in children is required.

Corticosteroids instilled intrarectally can provide beneficial relief from symptoms of colitis. Extemporaneous preparations of various salts of hydrocortisone in vehicles such as water, safflower oil or propylene glycol or commercially available preparations for retention enema are the most popular forms of local treatment used in colitis. Enemas can be given once or twice daily during active colitis or intermittently depending upon the severity of symptoms, response and clinical course. The major therapeutic effect appears to be local on the colonic mucosa. However, steroid levels in plasma have been recorded to reach similar magnitude as those following equivalent oral doses (1). Reports of the use of many different hydrocortisone salts in this manner show considerable variation in the amount of systemic absorption that occurs. Studies have reported 30 to 50% absorption for hydrocortisone; the variation for systemic absorption with prednisolone is even greater. Hydrocortisone hemisuccinate is absorbed significantly, and the acetate is less readily absorbed than the alcohol. Since there is no apparent correlation between the therapeutic effects of locally instilled hydrocortisone with the degree of systemic absorption and adrenal suppression, the acetate salt, having the least capacity for absorption, would be preferred (1). Patients with active colitis confined to the rectum and distal sigmoid colon respond well to this form of therapy. There is evidence that intrarectal hydrocortisone can spread as far proximally as the hepatic flexure and thus this spread may be greatest in patients with active disease (1, 18, 28). Patients with extensive colonic involvement therefore may benefit from this form of treatment. If improvement is not apparent soon after intrarectal administration of corticosteroids, systemic administration should be initiated. Sulfasalazine and intermittent courses of topical corticosteroids may induce a reasonable state of health in children and eventual remission where colitis involvement is limited to the left and transverse colon.

Ill afforded delays in the diagnosis and treatment of severe fulminant colitis may occur when corticosteroids are used because symptoms of peritonitis and perforation may unknowingly be masked by them. Opinions vary as to the contribution which corticosteroids make in increasing the operative mortality of colitis, but it appears that the complication rate reflects the severity of the disease and associated complications (22). The mortality rate is increased when surgical intervention is attempted late in the course of acute, severe colitis regardless of whether corticosteroids are used. It is also important to consider that normal adrenal responsiveness will be suppressed during long-term use of corticosteroids and will continue to be for many months even after complete withdrawal. Therefore, during periods of increased stress such as infection, sugery or exacerbation of colitis corticosteroids should be given in adequate amounts since pituitary and adrenal reserves may be partially or totally compromised. Judicious and rational use of corticosteroids will provide profound amelioration of the patient's symptoms, but it can never be curative. Therapy with corticosteroids is not a replacement for conventional therapy but is to be used concomitantly with rest, diet and supportive care. While corticosteroids have definitely been proven to be beneficial for the treatment of ulcerative colitis, their potential adverse effects and precautions which accompany their use should never be ignored or overlooked.

Some clinicians prefer to use adrenal corticotropin (ACTH) alone or in combination with corticosteroids in the management of ulcerative colitis. Although complications of adrenal and growth suppression are avoided, opinions remain divided as to the appropriateness of ACTH in the management of ulcerative colitis. There are no reliable or conclusive studies which demonstrate the superiority of ACTH over corticosteroids in the treatment of this disease (18). Stimulation of the adrenal gland with ACTH, either intermittently or concurrently as suggested by some clinicians, in attempts to restore or maintain adrenal cortical responsiveness is controversial. A greater suppression may be produced by such attempts than with steroids given alone. Any patient who has received corticosteroids on a long-term basis should not be administered ACTH since the secretory capacity of his adrenals are more likely to be impaired and unresponsive. In acute fulminating colitis, systemic corticosteroids are preferred over ACTH since high doses of corticosteroids can be given rapidly with good assurance of predictable and reliable results.

Immunosuppressants

Immunosuppressive agents have been used in selected cases of ulcerative colitis. There are reports which suggest that azathioprine used on a short-term basis improved the condition of colitis patients who were refractory to conventional medical management. Others have reported a reduction in steroid dosage when similar doses of azathioprine were used (18). The long-term effects of these agents used for colitis still remains to be evaluated. Controlled evaluation of immunosuppressants is lacking. Preliminary reports of encouraging results are based on experience with patients who were concomitantly receiving corticosteroids and sulfonamides. The dosage of azathioprine to produce clinical improvement remains a controversial issue. Patients in acute toxic dilation should definitely not receive immunosuppressants. A major drawback for their potential widespread use is that nearly all the patients receiving immunosuppressants reportedly developed some adverse effect. Therapy with 6-mercaptopurine for ulcerative colitis has largely been abandoned owing to the high incidence of toxic effects. Cyclophosphamide has also been utilized, but evidence suggesting it has any additional benefits over other immunosuppressants is equivocal. Disodium cromoglycate (DSCG) has been tried in the treatment of ulcerative colitis because of possible immune mechanisms. Doses of 200 mg taken orally 4 times daily have been used. Controlled trials comparing DSCG with sulfasalazine have failed to show a significant benefit and in fact have shown a greater relapse rate with DSCG than sulfasalazine (18, 29, 30). Until the role of autoimmunity and hyperimmune activity is better understood as an etiological factor in ulcerative colitis, the use of immunosuppressants is largely empirical.

Therapy of Anemia

The frequency with which ulcerative colitis patients experience iron deficiency anemia indicates that the body iron stores should be replenished. Transfusion of whole blood is preferred for patients in acute colitis who become extremely anemic because of blood loss. Iron therapy should be reserved until the acute inflammatory activity has subsided since bone marrow utilization of iron apparently is diminished during these episodes. After the acute attack, oral iron therapy can be initiated, provided there is no exacerbation of the condition. Therapy should be continued on a daily regimen until the depleted body stores of iron have completely been replenished. The course of iron therapy should be at least 3 to 6 months since the capacity for iron absorption returns to its preanemia state as the hemoglobin levels are restored and the deficiency is corrected. Continuous iron therapy should be considered for those patients who experience chronic relapses until successful remission is assured by either medical or surgical intervention.

Iron-containing products range from simple iron salts to combinations of iron, liver and vitamin B_{12} with concentrates of intrinsic factor. Ferrous sulfate tablets are the least expensive and the most efficient means of treating simple iron deficiency anemias. Since many patients often complain of unpleasant side effects from such treatment, many substances have been added to iron preparations supposedly to enhance the absorption of iron while minimizing the side effects. Claims that such fixed combinations are a more effective form of iron preparation should be examined very critically. There is little to choose between ferrous, lactate, carbonate, fumarate, glycine, glutamate, gluconate or sulfate with regard to absorption. Studies which have claimed the superiority of one iron preparation in many cases are based on poor experimental methods and uncritical evaluations. Iron therapy in any form will produce more side effects than placebo, and it is equivocal whether there are real differences in effectiveness and acceptability between the various forms of iron preparation. The gastrointestinal intolerance, which is the most common side effect, appears to be a function of the total amount of iron available in the preparation. Nausea, vomiting, epigastric pain and other gastrointestinal discomforts can be avoided or minimized by advising that these preparations be taken with meals or that dosing be gradually increased until side effects occur or optimal dose is attained. The drawback of such recommendations is that less than optimal or desired amounts of iron may be assimilated, delaying the time for total recovery of body iron stores. However, iron deficiency is rarely a life-threatening experience, and concern for its immediate correction in the majority of ulcerative colitis patients is not warranted.

Injectable iron can be considered when the patient is unable to tolerate oral iron preparations, is unreliable or noncompliant with medications or has impaired absorption of iron. Iron dextran is the most commonly used parenteral preparation. Side effects experienced following intramuscular injection of iron have included local pain, skin discoloration, gastrointestinal disturbances, weakness, headache, flushing and muscle and joint pains. Systemic toxicities reportedly occur in fewer than 1% of patients receiving parenteral iron. The onset of reactions such as urticaria, rash and, rarer bronchospasm, hypotension, tachycardia and anaphylaxis is rapid, usually within 10 min following administration. Iron dextran can also be administered by the intravenous route. Side effects following intravenous administration have not been shown to be of any greater severity or rate of occurrence than by the intramuscular route. The advantages of the intravenous over the intramuscular route are: the total dose can be given once; it is an acceptable route of administration for a debilitated patient with insufficient muscle mass, which is not uncommon in colitis; less local pain and discoloration is produced. Particular attention must be given to any history of eczema, asthma, hay fever or the presence of renal insufficiency, nephritis or urinary tract infection since these conditions have frequently been present in patients who develop complications following parenteral iron therapy, especially hypersensitive reactive patients should be observed for 1 hour following intravenous therapy for any signs of an anaphylactic reaction. Patients with a history of asthma or allergy should not be given iron by the intravenous route. Patients with rheumatoid arthritis have exacerbated joint pain and swelling following intravenous administration of iron dextran. The rate of hemoglobin synthesis and erythropoiesis following parenteral iron is not significantly different from that of oral iron. The average daily increase in hemoglobin is about 0.15 g/100 ml and rarely exceeds 0.30 g/100 ml. Therefore, the oral route of administration is indicated for these higher risk individuals. The amount of parenteral iron administered should always be calculated on the basis of body weight and the patient hemoglobin content since the body's capacity to excrete is limited. The induction of hemosiderosis should never serve as the clinical end point of therapy with parenteral iron. Experimentally, ascorbic acid has been demonstrated to act successfully as a reducing agent, converting ferric ions to ferrous ions which then can readily be assimilated. However, the amount of ascorbic acid necessary to accomplish this activity is far in excess of those quantities which have been incorporated into commercially available iron preparations. Until the role of ascorbic acid in deficiency anemias can be scientifically and clinically established, its presence in iron preparations on the basis that it may offer some preventive or prophylactic measure is unacceptable. There is also at present no clnically reliable evidence to suggest that the prolonged release or enteric-coated iron preparations are more effective.

Iron preparations are also available in combination with vitamin B_{12}, folic acid and dried stomach concentrates. These preparations are suitable for anemias which occur as a result of multiple deficiencies. Following gastrectomy or gastroenterostomy disorders such as gastric carcinoma or gastric ulcers, preparations containing iron and vitamin B_{12} with concentrates of intrinsic factor are appropriate choices for correcting deficiencies. The large number of iron preparations available suggest that they are often prescribed with little understanding of their proper or rational use. The patient must bear the burden of high costs of such preparations. These preparations must never serve as an excuse for poor or inadequate diagnosis or therapeutic management of any patient with symptoms of anemia.

Antispasmodics and Opiates

In mild to moderate cases of colitis, many clinicians will employ antispasmodics and opiates for purposes of diarrhea control. Toxic megacolon may be associated with the use of opiates and therefore these drugs must only be used sparingly, and long term chronic therapy with them should be discouraged (6, 8). During periods of severe diarrhea, oral intake should be restricted to medications and clear fluids until the diarrhea subsides. Antidiarrheal agents containing kaolin, methylcellulose, pectin or psyllium provide minimal benefit on such occasions. Antispasmodics and opiates should be avoided in acute fulminating colitis. Therapeutic amounts of these drugs are seldom successful in controlling diarrhea in severe cases since diarrhea is symptomatic of an inflamed, hyperemic and marginally motile bowel rather than the result of hypermotility.

Nutrition

Acute severe attacks of ulcerative colitis are usually more responsive to bowel rest and intravenous therapy. Since patients may be without oral nutrition for several days to months, total parenteral nutrition is sometimes indicated. Several reports have indicated weight stability as well as weight gain when total parenteral nutrition has been employed (1). Total parenteral nutrition usually takes the form of aminoacids, glucose, electrolytes and vitamins and should be designed to deliver daily caloric need. Following acute attack, the patient's nutritional deficiencies should be corrected by giving small frequent feedings which are high in calories and protein but low in residue. There is evidence that nearly 20% of patients with ulcerative colitis benefit from a milk-free diet as evidenced by a decrease in their incidence of relapses (10). It is unclear whether this is reflection of an allergic sensitivity to protein or a deficiency in the affected colon of the enzyme lactase. Egg albumin, oranges, potatoes, tomatoes and wheat have been suggested as foods which can exacerbate colitis; however, substantiation of this causal relationship continues to be equivocal. Children with ulcerative colitis who have milk products restricted from their diet should receive daily supplements of calcium and vitamin D, necessary in appropriate quantities in order to maintain biochemical function and physiological growth. Concurrent administration of corticosteroids in patients who have been restricted from milk further complicates the task of management since the effect of vitamin D on calcium absorption is antagonized. Therefore careful consideration should be given to recognizing the clinical manifestations of hypocalcemia. Adequate vitamin D as 25-hydroxycholecalciferol or dihydrotachysterol and calcium intake should be provided from sources other than milk products. Some clinicians advocate unlimited diet, while others recommend low residue diets and restricting certain foods which by patient experience and judgment have not been well tolerated. There is no universal agreement as to the benefits derived from dietary restraints for the ulcerative colitis patient. Decisions as to what constitutes a suitable dietary regimen should be individualized following an evaluation of the effect of diet on the patient's condition. The goal of dietary management for the ulcerative colitis patient is to overcome nutritional deficiencies and improve the patient's overall sense of well being.

Psychotherapy

Although it cannot be confirmed that there is an increased frequency of psychological or personality difficulties in patients with ulcerative colitis, an essential ingredient in the management of the disease is emotional assurance and support. The physician and pharmacist should endeavor to establish a meaningful professional relationship and rapport with the patient. It is acknowledged that emotional factors such as anxiety and stress influence the clinical course of the disease and the eventual outcome of management. Drugs such as the tricyclic antidepressants or phenothiazine tranquilizers should never be considered as appropriate substitutes for efforts at understanding and communicating with patients afflicted with ulcerative colitis. Nonspecific measures such as rest may be beneficial. Separation from emotionally stressful situation and even hospitalization for the patient may be justifiable during periods of disease activity. Medical management without conscientious, skillful and rational psychotherapy or emotional support from the physician does not meet the total needs of these patients.

Surgery

Indications for surgical management of ulcerative colitis include the following: toxic megacolon, perforation, acute and severe bleeding, colonic stricture with obstruction or reasonable suspicion of malignancy. The decision to intervene surgically in cases of intractable colitis where medical management has been unsuccessful should be made only after considering factors such as the effects of chronic invalidism, physical and developmental retardation, the drugs used, particularly corticosteroids and the risk of carcinoma. There is a lack of reliable clinical information regarding the outcome of continued medical management in these patients. In spite of maintenance therapy, the patient with near total colonic involvement or who is 60 years and older will most likely develop severe re-

current attacks eventually requiring surgery. Milder forms of colitis confined to the rectum and sigmoid colon rarely require surgery. Table 16.3 summarizes those surgical procedures which are commonly done for ulcerative colitis of the bowel. The management of toxic megacolon by medical means alone often is unsuccessful. The patient who recovers from a fulminating attack following intensive medical management usually will require surgery within a few years. The mortality rate of surgical procedures is significantly higher for emergency procedures than for elective ones. Early surgery is encouraged in the very ill patient with severe recurrent colitis. Intensive medical treatment should be started in acute fulminant cases in order to reduce the operative risk. Careful monitoring of patient response to treatment during this period must be conducted. Although the incidence of surgical intervention has not changed appreciably in recent years, the operative mortality has decreased as has the number of emergency procedures performed. The likelihood that this is indicative of the success of intensive medical treatment prior to surgery has been suggested.

Provision for restoring and maintaining adequate electrolyte, fluid, hemoglobin levels and corticosteroid coverage must be made prior to and after colectomy. The patient and his family should be advised on the nature of the surgery and sufficiently prepared emotion-

Table 15.3.
Surgical Basis for Treatment of Ulcerative Colitis

Procedure[a]	Comments
1. Total colectomy with ileostomy; also: panproctocolectomy	The surgical procedure of choice where colitis involvement is diffuse affecting extensive portion of colon and rectum; the entire colon is removed; an ileostomy or "artificial anus" is constructed from the ileum; this procedure does not offer opportunity for restoring the continuity of the bowel; the psychological adjustment to the impact of this procedure is important
2. Subtotal colectomy with ileorectal anastomosis	Suitable for right-sided or segmental colitis and Crohn's disease or granulomatous colitis; spares the rectum and variable amount of the distal colon; offers the opportunity for restoring continuity of the bowel; failure rate is significant where colitis is diffuse and extensive owing to continuing activity in remaining segment; risk of developing malignancies in the remaining rectal segment is considerable

[a] Twenty percent of patients with ulcerative colitis will require surgery. Prior to surgery, complete evaluation of vital signs, electrolyte levels, blood volume, hemoglobin, renal function and corticosteroid coverage must be considered. Postoperative complications (e.g., fistula, serious debilitation) contraindicating oral or tube feeding may necessitate hyperalimentation by intravenous administration of protein hydrolysates, hypertonic glucose, electrolytes and vitamin solutions for prolonged periods to provide positive nitrogen balance and calories.

ally to accept an ileostomy. The psychological adjustment required for the individual who has recently undergone an ileostomy is often facilitated by the improvement he or she experiences with respect to the quality of life. As health is restored, participation in normal activities for the patient is again possible. For most patients living with an ileostomy is invariably preferred to existing as a chronic invalid. The concerned pharmacist can often provide the ostomate patient psychological support and assurance by demonstrating an awareness and understanding of those problems which the patient might encounter. Groups have been formed in many cities and counties throughout the United States for the purpose of assisting in emotional and social rehabilitation and in dealing with those problems common to the ostomate patient.

Especially trained individuals known as enterostomal therapists have provided valuable assistance for many ostomate patients experiencing problems, many quite complex, which required attention or simply reassurance. Significant difficulties and complications have been noted to develop in many patients during the first 3 or 4 months following colectomy and ileostomy. Obstruction is the most frequent complication. It appears that proper understanding and use of judgment often are sufficient to overcome many such difficulties and complications. While servicing the ileostomy patient with the necessary appliances and supplies, the pharmacist should also make efforts to assist and inform the patient on their proper use and care. The pharmacist should also be aware that drug therapy in patients with an ileostomy may require specialized dosage adjustments due to absorption variabilities. The ostomate patient may absorb drugs to a lesser degree due to a shortened intestinal tract. Table 15.4 summarizes common complications from ileostomies.

PROGNOSIS

For patients with ulcerative colitis, the outlook for successful prognosis is encouraging as the quality of medical management improves. Particular attention given to intensive therapy during the onset of symptoms and a comprehensive approach to treatment with drugs, psychological support and diet have contributed to resolving the symptoms of the disease with better success. Since the therapeutic ap-

Table 15.4.
Complications from Ileostomies

Type	Comments
1. Obstruction	Most frequent; result of high residue and high bulk foods, e.g., popcorn; overeating should be avoided; scar formation and strictures can lead to obstruction; symptoms include: cramps, distention, vomiting, nonfunctioning ileostomy or diarrhea due to accumulation of pressure; contact patient's physician
2. Dehydration	Secondary to diarrhea; caution in recommending antidiarrheals since symptoms may be due to obstruction; abnormally liquefied and constant ileostomy drainage is hazardous; serious when complicated by electrolyte depletion, acid-base imbalance and hypoproteinemia
3. Electrolyte deficiency	
a. Hypokalemia	Potassium deficiency; loss from ileostomy can be considerable; symptoms include muscle weakness, numbness of fingers, toes, dyspnea, irregular pulse, bradycardia, metabolic alkalosis; of particular concern in patients on digitalis glycosides and/or taking diuretics; if hypokalemia is mild and only transient, dietary replenishment often is adequate
b. Hyponatremia	Sodium deficiency; symptoms include abdominal cramps, fatigue, oliguria, low blood pressure; should consider even in absence of diarrhea since excessive drainage and insensible loss of fluids and sodium need to be considered
4. Peri-ileostomy	Soreness around ileostoma and appliance; allergic reaction to adhesive improper fit should be ruled out; improper application or care of appliance; use of certain allergenic solvents or soaps around area should be ruled out
5. Bleeding	Contact patient's physician; cause should be determined

[a] Pharmacist considerations: enteric-coated medications are poor dosage form choices; also sustained release dosage forms; recommend liquids or soft gelatin preparations, e.g., vitamins.

Table 15.5.
Basis for the Management of Ulcerative Colitis

Area of Disease Involvement	Clinical Course	Treatment Considerations
Rectum	Acute	Local corticosteroids for short term
	Intermittent	Sulfonamides for long term; may require adjustment of dosage during exacerbations; local corticosteroids for short term during flare-ups may be useful
	Continuous	Maintenance sulfonamides, e.g., sulfasalazine 2 g daily; attempt to resolve possible etiological factors, e.g., stress, anxiety, diet, allergies, cathartic abuse, etc.
Rectum/sigmoid	Acute	Local or systemic corticosteroids for short term; concomitantly sulfonamides; i.e., sulfasalazine 2–4 g may be tried; replace blood loss if anemia severe
Rectum Sigmoid colon Descending colon	Intermittent	Maintenance sulfonamides; intermittent corticosteroids locally if symptoms are successfully treated in such a manner; may need to consider systemic corticosteroids on short-term basis during exacerbations; correct deficiency anemia; rule out contributing factors, e.g., milk products, stress, anxiety, diet
	Continuous	Maintenance sulfonamides; corticosteroids should not be used on a chronic basis, rather only when acute exacerbations occur; continuous iron therapy should be considered; rule out contributing factors; avoid long-term use of opiates for diarrhea in most patients
Rectum Sigmoid colon Descending colon Transverse colon	Acute	Same as rectum/sigmoid and descending colonic involvement; sulfonamide, i.e., sulfasalazine, dosage may have to be adjusted toward 6 g daily if patient can tolerate; unlikely treatment would be effective if given without corticosteroids concurrently; systemic corticosteroids may be more effective since enemas may be difficult to retain; concern for perforation, toxic megacolon and perforation; if not resolved medically within several days must consider surgery
	Intermittent	Same as for rectum/sigmoid and descending colonic involvement; if medical management is unsuccessful, surgery must be considered
	Continuous	Same as for rectum/sigmoid and descending colon; if intractable to medical management or contributing to chronic invalidism, surgery should be considered; deficiency states, e.g., anemia, vitamins, especially B_{12} and K, should be restored

Table 15.5.—*Continued*

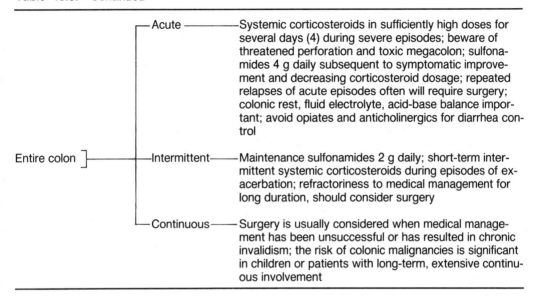

	Acute	Systemic corticosteroids in sufficiently high doses for several days (4) during severe episodes; beware of threatened perforation and toxic megacolon; sulfonamides 4 g daily subsequent to symptomatic improvement and decreasing corticosteroid dosage; repeated relapses of acute episodes often will require surgery; colonic rest, fluid electrolyte, acid-base balance important; avoid opiates and anticholinergics for diarrhea control
Entire colon	Intermittent	Maintenance sulfonamides 2 g daily; short-term intermittent systemic corticosteroids during episodes of exacerbation; refractoriness to medical management for long duration, should consider surgery
	Continuous	Surgery is usually considered when medical management has been unsuccessful or has resulted in chronic invalidism; the risk of colonic malignancies is significant in children or patients with long-term, extensive continuous involvement

proaches to treating ulcerative colitis are largely empiric and primarily directed at providing symptomatic relief, no single approach or regimen can be recommended as universally effective. The therapy plan must be individualized with a goal of providing the patient an opportunity to resume normal activity. Mild to moderate symptoms of short duration are most likely to respond favorably to medical management. Prognosis is also improved for the patient with disease limited only to the rectum and sigmoid colon. Nearly 75% of patient with ulcerative colitis respond to medical treatment and may remain symptom-free. For some patients there may be even complete remission and reversal of the disease on clinical evaluation.

Immediate and intensive therapy is required in acute fulminating colitis since the risk of mortality from such cases is significant. Hospitalization is necessary because it facilitates efforts to assess and evaluate the clinical course of the condition and its response to management. Management of the acute attack initially should be attempted by medical means. Supportive measures such as bed rest, fluid and electrolyte replacement, colonic rest by restriction of oral intake and correction of significant anemia should be undertaken to provide relief from symptoms. Corticosteroids may be initiated on the onset of an attack depending on its severity or several days after symptomatic treatment has not produced any

apparent improvement. Patients who received corticosteroids chronically prior to the acute episode or during previous attacks should be started on them immediately. One should always be aware that corticosteroids may mask symptoms of perforation. Continued evaluation for development of toxic dilation of the colon should be part of the therapy for these patients. Although not all acute attacks of colitis are terminated surgically, invariably a number of patients with recurrent severe episodes of colitis will require surgical intervention. If improvement following aggressive medical treatment is not satisfactory within several days, surgery must then be considered without further delay. Prognosis for successful recovery in such situations favors the patient whose conditions improved following medical treatment prior to surgery.

CONCLUSION

The therapeutic management of ulcerative colitis is a formidable task owing to the lack of complete understanding of its etiology, difficulty in evaluating the effectiveness of treatment and the unpredictable and chronic nature of its clinical course. The successful outcome of treatment is greatly dependent on the combined presence of psychological support, patient awareness of the lmitations of the therapeutic measures employed and adherence to prescribed drug and dietary regimens (Table 15.5). The pharmacist can contribute significantly to the total management of the patient with colitis. (S)He can serve as a reliable resource of information on matters such as ostomate appliances and medications prescribed as well as being available to provide often needed emotional reassurance by virtue of accessibility to the patient. Conscientious monitoring of the patient compliance to prescribed therapeutic regimen and participation with the colitis patient's physical therapist and nurse in evaluating the effectiveness of therapy are responsibilities which a pharmacist should assume. Success at such formidable tasks can only be achieved if the pharmacist is aware of the current concepts of the nature of the disease, problems associated with its management and the capabilities and limitations of available therapeutic approaches.

References

1. Smith GH, Tong TG; Ulcerative colitis. In Herfindal ET, Hirschman JL: *Clinical Pharmacy and Therapeutics.* Baltimore: Williams & Wilkins, 1979, pp 224–241.
2. Beeken WL: Transmissible agents in inflammatory bowel disease. *Med Clin North Am* 64:1021, 1980.
3. Sachar DB, Auslander MO, Walfish JS: Aetiological theories of inflammatory bowel disease. *Clin Gastroenterol* 9:231, 1980.
4. Campbell AC, Skinner JM, Maclellan ICM, et al: Immunosuppression in the treatment of inflammatory bowel disease. *Clin Exp Immunol* 24:249, 1976.
5. Jewell DP, Truelove SC: Azathioprine in ulcerative colitis: final report on controlled therapeutic trial. *Br Med J* 4:627, 1974.
6. Fazio VW: Toxic megacolon in ulcerative colitis and Crohn's colitis. *Clin Gastroenterol* 9:389, 1980.
7. Roys G, Kaplan MS, Jules GL; Surgical management of toxic megacolon. *Am J Gastroenterol* 63:161, 1977.
8. Brown JW; Toxic megacolon with loperamide therapy. *JAMA* 241:501, 1979.
9. Binder V, Bonnevie D, Gertz TCL, et al: Ulcerative colitis in children. *Scand J Gastroenterol* 8:161, 1973.
10. Goel KM, Shanks RA: Long-term prognosis of children with ulcerative colitis. *Arch Dis Child* 48:337, 1973.
11. Dobbins WA: Current status of the precancer lesion in ulcerative colitis. *Gastroenterology* 73:1431, 1977.
12. Bartlett JG,, Willey SH, Chang TW, et al: Cephalosporin-associated pseudomembranous colitis due to *Clostridium difficile. JAMA* 242:2683, 1979.
13. Bartlett JG, Chang TW, Garwith M, et al: Antibiotic-associated pseudomembranous colitis due to toxin-producing clostridia. *N Engl J Med* 298:531, 1978
14. George WL, Rolfe RD, Finegold SM: Treatment and prevention of antimicrobial agent-induced colitis and diarrhea. *Gastroenterology* 79:366, 1980.
15. Chang TW, Gorbach SC, Bartlett JG, et al: Bacitracin treatment of antibiotic-associated colitis and diarrhea caused by *Clostridium difficle* toxin. *Gastroenterology* 78:1584, 1980.
16. Saadah HA: Carbenicillin and pseudomembranous enterocolitis. *Ann Intern Med* 92:645, 1980.
17. Gantz NM, Zawacki MD, Dickerson J: Pseudomembranous colitis associated with erythromycin. *Ann Intern Med* 71:866, 1979.
18. Lennard-Jones JE, Powell-Tuck J: Drug treatment of inflammatory bowel disease. *Clin Gastroenterol* 8:187, 1979.
19. Klotz U, Maier K, Fischer C, et al: Therapeutic efficacy of sulfasalazine and its metabolites in patients with ulcerative colitis and Crohn's disease. *N Engl J Med* 303:1499, 1980.
20. Campieri M, Lanfranchi GA, Bazzocchi G, et al: Treatment of ulcerative colitis with high dose 5-aminosalicylic acid enemas. *Lancet* 2:270, 1981.
21. Dissanayake AS, Truelove SC: A controlled therapeutic trial of long-term maintenance treatment of ulcerative colitis with sulphasalazine (Salazopyrin). *Gut* 14:923, 1973.
22. Riis P, Anthonisen P, Wulff HR, et al: The prophylactic effect of salazosulphapyridine in ulcerative colitis during long-term treatment. *Scand J Gastroenterol* 8:71, 1973.
23. Palmer KR, Goepel JR, Holdsworth CD: Sulphasalazine retention enemas in ulcerative colitis: a double-blind trial. *Br Med J* 282:1571, 1981.
24. Azad-Khan AK, Howes DT, Piris J, et al: Optimum dose of sulphasalazine for maintenance treatment in ulcerative colitis. *Gut* 21:232, 1980.
25. Singleton JW, Law DH, Kelley ML Jr, et al: National cooperative Crohn's disease study: Adverse reaction to study drugs. *Gastroenterology* 778:876, 1979.
26. Halsted CH, Gandhi G, Tamura T: Sulfasalazine inhibits the absorption of folates in ulcerative colitis. *N Engl J Med* 305:1513, 1981.
27. Kristensen M, Koudahl G, Fischerman K, et al: High dose prednisone treatment in severe ulcerative colitis. *Scand J Gastroenterol* 9:177, 1974.
28. Farthing MJG, Rutland MD, Clark ML: Retrograde spread of hydrocortisone containing foam given intrarectally in ulcerative colitis. *Br Med J* 2:822, 1979.
29. Willoughby CP, Heyworth MF, Piris J, et al: Comparison of disodium cromoglycate and sulfasalazine as maintenance therapy for ulcerative colitis. *Lancet* 1:119, 1979.
30. Binder V, Elsborg L, Griebe J, et al: Disodium cromoglycate in the treatment of ulcerative colitis and Crohn's disease. *Gut* 22:55, 1981.

CHAPTER 16

Hepatitis: Viral and Drug Induced

WAYNE A. KRADJAN, Pharm.D.

A simple definition of hepatitis is "an inflammatory disease of the liver which may produce hepatic cell necrosis." There are multiple causes of hepatitis including viral and bacterial infections and exposure to chemicals (drugs). The pharmacist needs to be aware of the causes and treatment of viral hepatitis because of its relatively high prevalence and must understand drug-induced causes to help identify and eliminate their occurrence.

ETIOLOGY
Viral Hepatitis

On the basis of epidemiologic data, it is believed that there are at least three distinct types of viral hepatitis, each caused by a specific virus: hepatitis A (formerly called infectious hepatitis), hepatitis B (formerly called serum hepatitis) and hepatitis C (also called non-A, non-B hepatitis) (1, 2). Recent investigation has shown that other infectious diseases may mimic classic viral hepatitis including cytomegalovirus, Epstein-Barr virus, adenovirus and mononucleosis.

Hepatitis A virus (HAV) is an RNA virus usually contracted by oral-fecal exposure to an infected individual and with a short incubation period of from 15 to 50 days. The existence of this virus is now clearly identified with the presence of the hepatitis A antigen (HA Ag). The antigen is found in the blood 5 to 6 days before biochemical or clinical signs of disease occur and it disappears at the peak of disease symptoms. Fecal shedding of the antigen during the early course of the illness can lead to disease transmission, but no long term carrier state has been identified. Hepatitis A antibodies (anti-HAV or HA Ab) appear soon after the onset of clinical illness and remain elevated indefinitely. Once the antibody appears, the person is no longer infectious to others and the person is immune to further infections.

Hepatitis B virus (HBV) is a DNA virus generally acquired by parenteral exposure to contaminated blood products or infected hypodermic syringes and needles. Hepatitis B can also be transmitted by saliva, sputum, semen and contact with contaminated blood specimens. Those at high risk are laboratory and renal dialysis unit personnel, surgeons, dentists and oncologists. In contrast to hepatitis A, hepatitis B has a long incubation period of from 40 to 180 days.

Plasma rich in HBV contains several particles of different sizes and shapes. One of these, a 42-nm spherical particle called the "Dane particle," represents the true hepatitis B virus. A smaller particle, which is probably the external lipoprotein coat of the virus, is called the hepatitis B surface antigen (HB$_s$Ag). This antigen was formerly called the Australian antigen (because of its discovery in aboriginal natives in Australia) and the hepatitis associated antigen (HAA). The HB$_s$Ag can be further broken down into 10 distinct antigenic subtypes. HB$_s$Ag first appears in the blood 27 to 41 days after innoculation or about 7 to 46 days before clinical illness occurs. Antigen titers stay high throughout the course of the illness and for 1 to 13 weeks after the illness clears. Approximately 4% of patients have indefinite persistence of the HB$_s$Ag, often associated with continued infectivity to others (e.g., via blood contamination) and the presence of chronic active hepatitis. Antibody to the surface antigen (anti-HB$_s$ or HB$_s$Ab) develops in 80% of those infected, but its appearance may be delayed for several weeks to months after the clearance of the antigen. Therefore, a gap may exist where neither the antigen nor antibody can be detected in the patient's blood, but the person may still be infective to others. In contrast to hepatitis A, the antibody to the surface antigen may last for only short periods of time in some persons or indefinitely in others. As long as the antibody is present, the patient is immune to reinfections.

Disruption of the Dane particle also causes

release of a 7-nm inner core of antigenic DNA material referred to as hepatitis B core antigen (HB$_c$Ag). This antigen is more specific for infectivity than the surface antigen and may persist in the absence of surface antigen. Its presence denotes acute viral infection and replication. Antibody to the core antigen (anti-HB$_c$) may appear during infection and may even persist during chronic active hepatitis. Therefore, the presence of core antibody does *not* signify immunity or decreased infectivity. It usually appears 12 to 20 weeks after exposure or about 4 to 10 weeks after the appearance of the surface antigen. Core antibody may be found during the gap between HB$_s$Ag and anti-HB$_s$. Another core antibody, HB$_e$Ag, is associated with a chronic carrier state. Table 16.1 summarizes the significance of various antigen-antibody patterns found in the serum from HBV infections.

Much less is known about non-A, non-B hepatitis infections. They are most commonly transmitted via blood transfusions and have an incubation period intermediate to those of hepatitis A and B. The antigen is usually detected within 3 weeks of transfusion with clinical disease occurring another 3 to 6 weeks later. The antigen clears within 14 weeks, but may persist in a small number of individuals representing a chronic infectious state. Since screening for non-A, non-B antigens and antibodies is not readily available, a hepatitis reaction without known etiology and with an absence of hepatitis A or B antigen is usually diagnosed as non-A, non-B hepatitis by exclusion.

Drug-induced Hepatitis

Drugs can produce hepatic damage by three general mechanisms (3–5): (a) by acting as a vehicle for transmission of viral hepatitis, (b) by acting as direct (intrinsic) hepatotoxins or poisons, and (c) by inducing a hypersensitivity or idiosyncratic type reaction.

The first category, carriers of hepatitis virus, is composed primarily of blood and blood products. Table 16.2 lists some of these products and the relative risk from their use. To decrease the number of transfusion-related causes of hepatitis, many blood banks are now performing hepatitis associated antigen screening. In addition, blood from paid donors is being used less because of the high frequency of HAA in their sera.

Drugs affecting liver function by the latter two mechanisms are differentiated as follows. The direct hepatotoxins cause a reproducible

Table 16.1.
Summary of Hepatitis B Serum Findings

Antigen-Antibody Pattern	Significance
HB$_s$Ag alone	Acute infection or chronic active disease
HC$_c$Ag alone	Acute infection
HB$_s$Ag plus HB$_c$Ag	Acute infection or chronic active disease
Anti-HB$_s$ alone or with anti-HB$_c$	Convalescence, immunity, noninfective
Anti-HB$_c$ alone	"Serologic gap"—unknown infectivity
HB$_s$Ag plus anti-HB$_c$	Chronic active disease, chronic carrier state
HB$_s$Ag plus anti-HB$_s$ plus anti-HB$_c$	Fulminant infection or chronic active disease
HB$_e$Ag	Subtype of surface antigen with high correlation to chronic active disease

Table 16.2.
Risk of Hepatitis Transmission from Blood Products[a]

A. *High risk—multiple donors, cannot be heated*
1. UV-exposed pooled plasma (8 donors). If stored at room temperature for 6 mo, the risk may be less
2. Platelets
3. Antihemophiliac (AHF) concentrate
4. UV-exposed fibrinogen
5. Factor IX complex (Konyne)

B. *Moderate risk—single donors, cannot be heated*
1. Whole blood
2. Packed red blood cells (2–6°C)
3. Frozen red blood cells (may be safer than refrigerated only)
4. Single donor plasma
5. Platelets
6. AHF concentrate

C. *No risk*
1. Human serum albumin (sterilized at 57°C)
2. Plasma protein fraction
3. Immune and hyperimmune γ-globulin

[a] Drying, freezing or UV light will not kill the hepatitis virus. Heat at 55°C for 1 hour will kill the virus, but denature plasma proteins.

and predictable type of reaction. When given in sufficient quantities or for a sufficient length of time they will cause hepatocellular damage in all exposed individuals. Usually only zonal regions of the liver are destroyed, but in severe intoxication whole lobes and even the entire liver can be destroyed. Injury may be caused directly by the offending drug or indirectly through the drug's metabolite, or by decreasing bile flow. Alcohol is frequently included in this category and a special type of nonviral-induced hepatitis is considered under the title of alcoholic hepatitis (6).

In contrast, idiosyncratic or hypersensitivity type reactions are unpredictable. If they are immunologically mediated they require previous exposure or sensitization to the drug, but they can occur from very small doses once the person is sensitized. Idiosyncratic reactions can be further subdivided into two types: *hepatocellular damage* (cytotoxicity) where liver cells are actually destroyed due to focal necrosis and *cholestatic reactions* where there is merely swelling of the liver cells leading to compression of the bile ducts and thus stasis of bile flow with the formation of thickened bile plugs. Although cholestatic changes are not a true form of hepatitis, prolonged cholestatic injury may progress to hepatocellular damage.

Table 16.3 lists some of the drugs known to cause the various types of drug-induced liver changes. While it is not within the scope of this chapter to discuss all the drugs listed, a few are chosen as representative examples. Acetaminophen is a widely used aspirin substitute that is generally felt to be quite safe. However, overdoses with as little as 10 g can lead to fatal hepatic necrosis within 2 to 3 days after ingestion (7). Some evidence exists that

Table 16.3.
Drug-induced Hepatitis[a]

Intrinsic Toxicity	Idiosyncratic	
	Hepatocellulalar	Cholestatic
Acetaminophen (overdose)	Allopurinol	Acetohexamide
Acetone	Antipyrine	Aprindine
Alcohol (ethanol)	Azathioprine	Azathioprine
Antimony	Chloramphenicol	Butyrophenones (e.g. haloperidol)
Arsenicals	Dantrolene	Chloromazine (phenothiazines)
Aspirin	Disulfiram	Chlorpropamide
Carbon tetrachloride	Diocytl sodium sulfosuccinate	Erythromycin estolate
Chloroform	Ethionamide	Estrogens (contraceptives)
Cincophen	Fluroxane	Methimazole
Daunorubicin	Furosemide	Methyl testosterone (17 alkyl substituted androgens)
Halothane	Gold salts	PAS
Isoniazid	Halothane	Phenylbutazone
Phenothiazines	Isoniazid	Phenytoin
Phosphorus	6-Mercaptopurine	Propylthiouracil
Tetracyclines	Methoxyflurane	Tricyclic antidepressants
Toluene	Methyldopa	Valproic acid
	Oxacillin	
	Oxyphenisatin	
	Papaverine	
	PAS	
	Phenylbutazone	
	Phenytoin	
	Procaineamide	
	Pyrazinamide	
	Quinidine	
	Rifampin	
	Sulfonamides	
	Thiazole diuretics	
	Trimethadione	
	Valproic acid	

[a] Drug names appearing in more than one colume denote either a mixed type of reaction reported with the drug or poor documentation as to the mechanism of injury.

even chronic ingestion of greater than 3 g per day may be toxic (8, 9). The determinant of acetaminophen toxicity is felt to be a toxic metabolite. Normally, the majority of therapeutic dose is conjugated with glucuronates and sulfates, with a smaller portion being metabolized by the cytochrome P-450 system to intermediate metabolites. These intermediate metabolites are dependent upon conjugation with either cysteine or glutathione (sources of sulfhydryl groups) to form mercapturic acid which is excreted in the urine. Acetaminophen overdoses saturate both glucuronide and sulfate pathways and deplete hepatic glutathione stores allowing for a buildup of intermediate metabolites. These metabolites then bind (arylate) to sulfhydryl groups in liver cells and produce necrosis. Plasma acetaminophen concentrations of greater than 120 to 300 μg/ml at four hours after ingestion or an elimination half-life exceeding 4 hours has been correlated to hepatic toxicity (7, 10).

Isoniazid is an antitubercular drug used both as a prophylactic agent in patients with positive purified protein derivatives (PPDs) and for treatment of active tuberculosis. In contrast to other toxicities of this drug (e.g., pyridoxine deficiency) which are more prevalent in slow acetylators, the hepatotoxicity produced by this drug is more prevalent in fast acetylators. It is speculated that the hepatotoxicity is a result of rapid metabolism to isonicotinic acid and acetyl hydrazine, the latter being a potent hepatotoxin (11). Others claim that acetylator phenotyping provides no value for predicting hepatotoxicity (12).

Chlorpromazine provides an example of a hypersensitivity induced cholestatic reaction. The reaction is unrelated to dose and generally occurs within the first 4 weeks of treatment, but may appear as long as 3 weeks after the drug is discontinued. The incidence is low, probably affecting less than 0.5% of those receiving the drug. It is thought that the drug causes a direct impairment of biliary micelle formation thus causing insoluble complexes with bile salts. In addition, nonmetabolized chlorpromazine has caused precipitation of biliary proteins in vitro (13).

INCIDENCE

In 1982 viral hepatitis ranked only behind gonorrhea, syphilis and tuberculosis in the number of reported cases to the Center for Disease Control (CDC) in Atlanta (14). A total of 55,356 cases of hepatitis were reported to the CDC in 1982 including 22,652 cases of hepatitis A and 21,532 cases of hepatitis B. This probably only represents a fraction of total persons infected since many cases go undetected or unreported.

Hepatitis A occurs sporadically throughout the year and may assume epidemic proportions particularly under crowded living conditions such as in the military or in underprivileged populations. It is common in children and young adults, but an increasing number of adults are contracting the disease. There is a tendency toward cyclic recurrence in populations at 7-year intervals.

In the past, only a small fraction of the reported cases were due to hepatitis B, but with widespread intravenous drug abuse and the more sophisticated immunological techniques described above, the incidence of hepatitis B now rivals that of hepatitis A. The estimated lifetime risk of hepatitis B infection in the United States is approximately 5% for the population as a whole, but considerably higher in high risk groups such as hemodialysis unit personnel and patients, other health care workers with direct patient contact or who are frequently exposed to blood, children born to affected mothers, illicit IV drug abusers, homosexual males or prostitutes. An estimated 200,000 persons, primarily young adults, are infected annually. One quarter of them develop symptomatic disease. More than 10,000 patients are hospitalized with hepatitis B each year and an average of 250 die of fulminant disease. Between 6 and 10% of persons with HBV infection become carriers. The United States currently contains an estimated pool of 400,000 to 800,000 infectious carriers (15).

CLINICAL FINDINGS AND DIAGNOSIS

Viral Hepatitis

The majority of individuals exposed to viral hepatitis do not develop clinically overt disease or have changes in their liver structure or function. Others may have subclinical disease in the form of minor liver changes without jaundice (anicteric hepatitis).

In most patients with hepatitis A the onset of jaundice is preceded by nonspecific constitutional and gastrointestinal symptoms. From 2 to 14 days before the appearance of jaundice, the patient abruptly develops anorexia and fatigue, and often has nausea, fever, chills and occasionally arthralgias. Right upper quadrant or epigastric discomfort described as either a sense of fullness or pain is common. In contrast, hepatitis B usually begins insidiously with fever and flu-like symptoms being uncommon. Often the first evidence of hepatic involvement in hepatitis B is the appearance of jaundice.

One to 4 days before the onset of jaundice the urine darkens because of bilirubinemia and the stool color lightens. Transient pruritus may occur at this stage. Once jaundice appears, the clinical features of hepatitis A and B are identical. The prodromal gastrointestinal symptoms usually decrease in severity within a few days and fever rapidly subsides. The jaundice usually reaches a maximum between the first and second weeks and decreases steadily thereafter. In typical cases the duration of jaundice is variable but lasts less than 6 to 8 weeks. During the icteric phase the liver is often enlarged and tender to palpation. The liver may begin to decrease in size and tenderness in 1 to 2 weeks after the onset of jaundice and returns to normal size over several weeks. When necessary, definitive diagnosis is made by liver biopsy. It should be noted that in both forms the infective virus can be transmitted weeks before symptoms appear. There is no correlation between the histologic changes in the liver and the severity of jaundice.

Serum glutamic oxaloacetic transaminase (SGOT) and serum glutamic pyruvic transaminase (SGPT) levels may be elevated 7 to 14 days prior to the onset of jaundice reflecting hepatic cell necrosis and altered cell permeability within the liver, allowing these enzymes to leak into the blood. Serum alkaline phosphatase levels are generally normal or only slightly elevated unless cholestasis is also present (5% of cases). Protein (albumin) remains near normal or may decrease slightly if production is impaired. Globulin levels are commonly elevated and the bilirubin levels may reach 5 to 20 mg/dl. The prothrombin time may be prolonged due to inability to produce the vitamin K dependent factors II, VII, IX, and X.

Drug-induced Hepatitis

Drug-induced hepatitis may be indistinguishable from viral hepatitis. The diagnosis of drug-induced liver disease is usually made in the absence of known exposure to viral hepatitis and with documented exposure to a known hepatotoxic drug. A well-performed drug history by the pharmacist or careful scrutiny of a patient's profile may aid in diagnosing drug-induced hepatic reactions. Often drugs may induce slight, transient rises in the SGOT. These minor changes do not warrant stopping the drug if the patient is asymptomatic and not jaundiced. Drug-induced cholestatic changes usually lead to increased serum bilirubin levels as well as an increased serum alkaline phosphatase level since intrahepatic plugging prevents normal exocrine excretion of alkaline phosphatase. If alkaline phosphatase is not elevated, drug-induced cholestasis can generally be ruled out. Drug-induced hypersensitivity reactions are frequently accompanied by fever, rash, arthralgias and eosinophilia, whereas these symptoms are absent in direct hepatotoxic reactions.

COMPLICATIONS

Immediately following the icteric phase of acute viral hepatitis, the patient usually feels well, but recovery is seldom complete at this stage. Fatigue, mild liver enlargement and tenderness may still be evident. The duration of the posticteric phase varies from 2 to 6 weeks, but may be longer in some instances. Full clinical or biochemical recovery can be expected in 3 or 4 months in most cases. The mortality rate is quite low, 0.1 to 0.4% for hepatitis A and 10 to 12% for hepatitis B (2).

Rarely, the disease may run a prolonged course for several months or years. Two types of prolonged courses are recognized: chronic *persistent* hepatitis which is basically a delayed convalescence with eventual full recovery and chronic *active* hepatitis (CAH) which continues to produce active inflammatory disease and carries a poor prognosis. Table 16.4 contrasts the two types of chronic hepatitis. Some patients with CAH may have low grade symptoms for years and then get better; others progress into more serious stages including postnecrotic cirrhosis followed by death. CAH following hepatitis B infection with persistence of HB_sAg carries a poor prognosis. Another form of CAH is found predominantly in women who have positive serologic markers such as antinuclear antibodies (ANA). This latter group may represent an autoimmune form of hepatitis unrelated to viral infections. These people respond well to corticosteroids.

Chronic carriers of HB_sAg are a major source of infection for others and are also at risk for

Table 16.4.
Differentiation of Chronic Hepatitis States

Characteristic	Chronic Active Hepatitis	Chronic Persistent Hepatitis[a]
Onset like acute viral hepatitis	30%	70%
Recurrent acute episodes	Common	Infrequent, mild
Extrahepatic involvement (e.g. arthralgias, pleuritis, colitis)	Common	Rare
Prognosis	Poor	Good
Liver histology	Often necrosis with fibrosis, lobular changes and progression to cirrhosis	Preserved
Presence of HB_sAg	Present	Absent

[a] Chronic persistent is synonymous with "delayed convalescence." It occurs in 5 to 10% of cases of acute hepatitis and may be manifest as mild enzyme elevations without symptoms.

development of cirrhosis or primary hepatobiliary carcinoma. It is estimated that 4,000 deaths occur yearly in the United States due to cirrhosis secondary to hepatitis B infection and up to 800 deaths annually may be associated with hepatocellular carcinoma (15).

Approximately 5% of patients with acute hepatitis have an exacerbation within the first 6 months. The symptoms and course are identical with the first but may be milder. The relapse usually does not alter prognosis for the patient or increase residual liver damage unless it progresses into subacute (submassive) or massive hepatitis. The prodromal stage of submassive hepatic necrosis is similar to normal acute hepatitis, but the preicteric phase is usually longer than two weeks. Once jaundice is present the course of the illness is clearly different from that of typical acute viral hepatitis. The patient continues to feel ill and weakness and vomiting may persist. Serum bilirubin may still be increasing after 2 weeks and usually plateaus at higher than 20 mg/dl. Transaminase levels also remain elevated for several weeks. A liver biopsy is essential for diagnosis. Submassive hepatitis may progress to cirrhosis, portal hypertension and death after several months or years.

In massive hepatic necrosis one sees a sudden shrinkage of the liver over a period of several hours or days. The patient develops hepatic coma and fatality is 60 to 90%. The interval between the onset of illness and death is usually less than 2 weeks. Figure 16.1 summarizes the clinical course of the various stages of viral hepatitis.

TREATMENT

Viral Hepatitis

In the treatment of acute viral hepatitis drugs are of little value. Currently available antiviral drugs and antibiotics are ineffective. As a general rule most drugs, especially those that are metabolized in the liver, should be avoided during hepatic diseases to circumvent potential toxicity. In contrast to drug dosing in kidney failure, there is poor correlation between the magnitude of liver function test abnormalities and the rate of metabolism of drugs (16). Fortunately the liver has a large residual capacity that allows nearly normal metabolic processes to occur except under extraordinary conditions. For example, two drugs that are extensively metabolized, warfarin (17) and phenytoin (18), have been shown to have no change in their elimination rates in people with acute hepatitis.

Historically, strict bed rest for several weeks or months was advocated, but now people are encouraged to maintain a certain minimal amount of exercise. They should be cautioned not to overwork, but to ambulate as tolerated. During the acute stages of the disease, patients are very often fatigued and cannot tolerate more than a few hours out of bed. Adequate nutrition is advocated and if the patient is too sick to eat, parenteral feedings should be instituted. If the patient has contracted hepatitis due to poor living conditions, these conditions should be ameliorated and the patient encouraged to practice good hygiene thus protecting himself and other people with whom he has contact.

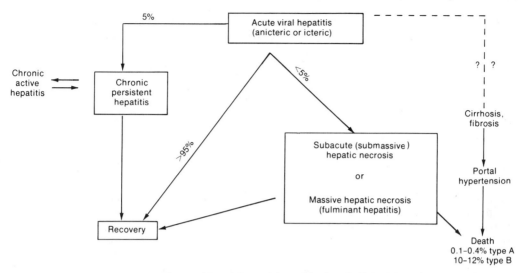

Figure 16.1. Complications of hepatitis. (Adapted from *Harrison's Principles of Internal Medicine*, ed. 6, New York: McGraw-Hill Book Co., 1970.)

Often the patient will complain of intense itching due to deposition of bile acids in the skin associated with biliary stasis. Cholestyramine (Questran) and colestipol (Colestid), both anion exchange resins, are occasionally given to relieve these symptoms. By forming an insoluble, nonabsorbable complex with bile acids, these drugs markedly increase the fecal excretion of the bile acids. However, if the biliary obstruction is severe, binding agents are of little value. It may take several days to get a response and it is difficult to separate drug effect from natural decreases in the disease process. The usual dose of cholestyramine is 4 g given 3 to 4 times daily for at least 2 weeks. An equivalent dose of colestipol is 5 g. Being resinous powders, these drugs are unpleasant to take; however, the flavor and texture are masked when suspended in a thick juice such as orange or apricot juice. Hot liquids and pureed fruits (such as applesauce) should not be used to mix these products due to lumping and dehydration, respectively. Carbonated beverages are difficult to use because of excessive foaming. Although Questran has a mild orange flavor that masks the normal fishy odor of the drug, colestipol is preferred by many patients. Both drugs are primarily indicated for treatment of hypercholesterolemia. Their main side effects are constipation and GI distress. This may be relieved by taking the drug with meals and using stool softeners. Absorption of certain fat soluble substances, e.g., vitamins A, D, E or K may be impaired by binding resins. Of more importance to the pharmacist is the fact that cholestyramine and colestipol will bind weakly acidic drugs such as thiazides, phenobarbital, phenylbutazone, tetracyclines and warfarin. The pharmacist should always recommend that all other drugs be spaced as far apart from cholestyramine and colestipol as possible.

Antihistamines such as diphenhydramine or hydroxyzine may have some antipruritic effect, but may cause excessive drowsiness due to slowed metabolism during the acute stage of liver disease. Likewise, antiemetics, especially phenothiazines, should be avoided due to decreased metabolism and a risk of hepatotoxicity due to cholestasis. Vitamin K as 10 mg of phytonadione or menadione may be given if the person has an elevated prothrombin time or excessive bleeding.

If the patient develops signs of encephalopathy or a liver flap, protein should be limited to 20 g per day and neomycin started at 2 to 4 g orally 3 to 4 times daily. By sterilizing the gut with neomycin and limiting protein intake, there is a reduction of bacterial breakdown of protein to ammonia products. Alternatively the person can be given lactulose, a nonabsorbable sugar solution that decreases lower bowel pH and causes ion trapping of ammonia. Often there is a dramatic recovery in the patient's mentation with the institution of either neomycin or lactulose therapy. Fortunately, hepatic failure due to hepatitis is rare. The treatment of hepatic encephalopathy is discussed more fully in the chapter on the treatment of cirrhosis.

CORTICOSTEROIDS

The area of greatest controversy in the treatment of hepatitis is with regard to the role of corticosteroids. While prednisone or prednisolone in doses of 40 to 60 mg daily may rapidly produce a feeling of well being in the patient and cause an increase in appetite, there is no proven decrease in morbidity or mortality in acute hepatitis. There may be a rapid initial fall in serum bilirubin during the first 3 days of steroid therapy, but these effects are only transient so that by the end of 2 weeks the bilirubin levels are not significantly different in patients treated with steroids compared to those not receiving therapy (19). The early reduction in bilirubin is not due to stimulation of bile secretion into the intestine, increased renal clearance of bilirubin or decreased bilirubin synthase. It is presumed that there is an enhancement of bilirubin excretion via alternate metabolic pathways. Since acute viral hepatitis is usually a benign, self-limiting disease, it can be concluded that the use of steroids is not warranted (20–22). In fact patients given steroids are at risk for developing unwanted complications such as GI ulceration, sodium retention, hypokalemia, psychotic reactions, hyperglycemia and an increased risk of infection. Rapid discontinuation of steroids may actually be associated with an increased risk of relapse of the hepatitis.

In contrast to acute hepatitis, there may be a place in therapy for corticosteroids in selected patients with chronic active hepatitis or life-threatening submassive or massive necrotic hepatitis. A number of investigators have shown that approximately 50 to 60% of patients with chronic active hepatitis will achieve remission of their symptoms, resolution of biochemical abnormalities, and histological improvement while receiving steroids (23–27). For some, the histology of the liver may convert from that of chronic active hepatitis to a picture more compatible with chronic persistent hepatitis. Once patients are begun on steroids they may be committed to long term therapy and the improvement may not be permanent. Attempts to discontinue steroid treatment may be successful in about one half of the persons who initially responded, but the other half will have a relapse within 6 months necessitating reinstitution of therapy. Only about 17% of all patients with chronic active hepatitis who respond initially to steroids will be able to achieve a permanent remission (24). Fortunately, most of those who relapse when steroids are stopped will again achieve a remission then steroids are reinstituted. At this time it is unresolved as to whether it is better to give long term steroid therapy without interruption or to use intermittent therapy for treatment of disease flares when needed.

There are no reliable predictors as to who will respond best to steroids, but those who develop cirrhosis while on steroids have a greater risk of relapse when the drugs are stopped (24). One study has shown that steroid therapy in patients who have chronic active hepatitis associated with a positive hepatitis B surface antigen may help to lower serum bilirubin levels, but there is an increased frequency of biochemical relapse, an increased frequency of complications and a higher death rate (28). Conversely, in populations of women with negative HB$_s$Ag, but with high titers of abnormal serologic markers, such as antinuclear antibodies, there is a much better prognosis with steroid treatment (23, 25). It is speculated that this latter group of patients has an immunologic basis for their chronic liver disease as opposed to a viral origin. They also respond well to other immunosuppressant drugs such as azathioprine. Since it is possible that corticosteroids may potentiate hepatitis B viral replication, it is now recommended that steroids not be given in cases where the HB$_s$Ag is positive.

Controversy also surrounds the issue of which corticosteroid is the most effective and what doses should be given. It is claimed by some that prednisolone is preferred over prednisone since prednisone must be converted to prednisolone in the body before it is active (21, 29). This conversion to the active moiety is dependent upon a functional liver metabolizing system. However, Uribe and others have found prednisone to be essentially 100% absorbed in patients with chronic active liver disease and the conversion to prednisolone was equivalent to that in healthy volunteers (30–32). In acute flairs, the prednisone or prednisolone dosage may be anywhere from 40 to 80 mg per day for several days followed by a slow taper to the lowest possible dose that maintains a remission. Decreasing the dose below 10 to 20 mg per day is often followed by an acute flair of the disease.

In a similar manner, high doses of corticosteroids have been tried in patients with alcoholic hepatitis (6, 33–35). In most instances there is no objective difference in the steroid treated group versus the nonsteroid treated group (34, 35). Only in those patients judged to have severe illness (e.g. markedly elevated bilirubin, prolonged prothrombin time, and presence of hepatic encephalopathy) do steroids have some possible benefit in improving caloric intake and decreasing short range mortality (6, 33). However, prednisolone does not affect the rate of histologic improvement or prevent cirrhosis.

Drug-induced Hepatitis

Acetaminophen is the only hepatotoxic drug for which a specific antidote is available (36). Since acetaminophen is rapidly absorbed, activated charcoal, forced emesis or gastric lavage are only of value if given within one to two hours of ingestion. Antidotes are based upon supplying exogenous sources of sulfhydryl groups to replace depleted body stores of glutathione. Cysteamine, cysteine and methionine have been utilized with equivocal results (36). Acetylcysteine (Mucomyst) is currently under investigation and appears to be effective if administered within 24 hours of ingestion (37). Available as 10 and 20% solutions for inhalation therapy, acetylcysteine should be diluted with water or juice to achieve a 5% solution. A loading dose of 140 mg/kg should be given followed by a maintenance dose of 70 mg/kg every 4 to 8 hours for a total of 3 days. The only reported toxicity of the antidote to date is nausea and vomiting.

PROPHYLAXIS AND PREVENTION

Attempts to prevent hepatitis viral infections center around use of γ-globulin and recently developed hepatitis B vaccine. Before discussing these modes of therapy, several principles need to be reviewed (38). Hepatitis B virus *infection* can be defined by the development of HB_sAg, while hepatitis B *disease* can be defined as an infection accompanied by clinical symptoms and biochemical abnormalities consistent with hepatitis. There are three mechanisms by which immune globulin or vaccines might be effective in preventing viral hepatitis: passive immunization, active immunization and passive-active immunization. In passive immunization, exogenously administered antibody neutralizes the virus thus preventing both infection and disease. In active immunization, noninfectious or inactive viral antigen is administered which induces production of antibody in the recipient thus preventing both infection and disease. In passive-active immunity, antibody is administered in a manner similar to passive immunity, but the antibody does not actually prevent the infection, it only acts to make the disease milder or subclinical. Active immunity is more likely to be conferred if the antibody is given before actual exposure to the virus or within a very short period of time after virus exposure. On the other hand, one might expect development of passive-active immunity if the antibody is given several days or weeks after viral exposure.

Regular commercially available γ-globulin (immune globulin, IG), available in 2- and 10-ml vials, contains 150 to 180 mg of protein per ml, 90% of which must be γ-globulin. The majority of γ-globulin is present as IgG, but contains some IgA and IgM. The antibodies present in IG are very effective in protecting against type A hepatitis by means of passive-active immunity. In other words the globulin prevents symptomatic type A hepatitis, although it is highly likely that the person who was immunized will have an asymptomatic or subclinical infection.

Unless very large doses are given, most commercially available lots of IG are ineffective in preventing or modifying hepatitis B, presumably due to minimal concentration of hepatitis B antibody in the general population. Hyperimmune globlin or hepatitis B immune globulin (H-BIG) is prepared from the serum of persons known to have anti-HB_s antibodies, and thus contains extremely high titers against hepatitis B surface antigen. Unfortunately, H-BIG is extremely expensive. Whether H-BIG induces passive or passive-active immunity is being debated (38–40). When given as preexposure prophylaxis, passive immunity may be imparted (40). However, the drug is usually given to persons known to have had accidental exposure to hepatitis B virus and in these cases one would expect passive-active immunity. In a large scale study conducted in the Veterans Administration comparing standard immune globulin to H-BIG after accidental needle-stick exposure, there was an equal frequency of infection (12%) in both groups. However, clinically active disease occurred in only 2% of the H-BIG treated individuals compared to 8% of persons in the IG group (38).

The Center for Disease Control recommends the following guidelines for use of IG and H-BIG (41). A 0.02 ml/kg IM injection of IG should be given within 2 weeks of exposure to hepatitis A. Such prophylaxis is not recommended for random contacts such as hospital personnel, office workers or school children in an area where a case is discovered. Only those with close personal contact such as household or sexual contacts, those handling fecal soiled clothing (e.g. diapers) or residents in custodial care institutions need be given treatment. Preexposure prophylaxis is recommended for travelers to high risk areas. In this case, a single 0.02 ml/kg dose of IG is given prior to travel with follow-up injection every 3 months while remaining in the endemic area.

For hepatitis B prophylaxis, IG or H-BIG can be given. For postexposure prophylaxis, the type of globulin selected depends upon the nature of the exposure and the knowledge of the HB_sAg status of the source. H-BIG is preferred when there is known percutaneous or mucous membrane exposure to blood containing HB_sAg. H-BIG 0.06 ml per kg should be given within 24 hours of exposure with a second dose 1 month later. If H-BIG is not available, IG should be used at the same dose and schedule. Prompt therapy is important since the value of treatment beyond 7 days of exposure is unproven. For a source whose HB_sAg status is unknown, where there is a high risk situation and where HB_sAg results can be known within 7 days, IG should be given immediately (0.06 ml per kg) and if results of the tests of HB_sAg are positive H-BIG (0.06 ml per kg) should be given at the time the results become available and one month later. If the HB_sAg cannot be known within 7 days, the decision for IG or H-BIG must be made on clinical and epidemiologic grounds. For a low risk source, such as an average hospital patient, prophylaxis is optional and HB_sAg testing is not recommended. IG, if used, should be given at 0.06 ml per kg within 24 hours. For those where both the source and HB_sAg status are unknown, prophylaxis is optional, with IG at 0.06 ml per kg given promptly within 24 hours and no other action necessary. For infants born to HB_sAg positive mothers, H-BIG is indicated, with a total dose of 0.5 ml as soon after birth as possible.

Even when H-BIG is used, the duration of immunity imparted is short and persons with high risk jobs or living in endemic areas may require multiple injections. A newly developed hepatitis B vaccine appears to impart a long lasting active immunity (42, 43). The vaccine is prepared by obtaining and purifying HB_sAg particles from the serum of asymptomatic long-term carries. To eliminate the possibility of residual live hepatitis B virus, the vaccine is inactiviated with formalin (44). Unfortunately, production of the vaccine is slow and expensive since each batch must be tested for 6 months for safety and immunogenicity in chimpanzees. Experience with the vaccine is limited, but early data show that two 20- to 40-μg injections separated by 1 month and followed by a 20–40-μg booster at 6 months leads to rapid development of anti-HB_s antibodies, usually without clinical illness or presence of HB_sAg. The effects are clearly seen within 10 weeks of the first injection and last at least 8 to 18 months. No long-term follow-up studies have been done at the time of this writing, but in some instances anti-HB_s titers have been shown to fall after 9 months. In cases where infection did occur after vaccination, it was usually within 4 to 5 months of the initial injection, suggesting that the person had already been exposed to the virus before immunization.

The high cost of the vaccine (approximately $100 per treatment course) plus initial limited supply raises ethical questions as to who should receive the drug and who should pay for it. On one hand, there is a need to protect health care workers such as emergency room, intensive care unit and dialysis unit physicians and nurses as well as laboratory personnel. On the other hand, high risk patients such as refugees from endemic regions and their children, persons receiving multiple blood transfusions or chronic hemodialysis, illicit IV drug users, homosexually active males and prostitutes are at high risk and also can benefit from immunization. Increased availability of the vaccine may help to answer these questions.

CONCLUSION

Acute viral hepatitis is not usually a life-threatening disease, with the mortality rate from hepatitis B being higher than that for hepatitis A. The rare case that progresses into chronic active hepatitis or into submassive or massive hepatic necrosis has a much poorer prognosis. The pharmacist can have input into the therapy of hepatitis by discouraging the use of drugs rather than to promote their use, especially making sure that corticosteroids are used appropriately. Prevention is the key to success by encouraging good hygiene and avoidance of high risk factors including illicit drugs. Finally, purification of hepatitis B vaccine may lead to a marked decrease in the incidence of hepatitis in the future.

References

1. Czaja A: Serologic markers of hepatitis A and B in acute and chronic liver disease. *Mayo Clin Proc* 54:721, 1979.
2. Anon: Hepatitis knowledge base. *Ann Intern Med* 93:191, 1980.
3. Zimmerman H: Drug induced liver disease. *Drugs* 16:25, 1978.
4. Maddrey W: Drug related acute and chronic hepatitis. *Clin Gastroenterol* 9:213, 1980.
5. Rosenoer V, Tormay A: Drugs and the liver. *Med Clin North Am* 63:405, 1979.
6. Helman R, Temko M, Nye S, et al: Alcoholic hepatitis natural history and evaluation of prednisolone therapy. *Ann Intern Med* 74:311–321, 1971.
7. Black M: Acetaminophen hepatotoxicity. *Gastroenterology* 78:382, 1980.
8. Johnson G, Tolman K: Chronic liver disease and acetaminophen. *Ann Intern Med* 87:302–304, 1977.
9. Barker J, Carle D, Anuras S: Chronic excessive acetaminophen use and liver damage. *Ann Intern Med* 87:299–301, 1977.
10. Prescott LR: Plasma paracetamol half-life and hepatic necrosis with paracetamol overdosage. *Lancet* 1:519–522, 1971.
11. Mitchell J, Zimmerman H, Ishak K, et al: Isoniazid liver injury: clinical spectrum, pathology and probable pathogenesis. *Ann Intern Med* 84:181–192, 1976.
12. Singapore Tuberculosis Service: Controlled trial of intermittent regimens of rifampin plus isoniazid for pulmonary tuberculosis in Singapore. *Am Rev Respir Dis* 116:807–827, 1977.
13. Berthelot P: Mechanisms and prediction of drug induced liver disease. *Gut* 14:332, 1973.
14. *Morbidity and Mortality Weekly Report:* Center for Disease Control, U.S. Department of Human and Health Services, Public Health Service, 31:702, 1983.
15. *Morbidity and Mortality Weekly Report:* Center for Disease Control. U.S. Department of Human and Health Services, Public Health Service, 31:317–322, 1982.
16. Bond W: Bond relevence of the effect of hepatic disease on drug disposition. *Am J Hosp Pharm* 35:400, April 1978.
17. Williams R, Schary W, Blaschke T, et al: Influence of acute viral hepatitis on disposition and pharmacologic effect of warfarin. *Clin Pharmacol Ther* 20:90–97, 1976.
18. Blaschke T, Jeffin P, Melmon K, et al: Influence of viral hepatitis on phenytoin kinetics and protein binding. *Clin Pharmacol Ther* 17:685–691, 1975.
19. Schiff L: The use of steroids in liver disease. *Medicine* 45:565–569, 1966.
20. Williams R, Billings B: Action of steroid therapy in jaundice. *Lancet* 2:392–396, 1961.
21. Tanner A, Powell L: Corticosteroids in liver disease: possible mechanism of action, pharmacology and rational use. *Gut* 20:1109, 1979.
22. Gregory P, Knauer C, Kempson R, et al: Steroid therapy in severe viral hepatitis. *N Engl J Med* 294:681, 1976.
23. Wright E, Seeff L, Berk P, et al: Treatment of chronic active hepatitis: an analysis of three controlled trials. *Gastroenterology* 73:1427, 1977.
24. Czaja A, Ammon H, Summerskill W: Clinical features and prognosis of severe chronic active liver disease (CALD) after corticosteroid induced remission. *Gastroenterology* 78:518, 1980.
25. Czaja A, Ludwig J, Baggenstoss A, et al: Corticosteroid treated chronic active hepatitis in remission. *N Engl J Med* 304:5, 1981.
26. Soloway R, Summerskill W, Baggenstoss A, et al: Clinical, biochemical and histological remission of severe chronic active liver disease: a controlled study of treatments and early prognosis. *Gastroenterology* 63:820, 1972.
27. Cook G, Mulligan R, Sherlock S: Controlled prospective trial of corticosteroid therapy in active chronic hepatitis. *Q J Med* 40:159, 1971.
28. Lam C, Lai C, Ng R, et al: Deleterious effects of prednisolone in HB_sAg positive chronic active hepatitis. *N Engl J Med* 340:380–386, 1981.
29. Schalm S, Summerskill W, Go V: Prednisone for chronic active liver disease: pharmacokinetics, including conversion to prednisolone. *Gastroenterology* 72:910, 1977.
30. Uribe M, Schalm S, Summerskill W, et al: Oral prednisone for chronic active liver disease-dose responses and bioavailability. *Gut* 19:1131, 1978.
31. Uribe M, Go V: Corticosteroid pharmacokinetics in liver disease. *Clin Pharmacokinet* 4:233, 1979.
32. Pickup M: Clinical pharmacokinetics of prednisone and prednisolone. *Clin Pharmacokinet* 4:11, 1979.
33. Maddrey W, Boitnott J, Bedine M, et al: Corticosteroid therapy of alcoholic hepatitis. *Gastroenterology* 75:193, 1978.
34. Blitzer B, Mutchnick M, Joshi P, et al: Adrenocorticosteroid therapy in alcoholic hepatitis. *Dig Dis* 22:477, 1977.
35. Campra J, Hamlin E, Kirshbaum R: Prednisone therapy of acute alcoholic hepatitis. *Ann Intern Med* 79:623–631, 1973.
36. Krenzelok E, Best L, Manoguerra A: Acetaminophen toxicity. *Am J Hosp Pharm* 34:391–394, 1977.
37. Anon: Symptoms and treatment of overdosage of selected McNeil products, update. McNeil Laboratories Inc., Fort Washington, PA 19034, Nov. 1, 1976.
38. Hoofnagle J, Seeff L, Bales Z, et al: Passive-active immunity from hepatitis B immune globulin. *Ann Intern Med* 91:813, 1979.
39. Surgenor D, Chalmers T, Conrad M: Clinical trials of hepatitis B immune globulin: development of policies and materials for the 1972–1975 studies sponsored by the National Heart and

Lung Institute. *N Engl J Med* 293:1060–1062, 1975 (three other articles in the same issue).

40. Szumness W, Prince A, Goodman M: Hepatitis B immune serum globulin in prevention of non-parenterally transmitted hepatitis B. *N Engl J Med* 290:701–706, 1974.

41. Anon: Guidelines for hepatitis prophylaxis with gamma globulin. *MMWR* 30:423, 1981.

42. Szumness W, Stevens C, Harley E, et al: Hepatitis B vaccine. *N Eng J Med* 303:833, 1980.

43. Dienstag J: Toward the control of hepatitis B. *N Engl J Med* 303:874, 1980.

44. Francis D, Hadler S, Thompson S, et al: The prevention of hepatitis B with vaccine. *Ann Intern Med* 97:362–366, 1982.

CHAPTER 17

Cirrhosis

WAYNE A. KRADJAN, Pharm.D.

Cirrhosis may be defined as a diffuse increase in the fibrous connective tissue of the liver usually associated with necrosis and regeneration of parenchymal cells imparting a nodular or glandular texture to the liver. In its later stages cirrhosis leads to such deformity of the liver that it interferes with liver function and the circulation of blood and bile to and from the liver. While no specific therapy exists for cirrhosis except prevention of its etiologic factors (e.g., alcohol abstinence), the pharmacist will be involved with providing drugs to treat the complications of this disorder.

ETIOLOGY

Several major types of cirrhosis have been described, but cirrhosis associated with alcohol abuse or Laennec's cirrhosis is by far the most commonly encountered in the United States (1). Cirrhosis usually begins with severe fatty changes in the liver. In the early stages this fatty infiltration is unassociated with fibrosis and scarring, while the late stages are marked by a progressive loss of fat, an increase of fibrous tissue and a progressive shrinkage and nodularity of the liver.

Dietary derangements, especially severe protein deficiencies (e.g. kwashiorkor), may induce fatty changes in the liver with subsequent development of cirrhosis in a small number of individuals. Thus, it is often claimed that dietary indiscretion in alcoholics may be the underlying cause of their cirrhosis. In support of this concept is the observation that when a chronic alcoholic is hospitalized and placed on an adequate diet, excess fat can be mobilized and the liver structure and function may return to normal. This reversibility is less clear if fibrosis has already occurred. More recent evidence implicates alcohol as a direct hepatotoxin. One group of investigators using the baboon as a model were able to demonstrate development of cirrhosis in experimental animals maintained on a balanced diet but given large daily doses of alcohol (2).

Biliary cirrhosis refers to cirrhosis following chronic obstruction of bile flow (cholestasis). Primary biliary cirrhosis follows long-standing cholestasis generally of unknown etiology, but may have an underlying immunologic basis with elevated IgM antibodies and the presence of circulating complement fixing immune complexes. Secondary biliary cirrhosis may be caused by stones or a tumor obstructing bile flow leading to an inflammatory reaction and scarring. Less common causes of cirrhosis are the aftermath of rapidly progressive hepatitis, hemochromatosis, tertiary syphilis or hemorrhage within the liver (Table 17.1).

INCIDENCE

Cirrhosis, although a common disease throughout the world, varies in incidence not only from country to country, but from one hospital or section of a city to another. For example, it is much more common in a county hospital or veterans' hospital than in a private community hospital. It is difficult to cite an incidence of cirrhosis since patients often do not exhibit any signs or symptoms. Autopsies at various hospitals have shown an incidence ranging from 3 to 15%. In 1977, cirrhosis was the seventh most common cause of death and the third leading cause in the age group of 25 to 65-year-olds (1). It also appears that cirrhosis has increased in frequency over the past 40 years. Various explanations for this increase have been proposed, including (a) better medical care enabling patients to live through an initial liver disease, (b) increased incidence of alcoholism, and (c) a greater exposure to hepatotoxic drugs and chemicals which cause diffuse liver toxicity leading to cirrhosis. Table 17.1 lists the relative incidence of the various types of cirrhosis encountered. The largest percentage is Laennec's cirrhosis which occurs principally in patients between 40 and 60 years of age and is found most often in male patients. A history of chronic alcoholism can be obtained in 50 to 90% of these patients in the

Table 17.1.
Types of Cirrhosis: Incidence and Etiology

Type	Incidence (%)	Etiology
Alcohol associated (Laennec's)	60–70	Alcohol abuse and protein deficiency inducing fatty changes in liver
Biliary (primary and secondary)	10–15	Obstruction to bile flow, e.g., immune complexes, stones and carcinoma; often secondary to long standing bacterial infection
Postnecrotic	10–15	Scarring following massive hepatic necrosis such as that seen in chronic viral hepatitis or after exposure to hepatotoxic drugs (*Note*: some contend that viral hepatitis cannot progress into cirrhosis)
Pigment	5	Excessive deposits of hemosiderin in hemochromatosis
Syphilitic	1–2	Tertiary syphilis
Cardiac	2–3	Hemorrhage within the liver or increased hepatic venous pressure from right-sided heart failure
Other		For example, α-antitrypsin deficiency

United States. In Africa and Asia children are frequently affected due to protein-deficient diets.

CLINICAL FINDINGS AND DIAGNOSIS

Cirrhosis is insidious in its development and often produces no clinical manifestations. In fact, as many as 50% of all cases are discovered only at the time of postmortem examination. Many patients present themselves to their physician complaining of vague, nonspecific symptoms such as weight loss, loss of appetite, nausea, vomiting and ill defined digestive disturbances. Others enter the hospital acutely ill with the full syndrome of acute alcoholic hepatitis (a precursor to cirrhosis). These patients present with deep jaundice (bilirubin levels from 2 mg/dl to greater than 40 mg/dl), elevated SGOT and alkaline phosphatase, impaired coagulation (manifest as a prolonged prothrombin time due to impaired production of clotting factors), and right upper quadrant pain. Finally another group presents with the more dramatic secondary effects of cirrhosis including ascites (accumulation of large amounts of fluid in the abdominal cavity), massive gastrointestinal (GI) bleeding and rapid mental deterioration.

COMPLICATIONS

While cirrhosis, per se, is a relatively benign situation the complications are many and must be fully appreciated. The first concept to be understood is portal hypertension. It will be recalled that the portal vein drains the arterial and capillary system of the entire GI tract. This system is unique in that while it is a venous system, it has a second set of capillaries (or sinusoids) that ramify throughout the liver and then rejoin to empty into the hepatic vein and the inferior vena cava. The main function of the portal system is not to provide oxygenated blood to the liver (this is done by the hepatic artery), but rather to function as a detoxifying and metabolizing system for substances entering the GI tract. It should be remembered that the portal system is responsible for "first pass" metabolism of such drugs as propranolol. As scarring and nodularity increase in the liver during cirrhosis, the blood flow through the portal system becomes obstructed. As a result the blood pressure in the portal vein and its tributaries in the GI tract rises dramatically. Blood may also be shunted around the liver to empty directly into the inferior vena cava. Some of the problems arising secondary to increased portal pressure are ascites, hepatomegaly, spenomegaly, and GI bleeding.

Ascites

Ascites is one of the most striking features of cirrhosis. The amount of fluid in the abdomen can vary from a few liters to 20 or more liters leading to large protuberant abdomens and umbilical hernias. A combination of factors lead to the formation of ascitic fluid. These factors must be understood to appreciate therapeutic intervention. In simple terms ascites can be thought of as an imbalance between normal hydrostatic pressure in the portal system and the colloidal (osmotic) pressure produced by albumin. As portal hypertension increases, the high pressure in the vessels forces fluid and electrolytes into the surrounding tissues, especially the abdominal cavity. Decreased hepatic synthesis of proteins, especially albumin, leads to a low osmotic pressure in the vessels and thus less ability to hold fluid in the vascular space. In addition, the ascitic fluid is generally high in protein due to obstruction of venous and lymphatic flow in the liver itself, further adding an osmotic pull of fluid into the extravascular space. Finally, the lowered osmotic pressure of the blood stimulates the renin-angiotension system of the kidneys to produce a relative hyperaldosteronism. The elevated aldosterone levels lead to further accumulation of vascular volume via sodium retention in the distal tubule of the kidney.

Bleeding Disorders

GI hemorrhage occurs with cirrhosis in about one fourth to one third of patients, and in about one third of these cases the patient dies from the initial hemorrhage. Even nonfatal hemorrhages tend to be massive. Only occasionally is there an insidious leakage of blood, with anemia and occult blood in the stools. Bleeding is partially secondary to portal hypertension with the most common sites being in the esophagus (esophageal varices), upper intestinal tract and hemorrhoids. These problems may be compounded by an impaired clotting system due to deficiencies in vitamin K dependent clotting factors and by gastritis induced by excessive alcohol intake. Esophageal varices account for about 50% of the bleeding, while peptic ulcer accounts for another 25%.

Hematologic Disorders

Anemias are common in cirrhotics. Chronic alcoholics tend to malabsorb folic acid (leading to macrocytic anemias) as well as iron (leading to microcytic anemias). In addition their diets may be deficient in both iron and folate. Iron deficiency may be further aggravated by inflammatory block of iron uptake into the bone marrow induced by chronic alcoholism and by slow GI bleeding due to gastritis. Thrombocytopenia and leukopenia may occur due to folic acid deficiency and due to hypersplenism secondary to portal hypertension.

Endocrine Disorders

Endocrine disorders are seen in far advanced cirrhosis due to the inability of the liver to metabolize the steroid hormones of the adrenals and gonads. Commonly seen are gynecomastia, loss of body hair, impotence, spider angiomas and palmar erythema due to an increase in circulating estrogen levels.

Fluid and Electrolyte Balance

Patients often demonstrate hyponatremia from retention of free water induced by elevated antidiuretic hormone (ADH) levels. ADH is elevated due to decreased hepatic metabolism. In addition these patients are often hypokalemic secondary to their hyperaldosteronism which is further aggravated by excessive vomiting.

Hepatic Encephalopathy

The ultimate result of far advanced cirrhosis or of severe hepatitis is liver failure and hepatic coma (hepatic encephalopathy). This is characterized by increasing personality changes and mental confusion with a characteristic flapping tremor of the fingers and hands (liver flap or asterixis), eventually followed by a deepening coma and death.

The pathogenesis of these central nervous system derangements is not well understood, but is correlated by many researchers with an increased arterial and CNS ammonium level. Although a direct cause and effect relationship has not been shown to exist between encephalopathy and blood ammonium concentration, it has been shown that by decreasing factors that influence ammonium production, the patient's sensorium is often cleared. One of the most common sources of increased ammonium content of the blood is the action of bacteria in the small intestine and colon to produce ammonia from protein and urea breakdown. This ammonia is then absorbed into the bloodstream and converted to ammonium ion. Normally these factors rarely lead to any CNS abnormalities since the liver converts the ammonium into urea, but when the liver is malfunctioning or the blood is being shunted away from it as in far advanced cirrhosis, encephalopathy ensues. It is theorized that the cerebrotoxicity of ammonia is due to inhibition of oxidative metabolism by the citric acid cycle in the brain. α-Ketoglutarate combines with ammonia to produce high CNS levels of glutamine (a by-product of ammonium metabolism) while at the same time robbing the citric acid cycle of the α-ketoglutarate needed for production of "high energy" adenosine triphosphate (ATP). Cerebrospinal fluid (CSF) glutamine and ammonium levels are sometimes measured to confirm the presence of hepatic encephalopathy.

An alternative explanation for the pathogenesis of hepatic encephalopathy is associated with derangements in plasma and brain amino acid patterns (3, 4). Characteristically, there appears to be an elevation in methionine and aromatic amino acids (e.g., phenylalanine, tyrosine, tryptophan, histidine, glutamine and aspartate) and a deficiency in branched chain amino acids (e.g., valine, leucine and isoleucine). These derangements lead to an imbalance of brain neurotransmitters causing elevated levels of serotonin, octopamine and phenylethanolamine and a decrease in dopamine and possibly norepinephrine. Serotonin is an end product of tryptophan metabolism while phenylethanolamine and octopamine are by-products of phenylalanine and tyrosine metabolism.

The arterial concentration of ammonium and other amines may be accentuated by excessive dietary protein consumption, GI hemorrhage (source of protein), overdiuresis leading to dehydration and other conditions that lead to severe electrolyte imbalances. Hepatic encephalopathy may also be induced by increased arterial pH (alkalosis) and abnormalities in various biochemical pathways.

Hepatorenal Syndrome

Significant azotemia (elevated BUN) sometimes occurs in patients who have liver or biliary tract disease. The concurrent impairment of renal function along with hepatic failure is designated as the hepatorenal syndrome. The exact cause for the progression to renal failure, if a cause and effect relationship exists, is unknown. Of interest is the fact that often no structural abnormalities can be found in the kidneys at postmortem examination and some have performed well when used as a donor for a renal transplant. It could may be that there is simply a functional change in the kidney due to fluid and electrolyte disturbances, shock or unmetabolized toxic substances. The use of neomycin to treat encephalopathy has also been implicated as a cause of the change in renal status.

TREATMENT

As with hepatitis, the management of cirrhosis is largely symptomatic (Table 17.2). In Laennec's cirrhosis the primary treatment is to encourage the patient to abstain from alcohol. Fluid and electrolyte balance should be maintained either by parenteral administration or a good diet. If the patient is vomiting, antiemetics such as prochlorperazine may be used. However, one should remember that the phenothiazine type antiemetics have been known to cause obstructive jaundice. For abdominal pain, analgesics may be administered, bearing in mind that aspirin-containing products may worsen gastritis or GI bleeding. Narcotics may lead to profound CNS and respiratory depression if the patient's liver status is significantly compromised or if he is already obtunded. Sedatives and hypnotics should be avoided if there is any danger of the patient developing hepatic coma. If there are no signs of impending hepatic coma the patient should be maintained on a 2000- to 3000-calorie diet with 1 g of protein per kg of body weight. If encephalopathy is present, dietary supplements rich in branched chain amino acids and low in aromatic amino acids (e.g., Hepatic Aid) may be used to prevent negative nitrogen balance.

Vitamin replacement is essential in a majority of cirrhotic patients, especially those with a recent alcoholic history. Replacement of thiamine at 50 to 100 mg per day along with a good diet often brings about remarkable increases in mentation in chronic alcoholics as well as a decrease in peripheral neuritis and improvement in gait disorders. Maintenance of thiamine therapy beyond 1 or 2 weeks is questionable since it is a water-soluble vitamin whose stores are rapidly replaced. Up to 1 g per day may occasionally be required if the patient displays severe nystagmus, Wernicke's encephalopathy or oculogyric crisis. Chronic alcoholics often malabsorb folate and their bone marrow does not adequately respond to the folate they do absorb, leading to the development of a megaloblastic anemia. Thus 1 mg

Table 17.2.
Drugs Used in Cirrhotic Patients

1. *Thiamine*
   a. Reason: reverse mental confusion secondary to thiamine deficiency (Wernicke's syndrome) and decrease peripheral neuropathies
   b. Dose: 100–200 mg per day. Occasionally higher dosage
   c. Monitoring parameters:
      (1) Mental status
      (2) Decrease in nystagmus, peripheral neuropathies
      (3) Greater than 10 days of therapy is unwarranted
2. *Vitamin K (phytonadione) (Aqua Mephyton preferred)*
   a. Reason: prevent bleeding secondary to decreased production of factors II, VII, IX, and X (vitamin K dependent factors)
   b. Dose: 10–15 mg per day, not to exceed 3 doses
   c. Monitoring parameters:
      (1) Hypersensitivity—fever, chills, anaphylaxis, flushing, sweating
      (2) Prothrombin time
3. *Spironolactone*
   a. Reason: diuresis in ascites. Specific for antagonism of preexisting hyperaldosteronism
   b. Dose: 200–400 mg per day, occasionally higher. May be given as a single daily dose
   c. Monitoring parameters:
      (1) Weight (avoid more than 1-kg weight loss per day)
      (2) Mental status
      (3) Serum K^+
      (4) Urine Na^+ and K^+ (Na^+ should exceed K^+ at therapeutic doses)
      (5) Abdominal girth
      (6) BUN (increases in dehydration)
      (7) Gynecomastia—prolonged use
      (8) Blood pressure
4. *Vasopressin*
   a. Reason: vasoconstrictor for esophageal bleeding
   b. Dose: 20 units IV over 20 min *or* infusion at 0.2 unit per min
   c. Monitoring parameters:
      (1) Rate of GI bleeding
      (2) Signs of ischemia—chest pain, elevated blood pressure, bradycardia
      (3) GI cramping
      (4) Serum Na^+
5. *Propranolol*
   a. Reason: prevent GI bleeding
   b. Dose: 40–320 mg/day
   c. Monitoring parameters:
      (1) Signs of GI bleeding
      (2) Mental changes
      (3) Signs of congestive heart failure, bradycardia
      (4) Signs of bronchospasm
      (5) Renal function
6. *Neomycin*
   a. Reason: hepatic encephalopathy. Sterilizes gut to prevent bacterial breakdown of protein and thus decreases serum NH_3 level
   b. Dose: 2–6 g per day, orally or rectally
   c. Monitoring parameters:
      (1) Mental status, liver flap
      (2) Diarrhea, bacterial overgrowth
      (3) Renal function
      (4) Signs of ototoxicity
7. *Lactulose*
   a. Reason: hepatic encephalopathy. Converted to lactic acid to lower bowel pH and prevent absorption of NH_3
   b. Dose: 30–45 ml q.i.d. or to 3–4 soft stools per day

Table 17.2.—Continued

    c. Monitoring parameters:
      (1) Mental status, liver flap
      (2) Diarrhea
8. *Magnesium citrate*
    a. Reason: cleanse bowel of bacteria and protein (including blood)
    b. Dose: 8 oz
    c. Monitoring parameters:
      (1) Mental status, liver flap
      (2) Fluid and electrolyte balance
9. *Dopamine*
    a. Reason: hepatic encephalopathy and hepatorenal syndrome
    b. Dose: 1–4 μg/kg/min
    c. Monitoring parameters:
      (1) Mental status, liver flap
      (2) Urine output
      (3) Blood pressure
10. *L-Dopa*
    a. Reason: hepatic encephalopathy. Restores normal neurotransmitter balance
    b. Dose: 500 mg t.i.d. to q.i.d.
    c. Monitoring parameters:
      (1) Mental status, liver flap
      (2) Nausea and vomiting
      (3) Pulse—tachycardia
      (4) Blood pressure—orthostatic drop

of folic acid is often administered daily. At the same time iron therapy with ferrous sulfate or gluconate is required if the patient is actively bleeding or if his hematocrit or hemoglobin counts are depressed and the bone marrow shows decreased iron stores.

Vitamin K, 10 mg daily for 3 or more days, IV, IM or orally, is given if the prothrombin time is elevated. If the prothrombin time is not reversed after 3 to 5 doses, further doses should be avoided as an occasional patient will demonstrate a paradoxical lengthening of the prothrombin time from excessive vitamin K. This paradoxical effect is theorized to be a result of "consumptive processes" induced by overstimulation of production of clotting factors leading to an eventual depletion of their body stores. Vitamin K_1, or phytonadione (Aquamephyton), gives a more rapid response when given parenterally than vitamin K_3 (menadione) or vitamin K_4 (menadiol) (5). When giving vitamin K parenterally, the subcutaneous or IM route is preferred but it may also be given by very slow IV infusion in 50 ml of 5% dextrose in water (D_5W) over 15 to 20 min. IM injections may be contraindicated if the patient has a prolonged prothrombin time or thrombocytopenia. Since the parenteral preparations are colloidal suspensions there is a small risk of development of fever, chills, and even anaphylactic reactions with rapid IV injection. If the patient is malabsorbing fats, menadiol is the vitamin K of choice for oral administration since it is water-soluble and absorbed independent of bile acids.

Ascites

Ascites is more than just a cosmetic problem being a good culture medium for bacterial growth (especially tuberculosis) and being quite painful as the abdomen becomes distended and tense. Respiratory distress may be induced by compression of the diaphragm and gastroesophageal reflux is common. Unfortunately, the reversal of ascites is a very time consuming process requiring weeks and even months of conservative management.

Paracentesis (aspiration with a needle), except for diagnostic purposes, is to be discouraged since there is a risk of abdominal perforation and introduction of infection. Moreover, 15 to 100% (mean 58%) of the fluid reaccumulates over the next 24 to 48 hours leading to transient hypovolemia and the possibility of shock or acute renal failure (6).

Conservative management consists of bed rest, salt restriction (500 mg to 2 g/day) and, in some cases, fluid restriction. Approximately 5% of patients will have spontaneous diuresis with bed rest alone and another 10 to 25% will respond to salt restriction (7). Fluid restriction is only warranted in cases of hyponatremia (water overload) since excessive fluid restriction may lead to azotemia secondary to decreased renal blood flow.

While the cornerstone of drug therapy of ascites is diuresis, one important rule must be remembered: the diuresis must be slow. In patients treated with sodium restriction alone, no more than 300 ml of ascites can be resorbed per day and even with the use of diuretic agents the maximum rate of reabsorption is 930 ml per 24 hours (6). Furthermore, the diuretic response seems to be more pronounced in those patients with peripheral edema in addition to ascites. Any greater diuretic response than 1 liter per day (equivalent to 1-kg loss in body weight) is either from mobilization of peripheral edema or depletion of vascular volume. It is imperative, therefore, to monitor diuretic therapy by observing rate of weight loss (not to exceed 0.5 to 1 kg/day), urine output, blood pressure (avoiding postural hypotension secondary to volume depletion), changes in BUN (elevated secondary to prerenal azotemia in volume depletion) and changes in mental status (encephalopathy from volume depletion).

The first diuretic that is generally started is spironolactone since it is a slow-acting diuretic and is specific for antagonizing the effects of the hyperaldosteronism that exists in these patients. In contrast to the small doses of this drug used as an adjunct in hypertension, the dose in ascites is often begun at 100 mg per day with 400 mg per day being needed in 75% of patients (8). Even greater doses, up to 1 g per day, have been used, but this is quite expensive and other diuretics are usually added before doses of this magnitude are tried. Although spironolactone is generally given on a divided dose schedule, it is a long-acting drug and once daily dosing is effective for most patients if they can swallow the required number of tablets without gastric distress. A 3- to 5-day lag period exists for maximum response from spironolactone and thus frequent dosage adjustments should be avoided. Triamterene or amiloride may be slightly more rapid in onset, but they are not specific aldosterone inhibitors. Clinically, they are probably equal in effect to spironolactone, although no one has specifically studied the response of ascites to these drugs in comparison to spironolactone.

Beside the general monitoring parameters cited above for diuretic therapy, serum and urine electrolytes, especially potassium, must be monitored. Because of the relative hyperaldosteronism existing in these patients, it is not uncommon to see very small or nonexistent urinary sodium excretion and exceedingly large urinary potassium losses. One measure of having achieved the desired spironolactone dose is a reversal of the urine electrolyte picture to normal (i.e., sodium loss greater than potassium loss). For the same reasons, these patients often have low serum potassium concentrations. While the use of spironolactone with potassium supplements is nearly always contraindicated in treatment of other disease states due to a high risk of hyperkalemia (9), this combination may be of necessity early in the treatment of ascites, especially if the patient has also had GI losses of potassium secondary to vomiting or diarrhea. Serum potassium must be monitored daily to prevent either hypo- or hyperkalemia. Long-term use of spironolactone can lead to gynecomastia, a problem which is frequently present in cirrhosis independent of use of diuretics.

While gentle diuresis is of necessity, high spironolactone doses may fail to produce the desired effects in many patients. In this case the addition (not substitution) of more potent diuretics such as thiazides and loop diuretics may be warranted. The dose should be started low (50 mg per day of thiazide or 20 to 40 mg per day of furosemide) and gradually increased. Some patients are especially refractory requiring several hundred milligrams per day of furosemide to obtain the desired 1 kg per day weight loss.

Infusions of 25 to 50 g of human serum albumin are occasionally used to raise the colloid pressure of the serum in an attempt to draw the ascitic fluid back into the circulation. This has the disadvantage of very high cost and a possibility of increasing portal hypertension precipitating a gastrointestinal bleed.

LaVeen has devised a peritoneo-venous shunt (LaVeen shunt) for use in refractory cases of ascites (10). This consists of a subcutaneous catheter that drains ascitic fluid into the venous system (e.g., inferior vena cava) through a one-way valve. As the diaphragm descends, the pressure in the intrathoracic veins drops and intraperitoneal pressure rises. This pressure differential pumps the ascitic fluid into the venous system. The results may be dramatic with urine flows as high as 15 liters occurring during the first 24 hours. Supplemental diuresis with furosemide may be required to prevent vascular overload. However, use of this procedure is limited by such complications as fever, shunt occlusions, hypokalemia, infection, shunt leaks, disseminated intravascular coagulopathy (DIC) and less frequently variceal hemorrhage, bowel obstruction, pulmonary edema and pneumothorax (11).

GI Bleeding

Bleeding from esophageal varices is a grave sign and is very difficult to stop, often requiring multiple transfusions. Even if the bleeding is stopped the chances of the patient hemorrhaging again are high. Placement of a Sengstaken tube and balloon in an attempt to slow the bleeding by compression is sometimes tried, yielding varied results. This procedure is complicated by vomiting and a high incidence of aspiration or recurrence of bleeding as soon as the balloon is deflated.

More often, the natural hormone vasopressin (ADH) is given IV in a dose of 20 to 40 units in 100 ml of 5% dextrose or saline over 20 to 40 min (8). This produces a significant decrease in portal blood flow and pressure by vasoconstriction of portal and other splanchnic arterioles. This vasoconstriction slows or stops bleeding long enough to allow thrombus formation at the site of bleeding. The dose may have to be repeated 3 or 4 times daily and even then the termination of bleeding may be transient. Some authors have described tachyphylaxis with continued use. Pharmacokinetically it would be better to give the drug more often since it has a very short half-life (about 20 min) but, due to its intense vasoconstrictor action, it decreases cardiac output and may cause coronary ischemia. This is especially a problem in patients with coronary artery disease or hypertension, but ECG changes have been reported in patients with no prior evidence of heart disease (12). Bradycardia is the most widely observed side effect of vasopressin due to stimulation of the vagus nerve (13–17). It also may produce GI cramping and even bowel necrosis due to stimulation of smooth muscle contraction. Women may experience uterine pain similar to menstrual cramps. Finally, it may lead to excess water retention and a dilutional hyponatremia (18).

In an attempt to reduce the toxicity of intermittent large dose vasopressin, continuous intravenous infusions at 0.2 to 0.4 unit per min (19) or direct intra-arterial infusion (13–16, 20, 21) via a catheter into the superior mesenteric artery at 0.05 to 0.4 unit per min has been tried. These infusions may be continued for up to 72 hours in some instances with a slow tapering of the dose over time. The results have been varied with some authors claiming up to 50 to 70% effectiveness (8, 15, 20). Others claim poor response and a high incidence of complications including bleeding from the site of catheter insertion and septicemia (21). An overall decrease in mortality rate has not been shown (15). In an attempt to prevent bradycardia, Sirinek advocates infusion of 0.002 mg/ml of isoproterenol at 50 ml/hr along with the vasopressin (17).

Bleeding from other GI sites, especially due to gastritis and peptic ulcer, is usually treated with nasogastric suction, iced saline, cimetidine and hourly antacids. Since these patients often tend to retain sodium due to a relative aldosteronism, a low sodium antacid should be used. Occasionally 20 units of vasopressin or 1 to 2 ampules of norepinephrine are used in a gastric lavage to cause localized vasoconstriction in an attempt to slow the bleeding.

It has been suggested that since propranolol decreases portal venous pressure, it may prevent gastrointestinal bleeding associated with portal hypertension. Lebrec (22) showed that oral propranolol in doses that reduced the heart rate by 25% significantly reduced the incidence of rebleeding compared to placebo during a 1-year study period. Only 4% of patients in the propranolol group had recurrence of bleeding compared to 50% in the placebo group. None of the patients showed deterioration of hepatic or renal function while taking propranolol, but because propranolol may decrease cardiac output and liver blood flow patients should be monitored closely.

Hepatic Encephalopathy

If the patient should develop signs of an impending hepatic coma (e.g., confusion, drowsiness, liver flap), neomycin, 1 to 2 g, 4 times daily, may be started and the dietary protein decreased to 20 to 30 g per day. Neomycin depresses the colonic bacterial count thus slowing the degradation of protein to ammonia. Diuretics should be held at this stage since hypovolemia and hypokalemia tend to aggravate the encephalopathy. If the above measures do not work and the patient lapses into a coma, the dose of the neomycin should be increased to 8 to 12 g per day and the protein restriction lowered to 0 to 20 g per day. When the patient improves the maintenance dose of neomycin may be lowered to 2 to 4 g per day. Duration of therapy is variable and may last less than a week for some patients, up to months and even years in patients with very tenuous balance. The importance of protein restriction cannot be overemphasized. Many patients who look well compensated can rapidly defervesce by eating just one hamburger or tuna fish sandwish.

If the patient is not able to take medications orally, a retention enema of 2 to 4 g of neomycin in 200 ml of saline and thickened with methylcellulose may be used morning and night. Neomycin is one of the "nonabsorbable" antibiotics and thus orally it is claimed to give only local effects in the gut. However it has been shown that from 1 to 3% (23) of a dose is absorbed and there are several reported cases of ototoxicity in patients on chronic oral neomycin therapy (24). Most of these patients had been taking the neomycin for at least 8 months and had coexisting renal dysfunction. In any case, periodic auditory testing should be performed and the patient observed for subjective changes in hearing status if the drug is to be used for prolonged periods.

Neomycin has also been implicated in the development of the hepatorenal syndrome since it is a known renal toxic drug when given parenterally. However, it is difficult to determine if the renal changes are due to the drug or just a progression of the disease process itself. The consensus is that the latter mechanism prevails.

Another problem encountered with neomycin therapy is diarrhea due to changes in the bowel flora. However, this may not be a deleterious consequence and in fact patients are often given cathartics to cleanse the bowel and thus eliminate excess ammonia production. Orders may be written for magnesium citrate (citrate of magnesia) or for 50 g of sorbitol in 200 ml of water. It should be noted that these agents are not effective to any great extent when used alone and should always be accompanied by neomycin therapy and protein restriction. The danger of the cathartic procedures is that fluid and electrolyte imbalances may occur, thus worsening the encephalopathy. It is imperative that adequate intravenous infusions of dextrose or saline with potassium supplements be maintained.

Lactulose

The marketing of lactulose has prompted some clinicians to avoid high dose neomycin by substituting lactulose instead. It is a synthetic disaccharide of galactose and fructose which is neither absorbed nor hydrolyzed in the small bowel. It is degraded by the colonic bacteria to lactic acid thus decreasing the pH of the colonic contents to about 5.5. The effect of lactulose was originally attributed to replacement of proteolytic bacteria such as *Escherichia coli*, *Proteus* and *Bacteroides* with organisms like *Lactobacillus* which thrive in a more acidic medium and which are lacking in urease and other enzymes used in the production of ammonia products. However, most investigators have not been able to demonstrate a marked change in the colonic flora and attribute the effects of lactulose solely to the pH changes that occur leading to a greater ammonium ion to ammonia concentration in the bowel lumen, and thus less absorption of the ammonia products. There may also be back diffusion of ammonia from the blood to the intestinal lumen under acidic pH conditions. In any event, the final outcome of lactulose therapy is a decrease in arterial ammonium levels (25–27). A recent well-controlled study (28) failed to show a clear superiority of either neomycin (83% effective) or lactulose (90% effective) in the treatment of acute encephalopathy. For long-term use lactulose has the potential advantage of less toxicity, but is considerably more expensive. A theoretical drug interaction that sterilization of the gut by neomycin may lead to decreased effectiveness of lactulose (29) appears to be of minimal consequences and in fact the two drugs may have some added effectiveness when used together (30).

Each 15 ml of lactulose contain 10 g of lactulose and it is usually given in a dose of 30 to 45 ml, 3 to 4 times daily. Use of retention enemas (31) of 300 ml of 50% lactulose diluted to 1000 ml with tap water has also been reported. Onset of effect by either route is 24 to 48 hours. When lactulose is not available, 20% lactose enemas at a dose of 1000 ml, 3 times daily may also be effective (32).

The most common complaint of patients

treated with lactulose is diarrhea due to osmotic effects of the drug in the bowel. This diarrhea may account for part of the therapeutic effects of lactulose (33, 34) but, when compared to sorbitol, lactulose is much more effective in overcoming the encephalopathy indicating other mechanisms are working (25, 26). In fact the dose that is usually given is adjusted so that the patient has two to three soft, semiformed stools daily avoiding watery diarrhea. The success rate at these doses has been reported to be around 85%. This includes some patients who had previously shown poor response to neomycin therapy. Unfortunately a few patients tend to become resistant after prolonged therapy and many patients die of other complications of the disease even though they are helped through the encephalopathy.

Dopamine and L-Dopa

Dopamine and norepinephrine are important mediators for normal sympathetic activity in both the central nervous system and in the periphery, especially in the kidney. Some of the neurological manifestations of hepatic failure, as well as the hepatorenal syndrome, may be due to accumulation of other β-hydroxylated phenylethylamines that replace normal transmitters and act as false neurotransmitters in sympathetic nerve terminals and granules. (See above, "Hepatic Encephalopathy".) One of these compounds, octopamine, has been found in higher than normal concentrations in patients in hepatic coma. These compounds can displace or coinhabit the adrenergic neuron with norepinephrine and be released in its place when sympathetic discharge is mediated. However, they are unable to elicit the normal responses that norepinephrine would mediate and may lead to some of the deficits seen in these patients.

Precursors of these false neurotransmitters, such as phenylalanine and tyrosine (Fig. 17.1), are produced from protein in the gut by the action of bacterial amino acid decarboxylases. Normally they are rapidly metabolized in the liver by monoamine oxidase (MAO) so that norepinephrine that is formed elsewhere in the body predominates. When hepatic function is impaired or when blood is shunted away from the liver these false neurotransmitters may replace the normal transmitter. Systemically this may lead to lowered peripheral vascular resistance and shunting of blood

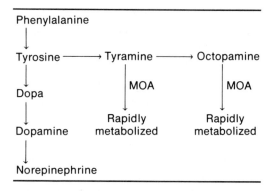

Figure 17.1. Synthetic pathway of neurotransmitters. Monoamine oxidase (MOA) action mainly in the liver. Depressed in hepatic disease and shunting.

away from the kidney. Similarly asterixis and other signs of hepatic encephalopathy might be the result of displacement of transmitters such as dopamine and norepinephrine in the basal ganglia and other areas in the brain.

If the displacement of normal central and peripheral transmitters by less active amines can account for hepatic coma and its cardiovascular complications, then the restoration of normal transmitter stores might restore normal function. For hospitalized patients this is accomplished by administering low dose infusions of dopamine (1 to 4 μg/kg/min). This helps restore central stores of dopamine and increases renal blood flow to help reverse the hepatorenal syndrome. By referring to Figure 17.1, it can be seen that dopamine is also a precursor to norepinephrine and thus helps to restore natural neurotransmitter balance in a second way.

In less emergent cases or when one wishes to wean the patient off of parenteral dopamine, oral administration of L-dopa can be given as a source of dopamine (35, 36). At this time, L-dopa therapy is investigational and its efficacy is unclear. In this author's experience the results have been varied. Three cases failed to respond, two cases responded after several days of therapy (concurrent with neomycin which had been started 1 week earlier) and a third case showed some response after 1 day and by the 3rd day the patient was able to communicate rationally for the first time in over 1 month. Doses have usually been 500 mg 3 to 4 times daily, or in the latter instance 1 g twice daily by rectal enema. Side effects of L-dopa (nausea, vomiting, hypotension, and tachycardia) are minimal because of the relatively small doses used compared to doses used for parkinsonism.

Branched Chain Amino Acids

One of the goals of management in progressive liver disease is to provide adequate nutritional support, including proteins and calories, to prevent negative nitrogen balance while at the same time preventing hepatic encephalopathy due to excess protein substrates. It has been found in experimental animals, and to a lesser extent in humans, that the administration of diets high in branched chain amino acids and low in aromatic amino acids and methionine may help restore normal amino acid balance and reduce encephalopathy (3, 4). One such dietary supplement is Hepatic-Aid, a suspendable powder containing essential and nonessential amino acids, carbohydrate and fat in a readily digestible form. One package of Hepatic-Aid mixed in a blender with 250 ml of water yields 340 ml of suspension for oral or nasogastric administration which contains 2.2 g of nitrogen (15 g protein), 98 g of carbohydrate, 12 g of fat and 560 calories (500 nonprotein calories). One to four packages may be given per day, but the administration rate should not be too rapid at first to prevent osmotic induced diarrhea and glucose overload. At this time, use of branched chain amino acids is still considered investigational in severe hepatic encephalopathy and is limited by high cost and a disagreeable taste.

Surgical Treatment

Surgical treatment may be required for patients who have repeated GI bleeding, especially esophageal varices, or who have bleeding that cannot be stopped by the more conservative measures already described. The surgery performed is called a portacaval shunt and involves an anastomosis of the portal vein directly to the inferior vena cava, thus bypassing the cirrhotic liver. This serves to decrease portal hypertension and thus the back-pressure on the abdominal venous system. Unfortunately these patients have a very poor prognosis since the only source of blood supply to carry toxins to the liver for detoxification is now the hepatic artery. Thus, if they survive the initial surgery, these patients often die of sepsis or develop hepatic failure and encephalopathy (37). The Warren shunt is a method of decompressing varices by shunting spleen blood flow to the renal vein (splenorenal shunt) and may be associated with less of a decrease in hepatic profusion.

PROGNOSIS

The outlook for patients with cirrhosis depends entirely upon the stage of advancement of the cirrhosis. If the liver is fatty with little fibrosis, remarkable improvement follows the initiation of a well-balanced diet. The fat can be mobilized, the liver decreases in size, evidence of hepatic cell necrosis disappears and liver function is much improved. Even when there is considerable fibrosis the forward progress of the disease can be halted by good dietary discretion although the existing fibrosis cannot be reversed. If the cause of the cirrhosis is alcoholism and the patient continues to drink and neglect a proper diet, the prognosis is poor. Such patients usually die of either liver failure in hepatic coma, massive bleeding from esophageal varices or infection. About 50% die within a year of the appearance of major complications and an additional 25% die within the next 3 to 5 years (8). In the United States cirrhosis has become one of the 5 most frequent causes of death in persons over the age of 40.

CONCLUSION

Despite the large amount of study done on the liver and a vastly expanding understanding of its functions and pathologies, effective therapy for liver disease does not exist. At best only symptomatic management of the complications of chronic liver disease is as yet possible. One redeeming factor is that although the lesions of advanced cirrhosis are irreversible, it is estimated that 70% or more of liver tissue must be destroyed before the body is unable to eliminate drugs and toxins via the liver. Unfortunately it is difficult to foretell just which patients have reached this stage of involvement so that when working with a patient with advanced liver disease the pharmacist should always be aware of the potential inability of the patient to excrete certain drugs and see that doses are adjusted accordingly.

References

1. Robbins S, Angell M, Kumar V: *Basic Pathology,* ed 3. Philadelphia: W. B. Saunders, 1981, pp 520–533.
2. Rubin E, Lieber C: Fatty liver, alcoholic hepati-

tis, and cirrhosis produced by alcohol in primates. *N Engl J Med* 290:128, 1974.

3. Freund H, Yoshimura N, Fischer J: Chronic hepatic encephalopathy, long term therapy with a branched-chain amino-acid-enriched elemental diet. *JAMA* 242:347, 1979.

4. James J, Ziparo V, Jeppson B, et al: Hyperammonaemia, plasma amino acid inbalance, and blood-brain amino-acid transport: a unified theory of port-systemic encephalopathy. *Lancet* 2:772, 1979.

5. Udall J: Don't use the wrong vitamin K. *Calif Med* 112:65, 1970.

6. Shear L, Ching S, Gabuzda G: Compartmentalization of ascites and edema in patients with hepatic cirrhosis. *N Engl J Med* 282:1391, 1970.

7. Reynolds T, Geller H, Kuzma O, et al: Spontaneous decrease in portal pressure with clinical improvement in cirrhosis. *N Engl J Med* 263:734, 1960.

8. Conn H: Cirrhosis. In Schiff L: *Diseases of the Liver*. Philadelphia: J. B. Lippincott, 1975.

9. Greenblatt D, Koch-Weser J: Adverse reactions to spironolactone. *JAMA* 225:40, 1973.

10. LaVeen H, Christoudias G, Ip M, et al: Peritoneovenous shunting for ascites. *Ann Surg* 180:580, 1974.

11. Epstein M: The LaVeen shunt for ascites and hepatorenal syndrome. *N Engl J Med* 302:628, 1980.

12. Beller BM, Trevino A, Urban E: Pitressin-induced myocardial injury and depression in a young woman. *Am J Med* 51:675, 1971.

13. Sirinek K: Peripheral vasopressin for safe and adequate control of portal hypertension during shunt operation. *Am J Surg* 131:103, 1976.

14. Marubbio A: Control of variceal bleeding by superior mesenteric artery pitressin perfusions—complications and indications. *Am J Dig Dis* 18:539, 1973.

15. Conn H, Ramsey G, Storer E: Intra-arterial vasopressin in the treatment of upper gastrointestinal hemorrhage. *Gastroenterology* 68:211, 1975.

16. Johnson W, Widrich W: Efficacy of selective splanchnic arteriography and vasopressin perfusion in the diagnosis and treatment of gastrointestinal hemorrhage. *Am J Surg* 131:481, 1976.

17. Sirinek K: Isoproterenol in offsetting adverse effects of vasopressin in cirrhotic patients. *Am J Surg* 129:130, 1975.

18. Marubbio A: Antidiuretic hormone effect of Pitressin during continuous Pitressin administration. *Gastroenterology* 62:1103, 1972.

19. Thomford N, Sirinek K: Intravenous vasopressin in patients with portal hypertension; advantage of continuous infusion. *J Surg Res* 18:113, 1975.

20. Baum S, Nusbaum M: The control of gastrointestinal hemorrhage by selective mesenteric arterial infusion of vasopressin. *Diag Radiol* 98:497, 1971.

21. Murray I, Pugh R, Nunnerley H, et al: Treatment of bleeding oesophageal varices by infusion of vasopressin into the superior mesenteric artery. *Gut* 14:59, 1973.

22. Lebrec O, Poynard T, Hillon P, et al: Propranolol for prevention of recurrent gastrointestinal bleeding in patients with cirrhosis. *N Engl J Med* 305:1371, 1981.

23. Breen K, Gryant R, Levinson J, et al: Neomycin absorption in man. *Ann Intern Med* 76:211, 1972.

24. Berk D, Chalmer T: Deafness complicating antibiotic therapy of hepatic encephalopathy. *Ann Intern Med* 73:383, 1970.

25. Bircher J, Haemmerli UP, Scollo-Lavizzari G: Treatment of chronic portal-systemic encephalopathy with lactulose. *Am J Med* 51:148, 1971.

26. Elkington SG, Floch MH, Conn HO: Lactulose in the treatment of chronic portal systemic encephalopathy; a double blind clinical trial. *N Engl J Med* 281:408, 1969.

27. Avery GS, Davies EF, Brogden RN: lactulose; a review. *Drugs* 4:7, 1972.

28. Conn HO, Leevy CM, Vlahcevic J, et al: Comparison of lactulose and neomycin in the treatment of chronic portal systemic encephalopathy. *Gastroenterology* 72:573, 1977.

29. Conn HO: Interactions of lactulose and neomycin. *Drugs* 4:4, 1972.

30. Pirotte J, Guffens JM, Devos J: Comparative study of basal arterial ammonia and of orally-induced hyperammonemia in chronic portal-systemic encephalopathy, treated with neomycin, lactulose and an association of neomycin and lactulose. *Digestion* 10:435, 1974.

31. Kersh ES, Rifkin H: Lactulose enemas. *Ann Intern Med* 78:81, 1973.

32. Uribe M, Berthier J, Lewis H, et al: Lactose enemas plus placebo tablets vs. neomycin tablets plus starch enemas in acute portal systemic encephalopathy. *Gastroenterology* 81:101, 1981.

33. Rodgers JB Jr, Kiley JE, Balint JA: Comparison of results of long term treatment of chronic hepatic encephalopathy with lactulose and sorbitol. *Am J Gastroenterol* 60:459, 1973.

34. Brown H, Trey C, McDermott WV Jr: Lactulose treatment of hepatic encephalopathy in outpatients. *Arch Surg* 102:25, 1971.

35. Fischer J, Baldessarini R: False neurotransmitters and hepatic failure. *Lancet* 2:75, 1971.

36. Fischer J, James J: Treatment of hepatic coma and hepatorenal syndrome, mechanisms of action of L-dopa and aramine. *Am J Surg* 123:222, 1972.

37. Garabedian M, Whitcomb F: Medical treatment of portal hypertension. *Surg Clin North Am* 51:749, 1971.

CHAPTER 18

Diarrhea and Constipation

PETER J. FORNI, Pharm.D.

Two of the most common problems that affect us throughout our lives are constipation and diarrhea. In this chapter these two problems will be discussed in the context of what is experienced in industrialized societies rather than specifics as related to less developed countries. Emphasis is placed on basic treatment approaches that health professionals should know and use. Other specific therapies are covered.

It is important to remember that simple constipation is usually easy to treat, self-limiting and nonlife-threatening. Diarrhea, on the other hand, is usually dibilitating to some degree in the best of circumstances and is often fatal in the worst cases. Furthermore, either condition may be symptomatic of a more serious medical problem which needs to be treated by medical specialists. Therefore, it is imperative that pharmacists become more cognizant about these problems so that they can better serve patients presenting with either one.

Drugs used to treat either symptomatic problems are very popular, especially in the nonprescription items. It is interesting to note that the World Health Organization (WHO) has only three products, aside from antibiotics, on its Model List of Essential Drugs (1). Senna is the only carthartic. Codeine and oral rehydration solution are the only antidiarrheals. Admittedly, the WHO List contains the bare minimums for Third World populations. It does provide food for thought for the high drug consuming industrialized nations trying to provide affordable health care services.

INTESTINAL PHYSIOLOGY

The physiology of the gut involves many complex processes (2, 3). For the purposes of this discussion, a brief review of fluid and electrolyte movement between the intestines and mucosal cells is warranted for a better understanding the problems of constipation and diarrhea.

In healthy individuals on a normal diet the stomach empties several hours after food is ingested. When the contents reach the ileoceal valve most of the carbohydrates, proteins and fats are broken down into digestible forms. This bolus moves slowly through the ileum unless the stomach empties. Defecatory reflexes are stimulated by distention of the rectal musculature followed by descent of the pelvic floor and inhibition of defecation is accomplished by relaxing abdominal muscle and contracting anal sphincter. The gastroileal reflex causes the ileum to empty into the cecum. Segmental contractions with occasional coordinated wave move the bolus along. Eating or walking may increase these contractions. Cholingergic nerves control motor and secretory functions.

Normal fecal weight in an adult is about 150 g daily. This results from the normal ingestion of food and drink. Daily fluid reaching the intestines includes approximately 2 liters from food and drink, 1 liter of saliva, 2 liters of gastric secretions and 2 liters from pancreatic secretion, 1 liter each from liver and small bowel secretions. About 8 liters are absorbed in the small intestines and 0.85 liter is absorbed in the large bowel leaving 150 ml for excretion in the stool. This occurs following absorption and secretion of glucose, fatty acids, and electrolytes along with water. Note that glucose, itself, facilitates sodium adsorption.

The normal jejunum absorbs water and small solutes until the luminal content is isotonic with interstitial fluids. Active absorption of glucose and amino acids create an osmotic gradient and a solvent drag effect on sodium, potassium and water. There are also carrier proteins which actively carry glucose and sodium into cells. Chloride ions are absorbed passively in the jejunum. Bicarbonate ions combine with hydrogen ions to form water to be absorbed against an electrochemical gradient. In the ileum chloride ions are exchanged for intracellular bicarbonate ions.

The colon gets an isotonic solution from which sodium and chloride ions are actively absorbed in exchange for bicarbonate ions. Potassium ions move passively down a gradient and are also secreted.

Hypotonic luminal contents cause water to be absorbed and electrolytes secreted. Hypertonic loads causes water to be secreted. Starches and sugars increase luminal osmotic load. As the luminal contents move down the colon, bacteria biodegrade disaccharides, e.g., lactose, into two molecules which increase the osmotic gradient. This is also seen in steatorrhea. If twice the sodium and potassium concentration is less than the measured stool osmolality then extra solute is causing the increased osmolality.

Adenyl cyclase stimulates the production of cyclic AMP in the intestinal epithelial cells. Cyclic AMP stimulates the secretion of chloride ions and water. At the same time sodium absorption is blocked. Fats, bile and enterotoxogenic bacteria stimulate this biochemical process.

This mechanism seems to be mediated by prostaglandins. Certain prostaglandin inhibitors block various intestinal secretory mechanisms. These agents include aspirin, indomethacin and phenothiazines.

Traditionally, diarrhea was thought to be due to hypermotility. Increased motility and decreased segmenting activity lead to faster transit time for luminal contents. Water and electrolyte malabsorption are now known to be the primary reason for diarrheal problems. Four mechanisms can contribute to this malabsorption. Decreased permeability of the intestinal mucosa or defective active transport processes resulty in more fluid being left in the gut lumen. Increased osmolality of the luminal content and increased intestinal secretion also can significantly increase fluid loss in stool.

CONSTIPATION

Tens of millions of dollars are spent each year in the United States by the general public for the treatment of constipation. Most of these expenditures are not justified on a medical or physiologic basis. Misguided beliefs about the need for "regular" bowel movements have led many people to overutilize or misuse laxatives resulting in not only the waste of consumer dollars but also in the development of cathartic dependency and associated medical problems.

Stedman's defines constipation as a "condition in which bowel movements are infrequent or incomplete." Simple irregularity of defecation of normal stool is not an indication for laxative use. Laxatives are routinely used in patients with certain medical problems in which straining at stool is not desirable. Bowel evacuation in preparation for radiographic or endoscopic procedures also warrants use of various cathartics. Short-term laxative therapy may occasionally be necessary, usually as adjunctive therapy, in correcting a simple constipation problem.

Etiology

Many causes of constipation (Table 18.1) can and should be treated by medical or surgical intervention and not with laxatives. When confronted with a patient complaining of constipation one should ascertain whether the problem is most likely a simple problem or possibly a more serious problem requiring referral to a physician for proper diagnosis and treatment. Disorders such as ulcerative colitis, colonic disorders, excessive parasympathetic nerve stimulation and even chronic laxative use are common causes of constipation. Other organic causes include benign and malignant bowel lesions, strictures, and hypothyroidism. A thorough history and physical, when possible, will help rule out these causes which

Table 18.1.
Common Causes of Constipation

Disorder Type	Cause
Metabolic	Hypokalemia, diabetes, porphyria, amyloidosis, hypothyroidism, hyperparathyroidism, milk-alkali syndrome, lead poisoning
Neurogenic	Parkinson's disease, multiple sclerosis, paraplegia, tabes dorsalis, cerebral tumors, cerebrovascular accidents, Chagas disease, meningocele
Structural GI	Tumors (benign or malignant), strictures, hernias, rectocele, rectal prolapse, chronic volvulus
Functional GI	Irritable bowel syndrome, diverticulitis, stenosis, proctitis, myotonic dystrophy, dermatomyositis

require appropriate medical or surgical intervention. If simple constipation requires laxative therapy, the treatment should be only for a few days. Long-term laxative use is usually unnecessary and may actually exascerbate the constipation, or worse, delay proper diagnosis and treatment (4).

Pharmacists must also be more aware of the possibility of drug-induced constipation. Table 18.2 lists the more common constipating agents. Many people do not realize that these can cause serious problems. Laxative abuse may be one of the most common causes and is often overlooked. Aluminum- and calcium-containing antacids are seldom considered to be medications by the consuming public. The continuous, casual use of "acid neutralizing" tablets and liquids can severely constipate. Iron-containing preparations are often used in children and women and may be missed as a contributing cause of constipation. Some medications combined with an existing condition can be enough to produce a clinical bowel problem. For example, a slightly dehydrated person placed on a diuretic for hypertension may lose enough additional fluids to produce abnormal bowel activity. This type of problem may be seen more often in the elderly and the very young (5).

Other medication combinations may be overlooked by health professions. The patient taking antihistamines for hay fever develops a cold and a cough which are treated with a codeine-containing antitussive. In this situation the additive anticholingeric activity and narcotic action on the gastrointestinal tract can be very significant. One particular group of patients has a high susceptibility to this type of polypharmacy induced constipation. These are the mentally ill patients seen in both institutions and the community. Many of these individuals may be on multiple drugs which have significant anticholinergic activity. The depressed patient on both a tricyclic antidepressant and a monoamine oxidase inhibitor or the schizophrenic individual receiving both a neuroleptic and antiparkinson agent will often need assistance in minimizing bowel problems. In these latter situations, selection of therapy may actually combine stool softeners and altering psychotherapeutic agents in minimize excessive anticholinergic action.

Incidence

Constipation affects everyone at some point in life. It is commonly seen in people who are bedridden for prolonged periods of time. Elderly individuals and children are particularly sensitive to developing constipation secondarily to other problems. For example, these two groups are susceptible to dehydration from a variety of causes. Dehydration is a leading cause of simple constipation. Also, as one ages there is a loss of sensitivity of various sensory reflexes necessary for normal bowel function, thus contributing to bowel irregularity. Use of laxatives is seen in over three quarters of individuals complaining of constipation.

Diagnosis and Clinical Findings

The complaint of constipation represents a myriad of symptoms. Straining at stool with or without abdominal pain or discomfort is common. Other common symptoms may include abdominal distention, nonspecific back pain, general lassitude, headache and anorexia. These constitutional complaints obviously have multiple causes. It is important to determine why the patient believes he or she is constipated. People vary greatly in the number of daily bowel movements. The consuming public has been led to believe that a daily bowel movement is necessary. This is not so. Normal bowel habits range from several stools daily to a stool every other day. Furthermore, the type of stool seen in a constipated patient is hard and dry. Many people use laxatives even though their stools have normal consistency and water content and are not difficult to pass. These patients usually have no other constitutional problems, other than they do not pass stool daily at a prescribed time. An-

Table 18.2.
Constipating Drugs

Laxatives
Narcotic analgesics
Aluminum/calcium antacids
Antihistamines
Antiparkinson agents
Tricyclic antidepressants
MAO inhibitors
Heavy metals poisoning
Neuroleptic agents
Anesthetic agents
Diuretics
Barium sulfate
Ganglionic blockers
Iron containing hematinics

other common sign of bowel problems is the continued use of laxatives and cathartics with inadequate results. This may well be a sign of laxative abuse, the "cathartic habit." In simple constipation requiring a laxative, therapy should show adequate results within a few days. Excessive laxative use leads to a vicious cycle of trying to treat constipation with the actual causative agent. Symptoms of laxative abuse include steatorrhea, osteomalacia, electrolyte imbalance, diarrhea and protein-losing enteropathy.

It must be remembered that constipation and associated symptomatology may be signs of more serious problems shown in Table 18.1. The astute pharmacist must recognize this and not hesitate to refer any patient with protracted constipation not responding to therapy or anyone with other signs and symptoms indicative of the disorders listed above.

Treatment

BASIC APPROACH

Constipation is best treated by educating the patient about the influence of dietary and physical activity on gastrointestinal function. Along with this, one should clearly explain where the various types of medications belong in the scheme for treating simple constipation. Table 18.3 outlines this basic approach. Note that most cases of simple constipation can be easily corrected by properly educating the patient and correcting dietary habits. Of course, reiteration of these steps may be necessary over time and should be routine anytime one is presented with the problem of simple, functional constipation. Use of simple explanation sheets may assist in simplifying the physiology aspects and clearly list key dietary items for inclusion and exclusion. Although misinformation may be forcing an individual to get his or her bowels "regular," most people appreciate tactfully presented information, especially if they can correct a problem with minimal expenditure of funds.

When confronted with a patient complaining of constipation, the pharmacist should obtain a detailed history from the patient to determine if the complaining is a simple functional syndrome. Determine whether or not the individual has recently been physically inactive, such as recovering from surgery. Remember, many simple surgical procedures are being done on an outpatient basis. These patients still are required to fast, to take consti-

Table 18.3.
Basic Treatment of Constipation

A. *Obtain patient history*
   1. Presenting symptomatology
   2. Medical history
   3. Medication history
   4. Dietary and physical activity habits
B. *Educate patient*
   1. Review in layman's terms normal gastrointestinal physiology
   2. Explain the variations in normal bowel habits
   3. Eliminate laxative and other constipating medications slowly if possible
   4. Remind the patient to allow time to defecate, i.e. "call to stool"
   5. Encourage patient to exercise regularly according to the individual's abilities and explain why physical activity is important
C. *Provide dietary information*
   1. Explain importance of adequate fluid intake—at least the equivalent of six 8-oz glasses of liquid daily
   2. Explain importance of roughage and bulk in foods with high residue such as unprocessed grains, vegetables and fruits
   3. Decrease intake of processed foods, e.g., white flour, sugar

pating preoperative drugs and to rest in bed. Obtain a clear dietary history, including fluid intake and food types. Be sure the patient does not have some obvious symptoms of a more serious problem. Ask if there is blood in the stool or other signs and symptoms indicative of a more serious problem. The patient should describe exactly what he is calling constipation. Very often the patient really will be concerned about "irregularity" with normal stools, rather than actually difficulty in passing stool that is hard and dry. A patient's dietary history is also very important. Inadequate intake of dietary bulk and fluids are major contributory factors. Changes in diet may also severely alter normal bowel function.

MEDICATIONS

After the basic treatment approach outlined above a laxative may still be needed on occasion. Since there is no perfect laxative, one must weigh the immediancy of the patient's needs and the relative toxicities of available agents when selecting or recommending any agent (4–6). If one must prepare a patient for surgery or radiological study, one would need an agent with more purgative action. On the other hand, such an agent may be harmful to a pregnant women needing only a mild laxative. Table 18.4 lists the basic types of available laxatives. All of these agents are available over-the-counter.

Bulk-producing laxatives are polysaccharide and cellulose derivatives and are often the laxative of choice for treating simple constipation. Derived from both natural and synthetic sources these compounds act similarly to other food sources of roughage, e.g., cereals, fruits and vegetables. Bulk laxatives appear to work by retaining water in the stool (6). They should be taken with adequate amounts of water. Onset of action is slow, usually over a 12- to 72-hour period. Although very safe to use, bulk formers should be used only for a few days while dietary changes are made to ensure more roughage.

Stimulant or irritant laxatives directly stimulate intestinal motor activity. Most of these agents work in the colon, with the exception of castor oil which works in the small intestines. Excessive use of stimulants can lead to dependency, the cathartic habit. Usual onset of action is between 6 to 10 hours. These are not agents of first choice because severe cramping, excessive fluid loss and electrolyte imbalance often occur. Phenolphthalein is slightly absorbed and will cause urine to color pink or red. It goes through enterohepatic recycling which may prolong its duration of action. Although generally nontoxic, phenolphthalein has been associated with cardiovascular and respiratory collapse. Very severe skin reactions have occurred, including toxic epidermal necrosis.

Glycerin suppositories are very fast acting, causing irritation to the exposed tissues through osmotic dehydration. Lower bowel evacuation occurs within 30 min.

Lubricant laxatives contain mineral oil or plant oils which lubricates the mucosal surface of the intestines and softens the stool (4). Onset of action occurs within 8 hours. Malabsorption of fat-soluble vitamins, nutrients and drugs may occur with prolonged use of mineral oil. Aspiration of mineral oil will cause lipid pneumonia. For this reason it is best not to give it at bedtime or to young children or elderly patients who have more likelihood to aspirate their gastric contents. Perianal problems also are seen with excessive use of lubricants. Pruritus ani, hemorrhoids and cryptitis are common. Lubricants can initially be helpful following abdominal surgery, myocardial infarc-

Table 18.4.
Laxative Agents

Agent	Daily Adult Dose
A. *Bulk-producing laxatives*	
1. Methylcelluose	4–6 g
2. Sodium carboxymethyl cellulose	4–6 g
3. Psyllium	4–30 g
4. Malt extract	12–64 g
5. Polycarbophil	4–6 g
B. *Stimulant laxatives*	
1. Cascara sagrada	200–400 mg
2. Danthron	75–150 mg
3. Senna	0.5–2.0 g
4. Phenolphthalein	30–270 mg
5. Bisacodyl	10–15 mg
6. Castor oil	15–60 ml
C. *Glycerin suppositories*	3 g
D. *Lubricant laxatives*	
1. Mineral oil	15–60 ml
E. *Stool softeners*	
1. Docusate sodium	50–240 mg
2. Docusate calcium	50–240 mg
3. Docusate potassium	240–300 mg

tion, cerebral vascular accidents and hemorrhoidectomy.

Stool softeners are surfactants which soften stool by retaining water within the stool (7). These emollient agents are effective on softening fecal masses in nondebilitated patients within 3 days of therapy. They may not be as effective in the inactive, elderly patients. When given alone these agents are nontoxic. However, they can promote absorption of other toxic substances like mineral oil and danthron. For this reason, a FDA advisory panel recommends that these not be taken with mineral oil or prescription medication. Obviously, stool softeners are given safely with other medications, but the pharmacist should be aware of potential problems and monitor and instruct such patients accordingly.

Saline laxatives contain poorly absorbed cations and anions which produce hyperosmolar condition in the intestinal lumen, thus promoting water secretion and retention. There also appears to exist other actions stimulated by these cathartics that promote water retention. They act very fast, usually within 30 to 120 min. Saline cathartics are indicated for acute bowel evacuations in preparation for endoscopic study. Their use in acute poisoning is not proven.

One should remember that magnesium is a CNS depressant. Accumulation of magnesium in the renally impaired patients and sometimes in the elderly or very young can cause hypotension, muscle weakness and cardiotoxicity. Saline cathartics can drastically alter fluid and electrolyte balance. Careful monitoring of electrolytes may be required even in seemingly healthy individuals.

Lactulose is a synthetic analog of lactose available by prescription. It is a disaccharide that is not metabolized by humans until it reaches the colon where bacteria produce enzymes which convert lactulose to lactic, formic and acetic acids plus carbon dioxide. These increase the osmotic pressure in the colon which increases the water content of the stool. Onset of action may take up to 48 hours. Lactulose is indicated for chronic constipation. Side effects are generally limited to cramps and flatulence. Long-term use of 6 months or more can cause electrolyte imbalance in debilitated individuals. It should be used cautiously in diabetics because of some digestible sugars in the product. There is no evidence to support this osmotic laxative is any more effective than less expensive agents (9).

ADVERSE REACTIONS,
CONTRAINDICATIONS AND WARNINGS

Known sensitivities to these agents are uncommon, except for phenophthalein as previously noted. Laxatives are generally contraindicted in patients with possible bowel obstruction, appendicitis, intestinal perforation, fecal impaction, acute hepatitis, abdominal pain of unknown origin, nausea or vomiting. Patients with known tartrazine sensitivity or who have salicylate allergies should determine which agents contain tartrazine and select another agent.

Sodium-containing laxatives should not be used in patients on low sodium diet, impaired renal function, congestive heart failure or megacolon. Pregnant women should not use castor oil or mineral oil. Danthron and cascara sagrada are excreted in breast milk. Discoloration of the urine occurs with cascara sagrada, senna, phenophthalein and danthron. Alkaline urine may cause a pink-red-brown color and an acid urine may cause a yellow-brown color. Biscodyl tablets should be swallowed whole to prevent severe stomach cramping. Also, antacids or milk should not be given concomitantly with biscodyl.

DIARRHEA

Simply defined diarrhea is a precipitous passage of poorly formed stools. Bowel movement frequency and fluidity increase significantly, resulting in fluid and electrolyte loss.

Worldwide diarrheal episodes affect at least three quarters of a billion people. Over five million deaths are the direct consequences of severe dehydration due to diarrhea. Young children under the age of 5 and elderly, debilitated individuals suffer the worse from dehydrating effects of diarrhea.

Probably the two most important things to remember are that diarrhea is not a disease but a sign of an underlying problem and that supportive therapy is critical in minimizing morbidity and mortality.

Etiology

Diarrhea is a symptom in literally dozens of disorders (3). Table 18.5 lists some of the more common causes of diarrhea. Note that many of these are treatable if an early and accurate diagnosis is made. It is most important to initiate medical follow-up whenever there is a suggestion that the diarrhea is not the simple, self-limiting variety. Aside from various endocrine and neoplastic disorders, the most frequently seen cases requiring treatment are infectious in origin. These infectious agents include various bacteria which either produce enterotoxins which adversely affect absorption or secretion of electrolytes and fluids in the intestines or cause mucosal damage by actually invading the gut walls.

Escherichia coli, Staphylococcus aureus, Vibrio sp. and *Clostridia* sp. produce enterotoxins which stimulate adenylcyclase and increase cyclic AMP. This causes chloride ions and

Table 18.5.
Common Causes of Diarrhea

Viral gastroenteritis
Bacterial gastroenteritis
Protozoan gastroenteritis
Medications, e.g., laxative abuse, antibiotics
Irritable bowel syndrome
Diverticulitis
Ulcerative colitis
Diabetic neuropathy
Malabsorption syndrome
Gluten enteropathy
Surgery
Uremia
Endocrine/metabolic diseases, e.g., hyperthyroidism
Neoplasms
Drug withdrawal, e.g., opiates, barbiturates

water to be secreted and sodium ion absorption to decrease. The net result is an increase in fluid and electrolytes in the stool. *Shigella* sp., *Salmonella* sp. and invasive *E. coli* actually invade the epitheleal mucosa and damage it so that absorption is greatly decreased. This invasive type infection leads to a severe dysentary syndrome (Chapter 8).

Traveler's diarrhea is the infamous "turista" many of us suffer when visiting foreign climes. Among the various agents causing "turista" enterotoxigenic *E. coli* is the most common. (10). Shigellae, salmonella and various viruses are less common causative agents. *Giardia lamblia* is often seen in delayed onset of traveler's diarrhea. *Entamoeba histolytica* is common among institutionalized people, migrant workers and among travelers. In all these cases the infection is usually the result of contaminated food and drink due to poor sanitation and lack of adequate hygiene.

Infantile diarrhea is a common pediatric problem, usually caused by rotoviruses (11). Adenovirus, parvovirus-like agents, coxsackievirus and echovirus are also seen. Bacterial agents are implicated in some instances.

Drug-induced diarrhea secondary to antibiotic therapy is well recognized (12). Many broad-spectrum antibiotics have been implicated, including chloramphenicol, neomycin, erythromycin, cephalosporins, tetracyclines, ampicillin, clindamycin, lincomycin, sulfonamides, trimethoprim and metronidazole. The primary cause is the secondary overgrowth of antibiotic resistant bacteria and fungi. The initial disruption of the gut flora occurs after several days of therapy. Usually, these episodes are self-limiting and do not require changing antibiotic therapy.

However, a more severe pseudomembranous colitis clinical picture can develop from the overgrowth of *Clostria difficile*, which produces a bacterial toxin. *C. difficile* and the cytopathic toxin can be detected in laboratory cultures.

Other drugs cause diarrhea. The most common culprits are the various laxatives, especially magnesium-containing antacids. Other common drugs associated with diarrhea are alcohol and caffeine. Bethanacol, reserpine, methyldopa and guanethidine are prescription items often causing diarrhea.

Drug withdrawal from alcohol, barbiturates, sedative-hypnotics and opiates usually presents with a myriad of constitutional complaints, including diarrhea. Many times these complaints are ignored by health professionals as they continue to unknowingly provide medications that are misused.

Food-induced diarrhea occurs when individuals cannot properly digest certain foods. Milk intolerance is very common among elderly people who have decreased lactase and cannot digest lactose or sucrose. These then produce an osmotic gradient and pH changes which lead to increased secretion of fluid and electrolyte into the gut. Similarly, steatorrhea may be due to a patient's inability to digest gluten in celiac disease or due to a lack of pancreatic enzymes.

Incidence

The incidence of diarrhea is higher in the very young, the elderly and the debilitated individuals. Obviously, poor sanitary conditions will increase the chances of exposure to causative infectious agents and compound the problems of instituting adequate treatment methods. Iatrogenic causes of diarrhea occur with different frequency rates depending on the causative agents involved. Laxative abuse and alcohol abuse are the most common drug-induced causes.

Diagnosis and Clinical Findings

Diarrhea can be acute or chronic. The former type is usually infectious or iatrogenic in origin, while the latter is usually associated with other medical disorder, such as Crohn's disease, ulcerative colitis, neoplasms or endocrine disorders.

Acute diarrhea has a sudden onset of frequent, liquid stools. There may be general weakness, abdominal cramping pain, muscle pain and flatulence. Fever may be present. Nausea and vomiting are common. Provided that severe dehydration is not present, these acute episodes are self-limiting and usually resolve after a few days. Unidentified infectious agents are the usual cause (3).

In chronic diarrhea one sees a functional syndrome with recurring episodes lasting several weeks in duration, although actual diarrhea may not be a daily event. When the actual cause is a chronic disease, like ulcerative colitis, psychogenic factors tend to be important. Chronic diarrhea with no medical findings of chronic disease or neoplasm suggests laxative abuse or drug withdrawal as possible causes.

Three different clinical pictures are seen in chronic diarrhea. One type involves frequent, small stools with tenesmus. A second type exhibits as large, oily and malodorous formed stools. The third type involves frequent and voluminous loosely formed stools. Chronic weakness, anorexia and weight loss are common.

With infectious diarrhea one sees either a cholera-type syndrome, suggesting small bowel involvement, or the invasive-type syndrome, suggesting large bowel involvement. The cholera-type syndrome shows large volumes of watery stools with a low grade fever. Nausea, vomiting and abdominal cramps may be present to varying degrees. With the invasive-type syndrome, one sees a dysentery condition with fever, painful abdominal cramps and tenesmus. The bowel movements will usually be small and frequent. Stools will often contain pus and blood.

In 90% of all infectious diarrhea no etiologic agent is identified. Stool cultures may be necessary in severe cases to identify causative agents so that proper treatment may be instituted. This is extremely critical whenever severe antibiotic-induced diarrhea is suspected.

Pseudomembranous colitis is a life-threatening iatrogenic disease requiring medical intervention (see Chapter 15, *Ulcerative Colitis*). It develops 4 to 10 days after initiating antibiotic therapy and presents with voluminous mucous fluid, fever and abdominal pain. Diagnosis can be made by an antitoxin neutralization test (*Clostridium sordellii*) which detects the presence of the cytotoxin produced by an overgrowth of *C. difficile*. On sigmoidoscopy and colonoscopy one finds an edematous mucosa with raised, yellow-white exudative plaques that are characteristic of this type of colitis.

Treatment

BASIC APPROACH

Assessing a patient presenting with a complaint of diarrhea requires obtaining a detailed history about past and current medical problems, medications, onset and duration of problem, exact symptoms and suspected precipitating factors. If the patient has used successful remedies in the past, ascertain what these were. Be sure to check for laxative or alcohol misuse. Be sure to assess dietary habits, especially any unusual ones. For example, health food advocates often drink unpasteurized milk which can be a source of salmonella.

If the current episodes appears to be a simple case of diarrhea, then institute basic therapy of rehydration, resting of the gut by taking only clear liquids and easily digested foods for a day or so. Tell the patient that if the problem does not clear up within a couple of days to contact a physician.

Patients presenting with diarrhea with blood in the stool, abdominal tenderness, high fever, significant dehydration, severe weight loss or protracted diarrhea of more than 2 days duration should be referred for medical evaluation. Likewise, infants and young children, elderly people with other medical problems, the chronically ill and pregnant women should be seen by their physician first.

Prevention of infectious diarrhea requires educating the public about the hazzards of poor sanitation and hygenic practices. Whenever one is in such an area, it is best to avoid unbottled water, including ice cubes. Drink carbonated beverages, wine, beer or bottled water. Do not use the tap or well water for brushing teeth. Peel all fruits and vegetables.

Non-drug treatment will often suffice. Primary emphasis should be placed on getting the intestines to function normally and minimize dehydration. Bed rest and resting the gut by withholding food and drink for 4 to 6 hours should be done, if possible. Then follow with clear liquids, e.g., soda, Gatorade, liquid gelatin, or one of the commercially or homemade electrolyte solutions. (See discussion under "Rehydration" and Tables 18.6 and 18.7.) Begin with small, frequent quantities. After 24 hours easily digestible foods may be given. Then gradually work up to a regular diet. One may

Table 18.6.
World Health Organization Recommendation for Oral Rehydration Solution

Ingredient	Concentration	Ingredient in 1 L of Water
Glucose	111 mmol/L (2%)	20 g (glucose)
Sodium	90 mmol/L (90 mEq/L)	3.5 g (NaCl)
Potassium	20 mmol/L (20 mEq/L)	1.5 g (KCl)
Chloride	80 mmol/L (80 mEq/L)	
Bicarbon-ate	30 mmol/L (30 mEq/L)	2.5 g (NaHCO$_3$)

Table 18.7.
Commercially Available Oral Electrolyte Solutions[a]

Electrolyte	Lytren (Mead Johnson) (Mixed Glucose Forms)	Pedialyte (Ross) (Glucose 5% (50 g))	Pedialite R.S. (glucose 2½%)	Oral Electrolyte Solution (Wyeth)	Hydra-lyte (Jayco) (Mixed Glucose Forms 2%)	Infalyte (Penn-walt) (Glucose 2%)
Sodium	30	30	60	30	84	50
Potassium	25	20	20	20	10	20
Chloride	25	30	50	30	59	40
Bicarbonate	0	0	0	0	10	30
Calcium	4	4	0	4	0	0
Magnesium	4	4	0	4	0	0
Citrate	36	28	0	23	20	0
Sulfate	4	0	0	0	0	0
Phosphorus	5	0	0	5	0	0

[a] Values are milliequivalents per liter (mEq/L).

need to avoid milk products and fruits for several days.

REHYDRATION

The major metabolic consequences of diarrhea are dehydration, metabolic acidosis and potassium deficiency. These are the consequences of altering the absorption and secretion functions of the intestines. Most commonly these alterations are the result of enterotoxins produced by bacteria or by the mucosal damage done by invasive bacteria.

It has been well established that proper rehydration will minimize problems in even the most severely dehydrated patient (13). Oral rehydration is recommended by the World Health Organization (WHO) in lesser developed countries and this technique has proven to be very effective. Table 18.6 describes the solution recommended by the WHO (14). Care must be taken not to use high sodium solutions in excess of 90 mmol/liter because severe hypernatremia can develop, especially in children. In comparison with commercially available solutions the WHO solution contains less glucose and more sodium, but is almost isotonic. Too high a glucose concentration can cause increased fluid loss. Sucrose may be substituted for glucose, using 40 g of sucrose per liter. It is equally efficatious except if the patient has disaccharidase or sucrase deficiency.

The basis for oral rehydration is the glucose facilitated sodium absorption in the small intestines. In severe diarrhea, passive sodium diffusion and the active sodium pump mechanism are not functioning properly. However, the glucose-facilitated sodium absorption remains intact. Glucose concentration should be between 80 to 120 mmol/liter to optimize this absorption process. Glucose concentrations in excess of 160 mmol/liter will create an osmotic gradient that results in a net loss of electrolytes and water.

Oral rehydration should be used in treating mild to moderate diarrhea. The volume of oral solution to use can be estimated by using approximately 7.5% of body water over about 4 hours. Minimum replacement and maintenance for an adult is 2 or 3 quarts per day. For children, an estimate of 2400 ml per square meter of body surface may be used initially. Decrease amounts as other electrolyte fluids and food are increased in diet.

Severely dehydrated patients with greater than 7.5% loss of body water should be hospitalized, if possible to minimize severe complications and death. These patients should receive electrolyte solution intravenously. Ringer's lactate solution has been recommended, but must be used carefully to avoid lactic acidosis. Adjustments in electrolyte composition should be based on blood chemistry evaluations. Monitoring either therapeutic technique should include periodic evaluation of hydration status, determination of approximate fluid loss, measurement of fluid intake and urine output.

DRUG THERAPY

Three types of drugs are used in the treatment of diarrhea (15, 16). The first type is used for treating the primary cause, e.g. certain infectious types of diarrhea. Table 18.8 lists some of the specific antiinfectives that are indicated in these cases. Note that antibiotics will not alter the natural history of acute gastritis.

Enterotoxigenic E. coli diarrhea may be prevented with doxycycline in 200-mg daily doses (19). Some of these E. coli may be resistant. Doxycycline can itself cause diarrhea. Trimethoprim-sulfamethoxazole (160 mg-800 mg) twice daily for 5 days may be effective against E. coli or Shigella. Rare skin reactions may occur, including Stevens-Johnson syndrome.

Iodochlorhydroxyquin was used worldwide to treat traveler's diarrhea. However, serious subacute myelo-opticoneuropathy is a common adverse effect. The FDA removed it from the U.S. market; however, it is still available overseas even though no clinical evidence supports its effectiveness.

Protozoan-induced diarrhea may be treated with metronidazole. Adult dose for giardiasis is 250 mg, 3 times daily for 7 days. The pediatric dose is 15 mg/kg per 24 hours in divided doses. Amebiasis is treated with 750 mg, 3 times daily for 10 days in adults and 35 to 50 mg/kg per 24 hours in children.

For antibiotic-induced diarrhea, oral vancomycin should be used if there is evidence of

Table 18.8.
Treatment of Acute Infective Diarrhea

Type	Treatment
Viral	Usually self-limiting: fluids, rest, diet
Bacterial	
Escherichia coli	Fluids/electrolytes Tetracycline 500 mg q.i.d.
Shigella (severe fevers, chills, shock)	Ampicillin 1 g q.i.d. Trimethoprim-sulfamethoxazole 2 tablets b.i.d.
Salmonella (septicemia)	Ampicillin 1 g q.i.d.
Campylobacter (severe)	Erythromycin 1 g daily
Yersinia enterocolitica	Tetracycline 500 mg q.i.d. for 7 days
Clostridium difficile	Vancomycin 500 mg q6h
Protozoal	
Giardia lamblia	Metronidazole 2 g daily for 3 days
Entamoeba histolytica	Metronidazole 800 mg t.i.d. for 5 days

staphylococcal enterocolitis. If no secondary staphylococcus infection is present, changing the antibiotic agent may be all that is necessary along with rehydration (20).

Drugs used to treat the various endocrine and gastrointestinal disorders are discussed in other chapters of this text. The second type of drug is that used for fluid and electrolyte replacement as already discussed.

The third group of drugs are those used to relieve specific symptoms. These can be divided into four categories: those that absorb water, those that absorb toxins, those that alter gut motility, and those that alter electrolyte transport and secretion. The FDA recognizes only opiates and derivatives and polycarbophil as safe and effective for the symptomatic relief (17). Other nonprescription antidiarrheal ingredients are safe but actual effectiveness has not been proven in controlled clinical trials.

The Medical Letter noted that calcium polycarbophil may be effective (18). It supposedly acts in a similar manner as do other bulk laxatives by retaining water in the bowel and acting as a "hydrophilic stool normalizer." Onset of action may take as long as 48 hours. The usual adult dose is 4 to 6 g daily. Polycarbophil is nonabsorbable and metabolically inert. The only adverse effects reported are epigastric discomfort, bloating and flatus. It should not be used in young children or in suspected bowel obstruction. Other absorbing agents (methycelluose or psyllium) modify frequency and stool consistency but do not significantly alter fluid loss.

Opiates appear to function primarily as antiperistaltics, decreasing propulsive movements of the small intestines and colon. They cause increased tone and segmenting activity which decreases luminal transit. This alleviates cramping and stool frequency, but does not necessarily decrease fluid loss. Furthermore, in infectious diarrhea these agents may actually prolong or worsen the problem by preventing expulsion of the causative agents and should probably not be used in these types of diarrhea (21). They must also be used cautiously in ulcerative colitis to prevent megacolon.

The effective dose of paragoric is 1 teaspoon which is equivalent to about 15 to 20 mg of opium. Equivalent dose for diphenoxylate is 1 to 2 tablets every 6 hours as needed. Codeine is effective in doses of 45 to 60 mg daily in divided doses. Although these agents are relatively safe, be alert for respiratory depression. As little as 4 Lomotil tablets can be lethal in a child. None of these increase anal sphincter tone so leakage may still occur with attendant problems (22).

Loperamide has similar action to diphenoxylate (23). It may also alter the sodium pump to decrease fluid secretion. The effective dose is 4 mg initially followed by 2 mg after each loose bowel movement up to 16 mg daily. There appear to be no opiate effects at these doses. It does increase anal sphincter tone and may be useful in the incontinent patient.

The most frequently used over-the-counter antidiarrheal are the absorbents. They are safe but not necessarily effective. Theoretically these agents adsorb the various enterotoxins. They may also adsorb other compounds including nutrients and medications. They are relatively inert. Included in this group are activated charcoal, aluminum hydroxide, attapulgite, pectin, kaolin, magnesium trisilicate and cholestryamine.

One adsorbent may be effective in treating "turista." Bismuth subsalicylate (Pepto-Bismol) in large doses (60 ml) can prevent traveler's diarrhea. In acute "turista" one should use 30 to 60 ml at 30- to 60-min intervals up to 8 doses (24–26). The only significant problems associated with this dosage is increased salicylate levels which could become toxic if a patient is already receiving high dose salicylates for arthritis. Significant drug interactions can occur in patients also taking coumadin, probenecid, sulfinpyraxone or methotrexate.

Anticholinergics like belladonna alkaloids decrease gut contractility and relieve cramping pain but they do not decrease fluid loss. Most over-the-counter products do not contain effective dosage. Approximately 0.6 to 1 mg atropine sulfate equivalent is necessary. This amount can be obtained only by prescription. Anticholinergics have a very narrow therapeutic index, especially in the very young and very old. They can also exacerbate glaucoma, cause drug-induced organic brain syndrome (OBS) and severe CNS depression in higher doses.

Lactobacillus has not been shown to be effective in controlled studies. The purported mechanism of action is the reestablishment of normal gut flora. One probably gets the same effect by eating yogurt and it is less expensive and more nutritious.

Cromolyn sodium may be effective in persistent diarrhea not responding well to other standard therapy. Speculation is that responding individuals may actually be suffering from a food-induced, allergic diarrhea, which responds to cromolyn sodium (27).

CONCLUSION

Constipation and diarrhea affect everyone at one time or another throughout life. Fortunately these problems are usually self-limiting and can be controlled by minimal medical and pharmacological intervention.

Pharmacists are afforded a key role in assisting consumers with simple bowel problems. First, the triage function by pharmacists to identify those complaints which warrant medical referral should not be overlooked. When bowel irregularity is a complaint resulting from a more serious condition, early detection and treatment will reduce both morbidity and mortality. Second, the pharmacist functioning as a health educator should take the opportunity to provide the dietary, hygiene and exercise information most consumers do not have regarding a more holistic approach to resolving and preventing simple bowel problems. Third, proper medication monitoring will allow the pharmacist to properly intervene and inform physicians about patients suffering from side effects of necessary drug therapy or detect other correctable medication problems. Finally, when a consumer must use a laxative or antidiarrheal product, the pharmacist should offer informed advice for selecting the right product for a given problem.

Perhaps the most important consideration for the practicing pharmacist is to be sure to intervene whenever presented with a complaint or question regarding gastrointestinal problems. Complacency will at best lead to inappropriate medication use or nonuse. At worse it will lead to serious medical consequences which could have been prevented.

References

1. Anon: The selection of essential drugs. *WHO Tec Rep Ser* 641, 1979.
2. Schedl HD: Water and electrolyte transport—clinical aspects. *Med Clin North Am* 58:1429–1448, 1974.
3. Phillips SF: Diarrhea: a current view of the pathophysiology. *Gastroenterology* 63:495, 1972.
4. Binder HJ: Pharmacology of laxatives. *Annu Rev Pharmacol Toxicol* 17:355–367, 1977.
5. Mercer RD: Constipation. *Pediatr Clin North Am* 14:175–185, 1967.

6. Binder HJ, Donowitz M: A new look at laxatives action. *Gastroenterology* 69:1001–1005, 1975.
7. Anon: Safety of stool softeners. *Med Lett* 19:45–46, 1977.
8. Goodman LS, Gilman A (eds): *The Pharmacological Basis of Therapeutics.* New York: Macmillan, 1980, pp 120, 513, 1002.
9. Anon: Lactulose (Chronulac) for constipation. *Med Lett* 22:20–4, 1980.
10. Anon: Traveler's diarrhea. *Med Lett* 21:41–43, 1979.
11. Hirschorn N: The treatment of acute diarrhea in children. *Clin Nutr* 33:637–663, 1980.
12. Anon: Antibiotic colitis—new cause, new treatment. *Med Let* 21:97–98, 1979.
13. Anon: Oral rehydration solutions. *Med Lett* 25:19–20, 1983.
14. Sack DA: Treatment of acute diarrhea with oral rehydration solution. *Drugs* 23:150–157, 1982.
15. Bradshaw MJ, Harvey RF: Antidiarrheal agents clinical pharmacology and therapeutic use. *Drugs* 24:440–451, 1982.
16. Anon: Immunizations and chemoprophylaxis for travelers. *Med Lett* 25:37–40, 1983.
17. Anon: Guidelines for the clinical evaluation of antidiarrheal drugs. *HEW (FDA)* 78:3049, 1977.
18. Anon: Calcium polycarbophil (Mitrolan). *Med Let* 23:52, 1981.
19. Sack RB, Froelich JL, Zulich AW, et al: Prophylactic doxycycline for traveler's diarrhea. *Gastroenterology* 76:1368–1373, 1979.
20. Tedesco F, Markham R, Gurwith M, et al: Oral vancomycin antibiotic-associated pseudomembranous colitis. *Lancet* 2:226, 1978.
21. Dupont HL, Hornick RB: Adverse effect of Lomotil therapy in shigellosis. *JAMA* 226:1525–1528, 1973.
22. Harford WV, Krejs GJ, Santa Ana CA, et al: Acute effect of diphenoxylate with atropine (Lomotil) in patients with chronic diarrhea and fecal inconsistence. *Gastroenterology* 78:440–443, 1980.
23. Corbett CL, Palmer KR, Holdsworth CD: Effect of loperamide, codeine phosphate and diphenoxylate on urgency and incontinence in chronic diarrhea. *Gut* 21:924, 1980.
24. Dupont HL, Sullivan P, Pickering LK, et al: Symptomatic treatment of diarrhea with bismuth subsalicylate among students attending a Mexican university. *Gastroenterology* 73:715–718, 1977.
25. Dupont HL, Sullivan P, Evans DG, et al: Prevention of traveler's diarrhea (emporiatric enteritis) prophylactic administration of subsalicylate bismuth. *JAMA* 243:237–241, 1980.
26. Anon: Salicylate in Pepto-Bismol. *Med Lett* 22:63, 1980.
27. Bolin JD: Use of oral sodium cromoglycate in persistant diarrhea. *Gut* 21:848–850, 1980.

SECTION 4
Cardiovascular Disorders

CHAPTER 19

Angina Pectoris

ARTHUR F. HARRALSON, Pharm.D.

Angina pectoris is a clinical syndrome characterized by substernal chest discomfort that is precipitated by effort and relieved by rest or nitroglycerin. This discomfort or pain may radiate to the neck, lower jaw, shoulder, or arm. Patients commonly decline to apply the word pain to their chest symptoms but will usually select words such as choking, heaviness, tightness, or squeezing to describe the sensation.

The manifestation of angina is usually due to ischemic heart disease and results from an imbalance in myocardial oxygen supply and demand. The pathologic lesion most frequently producing angina is an obstruction or narrowing of the coronary arteries caused by atherosclerosis. Other less frequently encountered causes may include coronary artery spasm, valvular heart disease, pulmonary hypertension, disease of the microcirculation, and myocardial hypertrophy.

TYPES OF ANGINA

Several types of angina pectoris have been identified based upon their clinical features. The "classical" type is often referred to as stable angina. This is the typical angina in which discomfort is precipitated by physical activity or emotional disturbance and is relieved by rest.

Another variety, unstable angina, is also referred to by several other names, such as crescendo angina, accelerated angina, preinfarction angina, and status anginosis. Angina of the unstable variety is characterized by an increase in duration, intensity, or frequency of symptoms and a decrease in responsiveness to treatment.

The term angina decubitis or nocturnal angina has been applied to the variant of angina pectoris which develops while the patient is in the recumbent position. The patient may report being awakened at night with pain or a sensation very similar to that experienced with exertion. The nocturnal angina syndrome is similar to that of paroxysmal nocturnal dyspnea, and dyspnea may often accompany the chest discomfort.

The terms prinzmetal or variant angina refer to the angina that occurs while the patient is at rest. An unusual characteristic of variant angina is S-T segment elevation on the electrocardiogram rather than S-T segment depression seen with "classical" angina. Variant angina is probably associated with coronary artery spasm and is usually less responsive to the usual forms of medical treatment (1).

NATURAL HISTORY AND RISK FACTORS

The general prognosis of patients who have been diagnosed as having angina pectoris has been shown to be progression to a fatal cardiovascular incident within 10 years. Mortality rates for specific types of angina, however, vary considerably. The mortality for patients with medically treated stable angina is about 4% per year, which is about twice the average mortality of the normal population (2). On the basis of coronary angiography, more diffuse disease is associated with poorer survival. The 5-year mortality rates for single, double, and triple vessel disease are 7%, 35%, and 45%, respectively (3).

Numerous risk factors associated with the developement of angina have been identified. Among the major risk factors that may contribute to the development of angina are high serum cholesterol, high blood pressure, cigarette smoking, diabetes mellitus, and certain electrocardiographic abnormalities (4–6). Anxiety, severe psychosocial problems, and so-called Type A behavior (hard driving, competitive, overly ambitious) may also be implicated as important risk factors (6, 7). Although modification of these factors may retard the development of angina, it is obvious that many of these factors cannot be easily changed.

HISTORY AND DIAGNOSIS

When a patient is encountered with the typical anginal discomfort, as described earlier, the diagnosis of angina should be seriously considered. Atypical features of the anginal pain syndrome are, however, common enough that additional evaluation is necessary to confirm the diagnosis. Other symptoms such as palpitations, lightheadedness, or breathlessness may occur in association with angina and may result from transient arrhythmias and ventricular dysfunction.

A previous history of myocardial infarction strongly suggests the presence of coronary atherosclerosis with ischemic heart disease. Histories of previous "heart attacks" require clarification by objective data or discussion with a reliable observer who was involved in the patient's care. A larger number of nonischemic cardiac episodes may referred to as "heart attacks." The diagnosis of a previous myocardial infarction may be missed on a historical basis because not all myocardial infarctions are painful.

PHYSICAL EXAMINATION

The physical examination of the patient thought to have angina pectoris is often normal. During an episode of pain, transient findings, such as as abnormal precordial bulge, atrial gallop, or heart murmur, may provide support for an ischemic origin of the symptoms. It is unlikely, however, that a physician will encounter an anginal episode during an examination, which represents the major shortcoming of the physical diagnosis of angina pectoris. The examination may, however, uncover other processes such as aortic stenosis, thyrotoxicosis, or anemia that may be responsible for anginal symptoms.

LABORATORY TECHNIQUES

There are numerous laboratory techniques available that may assist in the evaluation of patients thought to have angina pectoris. Each technique has certain advantages as well as disadvantages which will be reviewed.

Electrocardiography. The electrocardiogram is risk free, and is quick and easy to accomplish. Unfortunately, it is also found to be normal in many patients coronary heart disease. As many as 50 to 75% of patients with stable angina pectoris will have normal resting electrocardiograms at times when they are free from chest pain. An electrocardiogram recorded during an episode of chest pain will usually show displacement of the S-T segment (typically 1 mm of horizontal or downsloping depression) which returns to normal after re-

lief of discomfort. Variant angina may exhibit a paradoxical S-T segment elevation in association with pain. Other electrocardiographic abnormalities such as T-wave alterations, smaller S-T segment deviation, conduction disturbances, and arrhythmias are nonspecific and may occur in the absence of coronary heart disease. Single normal electrocardiograms are not sufficient to rule out acute ischemic episodes since changes may take hours to occur.

The findings of a previous myocardial infarction provide strong evidence for coronary obstructive disease. The classical electrocardiographic finding of a previous myocardial infarction is an abnormality of the initial portion of the QRS complex with forces directed away from the area of scarred myocardial tissue (usually a pathologic Q wave or negative deflection). In addition, S-T segments may become displaced and T-wave alterations may occur. In the presence of electrocardiographic changes, it is possible to determine the location of infarction by knowing which areas of the heart reflected by the various electrocardiographic leads.

Exercise Electrocardiography (Stress Testing). In view of the relative insensitivity of the electrocardiogram of a resting patient as a diagnostic test for ischemic heart disease, various exercise tests have been developed to provoke ischemic electrocardiographic changes. Exercise may be performed by walking on steps (Master's test), on a treadmill, or by pedaling a bicycle equipped with an ergometer.

The most commonly accepted criterion for ischemia is a 1-mm horizontal or downsloping S-T segment depression during, or immediately following, exercise. As a diagnostic tool, the exercise S-T segment response is of greatest value in male patients with normal resting electrocardiograms and exertional chest discomfort. In this group the test has a predictive accuracy of 95% and demonstrates that it is a highly reliable indicator of significant coronary heart disease. However, when exercise testing is used as a screening test for coronary disease in an asymptomatic population, its specificity is poor and there may be many false-positive tests. Further evidence indicates, however, that consideration of age, sex, duration of exercise before S-T segment change, and the depth of S-T depression may allow identification of certain subgroups within the asymptomatic population in which the exercise test may have greater predictive value.

False-positive tests are far more common in females than in males. The frequency of false-positive exercise tests in women with chest pain has been reported to be as high as 66% (8). Digitalis glycosides are a common pharmacologic cause of false-positive tests.

False-negative tests may also occur. The percentage of patients with significant coronary disease who have positive exercise tests is about 60%. This means that 40% of patients who have true coronary disease will have negative exercise tests. Among the pharmacologic agents that may produce false-negative exercise tests are nitrates and propranolol.

Obviously, patients with acute or very recent myocardial infarctions should not be exercise tested. Unstable angina, severe aortic stenosis, uncontrolled hypertension, or cardiac arrhythmias are other contraindications to exercise testing.

Radionuclide Imaging. Radionuclide imaging has only recently become widely available as a technique for evaluation of ischemic heart disease. The technique utilizes intravenous injection of radioactive tracer substances and precordial recording of radioactive emissions. Tracers such as thallium concentrate in myocardial cells in proportion to blood flow. Areas of ischemia or infarction appear as a zone of decreased tracer density in comparison with the surrounding myocardium (9).

Tracers such as technetium concentrate in areas of myocardial necrosis and appear as areas of increased tracer density. Patients with partial occlusion of coronary vessels may have normal perfusion of the myocardium at rest. These obstructive lesions, however, may now allow an adequate increase in blood flow to satisfy the metabolic demands of exercise and decreased tracer uptake may be uncovered only during exercise.

These studies may be particularly valuable in defining the significance of exercise-induced S-T segment depression in asymptomatic patients since a normal radionuclide scan during stress is unlikely to occur when there is a major obstructive coronary lesion. It may then be possible to differentiate true positive from false-positive exercise electrocardiograms when that procedure is used for screening asymptomatic populations.

Cardiac Catheterization. The role of cardiac catheterization in coronary heart disease is to confirm the diagnosis, estimate prognosis, and assist in establishing an optimal therapeutic plan.

One of the most common situations in which cardiac catheterization is of value is the evaluation of the patient with chest pain of uncertain etiology. Because of the many shortcomings of the noninvasive techniques previously discussed, cardiac catheterization remains the most definitive method of confirming or ruling out the diagnosis of angina pectoris due to obstructive coronary artery disease. When uncertainty exists regarding the etiology of chest pain, management of the patient may be vastly simplified by the presence of clear diagnostic information obtained by this technique.

Another indication for cardiac catheterization is the preoperative evaluation of symptomatic patients. Patients commonly considered for coronary bypass surgery include those with chronic anginal pain which cannot be satisfactorily controlled with medication, patients with unstable angina which continues despite bed rest and vigorous medical treatment, and patients with congestive heart failure due to mechanical complications of myocardial infarction.

Unlike the noninvasive techniques, there are definite risks associated with cardiac catheterization. These risks are generally less in laboratories where many studies are performed annually.

MANAGEMENT OF ANGINA: GENERAL

Although it is important to treat the underlying cause, this is possible in only a few circumstances, such as pulmonary hypertension, valvular heart disease, anemia, and thyrotoxicosis. Most patients with angina require primarily symptomatic treatment. The management objectives are not aimed at reversal of the disease process, but rather at slowing progression of the process. Successful management may be defined as a reduced frequency and severity of anginal attacks.

The first step is to avoid activities which can precipitate angina. These include eating heavy meals, getting emotionally upset, performing strenuous physical activity, and exposure to cold. Drinking beverages which contain caffeine (colas, coffee, tea) may precipitate angina in some patients. Cigarette smoking can increase heart rate and blood pressure in addition to impairing myocardial oxygen delivery in some individuals. Cigarette smoking should be stopped in all patients, if possible. Other contributory disease states such as hypertension, hyperlipidemia, anemia, hyperthyroidism, and cardiac arrhythmias should be adequately controlled.

Pharmacists should pay particular attention to the medications that the angina patient may use. Many over-the-counter (OTC) preparations contain sympathomimetic amines and can increase heart rate or blood pressure and may precipitate an anginal attack. Other drugs such as thyroid preparations, amphetamines, ergot alkaloids, methysergide, hydralazine, and diazoxide can all precipitate an anginal attack and should be avoided if at all possible (10, 11).

DRUG TREATMENT

The critical evaluation of agents used in the treatment of angina pectoris is complicated by the fact that objective evaluation of any syndrome is at best difficult and subject to any number of variables. Considering the large number of factors that may be involved in a patient's perception of their anginal distress, documenting the extent to which changes in this perception can reasonably be attributed to a particular drug regimen is extremely difficult. The development of sophisticated methods for evaluating hemodynamic alterations and improved electrocardiographic patterns with antianginal agents has dramatically improved our understanding of the pathophysiology of angina, but still has not solved all the problems encountered in the management of the angina patient. The ultimate value of any antianginal regimen still depends upon the patient's perception of a significant improvement in their angina-related distress.

Many agents have been tested for use in the treatment of angina, but few, if any, have been shown to be unequivocally superior to the nitrite group of drugs. The nitrite group (which includes nitrates, organic nitrites, and nitrite ion) has remained the mainstay of the medical treatment of angina pectoris through controlled clinical trials and extensive clinical use over many years. Other drugs that may be considered for use in some patients include β-adrenergic blocking agents and sedatives. Digitalis and diuretic agents have a role in the treatment of patients with angina that is exacerbated by congestive heart failure.

Nitrates and Nitrites (Table 19.1)

The term nitrate is often used generically when referring to any one or all of the compounds in the nitrite group. The principal pharmacologic action shared qualitatively by all of these agents is the direct relaxation of smooth muscle, including that of bronchial, gastrointestinal, and vascular sites.

The metabolic fate of these various organic nitrates has been extensively studied, but many questions concerning the pharmacology of these agents remain unanswered. All parent compounds in this group, as well as their active metabolites, are rapidly denitrated by the liver's glutathione reductase system. The activity of this glutathione reductase system is remarkably high and most active nitrates are quickly denitrated to comparatively inactive compounds. The metabolism of some of these compounds, such as the highly active trinitrate metabolite, is so rapid that little if any can be detected in the bloodstream. In contrast to the rapid clearance of active nitrate compounds, the substantially less active mononitrates and dinitrates can be found circulating in the blood for many hours and represent the major metabolite found in the urine. The amount of endogenous hepatic glutathione present appears to be the rate limiting step in the denitration of nitrates. Further evidence indicates that the circulation of large amounts of nitrates through the liver as with nitroglycerin infusion could result in depletion of glutathione and lead to marked impairment of the inactivation process.

Mechanism of Action. Despite the many years of continued and successful use of nitrates to treat angina pectoris, the specific mechanism of action responsible for the alleviation of anginal distress is still not completely understood and remains somewhat controversial.

There are currently two principal theories used to explain the therapeutic action of nitrates in the reduction of pain from stable angina pectoris. The first of these holds that nitrates improve the delivery of oxygen to ischemic tissue by producing a redistribution of regional myocardial blood flow in addition to augmenting total myocardial blood flow as a result of coornary vasodilation (12). The second theory asserts that nitrates are effective in improving the imbalance between myocardial oxygen supply and demand (10).

Table 19.1.
Nitrates

Generic Name	Brand Names	Dosage Forms	Usual Dosage
Nitroglycerin (glyceryl trinitrate)	Nitrostat	0.15, 0.3, 0.4, 0.6 mg sublingual tablet	1 tablet p.r.n. sublingually, but not more than 3 within 15 min
	Nitroglyn	1.3, 2.6, 6.5 mg oral (sustained release) tablet	1 tablet b.i.d./t.i.d.
	Nitrospan	2.5 mg oral (sustained release) capsule	1 capsule q12h
	Nitro-Bid	2.5, 6.5 mg oral (sustained release) capsule	2.5–6.5 mg q8–12h
	Nitro-Bid	2% ointment	2–5 inches applied to skin q3–4h p.r.n.
	Nitrol	2% ointment	2–5 inches applied to skin q3–4h p.r.n.
	Nitrong	2% ointment	2–5 inches applied to skin q3–4h p.r.n.
	Transderm-Nitro 5	10 cm^2 disc (25 mg)	Once daily (delivers 5 mg)
	Transderm-Nitro 10	20 cm^2 disc (50 mg)	Once daily (delivers 10 mg)
	Nitro-Dur 5	5 cm^2 disc (26 mg)	Once daily (delivers 2.5 mg)
	Nitro-Dur 10	10 cm^2 disc (51 mg)	Once daily (delivers 5 mg)
	Nitro-Dur 15	15 cm^2 disc (77 mg)	Once daily (delivers 7.5 mg)
	Nitro-Dur 20	20 cm^2 disc (104 mg)	Once daily (delivers 10 mg)
	Nitro-Dur 30	30 cm^2 disc (154 mg)	Once daily (delivers 15 mg)
	Nitrodisc 5	9 cm^2 disc (16 mg)	Once daily (delivers 5 mg)
	Nitrodisc 10	16 cm^2 disc (32 mg)	Once daily (delivers 10 mg)
Isosorbide dinitrate	Isordil, Sorbitrate	2.5, 5 mg sublingual tablet	2.5–5 mg q2–3h p.r.n.
	Isordil, Sorbitrate	5, 10, 20 mg oral tablet	10–20 mg q.i.d.
	Isordil Tembid	40 mg oral (sustained release) tablet/capsule	40 mg q6–12h
	Sorbitrate	40 mg (sustained release) tablet	40 mg q6–12h
	Sorbitrate Chewable	5 mg chewable tablet	5 mg p.r.n.
	Isordil	10 mg chewable tablet	10 mg p.r.n.
Erythrityl tetranitrate	Cardilate	5, 10, 15 mg sublingual and oral tablet; 10 mg chewable tablet	5 mg sublingual, 10 mg orally or chewed t.i.d.
Pentaerythritol tetranitrate	Peritrate	10, 20 mg oral tablet	10–20 mg q.i.d.
	Peritrate SA	80 mg oral (sustained release) tablet	80 mg q12h
	Duotrate	30, 45 mg (sustained release) capsule	30–45 mg q12h
Mannitol Hexanitrate	Nitranitol	30 mg oral tablet	1 tablet q.i.d.

The evidence substantiating the hypothesis that increased delivery of oxygen to the myocardium represents the primary in reduction of anginal pain is somewhat tenuous. Some investigators (using coronary arteriography) have reported nitroglycerin's ability to produce coronary artery dilation even in the presence of coronary artery disease (11). Others have demonstrated only moderate alterations in coronary blood flow in response to nitroglycerin (13). Clear-cut decreases in coronary resistance and increases in total blood flow can be demonstrated in laboratory animals and man, but these effects are considerably more transient than would seem compatible with duration of action of nitroglycerin assessed by peripheral vascular or therapeutic criteria. In most angina patients treated with nitroglycerin, coronary resistance is only transiently decreased or remains unaltered, and coronary blood flow in such individuals tends to decrease in parallel with any fall in blood pressure (14). Nitrates do produce a more persistent dilation of large coronary vessels, but the extent to which this effect interfaces with alterations in smaller vessels and ischemic tissue awaits more extensive investigation. Even if one acknowledges that nitroglycerin produces some increases in total coronary blood flow, evidence clearly demonstrating that increased flow reaches and substantially affects areas of ischemia appears to be lacking. It has also been suggested that if small arterioles do dilate in nonobstructed areas, a situation may arise in which there is a shunting of blood away from areas of ischemia, a so-called "coronary steal" (15). Some evidence that direct coronary dilation does not represent the primary mechanism for the relief of anginal pain can also be found in the action of the drug dipyridamole. Dipyridamole has been shown to be a very potent dilator of coronary arteries yet appears relatively ineffective in relieving anginal pain (16, 17). Likewise, direct injection of nitroglycerin into coronary arteries increases blood flow but appears not to provide relief from anginal pain, other than that associated with vasospasm unless accompanied by systemic administration of nitroglycerin (18).

The second hypothesis used to explain the relief of anginal pain by nitrates asserts that nitroglycerin favorably alters the relation between myocardial oxygen supply and demand by its effects on the principal determinants of oxygen consumption. Those favoring this second hypothesis appear to have the best supporting documentation at this time (19–21).

In patients with symptomatic coronary disease a significant restriction of myocardial oxygen supply often exists as a result of the presence of one or more stenotic lesions of the coronary arteries. The presence of substantial coronary artery stenosis represents practical and finite limits to the extent to which alterations in oxygen supply could reasonably be expected to improve unfavorable supply and demand situations. For this reason, the probability of achieving a beneficial alteration in the myocardial oxygen supply and demand

relationship would seem greatest with therapeutic strategies that focus on reduction of oxygen consumption.

Among the more important determinants of myocardial oxygen consumption that must be considered are heart rate, the contractile state of the heart, and the intramyocardial tension (the product of ventricular systolic pressure multiplied by a term representing ventricular volume) (Table 19.2). Most investigations into the mechanism of action of nitroglycerin have involved the analysis of one or more of the previously mentioned determinants of myocardial oxygen consumption by indirect methods. Any conclusions concerning nitroglycerin's effect on local myocardial oxygen consumption based upon indirect measurements of this type must be viewed with caution.

Direct quantitation of changes in myocardial oxygen consumption made by measurement of changes in oxygen content in arterial and venous blood leave many unresolved questions. Critical evaluation of this method of analysis reveals several problems that may serve to produce more confusion about myocardial consumption than it solves. As an example, the distribution of blood flow to the left ventricle of patients with coronary artery disease is known to be heterogenous and changes in total oxygen consumption cannot be assumed to reflect local alterations in oxygen consumption which may be of much greater importance.

When used in the usual therapeutic doses, sublingual nitroglycerin is known to reduce venous vascular tone which produces pooling of blood in peripheral veins. In patients without severe congestive heart failure, this peripheral pooling results in a decrease in cardiac output, ventricular volume, stroke volume, and left ventricular end-diastolic pressure (decreased myocardial preload) (19). The

Table 19.2.
Effects of Nitrates and β-Blockers on the Major Determinants of Myocardial Oxygen Consumption (MVO$_2$)

Determinants of MVO$_2$	Nitrates	β-Blockade
Heart rate	↑ (reflex)	↓
Contractility	↑ (reflex)	↓
Intramyocardial tension		
A. Vent. syst. pressure	↓	↑
B. Vent. vol. (factor)	↓	↑

resultant reduction in heart size lowers the intramyocardial tension which in turn decreases myocardial oxygen requirements. Nitroglycerin also produces a certain amount of arteriolar dilation which may lower arterial pressure. The resultant decrease in intraventricular pressure in conjunction with a decrease in resistance to left ventricular ejection (decreased myocardial afterload) lowers oxygen even further.

Nitroglycerin can also increase heart rate as well as the contractile state of the heart resulting in a detrimental increase in myocardial oxygen needs. The net effect of nitroglycerin is, however, to decrease myocardial oxygen consumption by a quantitatively more important reduction in ventricular wall tension. The decrease in ventricular systolic and diastolic dimensions occurs within minutes after the use of sublingual nitroglycerin. The temporal relationship between this hemodynamic response and the classical response to the administration of nitroglycerin is quite striking (19). When measured by the technique of precordial S-T segment mapping, nitroglycerin consistently shows reductions in magnitude in regions presumed to represent areas of myocardial ischemia (22).

The majority of evidence available to date appears to lend most support to the hypothesis that the reduction in anginal pain by nitroglycerin is primarily a result of reduced myocardial oxygen consumption secondary to the peripheral effects of the nitrate. However, the importance of regional distribution of myocardial blood flow to the survival of ischemic myocardium is not well understood and certainly should not be discounted on the basis of information available at this time.

Nitroglycerin. Nitroglycerin represents the oldest and probably the most important vasodilator agent used in the treatment of conditions involving tissue ischemia. It has been used for over 100 years and still maintains a dominant position in the traditional medical treatment of angina pectoris.

The well-recognized efficacy of nitroglycerin as an antianginal agent can be extensively documented by both objective and subjective evidence (23). The relief of anginal pain by nitroglycerin is thought to be so predictable by some investigators that they advocate its use as a diagnostic test for the presence of myocardial ischemia (24). When evaluated by parameters such as pain relief, increased work performance, and improvement in electrocardiographic patterns after standardized exercise stress testing, nitroglycerin has been found to be effective in 90% of patients in some studies (25). In other studies of patients thought to have ischemic heart disease, nearly all patients tested showed relief from anginal pain after administration of nitroglycerin (24). Of those patients who did not exhibit this classical response, either no coronary heart disease could be identified or the patient was found to have very severe disease.

Because of the extremely rapid onset of action, sublingual nitroglycerin is an ideal preparation for acute relief of angina pectoris due to myocardial ischemia. The desired therapeutic response to nitroglycerin as measured by pain relief and favorable alterations in electrocardiographic patterns can be seen almost immediately upon administration of the drug. A study involving 49 patients with documented significant coronary artery disease demonstrated that at least 80% of these patients experienced relief of their anginal pain less than 3 min after receiving a sublingual dose (24). One third of these patients reported significant relief of symptoms in less than 1 min.

Accurate assessment of the duration of action of nitroglycerin in the relief of anginal pain presents quite a difficult problem since most anginal episodes last only a few minutes and pain often ceases if the patient stops the precipitating activity. The development of improved hemodynamic and electrocardiographic techniques permits assessment of the duration of some of nitroglycerin's complex pharmacologic actions. In a study in which forearm venous capacitance was used as a measure of the peripheral effects of nitroglycerin, the onset of action did not occur until 3 min after administration. The time to peak effect and the duration of action as measured by this method were 6 and 8 min, respectively (26). In view of the evidence supporting a much more rapid onset of action, it appears that symptomatic improvement can occur before the peripheral effects of nitroglycerin can be detected. Using increased exercise tolerance and improved electrocardiographic patterns as measurement parameters, nitroglycerin appears to have a duration of action of less than 30 min with a dose of 0.4 mg sublingually. The hemodynamic alterations induced by the same dose occur rapidly but are relatively short lived, lasting only 5 to 15 min (21).

When a patient experiences an episode of acute anginal pain all physical activity should be immediately stopped, a sitting position should be assumed, and 1 tablet from the patient's most recent nitroglycerin prescription should be administered sublingually (the use of agents other than sublingual nitroglycerin is discussed later). Additional doses can be administered every 3 to 4 min until relief is obtained. Pain, however, that is not relieved by 3 consecutive doses or that is out of character with the patient's usual anginal pattern should prompt an immediate visit to the nearest emergency room. At least initially, patients should be encouraged to remain in a sitting position rather than assuming standing or supine positions. Undesirable hemodynamic effects are less likely to occur if the sitting position is maintained initially. If the patient does experience syncope or excessive dizziness, he or she should then be placed in a supine position with their feet slightly elevated. Subsequent administration of additional doses of nitroglycerin, or other drugs may produce vasodilation, should be approached with caution.

It is generally acknowledged that the prophylactic use of nitroglycerin on an intermittent or short-term basis can play an important role in the overall management of the patient with angina pectoris. Demonstration of the efficacy of nitroglycerin when used prophylactically is most convincingly illustrated by the technique of exercise stress testing. When nitroglycerin is administered just prior to the testing procedure many patients are able to significantly increase their usual level of exertion before the appearance of subjective and electrocardiographic evidence of myocardial ischemia is noted (27). Nitroglycerin has also been shown to reduce the frequency of exertional arrhythmias that occur in patients with ischemic heart disease (28). The most compelling support for the use of nitroglycerin on a prophylactic basis is the potential it may provide for a patient to freely undertake necessary tasks and experience pleasures that are otherwise so closely coupled with the anticipation of anginal pain. When used prophylactically, nitroglycerin should be taken just prior to an event that is either known to, or could be expected to, precipitate an anginal attack.

Essentially all untoward responses encountered with the therapeutic use of nitroglycerin occur as a result of its pharmacologic actions on the cardiovascular system and include headache, dizziness, weakness, palpitations, and occasionally syncope. This remarkably small list comprises nearly the entire range of adverse effects attributed to this drug despite its high level of use. Although very rare, drug rash can be produced by all organic nitrates. This rash appears to occur most commonly with pentaerythritol tetranitrate.

Headaches represent the most frequently encountered side effect of nitroglycerin, with the reported incidence varying from 3% to as high as 50% in some groups. The majority of these headaches are of short duration, typically lasting less than 5 min, and are usually not severe enough to preclude use of the drug. The headache pain usually decreases over a few days with continued use, but dosage reduction may be necessary is certain instances. Analgesics such as aspirin or acetaminophen may offer relief to some patients. Although generally tolerable, patients can experience severe, prolonged, and disabling headaches from the use of nitroglycerin.

Transient episodes of dizziness or syncope are occasionally encountered with the use of nitroglycerin and are associated with postural hypotension. These episodes occur more frequently in elderly patients, in those taking other vasodilators, and with concomitant ingestion of alcohol. Procedures that facilitate venous return such as body positioning are usually sufficient to minimize this type of adverse response.

"Long Acting" Nitrates

The therapeutic effectiveness of sublingual nitroglycerin in the treatment of uncomplicated angina pectoris has been recognized for many years. The brief duration of action, however, has limited its role in the treatment of angina to acute situations or for prophylaxis of a distinctly transient nature. The anticipated value of an agent that might provide more sustained prophylaxis prompted extensive efforts to prolong the effects of nitroglycerin through alterations in molecular configuration and modes of administration. As a result of these efforts, a variety of so-called long nitrates were introduced and many are now extensively prescribed for angina prophylaxis. Although regarded by some as a mainstay of medical treatment of angina, critical questions concerning their efficacy and duration of actin remain unanswered. A great deal of the difficulty encountered in resolving these efficacy questions appears to be related to critical differences in the evaluation techniques employed by individual investigators. This can be clearly seen in subsequent reevaluation of those agents claiming prolonged efficacy. The results of nearly all of these studies have been challenged on the basis of critical faults in experimental design. The recent introduction of transdermal systems may provide the only true "long acting" nitrate based on the measurement of nitrates.

More recently, however, investigators have sought to avoid previous methodologic pitfalls by restoring to the use of extremely rigorous protocols. Strict and unwavering adherence to such protocols has resulted in the establishment of measurement parameters that are very sensitive, reliable, and can be consistently reproduced. The crucial improvement over previous methods involves the use of very sensitive standardized exercise stress testing procedures, drug dosage selection based on individual physiologic response at rest, and continuous measurement of hemodynamic parameters closely related to myocardial oxygen demand which permits comparison of clinical performance with physiologic alterations (29). This method has already shown that some studies previously thought to be conflicting actually reflected only a lack of understanding of the nitrate's dose-response characteristics. In view of the previous problems encountered in the comparative evaluation of nitrates, cautious interpretation of these data is indicated. Care should also be taken to avoid unsubstantiated extrapolation of data among various agents.

Isosorbide Dinitrate (ISDN). The important pharmacologic effects of ISDN, as well as all other long acting nitrates, appear qualitatively the same as nitroglycerin. With sublingual ISDN, the onset of action appears to be very similar to that of nitroglycerin. As previously discussed, however, the duration of action and the appropriate indices of evaluation remain extremely controversial. Studies comparing the duration of action of ISDN and nitroglycerin in doses matched for physiologic potency consistently fail to show any significant differences with exercise testing. Other studies, however, show that ISDN has a substantially longer duration of action when measured by stress testing and hemodynamic alterations. A certain amount of this contradictory data can be accounted for by recognition that the doses employed in many studies are not equivalent. Thus, an agent may appear longer acting simply because the dose administered is larger. The doses of nitroglycerin and ISDN in the routine clinical setting are not physiologically equipotent and many clinicians routinely note differences in duration of action. As a practical matter, the expectation of prolonged action from ISDN exceeding 1 hour has no basis.

Topical Nitrates. The cutaneous absorption of nitroglycerin is a well documented phenomenon which has proved very useful for the sustained prophylaxis of angina pectoris. In recent years, studies of the efficacy of nitroglycerin ointment show that it is capable of producing an increased exercise capacity for least 3 hours. Electrocardiographic evidence of a reduction in ischemia as well as beneficial hemodynamic changes has also been documented with the use of nitroglycerin ointment (30). The onset of action is about 30 min and it may be applied every 3 or 4 hours as needed.

Although nitroglycerin ointment has been shown to provide relatively sustained antianginal effects for a prolonged period of time, there are a number of problems associated with its use. The ointment can be very messy to use and precise dose measurement and application are difficult to reproduce. Consequently, the amount of the dose reaching the systemic circulation may vary significantly with each application.

In an effort to overcome the problems associated with the use of nitroglycerin ointment while maintaining the prolonged effect, several transdermal delivery systems have been developed. These systems are designed to provide a constant amount of nitroglycerin in the systemic circulation for a period of 24 hours. The transdermal systems are composed of an impermeable backing, an adhesive attachment system, and one of several drug delivery systems. The method of delivery and the control of the rate are provided by incorporating nitroglycerin in either a polymer or a gel-matrix, or by using a drug reservoir and a semipermeable membrane.

Except for a few abstracts, there have been no independent studies published that adequately compare transdermal nitroglycerin with other forms of therapy. Information provided by the manufacturers, however, indicates that the transdermal systems reproducibly provide steady state plasma nitroglycerin concentrations within a few hours after application. They also appear to sustain relatively constant concentrations for a 24-hour period that are comparable to those obtained with repeated application of nitroglycerin ointment. Despite the lack of information available, the transdermal delivery systems probably represent a milestone in the treatment of angina by providing sustained therapeutic concentrations of nitroglycerin with once daily administration.

Other Long Acting Nitrates. Efficacy studies of all the other so-called "long acting" nitrates have produced conflicting results. Some clinicians have found oral nitrate preparations to be ineffective or less effective than sublingual products when evaluated in terms of reducing anginal episodes, or increasing work capacity. Many current studies, however, show that if given in appropriate doses, oral nitrates are effective when evaluated in terms of exercise testing and the production of hemodynamic alterations.

β-Adrenergic Blocking Agents (Table 19.3)

The efficacy of β-adrenergic blocking agents in the treatment of angina pectoris due to coronary artery disease has been well established. The therapeutic effect of these agents in the treatment of angina depends in part upon their ability to alter the normal sympathetic augmentation of myocardial contractility and heart rate. In those individuals who function on a marginally positive myocardial oxygen balance, even slight elevations in the level of adrenergic nerve activity can be implicated in the precipitation of anginal attacks. The use of β-blockade, in many instances, is directed at minimizing the effects of increased sympathetic nerve activity induced by exertion, stress, or any number of other factors. The relative degree of myocardial oxygen imbalance that must exist before the normal sym-

pathetic augmentation of the heart's functions becomes a potential liability instead of an asset is unknown.

The great variety of potential pharmacologic uses for compounds of this nature has prompted investigators to pursue the development of many closely related agents. There are currently at least six β-blocking-type drugs in clinical use in the United States including propranolol, metoprolol, naldolol, atenolol, pindolol, and timolol. These compounds differ with respect to several pharmacologic characteristics such as membrane stabilizing activity, intrinsic sympathomimetic activity (partial agonist activity), and relative selectivity for receptor subtype. These drugs also differ with respect to their pharmacokinetic and pharmacodynamic properties. They exhibit differences in completeness of absorption, lipid solubility, rate of hepatic metabolism, extent of first pass metabolism, and renal excretion.

β-Adrenergic receptors are known to be nonhomogenous and are generally divided into two distinct groups. Those receptors associated with cardiostimulation are considered to be of the β_1-type and those associated with bronchodilation and vasodilation are of the β_2-type. β-Adrenergic blocking drugs may consequently be classified as either selective or nonselective according to their relative ability to preferentially block either β_1- or β_2-receptors. β-Adrenergic blocking drugs such as atenolol and metaprolol which more selectively block β_1-receptors would be expected to be less likely to exacerbate bronchoconstriction than nonselective drugs. Clinical trials with β_1-selective agents in low doses do show a lower risk of inducing bronchospasm than with equipotent doses of nonselective agents. At higher doses, however, the distinction between selective and nonselective agents diminishes. This loss of specificity is due in part to the fact that

Table 19.3.
β-Adrenergic Blocking Agents

Generic Name	Brand Name	Half-life (hr)	Percent Absorbed	Percent Bioavailable	β_1 Selectivity	Equivalent Dose[a]
Atenolol	Tenormin	6–9	50	40–60	+	100–150
Metoprolol	Lopressor	3–4	95	50	+	150
Naldolol	Corgard	14–24	30	30–40	0	80–120
Pindolol	Visken	3–4	90	80–90	0	30
Propranolol	Inderal	3–6	90	30	0	120
Timolol	Blocadren	3–4	90	75	0	20

[a] Dose equivalent to 120 mg propranolol.

rather than being exclusively either β_1 or β_2, most organs have both subtypes in varying proportions. The clinical effects of selective agents appear to be influenced not only by the relative proportions of the two receptor subtypes, but also by the existing level sympathetic tone.

Some β-adrenergic blocking drugs, such as propranolol, possess membrane-stabilizing activity resembling that of quinidine. The effect on the cardiac action potential, however, is not seen except at very high concentrations. This membrane-stabilizing activity does not appear to be responsible for the cardiac depression produced by β-blocking agents. Naldolol, which has no membrane-stabilizing activity, depresses left ventricular function to the same extent as propranolol which does possess this activity. In the doses used clinically, the antiarrhythmic activity of β-blocking drugs appears to be due to β-blockade rather than membrane-stabilizing activity.

β-Adrenergic blocking drugs may also have intrinsic sympathomimetic or partial agonist activity. This property is reflected in slight activation of the β-receptor while at the same time blocking it from activation by catecholamine-like agents. The possible advantages of this type of activity may include higher resting heart rate for equivalent degree of blockade, less myocardial depression, and less bronchoconstriction. It is not clear, however, whether the presence of this partial agonist activity constitutes true advantage in clinical use.

The β-blocking agents can also be classified according to their pharmacokinetic characteristics. Propranolol and metoprolol are primarily metabolized by the liver, have highly variable bioavailability despite extensive absorption, and have short half-lives. Naldolol and atenolol, in contrast, are eliminated by the kidney, have poor bioavailability, and have much longer half-lives. Because of their longer half-lives, both atenolol and naldolol are well suited for once a day dosing. Both pindolol and timolol have an intermediate proportion of renal elimination (20 to 40%), good bioavailability, and short half-lives. These pharmacokinetic differences are important in determining the specific agent and appropriate dose for patients with renal or hepatic impairment.

Although these agents do differ with respect to selectivity and partial agonist activity, their therapeutic effects are remarkably similar. A therapeutic failure with one agent cannot, in general, be overcome by adding a second β-blocker or selecting a different one.

The two β-blocking drugs with the most extensive clinical use in the United States are discussed in more detail below.

Propranolol. When given in appropriate doses, propranolol favorably affects two of the most commonly employed methods of evaluating antianginal therapy. It has been shown to increase exercise test performance and decrease the frequency of anginal attacks in most patients with coronary artery disease (31). Propranolol acts to inhibit the physiologic effects of endogenously released catecholamines on the body's β-adrenergic receptors. The reduction in the influence of sympathetic discharge reduces myocardial oxygen demands through alterations in heart rate, contractility, and intramyocardial tension (32). The efficacy of propranolol in a particular patient's treatment depends upon their intrinsic level of sympathetic tone and the extent of direct myocardial depression encountered. Propranolol can also increase ventricular end diastolic pressure and mean coronary vascular resistance, both of which can impair myocardial oxygen supply and demand balance. The overall effect of propranolol in most patients, however, is a favorable net decrease in myocardial oxygen consumption.

The role of propranolol in the treatment of angina pectoris is primarily prophylactic. Peak adrenergic blockade (as defined by resistance to induction of tachycardia by isoproterenol) occurs 60 to 90 min following single oral doses, making its use in acute situations impractical. Propranolol is generally utilized when angina interrupts a patient's regular activities despite adequate nitrate therapy. A reduction in nitroglycerin requirements by half is considered the minimal therapeutic goal when β-blockade is employed. An additional benefit encountered with combined nitrate-propranolol therapy is that certain detrimental effects of each agent are counteracted by beneficial effects of the other. The β-blockade antagonizes nitrate-induced reflex tachycardia and the venous pooling of nitrates reduces the increased cardiac volume caused by propranolol.

The large number of contraindications to the use of propranolol should prompt careful evaluation of any patient in whom its use is contemplated. These contraindications are relative, but include overt congestive heart failure, heart block, bradycardia, diabetes mellitus, obstructive pulmonary disease, or asthma. Although occurring primarily in patients with very severe coronary artery disease, abrupt withdrawal of propranolol has been reported to cause severe exacerbation of angina or myocardial infarction.

The most common side effects associated with the use of propranolol include nausea, fatigue, and light headedness. Among the more serious problems encountered are bradycardia, impaired atrioventricular (AV) conduction, acute pulmonary edema, and hypotension.

Metoprolol. In patients with stable angina pectoris, metoprolol has been shown to be effective in reducing the frequency of anginal attacks, reducing nitroglycerin consumption, and increasing exercise tolerance. When the dosage is titrated to individual patient requirements, metoprolol and propranolol appear to be equally efficacious in the management of angina (33).

Although metoprolol is regarded as being relatively more selective in its β_1-adrenergic receptor activity, the extent and practical import of this selectivity has not been adequately defined. Some differences in β-adrenoreceptor selectivity between metoprolol and propranolol can be detected in their effects on hemodynamic response to sympathomimetic agents. For example, intravenous administration of epinephrine produces vasodilation in skeletal muscle which is attributed to predominance in activation of β_2-adrenergic receptors. Propranolol inhibits this action, producing increases in peripheral vascular resistance and blood pressure, presumably as a result of relatively unopposed α-adrenoreceptor stimulation. The skeletal muscle vasodilating action of epinephrine, however, is largely preserved when β-blockade is produced by metoprolol (34).

Further evidence for the relative selectivity of metoprolol is illustrated by its effects on bronchial adrenoreceptors. Although metoprolol causes a reduction in forced expiratory volume and vital capacity in asthmatic patients, the effect appears to be less than that produced by equipotent doses of propranolol (as measured by reduction in resting heart rate) (35). The degree and significance of the specificity of metoprolol, however, seems to be dose dependent. The selectivity attributed to metoprolol is not clearly evident even in the moderate dosage range. Asthmatics who exhibit clinically significant bronchoconstriction from metoprolol may benefit from combined treatment with β_2-adrenoreceptor stimulants such as terbutaline. The β_2-adrenergic stimulants do not markedly diminish the β_1-blocking action of metoprolol necessary for the treatment of angina, yet partially counteract bronchoconstriction. Counteracting bronchoconstriction from propranolol has been reported with β_2 stimulants as well, but the doses required are quite high.

Although most evidence available to date documents the differential effects of various β-blocking agents based on receptor selectivity, the concept of specificity remains relative and substantial β_1 and β_2 overlap exists. When absolutely necessary, small doses of metoprolol can be used to treat angina in patients with respiratory impairment.

Contraindications and precautions for the use of metoprolol are essentially the same as those reported with all β-blocking drugs despite the relative selectivity of its actions.

In therapeutic trials, metoprolol appears to be well tolerated and reported side effects are generally mild. Tiredness, dizziness, and gastrointestinal disturbance have been the most frequently reported side effects.

Calcium Channel Blocking Agents (Table 19.4)

The calcium channel blocking agents have been shown to be very effective in the treatment of angina pectoris. They are potent dilators of coronary arteries and appear to be of great value in the treatment of angina due to

Table 19.4.
Calcium Channel Blocking Agents

Generic Name	Brand Name	Dosage Form	Usual Dosage
Nifedipine	Procardia	10-mg capsule	10–20 mg t.i.d.
Verapamil	Calan, Iosptin	80-, 120-mg tablet	80 mg t.i.d. or q.i.d.
		5 mg per 2-ml injection	0.075–0.150 mg/kg
Diltiazem	Cardizem	30-, 60-mg tablet	30–60 mg q.i.d.

coronary vasospasm. Their efficacy in the treatment of classical angina, however, appears to occur through additional mechanisms. By reducing peripheral vascular resistance and myocardial contractility, they improve the balance between myocardial oxygen supply and demand. These beneficial effects are offset in part, however, by reflex increases in heart rate and contractility secondary to the peripheral vasodilation.

On a cellular basis, the calcium channel blocking agents interfere with excitation-contraction coupling in vascular smooth muscle by altering the slow inward calcium current and the transport of calcium among intracellular sites. The dilating effect is produced by inhibition of calcium influx which is a critical factor in the excitation-contraction process that produces sustained vascular tone.

The effects of nifedipine on exercise tolerance and the symptoms of stable angina have been extensively studied. Several double-blind controlled studies have shown significant reductions in exercise induced S-T segment depression using single doses of nifedipine (36, 37). With chronic therapy, similar results have been obtained in large groups of patients (38). The improved exercise tolerance appears to be primarily due to dose-dependant decreases in peripheral vascular resistance and systemic arterial pressure resulting in reduced afterload. Although nifedipine frequently produces a reflex tachycardia, the increased heart rate does not appear to be sufficient in most patients to offset the effect of decreased arterial pressure on myocardial oxygen consumption. Verapamil has also been shown to be effective in the treatment of angina in a number of double-blind studies (39, 40). In doses of 120 mg, 3 times a day, verapamil produces a significant reduction in nitroglycerin consumption and improvement in exercise tolerance. In addition to symptomatic relief, verapamil decreases the amount and duration of S-T segment depression during exercise. Verapamil, in contrast to nifedipine, dose not appear to produce reflex tachycardia.

Most of the side effects produced by nifedipine are mild and are a result of vasodilation. The most commonly reported side effects include headache, flushing, dizziness, and nausea. In most cases, side effects are not sufficiently severe to require discontinuation of therapy. In a small number of patients, nifedipine may cause an exacerbation of ischemic symptoms as a result of the reflex tachycardia.

Verapamil produces a similar range of side effects, excluding the reflex tachycardia. Serious effects encountered with verapamil include hypotension, disturbances of AV conduction, and bradycardia.

References

1. Higgins CP, et al: Clinical and arteriographic features of Prinzmetal's variant angina; documentation of etiologic factors. *Am J Cardiol* 37:831, 1976.
2. Scheidt S, et al: Unstable angina pectoris; natural history, hemodynamics, uncertainties of treatment and the ethics of clinical study. *Am J Med* 60:409, 1976.
3. Burggraf GW, Parker JD: Prognosis of coronary artery disease; angiographic, hemodynamic and clinical factors. *Circulation* 51:146, 1975.
4. Brand RJ, et al: Multivariate prediction of coronary heart disease in the Western Collaborative Group Study compared to the findings of the Framingham Study. *Circulation* 53:348, 1976.
5. Kannel WB, et al: Factors of risk in the development of coronary heart disease; six-year follow-up experience; the Framingham Study. *Ann Intern Med* 55:33, 1961.
6. Medalie JH, et al: Angina pectoris among 10,000 men; II. Psychosocial and other risk factors as evidenced by a multivariate analysis of a five year incidence study. *Am J Med* 60:910, 1976.
7. Kosenmann RH, et al: Multivariate prediction of coronary heart disease during 8.5 year follow-up in the Western Collaborative Group Study. *Am. J. Cardiol.* 37:903, 1976.
8. Sketch MH, et al: Significant sex differences in the correlation of ECG testing and coronary arteriograms. *Am J Cardiol* 36:196, 1975.
9. Pitt B, Strauss HE: Myocardial imaging in the noninvasive evaluation of patients with suspected ischemic heart disease. *Am J Cardiol* 37:797, 1976.
10. Greenberg H, et al: Effects of nitroglycerin on the major determinants of myocardial oxygen consumption. *Am J Cardiol* 36:426, 1975.
11. Likoff W, et al: Evaluation of coronary vasodilators by coronary angiography. *Am J Cardiol* 13:7, 1964.
12. Becker L, et al: Regional myocardial blood flow, ischemia and antianginal drugs. *Ann Clin Res* 3:353, 1971.
13. Parker J, et al: The effect of nitroglycerin on coronary blood flow and the hemodynamic response to exercise in coronary artery disease. *Am J Cardiol* 27:59, 1971.
14. Gorlin R, et al: Effect of nitroglycerin on the coronary circulation in patients with coronary artery disease or increased left ventricular work. *Circulation* 19:705, 1959.
15. McGregor M, Fam W: Effect of coronary vasodilator drugs on retrograde flow in areas of chronic myocardial ischemia. *Circ Res* 15:355, 1964.
16. Kinsella D, et al: Studies with a new coronary vasodilator drug: Persantine. *Am Heart J* 63:146, 1962.
17. DeGreff A, Lyon A: Evaluation of dipyridamole (Persantine). *Am Heart J* 65:423, 1963.

18. Ganz W, Marcus H: Failure of intracoronary nitroglycerin to alleviate pacing-inducing angina. *Circulation* 46:880, 1972.
19. Braunwald E, et al: Studies on cardiac dimensions in intact unanesthetized man; effects of nitroglycerin. *Circulation* 32:767, 1965.
20. Mason D, et al: Effects of nitroglycerin on left ventricular cavitary size and cardiac performance determined by ultrasound in man. *Am J Med* 57:754, 1974.
21. Amsterdam F, et al: Effects of nitroglycerin on left ventricular hemodynamics and regional contractile function (abstract). *Clin Res* 23:170A, 1975.
22. Mason D, et al: Reduction of ischemia injury by sublingual nitroglycerin in patients with acute myocardial infarction. *Circulation* 54:761, 1976.
23. Aronow W: Medical treatment of angina pectoris; IV. Nitroglycerin as an antianginal drug. *Am Heart J* 84:415, 1972.
24. Horowitz L, et al: Clinical response to nitroglycerin as a diagnostic test for coronary artery disease. *Am J Cardiol* 29:149, 1972.
25. Russek H: The therapeutic role of coronary vasodilators; glyceryl trinitrate, isosorbide dinitrate and pentaerythritol tetranitrate. *Am J Med Sci* 252:43, 1966.
26. Bunn W, et al: Clinical evaluation of sublingual nitrates. *Angiology* 14:48, 1963.
27. Parker J, et al: The effect of nitroglycerin on coronary blood flow and the hemodynamic response to exercise in coronary artery disease. *Am J Cardiol* 27:59, 1971.
28. Mikalick MJ, Rasmussen S, Knoebel SB: The effect of nitroglycerin on premature ventricular complexes in acute myocardial infarction. *Am J Cardiol* 33:157, 1974.
29. Goldstein R, et al: Clinical and circulatory effects of isosorbide dinitrate, comparison with nitroglycerin. *Circulation* 43:629, 1971.
30. Lee G, et al: Effects of long-term oral administration of isosorbide dinitrate on the antianginal response to nitroglycerin. *Am J Cardiol* 41:82, 1978.
31. Nutley R, et al: Efficacy of β-adrenergic blockade in coronary heart disease; propranolol in angina pectoris. *Clin Pharmacol Ther* 18:598, 1975.
32. Harrison DC: Beta-adrenergic blockade, 1972; pharmacology and clinical uses. *Am J Cardiol* 29:432, 1972.
33. Comerford MB, Besterman EM: An eighteen month study of the clinical response to metoprolol, a selective beta$_1$ receptor blocking agent in patients with angina pectoris. *Postgrad Med J* 52:481, 1976.
34. Van Herwaarden C, et al: Effects of adrenaline during treatment with propranolol and metoprolol. *Br Med J* 1:1029, 1977.
35. Skinner C, et al: Comparison of effect of metoprolol and propranolol on asthmatic airway obstruction. *Br Med J* 1:504, 1976.
36. Ebner F, Dunsched HB: Hemodynamics, mechanism of action and clinical findings of Adalat use on worldwide clinical trials. In *The Third International Adalat Symposium*. Amsterdam: Excerpta Medica, 1976, pp 283–300.
37. Stein G: Antianginal efficacy of different doses of Adalat in angina pectoris patients in a double-blind trial. In *The Third International Adalat Symposium*. Amsterdam: Excerpta Medica, 1976, pp 233–239.
38. Moskowitz RM, et al: Nifedipine therapy for stable angina pectoris. *Am J Cardiol* 44:811–816, 1979.
39. Sandler G et al: Clinical evaluation of verapamil in angina pectoris. *Br Med J* 3:224–227, 1968.
40. Bala-Subramanian V, et al: Verapamil in chronic stable angina; a controlled study with computerized multistage treadmill exercise. *Lancet* 1:841–844, 1980.

CHAPTER 20

Congestive Heart Failure

ROBERT M. ELENBAAS, Pharm.D.

Congestive heart failure (CHF) results from an inability of the heart to pump sufficient blood to meet the body's oxygen needs. Although generally a disease of the elderly, it may occur in essentially any age group as a consequence of cardiovascular disease. The estimated national incidence of CHF is between 0.5 to 2 per 1,000 per annum. Since this incidence increases with age, a growth in the size of the geriatric population will likely continue to make CHF one of the more commonly encountered clinical entities.

ETIOLOGY

The most common etiologic agents associated with the development of CHF are essential hypertension, coronary heart disease and rheumatic heart disease. Pulmonary embolism, thyrotoxicosis, peristent cardiac arrhythmias and myocardiopathies, although less common, may also play a role in the development of CHF. Hypertension appears to be the most important of these factors; 75% of patients who develop CHF have prior histories of hypertension and the risk of developing congestive failure in hypertensive patients is 6 times that of patients with normal blood pressure.

PATHOGENESIS

Although the biochemical abnormalities responsible for myocardial failure are yet incompletely understood, factors responsible for the development of the clinical manifestations of CHF are well defined. When the heart fails and cardiac output decreases, a complex scheme of compensatory mechanisms designed to raise output is brought into play. At least in the early stages of heart failure, cardiac output is not dramatically reduced and the patient's symptoms result from the presence of these compensatory mechanisms.

In the failing myocardium the strength with which the ventricle may contract is reduced.

The reduction in stroke volume which results causes a decrease in the ejection fraction and an increase in residual blood volume within the ventricle at the end of the systole. If the atria continue to deliver blood to the ventricles at the same rate, the end diastolic volume and pressure will increase and the ventricles will dilate. The increased length of myocardial fibers allows an increased force of systolic contraction to be developed (Fig. 20.1). As long as ventricular function is represented by the ascending portion of the Starling curve, progressive increases in end diastolic volume and myocardial fiber length will continue to provide an increase in contractility and cardiac output. However, with further increases in left ventricular end diastolic volume, the function curve may simply plateau (and occasionally even enter a "descending limb"). Thus, an increase in end diastolic volume would increase end diastolic pressure without augmenting cardiac output.

Failure of the heart to provide an adequate cardiac output produces several changes designed to restore output toward normal. A reflex activation of the sympathetic nervous system and an increase in circulating catecholamines exist (1). This increase in sympathetic activity is manifest by an increase in heart rate and a redistribution of blood flow from the skin, splanchnic, and renal vascular beds to the brain and heart (Fig. 20.2). The resulting decrease in renal blood flow and increase in renal vascular resistance initiate several compensatory processes which favor retention of sodium and water. Sodium reabsorption in the proximal portion of the renal tubule is increased, as is renin release from the juxtaglomerular cells. An increase in plasma renin leads eventually to an increase in angiotension II and III formation, both of which have effects facilitating sodium retention. Angiotension II is a potent vasoconstrictor which further increases renal vascular resistance; it also causes

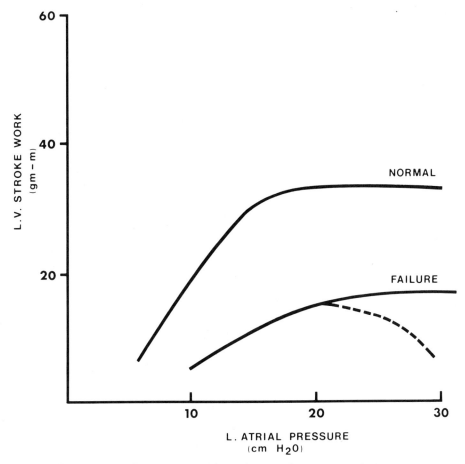

Figure 20.1. Starling curve for normal and failing heart (left ventricular (*L.V.*) stroke work may be equated to cardiac index and left atrial pressure to pulmonary capillary pressure, see Fig. 20.4.)

a redistribution of intrarenal blood flow so that glomerular filtrate is shunted to medullary nephrons having long loops of Henle where sodium and water reabsorption is more complete (5). Angiotension III, meanwhile, stimulates the zona glomerulosa of the adrenal cortex to secrete aldosterone, a potent mineralocorticoid which acts mainly on the distal convoluted tubule of the kidney to enhance sodium reabsorption. The net result of this increase in sodium and water reabsorption is an expansion of intravascular volume, performed in an attempt to restore cardiac output to normal (1). Unfortunately, the failing heart may not be able to accommodate normally to this increased blood volume (Fig. 20.1) and venous congestion results.

Failure of the heart as a pump results in congestion "behind" the failing ventricle. Thus, if the left ventricle is functioning inad- equately, the congestion occurs in the lungs; whereas, when the right ventricle fails, the congestion is found in the systemic venous circulation. Most patients who have had left heart failure for some time, however, will also develop right ventricular failure and thus present with both pulmonary and systemic congestion. This congestion results in an increased venous and capillary hydrostatic pressure, while simultaneously diluting the colloid osmotic pressure. Thus, a redistribution of fluid from the intravascular to interstitial spaces results in edema formation and most of the signs and symptoms of CHF.

CLINICAL FINDINGS

The manifestations and physical findings of CHF are easily predicted by considering the pathogenesis of the disease. Cardiac output is

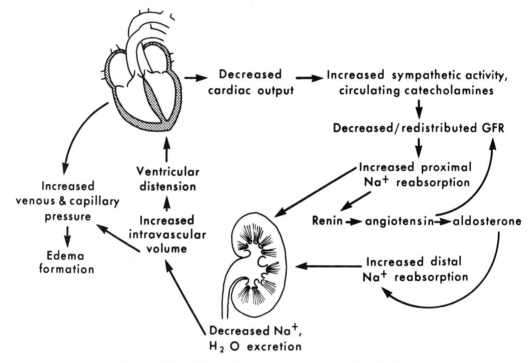

Figure 20.2. Edema formation in congestive heart failure.

not dramatically reduced in the initial phases of heart failure, and the patient's symptoms result from the presence of compensatory mechanisms outlined above.

Table 20.1 indicates the most common signs and symptoms found in patients with CHF. Most are the result of pulmonary or systemic venous congestion and edema formation. Dyspnea, orthopnea, and paroxysmal nocturnal dyspnea (PND) are signs of left-sided heart failure and represent pulmonary vascular congestion. Dyspnea on exertion (DOE) is the most common symptom of heart failure. As the myocardial failure advances, dyspnea appears with less strenuous activity until eventually it is present even at rest. Orthopnea is usually taken to be an indication of more advanced heart failure and occurs when the patient assumes a recumbent position. Blood from the lower extremities and splanchic bed redistributes to the lungs, resulting in an elevation of pulmonary venous pressure. PND (cardiac asthma) is characterized by severe shortness of breath which generally awakens the patient from sleep. PND is also the result of increased pulmonary vascular congestion which has been allowed to advance until pulmonary edema and bronchospasm develop. Rales, pleural effusions and chest x-ray find-

Table 20.1.
Common Symptoms and Physical Findings of Congestive Heart Failure

A. *Left ventricular failure*
  1. Dyspnea
  2. Orthopnea
  3. Paroxysmal nocturnal dyspnea (PND)
  4. Pleural effusion
  5. Rales
  6. S_3 gallop rhythm
B. *Right ventricular failure*
  1. Jugular venous distension
  2. Peripheral edema
  3. Positive hepatojugular reflux
C. *Nonspecific*
  1. Cardiomegaly
  2. Fatigue
  3. Tachycardia

ings indicating vascular congestion in the upper lung fields are also typical of left ventricular failure.

Ankle or pretibial dependent edema, congestive hepatomegaly, jugular venous distension, and hepatojugular reflux indicate systemic venous congestion and are signs of right-sided heart failure. Ankle and pretibial edema are common findings in ambulatory patients because fluid tends to localize in the dependent portions of the body secondary to gravitational forces. It should be noted, therefore, that sacral rather than ankle edema may be present in patients at bed rest. Venous congestion may also result in portal hypertension, hepatomegaly, and occasional ascites. Distension of the jugular veins as a sign of systemic venous congestion may also exist.

Cardiomegaly results from ventricular hypertrophy and distension. Tachycardia is often a very early sign of heart failure resulting from catecholamine excess. Peripheral cyanosis resulting from compromised respiration, decreased cardiac output, and shunting of blood away from the skin may be evident. Although nonspecific, fatigue and weakness are commonly found in patients with heart failure and are secondary to the reduction in cardiac output.

PRECIPITATING FACTORS IN CHF

CHF resulting from long-standing uncontrolled hypertension or valvular heart disease does not usually occur abruptly, but instead has a rather insidious onset. Acute ventricular failure is generally the result of myocardial infarction, cardiac arrhythmias, pulmonary embolus, or pulmonary infections. It is always prudent to search for factors which may precipitate or aggravate either acute or chronic heart failure in the patient who presents with myocardial decompensation. Important among these are uncontrolled hypertension, excessive dietary sodium intake, and certain medications.

Drugs which produce expansion of the intravascular volume (either through sodium retention or via their osmotic activity; Table 20.2) should be avoided or used with caution in patients with CHF. Medication preparations with extraordinarily high sodium contents must also be administered gingerly to these individuals.

TREATMENT—CHRONIC CHF

The principal considerations in the management of CHF include: eliminating precipitating factors, reducing workload on the heart, increasing myocardial contractility and decreasing renal sodium and water retention. Thus, modalities available for the medical management of CHF encompass correction of underlying disease states (e.g., hypertension), bed rest, a sodium-restricted diet, the use of positive inotropic drugs (e.g., digitalis), diuretics, administration of arterial and/or venous vas-

Table 20.2.
Drugs Which May Exacerbate/Precipitate Congestive Heart Failure

A. *Sodium retention*
 1. Androgens
 2. Corticosteroids
 3. Diazoxide
 4. Estrogens
 5. Guanethidine
 6. Licorice
 7. Lithium carbonate
 8. Methyldopa
 9. Minoxidil
 10. Phenylbutazone
 11. Nonsteroidal anti-inflammatory agents
 12. Salicylates
B. *Osmotically active substances*
 1. Albumin
 2. Glucose
 3. Mannitol
 4. Saline
 5. Urea
C. *Decrease contractility*
 1. Antiarrhythmic agents (e.g., quinidine, procainamide)
 2. β-Blockers—propranolol, metoprolol, nadolol
 3. Daunomycin
 4. Guanethidine (?)

odilators, and inhibitors of the renin-angiotension system. The ultimate goal of therapy is to abolish disabling symptoms and improve the quality of the patient's life. Unfortunately, none of the aforementioned measures are curative.

For years, clinicians have been plagued by the fact that therapeutic end points for CHF are rather subjective. The advent of hemodynamic monitoring with use of the Swan-Ganz catheter (see below) does provide objective end points and monitoring parameters for the hospitalized, usually unstable, patient. However, the direct measurement of pulmonary capillary pressure and cardiac index is not feasible or warranted in most patients, and in general the clinician must look for improvement of signs and symptoms of the syndrome. With therapy, the patient begins to improve subjectively and objectively: he is less dyspneic and complains less of orthopnea; venous distension and signs of pulmonary congestion diminish or disappear; and diuresis and decreased heart rate may also be observed. However, peripheral and pulmonary edema may not mobilize immediately; thus, aggressive therapy directed at these entities may lead only to side effects rather than benefit.

A general scheme for the management of CHF based upon the degree of myocardial decompensation is presented in Figure 20.3 (2).

Bed rest or restriction of physical activity decreases metabolic demands placed on the failing heart and minimizes gravitational forces contributing to edema formation. Renal perfusion is also increased in the supine position resulting in diuresis and eventual mobilization of edema.

A sodium-restricted diet may be instituted to offset the abnormal renal retention of sodium in CHF. Even though less than 1 g is required to meet physiological needs, the normal American diet contains 10 g of sodium chloride. Severe salt restriction (less than 500 mg Na or 1.3 g NaCl) is unpalatable and poorly followed. Moderate salt intake (2 to 4 g NaCl), which can be accomplished by restricting the addition of salt during cooking, is much more palatable. For convenience one should remember that 1 g of sodium is equivalent to 2.5 g of salt (NaCl), and that 1 level teaspoon of salt weights approximately 6 g.

DIGITALIS

The digitalis glycosides have provided the cornerstone of drug management in CHF for many years. Although their role has been questioned in patients with CHF and normal sinus rhythm (3, 4), digoxin and digitoxin will continue to hold a pivotal position in the chronic management of this entity (at least until orally available, catecholamine derivative inotropic agents with a wider therapeutic index are brought to the market) (5, 6).

Step 1. Restriction of physical activity
Restriction of sodium intake
Digoxin or digitoxin
Diuretics—hydrochlorothiazide or furosemide
Step 2. Above plus:
    Spironolactone if diuretic escape
    Vasodilators—
        Hydralazine if symptoms of low cardiac output
        Isosorbide dinitrate if symptoms of venous congestion
        Prazosin, or hydralazine and isosorbide, if symptoms of both
Step 3. Above plus:
    Captopril

Figure 20.3. Management strategy for chronic congestive heart failure.

The major therapeutic effect of digitalis in CHF is that of increasing the force and velocity of myocardial contraction (inotropic effect). It is thought that digitalis enhances excitation-contraction coupling by increasing intracellular calcium availability and that this effect may be mediated through its inhibition of Na-K ATPase, an enzyme required for the active transport of sodium and potassium across cardiac cell membranes. The mechanism of digitalis' electrophysiological effects (chronotropic, dromotropic) is also unclear but is more definitely related to an inhibition of the sodium-potassium pump. These effects account for the ability of digitalis to impair atrioventricular conduction and slow ventricular rate in atrial rhythms associated with a rapid ventricular response. Hence, the patient with congestive heart failure and atrial fibrillation may be especially benefited by digitalis.

It appears that the inotropic and electrical effects of digitalis are independent of each other (7). There are several important clinical implications of this fact: the practice of dosing a patient to toxicity to achieve the therapeutic benefits of inotropism is invalid since enhanced contractility may be observed before toxicity is reached; suppression of digitalis-induced arrhythmias does not simultaneously obliterate the inotropic effect of the drug; and because inotropic effects are observed at low doses, patients who are sensitive to the toxic effect of digitalis may still benefit from doses which were previously considered subtherapeutic.

The digitalis glycosides are most effective in the common forms of left or biventricular failure due to excessive hemodynamic burdens (e.g., hypertension, aortic or mitral insufficiency, ischemic heart disease). Unfortunately they are much less effective in diseases directly affecting the myocardial cell (e.g., myocarditis, alcoholic cardiomyopathy) and in heart failure secondary to anemia, cor pulmonale, thyrotoxicosis, or mitral or aortic stenosis. Digitalis is actually contraindicated in patients with idiopathic hypertrophic subaortic stenosis since any increase in contractility may actually reduce cardiac output by facilitating valvular obstruction (8).

COMPARISON OF DIGITALIS PREPARATIONS

Table 20.3 compares the digitalis glycosides most frequently encountered (9). The choice

Table 20.3.
Comparison of Digitalis Glycoside Preparations[a]

Agent	Gastrointestinal Absorption	Onset of Action (min)	Peak Effect (hr)	Average Half-life	Principal Route of Elimination	Average Digitalizing Dose		Usual Daily Oral Maintenance Dose
						Oral	I.V.	
Ouabain	Unreliable	5–10	½–2	21 hr	Renal; some GI excretion		0.3–0.5 mg	
Deslanoside	Unreliable	10–30	1–2	33 hr	Renal		0.8 mg	
Digoxin	50–75%	15–30	1½–5	36 hr	Renal; some GI excretion	1.25–1.5 mg	0.75–1.5 mg	0.25–0.5 mg
Digitoxin	90–100%	25–120	4–12	4–6 days	Hepatic; renal excretion of metabolites	0.7–1.2 mg	1.0 mg	0.1 mg
Digitalis leaf	About 40%			4–6 days	Similar to digitoxin	0.8–1.2 g		0.1 g

[a] Reprinted with permission from Ref. 9.

of which glycoside to use in a given situation would ideally depend upon the routes of administration available, the speed of onset desired, and the duration of action required. In the vast majority of cases, however, ouabain, deslanoside, digitalis leaf and, to some extent, digitoxin offer no real advantages over digoxin, which is considered the glycoside of choice by most practitioners.

Digitalis Leaf

USP digitalis leaf is composed primarily of three glycosides: digitoxin, gitoxin, and gitalin. Digitoxin is the most important of these compounds and is responsible for the majority of the pharmacological activities of the mixture. The onset and duration of action of digitalis leaf are therefore identical to those of digitoxin. The use of powdered digitalis leaf has been largely replaced by the purified crystalline preparations (digoxin, digitoxin). More accurate standardization of active drug content and an insignificant difference in cost have made these latter preparations the agents of choice; the use of digitalis leaf should be abandoned.

Ouabain/Deslanoside

Ouabain has the most rapid onset and shortest duration of action of the digitalis glycosides. It is often spoken of as having a "fast onset and short duration," which would lead one to believe that the effects of a single dose would terminate within minutes. However, such is not the case, and the "short" duration of action is actually a relative matter. Deslanoside is similar in its onset and duration to ouabain. While these two drugs are sometimes recommended in situations when a very rapid onset is desired, in actuality, their time to onset of action and peak effect following intravenous administration is not a great deal shorter than that for digoxin. Therefore, the latter agent can be used if initial parenteral therapy is desired, and oral therapy with the same drug easily begun when appropriate.

Digoxin

Digoxin is considered the glycoside of choice in the majority of situations. The availability of both intravenous and reliable oral routes of administration, relatively rapid onset of action, and intermediate duration of action are the main criteria which have resulted in the predominant use of digoxin.

Digoxin administered in a well-formulated tablet is rapidly absorbed and peak serum levels are usually achieved within 1 to 2 hours (10). Digoxin absorption, however, is far from complete, and tablet administration has been reported to yield about 50 to 85% (average = 70%) absorption (11). A marked variation in the bioavailability of digoxin from tablets produced by different manufacturers and from different lots of the same manufacturer had been reported in the past (10). This observation led to FDA regulations and USP standards concerning digoxin dissolution and bioavailability which have eliminated this problem. Nevertheless, it is advisable to evaluate bioavailability data if one is considering using a generic digoxin preparation.

Alteration of the absorption of digoxin following oral administration in patients with malabsorption syndromes has also been studied (12). Poor and erratic absorption occurs in patients with malabsorption states such as sprue, short bowel syndrome, and rapid intestinal transit. Bile salts and pancreatic enzymes are apparently not required for effective digoxin absorption.

Digoxin is available in injectable form for both intramuscular and intravenous use. However, it is recommended that the intramuscular route be avoided, since it produces severe local pain, muscle fasciculation, and marked creatine kinase elevations, and that digoxin be given intravenously if oral administration is not feasible. Previous concern that hepatic and splanchnic venous congestion present in patients with right-sided heart failure might decrease the oral bioavailability of digoxin may not be warranted (13). Therefore the intravenous route is principally indicated when a relativley rapid response is desired (e.g., selected patients with atrial fibrillation, moderate to marked pulmonary edema) or in patients incapable of taking oral medications. When given intravenously, digoxin should be administered at a maximum rate of 1 ml (0.25 mg) per min, or preferably it should be diluted with 10 ml of normal saline and given as a slow infusion over 10 min.

All digitalis glycosides are eliminated from the body following first order kinetics. In the case of digoxin, approximately 35% of the total amount of drug in the body will be lost during 1 day; the kidney is the main route of elimi-

nation (14). Glomerular filtration is primarily responsible for the renal excretion of digoxin and no significant tubular reabsorption or secretion occurs. Increased rates of urine flow caused by diuretic administration, water loading, or diabetes insipidus do not increase digoxin elimination. The average elimination half-life of digoxin in patients with normal renal function is between 1.6 and 1.9 days (14).

Since it is eliminated in large part as unchanged drug in the urine, digoxin kinetics are altered in patients with varying degrees of renal dysfunction. However, nonrenal mechanisms, principally hepatic metabolism, are also involved in digoxin elimination. It has been observed that anuric patients will eliminate approximately 14% of the total amount of drug in the body during 1 day and that the average half-life of digoxin in such patients is 4.4 days. Therefore, the daily maintenance dose must be decreased in patients with poorly functioning kidneys. It has been observed that the rate of digoxin elimination is directly proportional to creatinine clearance, and that if the creatinine clearance of a patient is known, it is possible to estimate the daily dose necessary to maintain body glycoside stores at a given level (14). The following relationship between creatinine clearance and percent of digoxin lost per day has been reported:

$$\% \text{ loss} = 14 + (\text{creatinine clearance})/5$$

For example, a patient with a creatinine clearance of 15 ml per min will eliminate approximately 17% of the total amount of digoxin in his body during a 24-hour period. If this patient had been digitalized intravenously with 1.0 mg of digoxin and it was desired to maintain his glycoside stores at that level, the daily maintenance dose should be 0.25 mg, assuming that digoxin is 70% absorbed when given orally. It should be recognized, however, that this formula provides only a guide to modifying the digoxin maintenance dose based on variations in renal function and that calculated doses simply represent sophisticated estimates. Clinical evaluation of patient status and response to digoxin continues to be the most important method of determining dosage.

Digitoxin

Digitoxin has the slowest onset of action, peak effect and half-life of all the digitalis glycosides. Digitoxin is essentially 100% absorbed following oral administration (15). However, alteration of absorption in patients with malabsorption syndromes or other gastrointestinal disease has not been studied. Digitoxin elimination occurs primarily via hepatic metabolism and renal excretion of the metabolic by-products; only about 30% of digitoxin is eliminated unchanged in urine or feces. Digoxin has been reported to be a minor metabolite of digitoxin; however, it is produced in such small amounts as to be of no significance. As far as is known, the balance of the digitoxin metabolites have little or no cardioactivity. Digitoxin undergoes some degree of enterohepatic recycling (15). The elimination half-life of digitoxin is approximately 6 days.

Since relatively little digitoxin is excreted unchanged in the urine, one would not expect that any significant alteration of digitoxin maintenance dose would be necessary in the presence of renal insufficiency. Clinical observations of patients with renal failure seem to indicate that no dose alteration is necessary (16). Despite this apparent advantage over digoxin, whether digitoxin should be the glycoside of choice for maintenance therapy is questionable. Its slow onset of action, long duration of action, somewhat interpatient variable elimination half-life and the need for a loading dose in essentially all patients (see below), constitute the primary disadvantages of digitoxin relative to digoxin. Nevertheless, digitoxin may provide an acceptable alternative in those few patients with renal insufficiency difficult to control on digoxin. Because digitoxin relies primarily on hepatic metabolism for its elimination, liver dysfunction may conceivably reduce the rate of metabolism and prolong half-life. To date no instances of this occurrence have been reported. Nevertheless, it would be advisable to avoid the use of digitoxin in patients with severe liver disease and administer digoxin instead.

DIGITALIZATION

The term "digitalization" refers to the loading dose of digitalis utilized to achieve a desired total body store of the drug. The size of this loading dose varies depending upon the therapeutic objectives; the speed with which digitalization is conducted depends primarily upon the clinical situation. The patient may be rapidly digitalized (i.e., over a 24-hour period), or he may be slowly digitalized over a week or more. CHF generally is not of such a severe nature that immediate improvement in cardiac function is necessary. In most instances there is no need to rapidly load the patient, and digitalization may actually be slowly and more safely accomplished over a week or more. Because there are many therapeutic modalities with a rapid onset of action and possibly greater therapeutic index than digoxin available for the management of acute congestive failure (see below), it should rarely be necessary to fully digitalize a patient within a 24-hour period. In acute cardiac failure due to myocardial infarction and in cardiogenic shock, for example, the results of rapid digitalization have been unimpressive and suggest that minimal clinical benefit is accrued (17). (It may be desirable, however, to rapidly digitalize a patient with a supraventricular tachyarrhythmia and fast ventricular response in order to control or prevent its adverse consequences.)

For a given patient, the total digitalizing dose will be independent of the rapidity of administration. On a mg-for-mg basis, digoxin and digitoxin are essentially equivalent with respect to their cardiac effects. Therefore, the digitalizing dose of each will be approximately equal. When fully digitalized, most patients will have 0.75 to 1.5 mg (0.01 and 0.02 mg per kg) of glycoside present in their bodies. Loading doses near the lower end of this range are associated primarily with an increase in contractility, while the higher dosages are generally necessary when treating supraventricular tachyarrhythmias and electrical effects to decrease AV nodal conduction are desired. It should be emphasized, however, that these figures represent average doses and that some patients may require much more. The initial phases of digitalis dosing are actually an exercise in titration (14).

Rapid Digitalization

Assuming that one wishes to initiate digoxin therapy rapidly, and that a total dose of 1.0 mg is desired, the following general procedure should be followed. An initial dose of 0.5 mg may be given. Six to 12 hours later the patient should be evaluated for clinical improvement and signs of digitalis toxicity. If no evidence of toxicity exists, he may be given a dose of 0.25 mg. In another 6 to 12 hours the patient should again be evaluated for signs of toxicity, and if there are no contraindications, a last dose of

0.25 mg may be administered. Thus, within a 12- to 24-hour period the patient may be digitalized to a level of 1 mg. Daily losses should be replaced by administration of a maintenance dose designed to sustain this level of digitalization (1 mg). This regimen can be administered either parenterally or orally. However, because orally administered digoxin is not completely bioavailable, it may be necessary to make a compensatory adjustment in the calculated daily oral dose for a patient digitalized intravenously if a given total body store must be sustained for continued achievement of the therapeutic effect.

Because digoxin and digitoxin have essentially equal potency, a similar digitalizing regimen could be used for the rapid institution of digitoxin therapy. It must be understood, however, that because of the slow onset of action and peak effect of digitoxin, dosages should be given less frequently (every 12 to 24 hours) and the total time for digitalization lengthened. Therefore, digitoxin is usually not an appropriate agent when a more rapid effect is desired (e.g., supraventricular tachyarrhythmias).

Slow Digitalization

Digitalization may be accomplished slowly simply by giving the patient a daily maintenance dose of digoxin without a prior loading dose. The main advantage of slow digitalization is that it does not require intensive monitoring of the patient and is thus very suitable to the ambulatory setting. The main disadvantage, however, is the length of time required to reach maximal body glycoside stores and therapeutic effect. Additionally, decreased renal function will prolong the time required to reach steady state drug concentrations.

The length of time required to achieve plateau concentrations of a drug administered on a maintenance basis is dependent on the elimination half-life of that drug. It will take essentially 5 half-lives to reach steady state. Thus, a patient with normal renal function placed on a daily dose of digoxin will require about 8 to 10 days to reach maximal glycoside concentrations (5 × 1.6 to 1.9 days). If, however, that patient were anephric ($t_{1/2}$ = 4.4 days) it would take 22 days to reach plateau (14). Administration of digitoxin in such a manner will require 20 to 30 days to reach steady state regardless of renal function. It is therefore impractical to

digitalize patients with digitoxin in this manner.

When using this method of digitalization, one must avoid increasing doses before maximal effects are observed. It would be inappropriate to increase a patient's maintenance dose after only 3 days, for example, if no clinical improvement were observed.

DIGITALIS TOXICITY

It is unfortunate that digitalis, the drug which forms the cornerstone of the current management of CHF, has an extremely narrow therapeutic index. This narrow therapeutic index, coupled with a relative lack of well-defined therapeutic endpoints, makes it regrettably easy to inadvertently produce intoxication. As many as 20% of patients taking digitalis eventually exhibit clinical and/or electrocardiographic evidence of toxicity. Up to 18% of these patients may die from digitalis-induced arrhythmias (18). A positive correlation between serum digoxin levels and toxicity has been noted (19, 20). Eighty-seven percent of digoxin-toxic patients had levels greater than 2 ng/ml while 90% of the nontoxic patients had levels of less than 2 ng/ml. Likewise, digitoxin plasma concentrations in excess of 35 to 40 ng/ml are more likely to be associated with toxicity than are concentrations less than 25 ng/ml (16). However, because a significant overlap exists between toxic and therapeutic levels, digitalis toxicity cannot be diagnosed solely on the basis of an elevated serum concentration; serum level determinations are currently most useful as an aid in confirming digitalis toxicity suspected on clinical grounds. Unfortunatley, digitalis-induced ECG changes (S-T depression and T wave flattening) do not correlate with toxic or therapeutic effects of the drug.

Signs and Symptoms of Digitalis Toxicity

Signs and symptoms of digitalis (digoxin and digitoxin) toxicity may be categorized as either cardiac or noncardiac; mortality is generally due to an uncontrollable cardiac arrhythmia. Noncardiac symptoms of digitalis toxicity may involve the central nervous system (CNS), gastrointestinal tract, and endocrine effects of the drug. Unfortunately, the clinical presentation of digitalis toxicity is highly unpredictable. Noncardiac symptoms precede cardiac symptoms in only about 50% of the cases, and cardiac arrhythmias may frequently be the only manifestation of digitalis toxicity (18, 21).

Neurologic (CNS) symptoms of digitalis toxicity are extremely common if patients are examined closely. Acute, extreme fatigue occurs in as many as 95% of digoxin-toxic patients, while approximately 80% may experience limb weakness and 65% suffer from psychic disturbances in the form of nightmares, agitation, listlessness, and hallucinations. Visual complaints (hazy vision, difficulty reading, impaired red-green color perception) may be present in about 95% of individuals. Other visual disturbances reported by toxic patients include glitterings, scotomata, photophobia, and a yellow-green tinge to the image (21).

Gastrointestinal symptoms, including anorexia, nausea, vomiting, abdominal pain, and diarrhea, occur in 80% of toxic patients (21). Of these symptoms, abdominal pain is the most common, being present in 65% of patients, while diarrhea is the least frequently noted. However, vague gastrointestinal symptoms characteristic of digitalis toxicity may be difficult to evaluate since anorexia and nausea are also part of the clinical picture of congestive heart failure. In fact, an equal frequency of anorexia and nausea has been observed in both toxic and nontoxic patients (19). The notion that gastrointestinal symptoms of digitalis toxicity are related to impurities in the drug preparations is no longer supported.

Additional unusual noncardiac adverse effects include rash and thrombocytopenia due to digitoxin, and unilateral or bilateral gynecomastia due to digoxin.

The arrhythmogenic action of digitalis is related to its complex effects on the electrophysiological properties of the heart. Toxic doses of digitalis may simultaneously depress the automaticity of the normal pacemakers and enhance the automaticity of ectopic foci. Conduction velocity is diminished in the AV node and other specialized conducting tissues of the heart while it is increased in the atrium and ventricles. Involvement of a central nervous system mechanism in digitalis toxicity has been proposed.

Digitalis-induced rhythm disturbances are often nonspecific, but are generally characterized by decreased conduction and/or increased automaticity. It is estimated that rhythm disturbances occur in 80 to 90% of digitalis toxic patients (18). The most common

rhythm disturbances observed in digitalis toxicity and their relative frequencies are indicated in Table 20.4 (22).

While it is commonly stated that digitalis intoxication may present as any imaginable cardiac arrhythmias, it should be noted that premature ventricular contractions represent that most frequently observed. Also, digitalis toxicity should be highly suspected in any patient exhibiting one of the following dysrhythmias: atrial fibrillation or flutter with an extremly slow ventricular response, atrial fibrillation with a completely regular ventricular response (actually representing a complete AV block with junctional escape), paroxysmal atrial tachycardia with 2:1 conduction, or ventricular bigeminy or trigeminy.

Factors Influencing Digitalis Toxicity

A number of factors may predispose patients to digitalis toxicity. Most important among these are the electrolyte imbalances hypokalemia, hypomagnesemia, and hypercalcemia; metabolic or respiratory acidosis; hypoxemia; and diminished renal function.

Twice as much digitalis is required to produce toxicity in patients with a serum potassium of 5 mEq per liter than in those with a serum potassium of 3 mEq per liter (27). Therefore drugs, diseases, and medical maneuvers

Table 20.4.
Common Arrhythmias Associated with Digitalis Toxicity

Type	% of Total Patients with Dysrhythmia	% of Type
Ventricular arrhythmias	71	
Ventricular premature contractions		90
Ventricular tachycardia		10
Atrioventricular block	29	
First degree		45
Second degree		30
Third degree		19
Atrial arrhythmias	26	
Atrial fibrillation		45
Paroxysmal atrial tachycardia with block		33
Sinoatrial arrhythmias	13	
Sinus tachycardia		34
Sinus bradycardia		31
Junctional arrhythmias	7	
Junctional tachycardia		70
Junctional rhythm		23

which induce hypokalemia or a drop in serum potassium from elevated to normal levels may potentially "unmask" digitalis toxicity or allow it to occur at lower doses. The mechanism of this potentiation is unclear; however, a low serum potassium has been observed to increase the uptake of digitalis by the myocardial tissue. Conversely, an increase in extracellular potassium results in a decrease in myocardial glycoside content and may slow the rate of binding of digitalis to myocardial Na-K ATPase (28). Some specific situations in which potassium depletion is likely to occur include diuretic therapy (with the exception of the potassium-sparing agents); administration of corticosteroids with mineralocorticoid activity; protracted vomiting or diarrhea; prolonged nasogastric suction or fluid losses from ileostomies or GI fistulas; and, potentially, glucose, insulin or bicarbonate administration.

Animal studies have demonstrated that the toxic dose of digitalis glycosides is reduced in the presence of hypomagnesemia, and clinical observations in patients support this observation (29). The long-term administration of magnesium-free fluids (e.g., hyperalimentation), diuretics and amphotericin B, chronic alcoholism, hemodialysis, and excessive upper GI fluid losses containing 10 to 20 mEq per liter have been associated with hypomagnesemia. Magnesium depletion should be considered as a cause of digitalis toxicity resistant to the usual therapeutic interventions.

The electrical and contractile effects of calcium on the myocardium are similar to those of digitalis. For this reason, rapid intravenous infusions of calcium are thought to facilitate the development of digitalis toxicity, and normal or low doses of digitalis to induce toxicity in patients with hypercalcemia. The clinical significance of calcium-induced digitalis toxicity has been questioned, although digitalis insensitivity has been shown to occur in hypocalcemia (30). There have been no reports of digitalis toxicity secondary to the oral administration of calcium-containing products.

Age may be an important predisposing factor in the production of digitalis toxicity. The same intravenous dose of digoxin administered to elderly and young patients produces higher serum concentrations in the elderly (31). It is proposed that the higher levels and prolonged half-life observed in these patients are due to diminished renal clearance of the drug and the smaller body size of this population.

Hypothyroid patients may be extremely sensitive and hyperthyroid patients quite resistant to the effects of digitalis. Although serum levels of digoxin have been noted to be higher in hypothyroid patients than in euthyroid individuals, half-life and tissue concentrations of the drug are probably unchanged. Other clinical studies have not demonstrated a difference in digoxin's pharmacokinetic properties among hyper-, hypo-, or euthyroid individuals (32). Whether the clinical differences in patient responsiveness to the drug are based on a pharmacokinetic abnormality or some other factor inherent to thyroid dysfunction has yet to be adequately determined. Nevertheless, the difference in sensitivity becomes clinically important when a hyperthyroid patient managed on high doses of digoxin becomes hypo- or euthyroid secondary to treatment; a hypothryoid individual becomes hyper- or euthyroid following replacement therapy; or when initially designing a dosage regimen for an individual with thyroid dysfunction.

An increased prevalence of digoxin toxicity has been observed in patients with advanced cardiac disease, chronic pulmonary disease, cor pulmonale, hypoxia, acid-base and electrolyte imbalance, and atrial fibrillation (19). Alteration in renal function from normal is probably the most common predisposing factor associated with digoxin toxicity. The specific influence of renal insufficiency on digoxin and digitoxin kinetics is discussed above. Diminished liver function may theoretically increase the half-life and serum levels of digitoxin because it is metabolized to a significant degree. Very little digoxin is metabolized by the liver and its elimination is unaltered in cirrhotic patients with normal renal function.

Treatment of Digitalis Toxicity

One's aggressiveness in management of digitalis toxicity is dependent upon its manifestations in a given patient. Noncardiac symptoms generally require only supportive therapy and will resolve without sequelae. Digitalis-induced cardiac dysrhythmias will usually require some sort of intervention, although simple drug withdrawal may be the only treatment needed if the arrhythmia is not life-threatening (e.g., sinus bradycardia, Mobitz I second degree AV block).

Potassium administration should be considered in patients with digitalis-induced ectopic beats who have low or normal serum potassium levels. The oral route of administration is generally adequate and should be used unless the patient cannot take medications by mouth. The following precautions should be considered when potassium is used to treat digitalis toxicity:

1. Potassium should be administered with caution in patients who have conduction disturbances characterized by second degree or complete AV block (18). Potassium also depresses conduction velocity in the distal AV node and its use may result in an augmentation of this cardiac arrhythmia;

2. Toxic doses of digitalis inhibit the uptake of potassium by myocardial, skeletal muscle and hepatic cells. Although seen principally in patients with acute intoxication following ingestion of a large dose, marked refractory hyperkalemia may occasionally develop (23);

3. Because potassium is eliminated by the kidneys, excessive potassium loads should be avoided in patients with compromised renal function;

4. Cardiac arrhythmias have been observed following the rapid intravenous administration of concentrated potassium solutions. If digitalis-induced arrhythmias occur in the presence of marked hypokalemia, potassium repletion should not exceed a rate of 0.5 mEq per min and solutions for IV administration should not exceed a concentration of 60 to 80 mEq per liter. When given at a rapid rate, the patient should be monitored for signs and symptoms of potassium toxicity with frequent ECG tracings (tall, peaked T waves, prolonged PR interval) and serum potassium determination. Generally, a less vigorous potassium repletion will suffice.

Virtually all of the antiarrhythmic agents have been used to treat digitalis-induced arrhythmias. Intravenous lidocaine, phenytoin, and propranolol have been used with the greatest success. Lidocaine and phenytoin have a theoretical advantage over propranolol and quinidine-like agents in the presence of hypokalemia in that they probably do not further depress AV or intraventricular conduction. Lidocaine is more easily administered than phenytoin and may thus be used as an initial drug in the management of digitalis-induced ventricular tachyarrhythmias or extrasystoles.

Reports regarding the efficacy of phenytoin as an antiarrhythmic have been variable; however, the drug appears to be particularly efficacious in the suppression of digitalis-induced supraventricular tachyarrhythmias with or without first or second degree AV block. It should probably be considered the drug of choice in this specific setting. A loading dose of up to 1 g (15 to 18 mg/kg) may be required before an antiarrhythmic effect is evident. The diluent for parenteral phenytoin contains 40% propylene glycol, which is cardiotoxic; for this reason the preparation should not be administered at a rate which exceeds 25 to 50 mg per min. Phenytoin is insoluble in many intravenous solutions and should therefore be given by direct IV injection, or alternatively diluted in 50 ml of normal saline and infused over 30 to 60 min (24).

Intravenous propranolol has been useful in abolishing digitalis-induced atrial tachycardia with AV block and ventricular premature contractions. One milligram of propranolol should be given IV over 1 min, and repeated every 5 min until a therapeutic response is achieved or a total dose of 0.1 mg/kg has been administered. Unlike phenytoin and lidocaine, propranolol is more likely to depress conduction velocity and may therefore augment AV and intraventricular block. It should not be used in asthmatic patients since it may induce bronchoconstriction.

Procainamide and quinidine have been used less frequently because their intravenous administration has been associated with hypotension and cardiotoxicity. Since conduction velocity is diminished by both of these drugs, their use should be avoided when AV or intraventricular block is present. Bretylium is currently believed to be contraindicated in patients with digitalis toxicity. Even though only animal data are available, bretylium administration in the presence of digitalis intoxication appears to precipitate ventricular tachyarrhythmias and profound hypotension (25).

Bradyarrhythmias and AV block resulting from digitalis toxicity are best managed with intravenous atropine or, if unsuccessful, a temporary electrical pacemaker. Magnesium depletion should be considered as a cause of digitalis toxicity resistant to the usual therapeutic intervention, and the ion repleted if hypomagnesemia is identified. Oral cholestyramine or colestipol may be useful as a means of enhancing glycoside elimination by interrupting enterohepatic recycling. This may be especially pertinent for digitoxin which normally undergoes more enterohepatic recycling than digoxin. However, preliminary evidence suggests that these binding resins enhance digoxin elimination and shorten its half-life as well (26).

DIURETICS

Role of Diuretics in the Management of CHF

Edema in CHF is a manifestation of abnormal retention of sodium and water, which occurs in response to a diminished cardiac output. Correction of the underlying disease process is most important to the removal of edema; therefore digitalis, which improves cardiac output and tissue perfusion, will usually abolish the need to increase intravascular volume. Not infrequently however, edema of moderate to severe cases of chronic CHF may be unresponsive to therapeutic doses of digitalis and sodium restriction alone and diuretic agents may be needed to reduce symptoms caused by excessive fluid accumulation. Additionally, individuals with more marked degrees of failure may receive an acute subjective and objective benefit from diuretic administration. The rate with which edema may be removed is limited by its mobilization from the interstitial to the intravascular compartment. If diuresis is too vigorous, intravascular volume depletion may occur, diminishing venous return and cardiac output. Hypotension may thus result. Patients most likely to acutely benefit from intravenous diuretic administration are those with marked left ventricular failure and an elevated pulmonary capillary pressure (i.e., elevated hydrostatic pressure in the pulmonary capillary bed) (33).

Diuretics have two effects of benefit to the patient with CHF. Following intravenous administration (furosemide), a reduction in pulmonary capillary pressure (PCP) can be seen within minutes, well before any increase in urine output is noted. This decrease in PCP is due to an increase in venous capacitance and a decrease in venous return (33). This would be of benefit to the individual with marked left ventricular failure and elevated pulmonary capillary pressure, since it will lessen the formation of pulmonary edema. By increasing renal sodium excretion diuretic administration will also directly reduce intravascular volume, thereby decreasing venous return and PCP and favoring the mobilization of peripheral edema.

Drug Selection

The thiazides are the most commonly employed diuretic agents in the chronic management of CHF. Aside from differences in duration of action there are essentially no differences in potency or toxicity among these compounds at maximal therapeutic doses. The choice of agent within this class, therefore is governed primarily by cost. A comparison of selected diuretics is presented in Table 20.5.

The effectiveness of diuretics is dependent upon the amount of sodium delivered to their site of action. Proximal tubular reabsorption of sodium is increased in patients with CHF, and in some instances the avidity for sodium at this site may render thiazide diuretics minimally effective. In these cases, the use of furosemide or ethacrynic acid, which work more proximally than the thiazides, should be considered. Used alone, spironolactone and triamterene are weak diuretics and are minimally effective in the treatment of symptomatic edema.

Loop diuretics (ethacrynic acid and furosemide) are the only agents which may be effective in the presence of any significant degree of renal failure (serum creatinine 3 to 8 mg/100 ml). This may be due to their ability to decrease renal vascular resistance and redistribute renal blood flow. It should be pointed out, however, that in the long run these agents are also capable of inducing azotemia secondary to contraction of the vascular volume and decrease glomerular filtration rate.

Spironolactone, triamterene, and amiloride should be avoided in patients with renal failure (BUN > 40 mg%) since hyperkalemia may develop from their use. Furosemide is the most commonly used agent when the intravenous route and a rapid response are desired. An initial dosage of 20 to 40 mg may be repeated (and doubled if desired) if no response is observed within 30 min.

Diuretic Escape

It is not uncommon for patients to "escape" from or become resistant to the diuretic effect of chronically administered thiazides. This may be attributed to one of the following:

1. Patient noncompliance with the prescribed regimen;

2. A decreased delivery of sodium to the site of action secondary to an increased proximal tubular reabsorption observed in patients with CHF and/or decreased glomerular filtration rates; or

3. An increased reabsorption of sodium at the distal tubule may result from increased

Table 20.5.
Selected Pharmacological Properties of Frequently Used Diuretics

Agent	Onset of Action	Peak Effect	Duration of Action	Usual Dosage (mg/day)	Commercial Availability	Relative Potency (Max Doses)	Comments
Chlorthalidone	2 hr	18 hr	48–72 hr	50–100	Tablets, 100 mg	1	Long acting diuretic with thiazide-like mechanism of action and toxicity.
Ethacrynic acid	0.5–1 hr	1–2 hr	6–8 hr	50 (IV/PO) max: 150–200	Tablets, 25, 50 mg; injectable 50-mg vials	5	Rapidly acting, extremely potent diuretic with greater potential for toxicity; should be reserved for patients refractory to minimum doses of thiazides; works in patients with renal failure; may have more GI irritant effects than furosemide; no more than 100 mg/dose parenterally to avoid ototoxicity
Furosemide	0.5–1 hr	1–2 hr	6–8 hr	40–80; may be much higher	Tablets, 40 mg; injectable, 20 mg, 10 mg/ml	8–10	Rapidly acting, extremely potent diuretic with greater potential for toxicity; should be reserved for patients refractory to minimum doses of thiazides; works in patients with renal failure; ototoxicity with IV use
Hydrochlorthiazide	1–2 hr	2–4 hr	4–8 hr	25–100	Tablets, 25, 50 mg	1	Ineffective in renal failure
Spironolactone	Delayed: 1–2 days	2–3 days	2–3 days after drug discontinued	100–200	Tablets, 25 mg	0.4	Potassium-sparing; avoid use in renal failure or in conjunction with potassium supplements
Triamterene	2	—	12–16 hr	100–200	Capsules, 100 mg	0.4	See spironolactone

levels of aldosterone due to diuretic-induced sodium loss (34).

The latter effect may be identified by monitoring urine electrolyte concentrations. Initially sodium excretion is enhanced, but as diuretic therapy progresses one may observe a drop in urine sodium and an increase in urine potassium concentration. In such cases, the effects of thiazide or loop diuretics may be enhanced by the concomitant use of triamterene, spironolactone, or amiloride. The initial onset of action of these latter agents may be delayed by 3 to 7 days so that one should not be discouraged if there are no immediate results.

Additional approaches to the management of diuretic escape may include administration of the drug at bedtime when recumbency normally increases GFR, administration of the diuretic every other day or only 5 days per week so renal compensatory mechanisms can be reset, or use of a short acting agent (e.g., furosemide) only once daily (34). Also, the addition of metolazone to the regimen of the resistant patient has been noted to produce a dramatic return of diuretic responsiveness (35).

Adverse Effects of Diuretic Agents

For the most part, the adverse effects of the diuretic agents can be seen to be simple extensions of their normal pharmacologic activities.

Loop diuretics, osmotic agents and the thiazides are all capable of producing intravascular volume depletion and hyponatremia if diuresis is too vigorous. It is important to emphasize that intravascular volume depletion may occur in the presence of peripheral edema or pulmonary congestion if the rate of diuresis exceeds the rate of edema mobilization. A drop in blood pressure with postural changes, diminished urinary output, and abnormal renal function tests may be observed. Rapid administration of osmotic diuretics such as mannitol and urea may also cause an acute volume expansion which may exacerbate CHF; this effect would be especially pronounced in patients with severe renal failure who are unable to eliminate these agents.

Hyponatremia may result when electrolyte-free fluid (water) is ingested and dietary sodium is restricted in the face of increased urinary losses of sodium. Additionally, thiazides and loop diuretics inhibit the formation of free water so that urinary sodium loss may exceed water loss. Symptoms of hyponatremia include lethargy, somnolence, muscle cramps, and weakness, which may be indistinguishable from hypokalemia without the aid of laboratory tests. Severe hyponatremia (usually less than 110 to 115 mEq/liter) is characterized by coma and focal or generalized seizures. Hypovolemia and hyponatremia may be minimized by dosing diuretics intermittently and by avoiding the use of long acting agents (chlorthalidone) or severely sodium-restricted diets (500 mg sodium or less). It has been proposed that chronic diuretic therapy be administered on an intermittent basis so that periods of diuresis are followed by rest periods during which diuretic-induced volume and electrolyte changes are allowed to recover and reequilibrate (see above). Such regimens must be individualized to the patient's response. Mild hyponatremia without coma or seizure activity may be treated by temporary discontinuation of diuretic therapy, liberalization of sodium intake, and fluid restriction. Severe hyponatremia must be treated aggressively with hypertonic saline, and potentially the addition of furosemide to promote free water excretion (36).

All diuretics, with the exception of the potassium-sparing agents, are capable of producing hypokalemia. The avoidance of potassium depletion is particularly important in patients receiving digitalis. Nevertheless, whether all patients administered diuretics should concomitantly receive potassium supplementation is uncertain, since the majority of individuals will not develop significant potassium depletion. While potassium supplementation does not need to be routinely given to patients receiving diuretics for treatment of hypertension, the prudent approach would be to provide potassium to the individual also receiving digitalis for CHF. Potassium supplementation (40 to 60 mEq per day) should be used with caution in patients with compromised renal function since they are frequently unable to eliminate large potassium loads. Administration of potassium with spironolactone and especially triamterene in renal failure patients should also be avoided since severe, life-threatening hyperkalemia may result. When diuretic-induced hypokalemia is accompanied by hypochloremic alkalosis, potassium must be repleted as the chloride salt. Low serum chloride levels perpetuate urine potassium losses so that replacement of potassium without chloride (e.g., gluconate and citrate salts) will be minimally effective.

With the exception of spironolactone, decreased renal clearance of uric acid and secondary hyperuricemia are potential complications of all diuretics frequently used in the management of CHF. In general, diuretic-induced hyperuricemia rarely induces gouty attacks, and gout or hyuperuricemia are not contraindications to use. If uric acid levels are in excess of 9 to 10 mg/100 ml or in patients with a history of gouty arthritis, probenecid or allopurinol may be used.

Diuretics may induce a diminished glucose tolerance and elevate blood sugar concentrations in the adult onset or latent diabetic (spironolactone excepted). Altered glucose tolerance probably results because of a diuretic-induced inhibition of pancreatic insulin release. Thus, persons with insulin-dependent diabetes should not experience this adverse effect. The use of diuretics is not contraindicated in noninsulin-dependent diabetics, and blood sugar can generally be controlled by adjusting the dose of diabetic medications if needed. Interestingly, in some patients blood glucose control may be reestablished by potassium choride supplementation; it is postulated that restoring pancreatic β cell electrolyte balance may normalize insulin release.

REFRACTORY HEART FAILURE
Peripheral Vasodilators

The introduction of peripheral vasodilators into the therapeutic regimen of patients with CHF has provided a major advance to the management of both acute and chronic heart failure. They may be dramatically effective in increasing cardiac output and improving the symptom complex of individuals with refractory failure. The digitalis glycosides still represent the agents of choice in the vast majority of patients with CHF. However, in some patients experiencing left ventricular failure as a complication of acute myocardial infarction (33) and in those with chronic CHF refractory to digitalis and diuretic therapy, the vasodilators may provide the most beneficial form of therapy (37).

Depending on the agent, the vasodilators are capable of arterial and/or venodilation; they will thus influence cardiac output, pulmonary capillary pressure, and systemic venous pressure through their effects on "preload" and "afterload" (Table 20.6). Preload is the extent of diastolic stretch of the ventricular myofilament (end diastolic ventricular volume, Fig. 20.1) and is directly determined by venous return. Afterload may be thought of as the impedance to ventricular ejection and in part is determined by the degree of peripheral vascular resistance. Arterial dilation will decrease peripheral vascular resistance and resistance to left ventricular ejection (afterload). Left ventricular ejection fraction thus increases, resulting in an augmented stroke volume and cardiac output and possibly a lessened left ventricular end diastolic volume. Thus, cardiac output is increased while pulmonary capillary hydrostatic pressure and edema formation may be decreased. Venodilation will increase venous capacitance, decrease venous return and thereby diminish left ventricular end diastolic volume and pulmonary capillary pressure. Formation of pulmonary congestion and edema is therefore decreased.

The goal of therapy with the peripheral vasodilators is to reduce left ventricular end diastolic volume and pulmonary capillary pressure and increase stroke volume and cardiac output. Such therapy is often accompanied by a fall in arterial pressure; fortunately, the desired hemodynamic effect can usually be achieved with only a slight reduction in the level of arterial pressure. The use of invasive hemodynamic monitoring to select the most appropriate vasodilator drug or dose in patients with severe heart failure (pulmonary edema) or left ventricular failure accompanying acute myocardial infarction is discussed below. In ambulatory patients, or those hospitalized but without invasive monitoring, the choice of vasodilator may be made with reasonable intelligence based on clinical assessment of the patient.

Those whose symptoms are principally due to low cardiac output (poor exercise tolerance) will benefit most from an agent with predominantly arterial vasodilatory properties. Those whose symptoms are primarily due to pulmonary or systemic venous congestion (pulmonary edema, rales, peripheral edema) will benefit most from an agent with venous dilating activity; while patients with symptoms of both low cardiac output and pulmonary/systemic congestion should be given a single agent or combination having both arteriolar and venous dilatory effects (38). Hydralazine,

Table 20.6.
Peripheral Vasodilators of Use in Congestive Heart Failure

Agent	Arterial and Venous Dilation Dose	Agent	Arterial Dilation Dose	Agent	Venous Dilation Dose
Nitroprusside	15–200 μg/min continuous IV infusion	Hydralazine	50–100 mg PO QID	Isosorbide dinitrate	10–40 mg PO QID
Nitroglycerin (IV)	10–100 μg/min continuous IV infusion	Phentolamine	0.25–2.0 mg/min continuous IV infusion	Nitroglycerin topical	½–4 inches QID
Prazosin	2–10 mg PO QID (average-20 mg/day)				

isosorbide dinitrate, and prazosin or an hydralazine-isosorbide combination, respectively, are the agents most studied and most commonly used in each of these settings (37, 38).

While questions of tolerance to the hemodynamic effects of the vasodilators have been raised, long-term benefit in the patient's functional level probably results (39). Evidence suggests that addition of an aldosterone antagonist (spironolactone) may restore drug sensitivity in those cases where it has been lost.

Other Therapeutic Modalities

Occasional patients will not be restored to an adequate functional level even with the aggressive use of digitalis glycosides, diuretics, and peripheral vasodilators. Since activation of the renin-angiotension-aldosterone arc may be important in maintaining the excessive fluid accumulation noted in these patients, captopril has been investigated and produced some benefit (40). Whether it will truly provide an effective long-term treatment, and its role compared to the vasodilators, remains to be determined.

A whole new spectrum of nondigitalis inotropic agents effective when given orally is currently under investigation (41). These compounds (e.g., pirbuterol, carbazeram, prenalterol) are hoped to provide effective alternatives to digitalis with a much wider therapeutic index.

ACUTE LEFT VENTRICULAR FAILURE

The problem of severe left ventricular failure, often of acute onset, is fairly common and is characterized by markedly reduced cardiac output and pulmonary edema. Pulmonary congestion may be so severe that gas exchange is impaired. The patient is extremely tachycardiac, tachypneic, and agitated. Such degrees of left ventricular failure may occur as a result of poorly controlled chronic CHF or as a complication of marked hypertension or acute myocardial infarction. Immediate, aggressive management is indicated.

For many years the classic approach to severe left ventricular failure with pulmonary edema was described by the acronym "MOST DAMP." Brief mention will be made of this regimen because of its importance in the initial (emergency) management of the patient with marked left ventricular failure, pending more patient-specific management outlined below:

M—Morphine. Morphine is useful in this setting because it relieves some of the patient's anxiety induced by air hunger and hypoxia; it decreases venous return, pulmonary hydrostatic pressures, and edema formation via peripheral vasodilation; it may also have a delayed, positive inotropic effect apparent 15 to 30 min after administration. A dose of 2 to 8 mg given intravenously at a rate of 1 mg per min is usually appropriate. Extreme care must be taken not to suppress the patient's respiratory drive; should this occur, naloxone should be immediately given to antagonize morphine's effects.

O—Oxygen. The presence of pulmonary edema impairs diffusion of oxygen from the alveoli to the pulmonary capillaries; increasing the concentration of oxygen in the inspired air helps to overcome this diffusion difficulty. Oxygen may be given by nasal cannula or mask if tolerated by the patient. It may often be necessary to perform tracheal intubation to gain control of the patient's respirations.

S—Sit Up. Having the patient sit in bed, possibly even with the legs dangling from the side, will cause blood to pool in dependent portions of the body and decrease venous return, pulmonary hydrostatic pressure, and edema formation.

T—Tourniquets. The use of tourniquets, rotated between the extremities and placed with enough pressure to decrease venous return, is another method of decreasing pulmonary pressure and edema formation. The tourniquets should be applied to three of the four extremities and rotated every 15 min (automated equipment is available though not truly necessary). Approximately 500 to 800 ml of blood may be captured in the extremities using this technique. The use of rotating tourniquets is not recommended in the presence of hypotension.

D—Digitalis. While part of the classic approach to the management of pulmonary edema, the current role of digitalis in this setting is unsettled. Digoxin is probably indicated in the patient with a rapid supraventricular tachyarrhythmia who has not previously been digitalized. However, in the absence of such an arrhythmia, digoxin is best avoided in the initial hours of management since its onset and maximal effects occur long after that of other available inotropic agents. The "D" of MOST DAMP may now be taken to represent either dopamine or dobutamine. It is best to consider digitalis a long-term treatment and institute its administraiton in a less dynamic setting.

A—Aminophylline. Aminophylline is capable of increasing myocardial contractility, heart rate, and cardiac output, thereby increasing renal blood flow and urine output. A decrease in left ventricular end diastolic pressure, secondary to its dilating action on the pulmonary and peripheral vasculature, follows aminophylline administration. Additionally, bronchospasm may occur occasionally as a result of pulmonary edema. Therefore, aminophylline is included in the classic approach to management of pulmonary edema. However, its use is particularly contraindicated in the patient with acute myocardial infarction; aminophylline may dramatically increase myocardial oxygen consumption and extend the size of an infarction.

M—Mercurial Diuretics. Although diuretics are still used beneficially in patients with pulmonary edema, furosemide is now considered the preferred agent.

P—Phlebotomy. Actual decrease of blood volume will, of course, decrease venous return, pulmonary pressure, and edema formation. Removal of 200 to 250 ml may provide substantial benefit in the patient unresponsive to other measures discussed above. Phlebotomy should not be utilized in the hypotensive patient.

Hemodynamic Monitoring

A notable advance in the management of patients with acute or severe left ventricular failure has been the introduction of convenient, bedside hemodynamic monitoring with the Swan-Ganz catheter (33). The Swan-Ganz catheter is a balloon-tipped catheter which may be advanced from a peripheral vein, through the right side of the heart and into a pulmonary artery. With the balloon "wedged" in a pulmonary artery of equal size, the transducer of the catheter tip no longer records pulmonary artery pressure but the "downstream" pressure, called pulmonary capillary pressure (PCP or pulmonary wedge pressure, PWP). Because there are no valves between the pulmonary capillaries and left atrium, during diastole when the mitral valve is open the left ventricle, left atrium and pulmonary venous bed become a common chamber. Therefore the pressure experienced by the left ventricle will be recorded by the catheter as PCP. Pulmonary capillary pressure is essentially equal to left ventricular end diastolic pressure. The normal PCP is 5 to 12 mm Hg. Those catheters equipped with a thermistor are also capable of measuring cardiac output. Cardiac index (cardiac output corrected for body surface area) is normally between 2.7 to 4.3 liters/min/square meter (7).

Correlation of pulmonary capillary pressure to the clinical findings of left ventricular failure in patients with myocardial infarction has demonstrated a very specific pattern: 5 to 12 mm Hg—normal; 18 to 20 mm Hg—onset of pulmonary congestion; 20 to 25 mm Hg—moderate congestion; 25 to 30 mm Hg—severe congestion; >30 mm Hg—frank pulmonary edema (assuming normal colloid oncotic pressure). Similarly, correlation of cardiac index to clinical findings has demonstrated the following: >2.7 liters/min/m²—normal; 2.2 to 2.7 liters/min/m²—subclinical depression; 1.8 to 2.2 liters/min/m²—onset of clinical hypoperfusion; <1.8 liters/min/m²—cardiogenic shock (33).

Using these criteria it has been possible to identify four "hemodynamic subsets" of patients with left ventricular failure (Fig. 20.4). While it is possible to place a patient into a subset based only on the results of clinical evaluation without invasive hemodynamic assessment, a direct correlation between clinical and hemodynamic subsets may exist only on initial patient examination and not in the early hours after therapy has been instituted. A fall in PCP following diuretic administration, for example, may occur acutely while clinical signs of pulmonary congestion may not resolve for 24 to 48 hours. One might have a tendency to overtreat the patient if only clinical signs are being monitored.

Although initially described and utilized in patients with complicated acute myocardial infarction, the concept of hemodynamic subsets provides a framework around which to organize one's approach to many patients with acute or severe left ventricular failure.

Subset I. Patients in Subset I do not have

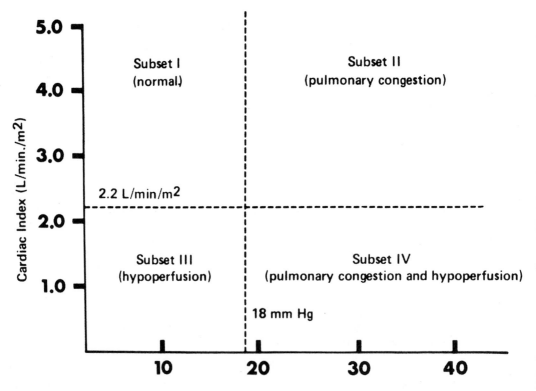

Figure 20.4. Cardiac index vs. pulmonary capillary pressure. Hemodynamic subsets of Forrester and corresponding clinical findings (33, 42).

any significant left ventricular dysfunction. In fact, patients with acute myocardial infarction who fall into Subset I based upon clinical criteria, would not be likely to receive a Swan-Ganz catheter in most institutions. No therapy specific to ventricular failure is indicated in these patients.

Subset II. The general goal of treatment for individuals in Subset II is to reduce PCP to a level not associated with pulmonary congestion. However, overzealous reduction is to be avoided because this would result in a significant fall in cardiac index. Therefore, a reduction in PCP to 15 to 18 mm Hg is considered optimal, assuming plasma oncotic pressure is normal. Furosemide is the preferred treatment for most patients in Subset II (42). A dose of 20 to 40 mg may be given intravenously and repeated in 30 to 45 min if needed. Depending upon the magnitude of the response, the dose may be doubled when repeated.

Patients who also have sustained hypertension (after diuretic administration) may benefit by use of a peripheral vasodilator, since these agents are capable of lowering both PCP and arterial pressure (42). Nitroprusside is the preferred agent in this setting because of its rapid onset of action, titratability of dose, and effects on both the venous and arterial circulation.

Subset III. Most patients in Subset III have a reduced cardiac index and compensatory tachycardia due to an absolute or "relative" hypovolemia. Therefore, they have a low peripheral perfusion with PCP in the normal or low range. Under these circumstances, cardiac output may be increased by expanding the intravascular volume, thus increasing venous return. Normal saline is usually chosen to accomplish this volume epxansion. A "fluid challenge" of about 250 to 300 ml should be given rapidly, with the goal to raise PCP to 15 to 18 mm Hg; additional saline can then be given to maintain this PCP. Elevating PCP above 15 to 18 mmHg is associated with very little additional increase in cardiac output and would favor edema formation (42).

A small proportion of individuals in Subset III have a normal stroke volume, but peripheral hypoperfusion on the basis of bradycardia. Therefore, measures to increase cardiac rate (e.g., atropine or electrical cardiac pacing) should be undertaken.

Subset IV. Unfortunately, even with currently optimal management the mortality rate of patients in this subset following acute myocardial infarction is quite high. The general goal of therapy is to reduce pulmonary capillary pressure and increase cardiac output. Combined vasodilator (nitroprusside, nitroglycerin) and inotropic (dopamine, dobutamine) therapy is usually required.

The peripheral vasodilators are usually the initial agents of choice in this setting; nitroprusside represents the most optimal drug because of its effects on both the arterial and venous circulations, the capability to closely titrate its dose to the patient's clinical response, and the widespread familiarity among clinicians with its use. The following guidelines should be followed when using nitroprusside in this setting:

1. PCP should be reduced to, but not allowed to fall below, 15 to 18 mm Hg;

2. In the hypotensive patient, diastolic pressure should not be allowed to decrease more than 10 mm Hg;

3. If systolic arterial pressure cannot be maintained at 90 to 100 mm Hg, an inotropic agent should be added and the nitroprusside dosage reduced.

Nitroprusside administration should be initiated as a constant intravenous infusion at a rate of 15 to 20 μg per min. Dosge may be increased by 5 to 10 μg per min every 5 to 10 min until the desired response is obtained. Since PCP may change acutely without an obvious improvement in clinical signs of pulmonary congestion, hemodynamic monitoring by use of the Swan-Ganz catheter is essential. Also, blood pressure measurements made with a sphygmomanometer may be very unreliable in the patient with diminished cardiac output; therefore, direct intra-arterial recording of arterial pressure may be necessary.

If an inotropic agent is needed to maintain arterial pressure at the appropriate level, dopamine is currently the most commonly used agent. An initial dosage of 3 to 5 μg per kg per min provides a good starting point. The infusion rate may be increased every 3 to 5 min until the desired effect on blood pressure, perfusion, and cardiac output is obtained. Infusion rates greater than 7 to 10 μg per kg per min will produce α-adrenergic vasoconstriction, while rates greater than 20 μg per kg per min produce intensive vasoconstriction. This may markedly increase blood pressure and offset the beneficial effects of nitroprusside.

Dobutamine may provide an effective alternative to dopamine in the patient requiring high infusion rates of the latter agent to achieve the needed intropic support. However, one must be aware that blood pressure may acutely fall if the patient is abruptly switched from dopamine to dobutamine, since the latter drug possesses essentially no vasoconstrictor activity. Dobutamine should be initiated at an infusion rate of 3 to 5 μg/kg/minute, and increased every 5 to 10 min to a maximum of 15 μg/kg/min.

CONCLUSION

Congestive heart failure is one of the more common cardiovascular diseases whose treatment may now be approached with a variety of therapeutic modalities. While digitalis, diuretics and dietary sodium restriction continue to represent the initial line of management in most patients with chronic CHF, the introduction of the peripheral vasodilators, inhibitors of the renin-angiotensin system, and newer inotropic agents is providing entirely new avenues for approaching therapy of this age-old condition. An understanding of the physiologic principles governing cardiac output is increasingly important to the optimal management of the patient with ventricular dysfunction and failure.

With the introduction of these additional therapeutic modalities for the treatment of CHF, the clinical pharmacist may have an increasingly significant role in helping to assure optimal patient management. Also, the incidence of toxicity in patients taking digitalis is alarmingly high. A good working knowledge of digitalis pharmacology, pharmacokinetics, and factors affecting its use may have a marked influence on decreasing the incidence of toxicity. Additionally, it has been shown that patients with CHF who understand their disease and the importance of properly taking prescribed medications have a much higher compliance rate than those that do not.

References

1. Cohn JN, Levine TB, Francis GS, et al: Neurohumoral control mechanisms in congestive heart failure. Am Heart J 102:509, 1981.
2. Braunwald E: Heart failure: pathophysiology and treatment. Am Heart J 102:486, 1981.
3. Johnston GD, McDevitt DG: Is maintanence digoxin necessary in patients with sinus rhythm? Lancet 1:567, 1979.
4. Guz A, McHaffie D: The use of digitalis glycosides in sinus rhythm. Clin Sci Mol Med 55:417, 1978.
5. Selzer A: Digitalis in cardiac failure. Do benefits justify risks? Arch Intern Med 141:18, 1981.
6. Sodums MT, Walsh RA, O'Rourke RA: Digitalis in heart failure. Farwell to foxglove? JAMA 246:158, 1981.
7. Mason DT, Braunwald E: Digitalis: new facts about an old drug. Am J Cardiol 22:151, 1968.
8. Duca P, Brest AN: Indications, contraindications, and non-indications for digitalis therapy. Cardiovasc Clin 6:131, 1977.
9. Smith TW, Haber E: Digitalis. N Engl J Med 289:1063, 1973.
10. Lindenbaum J, Mellow MH, Blackstone MO, et al: Variation in biologic availability of digoxin from four preparations. N Engl J Med 285:1344, 1971.
11. Greenblatt DH, Duhme DW, Koch-Weser J, et al: Evaluation of digoxin bioavailability in single-dose studies. N Engl J Med 289:651, 1973.
12. Geizer WD, Smith TW, Goldfinger SE: Absorption of digoxin in patients with malabsorption syndromes. N Engl J Med 285:257, 1971.
13. Applefeld MM, Adir J, Crouthamel WG, et al: Digoxin pharmacokinetics in congestive heart failure. J Clin Pharmacol 21:114, 1981.
14. Jelliffe RW: An improved method of digoxin therapy. Am Intern Med 69:703, 1968.
15. Smith TW: Digitalis. N Engl J Med 288:719, 1973.
16. Perrier D, Mayersohn M, Marcus FI: Clinical pharmacokinetics of digitoxin. Clin Pharmacokinet 2:292, 1977.
17. Loeb HS, Gunnar RM: Treatment of pump failure in acute myocardial infarction. JAMA 252:2093, 1981.
18. Chung EK: Digitalis-induced cardiac arrhythmias. Am Heart J 79:845, 1970.
19. Beller GA, Smith TW, Abelmann WH, et al: Digitalis intoxication, a prospective clinical study with serum level correlations. N Engl J Med 284:989, 1971.
20. Smith TW, Haber E: digoxin intoxication, the relationship of clinical presentation to serum digoxin concentration. J Clin Invest 49:2377, 1970.
21. Lely AH, Van Enter CHF: Non-cardiac symptoms of digitalis intoxication. Am Heart J 83:149, 1972.
22. Fisch C: Digitalis intoxication. JAMA 216:1770, 1971.
23. Ekins BR, Watanabe AS: Acute digoxin poisonings: review of therapy. Am J Hosp Pharm 35:268, 1978.
24. Cloyd HC, Bosch DE, Sawchuk RJ: Concentration—time profile of phenytoin after admixture with small volumes of intravenous fluids. Am J Hosp Pharm 35:45, 1978.
25. Heissenbuttel RH, Bigger JT Jr: Bretylium tosylate: a newly available antiarrhythmic drug for ventricular arrhythmias. Ann Intern Med 91:229, 1979.
26. Payne VW, Secter RA, Noback RK: Use of colestipol in a patient with digoxin intoxication. Drug Intell Clin Pharm 15:902, 1981.
27. Jelliffe RW: Factors to consider in planning digoxin therapy. J Chronic Dis 24:407, 1971.
28. Garrett L, Zelis R, Mason DT: Linear dose response and quantitative attenuation by potassium of the inotropic action of acetylstrophanthidin. Clin Pharmacol Therap 22:34, 1977.

29. Seller RH, Cangiano J, Kim KE, et al: Digitalis toxicity and hypomagnesemia. *Am Heart J* 79:57, 1970.

30. Chopra D, Jamson P, Sawin CT: Insensitivity to digoxin associated with hypocalcemia. *N Engl J Med* 296:917, 1977.

31. Ewy GA, Kapadia GG, Yao L, et al: Digoxin metabolism in the elderly. *Circulation* 39:449, 1969.

32. Lawrence JR, Sumner DJ, Kalk WJ, et al: Digoxin kinetics in patients with thyroid dysfunction. *Clin Pharmacol Ther* 22:7, 1977.

33. Forrester JS, Diamond G, Chatterjee K, et al: Medical therapy of acute myocardial infarction by application of hemodynamic subsets. *N Engl J Med* 295:1356, 1976.

34. Porter GA: The role of diuretics in the treatment of heart failure. *JAMA* 244:1614, 1980.

35. Ram CVS, Reichgott MJ: Treatment of loop-diuretic resistant edema by the addition of metolazone. *Curr Ther Res* 22:686, 1977.

36. Hautman D, Rossier B, Zohlman R, et al: Rapid correction of hyponatremia in the syndrome of inappropriate secretion of antidiuretic hormone. *Ann Intern Med* 78:870, 1973.

37. Mason DT, Awan NA, Joye JA, et al: Treatment of acute and chronic congestive heart failure by vasodilator-afterload reduction. *Arch Intern Med* 140:1577, 1980.

38. Lakier JB, Khaja F, Stein PD: Rationale and use of vasodilators in the management of congestive heart failure. *Am Heart J* 97:519, 1979.

39. Colucci WS, Williams GH, Alexander RW, et al: Mechanisms and implications of vasodilator tolerance in the treatment of congestive heart failure. *Am J Med* 71:89, 1981.

40. Vidt DG, Bravo EL, Fouad FM: Captopril. *N Engl J Med* 306:214, 1982.

41. Taylor CR, Baird JRC, Blackburn KJ, et al: Comparative pharmacology and clinical efficacy of newer agents in treatment of heart failure. *Am Heart J* 102:515, 1981.

42. Forrester JS, Diamond G, Chatterjee K, et al: Medical therapy of acute myocardial infarction by application of hemodynamic subsets, Part 2. *N Engl J Med* 295:1404, 1976.

CHAPTER 21

Thromboembolic Disease

STEVEN R. KAYSER, Pharm.D.

Despite the availability for 30 years of anticoagulant drugs, thromboembolism remains one of the major contributors to morbidity and mortality in the United States today. Venous thromboembolism is responsible for hospitalization of approximately 400,000 persons annually, 60,000 of whom die. The cost, excluding out of hospital management, is estimated at upward of $1 billion annually.

Arterial thromboembolism is a major contributor to death from acute myocardial infarction, stroke and renal disease, the numbers one, three and four causes of death in the United States. In addition, arterial thromboembolism is associated with other high risk illnesses such a rheumatic heart disease, congestive heart failure and peripheral vascular disease (1–3).

It is not yet known what impact the expanded indications for use of fibrinolytic agents like streptokinase and urokinase will have on these statistics, but with increased experience it is hoped that there will be a favorable impact.

ETIOLOGY

Many conditions may contribute to the development of thromboembolic disease (Table 21.1). Immobilization and bed rest, with resultant stasis, frequently contribute to thrombosis especially in the elderly and obese person. Prolonged partial occlusion of the veins in any person sitting for prolonged periods may also lead to stasis. A hypercoagulable state existing during the operative period may contribute to clotting. Trauma may initiate clotting and thus is a particular problem in patients suffering fractures of the hips and pelvis who may also require prolonged bed rest. Congestive heart failure, ulcerative colitis, myocardial infarction and other high risk medical illnesses are associated with an increased risk of thrombosis. Carcinomas, particularly pancreatic, bronchogenic, gastric and prostatic may produce procoagulant substances which initiate clot-

ting. The increased activity of many clotting factors during pregnancy contributes to an increased risk of thrombosis. Oral contraceptives have likewise been associated with an increased risk of clotting. Less frequently some unusual blood diseases and hereditary causes have been associated with thrombosis (4, 5).

PATHOGENESIS

When injury occurs to the vascular endothelium, platelets adhere to exposed collagen as well as to other exposed subendothelial tissue. Following platelet adhesion, release of adenosine diphosphate (ADP) by the injured platelets leads to platelet aggregation (Fig. 21.1).

Transformation of this temporary platelet plug to a permanent platelet fibrin clot is achieved through activation of the extrinsic or intrinsic blood clotting system (Fig. 21.2).

Throughout this process of platelet aggregation a balance is maintained between certain prostaglandins which occur naturally and may be synthesized in vivo. Thromboxane A_2 is found in platelets and is a potent stimulant to platelet aggregation as well as a potent vasoconstrictor. Prostacyclin, in contrast, is found in vessel walls and is an inhibitor of platelet aggregation as well as a vasodilator. Not only may the balance between prostacyclin and thromboxane be altered physiologically but various drugs and even doses of these drugs (e.g. aspirin) may alter this balance.

Each of the clotting factors exist in the blood as inactive proteins. Before clotting can occur, each must be converted to an active or enzymatic form. Exposure of subendothelial collagen, in addition to interaction with platelets, initiates the intrinsic pathway by stimulating activation of factor XII. Activated factor XII then stimulates conversion of factor XI to its active form which then stimulates activation of factor IX. Activated factor IX in the presence of calcium, phospholipids (platelet factor 3) and factor VIII, stimulates the conversion of factor X to its active form. Activated factor X

Table 21.1.
Conditions Associated with Venous Thromboembolism

1. Immobilization, especially in elderly and obese
2. Stasis
3. Surgical period
4. Trauma to lower limbs
5. High risk medical illnesses
   a. Congestive heart failure
   b. Ulcerative colitis
   c. Myocardial infarction
6. Carcinoma of the pancreas, lung, stomach and prostate
7. Pregnancy and contraceptives
8. Blood diseases
9. Heredity

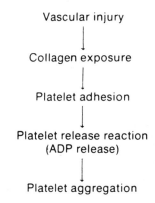

Figure 21.1.   Formation of the platelet plug.

in the presence of calcium, phospholipid (platelet factor 3) and factor V stimulates the conversion of prothrombin to thrombin.

The extrinsic clotting pathway may also stimulate the conversion of prothrombin to thrombin. The release of material extrinsic to the blood, such as tissue extract or tissue thromboplastin activates factor VII which stimulates activation of factor X. Factor X thus occupies a central position at the junction of the extrinsic and intrinsic systems.

Thrombin, which is generated by both pathways, stimulates the conversion of fibrinogen to fibrin in the presence of ionized calcium. The initial soluble fibrin clot is further converted to an insoluble fibrin polymer when factor XIII is activated by thrombin. In addition to stimulating the conversion of fibrinogen to fibrin, thrombin stimulates platelet aggregation and potentiates the activity of factors V, VIIa, VIII and Xa.

Once thrombin is formed, it is partly removed by absorption into fibrin. This, plus other naturally occurring inhibitors of clotting factors, play a role in localizing fibrin formation to the sites of injury and in maintaining the fluidity of circulating blood. Agents have been identified in normal blood which inhibit the activated forms of factors II, X, XI, and XII. Deposition of fibrin also activates plasmin or fibrinolysin, a fibrinolytic enzyme which also prevents excessive coagulation (Fig. 21.3).

Two types of thrombi are formed in response to appropriate stimuli. "White thrombi" or arterial thrombi are composed primarily of platelets although they also contain fibrin and occasional leukocytes. They generally occur in areas of rapid blood flow and are formed in response to an injured or abnormal vessel wall.

"Red thrombi" or venous thrombi are primarily found in areas of relative stasis where dilution of activated clotting factors by blood flow is prevented. They are almost completely composed of fibrin and erythrocytes with a small concentration of platelets.

The choice of an antithrombotic drug may thus be influenced by the most likely type of thrombus formed. Heparin and the coumarins are presently used in the treatment of both "red" and "white" thrombi. Drugs affecting platelet behavior are still being studied for their effect in preventing and treating "white thrombi." Fibrinolytic agents are effective in dissolving both types of thrombi.

INDICATIONS FOR THERAPY

Despite the association of thromboembolism with many different conditions, clear-cut indications with marked benefit from anticoagulant therapy exist only for treatment of pulmonary embolism, deep venous thrombosis, cerebral embolism, atrial fibrillation with rheumatic valvular disease, heart valve prostheses and acute peripheral arterial embolism (Table 21.2). Conditions with questionable benefit from anticoagulant therapy include acute myocardial infarction, transient ischemic attacks, hip fracture and disseminated intravascular coagulation. Despite several large scale investigations of the role of antiplatelet agents in the treatment of thromboembolism the indications for therapy remain unclear.

Deep Venous Thrombosis and Pulmonary Embolism

The clinical diagnosis of deep venous thrombosis is difficult and frequently misleading with most venous diseases occurring in the

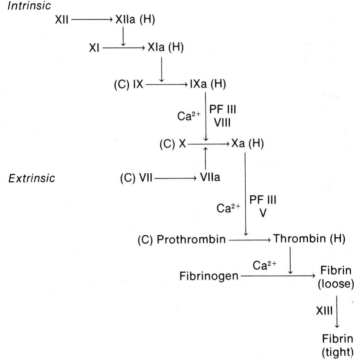

Figure 21.2. Soluble clotting cascade.

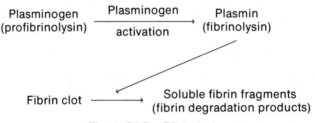

Figure 21.3. Fibrinolysis.

absence of significant findings. Nevertheless, the presence of certain clinical signs are helpful. In 80% of cases of deep venous thrombosis reviewed, unilateral ankle edema was present, followed by calf tenderness in 50% and a positive Homan's sign (pain upon dorsiflexion of the foot) in only 8%. Increased warmth and calf swelling are also consistent with deep venous thrombosis (5, 6).

Deep venous thrombi occur most frequently in the lower extremities in association with one or more of the previously discussed risk factors. The progression of thrombosis in the calf veins to the iliofemoral system in the thigh is associated with a greater risk of pulmonary embolism and prompts the early recognition and documentation of lower leg thrombosis in order to prevent pulmonary embolism.

The clinical manifestations of pulmonary

Table 21.2.
Indications for Anticoagulant Therapy

1. Marked benefit
   a. Pulmonary embolism
   b. Deep venous thrombosis
   c. Cerebral embolism
   d. Atrial fibrillation with rheumatic valvular disease
   e. Heart valve prosthesis
   f. Acute peripheral arterial embolism
2. Questionable benefit
   a. Acute myocardial infarction
   b. Transient ischemic attacks
   c. Hip fracture
   d. Disseminated intravascular coagulation

embolism, if present, may include fever, pleuritic chest pain, hemoptysis, tachypnea, tachycardia and shortness of breath. Electrocardiographic manifestations may include changes in the S-T segment and in T waves. Chest x-rays are usually not very helpful. Arterial blood gases generally show a reduced Po_2 as well as Pco_2 due to hyperventilation.

Objectively, the diagnosis of deep venous thrombosis may be confirmed by phlebography, Doppler ultrasound flow studies or by radionuclide labeled fibrinogen studies. Pulmonary embolism may be more specifically detected with the aid of pulmonary perfusion and ventilation scans, and pulmonary angiography (7).

The effectiveness of anticoagulant therapy in deep venous thrombosis of the iliofemoral area is well established. Treatment of deep vein thrombosis in the calf is usually initiated but not supported by all authors. Prompt anticoagulant therapy of pulmonary embolism is essential.

Cerebral Embolism

Thrombi dislodged from a fibrillating atrium or from a prosthetic heart valve are frequent causes of strokes. Strokes may also occur secondary to hemorrhage, thus it is imperative that an accurate diagnosis be made.

Anticoagulant therapy may be useful in preventing recurrence of emboli responsible for strokes, or in the treatment of evolving strokes or transient ischemic attacks. There is no place for anticoagulant therapy in the treatment of a completed stroke because of the risk of hemorrhage into an infarcted area which could then lead to extension of neurological damage (8).

Atrial Fibrillation

A high degree of correlation between atrial fibrillation and arterial emboli in patients with mitral stenosis has been recognized. Because of this, chronic anticoagulation is recommended. The presence of cardiomegaly (especially left atrial) or congestive heart failure in the presence of atrial fibrillation also is an indication for chronic therapy. Diagnosis of this condition is frequently preceded by symptoms of congestive heart failure, palpitations and occasionally syncope (9).

Myocardial Infarction

Since the early 1960s various clinical trials have been conducted in attempts to determine whether anticoagulants are beneficial in the treatment of myocardial infarction. There is still no agreement on this controversy (10, 11).

Many studies have failed to meet the criteria required for a good clinical trial. Although some studies have reported a decreased mortality in treated patients, it is now generally accepted that mortality is not altered by anticoagulant therapy. It has been shown in some studies that morbidity (strokes and nonfatal systemic emboli) may be decreased with anticoagulant therapy (12, 13).

If it is decided that a patient is to be treated with anticoagulants, a careful history of previous bleeding must be obtained so that a patient is not exposed to additional risk.

In summary, anticoagulants may be useful in the high-risk patient during hospital recuperation from a myocardial infarction, but anticoagulant therapy is not acceptable at present for all myocardial infarction patients (14). Early mobilization or treatment with low dose subcutaneous heparin may be more useful in prevention of thrombosis. Administration of streptokinase either intracoronary or intravenously within the first 6 to 8 hours following the onset of chest pain of myocardial infarction may prove useful in preventing loss of muscle tissue (15).

Heart Valve Prosthesis

Thromboembolism is one of the most frequent complications in survivors of prosthetic valve replacements. The greatest risk of embolism is to the brain. The development of porcine prosthetic valves holds great promise in decreasing the incidence of thromboembolism. All other valves, including the cloth-covered ones continue to carry a significant risk of thromboembolism.

It has been shown that patients receiving anticoagulants, who sustain an embolus, are likely to have had inadequate control of anticoagulant dosage.

The addition of an antiplatelet agent to an oral anticoagulant regimen may be useful in protecting against clotting. It has been recognized that the risk of thromboembolism is inversely proportional to the length of platelet survival and that platelet survival is decreased in many patients with prosthetic valves. Dipyridamole or aspirin plus dipyridamole will restore platelet survival to normal (16).

TREATMENT OF THROMBOEMBOLIC DISEASE

Measures other than pharmacologic intervention which contribute to the successful prevention or treatment of thromboembolic disease include proper education, the use of support garments and, infrequently, surgery.

Individualized patient education is important in an overall treatment plan. Prevention of stasis by avoiding prolonged sitting, crossing of legs or wearing of constricting garments is extremely important. Properly fitted and prescribed support stockings are important. Embolectomy or surgical placement of an inferior vena cava umbrella is occasionally performed.

Heparin and the oral anticoagulants (primarily coumarins in the United States) have been the major pharmacologic agents used in the treatment of clotting disorders. Recently the use of agents affecting either platelets or fibrinolysis have been added.

Prevention of the interaction of platelets with the arterial wall and subsequent microthrombosis and microembolization from these sites would prove useful. Drugs accelerating fibrinolysis would similarly prove useful adjuncts in increasing the rate of resolution of emboli but also preventing their extension.

LABORATORY ASSESSMENT OF ANTICOAGULANT THERAPY

Laboratory assessment of anticoagulant therapy was thought by some early clinicians to be superfluous. Since response to a given dosage of heparin or warfarin is highly variable, it is now recognized essential in monitoring for hemorrhage or recurrent embolization. Prolongation of the appropriate coagulation tests 1½ to 2½ times the control values provides the greatest protection against embolization with minimal risk of hemorrhage (17, 18).

Among the various tests available, the most commonly used ones are the Lee-White or whole blood clotting time (WBCT), the pro-

thrombin time (PT), the partial thromboplastin time (PTT), the activated partial thromboplastin time (APTT) and the activated coagulation time (ACT) (Table 21.3).

The whole blood clotting time or Lee-White clotting time is infrequently used today because of its lack of sensitivity. It is usually normal in the presence of factor VII deficiency, is insensitive in measuring prothrombin deficiency and is only moderately sensitive in measuring thromboplastin generation or fibrin formation. The normal clotting time is 9 to 14 min. The Lee-White clotting time is used primarily to measure heparin effect because of its insensitivity to the extrinsic clotting pathway.

The prothrombin time of Quick is prolonged by deficiencies of factors V, VII, X, and II and by low levels of fibrinogen and by high levels of heparin. The PT thus reflects alterations in the extrinsic and common pathways. The normal PT is approximately 12 sec. Prothrombin times are occasionally reported in percentage activity determined by dilution of plasma. This should be avoided due to the risk of confusing a protime in seconds with percentage activity. They are not the same and misinterpretation could lead to inappropriate changes in therapy. The PT is used to assess coumarin therapy.

The partial thromboplastin time is primarily a measure of the competency of the intrinsic and common clotting pathways. It is insensitive to factor VII and XIII. Its main use is in screening for deficiencies of the intrinsic clotting system in patients considered candidates for oral anticoagulation. The normal PTT is 60 to 85 sec. It can be used to assess heparin therapy; however, for this use it has generally been replaced by the activated partial thromboplastin time (APTT). The APTT differs from the PTT only in being performed on activated

Table 21.3.
Clotting Tests Used in the Management of Anticoagulant Therapy

Test	Factors Measured	Normal Value[a]	Drug Monitored
Whole blood clotting time (WBCT) (Lee-White)	All except VII	9–14 min (<15 min)	Heparin
Prothrombin time (PT)	II, V, VII, X	12 sec	Warfarin
Partial thromboplastin time (PTT)	All except VII	60–85 sec	Warfarin
Activated partial thromboplastin time (APTT)	All except VII	24–36 sec	Heparin
Activated coagulation time (ACT)	All except VII	80–130 sec	Heparin

[a] University of California, San Francisco.

plasma. It is generally a more sensitive test than the PTT and is widely used to monitor heparin therapy. The APTT, like the PTT, is performed with platelet poor plasma and thus it does not reflect the activity of platelets. Normal values for the APTT are between 24 to 36 sec.

The activated clotting time of whole blood is sensitive to all of the clotting factors except factor VII with undetermined sensitivity to factor V and II. The major advantages of this test are that it can be performed at the bedside and since it is a whole blood test, it does reflect the contribution of platelets in coagulation. The ACT is used to monitor heparin therapy and normal values are 80 to 130 sec (19).

Disadvantages associated with the ACT include relatively limited experience with this test in monitoring therapeutic heparin therapy and lack of correlation with the APTT. The APTT thus remains the standard for management of therapeutic heparin therapy.

DURATION OF ANTICOAGULANT THERAPY

Little agreement still exists regarding the optimal duration of anticoagulant therapy in the treatment of acute thromboembolic events such as deep venous thrombi or pulmonary embolism. The greatest risk for re-embolization is immediately after an initial event. The risk decreases over the next 6 to 8 weeks and it is during this period that adequate therapy is essential. In acute events most clinicians continue anticoagulants for 6 weeks to 3 months with little evidence supporting treatment for longer than this time (20–22).

Treatment of recurrent embolic events or prophylaxis of emboli in patients with prosthetic heart valves continues longer and may be for life.

PHARMACOLOGIC TREATMENT OF THROMBOEMBOLIC DISEASE— HEPARIN

Mechanism of Action

Heparin, a rapid-acting anticoagulant, exerts its antithrombotic effect by accelerating the action of a naturally occurring inhibitor of thrombin, an α_2-globulin, antithrombin III (AT III). This is also referred to as "heparin cofactor." AT III inhibits activated clotting factors which have a reactive serine residue at their enzymatically active center. Heparin, by binding at the lysine group of AT III (Fig. 21.4)

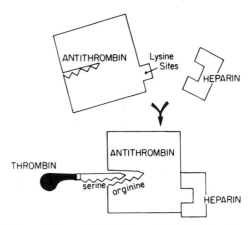

Figure 21.4.　Model of heparin-induced conformation change in antithrombin resulting in rapid inhibition of thrombin. (Reprinted with permission from *The New England Journal of Medicine*, 292:146, 1975.)

induces a conformational change in AT III which allows more ready access of the arginine residue to the serine group on the activated clotting factors. This forms an irreversible 1:1 stoichiometric complex (23).

Commercial heparin is obtained from hog mucosa or bovine lung. The anticoagulant activity of heparin from both sources appears to be equivalent. Differences may exist in the incidence of thrombocytopenia, which appears to be greater with heparin of bovine lung source. Because of this difference heparin sources within an institution should be standardized (24).

Pharmacokinetics

Heparin is not absorbed orally and therefore must be administered parenterally. It is usually administered intravenously with subcutaneous administration reserved for prophylactic, "low dose" use. Heparin should not be given intramuscularly because of the risk of hemorrhage.

Once absorbed, heparin is bound to a number of plasma proteins. It is metabolized primarily in the liver and reticuloendothelial system and is partly cleared by excretion into the urine.

The half-life of heparin's anticoagulant effect in normals and in patients with venous thromboembolism, as measured by changes in APTT, is approximately 1½ hours. The half-life, when plasma heparin activity is measured, is dependent upon the dose and increases with increased dose. It appears from limited studies that patients with pulmonary embolism have a greater heparin clearance and shorter half-life than those with venous thrombosis. This may be due to the continuing thrombin formation on the surface of the embolus, leading to an increased rate of heparin clearance (25–28).

Dosing and Administration

Intravenous administration of a large bolus dose of heparin assures that therapeutic anticoagulation is achieved without delay. Initial doses of at least 50 to 100 units/kg of body weight are needed to overcome the initial resistance which is present during early thromboembolic disease. Following an initial bolus dose, heparin is continued by intermittent intravenous or continuous intravenous administration.

In general, the maintenance of 35 to 50 units/kg of heparin in the body is required to anticoagulate blood to an acceptable level. General dosing guidelines can be applied to subsequent changes in the APTT (Table 21.4).

Prior to the initiation of heparin, baseline clotting studies must be performed and should include at least the prothrombin time (in anticipation of oral anticoagulant therapy) and the PTT, APTT or ACT.

Continuous infusion of heparin is the desired route of administration because it avoids the wide swings in heparin concentration, and thus the periods of supratherapeutic and subtherapeutic anticoagulation seen with intermittent administration. In addition, with continuous infusion, less heparin is required, and clotting tests may be performed at any time. Some disadvantages are that the rate must be controlled with an infusion pump. The usual dose needed to maintain the clotting time from 1½ to 2½ times the control is 1000 units per hour. This must, however, be adjusted based upon individual response.

Intermittent infusion, while not requiring an infusion pump, has numerous disadvantages. Larger doses and frequent injections are required. Clotting tests may be performed only at certain times for proper interpretation. In addition, Salzman et al. (29) have demonstrated that intermittent infusion with or without laboratory control is associated with more bleeding than continuous infusion to an APTT of 1½ to 2½ times the control.

The resistance to heparin therapy which is present initially, returns to normal within several days and reductions in dosage should be anticipated. Clotting tests should be performed frequently in the beginning and at least daily thereafter.

Heparin therapy should be continued for 7 to 10 days after the thromboembolic event, since it is during this time that the incidence of recurrence is greatest and also the time which a clot in the venous system requires for endothelialization. Oral anticoagulant therapy is usually initiated when heparin is started.

Subcutaneous heparin administration is normally reserved for "low dose" or "mini-dose" therapy. Small amounts of the initial coagulation enzymes (activated factors XII, XI, and IX) eventually lead to large amounts of thrombin. Heparin in relatively low concentrations can prevent this initiation of clotting, while much higher levels are required to inhibit fibrin formation once thrombin has been elaborated. Heparin in low subcutaneous doses especially augments the activity of an inhibitor of activated factor X. This inhibitor of factor Xa is probably the same as antithrombin III.

The greatest experience in the use of low dose heparin has been accumulated in prophylaxis of venous thromboembolism and pulmonary embolism during the surgical period. Publication of an International Multicentre Trial in 1975 has provided the strongest evidence for the efficacy of this route (30). The results showed clinically significant benefits in the reduction of venous thrombosis and pulmonary embolism. It is associated with a small, generally insignificant risk of bleeding.

It is most effective in elective gynecological and abdominothoracic surgery. Efficacy has not been clearly defined for orthopaedic procedures. It may also be useful in certain high risk medical patients such as those with congestive heart failure or myocardial infarction.

Administration regimens generally include 5,000 to 10,000 units subcutaneously from 12 to 2 hours preoperatively followed by 5,000 to 10,000 units every 8 to 12 hours postoperatively, or until the patient is ambulatory. While the APTT may be moderately elevated for several hours following administration, laboratory management is not necessary following initial assessment of clotting status. Adjusted subcutaneous heparin therapy has recently been compared to warfarin therapy in the treatment of deep vein thrombosis and pulmonary embolus. Heparin in doses ade-

Table 21.4.
General Guidelines for Heparin Administration[a]

This information for therapeutic intravenous heparinization of adult patients is intended as a general guide only

BEFORE BEGINNING HEPARIN THERAPY;

1. Order a STAT activated partial thromboplastin time (APTT); prothrombin time (PT), and platelet count
2. Review current medications for:
    a. *IM Injections:* Write an order that no IM injections be given while the patient is receiving anticoagulant therapy. If the patient is receiving a medication by the IM route, discontinue it and, if necessary, order the medication by another appropriate route or use an alternative
    b. *Drugs Inhibiting Platelet Function:* Avoid medications that may alter platelet function, especially aspirin, indomethacin, sulfinpyrazone and dipyridamole. If a patient is receiving a medication known to alter platelet function, discontinue it and, if necessary, select an appropriate alternative. There are occasional therapeutic situations where a drug affecting platelet function may be indicated, in this event a statement should be included in the chart documenting this
    c. Known meds which interact with heparin or warfarin

INITIATION OF HEPARIN THERAPY;

1. A typical bolus (loading) dose of heparin is 70–100 U/kg (dose to nearest 1000 U)
2. The initial bolus and infusion dose may require adjustment in the following conditions:

Increase	*Decrease*
Massive embolism	Recent bleeding history
	Age greater than 70
	Hematologic disorders resulting in bleeding tendencies
	Prior antithrombotic therapy
	Recent surgery (10 days)

3. Begin continuous infusion at the same time as the bolus administration. (See Maintenance Heparin Therapy No. 1 below for dosing information)

MAINTENANCE HEPARIN THERAPY:

1. The usual beginning maintenance infusion rate is 10–15 U/kg/hr for DVT and 25 U/kg/hr for pulmonary embolism. Order heparin as "Heparin Infusion —— units per hour." The IV additive service provides a standardized heparin concentration of 15,000 U/250 ml D_5W. All heparin infusions must be delivered with an infusion device. Dosing sheets are provided along with the solution
2. Obtain a second APTT 4–6 hr after the bolus dose and continuous infusion have begun
3. Aim to achieve a therapeutic APTT of 60–80 sec
4. Dependent on the APTT value, a change in regimen may be necessary. Typical adjustments are as follows:
    a. <40 sec, re-bolus 100 U/kg and increase infusion by 200 U/hr
    b. 40–60 sec, re-bolus 50 U/kg and increase infusion by 100 U/hr
    c. 60–80 sec, maintain the current rate of infusion
    d. 80–100 sec, decrease infusion by 100 U/hr
    e. 100–135 sec, stop infusion for 1–2 hr and decrease infusion by 200 U/hr
    f. >135 sec, stop infusion until APTT within 60–80 sec, and decrease infusion by 300 U/hr
    NOTE: If bleeding occurs at any time (regardless of APTT), discontinue heparin and treat appropriately
5. Obtain a repeat APTT approximately 6 hr after any dosage change
6. Obtain an APTT daily when patient is stable

GENERAL:

1. Obtain CBC and platelets every other day, and a stool guiaic and urinalysis every third day
2. Examine all sites (skin, nose, throat, urine, stool) for bleeding daily
3. Begin oral anticoagulant therapy, usually within the first or second day of heparin therapy (NOTE: continuous infusion of heparin may cause a 1–3-sec prolongation of the PT)

quate to prolong the mid-interval APTT to 1½ times the control value was administered to one group of patients while another group received warfarin in traditional doses. Both groups initially received high dose intravenous heparin for 14 days. Recurrent proximal vein thromboembolism was prevented in both groups, the incidence of bleeding was greater in patients on warfarin (31). More traditional low dose heparin (5000–10,000 units every 12 hours) without laboratory adjustment is equally effective in prevention of calf vein thrombosis when compared to warfarin, but is not as effective in prevention of recurrent proximal vein thrombosis as warfarin (32).

Adverse Reactions

Hemorrhage is the most frequent adverse reaction to heparin and is generally, but not always associated with clotting tests outside of the recognized therapeutic range. Spontaneous bleeding is rare (33).

Minor hemorrhage occurs in approximately 4% of courses of anticoagulant therapy and is usually into the skin, urine, or from the nose. Major hemorrhagic events occur in approximately 2% of courses and is usually in the gastrointestinal tract and/or the central nervous system.

Other more rare adverse effects include thrombocytopenia (34, 35), osteoporosis, hypoaldosteronism (36) and generalized hypersensitivity reactions. Thrombocytopenia secondary to heparin appears during the first 3 to 12 days of therapy, is unrelated to dose and reverses itself within 3 to 5 days following discontinuation. The exact mechanism has not been established. Osteoporosis has occurred with therapy of greater than 10,000 units per day for 6 months or longer. Hypoaldosteronism with resultant hyperkalemia and sodium diuresis is uncommonly associated with heparin therapy.

Drug Interactions

Heparin may interact with some antibiotics when mixed in the same intravenous solution. The most significant ones are erythromycin, gentamicin, kanamycin and tetracycline. Of lesser significance are the penicillins and cephalothin. Infusion of heparin in either 5% dextrose in water (D_5W) or normal saline appears safe if the solution does not stand for more than 24 hours.

Drugs impairing platelet function should be avoided in patients receiving heparin since they further impair hemostasis (Table 21.4).

Treatment of Overdose

Protamine sulfate, a strongly basic molecule is a specific antidote which will combine with, and inactivate heparin. The appropriate dose of protamine is dependent upon the dose of heparin, the time since administration and the route of administration. If administered immediately after intravenous heparin, 1 mg of protamine is given for every 100 units of heparin. If treatment is delayed, the dose of protamine must be decreased. Response can be assessed with the APTT or ACT.

In the event of significant hemorrhage, replacement of volume and clotting factors will need to be accomplished with whole blood or fresh frozen plasma.

ORAL ANTICOAGULANTS

Of the oral anticoagulants available in the United States, only warfarin and bishydroxycoumarin have found widespread use.

Oral anticoagulants exert their pharmacologic effect by interfering with synthesis of the vitamin K dependent clotting factors in the liver. These factors are II, VII, IX, and X. Early investigators assumed that a competitive antagonism existed to explain the relationship between warfarin and vitamin K. This has since been disproven. Presently it is felt that warfarin inhibits the effect of vitamin K at a postribosomal step in the hepatic synthesis of the vitamin K dependent clotting factors. Vitamin K is required in the conversion of nonactive precursor proteins (precursors of active clotting factors), which lack calcium binding capacity, to active precursor proteins (e.g., prothrombin) which have calcium-binding capacity. This calcium-binding capacity is needed to hold prothrombin onto phospholipid surfaces during its activation to thrombin. Vitamin K accomplishes this activation by carboxylation of glutamyl residues on the precursor protein to form γ-carboxyglutamic acid which allows for calcium binding. Vitamin K also probably carboxylates the glutamyl residues of factors VII, IX, and X. During the carboxylation of precursor proteins, vitamin K is converted to vitamin K epoxide. Vitamin K epoxide is then converted back to vitamin K. Warfarin prevents this reaction and thus produces a build-up of inactive precursor proteins. This effect of warfarin can be overcome by the administration of vitamin K (37, 38).

The onset of anticoagulant effect of the coumarins is not only dependent on this interaction with vitamin K, but also on the metabolic clearance of clotting factors already present in the blood.

Pharmacokinetics

Warfarin is the most frequently administered oral anticoagulant in the United States. There are few exceptions where other agents should be used, since the pharmacokinetics of warfarin have been most extensively studied. Warfarin is completely absorbed in the upper gastrointestinal tract with peak blood levels occurring in 60 to 120 min. The volume of distribution of warfarin is 12.5% of body weight. This small volume of distribution is consistent with the extensive binding of warfarin to albumin, since it is equivalent to the V_d of albumin, 2.6 times the plasma volume (39).

The mean half-life of warfarin is independent of dose and is 42 hours (40). Warfarin is highly protein bound; on the order of 99.5% to serum albumin. No apparent relationship exists between the extent of protein binding of warfarin and the concentration of albumin or total protein in the serum. Furthermore, there appears to be no correlation between prothrombin time and dose of warfarin, total warfarin concentration, or free warfarin concentration between individuals (41, 42).

Warfarin is metabolized in the hepatic microsomes by mixed function oxidase enzymes. It is administered as a racemate which contains equal parts of the R and S isomer. The S isomer is approximately 5 times more potent than the R isomer. S warfarin is oxidized to 7-hydroxywarfarin and reduced to alcohol 2 (SS alcohol) while R warfarin is metabolized primarily by reduction to alcohol 1 (RS alcohol). Both racemates are metabolized to 6-hydroxywarfarin in small amounts (43). The warfarin alcohols have minimal anticoagulant activity and are excreted renally. The hydroxylated products are inactive and are eliminated only by metabolism (44).

The reason why the R and S isomers differ in potency is unclear. The half-life of the R isomer is 45 hours while the half-life of the S isomer is 33 hours, and they both have the same volumes of distribution. It has been proposed that differences in permeability or affinity to the receptor site account for the differing potencies (45).

Knowledge of these two isomers is important because drugs interact with warfarin stereoselectivity. Phenylbutazone (43) and metronidazole inhibit the S isomer but have no effect on the R isomer. Long-term warfarin therapy of thrombotic diseases may be made safer in the future by the administration of the R isomer alone since it does not appear to interact with some other drugs to the same extent as the racemic mixture and the S isomer.

Dosing

Initiation of oral anticoagulant therapy should be accomplished without a loading dose. Many clinicians have traditionally started therapy with a large initial dose, followed by smaller doses over subsequent days. The belief was that therapeutic anticoagulation would be achieved more quickly.

The onset of warfarin effect is not only dependent upon the half-life of the parent drug but also upon the half-life of catabolism of the vitamin K-dependent clotting factors. These factors have half-lives of 5 hours for factor VII, 20 to 40 hours for factors IX and X, and up to 60 hours for factor II. Depression of any factor may predispose the patient to bleeding.

O'Reilly compared a loading dose of warfarin, 1.5 mg/kg, with two schedules without a loading dose of 10 mg and 15 mg daily. No significant difference was found in the rate of fall of factors II, IX, and X between the different schedules. However, there was a significantly faster decline in factor VII activity with the loading dose versus the other two regimens. Because the prothrombin time is most sensitive to factor VII, a more rapid prolongation of the PT with the loading dose lead many to believe that this was proof that loading doses achieved more rapid anticoagulation. Intrinsic coagulation is most dependent on factors IX and X and less so on factor VII. In summary, depression of factor VII offers little, if any, protection against thromboembolism and rapid depression may lead to hemorrhage (46). Because of the many factors contributing to anticoagulant response, prothrombin times should be obtained daily until therapy is stabilized.

In order to achieve a safe and rapid conversion from heparin to warfarin, it is recommended that both anticoagulants be administered concurrently, from the first day. Both agents are continued until a therapeutic prothrombin time is achieved. Heparin must be administered for a minimum of 7 to 10 days, and it usually requires this long for warfarin's effect to be stabilized. Once therapeutic prothrombin times have been achieved, heparin may be discontinued. When patients are on both agents, care must be taken to measure the prothrombin time when heparin's effect is at a minimum since heparin will interfere with it. With intermittent infusion the PT should be measured just before the next dose of heparin. With continuous infusion, the prothrombin time may be measured at any time since the interference is minimal.

It has generally been recommended that the degree of oral anticoagulant induced prolongation of the clotting tests should be the same as with heparin, i.e. prolongation of the prothrombin time 1½ to 2½ times the normal prothrombin time. Findings of a study have recently shown that in the treatment of proximal vein thrombosis less intense anticoagulant therapy is associated with a low frequency of recurrent venous thromboembolism (2%) and a reduced risk of hemorrhage (72). If these results can be confirmed and applied to treatment of other thromboembolic conditions, prothrombin times of only 15 to 16 sec may be effective in achieving therapeutic results.

Termination of Anticoagulant Therapy

When a therapeutic course of anticoagulant therapy is concluded, warfarin may be abruptly discontinued without risk of "rebound" thromboembolism. Since the half-life of warfarin is prolonged, a tapering of effect is evident.

Determinants of Response

Many factors may alter response to warfarin (Table 21.5) (47–49).

Diet. Excessive intake of foods rich in vitamin K may theoretically induce a relative resistance of warfarin. Clinically this is rarely a problem and patients may still eat foods such as spinach, kale, cabbage, cauliflower, peas, cereals and fish. Patients may occasionally be given nutritional supplements to improve their nutrition. Some of these (e.g., Ensure) contain vitamin K which may cause the development of resistance to warfarin, although recent reformulation of these products to decrease the amount of vitamin K minimizes this interference.

Conversely, poor nutrition may lead to an increased hypoprothrombinemic response. Fasting or malabsorption may lead to decreased vitamin K absorption and increased warfarin response. Any acute illness associated with diarrhea may quickly induce vitamin K deficiency and resultant potentiation of warfarin response.

Drugs. Many drugs may interfere with the effect of warfarin. The drugs which can cause a significant drug interaction with warfarin are listed in Table 21.6. Despite the small number of drugs that have been documented to interfere with warfarin, it is necessary to assume that all drugs have the potential for interaction unless proven otherwise.

Liver Function. Since the vitamin K-dependent clotting factors are synthesized in the liver, any disruption of normal liver function may lead to an increased prothrombin time without warfarin. In the presence of warfarin this prolongation will be exaggerated.

Hypermetabolic States. Fever or hyperthy-

Table 21.5.
Determinants of Warfarin Response

Diet
Vitamin K
Drugs
Liver function
Hypermetabolic states
Hereditary resistance
Other

Table 21.6.
Significant Drug Interactions with Warfarin

1. Drugs enhancing anticoagulant effect
   a. Cimetidine
   b. Clofibrate (gemfibrozil?)
   c. D-Thyroxine
   d. Disulfiram
   e. Glucagon
   f. Metronidazole
   g. Phenylbutazone (oxyphenbutazone)
   h. Sulfinpyrazone
   i. Salicylates
   j. Timethroprim-sulfamethoxazole
2. Drugs decreasing anticoagulant effect
   a. Barbiturates
   b. Cholestyramine
   c. Glutethimide
   d. Rifampin
   e. Vitamin K

roidism may result in increased sensitivity to warfarin due to increased catabolism of the vitamin K dependent clotting factors. This is the predominant effect since the handling of warfarin appears unchanged. The response to warfarin in myxedema is conversely diminished.

Hereditary Resistance. A hereditary resistance has been identified in animals and man. Findings consistent with an altered affinity of the receptor for the oral anticoagulants or for vitamin K have been reported. This is apparently mediated by a single autosomal gene and is very rare.

Others. Many other, less well documented, determinants have been proposed, including climatic changes, smoking, race, age, plasma lipids and renal function.

Adverse Reactions

Hemorrhage, the most significant adverse effect of warfarin is one of the most frequent reasons for admission to the hospital from adverse drug reactions. Patients should be instructed about the most common sites of bleeding and should routinely observe themselves for any signs.

Cutaneous. Warfarin may cause a hemorrhagic infarct especially into soft fatty tissues. This occurs 7 to 10 days after initiation of therapy and usually resolves with discontinuation of warfarin, but occasionally requires surgical intervention. Other skin lesions reported include urticaria, dermatitis and the "purple toes" syndrome, a nonhemorrhagic reaction occurring shortly after initiation of therapy.

Teratogenic. Warfarin crosses into the placental circulation and has been reported to cause chondromylasia punctata or stippling of the bones. Nasal bone deformities have been attributed to maternal consumption of warfarin during the first trimester (50, 51). While heparin does not cross the placenta and may be safer during pregnancy, it is not without risk and it has also been associated with increased fetal risk (52).

It appears from the limited studies that warfarin does not significantly cross into breast milk (53).

Treatment of Overdose

Excessive hypoprothrombinemia may be reversed by administration of vitamin K, or if associated with bleeding, with fresh frozen plasma or whole blood. Prolongation of the prothrombin time without evidence of hemorrhage may require no more than withholding further warfarin therapy until the prothrombin time returns to the therapeutic range. If there is evidence of minor bleeding or if the patient is at significant risk for bleeding, then administration of vitamin K is indicated. Vitamin K_1, or phytonadione, is the only vitamin K preparation that should be used because of its more rapid onset of action. It may be administered intravenously, subcutaneously or orally but should be avoided intramuscularly because of the risk of hematoma formation. Intravenously it should be administered slowly in order to prevent cardiorespiratory collapse. Administration of 5 to 20 mg results in a return of the prothrombin time toward normal in 6 hours after intravenous and in 24 hours after oral dosing (54, 55).

Patients who require continued anticoagulation may manifest resistance to subsequent warfarin administration for up to several weeks after vitamin K.

Drug Interactions

Drugs may interact with warfarin by different mechanisms (56). Pharmacodynamically, drugs may interfere by antagonizing warfarin at the site of action (e.g. vitamin K), by altering the synthesis of clotting factors (oral contraceptives) or clotting factor catabolism (thyroxine) and by altering the hemostatic process for example by inhibiting platelet function.

Pharmacokinetically, drugs may interfere with warfarin by altering its bioavailability, protein binding, metabolism and excretion.

It has been proposed for many years that the administration of antibiotics, by suppressing intestinal synthesis of vitamin K by intestinal bacteria, would result in enhanced hypoprothrombinemia. It is most likely, however, that dietary sources of vitamin K are more important and that gut production is insignificant. Interaction of broad spectrum antibiotics and coumarins has not been found of clinical significance except in debilitated patients or those on prolonged parenteral feedings. Cholestyramine has been shown to decrease the absorption of warfarin as well as the absorption of vitamin K. High doses of salicylates may depress prothrombin synthesis by a direct effect on the liver.

Many drugs have been reported to interfere

with coumarin absorption, protein binding and biotransformation. Few drugs interact significantly via these mechanisms. As mentioned above, cholestyramine impairs the absorption of warfarin. Phenylbutazone, oxyphenbutazone, glucagon, diazoxide, chloral hydrate, and perhaps some sulfonamides may potentiate the effect of warfarin by protein displacement (57). This effect should be transient if protein displacement is the mechanism since the increased free level of drug will be metabolized and the levels return to the predisplacement level.

Phenylbutazone, metronidazole, disulfiram, trimethoprim-sulfamethoxazole, sulfinpyrazone, and perhaps cimetidine may stereoselectively inhibit the metabolism of warfarin resulting in an enhanced anticoagulant effect.

Barbiturates, glutethimide, rifampin, and carbamazepine will reduce the effect of warfarin by inducing its metabolism by induction of microsomal enzymes.

Drugs affecting prothrombin complex concentration may do so by depressing clotting factor synthesis or by increasing the rate of catabolism of clotting factors. Hepatotoxic drugs may potentiate coumarin induced hypoprothrombinemia by destruction of the liver resulting in decreased synthesis of the vitamin K dependent clotting factors. Thyroid drugs may increase the response of clotting factors secondary to a hypermetabolic state.

Any drug interfering with hemostasis may increase the risk of therapy with warfarin. Drugs interfering with platelet function by further impairing hemostasis potentiate the hemorrhagic risk of warfarin and should be avoided. Occasionally the combination of warfarin with an antiplatelet agent may be useful therapeutically. In these situations close monitoring is essential.

The selection of a nonsteroidal antiinflammatory agent is a particularly difficult one because not only may these agents interfere with platelet function and cause gastric irritation, but some (like phenylbutazone) may pharmacokinetically interact with warfarin as well. Of the commercially available ones, ibuprofen and naproxen appear to be the safest.

ANTIPLATELET AGENTS

The role of platelets in thrombogenesis has been described in the discussion of the pathogenesis of thromboembolism. Drugs affecting platelet behavior may do so by various mechanisms. They may reduce platelet adhesiveness, decrease or inhibit platelet aggregation, alter platelet membranes, prolong platelet survival, or interfere with platelet factor 3 availability (16).

Many drugs have been identified which impair platelet activity but only a few have shown promise in treatment of clinical disease. These include aspirin, clofibrate, dextran, dipyridamole, and sulfinpyrazone (16, 58, 59).

Aspirin

Doses of aspirin as low as 80 mg or less have been shown to interfere with the arachidonate pathway of prostaglandin synthesis and result in an antiplatelet effect. Aspirin accomplishes this by acetylation on platelet membranes and results in an imbalance of prostacyclin and thromboxane. The ultimate dose required to achieve this effect is not clearly established but appears to be very low. Other salicylates such as sodium salicylate or choline salicylate do not affect platelets (60, 63).

A Canadian Cooperative Study has shown that aspirin in doses of 325 mg q.i.d. will reduce the incidence of stroke and death in men with a previous history of transient ischemic attacks. Other antiplatelet agents are ineffective (61).

A number of studies have looked at the value of aspirin in the secondary prevention of myocardial infarction. None have demonstrated a statistical benefit although some have shown a favorable trend toward a benefit (14, 62, 64).

Aspirin prophylaxis of venous thromboembolism following total hip replacement has been shown by Salzmann to be effective in men, but inexplicably not in women. Administration of 600 mg of aspirin twice daily revealed a statistically significant prophylaxis in males when assessed by radiographic phlebography (65).

Clofibrate

The mechanism of action of clofibrate in suppressing platelet function is unclear (16). In patients with ischemic heart disease it has been shown to reduce platelet adhesion and to suppress collagen induced platelet aggregation, as well as prolong platelet survival. The role of clofibrate in clinical medicine is unclear. Its efficacy has not been established in either the treatment of coronary artery disease or cerebrovascular disease.

Dextran

Dextran may interfere with platelet function by altering platelet membranes, interfering with platelet factor 3 availability or inhibiting the spreading capability of platelets. Some clinical evidence supports the efficacy of dextran in the prevention of venous thromboembolism while some contradict it. At the present time, not enough evidence exists to recommend the use of dextran in the treatment or prevention of thromboembolic disease.

Dipyridamole

Although high doses of dipyridmole (greater than 400 mg per day) have been shown to inhibit platelet aggregation in vitro, these effects cannot be demonstrated in man. Clinically, it has been noted in the prophylaxis of thromboembolism in patients with prosthetic heart valves that dipyridamole in doses of 400 mg per day restores platelet survival toward normal. This effect of dipyridamole can be potentiated by the addition of aspirin. The dosage of dipyridamole can be reduced to 100 mg per day with the addition of aspirin 600 mg per day.

Dipyridamole has been used in combination with warfarin in patients with prosthetic heart valves. The efficacy in venous thromboembolism, cerebrovascular disease and coronary heart disease has not been established. The results of the persantine-aspirin reinfarction trial (PARIS) demonstrated a trend toward benefit but no statistically significant effect (14, 16).

Sulfinpyrazone

Sulfinpyrazone inhibits the platelet release reaction as well as prolonging platelet survival. The duration of action, unlike that of aspirin is only as long as effective plasma concentrations of the drug is maintained.

The strongest evidence for an antithrombotic effect from sulfinpyrazone comes from positive results in reducing the frequency of shunt thrombosis in patients with arteriovenous fistulas used in chronic hemodialysis. Doses of 200 mg 4 times daily were well tolerated and resulted in a decrease in clot formation.

The results of the Anturane Reinfarction Trial (ART) have been the subject of extensive controversy (14, 16). Patients who received 800 mg (200 mg q.i.d.) of sulfinpyrazone within 25 to 35 days of infarct demonstrated a reduction in sudden death from 6.3 to 2.7% as well as a reduction in the annual death rate of 9.5 to 4.5%. These results have been questioned however because of questions in trial design and evaluation. Sulfinpyrazone is not presently approved for secondary prevention of infarct. The use of sulfinpyrazone in prevention of venous thromboembolism and cerebrovascular disease remains to be established.

FIBRINOLYTIC AGENTS (66–71)

Urokinase and streptokinase are both immediately acting fibrinolytic agents. If dosed properly, they have the capacity to interfere with the clotting process and actually dissolve clots. This is in contrast to heparin and warfarin which only prevent further clotting.

Streptokinase is approved for the treatment of massive, life threatening pulmonary embolism and deep venous thrombosis as well as acute coronary and arterial occlusion. Urokinase is approved for the treatment of pulmonary embolism and IV catheter clearance.

The use of streptokinase and urokinase in the treatment of pulmonary embolism is restricted to severe cases where accelerated resolution is desired. This is usually the case when pulmonary embolectomy is being considered. Therapy with streptokinase is initiated with a 250,000 IU loading dose over 30 min, followed by 100,000 IU per hour for 24 to 72 hours. Urokinase is initiated with a loading dose of 4,400 IU per kg over 10 min followed by 4,400 IU per kg per hour for 12 hours.

Hematologic status should be evaluated prior to administration of urokinase or streptokinase. The thrombin time, prothrombin time, activated partial thromboplastin time, CBC and platelets should be determined. Subsequent dosing is not usually based on clotting tests unless they indicate that an inadequate level of thrombolysis has been achieved. For this reason, a thrombin time is usually obtained shortly after therapy is initiated to determine the degree of thrombolysis and if it is between 2 and 5 times the normal level, the dosage is not increased.

Treatment of pulmonary embolism within 5 days of the onset of symptoms resulted in a more rapid resolution of angiographic and hemodynamic parameters than did heparin. Detectable differences one week after treatment were not present.

Treatment of deep vein thrombosis is usually reserved for cases where there is considered to be an increased risk of lifelong venous insufficiency. The loading and maintenance doses of streptokinase are the same with the exception that it is continued for 72 hours. In both pulmonary embolism and deep venous thrombi therapy is continued with heparin and oral anticoagulants following termination of fibrinolytic therapy. Heparin should not be started following fibrinolytic therapy until the APTT is 2 times normal or less. A loading dose is not used, but rather, a maintenance infusion is begun.

Treatment of acute coronary occlusion has recently been approved by the FDA. Generally streptokinase is administered directly into the occluded coronary artery following cardiac catheterization. A bolus dose of 50,000 units or more is administered followed by 2,000 to 6,000 units per minute for up to 2 hours or until resolution of the obstruction, whichever comes first. Administration must commence within 6 hours of symptoms to be effective in opening occluded artery. It is not known if there will be salvage of myocardium even if the artery is opened.

The mechanism of action of these agents is by activation of plasminogen (Fig. 21.3), urokinase by a direct mechanism and streptokinase by complexing with plasminogen. The half-life of streptokinase and urokinase is 10 to 15 min. Fibrinolysis induced by these drugs can induce widespread bleeding because they not only lyse thromboemboli but also hemostatic plugs. Therapy with these agents is contraindicated in patients who have had recent surgery, a kidney or liver biopsy or intra-arterial diagnostic procedures in the previous 10 days. In addition, a cerebrovascular accident within 2 months, previous bleeding problems or recent parturition preclude the use of these agents.

Adverse reactions other than bleeding include allergic and febrile reactions.

CONCLUSION

Thromboembolic disease contributes to significant morbidity and mortality in the United States. A recognition of the preventive measures which can be utilized and a knowledge and understanding of the pharmacology and clinical application of drugs affecting hemostases will go a long way in helping to decrease this.

References

1. Deykin D: Current status of anticoagulant therapy. Am J Med 72:659, 1982.
2. Rosenow EC, Osmundson PJ, Brown ML: Pulmonary embolism. Mayo Clin Proc 56:161, 1981.
3. Bell WR, Simon TL: Current status of pulmonary thromboembolic disease: pathophysiology, diagnosis, prevention, and treatment. Am Heart J 103:239, 1982.
4. Pitney WR: Clinical Aspects of Thromboembolism. Baltimore: Williams & Wilkins, 1972, p 23.
5. Goldhaber SZ, Savage DD, Garrison RJ, et al: Risk factors for pulmonary embolism. The Framingham Study. Am J Med 74:1023, 1983.
6. Stein PD, Willis PW, DeMets DL: History and physical examination in acute pulmonary embolism in patients without preexisting cardiac or pulmonary disease. Am J Cardiol 47:218, 1981.
7. Sassahara AA, Sharma GJRK, Barsamian EM, et al: Pulmonary thromboembolism. Diagnosis and treatment. JAMA 249:2945, 1983.
8. Genton E, Barnett HJM, Fields WS, et al: Report of the Joint Committee for Stroke Resources. XIV. Cerebral ischemia. The role of thrombosis and of antithrombotic therapy. Stroke 8:148, 1977.
9. Rogers PH, Sherry S: Current status of antithrombotic therapy in cardiovascular disease. Prog Cardiovas Dis 19:235, 1976.
10. Feinstein AR: More blood for the anticoagulant battle. N Engl J Med 292:1400, 1975.
11. Chalmers TC, Matta RJ, Smith H, et al: Evidence favoring the use of anticoagulants in acute myocardial infarction. N Engl J Med 297:1091, 1977.
12. Selzer A: Use of anticoagulant agents in acute myocardial infarction: statistics or clinical relevance (editorial). Am J Cardiol 41:1315, 1978.
13. Frishman WH, Ribner HS: Anticoagulation in myocardial infarction: modern approach to an old problem. Am J Cardiol 43:1207, 1979.
14. May GS, Eberlien KA, Furberg CD, et al: Secondary prevention after acute myocardial infarction. A review of long-term trials. Prog Cardiovasc Dis 24:331, 1982.
15. Mason DT (ed): Symposium on intracoronary thrombolysis in acute myocardial infarction. Am Heart J 102:1123, 1981.
16. Fuster V, Chesebro JH: Antithrombotic therapy: role of antiplatelet drugs. Mayo Clin Proc 56:102–112, 185–195, 265–273, 1981.
17. Basu D, Gallus A, Hirsch H, et al: A prospective study of the value of monitoring heparin treatment with the activated partial thromboplastin time. N Engl J Med 287:324, 1972.
18. Sevitt S, Innes D: Prothrombin time and thrombotest in injured patients on prophylactic anticoagulant therapy. Lancet 1:124, 1964.
19. Hattersly PG: Activated coagulation time of whole blood. JAMA 196:436, 1966.
20. O'Sullivan EF, Hirsch J, McCarthy RA, et al: Heparin in the treatment of venous thromboembolic disease. Administration, control and results. Med J Aust 2:153, 1968.
21. Acheson L, Speizer F, Tager I: Venous thrombosis; duration of anticoagulant therapy (letter). N Engl J Med 293:879, 1975.

22. Coon WW, Willis PW: Recurrence of venous thromboembolism. *Surgery* 73:823, 1973.

23. Rosenberg RD: Actions and interactions of antithrombin and heparin. *N Engl J Med* 292:146, 1975.

24. Coon WW: Heparin: a drug of varying composition and effectiveness. *Clin Pharmacol Ther* 23:139, 1978.

25. Estes JW: Kinetics of the anticoagulant effect of heparin. *JAMA* 12:1492, 1970.

26. Estes JW, Pelikan EW, Krugen-Thiemer E: A retrospective study of the pharmacokinetics of heparin. *Clin Pharmacol Ther* 10:329, 1970.

27. Nies DS: Pulmonary embolism. In Melmon K, Morelli H: *Clinical Pharmacology, Basic Principles in Therapeutics.* New York: Macmillan, 1972, p 230.

28. Hirsh J, Van A, Ken WG, et al: Heparin kinetics in venous thrombosis and pulmonary embolism. *Circulation* 53:691, 1976.

29. Salzman EW, Deykin D, Shapiro RM, et al: Management of heparin therapy. Controlled prospective trial. *N Engl J Med* 292:1046, 1975.

30. Kakkar VV: Prevention of fatal postoperative pulmonary embolism by low doses of heparin. An international multicentre trial. *Lancet* 1:45, 1975.

31. Hull R, Delmore T, Carter C, et al: Adjusted subcutaneous heparin vs. warfarin sodium in the long-term treatment of venous thrombosis. *N Engl J Med* 306:189, 1982.

32. Bynum LJ, Wilson JE: Low-dose heparin therapy in the long-term management of venous thromboembolism. *Am J Med* 47:553, 1979.

33. Kelton JG, Hirsh J: Bleeding associated with antithrombotic therapy. *Semin Hematol* 17:259, 1980.

34. Babcock RB, Dumper W, Scharfman WW: Heparin-induced immune thrombocytopenia. *N Engl J Med* 295:237, 1976.

35. Bell WR, Tomasulo PA, Alving BM, et al: Thrombocytopenia occurring during the administration of heparin: a prospective study in 52 patients. *Ann Intern Med* 85:155, 1976.

36. Wilson ID, Goetz FC: Selective hypoaldosteronism after prolonged heparin administration. *Am J Med* 36:635, 1964.

37. Stenflo J: Vitamin K prothrombin and gamma carboxyglutamic acid. *N Engl J Med* 296:624, 1977.

38. Suttie JW: Oral anticoagulant therapy, the biosynthetic basis. *Semin Hematol* 14:365, 1977.

39. O'Reilly RA, Aggeler PM, Leong LS: Studies on the coumarin antioagulant drugs; a comparison of the pharmacodynamics of dicumarol and warfarin in man. *Thromb Diath Haemorrh* 11:1, 1964.

40. O'Reilly RA, Aggeler PM, Leong LS: Studies on the coumarin anticoagulant drugs. The pharmacodynamics of warfarin in man. *J Clin Invest* 42:1542, 1963.

41. Yacobi A, Udall JA, Levy G: Serum protein binding as a determinant of warfarin body clearance and anticoagulant effect. *Clin Pharmacol Ther* 19:552, 1976.

42. Yacobi A, Lampman T, Levy G: Frequency distribution of free warfarin and free phenytoin

43. Lewis RJ, Trager WF, Chan KF, et al: Warfarin: stereochemical aspects of its metabolism and interaction with phenylbutazone. *J Clin Invest* 53:1607, 1974.

44. Lewis RJ, Trager WF, Robinson J, et al: Warfarin metabolites; the anticoagulant activity and pharmacology of warfarin alcohols. *J Lab Clin Med* 81:915, 1973.

45. Hewick DS, McEwen J: Plasma half-lives, plasma metabolites and anticoagulant efficacies of the enantiomers of warfarin in man. *J Pharm Pharmacol* 25:458, 1973.

46. O'Reilly RA, Aggeler PM: Studies on coumarin anticoagulant drugs: initiation of therapy without a loading dose. *Circulation* 38:169, 1968.

47. O'Reilly RA, Aggeler PM: Determinants of the response to oral anticoagulant drugs in man. *Pharmacol Rev* 22:35, 1970.

48. Fenech A, Winter JH, Douglas AS: Individualization of oral anticoagulant therapy. *Drugs* 18:48, 1979.

49. Breckenridge AM: Interindividual differences in the response to oral anticoagulants. *Drugs* 14:367, 1977.

50. Pettifor JM, Benson R: Congenital malformations associated with the administration of oral anticoagulants during pregnancy. *J Pediatr* 86:459, 1975.

51. Warkany J: A warfarin embryopathy. *Am J Dis Child* 129:287, 1975.

52. Hall JG, Pauli RM, Wilson KM, et al: Maternal and fetal sequlae of anticoagulation during pregnancy. *Am J Med* 68:122, 1980.

53. Orme ML'E, Lewis PJ, de Swiet MS, et al: May mothers given warfarin breast-feed their infants? *Br Med J* 1:1564, 1977.

54. Udall J: Don't use the wrong vitamin K. *Calif Med* 112:65, 1966.

55. Taberner DA, Thompson JM, Poller L, et al: Comparison of prothrombin complex concentrate and vitamin K in oral anticoagulant reversal. *Br Med J* 1:83, 1976.

56. MacLeaod SM, et al: Pharmacodynamic and Pharmacokinetic drug interactions with coumarin anticoagulant drugs. *Drugs* 11:461, 1976.

57. Koch-Weser J, Sellers EM: Drug interactions with coumarin anticoagulants. *N Engl J Med* 285:487, 547, 1971.

58. Gallus AS: Antithrombotic drugs. Part II. *Drugs* 12:132, 1976.

59. Mustard JF, Packham MA: Platelets thrombosis and drugs. *Drugs* 9:19, 1975.

60. Weksler BB, Pett SB, Alonso D, et al: Differential inibition by aspirin of vascular and platelet prostaglandin synthesis in atherosclerotic patients. *N Engl J Med* 308:800, 1983.

61. Canadian Cooperative Study Group: A randomized trial of aspirin and sulfinpyrazone in threatened stroke. *N Engl J Med* 299:53, 1978.

62. Mehta J: Platelets and prostaglandins in coronary artery disease. Rationale for the use of platelet-suppressive drugs. *JAMA* 249:2818, 1983.

63. Weiss HJ: Antiplatelet drugs—a new pharma-

cologic approach to the prevention of thrombosis. *Am Heart J* 92:86, 1976.

64. Aspirin Myocardial Infarction Research Group: An intervention study—the aspirin myocardial infarction study. *Lipids* 12:59, 1977.

65. Harris WH, Salzman EW, Athanasoulis CA, et al: Aspirin prophylaxis of venous thromboembolism after total hip replacement. *N Engl J Med* 297:1246, 1977.

66. Marder JT: The use of thrombolytic agents: choice of patient, drug administration, laboratory monitoring. *Ann Intern Med* 90:802, 1979.

67. Sharma GVRK, Cella G, Parisi AF, et al: Thrombolytic therapy. *N Engl J Med* 306:1268, 1982.

68. Sherry S: Thrombolytic therapy in thrombosis. A National Institutes of Health Consensus Development Conference. *Ann Intern Med* 93:141, 1980.

69. Anon: Streptokinase and urokinase. *Med Lett Drugs Ther* 20:37, 1978.

70. Genton E: Thrombolytic therapy of pulmonary thromboembolism. *Prog Cardiovasc Dis* 21:333, 1979.

71. Schröder R, Biamino G, Leiner ER, et al: Intravenous short-term infusion of streptokinase in acute myocardial infarction. *Circulation* 67:536, 1983.

72. Hull R, Hirsh J, Jay R, et al: Different intensities of oral anticoagulant therapy in the treatment of proximal-vein thrombosis. *N Engl J Med* 307:1676, 1982.

CHAPTER 22

Cardiac Arrhythmias

MARK A. GILL, Pharm.D.,
JEAN K. NOGUCHI, Pharm.D.

The appropriate treatment of arrhythmias requires an understanding of anatomy and electrophysiology. The frequency of serious adverse reactions from antiarrhythmic drugs must be compared to the morbidity associated with the particular arrhythmia under consideration. Once a drug is chosen, the principles of pharmacokinetics must be applied to tailor the regimen to each patient.

The electrical system of the heart consists of intrinsic pacemakers and conduction tissues. It is convenient to conceptualize the progression of normal cardiac rhythm in terms of its anatomical basis (Fig. 22.1). Figure 22.2 correlates the standard electrocardiogram with this normal electrical pathway.

The rate of electrical firing of the heart is dependent upon the most rapid pacemaker. Spontaneous electrical firing or automaticity can occur anywhere in the heart under certain conditions. Normally the sinoatrial (SA) node, which is located where the superior vena cava meets the right atrium, has the most rapid intrinsic rate (60 to 100 per min). Therefore, any electrical activity not initiated by a normal impulse generated by the SA node is considered an arrhythmia. Most arrhythmias are labeled as to anatomical location and rate.

Firing of the SA node initiates contraction in the atria. The electrical impulse is conducted through the atria via internodal tracts to the atrioventricular (AV) node near the coronary sinus, between the two atria. The AV node has pacemaker properties but normally serves to coordinate atrial and ventricular contraction.

The conduction system in the ventricles is more elaborate than the atria since the muscle mass is larger. Rapid and effective excitation is critical since the ventricles contribute the most to cardiac output.

Fibers leaving the AV node are called the bundle of His and separate into the bundle branches which traverse the septum between the ventricles. The final conducting components of the ventricles are the Purkinje fibers which emanate from the bundle branches to stimulate the ventricular cardiac muscle.

ELECTROPHYSIOLOGY

Conduction and electrical firing in myocardial cells may be analyzed by measuring the membrane potential of various tissues. The electrical potential of these membranes is established by the flow of ions. When electrodes are placed into these tissues, a characteristic repetitive pattern is seen called the action potential (Fig. 22.3). This action potential may be divided into five phases. Phase 0 is the period of depolarization. It is mediated by two ionic currents. The initial event is the rapid transfer of sodium ions into the cardiac cell. As the sodium depolarizes the tissues, the threshold for the slow response is reached. The slow response is dependent upon the transfer of calcium. Phase 1 is the rapid repolarization of the tissue and may be dependent upon the inactivation of the sodium current and activation of chloride flow. Phase 2 is a plateau maintained primarily by calcium flow. Phase 3 is the repolarization of the cells initially begun by inhibition of calcium flow. Repolarization is accelerated by potassium flow outward. The rate of fall of Phase 3 and its depth will determine the membrane responsiveness. Tissues may only depolarize after reaching a particular level of repolarization, at least -50 to -55 mV for Purkinje fibers. The tissue cannot be reactivated regardless of the stimulus until falling below the threshold potential (x in Fig. 22.3). This level of repolarization will therefore determine the end of the absolute refractory period (ARP). The ARP will vary in length depending upon the action potential duration (APD). Phase 4 is the depolarization of the cells. In Purkinje fibers, it is brought on by stimulation from the sinus node. Phase 4 may develop spontaneously if the slope is in-

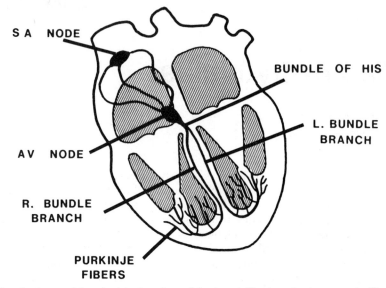

Figure 22.1. Anatomy of the electrical system of the heart. The impulse is generated by the sinoatrial (SA) node and is conducted through the atria to the atrioventricular (AV) node, which directs the current to the bundle of His, into the bundle branches and finally to the Purkinje fibers.

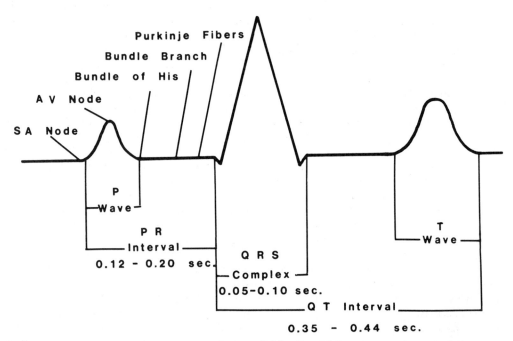

Figure 22.2. Stylized surface electrocardiogram (ECG). The ECG wave pattern is separated into its component parts and correlated with the anatomical sites that influence the pattern. The three intervals commonly measured (PR, QRS, and QT) have the normal durations noted. The duration quoted for the QT interval is corrected for the heart rate and is commonly referred to as QTc.

creased. The action potential of pacemaker tissue, such as the sinus node, differs from Purkinje fibers. The depth of repolarization is less dramatic and Phase 4 has a steeper slope that determines the rate of sinus firing and its automaticity. The precise ionic currents responsible for pacemaker cells are not entirely known.

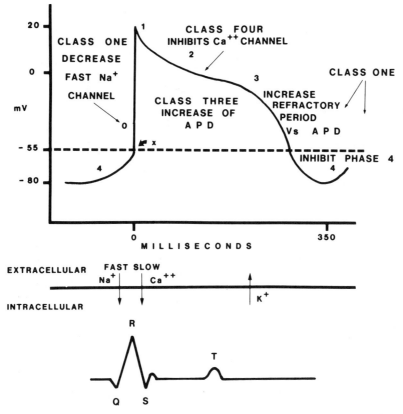

Figure 22.3. The action potential of a cardiac conduction cell correlated with electrolyte shifts and the ECG. *X* is the threshold potential. The effects of antiarrhythmic drug classes (see Table 22.1) are noted for the phases of the action potential.

ARRHYTHMIA GENESIS

In general arrhythmias may be described as abnormalities in electrical development as in ectopic tachyarrhythmias, in electrical conduction as in reentry arrhythmias, or in a combination of both mechanisms.

Ectopic beats may develop as pacemaking cells emerge when anoxia, stretch, catecholamine excess, or edema increase the slope of Phase 4. Reentry arrhythmias are dependent upon different velocity along adjacent fibers and unidirectional block in electrical conduction (Fig. 22.4). This allows for continuing excitation in a repetitive manner. This circus rhythm may develop as areas of infarcted tissue block or delay conduction. A single circuit of the fibers may induce a premature contraction while continuous cycling of impulses might produce sustained tachycardia. This process may occur in both atrial and ventricular tissue.

Antiarrhythmics have varying effects on reentry mechanics. One effect might be to inhibit membrane responsiveness in fiber 2 such that block is produced in both directions (Fig. 22.5A). Another effect might be to enhance conduction in the damaged portion of fiber 2 such that the impulse down fiber 1 will find depolarized fiber and cannot maintain the circuit (Fig. 22.5B).

Conduction velocity may decrease by blocking the fast response and allowing emergence of the slow response as in infarction or digoxin toxicity. In addition since ARP is dependent on the APD, if repolarization is accelerated, cardiac tissue may be more excitable. On the other hand, mechanisms (primarily drugs) that prolong the APD also lengthen the ARP and thereby reduce excitability. This prolongation of repolarization is associated with lengthening of the QT interval (called QTc when corrected for heart rate) (Fig. 22.2). Prolongation of depolarization also serves to lengthen the QRS duration.

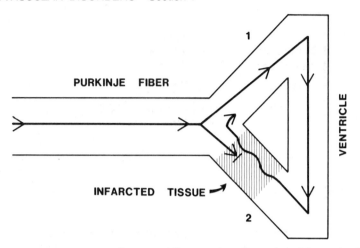

Figure 22.4. Reentry. A conduction fiber that bifurcates into fibers 1 and 2 to stimulate ventricular tissues. The normal pattern is for conduction through fibers 1 and 2 at similar rates. In this figure, fiber 2 was infarcted which slows conduction until it is blocked by refractory cells. The impulse is not impeded along fiber 1. Fiber 2 is activated by the impulse crossing the ventricular muscle tissue. The retrograde impulse finds fiber 2 repolarized and crosses, but at a slow rate. This circuit may be repeated or may terminate if fiber 1 is depolarized.

DRUG ACTION

Antiarrhythmic drugs are classified according to their electrophysiologic properties (Table 22.1). Class One drugs are depressants of myocardial membranes. The common and major property of this group is to increase the threshold of excitability (x in Fig. 22.3), which reduces ectopics and prolongs the refractory period which inhibits reentry. Class Two includes the β-blocking drugs. Many arrhythmias are produced or exacerbated by hyperactivity of the sympathetic nervous system. Class Three drugs prolong the APD thereby lengthening ARP. Class Four agents inhibit the slow response mechanism. Ectopic beats may develop if myocardial damage allows emergence of the slow reponse, coupled with inhibition of the fast response.

SINUS BRADYCARDIA

Sinus bradycardia is a rhythm having a rate of less than 60 beats/min, with impulses originating in the SA node. Sinus bradycardia may arise from a decrease in pacemaker activity in the sinus node (decreased automaticity) or improper impulse propagation out of the sinus node. In some situations (e.g. sleeping, or in well-conditioned athletes), sinus bradycardia has few adverse effects and is a normal occurrence, whereas in others (e.g. acute myocardial infarction), serious complications may arise.

The incidence of sinus bradycardia during acute myocardial infarction ranges from 10 to 41% (2). It occurs most commonly in inferior or posterior infarctions, reaching its peak incidence in the first few hours after infarction. In many instances, sinus bradycardia is transient, is not associated with any adverse hemodynamic consequences, and does not alter morbidity or mortality. (2, 3). Treatment of these patients is not necessary.

In some patients, hypotension, along with compromise of cardiac output and coronary perfusion, are associated with bradycardia. A low stroke volume may result from decreased left ventricular function, hypovolemia, or peripheral pooling of blood (vagal excess, or in some patients, drugs such as nitroglycerin or morphine), and in conjunction with a low heart rate, results in a very low cardiac output. Ventricular escape beats may occur, reflecting an increase in ventricular irritability from the slow rate. If the hypotension is mild and the patient is not symptomatic, elevation of the legs or infusion of fluids may be adequate. In the moderately to severely hypotensive or symptomatic patient, *atropine* is the drug of choice. Initial doses of 0.3 to 0.5 mg may be repeated every 3 min to a maximum of approximately 2.0 mg. The intravenous route should be used, as inadequate peripheral perfusion may result in unpredictable absorption from subcutaneous or intramuscular adminis-

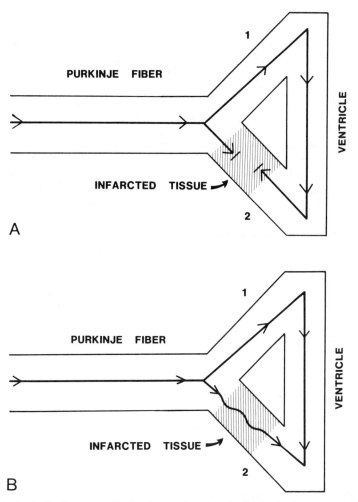

Figure 22.5. Antiarrhythmic drug effect on reentry. (*A*) Antiarrhythmics may inhibit reentry by slowing conduction in both directions in fiber 2 such that the cells are still refractory when the impulses arrive; (*B*) another mechanism to abolish reentry is to enhance conduction through fiber 2. Although conduction in fiber 2 is not normal, it is complete so that the impulse from fiber 1 finds refractory cells and cannot maintain the circuit.

Table 22.1.
Classification of Antiarrhythmic Drugs[a, b]

Class	Drug	Depression of Phase 0 (Fast Response)	Action Potential Duration	Depression of Slow Response	Sympatholytic Activity
ONE	Quinidine	4+	↑ +	0	0
	Procainamide	4+	↑ +	0	0
	Lidocaine	4+	↓ +	0	0
	Phenytoin	4+	↓ +	0	0
	Disopyramide	4+	↓ +	0	0
TWO	Propranolol	+	↓ +	0	4+
	Nadolol	+	↓ +	0	4+
	Atenolol	+	↓ +	0	4+
	Alprenolol	+	↓ +	0	4+
	Metoprolol	+	↓ +	0	4+
THREE	Bretylium	↑ Phase 4	↑ 4+	0	+
FOUR	Verapamil	↓ Phase 4	↑ Phase 1 and 2	4+	+

[a] From B. N. Singh et al. (1).
[b] 0 = no activity, + = slight activity, 4+ = major activity.

423

tration. Atropine's direct vagolytic action will increase sinus node automaticity, shorten SA conduction, and facilitate AV conduction (3). Because it has minimal effect on automaticity in patients with intrinsic sinus node dysfunction, atropine has little effect in these patients and pacemakers are frequently necessary.

Deleterious effects of atropine include excessive tachycardia (causing increases in myocardial oxygen consumption) and a possible increase in ventricular irritability, as well as other noncardiac effects (urinary retention, blurred vision, etc.). Because of the hemodynamic side effects, initial dosing in patients with acute myocardial infarction should be low, and repeated doses avoided if possible.

Isoproterenol has been recommended as a second line drug in patients unresponsive to atropine. However, this drug increases myocardial oxygen consumption, can increase ventricular irritability, and can aggravate venous pooling of blood in high doses. Therefore, in the setting of an acute myocardial infarction, this drug should be avoided.

Those patients not responding to atropine should have a *pacemaker* placed. In most patients, sinus bradycardia associated with an acute myocardial infarction is a transient problem and therefore only temporary pacemakers are necessary.

SINUS TACHYCARDIA

Sinus tachycardia is characterized by a rate of over 100 and usually less than 180 beats/min, with impulses originating in the sinus node. Sinus tachycardia is usually a normal physiologic response to a myriad of conditions, including exercise, anxiety, pain, fright, fever, hypoxia, anemia, hypovolemia, early congestive heart failure, drugs (sympathomimetics or vagolytics), hyperthyroidism or pheochromocytoma. The vast majority of patients with sinus tachycardia do not have symptoms except perhaps for palpitations. Patients with coronary artery disease may develop angina because of the increased myocardial oxygen consumption; those with poor cardiac reserve may not tolerate sustained tachycardia and develop congestive heart failure.

The treatment of sinus tachycardia consists of management of the underlying condition. Treatment of the tachycardia per se is not necessary and may even have deleterious effects, since decreasing the heart rate will decrease cardiac output and oxygen delivery to the tissues. In the rare instance where sinus tachycardia is sustained and causing palpitations or other symptoms (e.g. hyperthyroidism), *propranolol* or another β-blocker may be given as long as the patient is not in congestive heart failure.

PAROXYSMAL SUPRAVENTRICULAR TACHYCARDIA

Paroxysmal supraventricular tachycardia (PSVT) is a common cardiac arrhythmia, occurring at any age from infancy through adulthood. PSVT is frequently seen in healthy individuals with otherwise normal cardiovascular systems. Most cases of PSVT are abrupt in origin; termination also occurs abruptly, but the duration of PSVT is unpredictable, ranging from minutes to days.

Most cases of PSVT occur as a result of reentry at the level of the AV node. Requirements for AV node reentry include: (a) longitudinal dissociation of the AV node into two functional pathways, pathway 1 having slow conduction velocity and a short refractory period, and pathway 2 having rapid conduction velocity and a long refractory period; and (b) a premature atrial contraction (PAC). In reentry, a critically timed PAC enters the AV node at a time when pathway 1 will carry the impulse but pathway 2 is refractory and thus will not. Upon arrival at the His bundle, the His-Purkinje system is activated in a normal fashion; additionally pathway 2, now recovered, will transmit the impulse in a retrograde fashion (back toward the atria), resulting in an atrial echo. When the impulse arrives at the atria, if pathway 1 has had time to recover, the impulse will travel antegrade (back toward the ventricles) down pathway 1, and a sustained reentrant tachycardia will result. Thus, the impulse travels in a circuit antegrade down pathway 1 and retrograde up pathway 2 (Fig. 22.6) (4, 5). Clearly, in order to induce and maintain reentry, a fine balance between conduction and refractoriness must exist. The ventricular rate in PSVT ranges from 150 to 250/min.

Although some patients may be asymptomatic, many will almost immediately notice the very fast heart rate and will have symptoms such as light-headedness, syncope, weakness, dyspnea and chest pain. Congestive heart failure and shock may ensue in patients with tenuous cardiovascular status or in young otherwise healthy infants. Infants may be

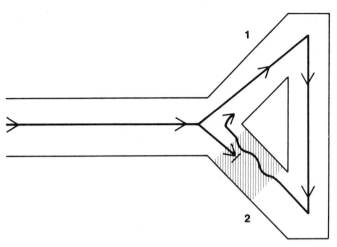

Figure 22.6.   Reentry at the level of the AV node. See text under "Paroxysmal Supraventricular Tachycardia" for explanation.

brought to the pediatrician for such nonspecific problems as "fussiness" or "won't eat," yet are frequently in florid congestive heart failure.

The goal of therapy for PSVT is to interrupt the critical relationship between conduction velocity and refractoriness so that reentry cannot occur. Initial treatment usually consists of maneuvers to increase vagal tone. This will slow AV conduction and increase AV nodal refractoriness, thus breaking the reentry circuit. *Carotid sinus pressure or massage* will stimulate the baroreceptors in the neck and are effective terminating procedures in many patients. Caution should be exercised in the elderly or others with signs of advanced atherosclerotic disease. In these patients, a temporary reduction in carotid blood flow may produce symptoms of cerebral ischemia, and a check of carotid pulses to ensure that both are strong, equal and without bruits should be done before pressure is applied. Other noninvasive vagotonic techniques which may be used include the Valsalva maneuver, and a "surprise" splash of ice water in the face. Vagotonic procedures of all types should not be used in patients with sinus node dysfunction, since a prolonged sinus node recovery time may result in a period of sinus arrest after the reentry circuit is broken.

The use of drugs which increase vagal tone, either directly (edrophonium) or indirectly (metaraminol or phenylephrine), in the termination of PSVT has been largely surpassed by the introduction of the calcium channel blocking agents.

The observation that the morphology of action potential curves of the pacemaker cells in the SA and AV nodes resemble those of the slow channel mediated by calcium, and the response of these nodal tissues to chemicals known to alter the calcium currents has led to the suggestion that excitation in these areas is mediated by the calcium channel. Other areas in the conduction system (such as the Purkinje cells) may also be calcium channel dependent under such abnormal conditions as ischemia, hypoxia or exposure to catecholamines (6, 7). Both cardiac and peripheral vascular smooth muscles are also calcium channel dependent (7–9). Therefore, drugs that block the calcium channel may have a variety of direct cardiovascular effects (on cardiac automaticity, cardiac conduction and peripheral and coronary vasodilation) with the net effect of each drug resulting from a complex interaction of direct and reflex actions.

Verapamil's direct effects on the heart produce a slower rate of spontaneous SA node discharge (negative chronotropic effect), a reduction in AV node conduction velocity (negative dromotropic effect), an increase in AV nodal refractoriness, and a reduction in contractility (negative inotropic effect). The peripheral vasodilating effects of the drug induce reflex increases in automaticity and contractility which largely offset the negative chronotropic and inotropic effects. Thus, the net cardiac effects of the drug occur predominantly at the AV node, with the other effects becoming significant only in diseased hearts (e.g. sinus node disease or myocardial dysfunction) (6, 9, 10). Nifedipine, the other currently available calcium channel blocker, is a much more potent vasodilator, and doses which are necessary to demonstrate a negative dromotropic effect will result in marked hemodynamic alterations (8, 9). Thus, verapamil is the only currently marketed calcium channel blocking agent used as an antiarrhythmic.

Although verapamil has well-documented efficacy in the management of PSVT and the other supraventricular tachycardias, its usefulness in ventricular arrhythmias is not well known at present. The lack of responsiveness of Purkinje cells to calcium channel blockers, except at very high doses or under abnormal conditions such as ischemia, points to a limited usefulness in these arrhythmias.

Intravenous verapamil will terminate PSVT in about 80 to 90% of patients (9–13), thus clearly surpassing other currently available drugs in efficacy and accounting for its emergence as a first-line drug for this arrhythmia. After a dose of 5 to 10 mg (0.075 to 0.15 mg/kg) IV over 1 to 2 min, a response is generally seen within 2 to 5 min. If no response is seen in 30 min, a repeat dose of 10 mg (0.15 mg/kg) may be given.

Following intravenous injection, serum levels of verapamil decline in a biexponential fashion, with an α-phase half-life of 18 to 35 min and a β-phase half-life of 3 to 7 hours (14). Rapid and extensive biotransformation to unknown metabolites occurs, with the majority (approximately 70%) of active drug and metabolites excreted in the urine (14). Verapamil is 90% protein bound. Discrepancies between serum level decay, timing of hemodynamic effect (peak 5 min, duration 10 to 20 min), and timing of AV nodal conduction effects (onset 1 to 2 min, peak 10 to 15 min, duration 6 hours) suggest that there may be preferential uptake of verapamil by the AV node, and that serum levels may not correlate well with pharmacologic effect.

Side effects after a single intravenous dose are minimal in most patients and reflect an extension of pharmacologic effect; a mild transient fall in blood pressure is the most common adverse reaction. Because of the action of verapamil on the SA and AV nodes, sinus node dysfunction and AV block may be worsened by verapamil and constitute absolute contraindications to its use. Patients taking β-blockers should be given this drug with caution and only under strictly monitored situations, since these drugs decrease AV conduction, SA node automaticity and contractility by an independent mechanism and thus may block the reflex increases in contractility and heart rate normally seen with verapamil. Suspected digitalis toxicity is another contraindication to verapamil, because it may further aggravate AV block, though in the absence of digitalis toxicity these drugs may be combined without problems (10, 12). Other contraindications are severe left ventricular dysfunction or severe hypotension; however in situations where *mild* congestive heart failure or hypotension are felt to be secondary to the PSVT, conversion to sinus rhythm with cautious verapamil administration frequently results in an improvement in hemodynamic status and thus resolution of these problems (10).

Verapamil does not aggravate bronchospastic or vasospastic disorders and thus is safe in patients unable to take β-blockers for these reasons.

If neither vagal maneuvers nor verapamil succeed in converting PSVT, *edrophonium* (5 to 10 mg IV over 1 to 2 min), *metaraminol* (0.5 to 1 mg IV over 2 to 3 min), or *phenylephrine* (0.5 mg IV over 1 to 2 min followed by 0.1 to 0.2 mg every 15 min as needed to a maximum of 1 mg) may be tried in an attempt to pharmacologically increase vagal tone. Each of these should be preceded and followed by vagal maneuvers. Caution should be used when giving edrophonium to patients on digitalis and when giving pressors to the elderly; all of these methods should be given only with caution to patients with sinus node dysfunction.

Digitalis has an overall lower response rate as well as a longer onset of action (up to several hours) than verapamil and vagotonic stimuli, making it a less useful drug for converting PSVT to sinus rhythm. However, it slows AV conduction by a different mechanism and thus failure to respond to these drugs or maneuvers does not necessarily imply a failure to digitalis. Therefore, digitalis retains its usefulness as an alternate drug for PSVT when verapamil and vagal stimulation (by maneuvers or pharmacologic therapy) fail. Specific aspects of digitalis therapy will be discussed in the section on atrial fibrillation.

Propranolol has in the past been recommended as another alternate drug in the treatment of PSVT. However, almost all patients will by this time already have received verapamil; in view of the deleterious effects of verapamil and β-blockers when given together, it would seem unwise to give propranolol in this situation and one should proceed directly to cardioversion.

The electrical management of PSVT is usually done with *DC cardioversion.* DC cardioversion works by simultaneously resetting all of the pacemakers in the heart and thus will abolish reentry and allow the sinus node to reestablish itself as the pacemaker. Because of its generally instantaneous action and its lack of intrinsic hypotensive effect, DC cardioversion is the maneuver of choice in a severely symptomatic patient. In contrast to ventricular arrhythmias, low voltage cardioversion is usually adequate for PSVT. A machine which synchronizes the discharge to the QRS complex will avoid the problem of ventricular fibrillation resulting from discharge on the T wave. Atrial pacing may also be attempted, but the need for individualized sophisticated electrophysiologic studies limits its usefulness in the acutely ill patient.

Patients with recurrent attacks of PSVT should be first instructed in *vagal maneuvers* such as carotid sinus massage, especially if attacks are infrequent and have been successfully managed in this manner in the past. When attacks occur often or are resistant to vagal maneuvers, pharmacologic prophylaxis may be initiated. This can be done with digoxin, propranolol or quinidine. Preliminary reports with verapamil are also encouraging.

Digoxin decreases conduction through the AV node, and may be successful as a single agent, especially in infants and children. The ideal digoxin dose should be one that controls the ventricular rate yet does not cause bradycardia when the patient is in normal sinus rhythm. For recommendations on dosing, see the section on atrial fibrillation.

Quinidine decreases atrial automaticity and therefore will decrease the number of premature atrial contractions (which are the initiating event in PSVT). Effects on the AV node are variable, because the direct action of the drug is modified by an independent vagolytic action. Therefore, it should be remembered that, once any supraventricular tachycardia has begun, quinidine has little effect on the arrhythmia and may in fact enhance AV nodal conduction (and thus ventricular rate) because of the vagolytic effect. Thus, all patients with PSVT or other supraventricular tachyarrhythmias should be fully digitalized before admin-

istration of quinidine. However, when given in conjunction with digoxin, quinidine may increase digoxin serum levels by up to 100%, resulting in digoxin toxicity in some patients (15).

In spite of these potential problems, quinidine remains a useful drug in the prophylaxis of PSVT. The usual dose of quinidine sulfate is 200 to 400 mg every 6 hours. Several different salts of quinidine are available; it is important to recognize that the actual quinidine content of these salts varies (quinidine sulfate = 82.9% quinidine base, quinidine gluconate = 62.3% base, quinidine polygalacturonate = 60.3% base), so that doses may be adjusted accordingly. Adjustment of dosage in patients with renal or hepatic insufficiency or congestive heart failure remains controversial; serum levels should be closely monitored in these patients.

After oral administration, quinidine sulfate is approximately 70% absorbed. Salts other than quinidine sulfate may have different absorption characteristics, especially when incorporated into sustained release forms. The drug is metabolized to several different active and inactive metabolites, and has a half-life in normal subjects of approximately 6 to 7 hours; 10 to 20% of the unchanged drug is excreted in the urine. Distribution, metabolism and excretion of quinidine are altered in the presence of congestive heart failure, hepatic or renal insufficiency, and old age (16).

Because some of the older assays for quinidine measured both active drug and metabolite, quotes of "therapeutic" serum levels have varied (16). The commonly used therapeutic range of 2 to 5 μg/ml is for those assays measuring active drug only; a check with the laboratory performing the assay would be prudent (Table 22.2).

A review of data from 652 patients taking

Table 22.2.
Therapeutic Plasma Drug Concentrations

Drug	Plasma Level
Procainamide	4–8 μg/ml
Lidocaine	1.5–5.5 μg/ml
Phenytoin	10–20 μg/ml
Disopyramide	3–6 μg/ml
Bretylium	0.5–1.5 μg/ml
Quinidine	2–5 μg/ml[a]
Digoxin	0.5–2 ng/ml[a]

[a] See text for qualifying statements.

quinidine in the Boston Collaborative Drug Surveillance Program (17) showed an incidence of adverse reactions of 14%. The most common adverse reactions were gastrointestinal (7.8%—nausea, vomiting and/or diarrhea), followed by arrhythmias (2.5%—sinus bradycardia, rapid ventricular rate during atrial fibrillation, ventricular tachycardia; the latter, with an incidence of 0.3%, was probably related to prolongation of the QTc interval, unrelated to dose but related to the phenomenon of quinidine syncope and sudden death), and fever (1.7%). Dermatologic and hematologic reactions and cinchonism each accounted for less than 1% of quinidine reactions.

Propranolol and the other β-blocking agents have a multitude of effects on cardiac conduction and contractility. A slowing of automaticity in sinus and ectopic pacemakers, a decrease in conduction velocity through the AV node, and an increase in the refractory period of the AV node account for their effectiveness in PSVT and the other supraventricular tachycardias. Although in theory the "quinidine-like" membrane stabilizing properties of the β-blockers may contribute to their antiarrhythmic properties, the doses required to produce these effects are substantially higher than those in clinical practice. Because its mechanism of action is by blockade of cardiac β-adrenergic receptors, propranolol is particularly effective in supraventricular tachycardias associated with excessive catecholamine release (hyperthyroidism, pheochromocytoma, exercise, emotional upset).

Dosage requirements for propranolol are difficult to predict, because of large variations in pharmacokinetics and physiologic responses to a fixed concentration of drug. This also accounts for the difficulty in establishing "therapeutic" serum concentrations. Individualization of dosage regimens is thus necessary.

Propranolol's effects on sinus node automaticity and cardiac contractility make its use in patients with sinus node dysfunction or congestive heart failure unwise. Selection of a β-blocking agent with intrinsic sympathomimetic activity could theoretically minimize these problems but may also attenuate the antiarrhythmic effects at the level of the AV node. The difficulties encountered when using propranolol in patients with chronic obstructive pulmonary disease or peripheral vascular disease may be reduced (although not necessarily eliminated) by the use of more cardio-selective agents such as atenolol or acebutolol. However, large scale studies with these agents are lacking.

In patients with recurrent PSVT resistant to drugs, *atrial pacing* may be attempted. This may be done with timed stimuli, in which a critically timed premature atrial stimulus breaks the reentry circuit by entering the circuit and creating a refractory zone ahead of the impulse, thus halting its transmission (18). This obviously requires prior individual electrophysiologic studies to determine that the patient will respond to pacing, as well as the placement and timing of the paced stimulus necessary to break the circuit. Overdrive pacing is a second technique where the atria are paced at a rate faster than that of the tachycardia. When symptoms occur, these pacemakers are activated by the patient, usually by placing a magnet over the generator pocket.

Automatic atrial tachycardia results from enhanced automaticity of an atrial ectopic focus. This type of PSVT is much less common than that caused by reentry. The management of automatic atrial tachycardia is similar to that of reentry PSVT, with a few exceptions. The success rate of verapamil is somewhat less than that for reentry, with about two thirds of patients converting to normal sinus rhythm (10, 11). Digoxin is of little use since it has no effect on ectopic focus automaticity. A search for and attempts at correction of such causes of this arrhythmia as hypoxia, ischemia or excess catecholamine secretion should also be undertaken.

An important example of an automatic atrial tachycardia is PSVT with block. PSVT with block is always a result of ectopic atrial activity, since the concept of reentry allows for only 1:1 AV conduction. In a patient taking digitalis, PSVT with block should be considered digitalis toxicity until proven otherwise. The principal management of a patient with digitalis induced PSVT with block is the administration of *potassium* since potassium counteracts the action of digitalis at the cellular level. Caution should be exercised in patients with oliguria or anuria as well as those who are already hyperkalemic at presentation. Verapamil is contraindicated in any patient with digitalis toxicity, as discussed above.

ATRIAL FIBRILLATION

Atrial fibrillation is characterized by very rapid atrial firing at a rate between 350 and 600/min ("auricular delerium"); the AV node prevents the majority of these impulses from reaching the ventricles, resulting in an average ventricular rate in untreated atrial fibrillation of 120 to 170 beats/min. Ventricular conduction in most cases is normal. Atrial fibrillation is the most common sustained arrhythmia in organic heart disease, and the second most common overall. It is frequently associated with rheumatic heart disease (particularly mitral valve disease), hyperthyroidism, and cardiomyopathies, and is seen more commonly in the elderly. Atrial fibrillation is also seen in 10 to 15% of patients with acute myocardial infarctions (2).

The hemodynamic effects of atrial fibrillation occur as a result of loss of synchronized atrial contraction (leading to a rise in mean left atrial pressure, a decrease in left ventricular end diastolic pressure, and a decrease in stroke volume), and a decrease in diastolic filling time of the ventricles (also leading to a decreased stroke volume). Thus the net effect is a decrease in cardiac reserve. The principal nonhemodynamic consequence of atrial fibrillation is embolism resulting from nonlaminar flow of blood through the ventricles and consequent formation of mural thrombi. Embolization may occur both during atrial fibrillation as well as during the immediate postconversion phase in sinus rhythm.

Clinical manifestations of atrial fibrillation are frequently the signs and symptoms of congestive heart failure, most commonly in the pulmonary system. Some patients may develop angina as a result of decreased coronary blood flow; palpitations are also sometimes seen. An irregularly irregular pulse is the classic physical finding of atrial fibrillation.

The primary goal of therapy in atrial fibrillation is to increase cardiac output. This is most commonly accomplished in the acute phase by pharmacologic slowing of the ventricular rate to allow for a longer diastolic filling time and thus a larger stroke volume. Attempts at conversion to normal sinus rhythm are preferably done when the patients cardiovascular status has been stabilized, and are limited in the acute phase to those patients who are grossly symptomatic with hemodynamic instability. Generally an arbitrary ventricular rate of less than 100 is chosen as a therapeutic goal, however the following considerations in therapy must be emphasized: (a) strict attention to ventricular rate should not be at the expense of objective and symptomatic relief or of drug intoxication; (b) allow-

ance should be made for any factors which may be independently increasing the heart rate, most notably excess catecholamine release as in infection or hyperthyroidism. If signs and symptoms improve, a rate of 100 to 120 may be acceptable in these patients, since strict adherence to a goal of a rate less than 100 may result in excessive bradycardia once the underlying problem is corrected. Rate titration should take into consideration the subjective and objective appearance of the patient as well as the anticipated rapidity of correction of catecholamine release; and (c) aggressive attempts at correction or improvement of coexisting problems such as infection, blood loss, hypoxia or hyperthyroidism should be undertaken.

Digitalis has traditionally been considered the drug of choice in atrial fibrillation, owing to its concomitant positive inotropic and negative chronotropic properties. Intravenous doses are generally indicated in patients with atrial fibrillation, because of their more rapid onset of action; oral dosing may be used in more stable patients. Intramuscular digoxin gives erratic absorption and causes excessive pain. Jelliffe (20, 21) has found that for most patients oral digitalizing doses of 10 to 20 μg/kg result in acceptable response without undue risk of toxicity. He also notes that those patients with supraventricular tachycardias frequently need doses in the higher range because of the need to block the AV node. For estimation of intravenous dosing, an adjustment downward is necessary in order to account for oral bioavailability of digoxin:

Intravenous dose

$$= \text{oral dose} \times \text{fraction absorbed}.$$

It must be emphasized that digoxin needs vary widely between patients, and this and other loading dose recommendations should be used only as rough guidelines to therapy, with the above goals and considerations being the primary determinant of dosing requirements. The use of serum levels as indicators of response to therapy or dosage requirement has been shown by several authors to be inaccurate (22, 23).

After oral administration, the fraction of digoxin absorbed (F) is currently estimated to range from 0.6 to 0.7 (note however that when using the Jelliffe method of digoxin dosing it is probably better to use his original estimation of 0.80 to 0.85 in order to validate his recommendations for dosing). Distribution into myocardial and other tissues requires about 4 to 6 hours, thus accounting for the recommendation that all doses of digoxin should be separated by at least this much time. Digoxin is primarily eliminated by the kidneys, with a smaller fraction metabolized in the liver. Hence, estimations of maintenance dosing is vitally dependent on renal function.

Many methods for estimation of maintenance digoxin doses have been proposed. After the intravenous loading dose (or its equivalent) to achieve the desired effect has been established in an individual patient, Jelliffe (21, 24) suggests an estimation of the maintenance dose as follows:

Maintenance dose

$$= \frac{\text{IV loading dose} \times \text{fraction lost each day}}{\text{fraction absorbed}}$$

Fraction lost each day

$$= \frac{14 + 0.2(\text{creatinine clearance})}{100}$$

However, it should be reemphasized that calculations of all digoxin dosing needs are only guidelines to therapy, and dosage requirements must be evaluated on an individual basis.

Evaluation of patients for digoxin toxicity is difficult because of the nonspecific nature of the symptoms. Anorexia, nausea, vomiting and lethargy are the most common symptoms, with vision changes seen in some patients as well. Elevated serum digoxin levels may help in the diagnosis. However, electrolyte abnormalities, most notably hypokalemia but also metabolic alkalosis, hypomagnesemia and hypercalcemia, may contribute to digoxin toxicity even in the presence of nontoxic serum levels. The earliest sign of digoxin toxicity on electrocardiogram is frequently a regularization of ventricular rate with continuation of atrial fibrillation, reflecting excessive AV block and a resultant dominance of the AV junctional tissue as the pacemaker of the heart (19). The ventricular rate in this situation generally slows to as low as 35 to 50, because of the slow intrinsic rate of the AV junction. As toxicity progresses, essentially all types of arrhythmias may be seen, including several tachyarrhythmias.

Numerous studies have demonstrated the usefulness of the calcium channel blocking agent verapamil in lowering ventricular rate in patients with atrial fibrillation (10–13). Verapamil has the advantage of being much faster than digitalis, with an onset of action generally less than 10 min. However, the effect in atrial fibrillation lasts only about 30 min, and therefore repeat boluses or a constant infusion as suggested by some authors (9, 10) may be necessary. Conversion to sinus rhythm with verapamil is rare, probably because of its negligible effects on atrial automaticity.

Verapamil may thus be useful in acute situations where rapid control of ventricular rate is desirable (e.g. while waiting for digoxin to take effect), but its precise role in other patients with atrial fibrillation has not been well established. The dose of verapamil for atrial fibrillation is the same as that for PSVT: 5 to 10 mg (0.075 to 0.15 mg/kg) IV over 1 to 2 min; if no response is seen a dose of 10 mg (0.15 mg/kg) may be repeated in 30 min. Side effects and precautions for use of verapamil have already been discussed in the section on PSVT.

An occasional patient will not have adequate ventricular rates on what are felt to be maximum digoxin doses, or will manifest toxic effects to digoxin before rate control is achieved. In these patients and in those in whom atrial fibrillation is induced by hyperthyroidism, propranolol and the other β-blockers may be a useful addition.

Because of the incidence of embolic phenomena in atrial fibrillation, chronic prophylactic anticoagulation is carried out in some patients. Clear-cut data on the exact risks of embolism in most patients with atrial fibrillation are lacking. Common candidates for anticoagulation include those patients with a history of embolism, those with large left atria, and those with mitral valve disease or idiopathic hypertrophic subaortic stenosis. The decision to anticoagulate these and other patients with atrial fibrillation must be made on an individual basis, taking into account both the potential benefit and the risks (which may be substantial in some patients).

Conversion to normal sinus rhythm is a second goal in the management of atrial fibrillation. Conversion may be of significant value, since it will increase cardiac performance (by adding synchronized atrial contraction) and will markedly decrease the incidence of embolism. Unfortunately, not all patients will sustain a sinus rhythm once converted. Therefore, although for some patients conversion to sinus rhythm may be crucial (e.g. DC cardioversion for severe unstable hemodynamic compromise), in others it may not be practical. Patients likely to revert to atrial fibrillation after conversion include those with cardiomegaly (particularly left atrial enlargement), those with atrial fibrillation of more than 1 year's duration, and those in functional classes III and IV (symptoms with minimal exertion or at rest) (19).

Cardioversion is most commonly accomplished with *DC countershock*. Morris and Hurst (19), in compiling data from a total of 824 patients, showed a conversion rate of 88%, with a 2.4% incidence of complications (emboli 1.3%, ventricular arrhythmias 0.4%, miscellaneous 0.6%). Because of the incidence of emboli, they recommend anticoagulation for several weeks before and 2 weeks after cardioversion, especially in patients with a history of embolism, valvular disease, or idiopathic hypertrophic subaortic stenosis. Digoxin should be withheld for 24 to 48 hours before cardioversion, since it may increase the incidence of arrhythmias.

Pharmacologic conversion to sinus rhythm, although less invasive than cardioversion, is also less successful. Digitalis and verapamil rarely convert patients with atrial fibrillation to sinus rhythm. This probably results from their minimal effects on atrial automaticity.

Quinidine is the most commonly used drug for cardioversion, and is also used as a prophylactic agent in maintaining sinus rhythm postcardioversion. Typical recommended dosage regimens for conversion are 300 to 400 mg orally every 6 hours for 72 hours, OR 200 mg orally every 2 hours for 5 doses, to be increased on successive days to 300 mg and 400 mg (no more than 5 doses in any 1 day); doses of 200 to 400 mg every 6 hours are commonly used for maintenance of sinus rhythm. Intravenous quinidine has traditionally been discouraged because of the incidence of hypotension. A recent study has critically reconsidered this problem (25). Additionally, this study and one by Hirschfeld et al. (26) have reported rapid achievement of therapeutic serum levels in 20 to 25 min using slow (0.3 to 0.4 mg/kg/min) infusions of quinidine. A reevaluation of intravenous quinidine may thus be in order.

The reported success rate with quinidine conversion has ranged from 53 to 89%, with a mean of 71% (19). Success rates for maintenance of sinus rhythm are variable, some of which no doubt relate to subtherapeutic serum concentrations and poor compliance. All patients with atrial fibrillation who receive quinidine should be digitalized first, to avoid enhancement of AV conduction and a consequent very rapid ventricular rate by quinidine. The pharmacology and side effects of quinidine have already been discussed under PSVT.

WOLFF-PARKINSON-WHITE SYNDROME

In Wolff-Parkinson-White (WPW) syndrome, there is an abnormal anatomical AV connection in addition to the AV nodal tissue. This accessory pathway allows the establishment of reentry circuits which may lead to various supraventricular tachycardias, including PSVT and atrial fibrillation. In the reentry circuit, antegrade conduction may be either down the AV node (more common) or down the accessory pathway (less common). WPW syndrome is frequently seen in young otherwise healthy children and adults. Characteristically, patients have recurrent paroxysmal attacks of supraventricular tachycardias interspersed on a baseline of sinus rhythm.

Although the clinical manifestations and hemodynamic consequences are the same, difficulty in the treatment of supraventricular tachycardias in these patients arises from the fact that the accessory pathway may not be affected by drugs in the same fashion as the AV node. Drugs such as *quinidine, procainamide* and *propranolol* decrease conduction velocity through both the AV node and the accessory pathway. Quinidine may slow accessory pathway conduction even more than AV nodal conduction because of its vagolytic effect on the AV node.

Vagal maneuvers, digitalis and *verapamil* will slow conduction through the AV node but have no effect on conduction via accessory pathways. In some patients, digitalis (and perhaps verapamil) may even shorten the refractory period in accessory pathways resulting in an increase in impulse transmission. These drugs can therefore be considered first line treatment in patients with antegrade conduction down the AV node, but potentially very dangerous in the unusual patient whose antegrade conduction occurs via the accessory pathway. This is particularly true in atrial fibrillation and flutter, where very rapid atrial firing may result in ventricular tachycardia or fibrillation.

As with the other supraventricular tachycardias, *DC countershock* is a very effective termination procedure and is the treatment of choice in patients with unstable hemodynamics. Permanent ventricular pacing may be necessary in patients needing large doses of drugs to control tachyarrhythmias (pacing will eliminate problems with excessive bradycardia while the patient is in sinus rhythm). Atrial pacing may be useful in patients with antegrade conduction down the AV node. Surgical division of the accessory pathway, a relatively new procedure, has also been effective in some patients with recurrent tachycardias unresponsive to pharmacologic management.

ATRIOVENTRICULAR BLOCK

Atrioventricular block is divided into three types, depending on the degree of transmission of sinus impulses into the ventricles. In first degree AV block, each sinus impulse formed is propagated completely (1:1 conduction ratio), but conduction through the AV node is delayed. This arrhythmia may be seen in otherwise healthy people, is common in the elderly, and may occur as a result of drug administration (digitalis, verapamil, propranolol, potassium). In most cases of first degree AV block, no therapy is required.

In second degree AV block, there is intermittent failure of impulse propagation from the sinus node to the ventricles. There are two types of second degree AV block: In Mobitz type I (Wenckebach), AV conduction time increases in successive impulses (variable PR interval) until a sinus impulse is not conducted; Mobitz type II AV block is characterized by a fixed conduction time for all conducted impulses (constant PR interval), with intermittent nonconduction.

Mobitz type I AV block is typical of AV block occurring within the AV node (proximal conducting system). It may be seen in acute inferior or posterior myocardial infarction, usually within the first 72 hours postinfarction (2). In the absence of bundle branch block (distal block), Mobitz type I block is usually a benign arrhythmia of short duration (2 to 3 days) that does not require treatment.

Mobitz type II AV block is suggestive of block in the distal conducting system (distal His bundle or below the trifurcation of the bundle branches). Distal conduction disturbances are usually the result of anteroseptal infarction, and also occur most commonly during the first 72 hours postinfarction. This type of block is frequently preceded or accompanied by bundle branch block. It is more dangerous than Mobitz type I, because it usually reflects damage to the bundle branches and Purkinje system, and progression of Mobitz type II block to third degree block frequently results in severe compromise of the cardiovascular system. First or second degree AV block, "new" bundle branch block and bilateral bundle branch block are not themselves causes of any major cardiovascular complications. However, because of their association with third degree distal conduction block and its adverse hemodynamic consequences, along with the fact that the development of third degree block may be unpredictable, some now advocate prophylactic *pacemaker* placement for those patients demonstrating two of these three criteria in the setting of an acute myocardial infarction (2, 27).

Third degree AV block represents complete failure of impulse propagation through the AV node, with ventricular contraction occurring as a result of an escape mechanism. If the level of block is within the AV node (proximal conducting system), the escape rhythm usually originates in the AV junction or proximal His bundle. Ventricular impulse conduction will thus be normal (normal QRS morphology and duration). Although the ventricular rate will be slow owing to the slower inherent rate of the AV junctional tissue, cardiac output is adequate for some patients because of the normal ventricular conduction. Treatment of these patients, if asymptomatic, is controversial, with some advocating nothing and others, pacemakers (2, 3). In the symptomatic patient (hypotension, persistent chest pain, syncope, congestive heart failure) or one with excessive ventricular irritability resulting from the slow rate, the ventricular rate can be increased with *atropine* (0.3 to 0.5 mg) or *isoproterenol* (1 to 4 μg/min). These drugs facilitate AV nodal conduction by decreasing refractory period of the AV node. Although these drugs are useful in the emergency situation, their potential adverse cardiac effects (increased myocardial oxygen consumption and excessive ventricular irritability) should be borne in mind and serious consideration be made to the placement of a temporary pacemaker. As with second degree AV block of the proximal conducting system, this type of third degree block is not usually a permanent problem.

Third degree AV block occurring in the distal part of the conducting system (distal His bundle or below the trifurcation of the bundle branches) will result in an escape rhythm with abnormal QRS morphology and duration (reflecting abnormal ventricular conduction), and a very slow rate (less than 30 beats/min, reflecting the very slow intrinsic rate of ventricular tissue). This is generally an unstable rhythm, may result in ventricular asystole, and is associated much more frequently with acute adverse hemodynamic effects (Stokes-Adams syncope, chest pain, congestive heart failure). Atropine is not effective in this arrhythmia, since it has little to no effect on ventricular automaticity, and may even worsen AV conduction in some patients. *Pacemaker* placement is thus the treatment of choice. AV block of the distal system associated with an acute myocardial infarction carries a high risk of sudden death and a poor long-term prognosis; this may be decreased in some patients by the placement of a permanent pacemaker (27).

PREMATURE VENTRICULAR CONTRACTIONS

Premature ventricular contractions (PVCs) are ectopic beats originating in the ventricular muscle. These beats are not initiated by the SA node but are stimulated by the spontaneous electrical firing of the local tissue. PVCs are the most common arrhythmia. Depending on the length of the observation, the frequency of PVCs in otherwise healthy subjects is variable. One half of young male subjects have PVCs with 24-hour monitoring (28). The frequency of PVCs increases with advancing age and the presence of cardiac disease. In most patients, this arrhythmia produces no symptoms whatsoever. However, it is also the most common arrhythmia (40 to 80%) seen with myocardial infarctions where it may adversely affect survival.

Not all PVCs require treatment. This arrhythmia in otherwise healthy persons, when it is asymptomatic, does not require suppression. PVCs may compromise cardiac output and produce syncope; even in a patient without a history of cardiac illness, these PVCs should be treated. Yet, many patients complain merely of palpitations. If this is the only symptom, the benefit of PVC suppression must be balanced against the cost and toxicity of treatment.

PVCs may be separated into simple and complex arrhythmias. PVCs seen in asymptomatic, noncardiac disease subjects are usually simple in that they are isolated beats, occurring singly, with a wave pattern on ECG that repeats itself, indicating that the beat originates from the same site. These appear to be well tolerated until their frequency compromises ventricular filling. Complex PVCs are uncommon in asymptomatic, noncardiac disease subjects but are frequent in patients with coronary artery disease. They may be subclassified as multiform or multifocal which means that the ECG wave form is different between ectopic beats suggesting more than one site in the ventricles is showing automaticity. Another complex classification refers to paired or runs of PVCs. These are consecutive PVCs without intervening sinus beats. The final type of complex PVC is one that is termed early or R-on-T, referring to the R wave of the PVC interrupting the T wave of the sinus beat. Complex PVCs are highly correlated with sudden death.

In the setting of coronary artery disease, a grading system has been proposed by Lown and Graboys (29) to separate patients according to risk of sudden death. This system gives a numerical grade from 0 to 5 with increasing risk of sudden death according to the following:

0 = no PVCs
1 = occasional simple, less than 30/hr
2 = frequent simple, greater than 30/hr
3 = multiform
4 = runs of PVCs
5 = early PVCs.

In an epidemiologic study over 7 months, the mortality rate varied from zero in class 0 to 30% in classes 3 to 5 (30).

Despite the fact that PVCs predispose to sudden death, the precise cause of death is not known. It may be a random event precipitated by the unfortunate timing of PVCs. Procainamide, lidocaine and quinidine are proven in their ability to reduce the frequency of, although not totally eliminate, PVCs. However, studies evaluating the response to these drugs do not demonstrate a significant decrease in mortality rate. On the other hand, death may be a result of acute ischemia which may not be altered by antiarrhythmic drugs. The agents shown to have an improvement in survival rate, the β-blockers may act on ischemia, not on the basis of their antiarrhythmic effects.

Lidocaine is the drug of choice for the parenteral treatment of PVCs. The therapeutic range for lidocaine is 1.5 to 5.5 μg/ml (Table 22.2). Lidocaine is usually initiated with a loading dose to produce rapid arrhythmia control. Any loading dose must account for the small central compartment, 0.5 liters/kg in normal subjects, reduced to 0.3 liters/kg in patients with congestive heart failure and increased to 0.6 liters/kg in liver disease (31). A minimum concentration in the central compartment must be reached, since the heart acts as if it belongs in this compartment, while limiting the maximum concentration, since the brain also is present in this compartment. The loading dose (LD) may be calculated to produce a plasma concentration (Cp) of 3 μg/ml, using the central volume (V_c) of 0.5 liters/kg as follows and administered over 1 to 2 min:

$$LD = Cp \times V_c$$
$$= 3 \ \mu g/ml \times 0.5 \ L/kg$$
$$= 1.5 \ mg/kg.$$

Since the loading dose will be rapidly distributed away from the heart and the central compartment with an α-phase half-life of about 10 min, arrhythmias may recur after the initial dose. Additional boluses, using one half the initial dose, may be given after 10 to 20 min or when ectopic beats recur. Unfortunately all bolus doses are only transiently effective due to rapid distribution. An alternative is to give the initial load, followed by a high dose infusion of 120 μg/kg/min for 25 min. This infusion avoids the subtherapeutic levels produced by multiple boluses (32). Most patients are placed on a constant infusion of lidocaine for ectopic suppression. This constant infusion, R, is dependent upon the therapeutic steady state serum level of about 3 μg/ml, Cp_{ss}, and the clearance of lidocaine, Cl, which is 10 ml/min/kg in normal subjects, 6.3 in congestive heart failure, and 6.0 in liver disease (33), as follows:

$$R = Cp_{ss} \times Cl$$
$$= 3 \ \mu g/ml \times 10 \ ml/min/kg$$
$$= 30 \ \mu g/kg/min.$$

Only 5% of lidocaine is eliminated unchanged in the urine and renal failure does not decrease the clearance of lidocaine. Certain metabolites of lidocaine are cleared by the kidneys and may contribute to lidocaine toxicity when lidocaine is administered for extended periods (34). Lidocaine blood concentrations may be obtained at any point during the first 12 hours of therapy. Levels of 1 to 2 μg/ml are only rarely effective. Many patients have arrhythmia control with concentrations of 3 to 5 μg/ml. Beyond 5 μg/ml neurologic toxicity may limit any further dosage increments. Paresthesias, dizziness, drowsiness and euphoria may be seen. Resistant arrhythmias may require concentrations of 6 to 8 μg/ml at the risk of further confusion, nausea, vomiting, dysarthria and psychoses. Pushing lidocaine beyond 9 μg/ml is rarely justified. Sweating, tremors and muscle fasciculations may precede seizures, respiratory arrest and coma. Lidocaine metabolites may contribute to the neurologic toxicity.

Prolonged infusions of lidocaine beyond 24 hours may require a downward adjustment. Steady state concentrations should be expected by approximately 4 times the normal lidocaine β half-life of 100 min. In patients with liver disease steady state may be further delayed due to the half-life of 300 min. Patients with uncomplicated myocardial infarction receiving constant infusions of lidocaine have developed progressive accumulation after 30 hours of lidocaine. Such patients have prolonged elimination half-lives of 3 to 4 hours after discontinuing their infusions. Despite an unknown mechanism for this phenomenon, lidocaine infusions beyond 24 hours should therefore be reduced by one half (35).

Procainamide is considered an alternative when toxicity or resistant arrhythmias to lidocaine develop. Lidocaine-resistant PVCs, on occasion, may respond to procainamide. Toxicity, not therapeutic inadequacy, has relegated procainamide to a secondary role. Still procainamide is the more versatile drug since it may be administered orally and parenterally. Systemic bioavailability after oral procainamide averages 75%, but certain patients may absorb as little as 10%. Procainamide displays two compartment kinetics similar to lidocaine. A rapid distribution phase with a half-life of 5 min is followed by an elimination half life of 2 to 5 hours. Rapid arrhythmia control may require intravenous bolus doses. The negative inotropic and hypotensive effects of procainamide limit the rate at which the drug may be given. Even in emergency situations procainamide should not be given at a rate exceeding 50 mg/min. The loading dose (LD) will be influenced by the therapeutic range for procainamide (Cp) of 4 to 8 μg/ml, the distribution volume (V_d) of 2 liters/kg, the procainamide content (S) of the hydrochloride salt, 0.82, as follows:

$$LD = \frac{Cp \times V_d}{S}$$
$$= \frac{6 \ \mu g/ml \times 2 \ L/kg}{0.82}$$
$$= 14.6 \ mg/kg.$$

In renal impairment and congestive heart failure the distribution volume may be decreased by 25%. Loading doses have been given as small boluses of 50 to 100 mg given every 5 min until arrhythmia control is seen or toxicity develops. Alternatively the entire estimated dose may be infused at a rate of 25 tc 50 mg/min.

The selection of maintenance doses of procainamide is intimately related to its metabolic fate. Procainamide may be excreted unchanged in the urine to the extent of 50%. The liver will transform 7 to 24% of procainamide to N-acetylprocainamide (NAPA). The extent of the metabolism depends on the rate of acetylation. Since NAPA has antiarrhythmic potency equivalent to procainamide, the maintenance dose of procainamide may differ in fast and slow acetylators.

The typical patient receiving intravenous procainamide is placed on a dose of 2 to 4 mg/min. This may be tailored to the patient using 2.8 mg/kg/hour as a standard, reduced in cardiac or renal impairment by one third for moderate impairment and two thirds for severe impairment (36). Calculations using population averages of kinetic variables for oral procainamide have not been particularly valuable or accurate. In general, patients may be started on 50 mg/kg/day given in 4 divided doses and titrated to response and toxicity. A lower dose is advised in renal impairment as the procainamide half-life may be prolonged to 5 to 10 hours while the NAPA half-life is greatly increased from a normal of 6 hours to as much as 42 hours.

The procainamide dose may be adjusted to maintain plasma levels of the drug as well as NAPA. When given alone, NAPA produces adequate PVC reduction at levels of 9 to 25 μg/ml (37). Procainamide and NAPA may be additive in certain patients yet the precise ratio of the two drugs for optimal therapy has not been established. The sum of the steady state trough concentrations equalling 10 μg/ml has been suggested as a guideline for the minimum effective concentration (36). The antiar-

rhythmic effects of NAPA coupled with its longer half-life allow for longer dosage intervals for procainamide dosing than the short half-life of the parent compound would suggest.

A sustained release preparation is available for procainamide. Since procainamide has such a short half-life, some references have suggested that the conventional release products must be given every 3 to 4 hours to limit fluctuation of plasma drug concentrations over the dosing interval. Using the sustained release product, the variation between maximal and minimal procainamide levels was slight at 35% when an 8-hour dosing interval was used (38). Patients may be started on 1 g every 8 hours. The dosage may be increased by 500 mg every day until toxicity or arrhythmia suppression is seen. Patients with renal impairment or heart failure have not been studied but may respond to lower initial doses and longer dosing intervals (every 12 hours). The European sustained release product has been used in myocardial infarction patients (without severe heart failure) in a dose of 1.5 g every 8 hours that produced therapeutic drug concentrations while a fixed dose of the standard preparation (375 mg every 4 hours) failed to produce therapeutic levels (39).

Adverse effects commonly seen with procainamide include gastrointestinal distress, weakness, dizziness, nervousness and blurred vision. These symptoms resolve if the dosage is reduced; however, many patients will develop tolerance to these effects with continued procainamide use without dosage reduction. Cardiac toxicity may be seen with procainamide levels exceeding 12 μg/ml such as progressive lengthening of the QTc interval and QRS duration, hypotension and myocardial depression. A lupus-like syndrome may develop in more than 20% of patients taking procainamide. Procainamide lupus differs from systemic lupus erythematosus in that arthritic features are more prominent while dermatologic, hematologic and renal changes are rare. Symptoms may develop as early as 2 weeks after initiating procainamide or as long as 2 years later. Risk factors include high dosages, high serum concentrations and slow acetylation status. Common signs and symptoms for monitoring include fever, skin rash, myalgias, arthralgias, pericarditis, pleuritis, hepatosplenomegaly and rarely tamponade. Many more patients will have positive serologic tests for lupus than will have symptoms.

Digitalis-induced PVCs: PVCs are the most frequent arrhythmia caused by digitalis. Generally this arrhythmia will resolve by simply discontinuing the digitalis. For frequent or symptomatic PVCs, potassium replacement in hypo- or normokalemic patients may suppress the arrhythmia. For sustained PVCs induced by digitalis, lidocaine or phenytoin have been used successfully. Phenytoin is considered to be an ideal drug to treat digitalis-induced arrhythmias since it improves AV conduction while it suppresses ventricular irritability. Unfortunately phenytoin is not nearly as effective in PVCs of different etiology.

For the treatment of digitalis-induced PVCs, phenytoin would most likely be given parenterally yet its hypotensive effects via this route are particularly troublesome. Phenytoin may lower blood pressure in 2 to 8% of patients given intravenous doses through vasodilation and myocardial depression (1). Parahydroxylation by the liver accounts for 50 to 76% of an administered dose of phenytoin while 5% is eliminated unchanged in the urine. Phenytoin is 93% protein bound, primarily to albumin. The degree of binding may be reduced in renal or hepatic disease where serum albumin concentrations may be reduced. In addition, in uremia the extent of binding is reduced. In such situations, the free drug may be adequate while the total measured phenytoin blood concentration may not be within the therapeutic range despite adequate arrhythmia suppression. The majority of arrhythmias are controlled by producing phenytoin plasma levels of 10 to 20 μg/ml. Phenytoin in most situations should be initiated with a loading dose. The propylene glycol diluent may cause cardiovascular collapse and central nervous system depression yet these complications may be reduced or avoided with rates of administration of 50 mg/min or less. Intramuscular injection may obviate this problem however absorption is erratic and slow due to precipitation of phenytoin. Phenytoin distributes into a volume, V_d, that approaches total body water (0.7 liters/kg) which may be used to estimate the loading dose (LD), based upon the desired plasma concentration, Cp of 15 μg/ml as follows:

$$
\begin{aligned}
LD &= Cp \times V_d \\
&= 15 \ \mu g/ml \times 0.7 \ L/kg \\
&= 10.5 \ mg/kg.
\end{aligned}
$$

The entire dose may be infused at a rate of 50 mg/min or by intermittent bolus infusions of 100 mg over 2 min given every 5 min until arrhythmia suppression, maximum dose of 1 g or toxicity occurs. Digitalis-induced PVCs may be eliminated by the loading dose of phenytoin and not require a maintenance dose. Sustained PVCs requiring maintenance doses of phenytoin will be influenced by the capacity limited metabolism of the drug. With therapeutic concentrations, the rate of metabolism is often near saturation. The Michaelis-Menton kinetic values of phenytoin suggest that changes in dose may lead to exponentially greater increases in serum concentration. As such, the typical patient should be given 300 to 400 mg/day as a single dose or divided into two doses. Subsequent adjustments should be made at 100 mg/day changes at approximately 2-week intervals. Additional bolus doses may be given to treat ectopic beats to avoid the delay to steady state conditions.

Parenteral therapy with phenytoin may produce bradycardia, hypotension and prolonged QTc interval and QRS duration related to rate of administration. Central nervous system toxicity may be related to blood concentrations. Nystagmus may be the initial sign of toxicity when levels exceed 20 μg/ml. Phenytoin levels beyond 30 μg/ml may produce ataxia. Mental changes are common with concentrations above 40 μg/ml. Toxicity such as gingival hyperplasia, folate deficiency, peripheral neuropathy, hypertrichosis and osteoporosis are seen with chronic therapy.

VENTRICULAR TACHYCARDIA

Ventricular tachycardia (VT) is a rapid (100 to 250 beats/min), regular ectopic rhythm of three or more consecutive ventricular complexes. VT is more serious than PVCs, producing more marked hemodynamic deterioration due to decreased diastolic filling and loss of coordinated ventricular contraction with atrial kick. The appearance of VT is also ominous since it often degenerates into ventricular fibrillation. VT may be seen in the prehospital phase of an acute myocardial infarction due to ischemic changes and often results in sudden death. VT may also appear in the early hospital stage, 12 to 24 hours after the onset of an acute myocardial infarction as a result of enhanced automaticity. At this stage the rhythm is somewhat more stable. The third phase of VT seen in ischemic heart disease is noted after several days to weeks.

There are two general types of VT. Isolated and infrequent episodes of VT may be seen in the setting of an acute myocardial infarction. These may require only close observation if they are asymptomatic. Sustained VT is another type which is often associated with hemodynamic instability. The drug therapy of recurrent VT may be defined by laboratory programmed electrical stimulation of the rhythm to determine the most efficacious drug, dose and plasma concentration. This laboratory model is reported to reflect clinical VT and indicate appropriate therapy (40). The successful drug concentration in the acute laboratory situation correlates well with the therapeutic level observed chronically for drugs such as quinidine and procainamide but not for propranolol, which is dependent upon prevailing sympathetic tone (41). Failures in the acute setting usually develop relapse of VT on chronic suppression therapy.

In the symptomatic patient with VT the therapy of choice is *electrical cardioversion*. VT seen in the late hospital phase of an acute myocardial infarction is often asymptomatic yet has a highly significant risk. Patients with VT may be 5 times more likely to die within 1 year than those without the arrhythmia (42). However, whether antiarrhythmics will influence the mortality rate is not known.

Lidocaine is the preferred agent for rapid control of VT. *Procainamide* is also effective yet many patients require plasma concentrations that are considered to be in the toxic range (greater than 8 μg/ml (43). *Quinidine*, *phenytoin*, and *disopyramide* are alternatives.

Disopyramide currently is available for oral use in the treatment of ventricular arrhythmias. It may also be as effective as quinidine in the management of atrial fibrillation. Parenteral disopyramide has been shown to be equally as effective as lidocaine in the treatment of ventricular arrhythmias (44), but is not yet available in the United States. Disopyramide is an effective agent in the prophylactic management of PVCs in patients with acute myocardial infarctions. The frequency of PVCs is reduced, ventricular fibrillation is prevented and overall mortality is decreased (45).

Disopyramide is well absorbed (83%). Variable amounts of disopyramide (36 to 71%) have been reported to be cleared by the kidneys as unchanged drug. The remainder is an N-dealkylated metabolite with some antiarrhythmic activity. In healthy subjects, half-life ranged from 4.4 to 8.2 hours. Renal impairment may prolong the half-life from 8.4 to 53 hours. The half-life may also be prolonged in patients with an acute myocardial infarction.

The therapeutic range for disopyramide appears to be 3 to 6 μg/ml. In some studies, atrial arrhythmias responded to lower concentrations than ventricular ectopics. Although steadily increasing the plasma concentration of disopyramide progressively reduces the frequency of ectopics, responders and nonresponders have similar mean levels. Therefore patients should be titrated to response rather than selecting an arbitrary drug plasma level.

Oral disopyramide may be initiated with a loading dose of 300 mg (200 mg for moderate renal impairment, liver dysfunction or decompensated heart failure). Maintenance doses of 100 to 150 mg may be given at 6-hour intervals (the lower dose is indicated for renal, liver and cardiac insufficiency). The recommended maximum daily dosage is 800 mg yet up to 1600 mg have been used under close monitoring. For patients with severe renal impairment the dosing interval may be prolonged to 12, 24, or 36 hours for creatinine clearances of 15 to 40, 5 to 15, or 1 to 5 ml/min. Intravenous doses (investigational) have been initiated at 2 mg/kg over 5 to 15 min, followed by 2 mg/kg over 45 min. Disopyramide may be maintained by 7 μg/kg/min.

Common adverse reactions observed with disopyramide have been anticholinergic symptoms of dry mouth, blurred vision, constipation, and urinary retention. Similar to quinidine, disopyramide may prolong the QTc interval and QRS duration. Initial reports on disopyramide were encouraging, indicating that quinidine produced more frequent adverse effects, yet the reports of acute heart failure developing during chronic disopyramide have dampened the enthusiasm. Disopyramide has a negative inotropic effect. The risk of developing symptomatic heart failure may be as high as 16% (46). The drug has been used without complications in patients with heart failure; however, such patients are at much greater risk for decompensation. The onset of symptoms is variable and there is no apparent correlation with dosage. Patients without any previous history of heart disease have developed acute heart failure associated with the use of disopyramide. Patients developing signs and symptoms of heart failure should be discontinued from disopyramide. Symptoms usually resolve over a few days; however, some patients may require diuretics or digitalis. As with other antiarrhythmics that prolong the

QTc interval, disopyramide may cause ventricular arrhythmias sometimes with symptoms similar to quinidine syncope. Many patients revert after discontinuing the disopyramide, yet others may require suppression with lidocaine.

VENTRICULAR FLUTTER/ FIBRILLATION (VF)

Some references consider ventricular flutter as a separate entity, a ventricular tachyarrhythmia of the vulnerable phase that responds to low energy cardioversion. Ventricular flutter, if sustained, may degenerate into ventricular fibrillation. In VF, the ectopic beat does not develop from a single area. Instead the firing is random and changing. Individual fibers or groups of fibers contract independently. When observed, the heart shows areas of twitching. Consequently, there is no effective net contraction and no pumping of blood.

Almost 50% of patients who develop VF do not have warning arrhythmias (see under PVC), especially during the early phase of acute myocardial infarction. Often the time period between warning arrhythmias and VF is very short (seconds). In the setting of an acute myocardial infarction, 88% of patients with VF will develop it within the first 6 hours of the infarct. Such patients in general have a good prognosis. VF associated with, or caused by, heart failure may occur at any time after an infarct and is associated with a higher mortality rate since myocardial damage is more extensive.

Since the warning criteria for predicting VF are not very accurate, some centers use prophylactic antiarrhythmics to prevent fatal VF. This therapy is highly controversial. Some studies, using relatively low dose infusions (2 mg/min) report that lidocaine does not prevent VF, particularly in the first few hours of the infarct (47). Higher doses of lidocaine (3 mg/min) have been shown to prevent VF at the expense of frequent toxicity (15%) in patients less than 70 years old without heart failure or block (48). This regimen is recommended for the first 24 hours after the infarct only.

The primary treatment of VF is *electrical cardioversion*. The likelihood of successful conversion is increased if coronary artery perfusion is maintained. In 80% of patients, a single shock is adequate to convert to a more stable rhythm. Nonresponders should receive cardiopulmonary resuscitation with repeated shock therapy and lidocaine. *Lidocaine* by consensus is the preferred pharmacologic agent for VF.

Bretylium is an alternative for patients resistant to lidocaine. This drug may produce chemical defibrillation without electric shock when it is given undiluted by rapid injection of 5 mg/kg. Rapid administration should be reserved for emergency use as in cardiopulmonary resuscitation. The average time to reversion after bretylium is 9 to 10 min. If after 15 to 30 min there is no response, another 10 mg/kg may be given up to a maximum of 30 mg/kg. For less serious arrhythmias, bretylium may be given over 8 to 10 min with 5 to 10 mg/kg as the loading dose. If the arrhythmia persists, the dose may be repeated at 1-hour intervals up to 30 mg/kg. For chronic suppression, bretylium may be given intramuscularly or by intermittent infusions (over 8 to 10 min), every 6 to 8 hours. Bretylium has also been given by constant infusion at 1 to 2 mg/min.

Elimination is primarily via the kidneys to the extent of 70 to 80%. Bretylium has a variable half-life of 4.2 to 16.9 hours. Oral absorption of bretylium is poor and unpredictable. The antiarrhythmic concentration of bretylium is 0.5 to 1.5 μg/ml.

Currently bretylium is not considered the drug of choice for any ventricular arrhythmia. Parenteral administration causes an initial release of catecholamines which is followed by sympathetic block. This temporary period of sympathetic excess may produce hypertension and arrhythmias particularly in patients with digitalis toxicity. In animals, bretylium given to treat digitalis-associated ventricular tachycardia produced a more rapid ventricular tachycardia is some and ventricular fibrillation in others. Pretreatment with bretylium, though, actually prevented digitalis toxicity. Bretylium may reduce the disparity in refractory periods between normal and infarcted tissues (felt to be responsible for reentry rhythms).

In addition, hypotension makes bretylium less attractive than lidocaine for use in the treatment or prophylaxis of ventricular tachyarrhythmias in the setting of an acute myocardial infarction. Postural hypotension develops in most patients (50 to 75%) but is usually a fall of less than 20 mm Hg. Volume expansion may resolve the hypotension. Additionally, the patient should be supine or in the reverse Trendelenberg position. Vasopressors should be used with caution since the adrenergic terminals will be supersensitive to sympathomimetics. For example, dopamine may be used with a starting dose of 0.5 to 1.0 μg/kg/min. Rapid injections of bretylium will produce nausea and vomiting.

SUDDEN DEATH

The predominant cause of sudden death is ventricular fibrillation. In approximately 25% of cases, sudden death (presumably via VF) is not preceded by a prior history of cardiac symptoms. Thus the prevention of VF with chronic antiarrhythmics becomes a question of patient selection. Sudden cardiac collapse via VF in ambulatory patients often (55%) is not associated with an acute myocardial infarction. These patients, after resuscitation have a very high (3 times greater than primary VF with an acute myocardial infarction) mortality rate. Chronic antiarrhythmics have produced mixed results in reducing sudden death.

When considering the choices for chronic management of VF and prevention of sudden death, β-blockers deserve a prominent role. Unfortunately a variety of conditions may preclude patients from the potential benefit of β-blockade such as uncontrolled cardiac failure, bradycardia, second or third degree heart block, SA block, insulin-dependent diabetes mellitus, peripheral vascular disease, and chronic obstructive pulmonary disease.

Propranolol has not met with exceptional results in ventricular arrhythmia suppression. It may not be effective in preventing ectopic beats after an acute myocardial infarction. In the treatment of VT, propranolol has been disappointing. However, it may be useful in exercise-induced arrhythmias, ventricular arrhythmias associated with mitral valve prolapse, digitalis-induced arrhythmias and arrhythmias associated with a long QTc interval.

Propranolol has been studied in post myocardial infarction patients with mixed results in lowering the risk of sudden death. The recent report from the National Heart, Lung and Blood Institute (49) revealed a 26% lower mortality rate for propranolol compared to placebo. The site of the infarct, age and sex had no influence on the response to propranolol. The initial dose of propranolol, 40 mg, 3 times daily, was adjusted to 60 or 80 mg, 3 times daily, depending upon serum propranolol concentrations.

Propranolol is felt to have the highest membrane-stabilizing potency of the β-blockers. Called a "quinidine-like" action, it is manifest, however, only in overdose situations. Propran-olol is a nonselective antagonist to β_1 (cardiac)- and β_2 (lungs and blood vessels)-receptors. It is well absorbed (more than 90%) yet first pass hepatic extraction may reduce bioavailability to about 30%. Protein binding is on the order of 90%. Propranolol is rapidly cleared with a half-life of 3.5 to 6 hours by hepatic metabolism.

Propranolol may be given intravenously under rare situations in doses of 0.5 to 0.75 mg and repeated every 2 min up to a maximum of 0.1 mg/kg. The effective dose may be repeated at 6- to 8-hour intervals. The oral propranolol dose is much higher, but variable. A typical starting dose may be 10 mg every 6 hours. The dosing interval may not correlate with the short half-life such that a twice daily regimen has been effective.

The most common adverse reactions seen with propranolol involve the central nervous system and include fatigue, hallucinations, weakness, insomnia and nightmares. These effects may not be related to β-blockade and differences between the various β-blockers have not been demonstrated. Since it is nonselective, propranolol may exacerbate bronchospasm. Although propranolol may precipitate or worsen congestive heart failure, if the arrhythmia is felt to have induced the symptoms, propranolol may not be contraindicated but could in fact relieve the symptoms as it suppresses the arrhythmia. The β-blockers with intrinsic sympathomimetic activity may produce less cardiac depression and may be indicated in patients prone to heart failure. Propranolol, by β_2-blockade, may allow α-vasoconstriction, producing cold or painful extremities. Gangrene, skin necrosis and claudication have been observed. Nonselective agents should be avoided after such symptoms develop while cardioselective or high intrinsic sympathomimetic agents are preferred.

Timolol is a nonselective antagonist with good absorption (over 90%) and bioavailability (75%). Protein binding is low at 10%. Timolol is cleared primarily by the liver with slight (20%) renal excretion. The half-life is short at 3 to 4 hours. Adverse effects are similar to propranolol.

Timolol has been compared to placebo in the chronic prophylaxis of post myocardial infarction patients (50). An interesting finding was that placebo patients had a nearly 3-fold increase in arrhythmias requiring treatment compared to the timolol group. Besides a decrease in overall mortality rate with timolol, the incidence of sudden death and presumably fatal VF was reduced by approximately one half. The study utilized a fixed dose regimen (5 mg twice daily for 2 days then 10 mg twice daily) which was associated with a significant reduction in resting heart rate. Whether beneficial effects in terms of mortality might be seen without bradycardia is not known.

Metoprolol, although currently limited to the treatment of hypertension, may be considered an alternative to propranolol for arrhythmias since it is somewhat selective for β_1-receptors and may be preferred over propranolol for patients with chronic or acute obstructive pulmonary disease. However, metoprolol should be used with caution since in high doses it may also block β_2-receptors.

Metoprolol is well absorbed, over 95%, with greater bioavailability than propranolol, about 50%. Protein binding is slight at 12%. Metoprolol is cleared hepatically with a short half-life of 3 to 4 hours. The typical patient is started at 20 mg, 4 times daily. Metoprolol has similar adverse effects as propranolol with less risk for patients with asthma or peripheral vascular disease.

Metoprolol has been compared to placebo in patients with an acute myocardial infarction treated for 90 days (51). It was initiated as 15 mg intravenously followed by an oral dose of 100 mg twice daily. The overall reduction in mortality was 36%. The beneficial effect of metoprolol was maintained in all age groups.

Nadolol offers little as an antiarrhythmic beyond propranolol. Absorption of nadolol is poor (30%). Protein binding is about 30%. Nadolol is cleared by the kidneys with a half-life of 14 to 17 hours.

There is little information regarding the use of nadolol as an antiarrhythmic. Presumably nadolol would retain its useful once daily dosing capability. The usual starting dose has been 40 mg, reduced in renal impairment, increased by 40 to 80 mg at 3- to 7-day intervals.

Atenolol is a selective β_1-antagonist. Absorption of atenolol is fair (50%) with 40% bioavailability. Protein binding is negligible. The predominant means of elimination for atenolol is renal. The half-life is 6 to 9 hours. The initial dose may be 50 mg as a single daily dose. The average dose is usually 100 mg.

Alprenolol is a nonselective β-blocker with intrinsic sympathomimetic activity. It is rapidly cleared by the liver with a half-life of 2 hours. The usual dose is 200 mg twice daily.

Alprenolol has produced a beneficial response in reducing sudden death. The reduction in sudden death has been limited to patients less than 65 years old (52).

As a class, β-blockers appear to be beneficial in the management of post acute myocardial infarction patients. The efficacy seems to be independent of intrinsic sympathomimetic activity, β_2-receptor blockade, and membrane-stabilizing properties. However, these properties may aid individual drug selection in certain patients. The duration of therapy has not been established. The onset of therapy has varied between the studies yet some evidence exists that immediate β-blockade (e.g. within 12 hours after the onset of pain) may limit the enzyme estimated infarct size.

References

1. Singh BN, Cho YW, Kuemmerle HP: Clinical pharmacology of antiarrhythmic drugs: a review and overview. *Int J Clin Pharmacol Ther Toxicol* 19:185, 1981.
2. Hindman MD, Wagner GS: Arrhythmias during myocardial infarction: mechanisms, significance and therapy. *Cardiovasc Clin* 11:81, 1980.
3. Schweitzer P, Mark H: The effect of atropine on cardiac arrhythmias and conduction. *Am Heart J* 100:119, 225, 1980.
4. Verz Z, Mason DT: Reentry versus automaticity: role in tachyarrhythmia genesis and antiarrhythmic therapy. *Am Heart J* 101:329, 1981.
5. Josephson ME, Kastor JA: Supraventricular tachycardia: mechanisms and management. *Ann Intern Med* 87:346, 1977.
6. Bailey JC, Elharrar V, Zipes DP: Slow-channel depolarization: mechanism and control of arrhythmias. *Annu Rev Med* 29:417, 1978.
7. Antman EM, Stone PH, Muller JE, et al: Calcium channel blocking agents in the treatment of cardiovascular disorders: basic and clinical electrophysiologic effects. *Ann Intern Med* 93:875, 1980.
8. Ellrodt G, Chew CYC, Singh BN: Therapeutic implications of slow-channel blockade in cardiocirculatory disorders. *Circulation* 62:669, 1980.
9. Stone PH, Antman EM, Muller JE, et al: Calcium channel blocking agents in the treatment of cardiovascular disorders: hemodynamic effects and clinical applications. *Ann Intern Med* 93:886, 1980.
10. Singh BN, Collett JT, Chew CYC: New perspectives in the pharmacologic therapy of cardiac arrhythmias. *Prog Cardiovasc Dis* 22:243, 1980.
11. Rinkenberger RL, Prystowsky EN, Heger JJ, et al: Effects of intravenous and chronic oral verapamil administration in patients with supraventricular tachyarrhythmias. *Circulation* 62:996, 1980.
12. Waxman HL, Myerburg RJ, Appel R, et al: Verapamil for control of ventricular rate in paroxysmal supraventricular tachycardia and atrial fibrillation or flutter. *Ann Intern Med* 94:1, 1981.
13. Gonzalez R, Scheinman MM: Treatment of supraventricular arrhythmias with intravenous and oral verapamil. *Chest* 80:465, 1981.

14. Schomerus, M, Spiegelhalder B, Eichelbaum M: Physiological disposition of verapamil in man. *Cardiovasc Res* 10:605, 1976.

15. Mungall DR, Robichaux RP, Perry W, et al: Effects of quinidine on serum digoxin concentration. *Ann Intern Med* 93:689, 1980.

16. Ueda CT: Quinidine. In Evans WE, Schentag JJ, Jusko WJ: *Applied Pharmacokinetics*. San Francisco: Applied Therapeutics, 1980, p 436.

17. Cohen IS, Jick H, Cohen SI: Adverse reactions to quinidine in hospitalized patients: findings based on data from the Boston Collaborative Drug Surveillance Program. *Prog Cardiovasc Dis* 22:151, 1977.

18. Wellens HJJ, Bar FW, Gorgels AP, et al: Electrical management of arrhythmias with emphasis on the tachycardias. *Am J Cardiol* 41:1025, 1978.

19. Morris DC, Hurst JW: Atrial fibrillation. *Curr Probl Cardiol* 5:1, 1980.

20. Jelliffe RW, Buell J, Kalaba R: Reduction of digitalis toxicity by computer-assisted glycoside dosage regimens. *Ann Intern Med* 77:891, 1972.

21. Jelliffe RW: An improved method of digoxin therapy. *Ann Intern Med* 69:703, 1968.

22. Goldman S, Probst P, Selzer A, et al: Inefficiency of "therapeutic" serum levels of digoxin in controlling the ventricular rate in atrial fibrillation. *Am J Cardiol* 35:651, 1975.

23. Chamberlain DA, White RJ, Howard MR, et al: Plasma digoxin concentrations in patients with atrial fibrillation. *Br Med J* 3:429, 1970.

24. Jelliffe RW: Administration of digoxin. *Dis Chest* 56:56, 1969.

25. Woo E, Greenblatt DJ: A reevaluation of intravenous quinidine. *Am Heart J* 96:829, 1978.

26. Hirschfeld DS, Ueda CT, Rowland M, et al: Clinical and electrophysiological effects of intravenous quinidine in man. *Br Heart J* 33:309, 1977.

27. Hindman MCC, Wagner GS, JaRo M, et al: The clinical significance of bundle branch block complicating acute myocardial infarction. *Circulation* 58:679, 689, 1978.

28. Brodsky M, Wu D, Denes P, et al: Arrhythmias documented by 24 hour continuous electrocardiography in 50 male medical students without apparent heart disease. *Am J Cardiol* 39:390, 1977.

29. Lown B, Graboys TB: Management of patients with malignant ventricular arrhythmias. *Am J Cardiol* 39:910, 1977.

30. Schulze RA, Strauss HW, Pitt B: Sudden death in the year following myocardial infarction. *Am J Med* 62:192, 1977.

31. Thompson PD, Rowland DM, Melmor KL: The influence of heart failure, liver disease and renal failure on the disposition of lidocaine in man. *Am Heart J* 82:417, 1974.

32. Salzer LS, Weinrib AB, Marina RJ, et al: A comparison of methods of lidocaine administration in patients. *Clin Pharmacol Ther* 29:617, 1981.

33. Benowitz NL: Clinical applications of the pharmacokinetics of lidocaine. *Cardiovasc Clin* 6:77, 1974.

34. Collinsworth KA, Strong JM, Atkinson AJ, et al: Pharmacokinetics and metabolism of lidocaine in patients with renal failure. *Clin Pharmacol Ther* 18:59, 1975.

35. LeLorier J, Grenon D, Latour Y, et al: Pharmacokinetics of lidocaine after prolonged intravenous infusions in uncomplicated myocardial infarctions. *Ann Intern Med* 87:700, 1977.

36. Lima JJ: Procainamide. In Schentag JJ, Jusko WJ: *Applied Pharmacokinetics*. San Francisco: Applied Therapeutics, 1980, p 404.

37. Roden DM, Reele SB, Higgins SB, et al: Antiarrhythmic efficacy pharmacokinetics and safety of N-acetylprocainamide in human subjects. *Am J Cardiol* 46:463, 1980.

38. Giardina EG, Fenster PE, Bigger JT, et al: Efficacy plasma concentrations and adverse effects of a new sustained release procainamide preparation. *Am J Cardiol* 46:855, 1980.

39. Birkhead J, Evans T, Mumford P, et al: Sustained release procainamide in patients with myocardial infarction. *Br Heart J* 38:77, 1976.

40. Wellens HI, Bar FW, Lie KI, et al: Effect of procainamide, propranolol and verapamil on mechanism of tachycardia in patients with chronic recurrent ventricular tachycardia. *Am J Cardiol* 40:579, 1977.

41. Horowitz LN, Josephson ME, Farshidi A, et al: Recurrent sustained ventricular tachycardia. *Circulation* 58:986, 1978.

42. Bigger JT, Weld FM, Rolnitzky LM: Prevalence, characteristics and significance of ventricular tachycardia detected with ambulatory electrocardiographic recording in the late hospital phase of acute myocardial infarction. *Am J Cardiol* 48:815, 1981.

43. Greenspan AM, Horiwitz LN, Spielman SR, et al: Large dose procainamide therapy for ventricular tachyarrhythmia. *Am J Cardiol* 46:453, 1980.

44. Sparbaro JA, Rawling DA, Fozzard HA: Suppression of ventricular arrhythmias with intravenous disopyramide and lidocaine: efficacy comparison in a randomized trial. *Am J Cardiol* 44:513, 1979.

45. Kidner PH, Carmichael D: The effects of disopyramide in the prevention of ventricular irritability following AMI. *J Ir Med Assoc* 70:22, 1977.

46. Podrid PJ, Schoenberger A, Lown B: Congestive heart failure caused by oral disopyramide. *N Engl J Med* 302:614, 1980.

47. Chopra MP, Thadami U, Portal RW, et al: Therapy for ventricular ectopic activity after acute myocardial infarction: a double blind trial. *Br Med J* 3:668, 1971.

48. Lie KI, Wellens HJ, Van Capelle FJ, et al: Lidocaine in the prevention of primary ventricular fibrillation. *N Engl J Med* 291:1324, 1974.

49. National Heart, Lung and Blood Institute: The beta blocker heart attack trial. *JAMA* 246:2073, 1981.

50. Norwegian Multicenter Study Group: Timolol induced reduction in mortality and reinfarction in patients surviving acute myocardial infarction. *N Engl J Med* 304:801, 1981.

51. Hjalmarson A, Elmfeldt D, Herlitz J, et al: Mortality of metoprolol in acute myocardial infarction. *Lancet* 2:823, 1981.

52. Andersen MP, Frederiksen, J, Bechsgard P, et al: Effect of alprenolol on mortality among patients with definite or suspected acute myocardial infarction. *Lancet* 2:865, 1979.

CHAPTER 23

Hypertension

ROBERT T. WEIBERT, Pharm.D.

Hypertension is one of the greatest challenges and opportunities in medical care. Millions of asymptomatic patients are at an increased risk of cardiovascular disease which is the leading cause of death in the United States. Despite the fact that the treatment of hypertension reduces mortality and morbidity, only 50% of patients with high blood pressure are adequately treated.

Antihypertensive drugs continue to be the cornerstone of therapy and patients often receive multiple drugs. Successful therapy requires consideration of the pathophysiology of hypertension; the pharmacology and adverse effects of the drugs; and most important, the individual needs of the patient.

Because of the large numbers of patients with hypertension, adequate detection and long-term treatment will require increased involvement by pharmacists and other health professionals. Pharmacists can cooperatively participate in the long-term management of patients with high blood pressure and provide the needed follow-up to keep patients on their antihypertensive drug regimens.

To work effectively in the area of hypertension, pharmacists must understand the disease and the rationale for therapy. Some of the important areas which should be understood include: How should blood pressure be measured? What are the criteria to define hypertension? Which patients should be treated? Which drugs should be used?

DEFINITION (1–3)

Hypertension is an abnormal elevation of arterial blood pressure. However, the definition and the rationale for treatment of hypertension is based on epidemiological data. In every individual, blood pressure varies from minute to minute and is influenced by measurement technique, time of day, emotion, pain, discomfort, hydration, temperature, exercise, posture, and drugs. Blood pressure also increases with advancing age.

A dividing line between normal blood pressure and hypertension is artificial and arbitrary. There is no evidence of a threshold level of blood pressure for the development of cardiovascular complications. Insurance actuarial data show a continuum where the higher blood pressure the greater the risk of developing complications. The World Health Organization has recommended that blood pressure less than 140/90 mm Hg be classified as normal. In 1980 the Joint National Committee on Detection, Evaluation and Treatment of High Blood Pressure set forth guidelines for establishing a diagnosis of hypertension:

After screening, the diagnosis of hypertension is confirmed when the average of two or more diastolic blood pressure measurements on at least two subsequent visits is 90 mm Hg or higher.

The Committee guidelines for rechecking blood pressure after screening are in Table 23.1.

Single, casual measurements of blood pressure may inaccurately classify individuals as having hypertension and cause unnecessary emotional, social and financial problems. The decision whether or not to employ drug therapy should be based on the extent of elevation of blood pressure, the presence of end organ damage and the presence of other cardiovascular risk factors.

ETIOLOGY (1, 4)

More than 90% of patients with high blood pressure have essential hypertension where no cause can be demonstrated. Fewer than 10% of patients may have potentially curable hypertension caused by renal disease, adrenal disease, coarctation of the aorta or other rare conditions. Essential hypertension is usually considered to be a disease of sustained elevation of diastolic arterial pressure.

Oral contraceptives are the single most important cause of drug-induced hypertension. Clinical hypertension occurs in up to 5% of patients taking the "pill" on a long-term basis.

Table 23.1.
Guidelines for Screening and Rechecking Blood Pressure

Blood Pressure (mm Hg)	Recommended Action
Diastolic:	
≥95	Confirm within 1 mo
90–95	Confirm within 3 mo
≥115	Immediate referral
Systolic:	
≥160	Confirm promptly
≥150	Confirm if age less than 35 yr

However, most women show small but measurable increases in blood pressure during the first 2 years on the "pill" (9/5 mm Hg). Oral contraceptives also increase the risk of myocardial infarction, stroke and other neurological catastrophies. The increased relative risk of death for oral contraceptive users vs. non-users is 2:1 for cerebrovascular disease, 3:1 for all cardiovascular disease, and 5:1 for hypertension and heart disease. Factors which may increase the likelihood of oral contraceptive hypertension include: older age, obesity and family history of hypertension. Although the estrogen is the most important component, the amount and type of progestin may further influence the effect on blood pressure. The mechanisms for contraceptive induced hypertension appear to include: sodium retention, increases in plasma renin activity (PRA) resulting in increased aldosterone, angiotensin II and renal vasoconstriction. Oral contraceptive hypertension may develop gradually over 1 to 2 years and is usually reversible within 1 to 8 months after therapy is stopped. However, if blood pressure does not normalize within 3 months, further evaluation and therapy is appropriate. Oral contraceptive-induced hypertension is best prevented by checking blood pressure every 6 months and using the agent with the lowest effective estrogen dose. Women who are at higher risk or who actually develop hypertension should be switched to other forms of contraception (see Chapter 4, "Obstetrics and Gynecology").

Other drugs which can contribute to high blood pressure include: corticosteroids, carbenoxolene, natural licorice, sympathomimetic drugs, tricyclic antidepressants and monoamine oxidase (MAO) inhibitors. Drug products which contain large quantities of sodium, for example, effervescent solutions (e.g., Alka-Seltzer) may also further elevate blood pressure.

INCIDENCE (5–8)

Hypertension is the most prevalent chronic condition affecting the adult population. Data on the frequency of occurrence of hypertension are presented in Table 23.2. The most recent screenings indicate that approximately 25% of the adult population will have a diastolic blood pressure greater than 90 mm Hg. The Health and Nutrition Examination Survey (HANES) data estimate this may approach 60 million people (5).

Several other population characteristics are also well described:

1. The incidence of hypertension increases with advancing age (HANES).

2. The incidence of hypertension is higher among black (34%) than white (24%) subjects (California survey) (7).

3. Hypertension occurs at a slightly lower rate in Asian (20%) and Hispanic (18%) populations (California survey) (7).

4. The prevalence of hypertension is similar between men and women of the same race (Hypertension Detection and Follow-up Program, HDFP) (6).

5. The criteria for the cutoff of blood pressure for inclusion as hypertension greatly influences the prevalence (HDFP) (6).

DBP mm Hg	≥90	≥95	≥110
% Hypertensive	25%	14.5%	3%

6. Blood pressures at an initial screening are widely variable and a substantial percentage (37%) of patients will have a diastolic blood pressure (DBP) <90 mm Hg at a follow-up recheck (HDFP) (6).

The major focus on hypertension by both the public and medical communities has resulted in improvement in the detection and treatment of hypertension over the past decade. Originally, only 1/2 hypertensive patients were aware of their disease; 1/4 were treated and 1/8 were controlled (classic pattern). Figure 23.1 demonstrates data showing the progress that has been made with control of greater than 70% of patients in some communities.

PATHOGENESIS (1, 2)

Hypertension is a disease of disordered autoregulation of blood pressure. A complex regulatory system maintains blood pressure within a relatively constant range despite changes in posture and wide variations in the demand for blood. The level of blood pressure is ultimately the result of the product of car-

Table 23.2.
Prevalence of Hypertension

Source[a]	Age (yr)	Diastolic Blood Pressure (mm Hg)	Population Estimate	Percentage Total
HANES (1971–1974)	18–74	>95	35 million	18%
		>90 or treated	57 million	
HDFP (1973–1974) (159,000)	30–69	>90 or treated		25%
California (1979) (8,350)	>18	>90 or treated		24%

[a] HANES = Health and Nutrition Examination Survey of the National Center for Health Science (BCHS); HDFP = Hypertension Detection and Follow-up Program.

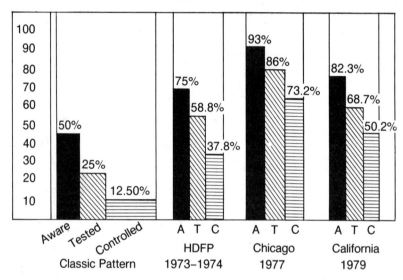

Figure 23.1. Awareness, treatment and control of hypertension (diastolic blood pressure ≥95 mm Hg or treated). HDFP = Hypertension Detection and Follow-up Program (6), Chicago 1977 (8), California 1979 (7).

diac output (CO) and peripheral vascular resistance (PVR). In many younger patients the initial change may be an increased cardiac output (hyperkinetic hypertension) with a rapid pulse, episodes of awareness of heart beat and increased sensitivity to beta-adrenergic stimulation. Over many years this hemodynamic picture may change to that seen in the majority of patients with fixed or established hypertension: a normal cardiac output and increased peripheral vascular resistance.

Many factors and mechanisms have been proposed as the pathogenesis of essential hypertension. Among the proposed models are:

1. *Classification by Plasma Renin Activity.* (a) patients with low plasma renin activity are hypervolemic and volume dependent; and (b) patients with high plasma renin activity are vasoconstricted.

Subsequent information has shown most patients have normal or reduced plasma volume and that few patients fit this model. However, the "normal" renin-angiotensin activity present in most hypertensives may well be inappropriate and contributory to the hypertension.

2. *Sympathetic Overactivity.* increased sympathetic nervous system activity may be induced by sustained psychogenic stress and increases cardiac output, heart rate, plasma renin and peripheral vascular resistance while decreasing plasma volume.

3. *Disordered Renal Salt Retention.* a relatively comprehensive model proposes that genetically predisposed patients after exposure to a high sodium diet retain salt/water, expand volume and increase cardiac output and blood pressure (Fig. 23.2). In normal subjects, elevation of blood pressure results in natriuresis. In hypertensive patients the natriuresis is inadequate and the resulting normal plasma volume is inappropriately high in the face of increased

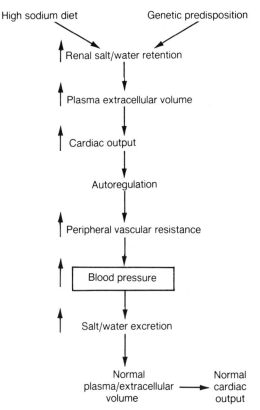

Figure 23.2. Hemodynamics of established essential hypertension.

peripheral vascular resistance. The final hemodynamics are elevated blood pressure and peripheral vascular resistance with normal plasma volume and cardiac output.

The present understanding indicates that hypertension is a multifactional disorder with excess dietary salt, heredity, renal handling of salt/water, increased sympathetic nervous activity and inappropriate renin and angiotensin contributing to the process. Further investigations are attempting to clarify the role of circulating vasodepressors such as prostaglandin A and kallikrein and to identify a possible natriuretic hormone. Despite these insights into the regulation of blood pressure, essential hypertension remains a process which must be controlled rather than a curable disorder.

DIAGNOSIS, SYMPTOMS AND CLINICAL FINDINGS (1, 2, 10–13)

Hypertension is usually an asymptomatic disease. Although headache, epistaxis and tinnitus are said to be symptoms of high blood pressure, a systematic study demonstrated no relationship between these symptoms and either systolic or diastolic blood pressure (10). Dizziness does occur more frequently in patients with very high diastolic blood pressure (>110 mm Hg). Occipital headaches occurring in the morning may be associated with severe hypertension.

Some patients may begin to complain of headaches after they have been told that they have hypertension. Emotional iatrogenic disease can be a common problem in patients with hypertension (11–13). The incidence of headache, pain and nervousness in hypertensive patients is similar to the frequency these complaints are found in normotensive, psychoneurotic patients. Mislabeled hypertensives (later found normotensive) were found to have more depressive symptoms, lower present perception of health and a worsening of health over the past 5 years (11). Caution is important in labeling patients as hypertensive, especially if treatment is not started. Work absenteeism can increase dramatically in newly labeled hypertensives (up to an 80% increase) (12, 13). Increased absenteeism is particularly likely in young, untreated patients with systolic hypertension and in patients noncompliant with treatment. Considerable care is needed to avoid frightening hypertensive patients.

The initial evaluation of the patients with possible hypertension is an important process with several objectives:

1. *Establishing a Diagnosis of Hypertension.* The average of 2 or more measurements of blood pressure with the subject seated and the diastolic pressure reported as the disappearance of sound (Phase V) on 2 subsequent visits after an elevated blood pressure at screening confirms the diagnosis of hypertension. Again, the diagnosis of hypertension should not be taken lightly as it can cause patients to view themselves as "sick" and thus increasing the number of workloss days and adversely affecting employment and insurance.

2. *Avoiding Early Dropout* (14–16). While this is usually not a specific objective that is listed in most approaches to the evaluation of the newly diagnosed patient with hypertension, it is the cornerstone for achieving long-term control. The problem of early dropouts from hypertension treatment programs is well documented. Dropouts from care during the first year of treatment frequently approach 50%. Examples include the Inner City Study

with a 83% dropout; the Australian Trial, 35% dropout, and a University of Chicago Study, 48% dropout. Therefore, the most important part of the initial visit is to insure that the patient will return for further followup.

3. *Evaluation for the Presence of Cardiovascular Risk Factors and Quantitation of Hypertensive Vascular Disease.* The medical history, physical examination and laboratory testing are directed to identifying risk factors, the extent of any existing vascular damage and the presence of concurrent diseases. The Joint National Committee has provided guidelines for evaluating patients (Table 23.3).

4. *Screening for Secondary Causes of Hypertension.* The vast majority of patients with elevated blood pressure have essential hypertension. Any patient whose medical history or physical examination suggests a possible cause of secondary hypertension warrants additional diagnostic evaluation (Table 23.4).

5. *Explanation of Findings.* To avoid early dropout and to work toward long-term control of hypertension, patients need to become active participants in their own care. To do so requires that patients understand: (a) the potential benefits and risks of therapy, (b) that their blood pressure exceeds normal limits, (c) the possible consequences of uncontrolled hypertension, (d) that hypertension is usually asymptomatic and that the presence or ab-

sence of symptoms does not reliably indicate the level of blood pressure, (e) prolonged follow-up and therapy are needed, (f) treatment will control but not cure high blood pressure, and (g) the presence of any other cardiovascular risk factors and how these indicate their own probability of developing cardiovascular disease.

In summary, the initial evaluation is to document the presence of hypertension, begin to establish long-term compliance, establish the extent of target organ damage and the existence of other risk factors. This allows a rational basis for planning treatment.

COMPLICATIONS (1–3, 9, 17–21)

Hypertension is the most important major risk factor for premature cardiovascular death. The life expectancy of a 35-year-old man with hypertension (150/100 mm Hg) is reduced by about 15 years or 40%. Complications of hypertension can be classified as being due to either the elevation of blood pressure or the acceleration of the atherosclerotic process (Table 23.5). High blood pressure increases the workload of the heart and congestive heart failure develops twice as often in hypertensive patients. Direct arterial damage can produce cerebral hemorrhage and malignant hypertension frequently results in renal failure.

Hypertension is additive with other risk fac-

Table 23.3.
Initial Evaluation of the Hypertensive Patient

Medical History	Physical Examination	Laboratory Testing
1. Family history of hypertension and its complications	Height/weight	Urinalysis: protein, blood, glucose
2. History of cardiovascular and cerebrovascular disease, renal disease or diabetes mellitus	Blood pressure seated and standing	Blood chemistry: potassium, creatinine, uric acid, glucose, cholesterol
3. Duration and level of elevated blood pressure	Fundoscopic Examination for arteriolar narrowing, hemorrhages, exudates and papilledema	ECG
4. Effectiveness and side effects of previous drug treatment	Neck examination for carotid bruits and distended veins	Complete blood count
5. Current medication history for drugs which may elevate blood pressure	Heart examination for increased rate, size, precordial heave, murmurs, arrhythmias and gallops	—
6. Health habits: exercise/lifestyle, sodium intake, smoking, alcohol excess	Abdominal examination for bruits, large kidneys or aortic dilation	—
7. —	Examination of the extremities for diminished or absent pulses	—

Table 23.4.
Clinical Finding Suggesting Potential Secondary Hypertension

Finding	Secondary Cause
Abdominal bruit	Renovascular disease
Abdominal/flank mass	Polycystic kidneys
Hypokalemia	Hyperaldosteronism
Headache, palpitation, sweating, spells	Pheochromocytoma
Delayed/absent femoral pulse	Aortic coarctation
Truncal obesity/striae	Cushing's syndrome

Table 23.5.
Complications of Hypertension

Hypertensive:
  Congestive heart failure
  Cardiomegaly, left ventricular hypertrophy
  Cerebral hemorrhage
  Renal failure
  Retinopathy
  Accelerated hypertension
  Aortic dissection
Arteriosclerotic:
  Ischemic heart disease
    Myocardial infarction
    Sudden death
    Angina pectoris
  Atherothrombotic stroke
  Peripheral vascular insufficiency

tors in the development of atherosclerosis. In white middle-aged men, hypertension (diastolic 95 to 104 mm Hg) doubles the incidence of death from myocardial infarction. If either smoking or elevated cholesterol are also present, the risk of death is tripled. When all three risks exist, the death rate from myocardial infarction is increased more than 5-fold.

Hypertension is also the major risk factor for cerebral thrombosis and infarction. The risk of stroke is 5 times as great in hypertensives compared to normotensives and is proportional to blood pressure. Systolic blood pressure appears to be the best predictor of the future risk of stroke.

The risk of complications is related to the degree of elevation of blood pressure. The Framingham study indicates that for each 10-mm Hg increment of blood pressure there is a 30% increase in cardiovascular mortality. One of the most important aspects is the dramatic interaction of hypertension and other cardiovascular risk factors. A modified method to use the *American Heart Association's Coronary Risk Handbook* has been incorporated into 2 tables to calculate the 6-year risk of heart disease based on: age, systolic blood pressure, serum cholesterol, glucose intolerance, left ventricular hypertrophy and cigarette smoking (22). This estimate of risk can be of assistance in planning therapy and in discussions with the patient.

TREATMENT (1, 2, 6, 9, 15, 23–33)

The goal in treating hypertension is to prevent the development of complications which cause morbidity and shorten life. A basic underlying question is: At what level of blood pressure should drug treatment be started?

Because drug therapy can be costly, inconvenient and carries some risk, the decision to begin antihypertensive drugs must be based on evidence that the patient is likely to benefit.

Evidence from the Veterans Administration Cooperative Study on Antihypertensive Agents has clearly demonstrated that reducing blood pressure to normal or near normal levels decreases the occurrence of complications (23–27). The study was conducted with compliant male veterans with clinic diastolic blood pressure of greater than 104 mm Hg and hospital diastolic blood pressure greater than 90 mm Hg. The results from the VA study provided the early evidence of the benefits of drug treatment. In the VA study, adequate treatment clearly decreased hypertensive complications and improved survival in patients with persistent diastolic blood pressures greater than 104 mm Hg (23, 24). Complications developed 3 times as frequently in untreated patients. The treatment of moderate hypertension (DBP ≥104 mm Hg) abolished hypertensive complications (congestive heart failure, accelerated hypertension, renal failure) and reduced cerebrovascular accidents by 75%. However, treatment did not decrease the incidence of myocardial infarction. Although some reduction in complications was seen in patients whose initial blood pressure was 90 to 104 mm Hg, the results were inconclusive. Finally, the VA study has shown that even partial reduction of blood pressure (DBP <105 >90 mm Hg) decreases cardiovascular complications (26). However, the VA Cooperative Study provided limited and inconclusive data regarding the benefits of treatments for female subjects, blacks, patients less than 50 years of age and patients with a DBP <105 mm Hg.

The largest completed study on antihypertensive therapy is the Hypertension Detection and Follow-up Program (HDFP) which followed almost 11,000 patients over a 5-year period (5, 28, 29). Patients in 14 cities were randomized to community care (referred care, RC) or a systematic hypertension treatment program (stepped care, SC). Seventy percent of the patients had "mild hypertension" (DBP 90 to 104 mm Hg). Strokes were reduced by 45% and death from myocardial infarction was decreased 26%. The 5-year mortality was 17% lower for the SC group compared to the RC group. Mortality was 20% lower for the SC subgroup with entry DBP of 90 to 104 mm Hg (5.9 vs. 7.4 per 100). The subgroup with DBP 90 to 140 mm Hg and no evidence of end organ damage at entry had 28.6% fewer deaths at 5 years. The treatment goal for HDFP patients was the lesser of a 10-mm Hg decrease from entry blood pressure or a DBP <90 mm Hg. The HDFP did not demonstrate a significant reduction on mortality for white women or for patients less than age 50 as the death rate was low in both groups.

From these results the HDFP Cooperative Group has concluded:

1. Patients with a DBP of 90 to 104 mm Hg benefit from drug treatment of hypertension and should be treated.

2. The treatment goal should be lowered to a DBP <90 mm Hg or a decrease of ≥10 mm Hg from the entry DBP. Thus for patients whose entry DBP is 90 mm Hg the target DBP is 80 mm Hg.

3. In patients with mild hypertension treatment should be considered early, before end organ damage occurs.

It is noteworthy that the 5-year DBP averaged 84 mm Hg for the SC group and 89 mm Hg for the RC group, a difference of only 5 mm Hg.

Other studies have also been completed:

1. *Australian Therapeutic Trial in Mild Hypertension* (15). A total of approximately 3400 men and women were followed for an average of 4 years after randomization to placebo or active treatment. The active treatment group had a ⅔ decrease in cardiovascular mortality with a 50% reduction in strokes and transient ischemic attacks. The excess mortality in the placebo group was concentrated in those with a DBP >100 mm Hg. Unlike the HDFP study there was not a significant reduction in ischemic heart disease. However, this study was not continued to further evaluate any effect on ischemic heart disease because of the reduction in cerebrovascular complications.

2. *The Oslo Study on the Treatment of Mild Hypertension* (30). Almost 800 men were randomized to placebo or active treatment and followed for 5 years. The treatment group maintained lower blood pressures throughout the study (17/10 mm Hg less than the control group). The study did *not* demonstrate any difference in cardiovascular mortality except in a subgroup whose entry DBP ≥100 mm Hg. There was a reduction in stroke, aortic aneurysm, left ventricle hypertrophy (LVH) and congestive heart failure. Coronary heart disease was slightly greater in the treatment group.

3. *Royal Sussex County Hospital Study* (31). This was a 5-year follow-up study of 961 patients. A well controlled group of hypertensive patients had mortality and morbidity equal to normotensives while uncontrolled patients had a pronounced increase in mortality (0.5% vs. 17.1%). The reduction in morbidity included both ischemic heart disease and cerebrovascular disease. Benefit was demonstrated in mild and moderate hypertension, in both sexes and at all ages. Even partial control had significant benefits.

4. *Multiple Risk Factor Intervention Trial (MRFIT)* (32). The MRFIT trial followed 12,800 men over 7 years. A special intervention group (SI) received stepped care treatment for hypertension, counseling for cigarette smoking, and dietary advice to lower cholesterol. Risk factors decreased compared to the usual care (UC) group. However, both total and cardiovascular mortality were the same for the two groups. The possibility that antihypertensive drug therapy had an adverse effect on some patients has been raised as a potential explanation for the similar mortality despite reduction of risk factors.

Summary of Treatment Studies

Based on HDFP findings the National Joint Committee has recommended that long-term reduction of blood pressure is needed for all levels of blood pressure (2). The arbitrary classifications are:

Class	DBP mm Hg
Stratum I (mild)	90–104
Stratum II (moderate)	105–114
Stratum III (severe)	≥115

While there is still controversy as to whether the treatment of hypertension reduced overall mortality in patients below age 50 years, treatment does decrease the incidence of hypertensive complications of stroke, congestive heart failure, LVH and hypertensive encephalopathy (33). Therefore, a reduction in blood pressure is recommended. In young patients with low short-term risk, nonpharmacologic measures may be tried. Alternatively, blood pressure could be controlled by drug therapy and then drug usage reduced if nonpharmacologic therapy is successfully implemented. Patients with an adverse prognosis (Table 23.6) may be more appropriately treated by early pharmacologic treatment of blood pressure.

NON-DRUG THERAPY

Nonpharmacologic methods to reduce blood pressure can be incorporated as a reasonable initial approach for young patients with mild hypertension and no other cardiovascular risk factors. Several of these measures can also be used to augment drug therapy.

Sodium Restriction (1, 34–37)

Sodium intake in the United States averages 4.0 to 5.0 g per day which is far in excess of the daily requirements of 400 mg. Moderate salt restriction can reduce DBP approximately 7 or 8 mm Hg (6%) and may normalize blood pressure in about 14% of patients. This approach requires no added salt and the avoidance of high sodium foods. Some home remedies (e.g. baking soda) and drug products (e.g. Alka-Seltzer) contain large quantities of sodium and should be avoided. Overnight urine collection followed by immediate analysis of urine sodium content improved dietary sodium restriction and reduced mean arterial blood pressure (MAP) by 11 mm Hg (37). Thus, a no added sodium diet allowed 80% of patients to stop or reduce the dose of antihypertensive medications. Severe sodium restriction (500 mg Na/day) can produce a greater reduction in blood pressure but is difficult to achieve.

The National Research Council has recommended that the American population reduce its average daily salt intake to 3 g/day. Salt restriction may have benefits by controlling blood pressure in some patients and augmenting drug therapy in others. Finally, a reduction in salt intake might help to reduce the development of hypertension in genetically susceptible individuals.

Table 23.6.
Adverse Prognostic Factors in Hypertension

1. Black race
2. Male
3. Youth
4. Persistent diastolic blood pressure >115 mm Hg
5. Elevated systolic blood pressure >160 mm Hg
6. Presence of target organ damage (retinopathy; cardiomegaly; ECG changes; proteinuria)
7. Previous or existing cardiovascular disease (angina pectoris; myocardial infarction; congestive heart failure; stroke, impaired renal function)
8. Family history of cardiovascular complications
9. Presence of other coronary risk factors (hyperlipidemia, smoking, diabetes mellitus; obesity; sedentary life)

Weight Reduction (38–41)

A large portion of hypertensive patients are overweight and underexercised. There is clear evidence that obesity is associated with an increased prevalence of hypertension. In hypertensive patients weight loss of 10% has produced a decrease of DBP of 10 mm Hg irrespective of salt intake in patients with or without concomitant drug treatment. Weight loss also reduces plasma renin activity and plasma aldosterone. Thus weight reduction is recommended for any overweight patient. It is well-recognized that long-term weight reduction is difficult to achieve especially by caloric reduction alone. For patients with significant cardiovascular risk it appears prudent to institute pharmacologic therapy while attempting to achieve weight reduction. Drug therapy can then be tapered if weight reduction is successful.

Exercise (42–45)

Exercise programs may have beneficial effects by reducing blood pressure, reducing weight, reducing triglycerides and increasing high density lipoprotein (HDL) cholesterol. Weight loss requires sustained aerobic exercise of at least 20 to 30 min duration with a frequency of at least 3 days per week. Two-day per week programs are ineffective in reducing body weight and fat.

The reduction of blood pressure in hypertensive patients who exercise may often be related to weight reduction. However, even a 2-day per week exercise program produced an 11.8-mm Hg reduction in DBP associated with only 1-kg weight loss (45). Finally, exercise programs (running in particular) reduce triglycerides, and increase HDL cholesterol and therefore modify two coronary risk factors. Thus an appropriate exercise program is desirable for hypertensive patients.

Stress Reduction (46, 47)

Various behavioral methods are proposed to lower blood pressure. These include biofeedback, relaxation, psychotherapy, environmental modification, placebo and suggestion. These methods which focus on emotional aspects may produce a modest decrease in blood pressure in selected patients and their effectiveness has not been substantiated in large clinical trials. Therefore, behavioral techniques should not be considered alternatives to pharmacologic therapy. These techniques may be useful in some patients but await further testing. Also, behavioral risk factors (e.g. stress, type A behavior) may increase risks of coronary disease independently of the effect on blood pressure.

Alcohol (48–50)

Alcohol consumption has an effect on blood pressure. The regular use of 3 or more drinks per day appears to be a risk factor for hypertension with higher blood pressures associated with increased alcohol consumption. Some studies suggest that there may be a threshold below which alcohol may have a beneficial effect on blood pressure (50). Regular alcohol consumption increases plasma renin activity, however, some evidence suggests that the alcohol-blood pressure relationship may be due in part to an alcohol withdrawal effect because of the usual timing of blood pressure measurements.

Also, patients who abuse alcohol (>6 drinks/day) have a high incidence (44%) of hypertension. This alcohol-induced hypertension correlates with markers of alcohol use (GGT and MCV); corrects after detoxification and blood pressure remains normal with continued abstinence. Patients with continued excessive alcohol consumption frequently fail to respond to conventional antihypertensive pharmacologic treatment.

Caffeine (51–53)

In non-coffee drinkers, caffeine increased blood pressure 10 to 14 mm Hg associated with increased plasma renin activity and increased plasma and urinary catecholamines. Chronic caffeine administration resulted in near complete tolerance and a lack of hemodynamic humoral effect. However, the combined effect of caffeine and cigarette smoking can produce a sustained increase in blood pressure in untreated or diuretic-treated patients with mild hypertension (52).

Cigarettes (1, 2, 17, 18, 22, 53)

Although smoking may increase blood pressure by a nicotine-mediated effect, little if any reduction of blood pressure occurs after cessation. However, smoking continues to be a major cardiovascular risk factor in treated hypertensive patients. Treated hypertensive patients who continue to smoke have a 2-fold increase in mortality over those who do not. So, cessation of smoking remains a high priority to reduce cardiovascular risk. As discussed, smoking plus caffeine can increase blood pressure.

DRUG THERAPY

When initiating drug therapy it is important to remember that hypertension is a disease of decades. Unless hypertension is severe, it is preferable to slowly approach a simple drug regimen which minimizes side effects and encourages long-term compliance.

Understanding the site and mechanism of action of the various antihypertensive drugs is the key to planning therapy. All current drugs impair normal homeostatic mechanisms and most reduce peripheral vascular resistance. Antihypertensive drugs act at several sites including: the peripheral sympathetic nerve endings, the vascular smooth muscle, the kidney, the central nervous system and the autonomic ganglia. Common side effects correlate with the site of action. A review of the pharmacology is presented in Table 23.7. The expected physiologic and hormonal actions of oral antihypertensive drugs are outlined in Table 23.8. Pharmacokinetic parameters are listed in Table 23.9.

Diuretics (1, 2, 54–66)

Thiazide and related diuretics have remained the mainstay of most antihypertensive regimens and are generally recommended as Step I therapy. About 40% of hypertensive patients may respond to diuretics alone. Even

Table 23.7.
Pharmacology of Antihypertensive Drugs

Drug	Available Sizes (mg)	Daily Dosage (mg)	Pharmacology	Adverse Effects
Diuretics				
Hydrochloro-thiazide	25, 50, 100	12.5–100	Distal renal tubule diuretic, naturetic, kaluretic	Hypokalemia, hyperuricemia, hypovolemia, hyperglycemia
Chlorthalidone	25, 50	12.5–50	As above	As above
Metolazone	2.5, 5, 10	2.5–20	As above	As above
Furosemide	20, 40, 80	20–320	Loop of Henle diuretic	As above
Ethacrynic acid	25, 50	50–200	As above	As above
Potassium-sparing Diuretics				
Amiloride	5	5–20	Potassium-sparing diuretic	Hyperkalemia
Spironolactone	25	50–200	Aldosterone antagonist	Hyperkalemia, gynecomastia
Triampterene	50, 100	50–200	Potassium-sparing diuretic	Hyperkalemia, nephrolithiasis
β-Blockers				
Atenolol	50, 100	50–100	β-Adrenergic blockade	See Table 23.16
Metoprolol	50	50–200	As above	As above
Nadolol	40, 80, 120, 160	40–320	As above	As above
Pindolol	5, 10	20–60	As above	As above
Propranolol	10, 20, 40, 60, 80	40–480	As above	As above
Timolol	10, 20	20–60	As above	As above
Central Sympatholytics				
Clonidine	0.1, 0.2, 0.3	0.2–2.4	Inhibits central sympathetic outflow (α_2-agonist)	Sedation, dry mouth, salt/water retention, sexual dysfunction, orthostatic hypotension, withdrawal syndrome, bradycardia (heart block)
Guanabenz	4, 8	8–32	As above	As above
Methyldopa	125, 250, 500	500–2000	Inhibition of sympathetic outflow false neurotransmitter, primarily central, some peripheral action	Sedation/fatigue, nasal congestion, forgetfulness, impaired concentration, depression, orthostatic hypotension, dry mouth, salt/water retention, sexual dysfunction, + direct Coombs test. *Uncommon:* drug fever, hepatitis, hemolytic anemia lactation, gastric distress
Reserpine	0.1, 0.25, 0.5	0.1–0.5	Sympathetic blockade by catecholamine depletion—central and peripheral	Sedation, nasal congestion, depression, nightmares, possible breast cancer, increased gastric distress

Table 23.7.—Continued

Drug	Available Sizes (mg)	Daily Dosage (mg)	Pharmacology	Adverse Effects
Peripheral Sympatholytics				
Guanethidine	10, 25	10–50	Peripheral sympathetic blockade, prevents storage and release of catecholamines	Orthostatic hypotension, sexual dysfunction, diarrhea, intestinal cramping, salt/water retention
Prazosin	1, 2, 5	3–40	Selective α_1 sympathetic blockade	Reflex tachycardia, salt/water retention, first dose syncope, headache, dizziness, drowsiness
Vasodilators				
Hydralazine	10, 25, 50, 100	20–200	Direct arteriolar vasodilator	Reflex tachycardia, aggravation of angina/heart failure, salt/water retention, headache/dizziness/flushing, lupus erythematosus reaction, gastric distress, nasal congestion
Minoxidil	2.5, 10	10–100	Direct arteriolar vasodilation	Reflex tachycardia, salt/water retention, hypertrichosis, aggravation of angina/heart failure
Converting Enzyme Inhibitor				
Captopril	25, 50, 100	75–450	Inhibition of angiotensin-converting enzyme	Proteinuria, rash, excessive hypotension, neutropenia/agranulocytosis

Table 23.8.
Hemodynamic and Hormonal Effects of Antihypertensive Agents[a]

Drug	Peripheral Vascular Resistance	Cardiac Output	Heart Rate	Plasma Renin Activity	Glomerular Filtration Rate	Plasma Volume
Oral diuretics (long-term)	↓	↔/↓	↔	↑	↔/↓	↓
Reserpine	↓	↓	↓	↓	↔/↓	↑
Methyldopa	↓	↓	↔/↓	↓	↔/↑	↑
Clonidine	↓	↓	↓	↓	↔	↑
Guanethidine	↔/↓	↓	↓	?/↓	↓	↑
β-Blockers	↔/↑	↓	↓	↓	↔	↔
Hydralazine	↓	↑	↑	↑	↔/↑	↑
Prazosin	↓	↔/↑	↔	↔	↔	↑
Minoxidil	↓	↑	↑	↑	↔	↑
Captopril	↓	↔/↑	↔/↑	↑	↔/↑	↑

[a] ↑ = increase; ↓ = decrease; ↔ = no change; ? = questionable.

when not completely effective alone, diuretics are usually continued to counteract salt and water retention from other drugs. During long-term therapy the initial decrease in plasma volume and cardiac output tend to correct but vascular resistance remains decreased. Whether thiazide diuretics have a direct vasodilating effect remains controversial but a functioning kidney is needed to lower blood pressure.

Diuretic therapy has been previously initiated with doses equivalent to 50 mg of hy-

Table 23.9.
Pharmacokinetics of Selected Antihypertensive Drugs

Drug	Absorption (%)	Protein Binding (%)	Elimination Half-Life (hr)	Elimination as Unchanged Drug (%)	Duration of Effect (hr)
Captopril	30–75	30	<2	66	8–12
Clonidine	75	<20	8	62	8–24
Guanethidine	20–50	—	75–150	50	Days
Hydralazine	30–50	87	3	14	12
Methyldopa	25–50	<20	2–4	63	12–24
Minoxidil	90	Minimal	3	<10	24
Prazosin	57	93	3	1	12
Reserpine	—	—	50–100	<1	Weeks

drochlorothiazide. Blood pressure usually decreases within 3 or 4 weeks or longer. Thus, doses should not be increased before 1 month of therapy has been completed.

Considerable evidence now suggests that diuretic doses greater than 50 mg of hydrochlorothiazide may be excessive (55, 56). The antihypertensive dose-response curve of oral diuretics is relatively flat and dose increases above 50 mg of hydrochlorothiazide produce little further reduction in blood pressure but substantially increase the incidence of biochemical abnormalities. Thus, the initial dose should be probably 12.5 to 25 mg of hydrochlorothiazide with a maximal antihypertensive dose of 50 mg.

The thiazide and related diuretics differ primarily in their duration of action (Table 23.10). To minimize the risks of hypokalemia and other abnormalities, a single morning dose of a diuretic of intermediate action, e.g. hydrochlorothiazide, offers the best balance of efficacy and safety at a reduced cost. Hydrochlorothiazide is effective in treating hypertension when administered once daily.

The major problem associated with the thiazide diuretics is hypokalemia (54, 57–60). Moderate hypokalemia (<3.5 mEq/liter >3.0 mEq/liter) may develop in 30 to 40% of patients. The degree of hypokalemia is clearly dose related (Table 23.11). Active younger or middle-aged patients without ischemic heart disease or the presence of multiple risk factors may tolerate asymptomatic moderate hypokalemia. However, evidence suggests that hypokalemia may pose a substantial risk for patients with or predisposed to ischemic heart disease (59, 60). The incidence of premature ventricular contractions (PVCs) both during exercise and at rest increases with diuretic-induced hypokalemia. Of importance is that hypokalemia develops more frequently with

Table 23.10.
Thiazide and Related Diuretics

Duration	Equivalent Dose (mg)
Less than 12 hr:	
Chlorothiazide	500
Hydrochlorothiazide	50
Hydroflumethiazide	50
Up to 24 hr	
Bendroflumethiazide	5
Benzthiazide	50
Methylchlothiazide	5
Metazolone	5
Quinethazone	50
Trichlormethazide	2
Longer than 24 hr	
Chlorthalidone	25–50
Cyclothiazide	2
Polythiazide	2

Table 23.11.
Dose-related Adverse Effects of Thiazide Diuretics

Dose of Hydrochlorthiazide (mg/day)	Serum Potassium (mEq/L)	Increase in Serum uric Acid (mg/100 ml)
0	4.5	—
50	3.9	0.8
100	3.4	3.1
200	2.4	4.3

larger diuretic doses, with long-acting diuretics like chlorthalidone and in patients with a high sodium intake (57). A diet with no added salt and no salty foods reduces potassium loss by 50%. Guidelines to reduce the risks of hypokalemia are presented in Table 23.12 (61, 62).

Increases in serum uric acid are also a dose-related adverse effect (Table 23.13). Hyperuricemia is usually asymptomatic, and most often does not require treatment. Allopurinol and probenecid have both been used to reduce thiazide-induced hyperuricemia but alternative antihypertensives should be considered. Patients who develop an increase in serum uric acid greater than 12 mg/100 ml and a serum creatinine greater than 3 mg/100 ml from thiazide therapy have a high probability of developing symptomatic gout.

Thiazide therapy also increases the serum

Table 23.12.
Techniques to Reduce the Occurrence and Risks of Diuretic-induced Hypokalemia

1. Limit diuretic dosage to 50 mg of hydrochlorothiazide in nonedematous hypertensive patients
2. Use a single morning dose of an intermediate-acting diuretic (e.g. hydrochlorothiazide). Avoid long-acting diuretics
3. Carefully instruct patients to follow a moderate sodium restricted diet (2–3 g/day) to reduce urinary potassium loss and enhance the diuretic hypotensive effects
4. Encourage some daily intake of potassium containing foods (fresh or dried fruits or juices). In overweight patients caloric restrictions may reduce the intake of these foods
5. Consider the use of potassium-containing salt substitutes (e.g. Lo-Salt, Diasal) to increase potassium and decrease sodium intake
6. Consider potassium chloride supplements (40–80 mEq/day) and/or a reduced diuretic dose in any patient with a serum potassium less than 3.0 mEq/L or with symptomatic hypokalemia (e.g. calf pain or muscle weakness)
7. Avoid even moderate hypokalemia (<3.5 mEq/L) in patients with an increased risk of myocardial irritability:
   a. Patients taking digitalis.
   b. Patients with angina or previous myocardial infarction. These patients should receive reduced doses of diuretics and prophylactic potassium supplements
8. Monitor the serum potassium at baseline, 3 mo, then 6–12-mo intervals when using diuretics
9. Patients with multiple cardiac risk factors may warrant more frequent monitoring to avoid even moderate hypokalemia

glucose an average of 9.6 mg/dl (63). Thiazide hyperglycemia is related to the extent of potassium loss and develops more rapidly in older patients. Clinical diabetes mellitus usually only develops in patients with preexisting borderline diabetes. Additionally, thiazide-type diuretics, in particular chlorthalidone, may adversely increase plasma cholesterol and triglycerides.

Furosemide generally produces a lesser reduction in blood pressure (approximately ½) and less potassium loss than thiazide diuretics (54). Furosemide should be reserved for patients unresponsive to thiazide diuretics who require its greater naturetic effect (e.g. patients with congestive heart failure or marked drug-induced sodium retention). Also, thiazide diuretics are ineffective in patients with reduced renal function (creatinine clearance <50 ml/min). These patients may require metazolone or furosemide.

POTASSIUM-SPARING DIURETICS

Three potassium-sparing diuretics are available: amiloride, spironolactone and triampterine.

Spironolactone (54)

Spironolactone is steroid competitive aldosterone antagonist which is used as a diuretic for patients with primary or secondary aldosteronism. Spironolactone may be an alternative diuretic for patients with gout or diabetes who are unable to tolerate thiazide diuretics. Finally, spironolactone has been used in combination with thiazide diuretics to prevent or treat hypokalemia.

The major adverse effect is hyperkalemia accruing in 3 to 9% of patients. Those at increased risk include patients with renal insufficiency or taking potassium supplements. Other adverse effects include gynecomastia, impotence and gastrointestinal irritation.

Triampterene (54, 64–66)

Triampterene has a direct action in the distal tubule with mild diuretic and hypotensive

Table 23.13.
Pharmacologic Properties of β-Blockers

	Atenolol	Metroprolol	Nadolol	Pindolol	Propranolol	Timolol
β_1-Selectivity	+	+	−	−	−	−
Intrinsic sympathomimetic activity	−	−	−	+	−	−
Membrane-stabilizing activity	−	−	−	+	++	−
β_1-Blockade potency ratio	1.0	1.0	1.0	6.0	1.0	6.0

effects. Its principal use is as adjunctive therapy to reduce the potassium loss from thiazide diuretics. Triampterene-hydrochlorothiazide combination (50/25 mg) produced hypokalemia (K <3.5 mEq/liter) in 6% of patients and hyperkalemia (K >5.4 mEq/liter) in 7% of patients (64). The higher percentage (22%) of hypokalemia in thiazide-only patients may well be related to the higher doses (hydrochlorothiazine 100 to 200 mg/day) used. Recent studies document an average serum potassium of 3.9 mEq/liter for patients treated with 50 mg of hydrochlorothiazide. Thus it appears that few if any patients will require the additional cost of combination triampterene therapy if the hydrochlorothiazide is limited to 50 mg daily or less.

The use of triampterene has additional risks. The major risk is hyperkalemia which may occur more frequently in diabetic patients. Triampterene can also produce hyperuricemia, hyperglycemia and nephrolithiasis (65). In addition, the combination of indomethacin and triampterene may cause reversible acute renal failure (66).

Amiloride (54)

Amiloride is the newest potassium-sparing diuretic which acts in the distal tubule similar to triampterene. Amiloride is excreted in the urine as unchanged drug, whereas triampterene undergoes extensive hepatic metabolism. Amiloride has a longer duration of action than triampterene and somewhat greater hypotensive effects.

The main adverse effects of amiloride are hyperkalemia, which may develop in 1 to 2% of patients with normal renal function and gastrointestinal disturbances. The presence of diabetes, cirrhosis, renal failure or potassium supplements increase the risk of hyperkalemia.

In general, combination therapy with potassium-sparing diuretics may not be needed for most hypertensive patients treated with 50 mg of hydrochlorothiazide or less. In high risk patients or when hypokalemia develops, the benefits, risks and costs of potassium sparing agents must be compared to the liquid or tablet potassium supplements.

β-Blockers (54, 67–78)

β-Blockers have gained a dramatic increase in use for the treatment of hypertension. This acceptance stems from a reasonable degree of effectiveness and a relatively low incidence of major side effects.

PHARMACOLOGY

β-Blockers competitively inhibit catecholamine neurotransmitters throughout the body at both cardiac receptors (β_1) and noncardiac receptors (β_2). Cardiac effects include a reduction in heart rate, cardiac output and cardiac work. In addition, β-blockers reduce plasma renin activity. Finally, it is believed the CNS effects of β-blockers are involved in control of blood pressure.

EFFECTIVENESS (67, 68)

The effectiveness of β-blockers is similar to other Step I and II antihypertensive drugs. Propranolol alone may reduce blood pressure about 11/8 mm Hg at doses up to 480 mg daily; it may control blood pressure in 40% of patients (67). Addition of a diuretic controlled 50% of patients and triple therapy (adding hydralazine) controlled 80% of the patients (67). Another factor that may favor the use of β-blockers in patients with ischemic heart disease is that they appear to be cardioprotective (68). Timolol, atenolol and propranolol all appear to provide secondary cardioprotection and reduce mortality and reinfarction following survival of an acute myocardial infarction (68). Further investigation is needed to establish whether β-blockers can prevent a primary infarction.

COMPARISON OF β-BLOCKERS (54, 69–75)

While the available β-blockers are similar in both efficacy and safety, there are some differences in both pharmacology and pharmacokinetics (Tables 23.13 and 23.14).

The major pharmacologic difference is the presence or absence of relative β_1-selectivity also called cardioselectivity. The cardioselective agents, atenolol and metoprolol, may produce a lesser degree of bronchospasm. They also may be better tolerated by patients with peripheral vascular insufficiency and produce less impairment in response to hypoglycemia in diabetic patients. Unfortunately cardioselectivity is relative, not absolute, and higher doses of these agents may produce a decrease in cardioselectivity.

The second pharmacologic difference is beta agonist activity or intrinsic sympathomimetic activity (ISA). Pindolol is currently the only β-

Table 23.14.
Pharmacokinetic Parameters of β-Blockers

	Atenolol	Metro-prolol	Nadolol	Pindolol	Propran-olol	Timolol
Absorption (%)	50	>95	30	>95	>90	90
Bioavailability (%)	40	50	30	100	30	75
Protein binding (%)	<5	12	30	57	93	10
Log partition coefficient (octanol/water)	0.23	2.15	0.71	1.75	3.65	2.10
Elimination half-life (hr)	6–9	3–4	14–24	3–4	3.5–6	3–4
Primary route of elimination	Renal	Hepatic	Renal	Hepatic, renal (40% unchanged)	Hepatic	Hepatic, renal (20% unchanged)
Equivalent dose (mg)	100–150	150	80–120	30	120	20
Dosing interval (hr)	24	12	24		12	12
Active metabolites	No	No	No	No	Yes	No

blocker with ISA and it may have some advantages for patients who experience bradycardia from other β-blockers. It may also be possibly less likely to exacerbate congestive heart failure or peripheral vascular disease.

The membrane stabilizing effect (quinidine-like antiarrhythmic effect) of β-blockers is not manifested except at plasma concentrations 50 to 100 times greater than usual concentrations which produce β-blockade and this property does not have clinical importance.

The β-blockers vary substantially in their pharmacokinetic properties (Table 23.14). Many differences are related to the solubility characteristic of the specific drug. Highly lipophilic drugs (e.g. propranolol and metoprolol) undergo extensive "first pass" metabolism; are primarily eliminated by hepatic metabolism; have a relatively short elimination half-life and more readily penetrate the blood-brain barrier. Conversely, the hydrophilic drugs, atenolol and nadolol are excreted by the kidney; have a longer elimination half-life; and are less able to penetrate the CNS. Because the antihypertensive effect of β-blockers appears to outlast the presence of the drug in plasma, all agents can be used on a twice daily schedule and the longer acting drugs can be given once daily. The bioavailability of propranolol and metroprolol is increased approximately 60% if the drugs are taken with food. Propranolol, in particular, has a wide dose range and plasma concentrations from a fixed dose may vary 20-fold between patients. The hydrophilic agents (atenolol and nadolol) have relatively flat dose-response curves but will accumulate in renal failure.

Several disease states contraindicate β-blockers or influence the selection of a β-blocker and the choice of agents should be individualized for patients (Table 23.15). Although pregnancy was once considered a contraindication, recent studies indicate that β-blockers improve fetal outcome when used to treat hypertension in pregnancy.

ADVERSE EFFECTS (54, 75–78)

The adverse effects of β-blockers can be divided into those caused by the β-blockade and all other adverse effects (Table 23.16). The most serious adverse effects are those related to β-blockade in predisposed patients. These major adverse effects tend to occur early in therapy and even at low doses. If initial doses are well tolerated it is uncommon for larger doses to produce adverse respiratory or cardiovascular effects. The major adverse effects are related to the dependence of some patients on stimulation of sympathetic nervous system rather than the specific β-blocker or dose. The CNS effects may be more common with lipophilic drugs like propranolol and frank depression or vivid visual hallucinations can occur. Dermatologic reactions have included a marked exacerbation of psoriasis. Other subtle hemodynamic and metabolic changes have been reported including a decrease on HDL cholesterol, a decreased cholesterol ratio and slight decrease in glomerular filtration rate (GFR). Overall, approximately 10% of patients may be unable to tolerate β-blockers.

The abrupt withdrawal of β-blockers, particularly in patients with ischemic heart disease,

Table 23.15.
Contraindications/Precautions with β-Blocker Therapy

Contraindication	Precautions
Bronchial asthma	Congestive heart failure
AV block with sinus bradycardia	Chronic obstructive pulmonary disease
Uncontrolled congestive heart failure	Diabetes mellitus
	Peripheral vascular disease

Selection of a β-Blocker			
Cardioselective agent	Intrinsic sympathomi-metic activity agent	Nonselective	Water-soluble
Angina	AV conduction defect	Migraine	Depression
Bronchitis	Bradycardia	Thyrotoxicosis	Adverse effects from lipophilic β-blockers
Impaired peripheral circulation	Congestive failure		
Diabetes mellitus			

Table 23.16.
Adverse Effects of β-Blockers

β-Blockade effects:
1. Bronchospasm
2. Congestive heart failure/acute pulmonary edema
3. Bradyarrythmias/AV conduction block/cardiac arrest
4. Aggravation of hypoglycemia
5. Impairment of peripheral circulation

Other adverse effects:
6. CNS effects (vivid dreams, nightmares, hallucinations, depression)
7. Withdrawal rebound syndrome (tachycardia and aggravation of ischemic heart disease)
8. Metabolic effects (lipid abnormalities, hyperglycemia)
9. Dermatologic reactions (includes exacerbation of psoriasis)
10. Gastrointestinal symptoms

Table 23.17.
β-Blocker Drug Interactions

Drug	Interaction
Antacids	Decreased propranolol absorption
Calcium channel blockers	Possible additive AV blockade and myocardial depression
Cimetidine	Decreased propranolol metabolism
Clonidine	Increased risk of "rebound" hypertension
Hypoglycemic agents	Increased risk of exercise hypoglycemia/masked warning symptoms
Lidocaine	Decreased lidocaine metabolism
Nonsteroidal anti-inflammatory drugs (NSAIDS)	Possible decreased antihypertensive effect
Prazosin	Increased "first dose" hypotension
Tricyclic antidepressant agents	Possible decreased antihypertensive effect
Phenothiazine	Possible increased β-blockade

may produce increased β-adrenergic sensitivity and has resulted in a withdrawal syndrome, usually at 2 to 6 days. This withdrawal syndrome can result in tachycardia, anxiety, tremors, increased blood pressure, angina pectoris and myocardial infarction and sudden death. β-Blockers should be discontinued by tapering over a 2-week period and should be continued up to the morning of cardiac surgery. β-Blocker drug interactions are listed in Table 23.17.

Sympathetic Inhibitors

Many antihypertensive drugs interfere with the sympathetic nervous system. These agents may act in the central nervous system, the peripheral nervous system or both.

CENTRAL ACTING SYMPATHOLYTICS

Clonidine (54, 79–87)

Clonidine is an imidazoline which stimulates α_2-adrenergic receptors in the lower brainstem decreasing sympathetic outflow to the cardiovascular system. Because clonidine has predominantly central effects, peripheral cardiovascular reflexes are preserved and there is a low incidence of orthostatic symptoms. Clonidine also acts as a peripheral presynaptic α_2-agonist, activating negative feedback inhibition of norepinephrine release from sympathetic neurons. It also appears to have a direct action on the kidney which in part produces the decrease in plasma renin activity. Clonidine usually decreases pulse rate but preserves GFR (Table 23.8).

Clonidine can be an effective agent at all levels of hypertension and monotherapy may normalize blood pressure in 50 to 60% of patients, producing a 25/15 mm Hg decrease in blood pressure (83). Clonidine can be effectively combined with diuretics, vasodilators and has been additive to "triple" therapy (β-blocker, diuretic, vasodilator). An oral clonidine loading regimen (0.2 mg followed by 0.1 mg/hour to a maximum 0.7 mg) has been effective in treating hypertensive urgencies (84). A clonidine suppression test also can aid in the diagnosis of pheochromocytoma (85).

Clonidine can be given on a twice daily dose schedule and in many patients a daily bedtime dose is effective and minimizes complaints of sedation. Initial doses of 0.1 to 0.2 mg at bedtime, gradually increased at 1- to 2-week intervals, also help to reduce sedation.

Sedation and dry mouth are the most frequent adverse effects (Table 23.7). They often disappear after the first few weeks. Saliva substitutes or sugarless gum/candy can provide relief from the dry mouth. About 7% of patients discontinue clonidine because of side effects.

Concern has been raised about an acute withdrawal syndrome (AWS) following the abrupt discontinuation of clonidine (86, 87). While exact incidence of AWS is not defined, the syndrome appears to be uncommon. AWS has also been described with other central acting sympatholytic and β-blockers. AWS is believed to be caused by a sudden increased concentration of plasma catecholamines, activation of renin, angiotensin, aldosterone and, if β-blockers have been used, a denervation hypersensitivity (87). Symptoms of AWS can include: nervousness, agitation, tremors, palpitations, insomnia, headache, flushing, nausea and vomiting. Signs can include: marked hypertension in excess of pretreatment blood pressure, tachycardia, diaphoresis, increased catecholamines and rarely malignant hypertension.

The risk of AWS appears to be higher in younger patients with severe hypertension who are treated with high doses and multiple antihypertensive agents. Combination with nonselective β-blockers appears to increase the risk of a hypertensive episode on discontinuation of clonidine. This combination should be avoided and if used the β-blocker should be tapered and stopped prior to decreasing the clonidine.

Avoiding excessive doses, encouraging patient compliance and tapering clonidine slowly may help to prevent an AWS. However, patients should be warned of the signs/symptoms of AWS so they can seek help if it occurs. Treatment by restarting medications, bedrest and sedation if required is usually effective in reversing an AWS.

Clonidine is additive to other sedating drugs including alcohol and patients should be cautioned about these combinations and driving. Other interactions are listed in Table 23.18.

Methyldopa (54, 79, 88)

Methyldopa has been an important antihypertensive drug for the past 20 years. The methyldopa metabolite, α-methyl norepinephrine, is a central acting α-agonist and like clonidine reduces CNS sympathetic outflow. α-Methyl norepinephrine may also have a peripheral effect by acting as a less potent false neurotransmitter competing with norepinephrine at α_1, postsynaptic receptors. The hemodynamic effects are described in Table 23.8. Methyldopa has an orthostatic effect greater than clonidine but less than guanethidine. Both cardiac output and renal function are usually preserved. Because salt/water retention can produce a "pseudotolerance," methyldopa is normally combined with a diuretic.

Methyldopa can be used with a twice daily dosing schedule despite a short plasma half-life (Table 23.9). In some patients a single bedtime dose can reduce side effects and help compliance. Adverse effects cause about 8 to 10% of patients to discontinue methyldopa. Sedation and fatigue (20%) are most frequent followed by postural/exercise dizziness (15%) and dry mouth (9%), and nasal congestion (4%). Sexual dysfunction and an acute withdrawal syndrome can occur. Again, some side effects regress with time and patient education can help to reduce the problems of postural dizziness and dry mouth. Methyldopa is also described to cause subtle CNS changes which impair complex mental function and increase forgetfulness.

More serious hypersensitivity reactions

have occurred with methyldopa including: drug fever, colitis, hepatotoxicity, a positive Coombs test and hemolytic anemia. The risk of serious toxicity and impaired mental function make alternative antihypertensive drugs preferable for many patients. Methyldopa drug interactions are listed in Table 23.18.

Reserpine (54, 79, 88, 89)

Reserpine has been used for more than 50 years. It acts in both the central and peripheral sympathetic nervous system depleting norepinephrine and serotonin stores in the brain and peripheral adrenergic nerve endings. Reserpine functions as an adrenergic antagonist rather than an agonist as with clonidine/methyldopa. Reserpine also increases vagal tone which contributes to the reduced heart rate and increased gastric acid secretions. Its cardiovascular effects are listed in Table 23.8.

Reserpine is rapidly but incompletely absorbed and is eliminated by hepatic metabolism. The elimination half-life of reserpine is longer than 11 days (Table 23.9). The onset of action of reserpine may take 3 to 6 days with maximal hypotensive effects taking 3 to 6 weeks. After discontinuing reserpine several weeks are required for its effects to disappear. Side effects usually limit the daily dose of reserpine to less than 0.5 mg. Doses of reserpine greater than 0.25 mg produce little additional decrease in blood pressure.

Adverse effects from reserpine necessitate discontinuation of therapy in about 5% of patients. Nasal congestion from cholinergic stimulation occurs frequently (22%). This may lessen with time and can be treated with a topical atropine solution (1:1000). Topical nasal decongestants must be avoided as they can result in rebound congestion and systemic decongestants may elevate blood pressure.

Reserpine-induced CNS changes include drowsiness/sedation (14%), dizziness (19%), weakness/lethargy (19%), sleep disturbances, difficulty in concentration or poor memory. Patients should be warned that drowsiness or dizziness may impair driving and alcohol may add to these problems. Depression can occur in 10 to 25% of patients and suicides have occurred. Higher doses (0.5 mg), a history of depression or recent emotional trauma are predisposing factors. Depression develops insidiously over months to years, responds poorly to antidepressants and requires drug discontinuation. Gastrointestinal symptoms (5%) and weight gain also occur. A possible association between reserpine and breast cancer was *not* substantiated in a large study (89). However, reserpine can increase prolactin secretion and cause galactorrhea and gynecomastia. Drug interactions are shown in Table 23.18.

Reserpine monotherapy is less effective than a diuretic and when combined with a diuretic or hydralazine doses should be limited to 0.25 mg. Despite success in some centers, other Step 2 agents are usually preferred because of greater efficacy and/or fewer adverse effects.

Newer Central Sympatholytics (54)

Guanabenz is a guanidine derivative which, like clonidine, blocks central sympathetic vasomotor impulses and also produces a guanethidine-like postganglionic blockade. Doses of 12 to 16 mg daily moderately reduce blood pressure (17 to 23 mm Hg); are additive with diuretics and are relatively well tolerated. The principal adverse effects are dry mouth and sedation which may occur in almost 50% of patients. Guanabenz is used on a twice daily dosing schedule. Guanfacine also stimulates vasomotor center α_2-receptors and reduces sympathetic outflow and plasma norepinephrine. Because of a longer duration of action it can be used once daily. Frequent side effects include dry mouth, constipation, fatigue, sedation, and weakness which often disappear after 3 to 4 months.

PERIPHERAL ACTING SYMPATHOLYTICS

Guanethidine (54, 60)

Guanethidine is actively transported into the peripheral adrenergic neuron where it depletes norepinephrine and produces a postural hypotension. Guanethidine decreases venous return to the heart, decreases cardiac output and interferes with the sympathetic reflexes which control the resistance (arteriolar) and capacitance (venous) vessels. Because guanethidine depletes myocardial catecholamines it can aggravate congestive heart failure.

Guanethidine is slowly and variably absorbed undergoing partial first pass hepatic metabolism. With chronic administration the half-life of guanethidine is 5 days with 50% of the drug excreted unchanged in the urine. Because of the long half-life, guanethidine can

Table 23.18.
Selected Antihypertensive Drug Interactions

Interacting Drug	Antihypertensive Drug							
	Clonidine	Methyldopa	Reserpine	Guanethidine	Prazosin	Hydralazine	Minoxidil	Captopril
Alcohol	Increased postural hypotension	Increased postural hypotension	Increased postural hypotension	Increased postural hypotension	Increased postural hypotension	Increased postural hypotension	Increased postural hypotension	Increased postural hypotension
Antipsychotics	Additive hypotension	Additive hypotension	Additive hypotension	Decreased antihypertensive effect	Additive hypotension	Additive hypotension	Additive hypotension	Additive hypotension
β-Blocker	Increased risk of rebound withdrawal hypertension	—	—	—	Increased first dose hypotension syncope	—	—	—
Digoxin	—	Possible bradycardia	—	—	—	—	—	—
Haloperidol	—	Possible haloperidol toxicity	—	Decreased antihypertensive effect	—	—	—	—
Indomethacin	—	—	—	—	—	—	—	Decreased antihypertensive effect
Levodopa	Decreased levodopa effect	Decreased levodopa effect/increased hypotension	Decreased levodopa effect	Increased hypotension	—	—	—	—
Lithium	—	Increased lithium effect	—	—	—	—	—	—
Monoamine oxidase inhibitor	Increased antihypertensive effect	Increased antihypertensive effect	Possible CNS excitation	Increased or decreased antihypertensive effect	—	—	—	—

	Potassium sparing diuretics	Sympathomimetics	Tricyclic antidepressant
	—	Decreased antihypertensive effect	Decreased antihypertensive effect
	—	Decreased antihypertensive effect	—
	—	Decreased antihypertensive effect	Possible CNS excitation
	—	Decreased antihypertensive effect	Decreased antihypertensive effect
	—	Decreased antihypertensive effect	—
	—	Decreased antihypertensive effect	—
	—	Decreased antihypertensive effect	—
Hyperkalemia	—	Decreased antihypertensive effect	—

be taken once daily and dosage adjustments should be made only after 2 to 3 weeks to allow for drug accumulation (Table 23.9). A 6-fold interindividual variation occurs between guanethidine dose and plasma level. Adrenergic blockade occurs when plasma levels exceed 8 ng/ml. This in part accounts for the wide range of effective doses (10 to 400 mg). In some cases, small doses of guanethidine (10 to 20 mg) are effective in mild or moderate hypertension without severe side effects. Used in this fashion, guanethidine has been substituted for reserpine.

Because the hypotensive effect of guanethidine is postural, it is augmented by standing, exercise and heat. Doses should be adjusted based on standing blood pressure. Blocks can be used to elevate the head of the bed to sustain a nighttime postural effect.

The major problem with guanethidine is postural and exercise hypotension, particularly with larger doses (>50 mg). Patients should be warned to rise slowly from supine or sitting positions; to flex their arms and legs before arising; and to avoid additive vasodilating factors such as prolonged standing, hot showers, and drinking alcohol. Postural effects are often most pronounced in the morning on arising. Guanethidine may be a poor choice for patients with autonomic insufficiency or who participate in vigorous physical activity. Other dose-related problems include sexual dysfunction and diarrhea which may require discontinuation of therapy. A "pseudotolerance" due to fluid retention may develop unless diuretic therapy is adequate. Because guanethidine diffuses poorly into the CNS, sedation and depression are infrequent problems.

Several drugs can interfere with the uptake of guanethidine into the adrenergic neuron and rapidly block its antihypertensive effects. Drugs included are: tricyclic antidepressants, phenothiazines, MAO inhibitors, amphetamines, and nonprescription sympathomimetics like ephedrine (Table 23.18).

Several investigational drugs have a mode of action similar to guanethidine. These include bethanidine, guanadrel, and debrisoquine.

Prazosin (54, 80, 90–92)

Prazosin selectively blocks postsynaptic α_1-adrenergic receptors producing both arterial and venous dilation (Table 23.8). It produces less tachycardia than hydralazine, an arteriolar vasodilator, but more postural hypotension. It produces about a 16/12 mm Hg reduction in blood pressure with a greater effect when standing. Prazosin is additive with diuretics and β-blockers.

The plasma half-life of prazosin is short, 2 to 3 hours. However, the antihypertensive effect lasts up to 24 hours and prazosin is effective when administered on a twice daily basis. Peak plasma levels occur 3 hours after oral doses and it is 97% protein bound. Prazosin undergoes hepatic metabolism with a significant "first pass" metabolism and some metabolites are active. The maximal antihypertensive effects of prazosin take up to 8 weeks and dosage should be increased accordingly.

About 9% of patients will discontinue prazosin from side effects. The adverse effects are most commonly cardiovascular (28%), central nervous system (24%), anticholinergic (10%) or gastrointestinal (8%). Prazosin can also cause a "first dose syncope." An episode of sudden collapse and unconsciousness can occur in patients taking 2 mg or more prazosin as a first dose. First dose syncope is most common in patients who have a depleted plasma volume (diuretics) or reduced ability to increase cardiac output in response to a decreased blood pressure (e.g. patients taking β-blockers). Syncope is usually preceded by palpitations and tachycardia. This is believed to be the effect of excessive postural hypotension and is most likely to occur in sodium-depleted patients. To avoid this problem the initial dose should be limited to 1 mg and taken at bedtime or when the patient can be observed. Fluid retention also occurs and prazosin should be administered in combination with a diuretic. Prazosin can also cause tachycardia which is most pronounced upon standing. Prazosin has also been used to reduce preload and afterload for severe chronic congestive heart failure (91). The development of "delayed tolerance" can often be overcome by increased diuretic doses, the addition of spironolactone or interruption of prazosin treatment followed by higher prazosin doses.

Vasodilators

Hydralazine (54, 90, 92–95)

Hydralazine has been used for over 30 years. It reduces blood pressure through direct relaxation of arteriolar smooth muscle. It does not interfere with autonomic reflexes nor produce postural hypotension. A baroreceptor-activated reflex sympathetic discharge increases heart rate, cardiac output and myocardial oxgyen demand (Table 23.8). Hydralazine also causes sodium and water retention. Both the increase in cardiac output and the fluid retention tend to blunt the antihypertensive effect. To avoid these problems hydralazine should be given in combination with a diuretic and a β-blocking agent in doses adequate to prevent the usual 10 to 30 beats/min increase in heart rate (triple therapy). Other sympatholytic drugs can be successfully substituted for β-blocking agents. The addition of hydralazine to a diuretic β-blocker can further reduce blood pressure by 10/14 mm Hg (54). Compared to prazosin when added to a diuretic, hydralazine produces less orthostatic dizziness, sexual dysfunction and nightmares (92). In elderly (>50 years) patients, reflex tachycardia did not develop to an important degree (92).

Hydralazine is rapidly and almost completely absorbed with peak plasma levels 1 to 2 hours after an oral dose. It is metabolized in the gut wall and during the first pass through the liver. The major pathway of elimination of hydralazine is hepatic acetylation. The acetylation rate is genetically determined and slow acetylators experience greater hypotensive effects and usually should not receive more than 200 mg of hydralazine daily. About 50% of blacks or whites are slow acetylators. The plasma half-life of hydralazine is 2 to 4 hours but antihypertensive effects persist much longer probably due to binding of the drug in the walls of arterial muscles (Table 23.9). Hydralazine is effective when taken only twice daily. The administration of hydralazine with food increases bioavailability. Uremia appears to slow biotransformation and produce drug accumulation and higher plasma levels. Only 10% of hydralazine is usually excreted in the urine as parent drug.

In combination therapy only about 4% of patients discontinue hydralazine because of side effects. Adverse effects of hydralazine are frequently related to the reflex sympathetic stimulation or its direct vasodilation. Side effects include headache (22%), nausea/vomiting (19%), tachycardia (18%), postural hypotension (16%), palpitations (15%), dizziness (6%), weakness (6%) and sleep disturbance (4%). The reflex tachycardia can produce palpitations and myocardial ischemia, and precipitate or aggravate angina pectoris. Hydralazine also causes a pyridoxine-deficiency induced peripheral neuropathy (3%).

The major question related to the safety of hydralazine is the development of an autoimmune response. About ⅓ of patients may develop a positive antinuclear antibody (ANA) (54, 95). The development of a positive ANA is much greater in slow acetylators (47%) than in fast acetylators (11%). Because autoimmune responses may take 6 to 12 months or longer to develop, it is recommended to monitor an ANA titer every 6 months. About 3 to 6% of patients will develop a hydralazine lupus-like syndrome. These patients are most often slow acetylators. Presenting symptoms can include arthalgia, arthritis, fever, malaise, rash and weight loss. Symptoms can resolve rapidly and often disappear within 6 months; however, rheumatoid symptoms and a positive ANA can persist for years.

Minoxidil (54, 96, 97)

Minoxidil is a potent vasodilator which markedly reduces peripheral vascular resistance (Table 23.8). It can produce blood pressure reductions of 30 to 40 mm Hg when combined with diuretics and β-blockers.

Minoxidil is well absorbed and undergoes hepatic metabolism (Table 23.9). Despite a relatively short half-life the antihypertensive effect persists 12 to 24 hours. Therefore, minoxidil is dosed twice daily.

Minoxidil produces marked sodium/water retention and adequate diuretic therapy, often furosemide in large doses is needed to control the edema. Reflex tachycardia and increased cardiac output are prevented by adequate β-blocker therapy. Hypertrichosis occurs in nearly all patients. This can be partly controlled with dipilatories but limits its used in women. An unproven possibility of cardiac lesions also exists. Because of these adverse effects minoxidil is often reserved for patients who have failed other agents. Oral minoxidil has also been used in combination with propranolol and furosemide in a loading dose regimen for the treatment of severe hypertension.

Diazoxide (54)

Diazoxide is a nondiuretic thiazide which dilates peripheral arterioles and is used to treat hypertensive emergencies. Rapid intravenous injection produces a profound decrease in both systolic and diastolic blood pressure which does not require continuous infusion and infrequently causes hypotension.

Diazoxide is metabolized hepatically and excreted in urine. Its duration of action varies from 2 to 24 hours. Diazoxide is usually administered as a rapid intravenous bolus (5 mg/kg over 10 sec) to exceed plasma protein-binding capacity (90%) and achieve a high initial concentration of free drug. However, controversy exists as to the need for bolus administration.

Some clinicians have suggested that the standard 300-mg initial dose is excessive for a few patients and recommend an initial dose of 75 mg followed by 100 mg every 5 min until a response occurs.

Diazoxide produces sodium and water diuretic therapy to maintain blood pressure control. Hyperglycemia and hyperuricemia are usually not problems except during prolonged use. Patients with renal failure or myocardial ischemia are predisposed to the adverse effects of diazoxide.

Nitroprusside (54)

Nitroprusside relaxes both arteriolar and venous smooth muscles. Controlled intravenous infusions of nitroprusside are highly effective in treating hypertensive emergencies. Initial nitroprusside infusions should be at a rate of 1 μg/kg/min (50 mg nitroprusside in 500 ml 5% dextrose in water). The onset and cessation of the hypotensive action is almost immediate. Nitroprusside is unstable and must be protected from light.

Nitroprusside is metabolized to thiocyanate which is slowly excreted by the kidneys (half-life 4 to 7 days), thus patients with impaired renal function may rapidly accumulate thiocyanate. Plasma thiocyanate levels greater than 10 mg/dl can produce intoxication and plasma levels should be measured if nitroprusside infusions are continued longer than 24 hours.

Nitroprusside is particularly useful in patients with decompensated myocardial function. In these patients dilation of capacitance vessels (venules) decreases cardiac preload and may increase cardiac output. Nitroprusside decreases peripheral resistance and can improve left ventricular function in patients with congestive heart failure or with impaired cardiac output after a myocardial infarction.

Other Antihypertensive Drugs

Captopril (54, 98–102)

Captopril inhibits angiotensin converting enzyme (ACE) which results in decreased conversion of inactive angiotensin I to the potent pressor peptide angiotensin II. The absence of normal angiotensin negative feedback results in a marked increase in plasma renin activity. ACE also inactivates bradykinin, a vasodilator. ACE inhibition leads to an increased bradykinin which in turn releases vasoactive prostaglandins. Bradykinin induced hypotension is attenuated by prostaglandin inhibitors like indomethacin. However, the hypotensive effects of captopril are largely from the inhibition of angiotensin II generation as there is little change in heart rate or cardiac output which are normally increased by vasodilators such as bradykinin.

Captopril is well absorbed after oral administration (75%) but food can reduce absorption by 30 to 40% (Table 23.9). Captopril undergoes both hepatic metabolism and renal excretion as unchanged drug. The half-life of captopril is less than 2 hours. About 66% of captopril is excreted unchanged in the urine and the dose should be reduced for patients with impaired renal function.

Captopril can be effective in severe or resistant hypertension, renovascular hypertension, and hypertension with renal failure. It appers no more effective than diuretics or β-blockers in milder forms of hypertension. The antihypertensive effect of captopril is likely to be greater in white than in black patients. Because of its potential adverse effects captopril is reserved for patients who have failed to respond or tolerate multiple drug regimens. Blood pressure is further reduced by combining captopril with a diuretic. Captopril can correct diuretic-induced hypokalemia and reduce the need for potassium supplements. The addition of a β-blocker or other sympathetic inhibitor can also be used when patients do not respond to captopril plus a diuretic. Neither delayed tolerance or rebound hypertension is associated with captopril. The usual starting dose is 25 mg, 3 times a day, increased at 1- to 2-week intervals to a maximum of 450 mg daily. Dosage increases often prolong rather than increase the antihypertensive effect. Low dose (75 mg/day) captopril monotherapy is relatively ineffective in mild to moderate hypertension, however, when combined with a diuretic they can be an effective regimen with few side effects (100). However, captopril can also produce beneficial hemodynamic changes in patients with congestive heart failure (101).

Captopril avoids most of the adverse effects common to other antihypertensive agents. However, other severe or serious adverse effects have occurred. Evidence suggests that some of the adverse effects of captopril, including rash and neutropenia, are dose related.

A generalized maculopapular rash with fever or transient pruritus can occur in about 10% of patients. This usually occurs within 2 weeks of starting therapy or an increased dosage. The rash resolves with 7 to 10 days of stopping treatment of reducing the dosage. Taste disturbances (6%) are often transient and may be improved by a temporary drug discontinuation. Captopril is also associated with neutropenia (0.3%) and rarely agranulocytosis. Blood counts should be monitored frequently during the first 3 months of therapy and patients should be instructed to report any signs of infection or oral ulcers. Captopril can also cause proteinuria (1.2% of patients) which may progress to a nephrotic syndrome in 1 of 4 patients. A membranous glomerulopathy is also reported. The initial dose of captopril can produce a profound hypotension particularly in patients who are volume depleted by diuretics. This may be avoided by discontinuing the diuretics for 7 days prior to starting captopril and using a low (6.25 to 12.5 mg) initial dosage. Because captopril can increase serum potassium via a reduction on aldosterone, the risk of hyperkalemia is increased in patients with renal failure or who take potassium supplements or potassium sparing diuretics (Table 23.18).

Saralasin (54, 103)

Saralasin is a chemical analog of angiotensin II with weak agonist activity. In the presence of high circulating levels of angiotensin II, saralasin will function as a competitive antagonist, lowering arterial blood pressure. At low levels of angiotensin II, saralasin will increase blood pressure. A saralasin test can be used as first-stage screening of patients suspected of renovascular hypertension. A positive test is a decrease of 7 mm Hg in DBP after a 30-min saralasin infusion in a sodium-depleted patient. Saralasin has also been used for hypertensive emergencies.

Calcium Channel Blockers (104–108)

An emerging theory in the pathogenesis of hypertension combines the effect of sodium and calcium on blood pressure. It proposes that high sodium consumption in genetically predisposed subjects leads to volume overload and the appearance of a naturetic hormone which increases membrane permeability. This increases intracellular sodium, inhibits sodium-calcium exchange and results in an accumulation of calcium in vascular smooth muscle cells. The increased intracellular calcium produces increased contractility, increased peripheral vascular resistance and raised blood pressure. An epidemiologic survey found a positive correlation between serum calcium and blood pressure (107). Also, hypertensive patients have been found to have a decreased serum concentration of ionized calcium (108).

Calcium channel blockers inhibit the inward passage of calcium in vascular and myocardial smooth muscle cells. The effect of calcium inhibitors is to uncouple the excitation-contraction process causing smooth muscle relaxation. Nifedipine reduces arterial blood pressure; increases cardiac output and causes a reflex tachycardia and increased plasma renin activity. The reduction of blood pressure appears related to the level of pretreatment of arterial pressure. Oral nifedipine appears to be a potentially useful antihypertensive agent with both the degree and duration of activity dose related. Combination therapy with a β-blocker also appears useful. Sublingual nifedipine has also been effective in acute hypertensive emergencies. Other calcium blockers, verapamil and diltiazem appear less useful as antihypertensive drugs. Currently, nifedipine is not approved for treating hypertension.

CLINICAL USE OF ANTIHYPERTENSIVE DRUGS

The initial goal of antihypertensive drug therapy is to achieve and maintain DBP at less than 90 mm/kg. The Joint National Committee further states that the ultimate goal is the lowest DBP consistent with safety and tolerance.

The Joint National Committee has proposed a Stepped-Care Approach to drug therapy (2). This approach is to start with a small dose of an antihypertensive drug and increase the dose until the goal blood pressure is reached; side effects become intolerable or a maximum dose is reached. Then additional drugs are added sequentially (Table 23.19).

Step 1 Therapy

In the majority of patients Step 1 therapy is a thiazide diuretic, usually hydrochlorothiazide. Both the initial and maximal dosage should be lower than previously recommended. These lower doses reduce adverse biochemical effects, particularly hypokalemia and maintain the most of the hypotensive effect of diuretics.

β-Blockers, specifically propranolol, have been advocated as being preferable (to thiazide diuretics) as Step 1 drugs. Direct evidence to clarify this controversy has been provided by two large studies (109, 110).

A Veterans Administration Cooperative Study compared propranolol to hydrochlorothiazide in both a short-term dosage titration and at 1 year (109). Hydrochlorothiazide (H) was found to be more effective than propranolol (P) and produced:

1. Greater reduction in BP: H (−17.5/13.1 mm/kg) vs. P (−8.3/11.3 mm/kg

Table 23.19.
Stepped Care Antihypertensive Drug Regimen

Step 1	Step 2	Step 3	Step 4
Thiazide diuretic	Add propranolol or atenolol or clonidine or guanebenz or methyldopa or metoprolol or nadolol or pindolol or prazosin or reserpine or timolol	Add hydralazine	Add or substitute: Guanethidine Minoxidil Captopril

2. A higher percentage of patients at goal BP: H (65.5%) vs. P (52.8%)

3. Fewer terminations

4. A lower systolic BP: H (129 mm Hg) vs. P (134 mm Hg)

5. A higher percentage of goal BP in blacks: H (71%) vs. P (53%)

6. Fewer dosage titrations.

A 6-year study found similar antihypertensive and side effects between propranolol and bendroflumethazide (110). In summary, hydrochlorothiazide can have a greater antihypertensive effect than propranolol with similar to fewer side effects.

Thiazide diuretics are clearly the drug of choice in blacks and have an additional advantage in that they potentiate the effects of Step 2 antihypertensive drugs. In addition, there is a substantial cost savings in using hydrochlorothiazide. Thus, for the majority of patients hydrochlorothiazide remains the preferred Step 1 agent.

However, β-blockers may be appropriate as Step 1 for the following patient groups: (a) younger patients with a rapid heart rate and/or a high pulse pressure, (b) patients intolerant of diuretic-induced biochemical changes, and (c) patients with previous myocardial infarction or angina pectoris.

Refractory Hypertension (111, 112)

Patients who do not respond to Step 1 therapy should be evaluated for potentially correctable courses of treatment failure particularly: (a) patient noncompliance, (b) excessive sodium intake, and (c) concurrent use of interfering drugs.

For patients failing to respond to full stepped-care therapy several therapeutic options can be considered: (a) substitute furosemide for hydrochlorothiazide if sodium/fluid retention exists, (b) increase Step 2 drug dosage beyond maximal recommendations or substitute an alternate Step 2 drug, (c) add a second Step 2 drug, (d) substitute minoxidil for hydralazine, and (e) switch to captopril.

Step Down Therapy (113)

Another important aspect of therapy is that after arterial blood pressure has been adequately controlled for a sustained period it may be possible to reduce antihypertensive drug therapy while maintaining blood pressure control. Elimination of at least one drug may be possible in 50% of patients and dosage reductions in up to 80% (113). Step down therapy has an increased chance of success in patients who have modified their health habits.

Borderline Hypertension (114–116)

An estimated 18 million patients have borderline hypertension with blood pressure readings that fluctuate above and below 150/90 mm Hg. About 30% of patients with borderline hypertension will have sustained hypertensive (DBP ≥ 90 mm Hg) blood pressure readings at home. These patients may benefit from drug therapy.

Hypertensive Emergencies (54)

Accelerated and malignant hypertension can rapidly damage target organs. Complications of hypertensive emergencies include left ventricular failure with pulmonary edema, hypertensive encephalopathy, dissecting aortic aneurysm, intracranial hemorrhage and renal failure. The goal is to promptly lower but not to normalize blood pressure. Acute reduction of blood pressure to near normal levels can decrease renal blood flow and induce oliguria and other complications.

The drugs most useful in treating hypertensive emergencies are diazoxide, sodium nitroprusside, and hydralazine. Nitroprusside is preferred for patients with cardiac decompensation while diazoxide offers the advantage of not requiring a controlled intravenous infusion.

COMPLICATED HYPERTENSION (1, 2, 54)

The presence of chronic or acute complications of hypertension or other coexisting diseases can also alter the selection of antihypertensive drugs (Table 23.20).

Congestive Heart Failure

Antihypertensive drugs which decrease cardiac output and cause fluid retention can aggravate congestive heart failure. Therapy should include adequate oral diuretics including "loop diuretics" such as furosemide, if needed. Vasodilators or prazosin can further improve cardiac function by reducing afterload. Captopril is also a useful therapy which can improve congestive heart failure.

Table 23.20.
Complicated Hypertension

Condition	Drugs to Avoid	Useful Alternative Drugs
Heart failure	Propranolol guanethidine reserpine, clonidine	Diuretics, prazosin, captopril
Renal failure	Thiazide diuretics, guanethidine	Furosemide, clonidine, methyldopa, hydralazine, prazosin, minoxidil, captopril
Angina pectoris, myocardial infarction	Hyralazine (unless also taking β-blocker)	β-Blockers
Peripheral atherosclerosis	Propranolol	
Cerebral vascular disease	Furosemide, guanethidine	Methyldopa, clonidine
Diabetes	Propranolol (thiazide diuretic effects usually mild)	

Renal Insufficiency

Patients with mild to moderate renal insufficiency do not appear to have a marked decrease in their ability to metabolize and excrete antihypertensive drugs. By starting these drugs in small doses and carefully titrating the dose upward most agents can be used. Drugs which decrease renal blood flow and glomerular filtration should be avoided. These include thiazide and related diuretics as well as guanethidine. Thiazide diuretics are often ineffective as creatinine clearance falls below 25 to 50 ml/min. A potent diuretic (furosemide) may be needed to excrete salt and water. However, other patients with salt-wasting nephropathies do not have a "volume dependent" hypertension and tolerate diuretics poorly. Drug therapy should be carefully individualized in patients with renal disease. Preferred drugs are listed in Table 23.20.

Coronary Artery Disease

Patients with angina pectoris or recovering from a myocardial infarction should avoid drugs which cause reflex tachycardia and increase myocardial oxygen demand. The two most important drugs to avoid are hydralazine and prazosin. Propranolol can be a useful drug for these patients because it decreases anginal attacks and β-blockers have decreased the mortality rate following myocardial infarction.

Cerebral Vascular Disease

High blood pressure should be treated in patients with cerebrovascular disease to decrease the risk of cerebral infarction. However, great caution is needed to avoid causing episodes of hypotension. Drugs which produce postural hypotension, particularly guanethidine, should be avoided. However, elderly patients who have cerebrovascular disease may be more likely to experience hypotension from all drugs, including diuretics and sympatholytics, which are recommended agents. Therefore, therapy should be started with small doses.

Alcoholism

Undiagnosed alcoholism contributes to the difficulty in managing many hypertensive patients. Patients abusing alcohol often are unreliable in taking medications, experience additive drowsiness and dizziness and are prone to postural hypotension.

Hypertension in the Elderly (117–119)

An estimated 40 to 50% of people over 65 years of age have either isolated systolic hypertension or systolic-diastolic hypertension. The Framingham study has shown that systolic blood pressure is equal or better than diastolic blood pressure in predicting hypertensive complications, particularly stroke. However, adequate documentation of the value of lowering blood pressure with drugs is lacking. The HDFP study suggests benefits in lowering blood pressure in patients up to age 69. The treatment goals are similar: to reduce DBP to below 90 mm Hg or at least 10 mm Hg. If isolated systolic hypertension is treated the initial goal is to reduce the SBP to an acceptable range (140 to 160 mm Hg) rather than normalize the blood pressure.

Several factors influence drug therapy in the elderly and affect the choice of drugs and the drug dosage. In general drugs should be started in smaller than usual doses because elderly patients often have an increased response and are susceptible to a higher incidence of adverse drug reactions. Factors contributing to this problem often include: (a) reduced renal elimination of drugs, (b) possible slowed hepatic drug metabolism, (c) diminished baroreflexes which potentiate postural hypotension, (d) an increased incidence of relative dehydration predisposing to diuretic complications, (e) a possible predisposition to central nervous system side effects including depression, (f) an inadequate dietary intake which may predispose to hypokalemia, and (g) a number of physical and psychological factors can predispose elderly patients to making medication errors or failing to comply with drug therapy. Again, small doses of diuretic should be used and potassium supplementation may be needed.

Because of a reduced number of β-receptors the elderly often have a minimal response to β-adrenergic blocking drugs. Thiazide diuretics which have a greater effect on systolic blood pressure are usually preferred for patients with good renal function (104). Because the elderly have a reduced baroreceptor-mediated increase in heart rate, vasodilators, like hydralazine, may be effective even when used alone (87).

Overall, evidence suggests that treatment of hypertension in the elderly may lower the high incidence of cardiovascular complications and hypertension in the elderly warrants active but cautious treatment.

Pregnancy (1, 120)

Hypertension is present in about 7% of pregnancies. Therapy must be designed to use agents with minimal maternal, fetal and neonatal risks. A goal DBP of 75 to 84 mm Hg has been recommended. Agents most commonly recommended for use in pregnant women are methyldopa, hydralazine, and furosemide.

COMPLIANCE (6, 7, 14, 121–136)

Long-term compliance is the single most important factor in the successful treatment of hypertension. Public education programs have greatly increased the awareness of hypertension and have brought the majority of patients into treatment (Fig. 23.1). However, the problems of patient dropouts and noncompliance with treatment still result in usually less than one half of patients with hypertension under adequate treatment with a controlled blood pressure. The major surveys have shown only about 40 to 50% of hypertensive patients with controlled blood pressure (6, 7) (HDFP, 37.8%; California, 50.2%).

The first problem is that of patient dropout from the treatment program which may be 20 to 60% in the first year and a decline in appointment keeping continuously in subsequent years (14).

A second problem is that patients may keep appointments, yet fail to properly take their antihypertensive medications resulting in inadequate blood pressure control. It has been estimated that a compliance threshold of 80% of prescribed medication doses must be exceeded for an adequate antihypertensive effect. Many studies have shown that noncompliance with drug therapy and salt-restriction is the major reason for uncontrolled hypertension. Prescribed drugs have been undetectable in 50 to 80% of patients with uncontrolled blood pressure.

The major problem in hypertension is now clear. Efforts must be directed toward preventing patient dropout and improving compliance life-style changes. Initial screening and evaluation occurs only once and is wasted effort unless compliance is achieved which results in long-term control of blood pressure.

Noncompliance is a complex problem without a simple solution. Many factors are known to influence patient medication taking behaviors. The best predictors of noncompliance on hypertensive patients appear to be social isolation, an unwillingness to begin treatment, and drug side effects (123). Because it is difficult to accurately predict which patients will be noncompliant, an overall effort to encourage treatment compliance should be undertaken for all patients. Then a system to detect noncompliance can identify those patients who need extra attention and special techniques implemented to achieve compliance and blood pressure control. A number of methods are important in improving compliance.

Beliefs (130, 132)

The starting point for achieving compliance is the patient. Each person has his or her own attitudes and beliefs about medical care, hypertension as a disease and the value of therapy. The health-belief model suggests that patients are more likely to be compliant if they: (a) believe that hypertension is serious, (b) believe that they are personally susceptible to hypertensive complications, (c) believe that the therapy is beneficial, and (d) do not believe that the problems and barriers to following the treatment plan outweigh the benefits.

The patient's health beliefs are helpful in predicting compliance and where appropriate, changing health beliefs by education and counseling can improve compliance behavior.

Education (121, 125, 130, 132, 133)

Patient education about hypertension and the benefits of treatment is an important initial step in improving drug compliance and may aid in establishing positive health beliefs.

Patients should clearly understand their role and responsibility which includes: (a) keeping appointments, (b) taking medications, and (c) calling to report problems.

However, education alone may be insufficient to promote compliance in some patients (126). But, by providing a background understanding of the disease and treatment the stage can be set to encourage patients to carry out explicit directions by using behavioral modification techniques.

A variety of educational techniques can be useful including: (a) individual verbal counseling, (b) group classes/interaction sessions, (c) audiovisual programs, and (d) written instructions/pamphlets.

Any education program should be individualized and have the flexibility to provide ongoing instruction in small amounts.

Regimen (127, 130, 132, 134–136)

The treatment regimen is known to have an important influence on compliance behavior. A complex regimen which must be taken for a long duration is more likely to lead to noncompliance, particularly when given for an asymptomatic disease. Several steps can be taken in planning and implementing a drug regimen which can help foster compliance:

1. Individualize drug selection to reduce side effects and improve the blood pressure control. In short, try to choose the "best" drug first.

2. Begin treatment with a low dose and titrate the dosage upward slowly to reduce annoying side effects.

3. Simplify the drug regimen by eliminating any drugs of questionable benefit.

4. Limit drug administration times to once or twice daily.

5. Provide clear and explicit directions on the prescription label and indicate the purpose of the medication (high blood pressure).

6. Ask the patient to explain the specific times the medication is to be taken to avoid confusion and medication errors.

7. For complex medication schedules, provide a written medication schedule on a drug calendar or color-coded medication vials.

8. Use "prompting" cues to remind patients to take their medical: decals, stickers, storing the medication in a visible place, drug calendars, etc.

9. Provide organizers for patients a complex regimens: pillboxes, egg cartons, or compliance packages.

10. Tailor the medication dose times to coincide with existing daily habits such as awakening, mealtimes or toothbrushing.

11. Anticipate and discuss potential problems including: (a) drug costs, (b) child-proof vial caps, (c) difficulty in swallowing tablets or capsules, (d) unpleasant tasting medication, (e) possible confusion of look-alike drugs, and (f) previous problems with drug therapy.

Relationship (124, 125, 127, 129, 132)

A positive relationship between the patient and provider is another important factor influencing compliance behavior. Patients who feel they are treated in a warm friendly concerned manner and whose expectations are met are more likely to be satisfied, keep appointments and comply with treatment.

Activating the Patient (127, 129, 132)

An important part of improving drug compliance is to increase patients' awareness of their responsibility to actively participate in their health care. This can involve several aspects:

1. *Treatment Goals/Feedback.* An initial step can be to set a target blood pressure as a goal and tell the patient what the blood pressure results are at each followup visit. Recording results and appointment dates on a card also helps compliance.

2. *Self-Monitoring.* A further step on the feedback process is for patients to begin self

monitoring their progress. This can involve monitoring the process (i.e., a drug calendar to follow medication dosing) or the outcome (i.e., home measurement of blood pressure). Home blood pressure measurement requires some caution to avoid having the patient becoming pre-occupied with day-to-day variations on blood pressure or attempting to self-manage drug therapy. Self-monitoring is a potentially useful method for selected patients.

3. *Reinforcement/Rewards.* Reinforcement in its simplest form is encouragement. Patients can respond to praise and approval of even a small success. At the minimum, patients can be given positive support for keeping appointments, taking medications and reductions in blood pressure. The concept is that a series of small successes will ultimately lead to long term control. Some investigators have also used a reward system (i.e., providing blood pressure equipment for compliance and/or decreased blood pressure) (122).

Social Support (129, 130, 132)

Another important element in compliance behavior is encouragement and reminders from family and friends. This support can be a major factor on medication compliance for some patients. Conversely, social isolation tends to increase noncompliance and patients in this setting warrant increased attention. In addition, patient discussion groups can also have a positive impact.

Professional Supervision (121, 123–129, 132, 137)

Careful follow-up and close professional supervision are needed to prevent or detect noncompliance. The prevention of noncompliance involves attention to the areas discussed above and providing convenient appointments with a short wait time in a pleasant setting. Appointment reminders or medication refill reminders are also helpful in promoting continued care.

DETECTION OF NONCOMPLIANCE

1. An active recall system to retrieve patients who fail appointments is critical. Patients must be rescheduled promptly. A telephone follow-up by the provider is the most effective procedure. Alternatively, a telephone follow-up by clerical staff or a postcard reminder can be used. Pharmacists can also develop files to identify patients who should be due for refills of antihypertensive medications and send reminders.

2. In addition to patients who fail appointments, those who do not attain an adequate reduction in blood pressures should be viewed as possibly noncompliant.

3. Patients compliance can also be evaluated by a simple nonjudgmental interview. Patients who admit they are noncompliant with medications should be believed. Occasionally, noncompliant patients may deny missing medication doses. In addition, estimates of refill frequency also help in judging compliance. Changes in biochemical or physical parameters also provide information as to compliance (i.e. pulse, serum potassium).

In summary, continued professional involvement to prevent, detect and correct noncompliance is needed. Studies have shown that noncompliance is a chronic relapsing condition and even after compliance has been achieved that the removal of the professional efforts to sustain compliance result in a substantial number of patients returning to poor compliance (132). Compliance improving measures must be individualized; address patient behaviors and be sustained.

PHARMACISTS AND HYPERTENSION (137–140)

Opportunities exist for pharmacists to assist in overcoming the problem of hypertension in many areas. In the community setting, pharmacists have been active in screening programs; blood pressure monitoring; patient education and improving compliance behaviors.

Community pharmacists have provided patient education and drug monitoring (137, 138). These services have improved compliance; improved blood pressure control and detected adverse drug reactions and interactions. Other programs involving the clinical pharmacist in managing hypertensive patients has demonstrated fewer dropouts and increased blood pressure control in one program (139) and fewer dropouts and increased patient satisfaction in another program (140). The successful impact of improved compliance and improved blood pressure control in pharmacist hypertension program is shown in Table 23.21.

PROGNOSIS

Patients whose blood pressure is normalized by therapy can substantially reduce their risk

Table 23.21.
Effect of Pharmacist Hypertension Program

Study	Compliance (%)		Blood Pressure Control (%)	
	Control	Experi-mental	Control	Experi-mental
McKenny (1973)	—	—	20	79
McKenny (1978)	35	63	58	74
Hawkins (1979)	58	73	—	—
Conte (1982)	—	—	16	86

of developing congestive heart failure, renal failure and other hypertensive complications as demonstrated in numerous studies. Evidence from the HDFP study suggested a possible reduction in myocardial infarction and atherosclerotic complications. Even partial reduction of blood pressure appears to produce some benefit. Thus the prognosis for patients who comply with therapy and reduce blood pressure appears to be favorable.

CONCLUSION

Recent investigations on hypertension suggest that millions of patients with hypertension can benefit from therapy. Drug therapy usually involves multiple drugs and must be individualized. In addition, efforts to encourage treatment compliance must be employed and sustained. The magnitude of the services needed and the health benefits which can be attained call for increased involvement by pharmacists.

References

1. Kaplan NM: *Clinical Hypertension.* Baltimore: Williams & Wilkins, 1978.
2. Joint National Committee on Detection, Evaluation, and Treatment of High Blood Pressure: The 1980 Report of the Joint National Committee on Detection, Evaluation, and Treatment of High Blood Pressure. *Arch Intern Med* 140: 1280, 1980.
3. Smith WM: Epidemiology of hypertension. *Med Clin North Am* 61:467, 1977.
4. Stokes GS: Drug induced hypertension; pathogenesis and management. *Drugs* 12:222, 1976.
5. High Blood Pressure Coordinating Committee, New Hypertension Prevalence Data and Recommended Public Statements, February 1978.
6. Hypertension Detection and Follow-up Program Cooperative Group: Five-year findings of the hypertension detection and follow-up program. I. Reduction in mortality of persons with high blood pressure, including mild hypertension. *JAMA* 242:2562, 1979.
7. Leonard AR, Igra A, Hawthorne A: Status of high blood pressure control in California: a preliminary report of a statewide survey. *Heart Lung* 10:255, 1981.
8. Berkson DM, Brown MC, Stanton H, et al: Changing trends in hypertension detection and control. The Chicago experience. *Am J Public Health* 70:389, 1980.
9. Borhani, NO: Epidemiology of hypertension as a guide to treatment and control. *Heart Lung* 10:245, 1981.
10. Weiss NS: Relation of high blood pressure to headache, epistaxis and selected other symptoms. *N Engl J Med* 287:631, 1972.
11. Bloom JR, Monterossa S: Hypertension labeling and sense of well-being. *Am J Public Health* 71:1228, 1981.
12. Haynes RB, Sackett DL, Taylor DW, et al: Increased absenteeism from work after detection and labeling of hypertensive patients. *N Engl Med* 299:741, 1978.
13. Charlson ME, Alderman M, Melchor L: Absenteeism and labeling in hypertensive subjects. Prevention of an adverse impact on those at risk. *Am J Med* 73:165, 1982.
14. Finnerty FA, et al: Hypertension in the inner city; I. Analysis of clinic dropouts; II. Detection and follow-up. *Circulation* 47:73, 76, 1973.
15. Management Committee: The Australian therapeutic trial in mild hypertension. *Lancet* 1:1261, 1980.
16. Rudd P: Hypertension continuation adherence: natural history and role as an indicator condition. *Arch Intern Med* 139:545, 1979.
17. Chobanian AV: Hypertension: major risk factor for cardiovascular complications. *Geriatrics* 31:87, 1976.
18. Alderman MH, Stanback ME: Preventive cardiology: the state of the art. *Cardiovasc Rev Rep* 2:247, 1981.
19. Kannel WB, Wolf PA, Verter J, et al: Epidemiologic assessment of the role of blood pressure in stroke. *JAMA* 214:301, 1970.
20. Kannel WB, Castelli WP, McNamara PM, et al: Role of blood pressure in the development of congestive heart failure. *N Engl J Med* 287:781, 1972.
21. Kannel WB, Wolf PA, McGee DL, et al: Systolic blood pressure arterial rigidity, and risk of stroke: the Framingham study. *JAMA* 245:1225, 1981.
22. Brittain E: Probability of coronary heart disease developing. *West J Med* 136:86, 1982.
23. Veterans Administration Cooperative Study Group on Antihypertensive Agents: Effects of treatment on morbidity in hypertension; results in patients with diastolic blood pressure averaging 115 through 129 mm Hg. *JAMA* 202:1028, 1967.
24. Veterans Administration Cooperative Study Groups on Antihypertensive Agents: Effects of treatment on morbidity in hypertension; II. Results in patients with diastolic blood pressure averaging 90 through 114 mm Hg. *JAMA* 213:1143, 1970.
25. Veterans Administration Cooperative Study Group on Antihypertensive Agents: Effects of treatment on morbidity in hypertension; III. Influence of age, diastolic pressure and prior cardiovascular disease: further analysis of side effects. *Circulation* 45:991, 1972.
26. Taguchi J, Freis ED: Partial reduction of blood

pressure and prevention of complications in hypertension. *N Engl J Med* 291:329, 1974.

27. Perry HM: Veterans Administration cooperative studies of hypertension. *Angiology* 29:804, 1978.

28. Hypertension Detection and Follow-up Program Cooperative Group: Five-year findings of the hypertension detection and follow-up program; II. Mortality by race, sex and age. *JAMA* 242:2572, 1979.

29. Hypertension Detection and Follow-up Program Cooperative Group: The effect of treatment on mortality in "mild" hypertension. *N Engl J Med* 307:976, 1982.

30. Helgeland A: Treatment of mild hypertension: a five-year controlled drug trial. The Oslo study. *Am J Med* 69:725, 1980.

31. Trafford JAP, Horn CR, O'Neal H, et al: Five year follow-up of effects of treatment of mild and moderate hypertension. *Br Med J* 282:1111, 1981.

32. Multiple Risk Factor Intervention Trial Group: Risk factors changes and mortality results. *JAMA* 248:1465, 1982.

33. Freis ED: Should mild hypertension be treated? *N Engl J Med* 307:306–309, 1982.

34. Beard TC, Cooke HM, Gray WR, et al: Randomised controlled trial of a no-added-sodium diet for mild hypertension. *Lancet* 2:455, 1982.

35. MacGregor GA, Markandu ND, Best FE, et al: Double-blind randomised crossover trial of moderate sodium restriction in essential hypertension. *Lancet* 1:351, 1982.

36. MacGregor GA, Smith SJ, Markandu ND, et al: Moderate potassium supplementation in essential hypertension. *Lancet* 2:567, 1982.

37. Kaplan NM, Simmons M, McPhec C, et al: Two techniques to improve adherence to dietary sodium restriction in the treatment of hypertension. *Arch Intern Med* 142:1638, 1982.

38. Sims EAH, Berchtold P: Obesity and hypertension: mechanisms and implications for management. *JAMA* 247:49, 1982.

39. Reisin E, Frohlich ED: Effects of weight reduction on arterial hypertension. *J Chronic Dis* 35:887, 1982.

40. Reisin E, et al: Effect of loss without salt restrictions on the reduction of blood pressure in overweight hypertensive patients. *N Engl J Med* 298:1, 1978.

41. Tuck ML, Sowers J, Dornfeld L, et al: The effect of weight reduction on blood pressure, plasma renin activity and plasma aldosterone levels in obese patients. *N Engl J Med* 304:930, 1981.

42. Franklin BA, Rubenfire M: Losing weight through exercise. *JAMA* 244:377, 1980.

43. Wilcox RG, Bennett T, Brown AM, et al: Is exercise good for high blood pressure? *Br Med J* 285:67, 1982.

44. Fischell T: Running and the primary prevention of coronary heart disease. *Cardiovasc Rev Rep* 2:238, 1981.

45. Boyer, J: Exercise therapy in hypertensive men. *JAMA* 10:1668, 1970.

46. Shapiro AP, Schwartz GE, Ferguson DCE, et al: Behavioral methods in the treatment of hypertension. *Ann Intern Med* 86:626, 1977.

47. Jenkins CD: Recent evidence supporting psychologic and social risk factors for coronary disease. *N Engl J Med* 294:987, 1976.

48. Larbi EB, Cooper RS, Stamler J: Alcohol and hypertension (editorial). *Arch Intern Med* 143:28, 1983.

49. Saunders JB, Beevers DG, Paton A: Alcohol induced hypertension. *Lancet* 2:653, 1981.

50. Klatsky AL, Friedman GD, Siegelaub AB, et al: Alcohol consumption and blood pressure. *N Engl J Med* 296:1194, 1977.

51. Robertson D, Frölich JC, Carr RK, et al: Effects of caffeine on plasma renin activity, catecholamines and blood pressure. *N Engl J Med* 198:181, 1978.

52. Robertson D, Wade D, Workman R, et al: Tolerance to the humoral and hemodynamic effects of caffeine in man. *J Clin Invest* 67:1111, 1981.

53. Freestone S, Ramsay LE: Effect of coffee and cigarette smoking in the blood pressure of diuretic-treated hypertensive patients. *Am J Med* 73:348, 1982.

54. McMahon FG: *Management of Essential Hypertension.* Mt. Kuco, N.Y.: Futura, 1978.

55. Berglund G, Andersson O: Low doses of hydrochlorothiazide in hypertension. *Eur J Clin Pharmacol* 10:177, 1976.

56. Tweedale MG, Ogilvie RI, Ruedy J: Antihypertensive and biochemical effects of chlorthalidone. *Clin Pharmacol Ther* 22:519, 1977.

57. Ram CVS, Garrett BN, Kaplan NM, et al: Moderate sodium restriction and various diuretics in the treatment of hypertension effects on potassium wastage and blood pressure control. *Arch Intern Med* 141:1015, 1981.

58. Harrington JT, Isner JM, Kassirer JP: Our national obsession with potassium (editorial). *Am J Med* 73:155, 1982.

59. Holland OB, Nixon JV, Kuhnert L: Diuretic-induced ventricular ectopic activity. *Am J Med* 70:762, 1981.

60. Hollifield JW, Slaton PE: Thiazide diuretics, hypokalemia and cardiac arrythmias. *Acta Med Scand Suppl* 647:67, 1981.

61. Kosman ME: Management of potassium problems during long-term diuretic therapy. *JAMA* 230:743, 1974.

62. Schwartz AB, Swartz CD: Dosage of potassium chloride elixir to correct thiazide-induced hypokalemia. *JAMA* 230:702, 1974.

63. Amery A, Berthaux P, Bulpitt C, et al: Glucose intolerance during diuretic therapy. Results of trial by the European working party on hypertension in the elderly. *Lancet* 1:681, 1978.

64. Hansen KB, Bender AD: Changes in serum potassium levels occuring in patients treated with triampterene and a triampterene-hydrochlorothiazide combination. *Clin Pharmacol Ther* 8:392, 1967.

65. Ettinger B, Oldroyd NO, Sorgel F: Triampterene nephrolithiasis. *JAMA* 244:2443, 1980.

66. Favre L, Glasson P, Valloton MB: Reversible acute renal failure from combined triampterene and indomethacin. A study in healthy subjects. *Ann Intern Med* 96:317, 1982.

67. Veterans Administration Cooperative Study

Group on Antihypertensive Agents: Propranolol in the treatment of essential hypertension. *JAMA* 237:2303, 1977.
68. Braunwald E, Muller JE, Kloner RA, et al: Role of beta-adrenergic blockade in the therapy of patients with myocardial infarction. *Am J Med* 74:113, 1983.
69. Holland OB, Kaplan NM: Propranolol in the treatment of hypertension. *N Engl J Med* 294:930, 1976.
70. Esler M, Zweifler A, Otelio R, et al: Pathophysiologic and pharmacokinetic determination of the antihypertensive response to propranolol. *Clin Pharmacol Ther* 22:299, 1977.
71. Waal-Mannering HJ: β-Blockers in hypertension: how to get the best results. *Drugs* 17:129, 1979.
72. Frishman WH: Nadolol: a new β-adrenoreceptor antagonist. *N Engl J Med* 305:678, 1981.
73. Frishman WH: Atenolol and timolol, two new systemic β-adrenoreceptor antagonists. *N Engl J Med* 302:1456, 1982.
74. Golightly LK: Pindolol: a review of its pharmacology, pharmacokinetics, clinical uses and adverse effects. *Pharmacotherapy* 2:134, 1982.
75. Greenblatt DJ, Koch-Weser J: Adverse reactions to β-adrenergic receptor blocking drugs: a report from the Boston Collaborative Surveillance Program. *Drugs* 7:118, 1974.
76. Rangno RE: Propranolol withdrawal. Practical considerations (editorial). *Arch Intern Med* 141:161, 1981.
77. Leren P, Foss PO, Helgeland A: Effect of propranolol and prazosin on blood lipids: the Oslo study. *Lancet* 2:4, 1980.
78. Ruben PC: Beta-blockers in pregnancy. *N Engl J Med* 305:1323, 1981.
79. Weber MA, Drayer JIM: Antihypertensive agents that act in the central nervous systems. *Cardiovasc Rev Rep* 3:255, 1982.
80. Hoffman BB, Lefkowitz RJ: Alpha-adrenergic receptor subtypes. *N Engl J Med* 302:1390, 1980.
81. Motulsky JH, Insel PA: Adrenergic receptors in man. Direct identification, physiologic regulation and clinical alterations. *N Engl J Med* 307:18, 1982.
82. Lowenstein J: Drugs five years later: clonidine. *Ann Intern Med* 92:74, 1980.
83. Thananopavarn C, Golub MS, Eggena P, et al: Clonidine, a centrally acting sympathetic inhibitor, as monotherapy for mild to moderate hypertension. *Am J Cardiol* 49:153, 1982.
84. Anderson RJ, Hart GR, Crumpler CP, et al: Oral clonidine loading in hypertensive urgencies. *JAMA* 246:848, 1981.
85. Bravo EL: Clonidine-suppression test. A useful aid in the diagnosis of pheochromocytoma. *N Engl J Med* 305:623, 1981.
86. Garbus SB: The abrupt discontinuation of antihypertensive treatment. *J Clin Pharmacol* 19:476, 1979.
87. Cummings DM, Vlasses PH: Antihypertensive drug withdrawal syndrome. *Drug Intell Clin Pharm* 16:817, 1982.
88. Finnerty FA, Gyftopoulos A, Berry C, et al: Step 2 regimens in hypertension an assessment. *JAMA* 241:579, 1979.

89. Labarthe DR, O'Fallar WM: Reserpine and breast cancer, a commentary-based longitudinal study of 2,000 hypertensive women. *JAMA* 243:2304, 1980.
90. Benet LZ, Sheiner LB: Appendix II. Design and optimization of dosage regimens; pharmacokinetic data. In Gilman AG, Goodman LS and Gilman A: *The Pharmacologic Basis of Therapeutics.* New York: Macmillan, 1980, pp 1675–1737.
91. Awan NA, Mason DT: Oral vasodilator therapy with prazosin in severe congestive heart failure. *Am Heart J* 101:695, 1981.
92. Veterans Administration Cooperative Study Group on Antihypertensive agents: Comparison of prazosin with hydralazine in patients receiving hydrochlorothiazide. A randomized, double-blind clinical trial. *Circulation* 64:772, 1981.
93. Koch-Weser J: Hydralazine. *N Engl J Med* 295:320, 1976.
94. O'Malley K, Segal JL, Israili ZH, et al: Duration of hydralazine action in hypertension. *Clin Pharmacol Ther* 18:581, 1975.
95. Bing RF, Russell GI, Thurston H, et al: Hydralazine in hypertension: is there a safe dose? *Br Med J* 281:353, 1980.
96. Smith GH: Minoxidil. *Drug Intell Clin Pharm* 14:477, 1980.
97. Alpert MA, Bauer J: Rapid control of severe hypertension with minoxidil. *Arch Intern Med* 142:2099, 1982.
98. Vidt DG, Bravo EL, Fovad FM: Captopril. *N Engl J Med* 306:214, 1982.
99. Ram CV: Captopril. *Arch Intern Med* 142:914, 1982.
100. Vlasses PH, Rotmensch HH, Swanson BN, et al: Low-dose captopril. Its use in mild to moderate hypertension unresponsive to diuretic treatment. *Arch Intern Med* 142:1098, 1982.
101. Vlasses PH, Ferguson RK, Chatterjee K: Captopril. Clinical pharmacology and benefit-to-risk ratio in hypertension and congestive heart failure. *Pharmacotherapy* 2:1, 1982.
102. Ferguson RK, Vlasses PH: Clnical pharmacology and therapeutic applications of the new oral angiotension converting enzyme inhibitor. *Am Heart J* 101:650, 1981.
103. Frohlich ED, Maxwell MH, Baer L, et al: Saralasin: a test for renovascular hypertension. *Arch Intern Med* 142:1437, 1982.
104. Karlsberg RP: Calcium channel blockers for cardiovascular disorders. *Arch Intern Med* 142:452, 1982.
105. Stone PH, Antman EM, Muller JE, et al: Calcium channel blocking agents in the treatment of cardiovascular disorders; II. Hemodynamic effects and clinical applications. *Ann Intern Med* 93:886, 1982.
106. Frishman W, Klein N, Beer N: Nifedipine in hypertension. Expanding applications of a new drug. *Arch Intern Med* 141:843, 1981.
107. Kesteloot H, Geboers J: Calcium and blood pressure. *Lancet* 1:813, 1982.
108. McCarron DA: Low serum concentrations of ionized calcium in patients with hypertension. *N Engl J Med* 307:226, 1982.

109. Veterans Administration Cooperative Study Group on Antihypertensive agents: Comparison of propranolol and hydrochlorothiazide for the initial treatment of hypertension; I. Results of short-term titration with emphasis on racial differences in response. *JAMA* 248:1996, 1982; II. Results of long-term therapy. *JAMA* 248: 2004, 1982.

110. Berglund G, Anderson O: Beta-blockers or diuretics in hypertension? A six-year follow-up of blood pressure and metabolic side effects. *Lancet* 1:744, 1981.

111. Gifford RW, Tarzi RC: Resistant hypertension: diagnosis and management. *Ann Intern Med* 88:661, 1978.

112. Raftos J: The difficult hypertensive. *Drugs* 11:55, 1976.

113. Finnerty FA: Step-down therapy in hypertension. Importance in long-term management. *JAMA* 246:2593, 1981.

114. Cottier C, Julius S, Gajendragadkar SV, et al: Usefulness of home BP determination in treating borderline hypertension. *JAMA* 248:555, 1982.

115. Jordan MJ, Kennedy HL, Padgett NR: Do borderline hypertensive patients have labile-blood pressure? *Ann Intern Med* 94:466, 1981.

116. Pickering TG, Harshfield GA, Kleinert HD, et al: Blood pressure during normal daily activities, sleep, and exercise. Comparison of values in normal and hypertensive subjects. *JAMA* 247:992, 1982.

117. O'Malley K, O'Brien E: Management of hypertension in the elderly. *N Engl J Med* 302:1397, 1980.

118. National High Blood Pressure Education Program Coordinating Committee: Statement of hypertension in the elderly. U.S. D.H.H.S., April 1980.

119. Greenblatt DJ, Sellers EM, Shader RI: Drug disposition in old age. *N Engl J Med* 306:1081, 1982.

120. Wilson AL, Matzke GR: The treatment of hypertension in pregnancy. *Drug Intell Clin Pharm* 15:21, 1981.

121. Caldwell JR, Cobb S, Dowling MD, et al: The dropout problem in hypertension. *J Chronic Dis* 22:579, 1970.

122. Working Group to Define Critical Behaviours in High Blood Pressure Control: Patient behavior for blood pressure control. Guidelines for professionals. *JAMA* 241:2534, 1979.

123. Nelson EC, Statson WB, Neutra RR, et al: Identification of the noncompliant hypertensive patient. *Prev Med* 9:504, 1980.

124. Anderson RJ, Kirk LM: Methods of improving patient compliance in chronic disease states. *Arch Intern Med* 142:1673, 1982.

125. Blackwell B. Treatment adherence in hypertension. *Am J Pharm* 148:75, 1976.

126. Sackett DL, Haynes RB, Gibson EJ, et al: Randomized clinical trial of strategies for improving medication compliance in primary hypertension. *Lancet* 1:1205, 1975.

127. Haynes RB, et al: Improvement of medication compliance in uncontrolled hypertension. *Lancet* 1:1265, 1976.

128. Zismer DK, Gillium RF, Johnson CA, et al: Improving hypertension control in a private medical practice. *Arch Intern Med* 142:297, 1982.

129. Nessman DG, Carnahan JE, Nugent CA: Increasing compliance: patient-operated hypertension groups. *Arch Intern Med* 140:1427, 1980.

130. McKenney JM: Methods of modifying compliance behavior in hypertensive patients. *Drug Intell Clin Pharm* 15:8, 1981.

131. Lowenthal DT, Briggs WB, Mutterperl R, et al: Patient compliance for antihypertensive medication. The usefulness of urine assays. *Curr Ther Res* 19:405, 1976.

132. Weibert RT, Dee DA: *Improving Patient Medication Compliance*. Oradell, N.J.: Medical Economics, 1980.

133. Weibert RT: Patient package inserts. Potential distribution problems 1. *Drug Information J Suppl* p 45, 1977.

134. Mazzullo JV, Lasagna L, Griner PF: Variations of interpretation of prescription instructions; the need for improved prescription habits. *JAMA* 227:929, 1974.

135. Haynes RB, Sackett DL, Taylor DW, et al: Commentary. Manipulation of the therapeutic regimen to improve compliance; conceptions and misconceptions. *Clin Pharmacol Ther* 22:125, 1977.

136. Rudd P: Medication packaging: simple solutions to non-adherence problems? *Clin Pharmacol Ther* 25:257, 1979.

137. McKenney JM, Slining JM, Henderson HR, et al: The effect of clinical pharmacy services on patients with essential hypertension. *Circulation* 48:1104, 1973.

138. McKenney JM, Brown ED, Necsary R, et al: The effect of pharmacist drug monitoring and patient education on hypertensive patients. *Contemp Pharm Pract* 1:50, 1978.

139. Conte R, Kersh E: Management of hypertensive patients by nonphysician providers. *Calif Pharmacist* 29:27, 1982.

140. Hawkins DW, Fiedler FP, Douglas HL, et al: Evaluation of a clinical pharmacist in caring for hypertensive and diabetic patients. *Am J Hosp Pharm* 36:1321, 1979.

SECTION 5
Respiratory Diseases

CHAPTER 24

Asthma

PETER M. PENNA, Pharm.D.

Asthma is a chronic disease which pharmacists frequently see in their community or hospital practices. While there are many definitions of the disease, one of the better has been developed by a joint committee of the American College of Chest Physicians and the American Thoracic Society. Asthma is a disease "characterized by an increased responsiveness of the airways to various stimuli and manifested by slowing of forced expiration which changes in severity either spontaneously or with treatment. The term 'asthma' may be modified by words or phrases indicating its etiology, factors provoking attacks, or its duration" (1). The most important aspect of the disease is that there is episodic widespread obstruction to airflow. The disease may cause a number of distressing symptoms including wheezing and dyspnea, and less commonly a cough with the production of a thick mucoid sputum. In some patients, the frequency of attacks increases until there is a state of chronic airway obstruction. This situation may be virtually indistinguishable from chronic bronchitis and emphysema, but classically, asthmatics respond more readily to bronchodilators and corticosteroids than do patients with these other conditions. As emphasized in Chapter 25, there is a great deal of overlap in these diseases, and the methods of treatment for each may be very similar. There are many deaths reported every year due to asthma and its complications, and a large number of hospital beds are occupied by these patients. Acute attacks, exacerbations, and even overzealous use of drugs produce a great amount of morbidity and mortality.

ETIOLOGY

Asthma is a heterogeneous disease, and as such, it is difficult to classify and define its etiology. The basic problem in asthmatics is that their bronchi overreact to specific or non-specific stimuli. The term "twitchy lungs" has been used to describe this phenomenon. There are several systems for classifying asthma, depending on the type of precipitating factors. One of the most popular has been a system in which the stimuli are classified as coming from either the external environment, producing "extrinsic" or allergic asthma, or from the internal environment, producing "intrinsic" or idiosyncratic asthma. Table 24.1 summarizes the properties of these two types. While some patients will fit exclusively into one category or the other, many will exhibit properties from both.

Another way to classify the stimuli, and therefore the asthma, is to separate them into: allergic stimuli, emotional stress, pulmonary infections, physical exertion, environmental irritants, and drugs.

Many asthmatics will demonstrate allergy to one substance or another, particularly those patients whose symptoms start in childhood and young adulthood. The types of responsible allergens vary greatly, and include such things as pollen and other plant material, fungi and mold spores, animal dander (especially cat, dog, and horse), and house dust. Other allergens can be found in food (e.g., eggs, chocolate), or a working environment (e.g., some bakery workers may become allergic to flour). Allergy is responsible for 25–35% of all asthma cases, and plays a part in approximately 30% more. Allergic asthmatic reactions are thought to be the immediate, or type 1, reactions.

Emotional stress is known to precipitate asthmatic attacks in predisposed individuals. The mechanism is probably reflex bronchoconstriction through the efferent vagus. The important point to remember here is that these patients have hyperresponsive bronchi just like other asthmatics, but their attacks may be precipitated by psychological stress rather than pollen, infections, etc. The debate over the cause and effect relationships of asthma and its psychologic aspects has been well summarized by T. L. Creer (2).

Pulmonary infections are a common cause

Table 24.1.
Common Features of Intrinsic and Extrinsic Asthma[a]

Feature	Intrinsic Asthma	Extrinsic Asthma[a]
Other names	Nonallergic; infective; nonatopic; idiosyncratic	Allergic; atopic
IgE levels	Normal	Elevated
Skin tests	Negative	Positive
History of family allergies	Negative	Positive
Age at onset	Usually over 35 (middle age)	Usually below 5 (childhood to young adulthood)
Nasal symptoms	Polyps	Hay fever
ASA sensitivity	Strong association	None

[a] *Note*: Many patients exhibit properties of both. For example, some children with extrinsic asthma are hypersensitive to aspirin.

of asthmatic attacks. There is good evidence that most of these are due to viruses rather than bacteria. Allergic, hypersensitivity, and metabolic mechanisms have been proposed, but proof of any is lacking.

Physical exertion, especially in cold dry air, precipitates attacks in many asthmatics. The immediate effects may be bronchodilation, followed by constriction. It is not unusual for a patient to have a full attack, even if they stop the exercise before wheezing and dyspnea develop.

A number of nonallergenic, nonspecific irritants, including dust, sulfur dioxide, cold air, smoke, and even inhaled bronchodilators, are well-known causes of attacks. The mechanism here is unknown, but it appears that any irritant, if present in sufficient quantities, may produce an attack once the patient has the hyperreactive bronchi which characterize asthma.

Regardless of the cause of asthma in a specific patient, it is important to remember that there is usually a degree of overlap, and many factors may be involved in precipitating attacks. In a study by Williams et al. (3), it was found that out of 487 cases, allergy was a factor in 64.1%, infection in 88.1%, and psychology in 70.2%. Thirty-eight percent were affected by all three conditions, while allergy alone was important in only 3.3%, infection alone in 11.3%, and psychological factors alone in only 1.2%. It would seem that once the bronchial tree had conditioned itself to an asthmatic response, a number of influences may be able to set the system off.

Drug-induced asthma is not uncommon, and is of particular interest to pharmacists. One of the most common pulmonary adverse effects following drugs is asthma, and the most frequently implicated drug is aspirin. The incidence is questionable, but it has been estimated that 2 to 5% of all asthmatics are hypersensitive to aspirin, and in many cases, other nonnarcotic analgesics. The typical aspirin-sensitive patient is an adult onset asthmatic with a history of nasal polyps. The reactions which occur are often severe and prolonged and may even be fatal. A reaction may start within a few minutes to several hours after ingestion of the aspirin, but it usually begins within 30 minutes. The patient will often first notice a profuse, watery rhinorrhea followed by a scarlet flush of the head, neck, upper chest, and extremities, then wheezing and cyanosis due to bronchoconstriction. The patient may go into shock and die. The mechanism of the reaction is questionable, but the best evidence to date indicates that it is due to aspirin's effects on prostaglandins. Aspirin and the related drugs mentioned below all inhibit the biosynthesis of the E series of prostaglandins, which have bronchodilating activity. It is thought that this allows the bronchoconstricting effects of the F series of prostaglandins to dominate. The evidence is still inconclusive, but allergy has been largely ruled out. Most other salicylates (e.g., sodium salicylate) will not produce a reaction in sensitive individuals. However, indomethacin, mefenamic acid, phenylbutazone, ibuprofen and other nonsteroidal antiinflammatory drugs, sodium benzoate, and certain yellow food dyes such as tartrazine or FD&C yellow No. 5 may precipitate asthma in these patients (4–6). Tartrazine is very commonly used as a coloring agent in drugs, although many manufacturers are beginning to delete it. Lists of tartrazine-containing drugs are periodically published (7). The "safest" mild analgesic to use in these aspirin-hypersensitive patients is acetaminophen. There have been a few case reports of acetaminophen hypersensitivity, but the vast majority of aspirin-sensitive patients can take it with no problems. It would be wise, however, for those patients who have not taken acetaminophen previously to take the first dose in the physician's office.

A number of other drugs have been reported to precipitate asthmatic attacks in sensitive individuals by allergic reaction. Any drug which can cause anaphylaxis might be considered to cause asthma because the changes which take place in asthma are among the many which take place in anaphylactic reaction Table 24.2 lists those which have been reported to cause asthma by allergic reactions. Other than aspirin, which is associated with a relatively high incidence of asthma, and which is probably not an allergic reaction, the reports concerning these drugs are not very common, and many are highly questionable.

Drug-induced asthma may also be the result of the pharmacological properties of the drug. In contrast to the preceding type of reaction, these are much easier to anticipate because they are an extension of the normal pharmacology of the agent. They usually precipitate attacks in preexisting asthmatics. The most commonly implicated drugs are the parasym-

Table 24.2.
Drugs Which Have Been Reported to Precipitate Asthmatic Attacks by Hypersensitivity Reactions

Acetaminophen	MAO inhibitors
Allergenic extracts	Mefenamic acid
Aminophylline	Mercurials
Antisera	Nitrofurantoin
Aspirin	Oral contraceptives
Azathioprine	Penicillins
Bromsulphalein	Phenylbutazone
Cephalosporins	Pituitary snuff (vaso-
Chloramphenicol	pressin)
Cromolyn	Polymyxin B
Erythromycin	d-Propoxyphene
Hashish and marijuana	Quinidine and quinine
Ibuprofen (and the	Radioopaque organic
other nonsteroidal	iodides
antiinflammatory	Reserpine
drugs)	Succinylcholine
Indomethacin	Tetracyclines
Iodides	d-Tubocurarine
Iron dextran	Vaccines
Local anesthetics (es-	
ter-type)	

pathomimetics, the anticholinesterases, histamine, β-blockers (including those applied to the eye), and the F series of prostaglandins. These should be used with great caution, if at all, in asthmatics.

Some of the bronchodilator aerosols, notably isoproterenol and epinephrine, have been implicated in causing a worsening of asthma in a few patients. Although the mechanism is unclear, it is thought to be due to metabolic products of the drugs, including 3-methoxyisoproterenol, which have a paradoxical β-blocking effect. It has been observed that in an asthmatic attack, these people will begin using or overusing their aerosols, and after an initial period of relief, they will have a worsening of their symptoms.

Finally, there are drugs used by asthmatics which can precipitate attacks because of their irritating effects. N-Acetylcysteine often causes bronchospasm because it releases hydrogen sulfide. When it is used in asthmatics, they should be pretreated with a bronchodilator. Cromolyn sodium, beclomethasone, and any inhaled substance may cause similar effects.

INCIDENCE

The overall incidence of asthma is about 1 to 3% of the population. It occurs in up to 5% of children, but there appears to be significant country-to-country variation. After age 7, there is a decrease in incidence, probably because the increased bronchial diameter make the bronchi less susceptible to obstruction. In adults, the rate is 0.5 to 1%, and women are affected more commonly than men.

PATHOGENESIS

The obstruction to airflow in asthma is due to three processes: bronchial smooth muscle contraction, thickening of the mucous membrane lining of the lung, and plugging of the bronchi and bronchioles with thick, tenacious mucus. Of these, the first is the most readily reversible. Examination of the lungs following death due to asthma reveals large numbers of eosinophils and goblet cells in the bronchial walls, as well as hypertrophied mucus glands and bronchial musculature. The lungs usually do not collapse when the chest cavity is opened because of the extensive mucosal edema and mucus plugging.

Several mechanisms for asthmatic attacks have been proposed. In those whose attacks are related to allergies, the antibody IgE is particularly important, although other antibodies (e.g., IgG) have been implicated in some cases. After exposure to allergens, IgE is formed in plasma cells in a number of areas in the body, including the lung. This IgE is attached to the surface of mast cells in the lung tissue. When an antigen (allergen) attaches to this cell-bound IgE, a series of reactions is set up which allows the cell to release the mediators of an asthma attack: histamine, slow-releasing substance of anaphylaxis, kinins, prostaglandins, etc. This results in constriction of the smooth muscle surrounding the airways in the lung (bronchoconstriction), and capillary vasodilation with increased permeability (mucosal edema and increased secretions) (8). Other stimuli may also cause the mast cell to release these mediators.

The mechanism(s) for reactions in nonallergen-precipitated asthma is still unclear, but it appears to be mediated through the autonomic nervous system. Briefly, this hypothesis states that in susceptible individuals, vagal (cholinergic) impulses will cause bronchospasm by direct end-organ effects, as well as the releasing of histamine, etc., from mast cells. Conversely, bronchodilation is mediated through β_2-adrenergic stimulation which decreases mediator release and end-organ response. In asthmatics, it is thought that the autonomic system is dominated by the vagus. It appears that this system may be involved to some extent in allergic asthmatics (8).

DIAGNOSIS AND CLINICAL FINDINGS

Classically, asthmatics suffer acute attacks of dyspnea and wheezing. These attacks may vary in length from a few minutes to several days, and the patient appears physically well between episodes. The symptoms usually begin a few minutes after exposure to the precipitating factor. The patient may first notice tightness in his chest followed by wheezing and coughing and then dyspnea. In some people, the constriction may be so great that there is no wheeze. As in chronic obstructive pulmonary disease, the patient will have more difficulty with expiration than inspiration. Other signs and symptoms which sometimes occur include orthopnea, cyanosis, tachycardia, agitation and confusion, overinflation of the chest with decreased respiratory movements, and thick, viscous sputum which may contain mucus plugs called Curshmann's spirals.

Skin tests if properly used, may be very beneficial as an aid in the diagnosis of allergic bronchial asthma. Patients may react to many injected allergens, especially if concentrated solutions are used. In this case, few of these are actually the cause of the asthma. Allergic asthmatics will also usually show an increased number of eosinophils in blood and sputum.

Pulmonary function studies show hyperinflation of the lung and elevated airway resistance. Hypoxia is usually present in attacks, but the carbon dioxide levels may be low, normal, or increased, depending on the severity of the asthma. Significant carbon dioxide retention is a grave prognostic indicator.

When attacks first occur, the patient usually has no abnormalities between episodes, and he may be able to participate in vigorous exercise with no problem. Fortunately, some patients never progress beyond this point, and many children even experience a diminished number of attacks as they grow into adulthood. Other patients, however, may find that although they begin having less severe, and even less frequent attacks, they begin to have chronic airflow obstruction, possibly as a result of concomitant emphysema or chronic bronchitis.

TREATMENT
General Principles

At present, there is no cure for asthma. Treatment involves various procedures and drugs which are used to prevent or treat the acute attacks and their complications. Depending on the patient, his life situation, and the severity of the disease, various combinations of the therapeutic regimens discussed below may be used in order to control the asthma. One of the first steps in developing a treatment regimen is to search for and eliminate or control, if possible, the precipitating factor(s) for the attacks.

Exposure to pollen is a common cause of allergic asthma. It can often be reduced by keeping the windows closed during pollen season, and by using air conditioners. If a pet is the cause of asthma, the pet may have to be removed from the home. There is good evidence that cigarette smoke is particularly troublesome for some people. Elimination of cigarette smoking in the homes of these patients *should* be relatively easy to accomplish.

If exercise precipitates asthma, the patient needs to try to determine which types of exercise cause problems, since it would be unwise to eliminate or reduce all exercise. It appears that exercising in a cold, dry environment may be more harmful than exercising in warm, moist surroundings. For this reason, swimming is often an excellent form of exercise for these asthmatics.

Medications play a major role in the control of asthma. Dolovich and Hargreave have prepared an excellent summary on the principles of the use of drugs (9):

1. The minimum treatment necessary to maintain control is the correct treatment.
2. Bronchodilator side effects are not acceptable.
3. When the asthma gets out of control, the patient must quickly increase treatment, and then slowly decrease it once control is achieved.
4. The appearance of new coughing or breathlessness in an asthmatic is a sign to increase treatment.
5. Use of several drugs simultaneously is more effective than single agents.
6. Use of several agents in suboptimal doses often gives good relief and leaves a therapeutic reserve for exacerbation.
7. Patients hospitalized for exacerbation of their asthma should receive adrenocorticosteroids.

Hyposensitization

If it is felt that there is an allergic component to the disease, the physician will search for the responsible allergens, and the patient will be cautioned to eliminate or avoid these if at all possible. Skin tests can be used in an effort to identify allergens, but interpretation may be difficult, and accuracy may be questionable. If dilute solutions of skin testing reagents are properly used, these tests can accurately identify provocative allergens. More concentrated reagents are likely to either induce general inflammatory reactions or identify clinically insignificant allergies. In either case, the results can be very misleading. Other laboratory tests, such as the radioallergosorbent test (RAST), offer the hope of more quantitatively accurate identification of allergens. The history of the occurrence of the episodes may provide some very good information. For example, if the patient is a child whose attacks occur when sleeping, a responsible allergen

may be found in the bedroom—pillow feathers, blanket wool, house dust, etc. In this case, replacement of the feather pillow or wool blanket, or daily vacuuming or damp mopping of the floor and walls, may be very beneficial. If there are allergens or irritants in the atmosphere, moving to an area free of these substances may provide relief. In this case, symptoms usually abate for a year or two, but the patient often develops allergies or sensitivities to things in the new environment.

In other cases, it might be possible to desensitize or hyposensitize the patient to the allergens. The mechanism of hyposensitization is still unclear, but it is thought that injections of very small amounts of allergen (antigen) cause a buildup of IgG or "blocking" antibodies to the antigen. (Levels of IgE will also increase, but with continued treatment will decrease, often to levels less than those prior to initiation of therapy.) Therefore, when the patient is exposed to naturally occurring antigen, the IgG will combine with it and prevent or block it from reaction with the "asthma-producing" IgE antibodies. There also appears to be a nonspecific decrease in reactivity of mast cells in patients undergoing hyposensitization. While there is controversy concerning hyposensitization, many patients do benefit from it, especially in pollen-induced asthma. The process may take several years to complete, and it does have some significant risks. Local reactions are not uncommon. Drugs for the treatment of anaphylaxis should be readily available wherever patients receive their injections. To summarize the place of hyposensitization in asthma therapy, if a small number of responsible allergens can be identified, and if the patient continues to have significant disability in spite of vigorous applications of the standard forms of therapy, then hyposensitization may be a worthwhile venture (10).

Sympathomimetics

Symptomatic treatment of asthma involves the use of bronchodilators, hydration, expectorants (and mucolytics), corticosteroids, and cromolyn. Bronchodilators are the mainstay of asthma therapy, both in acute attacks and in relieving chronic obstruction. A bronchodilator alone may be sufficient for mild asthma, but they are also used in combination with other classes of drugs in the more severe cases. There are two major classes of bronchodilators—the sympathomimetics and the methylxanthines. They cause bronchodilation by different mechanisms so that their effects are additive. Both inhibit mediator release, as well as having a direct relaxing effect on bronchial smooth muscle.

There are three categories of adrenergic effects: α, β_1, and β_2. Their actions are summarized in Table 24.3. Because the β_2 sympathomimetic effects produce the desired bronchodilation, while α and β_1 effects produce side reactions in asthmatics, there has been an intensive search for drugs which have only β_2 effects. No such agent has yet been discovered.

Mast cells, and probably other cells in the lung, have receptors for α, β_2, and cholinergic agents. These exert their influences by affecting levels of either 3',5'-guanosine monophosphate (cyclic GMP), and 3',5'-adenosine monophosphate (cyclic AMP). In addition, levels of cyclic AMP in the cell are controlled by phospho diesterase, the enzyme responsible for the breakdown of cyclic AMP into inactive 5'-AMP.

Increased levels of cyclic AMP cause inhibition of mediator release and has a direct bronchodilator effect. Increased levels of cyclic GMP enhance mediator release. Therefore, the two compounds are antagonistic and asthma may result when levels of cyclic AMP are reduced relative to levels of cyclic GMP.

Cellular levels of cyclic AMP are enhanced by β_2-adrenergic stimulation which activates adenyl cyclase, the enzyme responsible for the conversion of adenosine triphosphate into cyclic AMP. The methylxanthines also produce increased levels of cyclic AMP by their effect of inhibiting phosphodiesterase, the en-

zyme responsible for the breakdown of cyclic AMP into 5'-AMP.

α-Adrenergic agents will cause a decrease in cyclic AMP, while cholinergic stimulation causes an increase in cyclic GMP. Therefore, α stimulation or cholinergic agents would be expected to enhance asthmatic attacks (8, 11).

The sympathomimetics available for the treatment of asthma are summarized in Table 24.4. Isoproterenol and epinephrine have been available for many years, and have been considered the standard for comparison of the other newer agents. Isoproterenol has almost pure β activity, although it does not discriminate between the two types of β-receptors. As such, it has very potent bronchodilating effects, along with some side effects, including tachycardia and other arrhythmias, precipitation of angina, headaches, muscle tremors, etc. A number of deaths have been attributed to the cardiac side effects of isoproterenol and other nonspecific sympathomimetics, especially when they are overused or abused. It was reported in several European countries in the 1960s that there appeared to be a rise in the mortality rate to asthma which correlated very well with the sales of the metered aerosols, which contained five times as much active drug as those aerosols in use in other countries. While it is easy to blame the increased death rate on the more potent inhalers, the correlation did not always hold true, i.e., there was a modest rise in the death rate in some countries which used the less potent preparations. In an effort to explain these findings, several possible mechanisms have been proposed:

1. The increased death rate was due to the cardiac toxicity of the sympathomimetic;
2. One of the metabolites of isoproterenol has mild β-blocking effects which might become significant if the patient overused the drug;
3. The propellants used in the aerosols are cardiotoxic, and may have caused fatal arrhythmias;
4. The patient became tolerant to the sympathomimetic, probably due to overuse, so that when it was needed for a severe attack, it no longer worked;
5. The aerosols provided a false sense of security for the patient, so that they delayed seeing a physician for an attack that proved to be particularly severe.
6. The aerosol actually kept the patient alive months or years longer than ex-

Table 24.3.
Common Reactions of Adrenergic Stimulation (12, 13)

α	β_1	β_2
Bronchoconstriction	Increased heart rate and conduction velocity	Bronchodilation
GI and bladder sphincter constriction		Arteriolar dilation
	Lipolysis	Muscle glycogenolysis
Vasoconstriction		
Hepatic glycogenolysis		Fine muscle tremor

Table 24.4.
Sympathomimetics Used to Treat Asthma

Drug	Activity			Route	Dose	Duration (hr)
	α	β_1	β_2			
Isoproterenol	0	+3	+3	Aerosol	1–2 puffs (0.075–0.150 mg)—repeat in 5 min if not relieved by first dose	0.5–1.5
Epinephrine	+3	+3	+3	SC	0.1–0.5 mg	0.5
				Aerosol	1–2 puffs (0.2–0.4 mg)—repeat in 5 min if not relieved by first dose	0.5–1
Isoetharine	0	+2	+3	Aerosol	1–2 puffs (0.34–0.68 mg) q3–4 hr, or 0.5 cc of the solution diluted to 2 cc with saline via hand-held nebulizer q4 h	1–2
Metaproterenol	0	+1.5	+3	PO	20 mg q6–8 hr	4
				Aerosol	1–3 puffs (0.65–1.95 mg) q4 h	3–4
				Aerosol	or 0.3 cc of the solution diluted to 2 cc with saline via hand-held nebulizer q41 h	
Terbutaline	0	+1	+3	PO	2.5–5 mg q8 h	4–6
				SC	0.25 mg; repeat in 30 min prn, but no more than 0.5 mg/4 hr	1.5–4
Albuterol	0	+1	+3	Aerosol	1–2 puffs (0.09–0.18 mg) q4–6 h	4–6
				PO	2–4 mg q6–8 h	4–6
Ephedrine	+3	+2	+2	PO	25–50 mg q3–4 h	4
Fenoterol (not yet available in U.S.)	0	+0.5	+3	Aerosol	1–2 puffs (0.2–0.4 mg) q8 h	6–8
				PO	5 mg q8 h	6–8

pected, and death occurred only when the patient experienced an especially severe attack; or

7. The lowering of the arterial oxygen levels which sometimes occur following isoproterenol may have left the patient so hypoxic that death occurred.

Whether one (or several) of the above is the real cause for the increased death rate is not known. There are other hypotheses, and even more questions which have been raised about these reports; nevertheless, at least one conclusion seems evident: metered aerosol sympathomimetics have been a great boon to the asthmatic, but misuse of these preparations can cause significant problems. It should be vigorously stressed to asthmatics and their families that these drugs do have their limitations and toxicities. They must not be used more often than directed, and if it appears that the patient is not responding to the appropriate number of doses, medical aid should be sought immediately (14, 15).

Isoproterenol is well absorbed by inhalation, but sublingual and oral administration pro-duce unreliable results, due in part to rapid hepatic metabolism. For this reason, oral and sublingual isoproterenol should not be used. The usual dose in adults is 0.1 mg (range of 0.05 to 0.25 mg) by aerosol. One or two puffs of a metered aerosol provide a "normal" dose. In order for an isoproterenol inhaler or any of the other pressurized metered inhalers to be effective, the patient must use them properly. The pharmacist needs to assure that patient not only understands the proper method of using these inhalers, but is, in fact, able to use them correctly. Some patients, especially young children, may not have the necessary coordination to effectively dose themselves. There have been several methods proposed for using them. While it can be argued that one method may be more effective than another, what really matters is that a patient gets relief with the method he or she uses, and they are consistent in the use of that method. The basic way to use these is:

1. Shake the container well and then hold it upside down.
2. Exhale slowly as completely as possible.

3. Place the mouthpiece of the inhaler between the lips.
4. Start inhaling slowly, and dispense one dose.
5. Complete inhaling slowly and hold the breath for about 10 seconds.
6. Exhale.
7. Generally, the dose may be repeated in 1–2 minutes if the attack has not been relieved. This procedure (1–2 puffs) may be repeated in 5 minutes if needed. If the attack is still not relieved in 10–15 minutes after a second dose, a physician should be consulted.

Some brands of inhalers dispense a very "tight bolus" of spray which may hit and deposit on the pharynx. These may require several more centimeters to disperse to the point where they can effectively inhaled. For this reason, it has been recommended that in step 3 of the above procedure, patients hold the mouthpiece several centimeters from their wide open mouth and fire the device while slowly inhaling.

The doses mentioned above for isoproterenol are the standards which have been used for many years. There is some evidence that perhaps these are too high. One study has been published in which 0.02 mg by aerosol provided as much relief in asthmatics as the standard doses (16). With the advent of the "selective" β_2 sympathomimetics, this finding may not be of that much clinical significance because isoproterenol inhalers are no longer the sympathomimetic of first choice. It should be mentioned here that IV isoproterenol has been used experimentally with some good results, but the newer agents now available may be as effective, with fewer side effects.

Epinephrine is another sympathomimetic which is commonly used by asthmatics who are having very severe attacks. Its actions are similar to those of isoproterenol except that it does affect the α-receptors, thereby causing vasoconstriction in the bronchial mucosa, which helps relieve edema of this tissue (the α activity theoretically may also facilitate release of the mediators of the attacks). In severe cases, it has been postulated that the α effects could be deleterious because it may lead to thickening of the mucus. Adequate hydration of the patient should help to avoid this problem. The overall significance of the α effects of epinephrine are questionable. The toxicities of the drug are essentially the same as those of isoproterenol. Epinephrine may be given by inhalation, but is more commonly injected subcutaneously for severe episodes. The SC dose is 0.1 to 0.5 ml of a 1:1000 solution, repeated in 5 to 10 minutes if needed, up to a maximum of 2.0 ml (17). Massage of the site of injection hastens absorption. Epinephrine is also very popular as the main ingredient in over-the-counter asthma inhalers.

As mentioned above, a pure β_2 agonist would make a most desirable sympathomimetic. While no such drug exists, there are a number in which the β_2 effects predominate. While β_1 effects are less with these drugs, they can and do occur. Thus, they are not entirely devoid of cardiac and other side effects.

Isoetharine was the first of this class to be introduced. While it does have more β_2 activity than β_1, and a slightly longer length of action than isoproterenol, controlled studies and editorials question any significant advantages over that drug (13, 18, 19).

Albuterol (salbutamol) was recently released for use in the U.S., following extensive use in other countries. It has a much longer length of action than isoproterenol, and seems to have significantly less cardiac side effects. Terbutaline and metaproterenol appear to be very similar to albuterol, but with a slightly shorter length of action. In addition, many patients report that there seem to be more muscle tremors with terbutaline. At the present time, it would be difficult to rank the "selective" β_2 stimulants other than by dosage form availability and length of action. While they probably have fewer cardiac side effects than isoproterenol and epinephrine, they are longer acting, so that if toxicity does occur, the patient will be toxic longer (13, 18, 21).

Patients who suffer from mild chronic asthma may obtain relief with oral ephedrine. It is not very effective in the more severe states of the condition. Tolerance can develop, and it can cause urinary retention, CNS stimulation, and the side effects seen with isoproterenol. Both metaproterenol and terbutaline are available for oral use, and are probably more effective than ephedrine, with fewer side effects. Nevertheless, ephedrine is an effective, inexpensive agent, and when properly used, will benefit many patients (13, 20, 21).

Sympathomimetics are very effective bronchodilators when given by inhalation, especially in acute attacks, and prevention of exercise-induced asthma. Using this route, side effects may be minimized because less drug is used, and therefore absorbed, to produce actions. The metered dose inhalers are convenient, relatively easy to use, and very effective for many asthmatics. For those patients who cannot use these, a compressor-powered hand-held nebulizer may be a very good way of providing adequate dosing, although they are expensive and bulky, and are time-consuming to use. It may take 10 to 15 minutes to administer a full dose. Nebulizers activated by compressing a rubber bulb by hand are also used. Because they also require 10 to 15 minutes to administer a full dose, patients tend to tire, and often split their doses in half with these units. For this reason, they may be very useful in those patients who overuse bronchodilators because they are tiring and time-consuming.

When used for chronic asthma, sympathomimetics are less effective, and tolerance may develop. Some patients may appear to be refractory to inhaled sympathomimetics, especially in severe attacks. There are several possible causes for this, and each must be evaluated. First, the patient's airways may be so severely plugged with mucus that the inhaled drug may not be able to reach the constricted area. Even if the drug is given parenterally, the patient will have difficulty breathing as long as the mucus is present. Removal of the mucus and mucus plugs by hydration, suction, etc., should restore the effectiveness of the drug. Second, the particles or droplets from the aerosol may not reach, or may not be retained in the bronchi and bronchioles if the drops or particles are the wrong size. This is rarely a problem with the metered aerosol sprays, but can occur with hand-held nebulizers. Third, a patient may continue to wheeze after aerosol administration because the mucus is being mobilized. As it reaches the larger diameter airways, it may cause wheezing. Humidification, controlled coughing, and deep breathing should help resolve this problem. Finally, and perhaps most important, some patients have become refractory to their sympathomimetics because of respiratory acidosis or overuse of the drug. Respiratory acidosis occurs in severe attacks, and diminishes the effect of sympathomimetics. Reversal of the acidosis or enhancing ventilation by other means will restore the effectiveness of the adrenergics. Also, patients who overuse these drugs may become less responsive to them. Withdrawal for a few days may restore effectiveness.

The Methylxanthines

The methylxanthines are the other major class of bronchodilators. The various theophylline salts (Table 24.5) are the most popular agents in this group because they have very pronounced peripheral effects with minimal CNS effects when compared with other methylxanthines.

Theophylline has been available for many years, but it fell into disrepute shortly after its introduction because of its significant toxicities. In the early 1970s, the principles of pharmacokinetics were applied to his drug, and the resulting scientific data base has greatly clarified its dosing parameters. While the dosing of theophylline and its salts still is not completely defined, our understanding of the drug is such that toxicities can be minimized while optimizing its bronchodilator effects. The drug is now one of the mainstays in the treatment of chronic and acute asthma.

The effectiveness of theophylline is related to its serum concentration. It is generally accepted that 10 to 20 $\mu g/ml$ is the optimum range for improvement of bronchoconstriction, although there are some patients who may require more or less drug for best effect. Similarly, toxicities correlate well with higher serum levels [21]. The half-life of the drug is significantly prolonged in patients with cardiac decompensation, cor pulmonale, severe pneumonia, cirrhosis, and in those taking enzyme-inhibiting drugs such as cimetidine, erythromycin, and troleandromycin. On the other hand, the half-life is decreased in patients who smoke, in infants, and in those

Table 24.5.
Theophylline Salts and Related Drugs

Drug	Theophylline (mg/100 mg Salt)	Equivalent Dose (mg)
Theophylline		
Anhydrous	100	100
Monohydrate	91	110
Aminophylline		
Anhydrous	85	118
Hydrous	80	125
Theophylline monoethanolamine	75	133
Dyphylline	70	143
Oxtriphylline	64	156
Theophylline sodium glycinate	50	200
Theophylline calcium salicylate	48	208

taking phenobarbitol. For those reasons, and because of other causes of patient-to-patient variability in requirements of the drug, the previously accepted guide to use 0.9 mg/kg/hr as a maintenance infusion should be avoided. Therapy must be titrated for each individual patient.

In acute situations, theophylline is usually given intravenously. A loading dose of 5 mg/kg given over 20 to 40 minutes should give a serum level of 10 mg/ml. This should be followed by a constant infusion of the drug. The recommendation in Table 24.6 has been shown to be safe and effective, although blood levels should be checked in 24 hours, and ultimately, patient response is the determining factor. If the patient has had any theophylline in the previous 24 hours, a blood level determination should be done prior to giving any more drug. In acute emergencies, when it is not possible to get a plasma level, it has been suggested that the patient could be cautiously given 2 to 2.5 mg/kg of theophylline over 30 to 40 minutes as a loading dose. In this case, any information that can be provided by the patient and/or family concerning recent doses and the presence or lack of signs of toxicity should be in the decision to reload the patient (21). For an excellent discussion of theophylline dosing kinetics, refer to *Applied Pharmacokinetics* by Hendeles et al. (24).

There are a number of methylxanthine preparations available for chronic therapy. Theophylline, its salts, and related compounds are available as coated and uncoated tablets, sustained release tablets and capsules, sup-

Table 24.6.
IV Theophylline and Aminophylline Requirements (after Loading) to Keep a Patient at a 10 mg/ml Serum Theophylline Concentration (21–23)

Age or Condition	Infusion Rate (mg/kg/hr)	
	Theophylline	Aminophylline
Neonates	0.13	0.16
Infants 2–6 mo	0.4	0.50
Infants 6–11 mo	0.7	0.87
Children 1–9 yr	0.8	1.0
Children over 9 yr	0.6	0.75
Adults who smoke	0.6	0.75
Otherwise healthy, non-smoking adults	0.4	0.50
Cardiac decompensation or hepatic cirrhosis	0.2	0.25

positories, enemas, and solutions. Theophylline in uncoated tablets, in either aqueous or hydroalcoholic solutions, and in retention enemas, is quickly and completely absorbed. Theophylline in suppositories is erratically absorbed, but this appears to be due to total time of retention of the suppository. For this reason, suppositories should not be used. There are many sustained release theophylline preparations available. Many of these provide complete and reliable absorption such that 12-hour dosing would provide effective blood levels over the full 12 hours in nonsmoking adults. Since children, adults who smoke, and those receiving phenobarbital eliminate the drug more rapidly, most of these drugs would have to be given every 8 hours. One product, Theo-Dur, has been shown to produce therapeutic blood levels consistently when dosed every 12 hours in children (25–27).

When switching from IV therapy to oral dosing, if the total oral dose per day is the same as the total IV dose given per day, the resultant blood levels will be the same.

To start a patient on oral theophylline who has not received it recently, the dose is 16 mg/kg of lean body weight/day, or 400 mg/day (whichever is less) for 3 days. This may be increased every 3 days by 25% if tolerated, to the desired effect, or until the following doses are reached:

16 years old and older	13 mg/kg/day or 900 mg/day (whichever is less)
12 to 16 years old	18 mg/kg/day
9 to 12 years old	20 mg/kg/day
1 to 9 years old	24 mg/kg/day

Depending on serum levels and the patients clinical response, these levels may require further adjustment (21).

As indicated in Table 24.5, there are a number of theophylline salts and derivatives available. When comparing doses of these drugs, the actual amount of theophylline in the preparation must be considered, rather than the total amount of the salt.

Most of these were developed in an effort to decrease the GI irritation of theophylline and to enhance absorption. Since most of the GI effect is centrally mediated, and since theophylline is very well-absorbed orally, none of these agents offers any advantage over theophylline.

The side effects and toxicities of theophylline are related to its serum level. These usually become evident at levels greater than 20 $\mu g/ml$, and include GI effects (nausea, vomiting, diarrhea), cardiac effects (hypotension, extrasystoles, tachycardia, and other arrhythmias), and CNS effects (irritability, headaches, insomnia, and seizures). Death from cardiac effects and seizures have been reported all too frequently. Rapid IV administration (over less than 20 minutes) has caused death due to cardiac effects. High blood levels (above 40 $\mu g/ml$) have been associated with seizures. In many cases, seizures are preceded by GI effects or irritability; however, there are cases on record where fatal seizures were the first sign of toxicity. Approximately 50% of patients who experience theophylline seizures will die (21).

Corticosteroids

While the corticosteroids are extremely effective in controlling asthma, their side effects have greatly limited their usefulness until the introduction of beclomethasone dipropionate. The use of steroids in asthma is largely empirical, since the mechanism(s) of action is questionable. Some of the proposed antiasthma mechanisms are: 1) direct bronchial smooth muscle relaxation, 2) suppression of the immune system, 3) beneficial changes in the cyclic AMP:cyclic GMP ratio, 4) alteration in the synthesis and release of the mediators of the attack, and 5) inhibition of prostaglandin synthesis.

Systemic steroids are generally indicated in the more severe forms of chronic asthma when the patient has not responded to other less toxic forms of therapy, and in status asthmaticus. Often, steroids are the only agents which can reverse bronchospasm which does not respond to the sympathomimetics and theophylline.

A patient should be placed on steroids only after careful reevaluation of previous therapy. If a patient is to be placed on continuous steroids, there are two methods which may be used: oral or inhaled. Patients placed on continuous oral steroids should be placed on the lowest dose possible, and every effort should be made to use alternate day therapy to decrease the incidence and severity of side effects. This requires the use of shorter acting agents such as prednisone, prednisolone, or methylprednisolone. With alternate day therapy, the patient may have some asthma symptoms on the "off" day, but these may be more tolerable than the side effects pursuant to daily steroid therapy. Typical doses are 20 to 40 mg of prednisone, or equivalent, every other day. Daily oral therapy has been used for short-term therapy of acute situations, often following a course of IV steroids. If the duration is less than 3 or 4 weeks, few side effects will occur, and tapering the dose is not really necessary (21, 28).

Because of the severe side effects of prolonged daily steroid therapy, a great deal of work has been done with inhaled steroids. Results had been disappointing until the introduction of beclomethasone dispropionate in 1976. Several other effective inhaled steroids, including triamcinolone acetonide, are available in other countries, and may soon be introduced in the U.S. These agents are very effective in controlling asthma with a minimum of steroid side effects. Results of tests of pituitary-adrenal function show little or no suppression in patients at recommended doses. As the dose is increased, however (above 800 $\mu g/day$ of beclomethasone), some suppression and side effects may become evident. At high inhaled doses, there appears to be little difference between beclomethasone and alternate day therapy. In many oral steroid-dependent patients, the dose of the oral agent can be reduced or completely withdrawn when beclomethasone is started (29, 30).

Effects of a first dose are measurable within several hours, although it usually takes about 7 days to achieve maximal effects of beclomethasone. The drug is ineffective for individual acute attacks. If an attempt is made to reduce the dose of oral steroids when a patient is placed on beclomethasone, it should be done very gradually. Frequent evaluation of adrenal status is highly recommended. In periods of stress, supplementary oral or parenteral steroids may have to be given in these cases because the adrenals may be unable to respond adequately. Deaths have been reported due to this problem. Patients who have switched must be made aware of this, and should have a supply of oral prednisone, prednisolone, etc., available for use (29).

The usual dose of beclomethasone is two puffs (100 μg) 3 to 4 times a day. In some patients, up to 1000 μg per day may be required. The major side effects include hoarseness and *Candida* overgrowth in the oropharynx. The infection may resolve spontaneously, or may have to be treated with nystatin. There are concerns that the drug may have long-term effects on the lung, but none have become evident thus far.

In acute situations, such as status asthmaticus, extremely high doses of parenteral steroids may be life-saving. Dosage regimens are empirical; essentially, enough drug is given as frequently as needed in order to reverse the attack. A typical regimen calls for 4 to 10 mg/kg/day of methylprednisolone intravenously, given in four to six divided doses. This dose may have to be continued for several days, after which it is tapered over a period of several more days. Tapering is done, not to prevent withdrawal, which is virtually nonexistent after short-term therapy, but to help assure that the patient does not suffer a relapse. Side effects from these short-term high dose regimens are very rare, other than sodium retention, if hydrocortisone is used (31).

Cromolyn Sodium

Cromolyn prevents degranulation of mast cells and, therefore, the release of the mediators of asthma in both allergic and nonallergic asthmatics. It has no bronchodilating or antiinflammatory effects; it is strictly prophylactic and has no benefit in acute attacks. Clinically, it appears to be more effective in extrinsic asthmatics and in those with exercise-induced asthma. In this latter condition, some patients find that premedicating themselves with cromolyn prior to exertion is very beneficial. They should also administer the drug on a routine basis. It may take up to several weeks to exert its effects, although a few patients have an almost immediate response (21, 32).

Cromolyn is inhaled as a dry powder from capsules which contain 20 mg of cromolyn in an inert powder (lactose) base. Generally, this is given 4 times a day until a favorable response is noted. After stabilization of the response, an attempt can be made to reduce it to the lowest effective maintenance dose. Of a 20-mg dose, only 1 to 2 mg gets into the lung. The rest is deposited in the mouth and throat and is swallowed. A small portion of the dose (inhaled and swallowed) is absorbed, but is quickly eliminated unchanged.

When dispensing cromolyn, the pharmacist must assure that the patient understands how to use and is capable of using the spinhaler device.

Cromolyn is not a first-line drug for asthma. It generally is used if the bronchodilators do not provide adequate relief. Some patients who have been on steroids may be able to reduce the dose when placed on cromolyn. Children may go through a phase of catch-up growth.

Cromolyn seems to have few toxicities. The most common problem is irritation from inhaling a dry powder. During the first few weeks of use, this can precipitate asthma attacks and, therefore, some patients premedicate themselves with a sympathomimetic prior to dosing with cromolyn. There have been a few cases of urticaria and angioedema reported. The most severe side effects are several reports of pulmonary eosinophilia (33).

Hydration and Expectorants

Adequate hydration is very important in the treatment and prevention of attacks. Dehydration may be responsible for recurring asthma by producing viscous mucus and mucus plugging which can cause bronchospasm. Therefore, patients must realize the importance of an adequate fluid intake. Some may benefit from humidification of their homes, or by breathing in steam or cool water vapor. If oxygen therapy is used, the oxygen must be humidified because gases can be very drying.

A few patients benefit clinically from expectorants, including guaifenesin and the iodides. Generally, these drugs cannot be recommended because of their toxicity (iodides) and lack of proof of efficacy (guaifenesin). N-Acetylcysteine is an effective mucolytic agent in vitro, but in vivo efficacy is questionable. Because of this questionable efficacy, and significant bronchospasm when it is used, it cannot be recommended. Generally, plain water, either as an increased fluid intake, steam, or mist, will very nicely liquify a patient's mucus. In severe situations, fluids given intravenously may be required.

Sedatives

Psychological factors can greatly affect asthmatics. For this reason, control of the emotional state of the patient with drugs has been tried in an effort to control the asthma. "Tranquilization" may be of benefit in a few patients, but can also cause significant problems. Any drug with respiratory depressant action, including barbiturates, benzodiazepines, phenothiazines, tricyclic antidepressants, narcotics, etc., must be used with extreme caution, if at all, in patients who are hypoxic. Their respiratory depressant effects can worsen the hypoxia and cause death. Also, many of these drugs have antihistaminic side effects which cause drying of the mucus membranes. Since one of the problems in asthmatics is thick tenacious mucus, it is best to avoid any drug which is drying.

Miscellaneous Drugs

Antihistamines, it would appear, should be beneficial in asthma since histamine is involved in the reaction. There are two basic problems, however: first, histamine is only one of the mediators of the attack (antihistamines have no effect on the others); and second, antihistamines are drying. For these reasons, they are contraindicated in asthma. Any beneficial effects caused by the antihistamines in asthmatics are probably due to their anticholinergic effects.

The new understanding of the role of the cholinergic system in the pathogenesis of asthma has caused renewed interest in anticholinergic drugs, including atropine and ipatropium bromide. These agents do have a beneficial effect in asthmatics, but may be even more effective in patients with bronchitis (34–36).

Combination products are a relatively popular item prescribed for asthmatics. Most of these contain ephedrine, a methylxanthine, a sedative, and sometimes expectorants, antihistamines, or other sympathomimetics, etc. Most of these preparations owe their efficacy to the ephedrine because the doses of sedative or xanthine are often subtherapeutic. While these preparations offer a simple method for a patient to dose himself with a number of drugs, best results are obtained if the patient is individually titrated with the necessary drugs so that he could obtain the best therapeutic response.

COMPLICATIONS

Status asthmaticus is an unrelenting asthmatic attack, lasting more than 24 hours, which does not respond to the bronchodilators. This is considered a medical emergency and requires hospitalization for the most effective treatment. Most deaths due to asthma are the result of status asthmaticus. The usual causes of death in these patients include: respiratory depression due to the overuse of either sedatives or oxygen, xanthine or sympathomimetic toxicity, extensive plugging of the bronchi with thick mucus due to dehydration and poor coughing effects, and cardiac failure. The usual precipitating causes include pulmonary infection, dehydration, massive exposure to allergen, or misuse of medication.

The treatment of this condition is similar to that for milder forms of asthma except that it is more vigorous, and the corticosteroids are almost always used intravenously in high doses for short periods. They are rapidly tapered after a few days. The sympathomimetics, by definition, are ineffective in status asthmaticus, possibly because of acidosis. This acidosis is best treated by improving ventilation, or if this fails, by IV sodium bicarbonate. This may restore responsiveness to the sympathomimetics, but care must be taken to avoid overtreatment. To correct dehydration, IVs should be started, and the patient should receive 3 to 5 liters the first 24 hours, depending on cardiac and renal function. Xanthines probably should be administered also, by the IV route. After a loading dose of aminophylline, it is best to give the drug as a continuous infusion.

Oxygen therapy should be considered in these patients, but it is important that blood gases be monitored before and during treatment. It is desirable to keep the pO_2 above 60 mm Hg. It may be necessary to perform a tracheostomy and use ventilation and bronchial lavage. Patients who are on assisted ventilation may be given sedatives safely. Deaths have been reported in patients with compromised respiratory function who were given even low doses of depressants. However, a patient in status asthmaticus may be in a state of exhaustion and may desperately require rest. Once his ventilatory functions are being handled by an external force, it is safe to give a sedative to allow rest (37, 38).

If there are signs of pulmonary infection, antibiotics should be started after material for culture and sensitivity is obtained. A Gram stain of the sputum may aid in narrowing the choice of antibiotics. Also, the experience of the physician, the patient's history, and consultation with the medical laboratory may give a clue to the most likely infecting organism.

PROGNOSIS

The prognosis of asthmatic patients is extremely variable. In those whose symptoms

Table 24.7.
Drug Therapy of Asthma: Preferential Order of Usage in Various Stages[a]

Class	Progressive Order of Drug Administration				
	First	Second	Third	Fourth	Optional
1. Minimal	B	T	C	—	H
2. Moderate	B	T	C	Sb	H, A
3. Severe	T	C	Sb	Sl	H, A
4. Severe (refractory)	T	Sl	—	—	H

[a] B = β-adrenergic agonists; T = theophylline; C = cromolyn sodium; Sb = corticosteroids, burst; Sl = corticosteroids, long term; H = hydrating agents; A = atropine, short term. (From Bernstein.[29])

begin in childhood, the outlook is very good. Fifty to 95% have a remission of symptoms when they reach adulthood. Five to 10% of the remainder, especially those who have associated eczema, will continue to have severe disability. In asthmatics whose symptoms started in adulthood, a study of Rachemann showed that after 15 years, 22% of patients were free of symptoms, 44% had improved, 33% remained the same, and 3% had died. There is no doubt that in either group chronic asthma has a poorer prognosis than the intermittent type (39).

SUMMARY

Asthma is the result of constriction of bronchi, edema of the mucosal walls, and production of viscous mucus. A number of factors are known to precipitate attacks, including allergens, irritants, physical exertion, emotions, and infections. Adequate treatment involves, first, the recognition and removal, if possible, of causative factors. Next, the patient should be taught to keep himself adequately hydrated and to properly use sympathomimetics and/or xanthines, if needed. If these things do not afford significant relief, the use of cromolyn should be considered, followed by steroids. Asthma rarely can be treated by a single procedure or drug. It must be approached from several different directions, using different agents and methods to gain the maximal benefit at the least therapeutic cost. Berstein has summarized this very nicely in Table 24.7 (40). Pharmacists come in contact with asthmatics daily and can be of considerable help by monitoring therapy and making sure that they understand the proper use of their drugs.

References

1. ACCP-ATS Joint Committee on Pulmonary Nomenclature: Pulmonary terms and symbols. *Chest* 67:383, 1975.
2. Creer TL: Asthma: Psychologic aspects and management. In Middleton E Jr, Reed CE, Ellis EF: *Allergy Principles and Practice.* St. Louis, Mosby, 1978.
3. Williams DA, Lewis-Faning E, Rees L, et al: Assessment of the relative importance of the allergic, infective, and psychological factors in asthma. *Acta Allergol* 12:376, 1958.
4. Settipane GA: Adverse reactions to aspirin and related drugs. *Arch Intern Med* 141:328, 1981.
5. Speer F, Denison T, Baptist J: Aspirin allergy. *Ann Allergy* 46:123, 1981.
6. Merritt GJ, Selle RI: Cross-reactivity between aspirin and ibuprofen in an asthmatic—a case report. *Am J Hosp Pharm* 35:1245, 1978.
7. Lee M, Gentry AF, Schwartz R, et al: Tartrazine-containing drugs. *Drug Intell Clin Pharm* 15:782, 1981.
8. Daniele RP: Pathophysiology of asthma. In Fishman AP: *Pulmonary Disease and Disorders.* New York, McGraw-Hill, 1980, p. 567.
9. Dolovich J, Hargreave FE: Strategies in the control of asthma. *Med Clin North Am* 65:1033, 1981.
10. Patterson R, Lieberman P, Irons JS, et al: Immunotherapy. In Middleton E Jr, Reed CE, Ellis EF: *Allergy Principles and Practice.* St. Louis, Mosby, 1978, p. 877.
11. Kaliner M: Immunologic mechanisms for release of chemical mediators of anaphylaxis from human lung tissue. *Can Med Assoc J* 110:431, 1974.
12. Lands AM, Lunduena FP, Buzzo JJ: Differentiation of receptor systems activated by sympathomimetic amines. *Nature* 214:597, 1967.
13. Alexander MR, Hendeles L, Guernsey B: The beta-2 against bronchochilators. *Drug Intell Clin Pharm* 11:526, 1977.
14. Stolley PD: Asthma mortality: Why the United States was spared an epidemic of deaths due to asthma. *Am Rev Respir Dis* 105:883, 1972.
15. Harris MC: Symposium on isoproterene therapy in asthma. *Ann Allergy* 31:19, 1973.
16. Williams MH, Kane C: Dose response of patients with asthma to inhaled isoproterenol. *Am Rev Respir Dis* 111:321, 1975.
17. Brandstetter RD, Gotz VP, Mar DD: Optimal dosing of epinephrine in acute asthma. *Am J Hosp Pharm* 37:1326, 1980.
18. Campbell AB, Soyka LF: Selective beta-2 receptor agonists for the treatment of asthma—therapeutic breakthrough or advertising ploy? *J Pediatr* 89:1020, 1976.

19. Kaimal J, Schwartz HJ, Chester EH: Aerosol bronchodilator therapy: A comparison of the effects of bronkometer with isoetharine, isoproterenol and phenylephrine. Ann Allergy 43:151, 1979.

20. Tinkelman DG, Arner SE: Ephedrine therapy in asthmatic children. JAMA 237:553, 1977.

21. Weinberger M, Hendeles L, Ahrens R: Pharmacologic management of reversible obstructive airways disease. Med Clin North Am 65:579, 1980.

22. Hendeles L: Poisoning with intravenous theophylline. Am J Hosp Pharm 37:49, 1980.

23. Hughey MC, Yost RI, Robinson JD, et al: Investigation of a dosage regimen for intravenous theophylline. Drug Intell Clin Pharm 16:301, 1982.

24. Hendeles L, Weinberger M, Johson G, et al: Theophylline: Counterpoint discussion. In Evans WE, Schentog JJ, Jusko WJ: Applied Pharmacokinetics. San Francisco, Applied Therapeutics Inc., 1980, pp. 95, 139, 167.

25. Weinberger M, Hendeles L, Wong L, et al: Relationship of formulation and dosing interval to fluctuation of serum theophylline concentration in children with chronic asthma. J Pediatr 99:145, 1981.

26. Kelly HW, Murphy S: Serum theophylline levels in asthmatic children receiving sustained-release theophylline tablets. Am J Hosp Pharm 36:1968, 1979.

27. Dasta J, Mirtallo JM, Altman M: Comparison of standard and sustained-release theophylline tablets in patients with chronic obstructive pulmonary disease. Am J Hosp Pharm 36:6131, 1979.

28. Spiegil RJ, Oliff AI, Burton J: Adrenol suppression after short-term corticosteroid therapy. Lancet 1:339, 1979.

29. Williams MH: Beclomethasone dipropionate. Ann Intern Med 95:464, 1981.

30. Wyatt R, Washels J, Weinberger M, et al: Effects of inhaled feclomethasone dipropronate and alternate-day predmious on pituitary-adrenal function in children with chronic asthma. N Engl J Med 229:1387, 1978.

31. Krouse HA, Santiago SM, Klaustermeyer WB: Intravenously given methylprednisolone in refractory asthma. West J Med 132:106, 1980.

32. Hermance WE, Brown EB: Cranolyn sodium (disodium cromoglycrate) in treatment of asthma. N Y State J Med 73:430, 1973.

33. Godfrey S, Balfour-Lynn L, Konis P: The place of cromolyn sodium in the long-term management of childhood asthma based on a 3- to 5-year-old follow-up. J Pediatr 87:465, 1975.

34. Harnett J, Spector SF: Blocking effect of Sch 1000, isoproterenol, and the combination of methacholine and histamine inhalation (abstract). J Allergy Clin Immunol 57:261, 1976.

35. Cropp G: The role of the parasympathetic nervous system in the maintenance of chronic airway obstruction in asthmatic children. Am Rev Respir Dis 112:599, 1975.

36. Petrie GR, Palmer KNV: Comparison of aerosol ipatropium bromide and salbutamol in chronic bronchitis and asthma. Br Med J 1:430, 1975.

37. Franklin W: Asthma in the emergency room. N Engl J Med 305:826, 1981.

38. Easton J, Hilman B, Shapiro G, et al: Management of asthma. Pediatrics 68:874, 1981.

39. Rachemann FM, Edward MC: Asthma in children: A follow-up study of 688 patients after an interval of 20 years. N Engl J Med 246:815, 1952.

40. Berstein IL: Asthma in adults. In Middleton E Jr, Reed CE, Ellis EF: Allergy Principles and Practice. St. Louis, Mosby, 1978, p. 743.

CHAPTER 25

Chronic Obstructive Pulmonary Disease

PETER M. PENNA, Pharm.D.

Chronic obstructive pulmonary disease (COPD), which is sometimes referred to as chronic obstructive lung disease (COLD), encompasses a number of disease entities. In this chapter, the major emphasis will be on the most common of these: emphysema and chronic bronchitis. Chronic bronchial asthma, which is a form of COPD, is discussed in Chapter 24. All of these conditions are characterized by resistance to the outflow of air from the lungs due to intrapulmonary lesions or processes. This is usually accompanied by dyspnea, a productive cough, and wheezing. These diseases cause either a narrowing of the bronchi and bronchioles, or destruction of the smaller units of the lung (alveoli, alveolar sacs, and respiratory bronchioles), causing enlargement of the terminal air spaces in the lung. In many patients, destructive changes may take place in both areas.

There have been many attempts to define these diseases. For our purposes, we will use the following: (1) Emphysema, according to the World Health Organization, is "a condition of the lung characterized by an increase beyond the normal in the size of the air spaces distal to the terminal bronchiole, with destructive changes in their walls" (1). The important points to remember here are that there is destruction of lung tissue (especially alveolar septa), and loss of pulmonary elasticity, with resultant enlargement of distal air spaces. The process is irreversible but not necessarily progressive. (2) Chronic bronchitis is defined as the continuous excessive production of mucus in the bronchi due to chronic inflammation, resulting in a productive cough. Also, by accepted definition, this process must occur for at least 3 months out of the year for 2 or more successive years (1). The obstruction which occurs in chronic bronchitis may be reversible at first, but with continued obstruction, irreversible damage to lung tissue will occur. The definition of emphysema is based on pathological findings, whereas chronic bronchitis is based on clinical features in which the patient's history is very important. As such, it is sometimes difficult to delineate which disease a patient has. Some patients who are told that they have emphysema may, in fact, have chronic bronchitis, and vice versa. While there are distinct differences in classic cases of these diseases, they are often of academic interest only. This may be due to the overlap that may exist among these diseases in individual patients. For example, a given patient may have chronic bronchitis and emphysema concurrently, emphysema and chronic asthma, etc.

There are several important generalities that can be made about these conditions:

1. The disease processes usually begin years before the onset of signs and symptoms.
2. The symptoms are usually slowly progressive, with acute exacerbations which can cause respiratory failure.
3. Exacerbations may be caused by such things as air pollution, infections, alcoholism, diabetes, anemia, or any debilitating disease.
4. Finally, the treatment regimens have a great deal in common.

ETIOLOGY

There are four major causative factors in COPD: cigarette smoking, atmospheric pollution, infection, and heredity. There is little doubt that cigarette smoking has contributed to these disease processes. Smoking is the most important cause of COPD in this country (2, 3). The mechanism by which smoking produces COPD is unclear. The best hypothesis is that smoke causes impaired ciliary and macrophage function, hypertrophy and hyperplasia of mucus glands, and preliminary obstruction due to inflammation, infection, edema, and fibrosis. Finally, lysosomal enzymes released from leukocytes and macrophages damage the elastic component of connective tissue in the lung (4). In a similar manner, it is felt that increases in environmental and occupational pollutants (e.g., smog, dust in mills and factories, etc.) have played a role in the increased incidence of these diseases. The evidence, however, is more circumstantial than that linking smoking to COPD. For example, the incidence of chronic bronchitis is twice as high in male inhabitants of London as in a matched group of men from rural areas. Also, a corresponding decrease in the amount or severity of COPD has been noted in those areas where air pollution has been diminished.

Pulmonary infections play a role in the course of COPD, although the relationship between pulmonary infection and initiation of the disease is unclear. It is generally felt that infections are infrequently the initiating cause, but that they can deal significantly in the process once it has started. Infections cause the majority of exacerbations of COPD, and are most often due to viruses, especially the respiratory syncytial virus. Other common agents are the influenza virus, mycoplasma, *Streptococcus pneumoniae*, and *Haemophilus influenzae*. The excess mucus that is present in COPD, and which is not easily cleared from the tracheobronchial tree, is a good medium for the proliferation of bacteria. Eventually, these bacteria can cause scarring of the walls of the bronchial tree. The symptoms produced during this infection process—severe cough, wheezing, purulent sputum, and exertional dyspnea—very often bring the person to a physician, who then discovers underlying COPD. In some types of COPD, e.g. bronchiectasis, infection of the bronchi may produce weakening of the wall which allows it to bulge in and out during expiratory movements, causing obstruction. When any pulmonary infection occurs in a COPD patient, large amounts of mucus are produced which helps to cause obstruction to airflow. It is also a well-known fact that infections are often responsible for exacerbation of a patient's symptoms of COPD. It is for this reason, as shall be discussed later, that part of the therapy used in an attempt to control these diseases is aimed at protection against pulmonary infection (1, 5, 6).

In 1963, it was reported that there was a correlation between the development of em-physema and the existence of an inherited deficiency (carried by an autosomal recessive gene) of the enzyme α_1-antitrypsin. Deficiency of this enzyme has been associated with disease of several organs, including the liver and pancreas, but the most common and severe disease seen is pulmonary emphysema. This low molecular weight glycoprotein is normally found in human serum, and it has the property of inhibiting proteolytic enzymes. The type of emphysema produced by deficiency of this enzyme occurs mainly in the lower lobes of the lung, causing diffuse panacinar destruction in these areas. In addition, the onset of the symptoms is usually earlier (third or fourth decade) than with the other types of emphysema, and it affects women much more commonly than the others. Finally, there is a very distinct familial history of the disease because deficiency of the enzyme is genetically determined. It should be noted, however, that some familial distribution of emphysema has been found where no deficiency of this enzyme could be demonstrated.

The mechanism whereby this deficiency leads to emphysema is unclear. α_1-antitrypsin inhibits a number of enzymes, including collagenase and elastase. Perhaps it is necessary to protect the lung from such enzymes. It is also possible that proteases from bacteria (and the leukocytes called forth to combat the bacteria) may be able to more easily attack the pulmonary tissue in those individuals with this deficiency state (1). It appears that smoking hastens the development of disease in individuals (1, 5, 7).

INCIDENCE

The incidence of COPD has been increasing in the U.S. due to two factors. First, air pollution and cigarette smoking have been increasing, especially after World War II. It is gratifying to note that there is a decrease in morbidity and mortality in areas where pollution is decreased. The second reason for the general "increase" in COPD is that diagnostic procedures have improved to the point where it is easier to diagnose patients with minimal disease.

It is estimated that approximately 20% of adult males have significant chronic bronchitis. Emphysema is also very common. Most adults will have some emphysema, especially after the fifth decade, but it is not clinically evident in most cases.

The mortality rate for COPD has also been increasing. In the 1960s, the mortality rate due to emphysema and chronic bronchitis increased by 145 and 72%, respectively. In 1950, the ratio of deaths due to emphysema and lung cancer was 1:15. In 1967, it was 1:2.6. In the U.S., COPD is second only to heart disease as a cause of disability among workers. In a study in Britain of people 40 to 54 years old, 17% of the men and 9% of the women had signs and symptoms of chronic bronchitis. Some authorities anticipate that the mortality rate due to emphysema will double every 5 years. In the U.S., in 1974, there were 25,000 deaths due to COPD; however, the figure is 100,000 when COPD is considered as a secondary cause of death (8, 9).

PATHOLOGY

In order to have an understanding of COPD, it is necessary to review briefly some of the anatomy of the respiratory tract. Starting from the trachea, there is a continuous branching of the bronchial tree through about 50 generations until it reaches the alveolar sacs and alveoli. The important structures, in descending order of size, are the following:

1. The bronchi, which are lined by ciliated cells and contain a large number of mucus glands. The bronchi are also lined by a diagonal layer of smooth muscle;
2. The bronchioles, which are simply bronchi less than 1 mm in diameter and which contain no mucus glands;
3. The terminal bronchioles, which contain no ciliated cells but still retain the smooth muscle layer;
4. The respiratory bronchiole, which has an incomplete layer of smooth muscle, such that the walls may bulge out to form alveoli;
5. The alveolar ducts, which are simply ducts completely lined with alveoli;
6. The alveolar sac, which contains many alveoli and forms the tip of the pulmonary tree;
7. The alveolus, which is the functional unit of the lung, where gas exchange takes place.

As mentioned previously, the basic problem in COPD is resistance to airflow, especially flow out of the lungs, due to an abnormality in one or more of the above structures.

In chronic bronchitis, the smaller bronchi (less than 2 mm in diameter) are affected the most. In this case, the bronchial tree responds to irritation from smoke, infection, etc., with an increase in the amount of mucus production accompanied by edema of the mucosal lining of the bronchi. If the irritation is removed, the process is entirely reversible. However, if the source of irritation remains, the mucus glands in the large airways hypertrophy and the goblet cells in the smaller airways increase in number. The increased amount of sputum, which usually must be removed by coughing and ciliary action, makes a very fertile medium for bacterial growth. Undoubtedly, infections of the smaller air passages extending into the alveolar sacs are responsible for breakdown of lung tissue and scarring in some individuals. A more significant finding, however, is that the mucus is often thick and difficult to remove and, therefore, it may act to cut down the effective diameter of the bronchi and cause turbulence in air flow. Also, the bronchi normally expand on inspiration and contract (or relax) on expiration. Therefore, a glob of mucus lining the bronchi will not have much effect on inspiration, but it may significantly hinder expiration. In this situation, expiratory effort will be increased. In addition, excess mucus lining the wall may act as an irritant and cause bronchospasm, thereby reducing the diameter even further.

As more mucus is produced, it may coalesce and consolidate to produce a mucus plug, especially in the smaller bronchi and bronchioles. These plugs very effectively trap air in the distal areas of the lung (alveoli, alveolar sacs, terminal bronchioles, and respiratory bronchioles). As pressure is built up in the thoracic cavity in the process of expiration, this trapped air exerts pressure on the walls of the alveoli, etc., and may cause a breakdown in tissue in these areas. In many instances, all of the alveoli in an alveolar sac may be broken down so that there is only one large air space left. There is much less functional surface area left for gas exchange in this large air space than in the normal structure. Another complication of the obstructive and destructive processes that take place here is that elastic fibers in the alveolus are lost. They are necessary in aiding the expulsion of air from the alveolus.

Essentially what is happening with chronic bronchitis in many patients is that the obstruction caused by the mucus eventually leads to emphysematous changes in the lung (destruction of tissue and expansion of air spaces). At autopsy, it is not at all uncommon to find bronchitic and emphysematous changes in the same patient (1, 5, 8).

In emphysema, the basic problem is destruction of tissue with resultant expansion of air spaces. There are several pathologically distinct forms of emphysema. The more important are:

1. Centrilobular emphysema, in which the walls of the respiratory bronchiole are weakened and will collapse during expiration;

2. Panacinar (panlobular) emphysema, in which there is diffuse destruction of all the smaller bronchi of the lung, from the respiratory bronchiole down; and

3. Senile emphysema, which is not a pulmonary disease at all. This condition can result when kyphotic changes in the spine cause the chest to bow outward, producing the so-called classic "barrel chest" sometimes seen in true COPD patients. It should be noted that in persons over 50 years old, there are frequently emphysematous changes in the lung which apparently result as the normal process of aging.

As mentioned previously, the elastic recoil of the lung is a major force in expiration, along with the work of the diaphragm and chest wall muscles. This elastic recoil keeps the pressure inside the lung higher than that in the thoracic cavity. If the elastic fibers in the lung are destroyed (infection, smoking, α_1-antitrypsin deficiency, etc.), the intraalveolar and intrabronchial pressure will be reduced. Since the pressure inside the thoracic cavity during expiration (generated by the diaphragm and intercostal muscle) would then be greater than that inside the airways, any structure or airway with a weak wall will collapse during expiration. This is one of the major reasons for obstruction to airflow in emphysema (1, 5, 10).

DIAGNOSIS AND CLINICAL FEATURES

The diagnosis of emphysema during life is difficult because emphysema is defined by its pathology and the changes that occur in the lung. While these changes will in time produce signs and symptoms of COPD, it is difficult to say that the clinical state of the patient is due, for example, to panacinar empnysema, rather than centrilobular. It is also difficult in many cases to differentiate a patient with chronic bronchitis from one who has emphysema because in most situations patients have components of both conditions or mixed COPD. In an effort to clarify this, patients have been grouped into two classes, depending on their presenting signs and symptoms. Dornhorst, in 1955, used the terms "pink-puffer" and "blue-bloater" to describe the typical patient in each of these classes. Generally speaking, pink-puffers (also referred to as emphysematous types or type A) are thin, anxious, and dyspneic on exertion. There is usually no cyanosis (hence, the term "pink") and they appear to be well-oxygenated when activity is minimal. However, they may develop shortness of breath (SOB) very easily when required to perform even the lightest tasks.

The blue-bloater (also called type B or bronchitic types) is typically obese, quiet, cyanotic at rest, and has a cough which produces a great deal of mucus. Table 25.1 summarizes the findings in these two classes of patients. It should be remembered that most COPD patients actually have mixed disease and will exhibit components of both classes.

The typical patient with COPD is a 50- or 60-year-old cigarette-smoking male. He usually complains of chronic, often productive cough, particularly in the winter. He becomes breathless very easily and may suffer from dyspnea, orthopnea, and wheezing.

Very often these patients will present with SOB, due in part ot a pulmonary infection. Upon questioning, it becomes evident that many of them have a long history of cigarette cough and excess sputum production, particularly in the winter months. Gradually, the cigarette cough worsens and the patient may suffer from it continuously. Mild upper respiratory tract infections become more severe and the mucus may appear purulent. Wheezing will often be noticed at this time.

In other cases, however, the patient is experiencing dyspnea, but accepts it as a result of the aging process and, therefore, does not seek medical attention. Eventually, he gets to a point where even the slightest physical exertion leaves him breathless, at which time he will seek aid. In either of these cases, a great deal of damage already may have occurred in the pulmonary system.

TREATMENT

Unfortunately, there is no one specific treatment or cure for COPD. With multiple causes

Table 25.1.
Findings in Patients with Chronic Obstructive Pulmonary Disease

Clinical Attribute	Chronic Bronchitis: Type B ("Blue-Bloater")	Emphysema: Type A ("Pink-Puffer")
Age at onset of symptoms	Younger (+45 years)	Older (55 years)
Body type	Obese	Thin (weight loss may indicate advanced disease)
Sputum	Copious; purulent	Scanty
Cough	Long duration	Late in course of disease
Major onset symptom	Tussive	Dyspnea
Shortness of breath	Absent initially; severe in advanced disease	Very common
Cyanosis	Very common	Usually absent, even with low pO_2
Recurrent infection	Severe problem; prophylactic antibiotics useful	Mild problem
Heart	Enlarged	Normal
Hematocrit	Increased	Normal, except in advanced disease
Chronic hypercarbia	Common	Rare, except in advanced disease
Chronic hypoxia	Often severe	Mild
Vital capacity	Decreased	Low normal
Total lung capacity	Low normal	Low normal
Expiratory flow rates	Decreased	Decreased
Enhanced VC and flow ranges following bronchodilator	Significant	Minimal
Diffusing capacity	Normal	Decreased
Residual volume	Increased	Increased
Cor pulmonale	May be found in moderate disease	Only in far advanced disease

for this condition, it is doubtful that there will ever be a single cure to cover the various types of these diseases. Perhaps the best treatment is prevention by reducing, avoiding, or eliminating such things as cigarette smoking and atmospheric and industrial pollution. It has been demonstrated that control of these things at an early age before pulmonary damage occurs would definitely decrease the incidence of COPD. Elimination at a later age would significantly decrease morbidity and mortality, although some damage remains. It should be noted that not all smokers will sustain pulmonary damage. The reasons are unclear and as yet, it cannot be predicted which smokers will be affected (11).

The treatment of COPD is such that a number of different measures are employed in order to stop or slow down the disease process and to make life more comfortable for these patients. Essentially, the goal of management is to allow these patients to lead as productive and normal lives as possible. There are three objectives in the management of COPD: pre-

vention or minimization of irreversible decreases in pulmonary function; decreasing symptoms of the disease; and prevention of death from respiratory insufficiency (5). There are six different strategies which are used to reach these goals and objectives: to prevent, eradicate, or reduce bronchial and alveolar inflammation; to alleviate bronchial obstruction; to train the patient to breathe properly; to rehabilitate the patient physically; to manage complications (e.g., respiratory failure brought on by an infection); and, finally, to educate the patient concerning his disease, and how he can live with it and treat it. It has been demonstrated that the development and initiation of a therapeutic program for the COPD patient will decrease hospitalization, reduce the emotional impact of the disease, and allow patients to lead more normal lives (12, 13).

As shall be demonstrated, these strategies and the means by which they are achieved have a great deal of overlap.

1. In order to eliminate or decrease inflam-

mation and irritation in the pulmonary tree, several things can be done. First of all, these patients should stop smoking. Often, this is enough to cause significant improvement in early chronic bronchitis. In early emphysema, the diminished elastic recoil of the lung is not regained upon cessation of smoking. Nevertheless, the disease may still be subclinical, and the other obstructive stimuli due to smoking (i.e., bronchospasm) will certainly cease when patients give up cigarettes (14, 15).

Another thing that can be done is to avoid air pollution if at all possible. If it is mainly industrial pollution, a change in jobs and/or training in a new career can be considered. If general atmospheric pollution is responsible, moving to a new area can be considered. Obviously, there are many patients for whom these possibilities are unacceptable.

Many people are able to relieve pulmonary inflammatory problems by adjusting the atmospheric environments in their homes. It is desirable to keep the rooms well humidified (30 to 50% humidity is optimal) and to have the temperature stabilized. Proper humidification helps in liquefying and removing the tenacious mucus secretions which often lead to the destructive changes, and exacerbation in the disease processes.

Finally, control of extreme temperature variations is important because extremes can cause increased mucus production.

2. The relief of bronchial obstruction is often referred to as "bronchial hygiene." Bronchodilators should be tried in virtually all patients with chronic obstruction. They work very well in COPD patients who have bronchospasm playing a part in their disease, but generally they are not as effective as they are in patients with asthma. A decision to use or not use bronchodilators should not be made based on spirometric evidence following a single dose of bronchodilator. Some patients will show a response only after several doses are given. Others may respond to theophylline, but not a sympathomimetic, or vice versa (16).

Sympathomimetics

The sympathomimetics may be given orally, or by inhalation with pressurized aerosols, hand-held nebulizers, or pump-driven nebulizers. The drugs used in this country traditionally have included epinephrine, isoproterenol, and ephedrine. Over the last few years, the use of these has been decreased due to the advent of the newer "selective" β_2-stimulants such as isoetharine, terbutaline, metaproterenol, and albuterol. There are numerous recommendations for specific drugs and doses to use in COPD patients. Many of these are based on empirical findings rather than on a large body of scientific data. Nevertheless, most authorities recommend the trial of a sympathomimetic for at least several weeks in an effort to control any of the reversible obstruction of COPD. Spirograms before, during, and after use usually demonstrate any beneficial effects in individual patients (17).

Ephedrine has been widely used for chronic oral therapy. Its side effects, especially in elderly males, restricts its use. If it is used, the dose is 25 mg four times daily. A "selective" B_2-stimulant, such as metaproterenol (20 mg orally three or four times a day) or terbutaline (2.5 to 5 mg orally three times a day), are considered a somewhat better choice for oral therapy, although they are more expensive. For inhalation therapy, isoproterenol has lost a significant amount of its popularity to the newer more selective β_2-stimulants. The problems with abuse of isoproterenol and related sympathomimetics, discussed in Chapter 24, have limited its use. There are fewer cardiac problems with the newer agents. The dosage recommendations for the sympathomimetics given in Chapter 24 for asthma apply equally well for use in COPD. A general guide to dosage adjustment is to use that amount of drug which produces the best objective improvement without cardiac side effects, tremors, or other untoward effects. As in asthmatics, tolerance can develop, and abuse with its sequelae should be monitored. These patients must be taught the proper use of their inhalers and consequences of overuse, to avoid these problems. The following procedures should be used for inhalation: (a) exhale slowly and completely, (b) activate the aerosol or nebulizer while inhaling deeply, (c) hold the breath for several seconds, and, then, (d) exhale slowly against pursed lips. Refer to Chapter 24 for a more detailed discussion of dosing techniques.

Methylxanthines

Theophylline and other methylxanthines may be used as an alternative, or in addition, to the sympathomimetics. Dosing guidelines are essentially the same as those detailed for asthma in Chapter 24. There are many salts and dosage forms available which can cause some confusion. For chronic oral administration, plain theophylline tablets are probably the best choice for an initial trial. Rectal administration produces erratic results. The blood levels associated with an adequate therapeutic response are 10 to 20 μg/ml. The clinical response, however, should be used as the final guide in dosing. Since CHF causes prolongation of the clearance of theophylline, dosage adjustments are likely to be required when a patient stabilized on theophylline develops cor pulmonale.

Corticosteroids

The corticosteroids, in general, appear to be less effective in COPD than in asthma. Most patients feel better subjectively, but objective evidence of improvement based on spirometric measurement is difficult to demonstrate (18, 19). The most likely responders are those patients with a history of allergy and sputum eosinophilia. In addition, corticosteroids may be lifesaving in the critically ill patient in whom the sympathomimetics and methylxanthines have not worked when given in appropriate doses. They may be very effective in some patients in relieving bronchospasm, but they should not be used casually or chronically in patients who benefit from other modes of therapy. In the acutely ill patient, large doses may be required (e.g., 300 mg of hydrocortisone daily, or equivalent doses of other corticosteroids). They may be continued at high doses for 3 to 5 days, then tapered over 7 to 10 days.

In patients whose obstructive symptoms are progressive, and which are not controlled by adequate doses of the bronchodilators, a trial of corticosteroids is justified. The patient should be monitored with pulmonary function tests to see if there is any objective improvement, which may take several weeks to develop. Routine bronchodilator treatment should be continued during this time. If there is improvement, the dose should be tapered to the least amount which sustains the improvement. Since the steroids have a known "euphoric" effect, subjective feelings of improvement voiced by the patient may be very misleading. In patients on chronic steroid therapy, consideration should be given to an alternate day dosing regimen. As with the methylxanthines, the effects of the corticosteroids on the gastrointestinal tract must be considered.

Inhaled corticosteroids have been shown to be very effective in the treatment of asthma. Evidence showing their efficacy in COPD is still lacking.

Atropine

Atropine and related drugs have been shown to be potent bronchodilators in some COPD patients. The role of the parasympathetic system in the development of bronchospasm is unclear (see Chapter 24). Nevertheless, atropine, given by inhalation, subcutaneously, or orally, seems to possess significant bronchodilatory effects on large and small airways in some chronic bronchitis patients. Further experimentation is needed to define the benefits and risks of this drug (20, 21).

N-Acetylcysteine

The mucolytic agent N-acetylcysteine has been used with varying degrees of success in COPD. It is certainly effective *in vitro*, but *in vivo* studies give conflicting results. It appears that inhalation of the drug may be an ineffective method of using it. Direct instillation with a catheter into segments of the bronchial tree blocked by mucus plugs is an effective way of using the drug. Also, the catheter would aid in suctioning off the liquified secretions. Two to 5 cc of a 20% solution are used for this purpose. Postural drainage following use will help in removing the mucus (22, 23).

There are three undesirable side effects from N-acetylcystine: the first is that it has a foul odor and frequently causes nausea. Second, a number of patients, especially asthmatics, are hypersensitive to it and develop bronchospasm with the drug. If it is to be used in asthmatics, they should be pretreated with a bronchodilator. The third problem is that some patients may experience a massive liquefaction of mucus, and they may have trouble removing this mucus by coughing and ciliary motion. Suction will be required in these cases.

Another method to improve bronchial hygiene is to humidify the atmosphere so that the excess mucus causing bronchial obstruction can be removed. Besides installing a humidifier in their homes, many patients benefit from directly inhaling highly moisturized air (e.g., from a vaporizer or nebulizer) for about 10 minutes after each use of a bronchodilator. They may follow this with careful coughing or postural drainage to aid in the removal of the mucus.

Miscellaneous Agents

There are several other agents which have been used to help remove mucus in COPD patients. Nebulized saline (0.5 to 1%), 2.5 to 5% propylene glycol, or 1.3 to 3% sodium bicarbonate are bland, and may be helpful in removing mucus. The expectorants (saturated solution of potassium iodide (SSKI) and guaifenesin) are of questionable efficacy. SSKI causes significant hypersensitivity reactions. Guaifenesin, in the doses commonly used (400 to 600 mg/day) has no effect, but as the dose is increased to 800 mg/day, there appears to be some response (24). Detergent aerosols have not been shown to be more effective than nebulized saline or water (25). At this time, the use of expectorants, mucolytics, and detergents cannot be recommended.

In general, the most effective way to help remove these secretions is to make sure that the patient is well-hydrated from an adequate oral fluid intake. This, along with inhalation of water or saline mist or with supplemental IV fluids, is the most efficient way to liquefy and remove mucus.

3. Training these patients to breathe properly can add greatly to their enjoyment of life. They must be taught to breathe in a slow and relaxed manner, emphasizing diaphragmatic breathing. Dyspnea can be terrifying, and many patients, when they become dyspneic, try to increase their inspiratory and expiratory efforts. Because of the nature of COPD they have no trouble with inspiration, but they are unable to exhale properly. Therefore, they are taught to breathe slowly, preferably inspiring through the nose and expiring through pursed lips. Many patients have adopted this technique spontaneously. Breathing control is essential to prevent overdistention and dyspnea (26). Patients are taught to let the natural rhythm of their breathing determine the amount of activity they can undertake. In normal individuals, the opposite occurs.

Finally, they are taught to cough properly. Coughing is one of the main mechanisms whereby sputum is removed, and it is rarely, if ever, justified to suppress the cough in these patients. On the other hand, it is important that they be taught to cough moderately and not too forcefully, since vigorous coughing can cause further breakdown of alveolar walls.

4. Physical rehabilitation, like breathing training, can improve the amount of work that these patients can do. In the usual patient, shortness of breath upon exertion removes the desire to attempt that type of exertion again. This leads to atrophy of the skeletal muscle which causes an even greater decrease in tolerance to exertion or exercise. This sets up a vicious circle which eventually results in a state of invalidism which may not be really warranted, if the actual amount of disease is considered. Therefore, many of these patients are placed on a series of graded exercise in an effort to enhance their stamina. Patients who are unable to do any exercises because of severe hypoxemia may be benefited by supplemental oxygen (30 to 50%) (5, 12, 27).

Oxygen therapy is very important in the treatment of COPD. Hypoxia can be severe and sudden in onset, or it can develop slowly over a long period of time. Many patients will tolerate chronic hypoxia and hypercarbia with no major problems. Oxygen should be used in anyone with an arterial pO_2 of less than 50 mm Hg at rest. The rate should be adjusted to provide an arterial pO_2 of 60 to 80 mm Hg. It has been well-documented that continuous oxygen therapy (e.g., 1 to 2 liters/min by nasal cannula) is effective in reducing morbidity and mortality in severely ill patients (1). When oxygen is administered, there are several problems which may occur. First of all, if the gas mixture is improperly humidified, it may be drying to the mucous membranes. Secondly, if the concentration of administered oxygen is too high, it may depress the respiration by suddenly removing CO_2 and saturating the blood with oxygen. This problem has probably been overemphasized. In exacerbations, oxygen therapy must be carefully monitored and controlled. It is important, therefore, to monitor blood gases carefully during oxygen therapy (8).

Many patients will react to hypoxia by becoming agitated, restless, etc. When a patient with COPD exhibits these symptoms, it is vitally important to make sure that he is not hypoxic before initiating therapy with a "tranquilizer." Obviously, if hypoxia is the cause of the agitation, oxygen therapy is indicated. Hypoxic patients are extremely sensitive to even low doses of the commonly used "tranquilizers." These include phenothiazines, barbiturates, and benzodiazepines. In hypoxia, these drugs (and any CNS depressant) can depress the respiratory center enough to completely obliterate respiratory drive, resulting in death. In the absence of hypoxia, these same drugs may be safe in normal doses in COPD patients. However, it would be wise to use depressants very cautiously, if at all.

5. Managing complications as they occur is one of the most important aspects of controlling COPD. The major problem here is pulmonary infection. Obviously, many of the other things that have been mentioned (e.g., bronchial hygiene) will aid in preventing infections. There are a few specifics, however, which should be mentioned. First of all, these patients should try to avoid crowds when respiratory infections are prevalent. Secondly, they should receive polyvalent influenza vaccine yearly. Thirdly, they should be very careful to practice proper oral hygiene since this may be a portal of respiratory infection.

When bacterial infections do occur, they should be treated vigorously, preferably with a bacteriocidal agent. Also, the treatment may need to be prolonged when compared with treatment in a normal individual. Material for culture and sensitivity should be collected before treatment is started. However, treatment must be started before the results are back. In many situations, past experience with a given patient or experience with many patients in the area may give a clue to the most likely offending organism. Also, a Gram stain of the mucus may provide some information. Recurrent infections are often due to viruses, S. pneumoniae, or H. influenzae. In diplococcal infections, penicillin is the drug of choice, followed by erythromycin; with Haemophilus, ampicillin would be the drug of choice. A good choice for initial treatment before results of culture and sensitivity tests are back, if Gram-positive cocci are predominant, would be ampicillin, 500 mg every 6 hours. In patients who do not practice good bronchial hygiene or who have been on prophylactic antibiotic therapy, it is not uncommon to see infections caused by Klebsiella, Escherichia coli, anerobic streptococci, etc. (11, 28).

Use of prophylactic antibiotics in patients with chronic bronchitis is well documented and is clinically beneficial (5, 29). Drugs commonly used include tetracycline, penicillin, erythromycin, trimethoprim-sulfamethoxazole, and ampicillin/amoxicillin. In some cases, patients take low doses daily continuously or during those months when respiratory infections are particularly common. In other cases, patients are given a supply of an antibiotic and instructed to begin dosing themselves at the first sign of an infection.

There are several other complications which can occur. Congestive heart failure, especially right-sided failure (cor pulmonale) is a fairly common finding. Cor pulmonale occurs when alveolar hypoxia causes pulmonary vasoconstriction and pulmonary hypertension. Therapy therefore consists of steps to correct alveolar hypoxia (bronchodilation, oxygen, and removal of secretions). Diuretics are useful if the above step does not completely reverse the process. Methylxanthines and sympathomimetics commonly used in these cases may have a beneficial inotropic effect. The use of digitalis is a more controversial topic. These patients develop digitalis toxicity more frequently than other patients, probably because of hypoxemia, and electrolyte imbalance (30). Polycythemia occurs frequently and may cause problems if the hematocrit gets too high. In these cases, venesection may be required to keep it at 55% or less. Oxygen therapy is often beneficial in helping to reduce the hematocrit. Acute respiratory failure and respiratory acidosis may occur, often as a result of pulmonary infections. The aim of treatment is to reduce bronchospasm, remove mucus secretions, treat infection (if present), and correct hypoxemia, hypercapnia, and heart failure. This involves the vigorous use of some of the things already mentioned, including oxygen, humidification, bronchodilators, mucolytics, corticosteroids, antibiotics, etc.

6. It is vitally important that the patient be educated concerning his disease. He should have an understanding of what is happening to him and how the disease process can be slowed or halted. The treatment of COPD involves many processes, procedures, and drugs. If the patient is to comply with all of this, he must understand why it is important that he do so. Also, the patient must learn to recognize problems or potential problems which might arise. For example, it is extremely important that infections be treated promptly and vigorously. For this reason, the patient has to be aware of not only the first signs and symptoms of the infection, but also what might happen if he delays seeking proper treatment. The pharmacist should make certain that his COPD patients have a thorough understanding of the use and limitations of their drugs.

PROGNOSIS

The prognosis of COPD is extremely variable. Death due to the disease may occur within several years after the onset of symptoms; likewise, some patients will live for many decades and will eventually die from some unrelated cause. The usual case is slowly progressive with acute exacerbations which may cause death. The average 5-year mortality rate is 50%.

There are several processes which relate particularly to a poor prognosis. These are: a sudden loss of weight, severe dyspnea, and one or more episodes of right-sided heart failure. In addition to these, the following may affect or give a clue to the prognosis:

1. The height above sea level at which the patient lives is important. Generally speaking, the higher the elevation, the shorter the life span. This is thought to be due to an increased hematocrit which will occur at higher elevations and which may precipitate heart failure.
2. Women seem to fare better than men.
3. Patients in whom the disease develops later in life do better than patients in whom the signs and symptoms occur earlier in life.
4. Patients who must work at physically taxing jobs do not fare as well as those who have less demanding work.
5. Patients who continue to smoke do not do as well as those who quit.
6. Finally, the type of onset of this disease can be important. Those in whom the first symptoms were related to dyspnea have the poorest prognosis; those in whom overproduction or mucus was the first sign do moderately well; and those in whom the first signs were asthmatic do the best.

CONCLUSION

COPD involves a number of interrelated disease processes. The basic abnormality is resistance to flow of air in the lungs, especially on expiration. Recognition of the etiological factors is important because it allows us to institute programs to reduce the very high incidence of these diseases. The treatment program involves a number of related processes which may aid the slowing or stopping the progression of the disease. The usual case, however, is slowly progressive, and death may result within 5 to 20 years after onset of symptoms. As pharmacists, we have the responsibility of not only providing the drugs used by these patients, but also making sure that appropriate drugs are used, and that the patient understands how best to use these drugs.

References

1. Hodgkin JE: Diagnosis and differentiation. In *Chronic Obstructive Pulmonary Disease*. Park Ridge, Illinois, American College of Chest Physicians, 1979, p. 5.
2. U.S. Public Health Service: Smoking and health: A report of the Surgeon General: I. The health consequences of smoking. U.S. Department of Health and Welfare, No. 79-50066, 1979.
3. Auerbach O, Hammond EC, Garfinkel L, Benante C: Relation of smoking and age to emphysema. *N Engl J Med* 285:855, 1972.
4. Ayres S: Cigarette smoking and lung diseases: An update. *Basics of Respiratory Disease*. American Thoracic Society, New York, 1975, vol. 3.
5. Welch MH: Obstructive diseases. In *Pulmonary Medicine*, ed. Philadelphia, Lippincott 1982, p. 664.
6. Levowitz MD, Burrows B: The relationship of acute respiratory illness history to the prevalence and incidence of obstructive lung disorders. *Am J Epidemiol* 105:544, 1977.
7. Talamo RC: Alpha-1-antitrypsin deficiency and emphysema. *Chest* 72:421, 1977.
8. *Chronic Obstructive Pulmonary Disease: A Manual for Physicians*, ed. 3. New York, National Tuberculosis and Respiratory Disease Association, 1972.
9. Dodge, RR, Burrows B: The prevalence and incidence of asthma in a general population sample. *Am Rev Respir Dis* 122:567, 1980.
10. Duffell GM, Marcus JH, Ingram RH: Limitation of expiratory flow in chronic obstructive pulmonary disease. *Ann Intern Med* 72:365, 1970.
11. Pride NB: Chronic bronchitis and emphysema: Recent trends. *Practitioner* 219:640, 1977.
12. Petty T: Does treatment for severe emphysema and chronic bronchitis really help? *Chest* 65:124, 1974.
13. Fishman DB, Petty T: Physical, symptomatic and psychological improvement in patients receiving comprehensive care for chronic airway obstruction. *J. Chronic Dis* 24:775, 1971.
14. Dosman JA: Preventive diagnosis in occupational pulmonary disease. *Ann Intern Med* 83:274, 1975.
15. Fletcher C, Peto R: The natural history of chronic airflow obstruction. *Br Med J* 1:1645, 1977.
16. Hudson LD, Pierson DJ: Comprehensive respiratory care for patients with chronic obstructive pulmonary disease. *Med Clin North Am* 65:629, 1981.
17. Paterson JW, Woolcock A, Shenfield GM: Bronchodilator drugs. *Am Rev Respir Dis* 120:1149, 1979.
18. Sahn SA: Corticosteroids in chronic bronchitis and pulmonary emphysema. *Chest* 73:389, 1978.
19. Albert RK, Martin TR, Lewis SW: Controlled clinical trial of methylprednisolone in patients with chronic bronchitis and acute respiratory insufficiency. *Ann Intern Med* 92:753, 1980.
20. Klock LE, Miller TD, Norris AH: A comparative study of atropine sulfate and isoproterenol hydrochloride in chronic bronchitis. *Am Rev Respir Dis* 112:371, 1975.
21. Chick TW, Jenne JW: Comparative bronchodilator responses to atropine and terbutaline in

asthma and chronic bronchitis. *Chest* 72:719, 1977.

22. Lieberman J: The appropriate use of mucolytic agents. *Am J Med* 49:1, 1970.

23. Barton AD: Aerosolized detergents and mucolytic agents in the treatment of stable chronic obstructive pulmonary disease. *Am Rev Respir Dis* 110: 104, 1974.

24. Thomson ML, Pavia D, McNicol MW: A preliminary study of the effect of guaiphenesin or mucociliary clearance from the human lung. *Thorax* 28:742, 1973.

25. Lourenco RV: Aerosol therapy: Introduction. *Am Rev Respir Dis* 110:85, 1974.

26. Grimby G: Aspects of lung expansion in relation to pulmonary physiotherapy. *Am Rev Respir Dis* 110:145, 1974.

27. Bass H, Whitcomb JF, Forman R: Exercise training therapy for patients with chronic obstructive pulmonary disease. *Chest* 57:116, 1970.

28. Anonymous: Antimicrobial treatment of chronic bronchitis. *Lancet* 1:505, 1975.

29. Burrows B, Nevin W: Antibiotic management in patients with chronic bronchitis and emphysema. *Ann Intern Med* 77:993, 1972.

30. Green LH, Smith TW: The use of digitalis in patients with pulmonary disease. *Ann Intern Med* 87:459, 1977.

SECTION 6
Endocrine and Metabolic Diseases

CHAPTER 26

Thyroid and Parathyroid Disorders

BETTY J. DONG, Pharm.D.

THYROID DISORDERS

Hypo- and hyperthyroidism are well-known disorders of the thyroid gland which affect a large proportion of the population. Since drugs constitute a major form of medical management, it behooves the pharmacist to have a basic understanding of the physiology, pathophysiology, and hormone biosynthesis of the thyroid, the laboratory and clinical manifestations of each disease state, and the numerous pharmacological and medical interventions available. The knowledgeable pharmacist, irrespective of location and practice, be it hospital, retail, or clinic, can optimize long-term care by participating in patient education, in the achievement of therapeutic indices, in the recognition of toxicity, in the interpretation of laboratory-drug and drug-drug interactions, and in the selection of appropriate proprietary and prescription preparations.

Physiology

REGULATION OF THYROID FUNCTION

The thyroid gland, a highly vascular organ lying on top of the trachea, consists of two lobes connected by a middle lobe known as the isthmus. The gland synthesizes, stores and releases two major metabolically active hormones: triiodothyronine (T_3) and thyroxine (T_4). T_3 may be the more active thyroid hormone since the receptor protein for thyroid hormone within the cell nucleus has about a 10-fold higher affinity for T_3 than for T_4 (1, 2). Regulation of hormone synthesis is achieved via an intricate negative feedback mechanism involving the gland and the hypothalamic-pituitary axis (Fig. 26.1), as well as through autoregulation of iodide uptake (3, 4).

Low circulating levels of thyroid hormone initiate the release of thyroid-stimulating hormone (TSH) from the pituitary and possibly the secretion of thyrotropin-releasing factor (TRF) from the hypothalamus. Rising levels of TSH promote increased iodide trapping by the gland with a subsequent increase in synthesis and in circulating hormone levels which feed back on the pituitary and hypothalamic centers to shut off TRF, TSH and further hormone biosynthesis. As the hormone levels drop, the hypothalamic-pituitary centers are once again responsive with release of TSH and TRF. Loss of this negative feedback mechanism can result in hypo- or hyperthyroidism.

The gland also has an inherent ability to regulate its uptake of iodide so that excessive formation of thyroid hormone does not occur even though a large iodide load may be present, i.e., dye for intravenous pyelography (IVP). This autoregulatory effect of the gland to prevent iodine organification is known as the "Wolff-Chaikoff block" (5). This effect is dependent upon establishment of a critical intrathyroidal iodide concentration beyond which hormone synthesis is impaired and is not overcome by TSH stimulation. The normal gland "escapes" from the "Wolff-Chaikoff block" within 7–14 days so that hypothyroidism and goiter does not occur. "Escape" is postulated to occur by a decrease in iodide transport or an "iodide leak," both which tend to decrease the intrathyroidal iodide concentration and remove the block to organification. Certain thyroid disorders, i.e., Hashimoto's, are unable to escape from the "Wolff-Chaikoff block," so that hypothyroidism occurs.

HORMONE SYNTHESIS/TRANSPORT

Both T_4 and T_3 are produced within the gland. However, the majority of T_3 production results from peripheral conversion of T_4.

Dietary inorganic iodide trapped by the gland is promptly oxidized by peroxidase to iodine before its incorporation with tyrosine molecules to form monoiodotyrosine (MIT) and diiodotyrosine (DIT). Subsequently, the formation of T_4 occurs with the coupling of

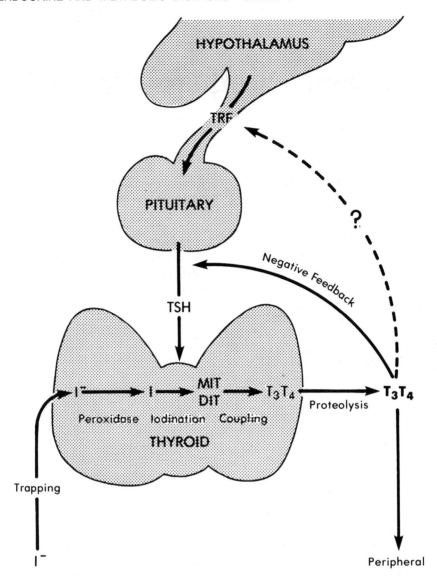

Figure 26.1. Hormone synthesis via negative feedback control on the hypothalamic-pituitary-thyroid axis.

two diiodotyrosyl residues and of T_3 by coupling a diiodotyrosyl and monoiodotyrosyl residue. The synthesized hormones are then stored within thyroglobulin until their release into the circulation through enzymatic cleavage.

In the circulation, the hormones exist in both the active-free and inactive protein-bound forms. Thyroxine is 99.89% bound while only 0.02% is free. This high affinity for the plasma proteins: thyroxine-binding globulin (TBG) 80%, thyroxine-binding pre-albumin (TBPA) 10 to 15%, and albumin 4 to 5%, accounts for the high serum concentration and

the slow metabolic degradation ($t_{1/2}$ = 7 days) of thyroxine. On the other hand, triiodothyronine is three times more potent metabolically than T_4, but the biologic activity is similar since T_3's lesser affinity for the plasma proteins results in a lower serum concentration and greater clearance ($t_{1/2}$ = 1.5 days). About 0.2% of T_3 is free and active.

THYROID HORMONE METABOLISM

About 35–40% of the secreted T_4 is peripherally monodeiodinated to active T_3 while about 40% is converted to reverse T_3 (rT_3)

which has little or no thyroidal activity (1). This extrathyroidal conversion of T_4 to T_3 accounts for about 80% of the total daily production of T_3. Much less information is available regarding the significance of rT_3, although there are some interesting findings. Certain acute and chronic nonthyroidal disorders (i.e., starvation, acute infection, chronic cardiac, pulmonary, renal, hepatic, and neoplastic diseases) have been associated with impaired conversion of T_4 to active T_3 secondary to increased conversion to rT_3 (6). Certain drugs such as propranolol (see Table 26.2) can also impair conversion. These "euthyroid sick" patients are not hypothyroid as evidenced by normal TSH and TRH tests, although the T_4 (RIA), RT_3U, T_3 (RIA), and FTI may be low (3, 6). Treatment is not indicated.

Thyroid Function Tests

Laboratory tests have been devised to evaluate thyroid homeostasis and metabolic function, as well as aid in the confirmation and diagnosis of circulating hormone levels, glandular activity, hypothalamic-pituitary function, autoimmunity, and various nonspecific metabolic indices. Initial screening for thyroid disorders should include the T_4 (RIA), RT_3U, and FT_4I (see Table 26.1).

CIRCULATING HORMONE LEVELS

Circulating hormone levels are determined by measuring total free and protein-bound concentrations of T_4 and T_3. These thyroid function tests (see Table 26.1) include the T_4 (RIA), RT_3U, T_3 (RIA), FT_4I, FT_3I, and PBI.

Resin T_3 Uptake

The resin T_3 uptake (RT_3U) provides an indirect assessment of the concentration and saturation of TBG by T_4. In this test, a fixed amount of labeled T_3 and a resin sponge is added to the serum and allowed to equilibrate. At equilibrium, the radioactive T_3 will bind to the unoccupied sites on the patient's circulating TBG and the remaining unbound radioactive T_3 will be picked up by the resin sponge. The amount of radioactivity remaining in the sponge will be inversely proportional to the number of unbound sites on the TBG. Therefore, the radioactivity in the resin will be greater when most sites on the patient's TBG are occupied as in hyperthyroidism (increased

RT_3U). Conversely, when there are more unoccupied TBG sites, as in hypothyroidism, most of the labeled T_3 will bind to the patient's TBG and a smaller proportion removed by the resin (decreased RT_3U).

Free Thyroxine Index, Free T_3 Index

Since the T_4 (RIA), RT_3U, and the T_3 (RIA) are dependent upon TBG, any changes in the amounts of TBG or the degree of TBG saturation will influence the results (see Table 26.2). If TBG levels are increased, as in pregnancy or with oral contraceptive use, there will be increased binding sites with resultant increased T_4 (RIA) concentrations and decreased RT_3U. However, the free T_4 levels and thyroid status are unchanged. Conversely, if TBG levels and, therefore, TBG binding sites are decreased as a result of androgen therapy, nephrosis, or cirrhosis, a depressed T_4 (RIA) and an elevated RT_3U will be seen. Displacement of T_4 from TBG by phenytoin or by large doses of salicylates (levels >15 mg/100 ml) will result in decreased T_4 (RIA) levels and unchanged RT_3U levels since the sites are occupied by phenytoin or salicylates.

The fluctuations in TBG do not accurately reflect the active-free thyroxine levels which remain unchanged in a euthyroid state. Multiplying the results of the T_4 (RIA) or T_3 (RIA) by the RT_3U gives the FT_4I or FT_3I which compensates for changes in binding sites and accurately reflects the biologically active fraction as could be measured directly by dialysis.

GLANDULAR ACTIVITY

Radioactive Iodine Uptake

The radioactive iodine uptake (RAIU) measures only the iodine trapping ability of the gland without regard to its ultimate fate (see Table 26.1). Thus, a high uptake may occur despite low circulating hormone levels which indicate defective synthesis or release as in Hashimoto's thyroiditis. A thyroid scan is often obtained concurrently. A scan and uptake are often helpful when discrete thyroid nodules and irregularities are palpable, when there is a history of prior neck irradiation, and when ablative radioactive iodine therapy is indicated.

Difficulty with accurate interpretation of the RAIU has caused it to be used as an adjunct rather than as a primary diagnostic tool. Fluc-

Table 26.1.
Thyroid Function Tests

Tests	Normal Values[a]	Measures	Hyperthyroidism	Hypothyroidism	Comments
PBI (protein-bound iodine)	4–8 μg/100 ml	Precipitated iodine content of thyroxine	↑	↓	Interference by iodide contamination has led to replacement by newer techniques
BEI (butanol-extractable iodine)					
T$_4$ by column (thyroxine by column)					
T$_4$ (RIA) (total thyroxine by radioimmune assay)	5–12 μg/dl	Total T$_4$ both free and bound	↑	↓	Altered by changes in thyroxine-binding globulin (TBG)
RT$_3$U (resin T$_3$ Uptake)	25–35%	Indirect measure of degree of saturation of TBG sites by T$_4$	↑	↓	Altered by changes in TBG
FT$_4$I (free thyroxine index)	1.3–4.2	Product of RT$_3$U × T$_4$ (RIA); estimation of active free T$_4$ levels	↑	↓	Compensates for changes in TBG concentration; usually reflects true thyroid status
T$_3$ (RIA) (T$_3$ by radioimmune assay)	80–180 ng/dl	Total T$_3$ both free and bound	↑	↓	Altered by changes in TBG
FT$_3$I (free T$_3$ index)	20–63	Product of RT$_3$U × T$_3$ (RIA) estimation of active free T$_3$	↑	↓	Compensates for changes in TBG concentration, usually reflects true thyroid status
RAIU (^{123}I radioactive iodine uptake)	At 5 hr = 5–15% At 24 hr = 10–35%	Iodine trapping ability of gland without regard to ultimate fate of iodine	↑	↓	Normals will vary depending on the degree of dietary iodide intake and on geographical locale; interfered by iodine intake
TSH (thyrotropic stimulating hormone)	0–10 μU/ml	Pituitary TSH; most sensitive indicator of adequate circulating thyroid levels	↓	↑	Interfered by pregnancy HCG (not at UC)
Antibodies: TgAB (thyroglobulin)	0–8%	Autoimmune process, i.e., Hashimoto's, Graves	Often +	Often +	
AntiM (microsomal)	<1:100 titer		Often +	Often +	Microsomal more sensitive, elevated even with remission

Test					
T_3 suppression test	Suppression of RAIU to 50% or less of baseline RAIU after 10 days of T_3 therapy	Autonomous functioning tissue (not under negative feedback control)	Nonsuppression	Suppression	Often seen in Graves' and hot nodules; non-suppression
TRH test (thyrotropin-releasing hormone test)	2–5-fold rise in serum TSH 15–60 min after injection of 200 μg TRH	Ability of pituitary to respond appropriately to TRH, as well as to endogenous thyroid levels	No response	Exaggerated response if primary hypothyroid; no response in pituitary	Very sensitive test to determine hyperthyroid state if other tests do not indicate such
Thyroid scan	Isotopes scan with ^{123}I or $^{99}TcO_4$	Areas of hypofunctioning (cold) and areas of hyperfunctioning (hot), as well as size of gland	Diffusely enlarged; can have hot areas	Not usually done unless discrete nodules are felt on physical examination	

[a] Normal values will vary with laboratories.

tuations in the total iodide pool, either through dietary or therapeutic maneuvers, will alter the true value of the RAIU (see Table 26.2).

HYPOTHALAMIC-PITUITARY FUNCTION

The following tests measure the function and regulation of the negative feedback hypothalamic-pituitary axis: the triiodothyronine (T_3) suppression test, the serum thyrotropin (TSH), and the thyrotropin-releasing hormone test (TRH) (see Table 26.1).

T_3 Suppression Test

The T_3 suppression test determines whether there is autonomy of any thyroidal tissue (not under negative feedback control). Most hyperfunctioning tissues operate independently of TSH stimulation; Graves' disease being the prime example.

First, a baseline RAIU is obtained. Then suppression doses of T_3 (25 μg q.i.d.) is administered for 7 days, after which a repeat RAIU is obtained. Normally, TSH suppression by T_3 administration will result in a decrease of the RAIU 30 to 50% from baseline. Little or no change in RAIU as compared to the baseline RAIU indicates autonomous function.

The presence of early asymptomatic Graves' disease and the prognosis of thionamide therapy may be clarified with the T_3 suppression test (7).

TSH Levels

TSH levels by radioimmune assay provide one of the most sensitive indices of hypothyroidism and can be used to monitor adequate response to replacement therapy. Elevations in serum TSH occur early in the course of thyroid failure and may be present before overt clinical and laboratory manifestations of hypothyroidism appear from disease or from treatment with antithyroid therapy, radioactive iodine, or surgery. TSH concentrations do not provide valuable information in hyperthyroidism.

The serum TSH can also be used to differentiate primary thyroid failure from diminished pituitary TSH reserve (secondary). TSH measurements are falsely elevated in pregnancy where high levels of human chorionic gonadotropins (HCG) can interfere with TSH determinations. The TSH is valuable in excluding primary thyroid failure but not sec-

Table 26.2.
Summary of Laboratory Alterations by Drugs/Disease States[a]

Drugs/Disease	Mechanism	T_4 (RIA)	RT_3U	FTI	Serum T_3	^{131}I Uptake	TSH	Comment
Estrogens, oral contraceptives, clofibrate, heroin addicts, methadone maintenance, genetic, pregnancy, acute and chronic active hepatitis	Increase serum TBG concentrations	↑	↓	No change	↑	No change	No change	FTI corrects for alterations in TBG, reflects true thyroid status
Androgens, anabolic steroids, danazol, glucocorticoids, L-asparaginase, nephrotic syndrome, cirrhosis, genetic	Decrease serum TBG concentration	↓	↑	No change	↓	No change	No change	FTI corrects for alterations in TBG, reflects true thyroid status
Phenytoin, high dose salicylates (4–5 g), phenylbutazone, Fenoclofenac, Halofenate, mitotane, chloral hydrate, 5-fluorouracil	Displacement of T_4, T_3 from TBG	↓	↑ or little to no change	No change *↓ free T_4 with phenytoin	↓	No change, ^{131}I ↓ with phenyl butazone	No change	FTI corrects for alterations in TBG, reflects true thyroid status
Iodide-containing compounds—contrast medium, Providone-iodine, kelp, tincture iodine, saturated solution potassium iodide (SSKI), Lugol's solution	Dilution of total body iodide pools	No change if test done by radioimmune assay	No change	No change	No change	↓	No change	No change in thyroid status
Strong diuresis by furosemide, ethacrynic acid; iodine deficiency	Decrease total body iodide pools	No change	No change	No change	No change	Variable	No change	No change in thyroid status
Phenytoin (also see section on displacement)	Alter cellular uptake and metabolism of T_4	↓	↑ or no change	↓	No change	No change	No change	No change in thyroid status

Drug	Mechanism				Comments
Phenobarbital	Hepatic enzyme inducer of T$_4$ metabolism	↓ in hypothyroid patients, no change in euthyroid	Normal or ↓	No change	Patient is clinically euthyroid. Free T$_4$ is normal or slightly elevated In severe illness T$_4$ binding to TBG is impaired
Propranolol, glucocorticoids, old age, fasting, malnutrition, acute and chronic systemic illness	Impair peripheral conversion of T$_4$ to T$_3$; ↑rT$_3$	Normal or ↓	Normal or ↑	→	
Amiodarone, iopodate, iopanoate	Impair peripheral and pituitary conversion of T$_4$ to T$_3$	Normal or ↑	→	↑	Patient is clinically euthyroid; but can cause hyper- or hypothyroidism in patient with underlying thyroid disorders

[a] See Table 26.1 for use of abbreviations.

ondary failure in patients with the "euthyroid sick syndrome."

Thyrotropin-releasing Hormone (TRH) Test

The TRH stimulation test is an easy and safe test that can be done on an outpatient basis with the availability of the synthetic TRH, protirelin. Rarely, reversible hypotension and shock have been reported (8).

Normally, when TRH 200 to 400 μg is administered to euthyroid patients, a 2- to 4-fold increase in TSH levels is expected within 15 to 30 min. Greater TSH responses are seen in women than in men (Table 26.3).

The value of the TRH test is in the diagnosis of strongly suspected thyrotoxicosis when other clinical and laboratory indices are not confirmatory, i.e., ophthalmic euthyroid Graves'. Since exogenous hormones are not administered, it is a much safer test and preferred diagnostically over the T$_3$ suppression test which exposes potentially toxic patients to even greater hormone elevations and toxicity. In thyrotoxic patients, a flat TSH hormone would be expected since high circulating thyroid hormone levels should block further rises of TSH after TRH administration.

The TRH test can be used to document nonprimary forms of hypothyroidism, but has limited value in differentiating secondary (pituitary) from tertiary (hypothalamic) hypothyroidism, since results may not always be consistent.

Pituitary hypothyroidism is highly likely with an absent TSH response to TRH, whereas an hypothalamic etiology would be suspected if a delayed sluggish TSH rise to TRH is seen. In primary (thyroid) hypothyroidism, the TRH is of little value since basal TSH levels are already elevated.

A blunted TSH response may occur with increased age, renal failure, depression, starvation, and high circulating cortisol levels (9).

Tests of Autoimmunity

ANTIBODIES

Two main antigens have been identified in the thyroid gland: thyroglobulin and the microsomal component. The presence of thyroglobulin (TgAb) and microsomal antibodies (Anti-M) suggest the presence of an autoimmune process as seen in Graves' disease and Hashimoto's thyroiditis (10). However, since positive antibodies may also occur in other

Table 26.3.
Factors Affecting Thyrotropic Releasing Hormone (TRH) Response

Dysfunction	TSH Level before Thyrotropin-releasing Hormone (TRH) Administration	TSH Response after TRH Administration	Comments
Hyperthyroidism	Low	No/impaired response	Useful for diagnosis in elderly or cardiac patients where T_3 suppression test may produce toxicity
Pituitary hypothyroidism (secondary)	Low/absent	No/impaired response	
Hypothalamic (tertiary) hypothyroidism	Low	Sluggish response; delayed up to 60 min	
Primary (thyroid) hypothyroidism	High	Exaggerated	Offers no extra information

disorders, such as collagen vascular diseases and in an asymptomatic patient population, their presence is not diagnostic of thyroid disease. The levels of thyroglobulin and microsomal antibodies are consistently higher during the acute phases of the disease and decline with remission and treatment. The microsomal antibodies may be the more sensitive of the two as detectable levels may remain during remission while antithyroglobulin levels are undetectable.

LONG ACTING THYROID STIMULATOR (LATS)

LATS is an abnormal gamma globulin which is capable of stimulating the thyroid for up to 10 hours. It is immunologically distinct from TSH although it can displace TSH from its receptor sites and activate adenylcyclase to increase thyroid response. The presence of LATS in a patient's serum is detected through its ability to stimulate the mouse thyroid (LATS bioassay). Although LATS is pathognomonic for Graves' disease, only 40% of patients with Graves will produce a positive mouse reaction. Thus, the specific role of LATS in Graves' disease is unsettled.

THYROID STIMULATING ANTIBODY (TsAb)

Another stimulating IgG immunoglobulin has been uncovered in patients with Graves' and a negative LATS bioassay. This immunoglobulin is almost always found in the serum of patients with Graves' disease. This activity has several acronyms although thyroid stimulating immunoglobulin (TSI) is common. Its presence and disappearance in the serum of patients with treated Graves' disease may be useful as a prognostic indicator of relapse and remission (11).

There are two main techniques for the assay of TsAb. One measures the ability of this antibody to inhibit the binding of TSH to its receptor, although inhibition of TSH to its receptor is not necessarily equivalent to thyroid stimulation. The other is a direct measurement of the stimulation of the human thyroid *in vivo* as indicated by an increase in the concentration of cyclic AMP (10, 11).

NONSPECIFIC INDICES

A number of nonspecific tests are related to changes in thyroid function. Serum cholesterol, carotene, SGOT, creatine phosphokinase (CPK), and LDH levels may be elevated with hypothyroidism while cholesterol and carotene levels may be depressed in hyperthyroidism.

HYPERTHYROIDISM

SYMPTOMS

Hyperthyroidism or thyrotoxicosis is characterized by increased metabolism of all body systems due to excessive quantities of thyroid hormone. The clinical symptoms are listed in Table 26.4 and reflect increased adrenergic activity, primarily cardiovascular and neurological. Not all manifestations will be present in the same patient.

Thyrotoxicosis-induced increases in heart rate (HR), stroke volume (SV), and cardiac output may present as new onset or worsening angina, atrial fibrillation, extrasystoles, or con-

Table 26.4.
Signs and Symptoms of Hyperthyroidism and Hypothyroidism

Body System	Hyperthyroidism	Hypothyroidism
General	Heat intolerance; weight loss despite increased appetite; increased sweating	Cold intolerance; weight gain despite decreased appetite; hoarseness and lowering of the voice pitch; decreased sweating, easy fatigability
Head	Thinning of the hair; fine texture	Dry, brittle, and sparse hair; thinning of the lateral aspects of the eyebrows; puffy facies, large tongue
Eyes	Prominence of the eyes, lid lag, lid retraction, can proceed to loss of visual acuity	Edematous eyelids; ptosis
Neck	Soft diffusely enlarged goiter with or without bruits/thrills	Goiter in primary hypothyroidism none found in pituitary disorders
Cardiac	Palpitations; high output failure; edema; increased pulse and systolic pressure; wide pulse pressure; presence of systolic murmurs	Cardiac enlargement; poor heart sounds; precordial pain; low output failure; dyspnea
Gastrointestinal	Diarrhea, loose bowels, or hyperdefecation	Constipation
Genitourinary	Amenorrhea or decreased in length of menstrual flow	Menorrhagia, dysmenorrhea
Extremities	Pretibial myxedema; Plummer's nails; hot, flushed and moist skin; palmar erythema	Broad hands and feet; pretibial myxedema; cold and dry skin; brittle nails, yellowish
Neuromuscular	Fatigue, weakness, tremor, rapid deep tendon reflexes	Muscle pain and weakness, paresthesias; delayed deep tendon reflexes
Emotional	Nervousness, irritability, emotional liability; insomnia or shortened sleep cycles	Emotional instability, depression, lethargy, decreased energy and increased sleep requirements; mental sluggishness

gestive heart failure; these will usually be unresponsive to further treatment until an euthyroid state is achieved. Clinically, a rapid bounding pulse, an elevated systolic blood pressure, a wide pulse pressure, cardiomegaly, and a systolic murmur are seen. Tachycardia, increased voltage, and a prolonged P-R interval may be seen on electrocardiogram (ECG). It is important to eliminate thyrotoxicosis as a cause or exacerbation of cardiac disease before definitive pharmacologic treatment is instituted, since drug action, as with digitalis, may be altered.

Occasionally, a severely toxic patient may not present with any of these described manifestations. This is known as "apathetic" or masked hyperthyroidism, and is commonly seen in the elderly patient after long-standing thyrotoxicosis (12). The presenting symptoms of fatigue, apathy, listlessness, dull eyes, extreme weakness, congestive heart failure, delayed speech and mentation, and low grade fever may obscure the diagnosis. Premature atrial contractions, atrial fibrillation, or tremor may be the only presenting symptom. Untreated, coma and death are assured. The presence of such a state can be confirmed by standard laboratory tests.

ETIOLOGY

Thyrotoxicosis is a disorder of various etiologies despite the common denominator of accelerated metabolism and excessive quantities of thyroid hormone. The primary causes of hyperthyroidism are listed in Table 26.5.

Graves' Disease

Graves' disease is characterized by symptoms of hyperthyroidism, a diffusely enlarged

Table 26.5.
Etiology of Hyperthyroidism

Graves' disease:	Toxic diffuse goiter
Toxic nodules:	Single and multinodular
Jod-Basedow:	Iodine-induced
Factitious	Self-administration
Tumors	Secretion of thyroid stimulating substance
Subacute thyroiditis:	Viral inflammatory condition
Hashitoxicosis	Early phase of Hashimoto's
T_3-toxicosis	Often precedes onset of T_4-toxicosis

Table 26.6.
Characteristics of Graves' Disease

1. Triad of hyperthyroidism, goiter, and ophthalmopathy
2. Laboratory findings:
   Elevated T_4 (RIA), RT_3U, FTI, RAIU, T_3-RIA; presence of antimicrosomal and antithyroglobulin antibodies, negative T_3 suppression tests, presence of LATS/TSI, flat TRH response curve

goiter, infiltrative ophthalmopathy, dermopathy, and acropachy, although all of these findings are not usually found at one time.

The diagnosis of Graves' is confirmed by elevated levels of T_4 (RIA), RT_3U, FT_4I, T_3-RIA and RAIU, positive assays for TsAb, presence of antibodies in 95% of patients with Graves', a nonsuppressible T_3 suppression test, and a negative response to TRH (Table 26.6).

Although the exact etiology of the disease is unknown, certain observations can be made: it is predominantly a disease of females (5:1 ratio) with its peak onset occurring between the ages of 30 to 40; it has a strong familiar association although the exact mode of genetic transmission has not been determined; precipitation of the disease has been associated with severe emotional stress, weight reduction involving severe diet restriction, use of stimulants, use of thyroid hormone, trauma, and with the administration of iodides in endemic goiter areas (Jod-Basedow).

The pathogenesis of Graves' disease, as well as Hashimoto's thyroiditis, appears to be an autoimmune phenomena related to genetic defects in immunological surveillance or control due to disorders of the regulatory suppressor T lymphocytes. The major subsets of T lymphocytes are helper and suppressor T lymphocytes. Normally, helper T lymphocytes interact with B lymphocytes to produce appropriate immunoglobulins, while suppressor T lymphocytes exercise immunological surveillance by preventing T lymphocytes from inappropriately producing immunoglobulins. In Graves' disease, a defect in suppressor T lymphocytes may be responsible for formation of the abnormal thyroid-stimulating immunoglobulin (TSI) found in the blood of most patients with active disease (10, 13, 14). The

presence of lymphocytic infiltration of the thyroid gland, IgG immunoglobulins, and antibodies directed against both thyroglobulin and microsomal tissue strongly support an autoimmune basis for Graves' disease.

The Graves' gland is usually diffusely enlarged and symmetrical with a firm but rubbery consistency. Thrills and bruits may be found in a hyperfunctioning goiter. A thrill, which is less common, is likely to be felt in the region of the superior thyroid arteries. Bruits are usually audible over the entire thyroid gland. Both will disappear as a euthyroid state is reached.

OPHTHALMOPATHY

The ocular manifestations consist of the noninfiltrative and the characteristic infiltrative ophthalmopathy of Graves' (15). The noninfiltrative ocular abnormalities result from hyperactivity of the sympathetic system and can be found in any thyrotoxic condition. Increased sympathetic stimuli on Muller's superior palpebral muscle result in spasm and retraction of the upper lid to produce widening of the palpebral tissue to give the characteristic stare or frightened expression. On physical examination, lid lag (lid falls behind movement of the eye and a narrow white rim of sclerae becomes visible between upper lid and cornea) is apparent. These types of ocular changes are nontoxic to ocular function and are reversible with control of the thyrotoxicosis.

The infiltrative ocular findings are the most striking abnormality of Graves' disease. They may appear before the presence of thyrotoxicosis, during the acute phases, or even years after successful treatment. The ocular involvement may be unilateral or bilateral and may not be reversible despite achievement of a euthyroid state. Interestingly, the most severe manifestations are often encountered in patients who are euthyroid or hypothyroid after radioactive iodine ablation (15–17).

It is not known why the eyes and associated muscles are attacked while other organ systems are exempt. Histological examination reveals lymphocytic infiltration, deposition of mucopolysaccharides, fat, and water in all retrobulbar tissues, which accounts for the unique symptomology.

Mild eye symptoms are found in 50% of patients while the more severe forms occur in less than 5% (15). Various degrees of the following signs and symptoms may be seen:

1. Edema and swelling of the lids and periorbital tissue, resulting in chemosis, excessive lacrimation, photophobia, and conjunctivitis.
2. Proptosis: Increase in the orbital contents causes the proptosis or protrusion of the cornea more than 18 mm beyond the lateral margin of the orbit. This may result in a wide-eyed staring expression. The globes are firmer and harder than normal. Increased tearing and irritation may occur from the exposed conjunctiva. Cornea scarring and ulceration occurs if severe proptosis prevents lid closure during sleep.
3. Paralysis of the extraocular muscles, resulting in loss of upward gaze; and convergence is most common. Diplopia and complete loss of extraocular movement can occur.
4. Blindness may result in venous congestion and hemorrhage of the retina and optic nerve.

DERMOPATHY

The dermopathy of Graves' disease, also known as pretibial myxedema, can be associated with infiltrative exophthalmos. Mucopolysaccharide infiltration of the skin accounts for the thickening and hyperpigmentation of the skin usually seen over the tibial aspect of the leg, although similar lesions can appear on the dorsum of the feet and hands. Pretibial myxedema usually cause no symptoms but at times may be painful or frequently the source of much itching. Like the exophthalmos, it can occur at any time in the course of the disease, with or without exophthalmos, goiter, or thyrotoxicosis. A clinical diagnosis can be confirmed by tissue biopsy if necessary. Treat-

ment with topical corticosteroids is often effective.

Toxic/Multinodular Disease

Toxic nodule (Plummer's disease) is characterized by a single autonomous hyperfunctioning nodule (18). The nodule, usually 3–5 cm in diameter, produces supraphysiological doses of hormone with suppression of normal thyroid tissue. Patients can either be euthyroid or toxic. A toxic nodule appears on scan as an area of increased iodine concentration. This is the least common of the three major types of hyperthyroidism.

Patients who have a large firm multinodular gland (more than one nodule) can remain completely asymptomatic for many years. The new onset of thyrotoxicosis in patients in their 5th or 6th decade of life often results from activation of many autonomous nodules within the multinodular gland (18). This is the most common form of thyrotoxicosis in the elderly.

Subacute Thyroiditis

Subacute thyroiditis (DeQuervain's thyroiditis) is a spontaneous remitting inflammatory condition of the thyroid which is believed to have a viral etiology (19). The clinical features include a diffuse or localized swelling of the gland associated with tenderness or difficulty in swallowing, flu-like symptoms of fever and malaise, and symptoms of hyperthyroidism. Laboratory manifestations include elevated erythrocyte sedimentation rate (ESR), low or undetectable RAIU, leukocytosis, and often a high T_4 and PBI level due to leakage of iodoproteins from the damaged gland in the early stages of the disease. Hypothyroidism can occur if the process is long standing, although spontaneous recovery is most common. Treatment is symptomatic and consists of heat, rest, and analgesics. In the nontoxic hypothyroid phase, thyroid administration is required to suppress further TSH stimulation and activation of a tender and enlarged gland.

T_3 Toxicosis

Hyperthyroidism of any etiology usually suggest excessive levels of T_4. However, the role of T_3 in thyrotoxicosis is just beginning to be understood.

T_3 thyrotoxicosis is characterized by normal levels of T_4 and elevated levels of T_3. It has been associated with Graves' disease, toxic goiters, carcinomas, and has been reported in children. Preferential T_3 secretion and toxicity may be more prevalent in iodine-deficient areas. Elevated T_3 levels in asymptomatic patients often precede the onset of frank T_4 toxicosis and can be used as a prognostic sign of relapse/remission after the withdrawal of antithyroid medications (20).

Drug-induced Thyrotoxicosis

Iodine-induced thyrotoxicosis (Jod-Basedow) was first described in the 1800s in residents of iodine-deficient areas who became symptomatic after adequate iodine supplementation. The most widespread epidemic of thyrotoxicosis occurred in Tasmania following iodization of bread. Most cases appeared in patients with multinodular goiters and autonomous nodules which were activated by the increased iodine supplements (4). Although it is believed that iodides only induce thyrotoxicosis in patients with abnormal glands residing in iodine-deficient areas, reports have appeared stating that this is not so (21). Thyrotoxicosis following injection of radiocontrast material has also been reported (22, 23).

The withdrawal of lithium, paradoxically, has been associated with the development of hyperthyroidism. Since lithium acts like iodides in preventing hormone release, it is likely that lithium may be suppressing frank hyperthyroidism which became evident after its withdrawal. Therefore, lithium has been advocated for the treatment of hyperthyroidism (24).

Rarely, thyrotoxicosis results from thyrotropin-secreting pituitary tumors, from ectopic thyroid tissue (e.g., struma ovarii), from TSH-like substances produced by hydatidiform moles and choriocarcinomas, from self-administration of thyroid (factitious hyperthyroidism), from posttraumatic or radiation injury to the thyroid, and from the initial transient stages of Hashimoto's thyroiditis.

Treatment of Thyrotoxicosis

The major treatment modalities for the management of thyrotoxicosis are the antithyroid drugs, radioactive iodine (RAI), and surgery (Table 26.7) (25). Each has its own advantages and limitations, so that treatment must be individualized. The type of hyperthyroidism, the severity, the patient's age, the existence of thyroidal and nonthyroidal complications, and

social and economic issues will also influence this decision-making process. For example, patients with Graves' disease may be managed medically until remission hopefully occurs. However, patients with toxic multinodular disease usually require definitive treatment with radioactive iodine or surgery. Thyrotoxic women who plan to be pregnant in the near future may wish to have their thyrotoxicosis permanently controlled prior to pregnancy with surgery or radioactive iodine since a high degree of relapse may occur during early pregnancy and postpartum (26). Regardless of later forms of therapy, most patients and definitely all severely thyrotoxic patients should be started initially on antithyroid medications to reduce their hypermetabolic rate before treatment with RAI or surgery is instituted. However, often the final decision in the uncomplicated patient is empiric, depending upon available resources and the physician's experience. In such patients, the final selection should be a joint patient-physician decision after discussion of the benefits and risks of each method.

Pharmacologic Management

THIOAMIDES

The thioamides, propylthiouracil (PTU), and methimazole prevent thyroid hormone synthesis by inhibiting the oxidation binding of iodide and its coupling to tyrosine residue. PTU, but not methimazole, inhibits the peripheral deiodination of T_4 to T_3. In addition, an immunosuppressive mechanism of action has been postulated.

Thioamides have been preferred over radioactive iodine and surgery since they do not destroy the gland but control the disease until remission occurs, so that long term thyroid replacement is not necessary. However, this advantage of thioamides may be less important since the natural history of Graves' disease is the development of hypothyroidism even if no glandular destruction occurs (27).

Biopharmaceutics

Methimazole is 10 times more potent than PTU (100 mg of PTU = 10 mg of methimazole); they are clinically equally effective when given in equipotent doses. Theoretically, PTU rather than methimazole may be the preferred agent since it can block the peripheral conversion of T_4 to T_3 (28). Both drugs are rapidly absorbed from the gastrointestinal tract and

Table 26.7.
Management of Thyrotoxicosis

Method	Drug	Dose	Mechanism of Action	Toxicity	Comments
Thioamides	Propylthiouracil (PTU) 50-mg tablets	100–200 mg every 6 hr initially, maintenance of 50–150 mg daily	Blocks organification of hormone synthesis, also inhibits peripheral conversion of T_4 to T_3. Immunosuppressive?	Skin rashes, agranulocytosis, gastrointestinal symptoms, hepatitis	Poor remission rate of 20–30%. Onset of action approximately 2–4 weeks
	Methimazole (Tapazole) 5- and 10-mg tablets	10–30 mg every 8 hr initially, maintenance of 10–30 mg daily	Blocks organification of hormone synthesis. Immunosuppressive?	Same as PTU. Secreted in breast milk, tetratogenic	Appears to have no cross sensitivity to PTU with regard to rashes. Longer duration of action than PTU
Iodides	Lugol's solution 8 mg iodide/drop Saturated solution of potassium iodide (SSKI) 50 mg/drop	6 mg iodide/day although larger doses are given	Blocks release of hormone from the gland; decreases the vascularity of the gland and increases the firmness—facilitates easier removal of the gland during surgery	Hypersensitivity reactions—rashes, rhinorrhea, parotid and submaxillary swelling	Can be used to control hyperthyroidism in patients with small glands and mild disease, Used in thyroid storm
Adrenergic antagonist	Propranolol (Inderal) 10-, 40-, 80-mg tablets, 1 mg/cc IV	20–40 mg orally every 6 hr	Blocks the peripheral action of thyroid hormone, no effect on underlying disease state	Bradycardia, congestive heart failure, asthma, inhibits hyperglycemic response to hypoglycemia	Acute onset provides symptomatic relief of symptoms while awaiting onset of action of thioamides, RAI, or surgery
Radioactive iodine	^{131}I	80 to 100 μCi per gram of thyroid tissue	Destruction of the gland	Hypothyroidism, fear of malignancy, leukemia, and genetic damage	Slow onset of action-approximately 2–4 weeks, full effects seen within 3–6 months
Surgery	Iodides, thioamides, or propranolol preoperative to induce relief of symptoms	5–10 drops/day of iodides for 10–14 days prior to surgery. See above doses for propranolol and thioamides	Total or subtotal removal of the gland	Hypothyroidism, hypoparathyroidism, complications of surgery and anesthesia	Should not perform a second thyroidectomy due to higher incidence of complications in a second operation. Total thyroidectomy is treatment of choice

peak plasma concentrations are reached within 30 min of ingestion.

The serum half-lives of 4 to 6 hours for methimazole and 1 to 2 hours for PTU do not change as the thyroid status changes. Despite the short half-lives, it appears that the duration of action is much longer so that PTU is effective if given every 6 hours and methimazole is given every 8 hours (28).

Treatment

Therapy is initiated with either 400 to 1200 mg/day of PTU given in four divided doses or 40 to 120 mg/day of methimazole given in three divided doses, depending on the degree of thyrotoxicosis. In very severe disease where the gland may be larger than four times the normal size, doses as high as 1200 mg/day of PTU or its equivalence given in divided doses may be required. The initial dose should be gradually reduced on a monthly basis to a maintenance dose of 50 to 300 mg/day of PTU or its equivalence given in either divided or a single dose regimen. Tapering of the antithyroid dosage should not begin until reduction of symptoms and normalization of circulating thyroxine levels are achieved, usually 4 to 8 weeks (dependent on elimination of existing thyroid stores; $t_{1/2}$ = 7 days). If alleviation of symptoms is not seen within the specified time, then factors such as patient noncompliance, incomplete blockage of synthesis by insufficient dosage, or inadequate dosing interval should be ascertained as causes of failure. Although it is not recommended here, some clinics advocate the concomitant use of thyroxine during antithyroid therapy to prevent hypothyroidism and suppress goiter formation resulting from excessive PTU or methimazole dosage.

Prior to administration of the thioamides, a baseline T_4 (RIA), RT_3U, FT_4I, and WBC with differential should be obtained. The therapeutic response is monitored by a repeat T_4 (RIA), RT_3U, and FT_4I after 1 month of therapy and 1 month after any change in dosing regimen. The laboratory results should parallel the clinical response. A baseline WBC with differential is helpful in ascertaining the development of agranulocytosis since hyperthyroidism per se can be associated with a relative reduction in neutrophil count.

Therapy is empirically recommended for 12 to 18 months although short-term treatment of 3 to 4 months has produced similar remission rates (29). However, short-term therapy needs further evaluation before becoming the recommended standard of practice, especially since therapy of greater than 1 year's duration has been associated with a greater frequency of long-term remission after treatment is discontinued (30, 31).

Hyperthyroid patients on thioamides can be managed by the pharmacist using a protocol (see Fig. 26.2).

Single-Daily Dose. A single-daily dose regimen of PTU or methimazole has been shown to be effective in selected patients (32–34). Although a single dose regimen throughout the entire treatment period may be effective for patients with mild disease, the best results are obtained by achievement of a euthyroid state through multiple dosing before changing to a single dose schedule. Methimazole is preferred because of its longer duration of action of 24 to 36 hours. The potassium perchlorate discharge test may predict which patients can be successfully managed by a single dose regimen. By administration of this test 12 hours after the last thioamide dose, Barnes and Bledsoe (35) were able to predict an optimal dosing schedule with 91% accuracy. The availability of such a therapeutic regimen allows for better patient acceptability, compliance and greater success. This schedule awaits further research.

Prognosis

The success rate of 30 to 40% (36, 37) or less for remission had led to the progressive disenchantment with the antithyroid drugs as a definitive form of therapy. However, a high rate of remission (67%) was noted in patients receiving 1 to 5 years of thioamide therapy (30, 31). The low success rate has been attributed by some to increased dietary iodine intake (38). A higher rate of permanent remission is achieved in those patients with small goiters, a short and mild duration of symptoms and disease, a reduction in goiter size during treatment, positive evidence of suppression with the T_3-suppression test and absence of TsAb after withdrawal of antithyroid agents (7, 11, 25, 39, 40). Analysis of HLA specificities (HLA-B8 and DW3) combined with level of IgG Immunoglobulin may be highly predictive of remission or relapse after withdrawal of thioamides (41, 42).

Adverse Reactions

Toxic reactions to PTU and methimazole range from 3 to 12% of patients depending on the dose and the drug.

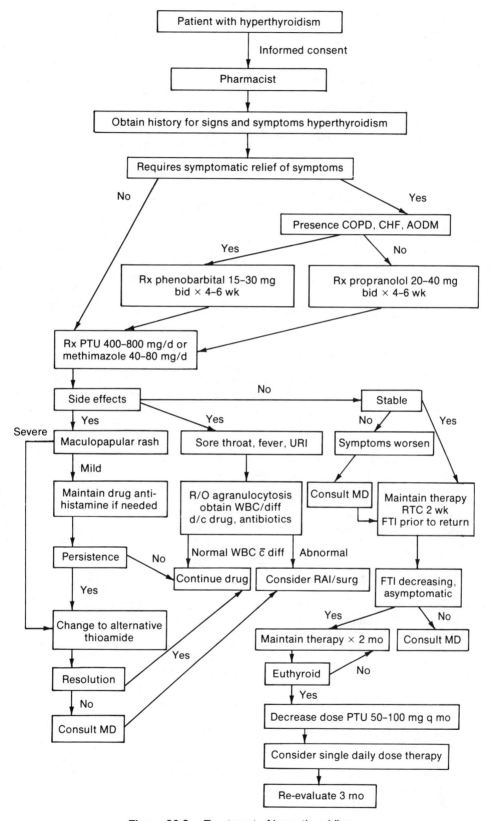

Figure 26.2. Treatment of hyperthyroidism.

Pruritic maculopapular skin rashes without other systemic manifestations are the most frequently encountered reactions and often disappear spontaneously despite continued therapy. If the rash persists, another thioamide can be substituted since there is little cross-sensitivity with regard to this side effect. However, if there is concomitant systemic symptoms, i.e. fever, substitution with another thioamide is not recommended.

Agranulocytosis constitutes the most serious reaction of the thioamides (43). The onset of fever, malaise, gingivitis, and sore throat is so abrupt that routine WBC counts are useless. Therefore, patients should be instructed to report the acute onset of such symptoms immediately to a pharmacist or physician. The incidence is variable between 0.5 to 6% and is higher in older patients (over age 40) receiving larger amounts of methimazole (greater than 40 mg/day) although the reaction is not necessarily dose-related, i.e. 2 cases out of 25 (8% incidence) in patients taking 120 mg/day of methimazole (44, 44a). Low dose (<30 mg/d) methimazole may be safer than high dose therapy or treatment with PTU (44a). Sex is not a predilectory factor. This type of reaction may be more frequent during the first 6 weeks of therapy although it can occur at any time in the course of treatment. Fortunately, complete reversal is often seen after withdrawal. If infection occurs, antibiotics, adrenal steroids, and possibly hospitalization (bacteria-free room) is indicated. After return of granulocyte counts within a few days to three weeks, rechallenge with the same drug or a different drug may or may not produce the same reaction since little information is available regarding cross-sensitivity in this area.

The thioamides have been associated with the development of serological abnormalities (lupus erythematosus (LE), antinuclear antibody (ANA)), lupus, and lupus-like syndromes. Recovery occurs upon withdrawal or institution of steroids. Hepatitis of an obstructive nature and hypoprothrombinemia are rare.

MONOVALENT ANIONS

Potassium perchlorate is the only member of the monovalent anions with sufficient antithyroid action to be clinically useful. In doses of 1 g/day perchlorate is concentrated by the gland, interferes with the gland's iodide binding, and causes the discharge of nonorganified iodide from the gland. Since perchlorate is a competitive inhibitor of iodide its antithyroid effect can be overcome by iodine administration. The severe toxicity of irreversible aplastic anemia and nephrotic syndrome has limited the usefulness of the monovalent anions.

IODIDES

Although iodides have been noted since the 1920s to relieve the symptoms of thyrotoxicosis, their clinical usage has largely been superseded by the introduction of the thioamides and the β-blockers. Several effects have been recognized when iodides are administered: inhibition of organification ("Wolff-Chaikoff" effect), inhibition of hormone release, and a decrease in gland size and vascularity (4). However, the rapid relief of thyrotoxic symptoms within 2 to 7 days of iodide administration suggest that inhibition of hormone release is the predominant mechanism of action rather than a block in organification which would not be apparent for several weeks. This rapid response has been beneficial in the therapy of thyroid storm and while awaiting the therapeutic effectiveness of thioamide therapy. However, they should not be used prior to RAI therapy or if RAI is to be eventually considered since iodide administration can block effective RAI concentration by the gland for several weeks after its discontinuation.

Iodides have routinely been used 10 to 14 days prior to surgery since the observation that they decrease the vascularity and increase the firmness of the hyperplastic gland so that surgical removal is easier. The combination of propranolol and iodides preoperatively has been recommended (45) although the established regimen of thioamides and iodides is preferred.

Stable iodine is available as either Lugol's solution (5% iodine and 10% potassium iodide) containing 8 mg of iodide per drop, or as the more palatable saturated solution of potassium iodide (SSKI) containing 50 mg/drop. A parental preparation, sodium iodide is also available.

The major toxicity from iodides are hypersensitivity reactions including skin rashes, drug fever, sialadenitis, conjunctivitis, rhinitis, and collagen vascular disorders. In susceptible individuals iodides can induce either hyperthyroidism or precipitate goiter and hypothyroidism as a result of failure of the Wolff-

Chaikoff block or failure to escape from the Wolff-Chaikoff block respectively (4).

Advantages of iodide therapy include simplicity, low cost, low toxicity, and no gland destruction. Limitations of treatment include gland escape, treatment relapse, allergic reactions, and interference with subsequent RAI therapy.

LITHIUM

Lithium, which acts like iodides in inhibiting hormone release, has been used in the treatment of thyrotoxicosis in doses of 800 to 1200 mg/day. Lithium serum levels must be closely maintained between 0.5 and 1 $\mu g/ml$ to avoid side effects of tremor, ataxia, dizziness, confusion, coma, nausea, vomiting, diarrhea, cardiac arrhythmias and circulatory collapse. Hyponatremia or sodium depletion through the use of diuretics will increase lithium toxicity. For these reasons lithium is not a first line drug but should be reserved for special circumstances where iodides are contraindicated (24).

ADRENERGIC ANTAGONISTS

Since many of the signs and symptoms of thyrotoxicosis are mediated through sympathetic overactivity, drugs that deplete or block the effects of thyroid on tissue catecholamines can provide symptomatic relief prior to the onset of thioamide action or while awaiting RAI or surgery. Such agents do not affect the underlying fundamental process. Reserpine (0.25 mg to 4.0 mg PO or IM) and guanethidine (80 mg/day PO) have been used successfully. However, their slow onset (up to several weeks) and frequent side effects, especially marked hypotension have resulted in their replacement by propranolol or other β blockers. Since propranolol has been the most widely used and studied in the therapy of thyrotoxicosis, it will be recommended here in lieu of other β-blockers although all are effective. When propranolol is given orally in doses of 20 to 40 mg, 4 times a day, relief of most symptoms of palpitations, anxiety, sweating, tremor and diarrhea is seen, although weight loss remains unaffected (46). Younger and severely toxic patients may require as much as 240 to 480 mg/day to achieve relief of symptoms and β-blockade (47). Propranolol is surprisingly effective in controlling the neuromuscular manifestations, especially periodic paralysis. It is useful as an adjunct to thioamides and RAI therapy, as a preoperative medication for surgery, in neonatal thyrotoxicosis, in pregnancy and in thyroid storm. Caution should be used when giving any beta blockers to patients with chronic pulmonary obstructive disease (COPD), asthma, congestive heart failure (CHF), or insulin dependent diabetes. Propranolol should not be used alone since inadequate control of severe thyrotoxicosis may result in storm (48, 49).

The kinetics and blood levels of propranolol in euthyroid patients are subject to large interindividual variation. This has been attributed to the variable degree of a significant first pass effect seen with oral doses as well as to the presence of an active metabolite, 4-hydroxypropranolol. Data on the kinetics of propranolol in thyroid disease are limited and subject to criticism since little information is available about the metabolite. A shortened half-life and an increased volume of distribution may account for the lower plasma levels and the increased rate of clearance seen in toxic versus euthyroid patients. Although these changes may be due to alterations in hepatic blood flow or to individual variations, data suggest that higher propranolol doses may be acutely necessary in toxic patients due to the increased clearance rate. The converse is true in hypothyroidism (50, 51).

RADIOACTIVE IODINE (^{131}I)

Radioactive iodine is indicated in patients past adolescence, in patients with a history of prior thyroid surgery, in patients who are poor surgical risks because of complicating diseases, and in patients who have failed or had drug toxicity on thioamide therapy. It is absolutely contraindicated in pregnancy. It is the treatment of choice in thyrotoxicosis due to multinodular goiters.

The isotope most frequently used is ^{131}I which has a half-life of 8 days and delivers high energy β-radiation to a maximal depth of 2 mm. ^{125}I, which has a half-life of 60 days, has been used as an alternative to ^{131}I, in hopes of decreasing the incidence of hypothyroidism, without much success. ^{125}I emits γ-rays which penetrates only a few microns so that larger therapeutic doses are needed which considerably increase the total body radiation without decreasing the incidence of hypothyroidism.

The formula for calculation of the administered dose depends on an estimate of gland size, the amount of ^{131}I taken up, and the standard microcurie of iodine given per gram of thyroid tissue. At the University of California patients receive approximately 80 to 100 $\mu Ci/g$.

Millicuries (mCi) given

$$= \frac{\text{estimated gland weight (g)} \times 100 \ \mu Ci/g \times 100}{24\text{-hour RAI}}$$

Despite use of a formula the proper dose of RAI is difficult to calculate or predict. The optimal dose is one which prevents recurrent hyperthyroidism as well as hypothyroidism.

Pretreatment prior to RAI therapy with thioamides or propranolol to prevent exacerbation of thyrotoxicosis is recommended in patients with severe heart disease or large stores of hormones. Iodides should not be used prior to RAI therapy since the uptake of ^{131}I will be significantly blocked. If thioamides are used they should also be discontinued 1 week prior to and after RAI therapy to facilitate optimal ^{131}I uptake and retention. Propranolol can be used without fear of compromising RAI therapy.

The therapeutic response should be apparent in 2 to 3 weeks with peak effects occurring in 3 to 6 months after an ablation dose. The slow onset is a disadvantage but symptoms can be controlled by the use of iodides, thioamides, or propranolol. If a second dose is required, a larger dose of RAI must be given to optimize thyroidal uptake, thereby exposing the body to greater radiation.

The appropriate age limit for radioactive iodine therapy is controversial although increasing clinical experience has lowered the age limit from the initial 35. After more than 25 years of experience with RAI it is generally accepted as safe for most adults. Adolescents have also been safely treated with RAI although this is not recommended (52, 53).

The major fears regarding RAI therapy include carcinogenesis, leukemia, and genetic damage. So far, verification of any of these hazards has been undocumented but further study is needed (54–56). The radiation dose to the gonads in patients treated with ^{131}I is usually less than 3 rads which is not significantly different from gonadal irradiation received from commonly used diagnostic tests such as barium enemas or pyelograms (55). The major known complication of RAI is hypothyroidism,

which occurs in 10% of treated patients the first year and increases at a constant rate of 2.5%/year thereafter, accounting for 20-year incidence of 30 to 70% (57, 58). The immediate side effects of ^{131}I therapy are minimal but may include mild thyroidal pain and tenderness, dysphagia rarely, some temporary thinning of the hair, and also transient thyroiditis rarely.

RAI therapy is effective, quick, easy, painless, and relatively nontoxic.

IPODATE

The most promising agent in the clinical treatment of hyperthyroidism appears to be the iodinated contrast medium, sodium ipodate (Oragrafin) which contains 61.4% iodine. Although similar inhibition of T_3 production was seen with other iodinated contrast media such as iopanoic acid (Telepaque), ipodate was the most potent. Changes in T_3, T_4 and rT_3 which are consistent with inhibition of peripheral deiodination was demonstrated in euthyroid, hypothyroid patients on replacement therapy, and in hyperthyroid patients. When administered in a dose of 3 g orally every 3rd day to thyrotoxic patients, improvement in both subjective and objective symptoms, i.e. decreased pulse and increased weight were noted rapidly (59, 60). The laboratory findings were the most significant. Reduction in T_3 levels were apparent within 6 hours of ipodate administration; reaching 50% of baseline at 24 hours and 70% of baseline (nadir) at 48 hours. T_3 levels remained suppressed for up to 3 to 5 days after administration. Similarly, decline in T_4 levels reached their nadir 3 days after administration and remained depressed as long as 6 days after the last dose. When compared to propylthiouracil, ipodate produced earlier symptomatic and objective improvement in symptoms as well as decreases in T_3 hormone levels (61, 62). The prolonged effect on suppressing T_3 and T_4 levels suggest that inhibition of hormone release due to the iodine released may be an additional ipodate mechanism of action. Since ipodate is relatively nontoxic while causing a dramatic improvement in symptoms and hormone levels it may prove to be very useful in the adjunctive treatment of thyrotoxicosis.

Surgery

Thyroidectomy is an effective method of therapy for patients in whom RAI or thioamides are contraindicated; for patients with large goiters causing cosmetic disfigurement, respiratory embarrassment, or swallowing difficulties; for patients with a suspected malignancy; and for selected pregnant and pediatric patients. Prior thyroid surgery should be considered a strong deterrent to further surgery since reoperation increases the hazard of vocal cord paralysis and hypoparathyroidism 10-fold and 30-fold, respectively (63). Other contraindications include presence of severe cardiac, respiratory or debilitating diseases or third trimester pregnancy since spontaneous labor can be precipitated.

The ideal surgical endpoint is a remnant of thyroid tissue left after surgery that results in neither recurrence of disease or hypothyroidism. Although this is often unobtainable one series reported a 94% euthyroid success rate using a modified subtotal thyroidectomy (64). Although subtotal thyroidectomy is the most common form of surgery for hyperthyroidism, total thyroidectomy is recommended since recurrence of thyrotoxicosis is high if any thyroid remnant is left behind. Furthermore, it appears that hypothyroidism is inevitable due to the natural course of the disease so that subtotal procedures offer no advantage in decreasing the incidence of hypothyroidism.

Surgery appears to be as safe as other nonsurgical treatments for hyperthyroidism if it is performed by experienced hands in a patient who has been adequately prepared prior to surgery by the standard combination of thioamides, iodides or propranolol. In the aforementioned patients, numerous studies have consistently shown an absence of operative mortality and thyroid storm, and occurrence of vocal cord paralysis and permanent hypoparathyroidism in fewer than 1% of patients after a subtotal thyroidectomy.

The major complication, however, is hypothyroidism which can develop insidiously as late as 10 years postoperatively. Incidences ranging from 5 to 75% have been described. The incidence of hypothyroidism is inversely proportional to the remnant of thyroid tissue left; remnants of 2 to 4 g gave an incidence of 70% (65). Because of the catastrophic nature of these complications, only surgeons experienced in thyroid surgery should perform such operations.

The disadvantages of fear of surgery, expense, and postoperative complications may outweigh the advantages of rapid definitive surgical treatment.

Special Considerations

PREGNANCY

The combination of pregnancy and thyrotoxicosis is rare (0.02 to 1.4% of the pregnant population) since most hyperthyroid patients are relatively infertile. Usually the thyrotoxicosis and treatment antedates the pregnancy. The clinical manifestations of hyperthyroidism during pregnancy may be difficult to recognize since similar symptoms are inherent to both conditions. Also pregnancy appears to ameliorate the symptoms of thyrotoxicosis so that spontaneous remission may occur till after delivery. The basis for this improvement may be the fall in both the concentrations of thyroid-stimulating immunoglobulins (TSI) and titers of thyroid antibodies in pregnancy (66).

Pregnancy and hyperthyroidism create special problems for management of the mother since the fetal thyroid which begins functioning during the 12th to 14th week will also be at risk. If fetal thyroid function is an important consideration in the outcome for the child, then measurement of the levels of rT_3 and TSH in amniotic fluid (67) which reflect fetal thyroid function would be helpful in management of pregnant women with Graves' disease.

However, maternal thyrotoxicosis if untreated results in a high incidence of abortion, perinatal death, and prematurity so that treatment is indicated. Both surgical and medical management may be used but the final decision is likely to be governed by the physician's personal experience and the patient's decision.

Radioactive iodine is absolutely contraindicated since transplacental passage of ^{131}I will destroy the fetal thyroid. Chronic iodide administration should be avoided since the ingestion of as little as 12 mg of iodine throughout pregnancy has resulted in fetal goiter and asphyxiation (68). Use of vaginal povidone iodine should also be avoided since the high serum concentrations of iodine attained has resulted in hypothyroidism and transfer into breast milk (69–71).

Surgery can be performed in the second trimester after suitable preparation with thioamides or short-term administration of iodides. During the last trimester surgery is not recommended since spontaneous abortion can be precipitated.

Thioamides which cross the placenta can be used if certain precautions are followed. The danger of fetal goiter and hypothyroidism is negligible if initial doses of PTU or its equivalent are less than 300 mg/day given in divided doses and maintenance doses of 100 to 150 mg/day are employed throughout pregnancy. Clinically, the mother should be maintained in a comfortable "mildly hyperthyroid" state with the FTI in the upper ranges of normal to prevent fetal thyroid suppression (72). The appearance of an enlarged maternal goiter during therapy is alarming since it implies maternal and fetal hypothyroidism. The concomitant use of thyroid hormone is not recommended since it does not cross the placenta and may make maternal management more difficult.

Propylthiouracil is recommended over methimazole since it blocks the conversion of T_4 to T_3 and has not been associated with congenital deformities, i.e. aplasia cutis (73). Additionally, PTU may be preferred over methimazole in the breast-feeding mother since insignificant amounts of PTU are excreted in the milk while 7 to 16% of a methimazole dose is recovered in breast milk (74, 75).

Propranolol may be a reasonable alternative to propylthiouracil and iodides in the pregnant female. However, long-term usage of propranolol during pregnancy, especially in the last trimester, has been associated with fetal respiratory depression, small placenta, intrauterine-growth retardation, impaired responses to anoxic stress, postnatal bradycardia, and hypoglycemia (76). Propranolol is also excreted in breast milk and should not therefore be given to lactating mothers. Such findings indicate that propranolol, like iodides, should be used only on a short-term basis in pregnancy.

EXOPHTHALAMOS/OPHTHALMOLOGIC COMPLICATIONS

The pathogenesis and progression of the ocular symptoms are not well understood so that treatment is symptomatic and empiric once thyroid ablation and achievement of a euthyroid state has taken place. Progression of exophthalmos may be greatest in euthyroid patients treated with antithyroid agents as compared to radioactive iodine and surgery (16). Therefore, thyroid ablation is recommended before further treatment of the exophthalmos is pursued.

Periorbital edema and chemosis are best handled by elevation of the head of the bed to promote diuresis. Protective glasses, methylcellulose, and hydrocortisone drops as well as avoidance of smoke and dust may alleviate photophobia and external irritation. Taping the eyelids shut at night may be necessary to prevent corneal scarring and drying (17).

Systemic corticosteroids are considered to be beneficial in progressive exophthalmos associated with decreasing visual acuity. High doses of 80 to 120 mg/day of prednisone is administered for 1 to 2 weeks and then gradually withdrawn. The therapeutic effect is unpredictable and can be dramatic or absent. The mechanism is unclear although there is decreased conversion of T_4 to T_3 resulting in lowered levels of T_3 and LATS.

X-ray therapy to the orbits and pituitary with or without steroids may also be effective.

If none of the above medical measures halt the progression of the exophthalmos then surgical orbital decompression is warranted.

NEONATAL THYROTOXICOSIS

Neonatal thyrotoxicosis results from stimulation of the fetal thyroid through transplacental passage of LATS from the maternal circulation. The infants are extremely ill and require ancillary measures including sedation, cooling, oxygen, fluid and electrolyte replacement, as well as management of the thyrotoxicosis by thioamides, iodides, or propranolol. Fortunately, the disease is self-limiting and symptoms disappear in 1 to 2 months as the level of LATS falls. Antithyroid drugs should be withdrawn at this time (77).

PEDIATRICS

Hyperthyroidism in children is rare, accounting for about 1 to 5% of cases. It is unusual in the first 5 years of life; the peak incidences occur between the ages of 10 and 12 years. Similarities to the adult form include preponderance of females over males and precipitation of the disease by acute infections, trauma, and stress. The presenting signs and symptoms are similar in most respects, i.e. nervousness, weight loss, tremor, eye signs but with the notable exception of cardiovascular manifestations. Excessive thirst, behavioral manifestations of restlessness, and inability to concentrate incur difficulties in school and in family relationships.

Optimal management of the disease in children is controversial although all three methods, surgery, RAI, and thioamides, have been advocated.

Radioactive iodine is usually not employed

in most clinics due to the high risk of hypothyroidism and the fear of genetic damage, leukemia and carcinogenesis, although unsubstantiated (52, 53). External radiation to the head and neck of children is associated with a high risk of subsequent thyroid carcinoma and disease although the same results have not been shown with internal radiation (78).

The usual choice for treatment is between the antithyroid drugs and subtotal thyroidectomy. The risks of surgery, mortality, scar, recurrence of thyrotoxicosis with subtotals, hyothyroidism, laryngeal and parathyroid damage, must be weighed against its benefits of speedy correction of thyrotoxicosis and the lack of need for compliance to the rigid dosing schedules of the thioamides.

The use of thioamides in children is similar to the regimen of adults and may be the method of choice in patients with small goiters and mild disease where a high rate of remission is likely. The limitations of medical management include noncompliance, strict parental and physician supervision, and the possibility of adverse reaction as weighed against the advantages of treatment until spontaneous remission occurs without damage to the gland.

The appropriate method will depend upon the circumstances and individuals involved.

THYROID STORM

Thyroid storm is a medical emergency characterized by the following clinical features: (a) acute onset of high fever (sine qua non); (b) cardiovascular: tachycardia, tachypnea, shock, congestive heart failure, and arrhythmia; (c) gastrointestinal: diarrhea, vomiting, abdominal pain, and liver enlargement; and (d) central nervous system: agitation and psychosis progressing to apathy, stupor, and coma.

The pathogenesis of storm is not well understood but appears to be an exaggerated form of thyrotoxicosis which has been precipitated by childbirth, stress, infection, trauma, diabetic acidosis, RAI treatment, and the abrupt discontinuation of antithyroid medication.

Prompt recognition and immediate treatment has decreased the mortality from a high of 100% to 7% or better. Treatment is aimed at five major areas:

1. Support of vital functions including sedation, oxygen, fluids, use of antipyretics, treatment of infection, correction of electrolyte abnormalities, and the use of corticosteroids (hydrocortisone 100 to 200 mg IV) in case of unsuspected hypoadrenalism. T_3 levels are also lowered by steroids.

2. The use of thioamides and iodides to block synthesis and release of hormones. Large doses of PTU 600 to 1200 mg/day or of methimazole 30 to 60 mg every 6 hours should be given. Iodides should be given 1 hour after thioamide administration so as not to block the latter's effect and not to iodize existing hormone stores which will be released before the onset of thioamide effect and therefore aggravate existing storm. Iodides (NaI 1 to 3 g IV drip/24 hours or Lugol's solution 30 to 60 drops PO daily) and the combination of thioamides may relieve symptoms within 1 day. Lithium which is similar to the effect of iodides may be used in doses of 500 to 1500 mg/day but has no advantage over iodides.

3. Blockage of the metabolic effects can be accomplished by reserpine 1 to 3 mg IM every 8 hours, guanethidine 20 to 50 mg PO every 8 hours or by propranolol 20 to 80 mg PO every 6 hours or 0.5 to 2 mg IV every 4 hours.

4. Elimination of the precipitating factors.

5. Removal of circulating hormone by plasmapheresis, exchange transfusion, and dialysis when more routine measures fail (79, 80).

HYPOTHYROIDISM

Hypothyroidism or myxedema is characterized by a slowing down of all body processes due to a deficiency of thyroid hormone. Thyroid hormone stimulates oxygen consumption and is essential for normal growth, maturation, and regulation of all organ systems.

CLINICAL FEATURES

Since the symptoms are often nonspecific, insidious, and obscure, a diagnosis of hypothyroidism, especially in the elderly (12) can be missed unless considered in the differential diagnosis. The signs and symptoms of hypothyroidism are listed in Table 26.4. Patients often will complain of weakness, lethargy, cold intolerance, and weight gain while the physical changes of hypothyroidism are often late findings. A puffy and masklike facies, edematous eyelids, myxedematous skin changes, especially over the pretibial aspects of the leg, loss of hair from the lateral aspects of the eyebrows, a large tongue, and a yellowish tint to the skin may be found.

The cardiovascular manifestations of hypothyroidism may appear as or exacerbate existing low output congestive heart failure and angina. The presenting symptoms include cardiomegaly resulting from loss of muscle tone and mucopolysaccharide deposition, dyspnea, edema and pleural effusions as a result of decreased cardiac output, decreased stroke volume, and decreased myocardial contractibility. The following characteristic changes may appear on the ECG: slow rate and low voltage, flattened or inverted T waves, and occasionally increased PR interval and widened QRS complex.

The exact relationship between accelerated atherosclerotic changes and hypothyroidism remain unclear although there appears to be a strong association.

Due to decreased cardiac output and blood volume, glomerular filtration rate (GFR) and renal plasma flow (RPF) are decreased despite no evidence of renal failure. A delay in water excretion in response to water loading in severe myxedema may result from changes in GRF or inappropriate antidiuretic hormone secretion.

COURSE

The onset of naturally occurring hypothyroidism is an insidious and nonspecific process which may go unnoticed by the patient or be attributed to other things. It is such a slow process that several years may pass with amazing placidity before the appearance of a terminal state. Myxedematous cachexia is characterized by intensification of all signs and symptoms and often precedes the onset of myxedema coma.

LABORATORY PARAMETERS

Laboratory manifestations include decreased T_4 (RIA), decreased RT_3U, decreased FT_4I, decreased RAI uptake, and elevation of TSH levels unless a pituitary etiology is suspected. Delayed metabolism of enzymes result in elevations of serum SGOT, LDH, CPK, cholesterol and triglycerides. Positive antibodies indicative of an autoimmune disorder may be present.

ETIOLOGY

No matter what the etiology of the deficiency the manifestations of the disease are relatively constant depending on the age of the patient and degree of deficiency. Hypothyroid-

ism can be classified as either nongoitrous (no goiter) or goitrous. Goiters (enlargement of the thyroid) result from excessive TSH stimulation in response to low levels of circulating hormone. Nongoitrous causes include secondary hypothyroidism either of pituitary or hypothalamic origin, cretinism (congenital hypothyroidism), iatrogenic and idiopathic atrophy. Goitrous forms include Hashimoto's thyroiditis, drug-induced dyshormonogenesis, endemic and multinodular. Despite the presence of a goiter, a euthyroid state as evidenced by a normal T_4 (RIA) and FTI can occur if increased thyroidal demand is compensated by increased thyroidal secretion (increased TSH levels) and enlargement of the gland; otherwise hypothyroidism ensues.

Secondary Hypothyroidism

Hypothalamic hypothyroidism arising from inadequate secretion of thyrotropin-releasing factor (TRF) appears to be rare. Low or absent levels of TSH suggest the possibility of pituitary hypothyroidism which can result from postpartum hemorrhage (Sheehan's), head injury, pituitary tumors, or idiopathic atrophy of the hypophysis. Concomitant disorders of the adrenals and gonads may also be seen (Simmonds' disease or panhypopituitarism). Primary, pituitary, and hypothalamic hypothyroidism can be differentiated by the use of the TRF and TSH tests.

Iatrogenic

Iatrogenic hypothyroidism from radioactive iodine and surgery constitutes one of the most common causes of hypothyroidism today. As previously discussed, virtually all patients receiving iodine will become myxedematous while about 50 to 75% of patients who undergo thyroidectomies develop hypothyroidism (57, 58, 65).

Idiopathic Atrophy

Idiopathic atrophy of the thyroid associated with hypothyroidism may constitute the end stages of Hashimoto's thyroiditis; antibodies, presumably the etiology of a destructive immune process, are frequently found.

Cretinism (Congenital Hypothyroidism)

Congenital nongoitrous hypothyroidism, produced by a deficiency of thyroid in utero and in the neonate may result from defective hormone synthesis, from iodine deficiency because of pituitary or hypothalamic dysfunction and from incomplete growth of the gland (agenesis) (67). Ectopic thyroid tissue and destruction of the gland by maternal auto antibodies and by RAI therapy, are possible causes of agenesis. Neonatal goitrous hypothyroidism has been reported after the maternal ingestion of iodides or antithyroid agents (68–72).

The clinical presentations vary in relation to the degree, the age of onset, and the duration of thyroid deficiency. The earliest manifestations are a heavy expression, a piglike appearance of the eyes, hypothermia, prolonged jaundice, umbilical hernia, hoarseness, thick tongue, protuberant abdomen, constipation and drooling. Delayed developmental characteristics, failure to thrive, poor appetite, and cretinoid facies may not appear until 3 to 6 months when neurological damage may be irreversible. In a child the clinical features are similar to that of an adult, along with growth retardation and development.

Radiologic examination revealing epiphyseal dysgenesis is pathognomonic of neonatal hypothyroidism. The early recognition is now made possible by radioimmune assay of TSH in cord blood. Levels of TSH greater than 20 microunits/ml are suspicious while levels of TSH greater than 50 μU/ml are diagnostic of congenital hypothyroidism.

Endemic Hypothyroidism

Endemic goiter is a descriptive term for thyroid enlargement due to iodine deficiency in a large fraction of the population residing in areas such as the Himalayas and the European Alps (81). Females are more often affected than males as with other thyroidal disorders. The amount of dietary iodine will determine the degree of enlargement which becomes nodular with advancing years. Laboratory manifestations include elevated RAIU, normal or low T_4 (RIA), RT_3U, FTI, and normal or elevated TSH levels.

Dyshormonogenesis

Dyshormonogenesis refers to a specific group of familial thyroid disorders resulting from abnormalities in the synthesis, delivery, or peripheral action of thyroid hormones. Impaired hormone synthesis can result from a defect in iodine accumulation, in iodide organification as a result of dehalogenase deficiency, and from a coupling abnormality. Patients with impaired thyroglobulin synthesis, release of abnormal iodopeptides, and peripheral tissue resistance to thyroid have also been described.

Since specific tests are not available, diagnosis is dependent on elimination of other goitrous causes of hypothyroidism. Laboratory manifestations include low or normal circulating hormone levels, increased TSH, and absence of antibodies. A defect in organification may be documented by the use of the potassium perchlorate discharge test.

Drug Induced

Goiters may occur from the use of certain agents with antithyroid activity. Drugs such as the thioamides and the monovalent anions which are used therapeutically in the treatment of hyperthyroidism may produce goiter if excessive doses are used (goitrogenic).

The iodides were first recognized as being goitrogenic after the induction of goiters in asthmatics. Certain types of patients have been found to be inordinately sensitive to the blocking effects of the iodides so that hypothyroidism results (4). These include patients with cystic fibrosis, patients with untreated Hashimoto's thyroiditis, and patients with euthyroid Graves' previously treated with RAI or surgery. The goiter or hypothyroidism is reversible after discontinuation of the iodides.

Lithium has also been reported to be a goitrogen when given to patients with abnormal thyroid glands. This antithyroid effect was first demonstrated in manic depressives as a side effect of lithium therapy. The onset of a nontender diffuse goiter with or without hypothyroidism may appear within 5 months to 2 years of treatment (82). The goiters are responsive to T_4 therapy or discontinuation of lithium. The tricyclics, especially imipramine, have been associated with the development of goiter.

The sulfonyurea antidiabetic agents, tolbutamide and possibly chlorpropramide may inhibit formation of thyroid hormone by inhibiting iodine binding. Depression of ^{131}I uptake and PBI is seen with large doses of chlorpropramide (3 to 7 g) and tolbutamide but does not seem to occur with the usual therapeutic doses.

Thiocyanate is a well-known inhibitor of iodide trapping when high concentrations are present in blood. Plants such as rutabagas, cabbage, and turnips contain thioglucosides which is metabolized in the body to thiocyanates. These dietary goitrogens do not produce any significant degree of hypothyroidism unless large amounts are ingested raw over a long period.

Multinodular Goiters

Multinodular goiters refer to an enlarged thyroid gland with more than one nodule. It is a common disorder affecting women more than men and occurs in about 4% of all adults beyond age 30. It appears to be the result of long-standing TSH stimulation and to be exacerbated by iodide deficiency, dietary goitrogens and enzymatic defects.

Clinically the patient can remain euthyroid, develop hyper-, or hypothyroidism after a few decades. The presence of pressure symptoms produced by compression of the trachea or esophagus by the enlarged gland is an indication for surgical removal. The possibility of malignancy must be eliminated, especially if a history of irradiation is present. Cold nodules in a multinodular goiter are rarely malignant.

Hashimoto's Thyroiditis (Chronic Thyroiditis, Lymphocytic Thyroiditis)

Hashimoto's thyroiditis is characterized by diffuse enlargement and lymphocytic infiltration of the thyroid, an immunological disturbance, and hypothyroidism although euthyroidism may occur if adequately compensated. This is probably the most common cause of goitrous hypothyroidism today and is similar to Graves' disease in frequency (3 to 6/10,000/year). It is 15 to 20 times more common in females than males with its peak occurrences in the middle ages although any age group can be affected. Like Graves' disease, there is a strong genetic predisposition.

PATHOPHYSIOLOGY

An autoimmune process due to defects in suppressor T lymphocytes is strongly suspected since antibodies against thyroglobulin, a microsomal component, and a colloid component as well as cell mediated immunity against thyroid antigens are found (13, 14). Furthermore, Hashimoto's disease often coexists with other autoimmune disorders including Graves' disease, rheumatoid arthritis, and other collagen vascular diseases. Pernicious anemia secondary to gastric antibodies can be found in about half of the patients with Hashimoto's disease and vice versa. Some postulate that Graves' and Hashimoto's thyroiditis may be different ends of the same disease since mild thyrotoxicosis may precede the onset of hypothyroidism. The onset of the process begins with gradual enlargement of the thyroid and maintenance of euthyroidism and progresses to hypothyroidism. Like the Graves' gland, the Hashimoto's gland is unable to bind iodide effectively and is inordinately sensitive to the antithyroid effects of iodides. This ineffective utilization of iodide results in the release and formation of inactive nonhormonal iodoproteins into the circulation which further increases TSH secretion and goiter formation. Once the gland is no longer able to increase production of the T_4 and T_3 through TSH stimulation, hypothyroidism results. Clinically the spectrum of Hashimoto's thyroiditis can present as early thyrotoxicosis, euthyroidism with goiter, hypothyroidism with goiter, or hypothyroidism without goiter. Asymptomatic thyroiditis characterized by euthyroid status, absence of goiter, normal levels of circulating hormones, but presence of antithyroid antibodies may precede clinical manifestations of overt hypothyroidism and goiter (83).

LABORATORY PARAMETERS

Laboratory manifestations include low or normal T_4 (RIA), RT_3U, FT_4I, normal or elevated RAI, normal or elevated TSH, normal T_3 suppression test and positive antithyroglobulin and antimicrosomal antibodies.

Treatment of Hypothyroidism

The administration of thyroid hormones provides adequate replacement therapy for hypothyroidism as well as shrinkage of the goiter by suppression of TSH production (see Fig. 26.3). The average replacement dose often quoted in medical textbooks is 200 to 300 μg/day of T_4 which parallels the normal thyroidal production. However, Stocks et al. (84) found that the average maintenance dose was 160 μg/day of L-thyroxine which correlated with a body weight of 2.25 μg/kg. When doses of 300 μg/day of L-thyroxine were given, symptoms of overt hyperthyroidism were produced. In the elderly, less T_4 (2.0 μg/kg or less) was needed to achieve euthyroidism (85, 85a). However, these doses may actually be higher than necessary since these values precede the reformulation of thyroxine by Flint Laboratories (Synthroid). The new bioavailability is now 100% versus 78% so that in some patients a 20% reduction in dosage may be necessary to prevent toxicity (127).

DOSING

The initial dose of T_4 (or its equivalent) administered will depend on the patient's age, the severity and duration of the disease, and the coexistence of cardiac manifestations. In young, healthy patients with disease of short duration, thyroxine (or its equivalent) can be administered in doses of 100 to 150 µg daily and adjusted as needed. However, patients with long-standing and severe myxedema, elderly patients, and patients with cardiac disease (i.e. angina, CHF) are extremely sensitive to the metabolic effects of thyroid hormone so that therapy must be started with minute doses of thyroid in order to avoid cardiovascular complications of failure, angina, tachycardia, and myocardial infarction. In these pa-

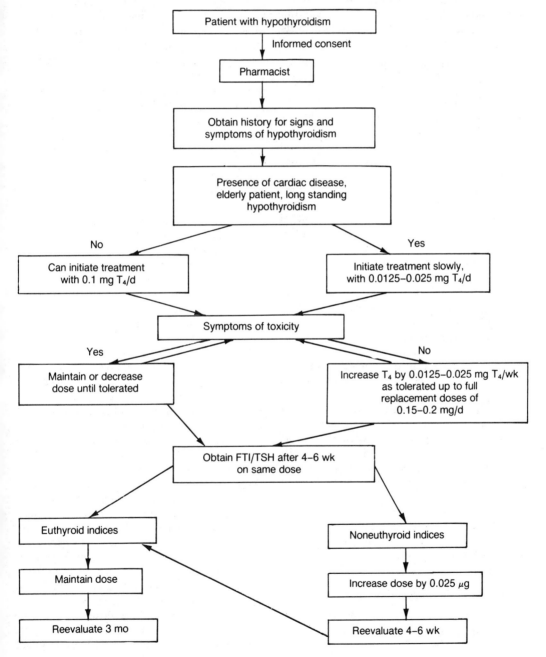

Figure 26.3. Treatment of hypothyroidism.

tients initial doses of 12.5 to 25 μg of T_4 given daily for 1 to 4 weeks can be increased by 12.5 to 25 μg increments every 2 to 4 weeks as tolerated or until therapeutic levels are achieved (86). In such patients complete euthyroidism may never be achieved. T_3 has been suggested by some as the drug of choice for patients with cardiovascular problems since its effects can be terminated rapidly within 3 to 5 days because of its short half-life as opposed to 7 to 10 days for T_4. However, the greater cardiotoxicity of T_3 may outweigh its advantage of rapid elimination from the body.

MANAGEMENT OF CONGENITAL HYPOTHYROIDISM

In congenital hypothyroidism normal growth and development is determined by the age treatment is instituted, continued maintenance of a euthyroid state, and the degree of initial athyreosis. The earlier the treatment the better the prognosis for normal mental and growth development although there is no assurance. Mäenpää (87) reported achievement of normal intellect in 81% of the patients if treatment was started before age 3 months. Likewise, mental impairment was seen if treatment was detained until 6 months to 1 year despite initiation of subsequent treatment. Treatment started late such as in an adolescent 5 years or older does not appear to improve intelligence although growth may be accelerated. With the severely myxedematous child, treatment may produce such undesirable symptoms as psychosis or unmanageability. In such cases it may be desirable to maintain a mild hypothyroid state.

Like the adult, the infant with long-standing and severe myxedema will be extremely sensitive to thyroid replacement so that very small doses are necessary to prevent hyperactivity and irritability. In such cases 25 μg/day initially is increased by 12.5 μg increments every 2 weeks until full maintenance doses of 75 to 150 μg or toxicity is reached.

Otherwise, half of the estimated replacement dose can be given initially and achievement of full therapeutic doses can be accomplished in a few days.

Dose of T_4 for Infants/Children:

Age	Dosage (μg/day)
0–12 mo	50–75
12–24 mo	75–125
2–4 yr	100–150
4–12 yr	100–300

The optimal replacement dose can be determined by monitoring TSH levels.

THYROID PREPARATIONS

All of the commercially available preparations of thyroid hormone are effective (88). However, there are a number of qualities of each drug that should be considered before a selection is made (Table 26.8).

Desiccated thyroid (USP) is obtained from hog thyroids although beef and sheep are also used. This preparation is standardized only with respect to iodine content (0.17 to 0.23% iodine) so that the ratio of hormones may vary from 2:1 (hog) while a ratio of 3:1 may be seen with beef or sheep. Therefore, variability in potency may result from changes in the ratio of the two hormones or from the quantity of organic iodine present. Loss of potency due to improper or prolonged storage can also contribute to an unpredictable response. Desiccated thyroid appears to be stable for five years or longer if it is kept dry. Inactive preparations containing small amounts of T_4 and T_3 or even iodinated casein as well as higher than reported biological activity have been observed (89). Allergic reactions to the protein component may also occur. Laboratory values of PBI, T_4 (RIA) and RT_3U remain within normal limits. Desiccated therapy may be continued if the person is well-maintained in a euthyroid state, although this would not be a first line choice.

Thyroglobulin is a purified hog extract which is standardized biologically to give a $T_4:T_3$ ratio of 2.5:1. It has no advantages over desiccated thyroid but is slightly more expensive. One grain of thyroglobulin is equivalent to one grain of thyroid USP.

L-Thyroxine is the most commonly prescribed synthetic thyroid hormone preparation. Its popularity stems from its stability, its uniform potency, its relatively low cost and its lack of foreign protein antigenticity. Its long half-life of 7 days makes it amenable to once-a-day dosing which may increase patient compliance. The only limitation is its variable absorption of 35 to 78% although most patients absorb 60 to 65%. This may be significant when changing from PO to IV or IM dosing regimen. Although 0.1 mg of L-thyroxine is equivalent to one grain of desiccated thyroid such equivalents may not be valid if higher amounts of desiccated thyroid were required to achieve euthyroidism due to less active desiccated thyroid preparations. In one study

Table 26.8.
Thyroid Preparations in Treatment of Hypothyroidism

Preparation[a]	Content	Advantages	Disadvantages	Effect on Thyroid Tests	Comments
Desiccated thyroid USP ½, 1, 2, 3, gr	Defatted, dried pig thyroid powder, containing 0.17–0.23% iodine	Inexpensive	Poor standardization with variable hormonal content and T_4/T_3 ratios; deterioration with storage	Normal T_4 (RIA), RT_3U, TSH	Potency may vary from batch to batch
Thyroglobulin ½, 1, 2, 3 gr	Partially purified pig thyroglobulin	Standardized biologically	More expensive than desiccated thyroid	Normal range for thyroid function tests	No real advantage over thyroid extract
Sodium L-thyroxine[b] 0.05, 0.1, 0.15, 0.175, 0.2, 0.3 mg	Synthetic, pure T_4	Stable, smooth action, relatively inexpensive; long half-life ($t_{1/2}$ = 7 days)	Variable absorption between 40–70%; cumulative effect	Normal thyroid function tests	May be more potent than desiccated thyroid, should lower the T_4 dose by ½ gr to avoid toxicity when changing from desiccated thyroid to L-thyroxine
Sodium L-thyronine, 25, 50 µg	Synthetic, pure T_3	Uniform absorption, fast onset of action	Expensive, short half-life (1.5 days) difficult to monitor—need to use TSH levels	Low T_4 (RIA) and RT_3U normal TSH	Requires multiple daily dosing schedule
Liotrix	Contains T_4 and T_3 in a ratio of 4:1 (mimics natural secretion of hormone)	Both short and long acting effects	Expensive	Normal thyroid function values	No real need for liotrix since T_4 is peripherally converted to T_3

[a] Dose equivalence: 1 gr desiccated thyroid = 1 gr thyroglobulin = 0.1 mg L-thyroxine = 25 µg L-thyronine = liotrix-1 (see "Comments" column).
[b] Reformulation of thyroxine (Synthroid, Flint) resulted in 100% bioavailability (older formulation had 78% bioavailability).

L-thyroxine 60 μg was equivalent to desiccated thyroid 1 grain (90). This disparity in equivalence should be especially noted when changing to L-thyroxine in patients previously requiring more than 2 grains/day of desiccated thyroid. Therapy can be monitored by use of TSH levels. Adequate thyroid replacement usually produces T_4 levels in the upper limits of normal, approximately 9 (T_4 (RIA) = 5 to 12). Generic thyroxine may not be bioequivalent to brand forms of thyroxine (91, 92).

L-Triiodothyronine or T_3 is a chemically pure agent with predictable potency and a half-life of 1.5 days. However, it is not usually employed as a chronic drug for routine replacement because of its high cost, the need for multiple daily dosing (because of its short half-life) to ensure uniform response, its greater ability to induce cardiotoxicity, and the difficulty in monitoring therapeutic/toxic responses. T_3 administration results in pretreatment plasma T_4 levels despite adequate replacement doses and must be monitored by the use of TSH concentrations. The main use of T_3 is as a diagnostic agent in the T_3 suppression test. Because of its rapid onset of 1 to 3 days, T_3 has been recommended by some as the drug of choice for myxedema coma but its routine use is limited by the unavailability of a commercial preparation as well as its greater risk of cardiovascular manifestations in such patients. A dose of 25 μg of T_3 is equivalent to 0.1 mg of thyroxine.

Liotrix is a combination of synthetic T_4 and T_3 in a ratio of 4:1 which mimics the natural secretion of hormones and is available commercially as Euthyroid and Thyrolar. Since these preparations approximate the normal thyroidal production they were once considered to be the agents of choice before it was recognized that a significant amount of T_4 is converted peripherally to T_3. These products are stable, chemically pure, have a predictable potency and produce laboratory values of T_4 (RIA) and RT_3U within the normal range.

In Euthroid-1, 60 μg of T_4 and 14 μg of T_3 are equivalent to 1 grain of thyroid, while in Thyrolar-1, 50 μg of T_4 and 12.5 μg of T_3 represent the same equivalency. Since Euthroid is 20% more potent than Thyrolar, it should be recognized that substitution may alter the patient's response. Due to its high cost and lack of therapeutic rationale, there appears to be no real advantage or need for such a preparation.

Special Considerations

PREGNANCY

Myxedema in the mother has been associated with congenital defects, hypothyroidism, spontaneous abortions, still births, and mental retardation. However, the exact significance of the effect of the maternal thyroid function on the fetus requires further clarification since normal children have been reported in women who remained hypothyroid throughout pregnancy (93). Infants of hypothyroid mothers may be normal because their hypothalamic-pituitary axis develops independently from the mother. In mothers with Hashimoto's thyroiditis, congenital hypothyroidism may result from the maternal transfer of destructive antibodies into the fetal circulation. Thyroid replacement in the mother does not affect the fetus since thyroid hormone does not cross the placental barrier. In the absence of risk factors, i.e. cardiac diseases, 0.15 to 0.2 mg L-thyroxine can be initiated and increased as tolerated to a euthyroid state. Despite increased binding of T_4 by TBG higher doses of T_4 are not needed since a new equilibrium is reached. Adequate replacement which is reflected by a normal T_4 (RIA) and FTI level usually results in a normal baby although abortions and congenital deformities may still occur due to poor placenta development. Pregnant hypothyroid patients on replacement T_4 therapy should have T_4 (RIA) and FTI checked every month for the first 3 months to insure adequate replacement. TSH levels are not helpful since HCG will interefere with this assay.

MYXEDEMA COMA

Myxedema coma is the end stage of long-standing uncorrected hypothyroidism. The clinical manifestations are hypothermia, an advanced state of hypothyroid symptomology, delayed deep tendon reflexes, and altered sensorium which may range from stupor to coma. Other predominant findings include carbon dioxide narcosis, hyponatremia, hypoglycemia, shock and paranoid psychosis (79).

Coma can be precipitated by cold weather (hypothermia), stress (surgery), infection, trauma, acid-base disturbances and the presence of uncontrolled coexisting disease, i.e. diabetes, arterosclerotic cardiovascular disease (ASCVD). Respiratory depressants of any kind which are metabolized slowly in the hypothyroid patient, i.e. anesthetics, narcotics, phenothiazines, sedative-hypnotics, can aggravate preexisting hypothermia and carbon dioxide retention; thereby precipitating coma.

Immediate and aggressive therapy is needed to prevent the high mortality (60 to 70%) seen.

Treatment is directed at three main factors: Replacement therapy with L-thyroxine 500 μg IV stat should be given to saturate the TBG. The dose can be decreased or increased depending on the size and number of restricting factors. T$_3$, 20 to 50 μg every 8 hours, although not commercially available, can be administered IV. Maintenance doses of 5 μg T$_3$ or 50 μg T$_4$ IV daily should be instituted until achievement of euthyroid state. Hydrocortisone 50 to 100 mg IV every 6 hours must be administered concomitantly since it is essential in cases of hypopituitarism presenting as myxedema.

Supportive measures should include assisted ventilation, glucose for hypoglycemia, restriction of fluids for hyponatremia and use of plasma expanders for shock and circulatory collapse. Cooling blankets which may further compromise shock through vasodilation are not recommended.

Last, precipitating factors should be eliminated or corrected.

If the proper treatment and support has been provided, consciousness and decreased TSH levels should be evident within 24 hours along with restoration of normal vital functions.

THYROID NODULES

The discovery of asymptomatic single or multiple nodules in a normal or enlarged thyroid gland is a very common occurrence which is of concern because of the risk of malignancy. It is often difficult to determine clinically if any nodule has the cancer or which cancer is in the nodule. In general 10 to 20% of cold nodules are cancers while "hot" nodules are rarely carcinogenic (94).

However, a high index of suspicion for thyroid carcinoma based on several high risk characteristics requires surgical intervention. These high risk factors are listed in Table 26.9 (95). In euthyroid nonirradiated patients with a low risk of suspicion for cancer, therapy with thyroxine 0.15 to 0.3 mg q.d. is recommended to suppress TSH stimulation and further growth of the nodule. If significant regression of the nodule(s) is seen after 3 to 6 months on thyroxine therapy, therapy is continued indefinitely. Any growth of the nodule while on thyroid suppression requires surgical removal to rule out malignancy.

A significant increase in thyroid abnormalities (20 to 33%) and thyroid cancers (6 to 9%) are observed in adults who had radiation to the thyroid 20 to 25 years ago (96). Patients receiving radiation to the thymus, tonsils, adenoids, or upper head and neck region are at risk. Benign abnormalities in radiated glands have included focal hyperplasia, Hashimoto's thyroiditis, adenomas, Graves' disease and colloid nodules. Malignancies have been papillary, mixed papillary-follicular and follicular. Since these tumors are slow growing, the prognosis is good if no evidence of metastases is present.

All patients with a history of childhood ir-

Table 26.9.
Risk Factors for Thyroid Cancers[a]

Evidence	Low Index of Suspicion	High Index of Suspicion
History	Familial history of thyroid disease or endemic goiter	Previous history of neck or head irradiation
Patient characteristics	Older women; soft nodule; multinodular goiter	Children, young adults, males; solitary firm dominant nodule; vocal cord paralysis; enlarged lymph nodes; hoarseness
Laboratory Characteristics	High levels of antithyroid antibodies; "hot" nodules on scan; cystic lesion on echo; negative thin needle biopsy (although does not rule out malignancy)	Elevated thyroglobulin; elevated serum calcitonin; "cold" nodule on scan; solid lesion on echo; positive thin needle biopsy
Thyroxine therapy (not recommended in patients with history of irradiation)	Regression after 0.2–0.3 mg/day for 3–6 months	No regression

[a] Adapted from F. S. Greenspan (95).

radiation should be evaluated by a physician skilled in thyroid examinations. Baseline T_4 (RIA), FTI, thyroid scan and uptake, and antibodies should be obtained even if physical exam of the thyroid is benign since microscopic nonpalpable thyroid cancer have been found during surgery. If no abnormalities are found, treatment with thyroxine suppression or routine yearly examination are recommended. Any palpable nodules are strong indications for needle biopsy and eventual surgery. For a more detailed discussion of this subject matter see Korff and Degroot (97).

DRUG INTERACTIONS (DRUG KINETICS AND THYROID FUNCTION)

A number of drugs and disease entities can alter laboratory values and make interpretation of thyroid status difficult. Conversely, the thyroid dysfunction can affect the metabolism and clinical effectiveness of several therapeutic agents (see Table 26.11).

Major drugs and disease states which may falsely alter laboratory values are listed in Table 26.2 (98). Since these patients are clinically and chemically euthyroid no treatment is indicated and may be dangerous. Major

agents which can alter thyroid activity are listed in Table 26.10 (99).

It has been observed clinically that hyperthyroid patients tend to be "resistant" to glycosides, whereas hypothyroid patients are more sensitive. This may be explained by the altered kinetics seen with thyroid dysfunction. Both the volume of distribution (V_d) and clearance are decreased in hypothyroidism; an increased V_d and clearance occurs in hyperthyroidism. The half-life is not changed. Since V_d determines the loading dose and clearance the maintenance dose, both a smaller loading and maintenance dose should be given in hypothyroidism while a larger loading and maintenance dose of digoxin will be required for therapeutic effectiveness in thyrotoxicosis. It is especially important that doses of digoxin are adjusted as euthyroidism occurs to prevent toxicity and obtain maximal therapeutic effects (100, 101).

Similar changes are required with warfarin therapy (102). In thyrotoxicosis both the synthesis and catabolism of vitamin K dependent clotting factors are increased so that there is no net change in level of clotting factors. However, an enhanced anticoagulant response is seen when the warfarin-induced decrease in

Table 26.10.
Alteration of thyroid hormone effects

Drug	Mechanism	Laboratory	Comments
Cholestyramine, Colestipol	Binds T_4 in gut, decrease absorption of T_4	↓ T_4, ↓ free T_4, ↑ TSH in hypothyroidism	Administer at least 4–5 hr apart
Nitroprusside	Metabolized to thiocyanate, an anion inhibitor	↓ T_4, ↓ free T_4, ↑ TSH	Increased risk with renal failure
Lithium	Inhibits hormone release	↓ T_4, ↓ free T_4, ↑ TSH	Usually in patients with underlying thyroid disease
Iodides	Inhibit organification Decrease release T_4, T_3	↓ T_4, ↓ free T_4, ↑ TSH	Usually in patients with underlying Hashimoto's or with Graves' previously treated with RAI or surgery
	Provides substrate to iodide deficient autonomous thyroid tissue; loss of Wolff Chaikoff control	↑ T_4, ↑ free T_4, ↑ T_3, ↓ TSH	Usually in nontoxic multinodular goiters with autonomous function (Jod-Basedow)
Sulfonylureas, sulfonamides, PAS, resorcinol, phenylbutazone	Inhibit organic binding and organification	↓ T_4, ↓ free T_4, ↑ TSH	Rare
Natural goitrogens cabbage, etc.	Contain thiocyanate and other goitrogens	↓ T_4, ↓ free T_4, ↑ TSH	Rare, need large consumption of raw vegetables

Table 26.11.
Effect of Thyroid Status on Drug Action

Drug	Thyroid Status	Mechanism of Action	Clinical Effect as Compared to Euthyroidism
Sympathomimetics, i.e., asthma and cold preparations	Hyperthyroidism	Increased sensitivity to catecholamines	Exacerbation of thyrotoxic symptoms, especially cardiac
Digitalis	Hyperthyroidism	Increased volume of distribution; ?increased renal clearance of digitalis	More resistant to digitalis effect; may necessitate increased doses to achieve therapeutic effect
	Hypothyroidism	Decreased volume of distribution of digitalis, ?decreased renal clearance	Increased sensitivity to digitalis effect, requires less digitalis to achieve therapeutic effect
Insulin	Hyperthyroidism	Increased renal clearance/ metabolism of insulin	May need more insulin to control diabetes
	Hypothyroidism	Delayed turnover	Need less insulin to control diabetes
Coumadin	Hyperthyroidism	Increased metabolism of clotting fctors—decreased half-life of clotting factors	Require less coumadin to achieve anticoagulation
	Hypothyroidism	Delayed turnover of clotting factors—increased half-life of clotting factors	Require more coumadin to achieve anticoagulation
Respiratory depressants (barbiturates, phenothiazines, narcotics)	Hypothyroidism	Increased sensitivity to the respiratory depressant effects of these agents	Increased CO_2 retention, may precipitate myxedema coma

clotting factor synthesis is combined with hyperthyroidism-induced increase in factor catabolism. The opposite occurs in hypothyroidism; the anticoagulant response is delayed due to slower catabolism of clotting factors. Therefore, thyrotoxic patients will need less warfarin while myxedematous patients will require more warfarin to achieve the same hypoprothrombinemic response. As thyroid status changes appropriate dosage adjustments should be made to maintain therapeutic effectiveness. The kinetics of a number of hormones including thyroid hormones themselves may be influenced by the thyroid status. This may be due to alterations in hepatic blood flow and metabolism.

T_4 has a normal half-life of 6 to 7 days but in hyperthyroidism this is shortened to 3 to 4 days and in hypothyroidism prolonged to 9 to 10 days. Similar changes for T_3 have been documented. The half-life, secretion and metabolism of cortisol are also affected. Infused cortisol had a half-life of 110 min in euthyroid patients, 155 min in hypothyroid patients and 50 min in thyrotoxic patients. Although the clearance of cortisol is changed in relation to thyroid function the plasma levels remained constant due to compensatory changes in secretion rates to maintain homeostasis.

Changes in metabolism of the sex hormones were opposite of what was expected. Decreased clearance and higher plasma level of testosterone and estrogens and androgens were found in hyperthyroidism; the converse in hypothyroidism. It appears that higher plasma levels seen in toxic patients may be due to changes in binding protein so that clearance was delayed.

Evidence for altered insulin kinetics as opposed to altered glucose metabolism with altered thyroid status is minimal in man. In hyperthyroid rabbits insulin degradation rates are increased although in man no such changes are observed. Clinically, hypoglycemia is more prevalent in hypothyroidism which suggests that insulin degradation may be delayed. Catecholamine levels are not changed by thyroid dysfunction although many of the thyrotoxic symptoms mimic catecholamine excess and hypothyroid symptoms mimic catecholamine deficiency.

There is definite evidence of hepatic enzyme induction in thyrotoxicosis and reduced metabolism in hypothyroidism (103). This is evidenced by increased clearance in hyperthyroidism of antipyrine, a drug widely used as an index of hepatic microsomal function. In hypothyroidism a decreased clearance of antipyrine occurs. Nevertheless, it is not possible to extrapolate such changes to the metabolism of other drugs cleared hepatically. Phenytoin is an example. Even though phenytoin can induce hepatic microsomal enzyme metabolism of thyroid hormones, changes in thyroid function do not appear to affect its metabolism. On the other hand, hypothyroid patients are inordinately sensitive to respiratory depressants such as anesthetics, narcotics, phenothiazines and sedative hypnotics, all of which undergo hepatic metabolism.

Absorption of agents such as riboflavine, ethanol, and acetaminophen appear to be increased in thyrotoxicosis and delayed in hypothyroidism. Significance in man is not clear since most of data was obtained by animal studies.

PARATHYROID DISORDERS

To understand the treatment of common parathyroid disorders, the pharmacist must first understand the effects of parathyroid hormone, the consequences of excessive secretion or lack of end organ response, and its relationship to calcium metabolism (see Fig. 26.4).

Parathyroid hormone (PTH) is the principal regulator of extracellular ionic calcium and is released from the parathyroid glands via a negative feedback system in response to plasma calcium levels. Normal plasma ionic calcium is maintained through the action of PTH on kidney, bone, and intestine. Magnesium is required for normal release of PTH from parathyroid glands and hypocalcemia can occur unless hypomagnesemia is corrected.

PTH protects against hypocalcemia by the following mechanisms: (a) increasing release of calcium as well as phosphate from bone

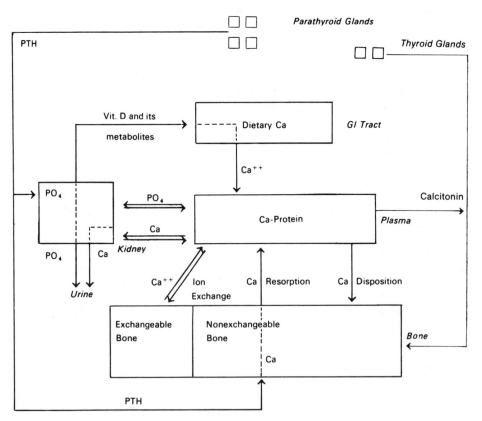

Figure 26.4. Simplified diagram of some of the normal relationships of parathyroid hormone (PTH) and calcium metabolism (126).

(resorption), (b) increasing reabsorption of calcium (also magnesium) by the kidney, (c) increasing intestinal absorption of calcium indirectly via vitamin D, (d) increasing conversion of the metabolite 25-hydroxycholecalciferol to active vitamin D_3 (1-α-25-dihydroxycholecalciferol or 1 α-25-$(OH)_2D_3$) through stimulating the activity of renal tubular 25-OH-1-α-hydroxylase, and by (e) increasing the renal excretion of bicarbonate (bicarbonaturia) producing an acidosis which decreases the ability of circulating albumin to bind calcium, thus increasing calcium by physiochemical means. PTH also acts on the kidney to increase phosphate excretion (hyperphosphaturia) to prevent elevations in plasma phosphate resulting from increased bone resorption.

Thus, a reciprocal relationship between calcium and phosphate exists. In hyperparathyroidism, serum calcium is elevated and hypophosphatemia occurs while in hypoparathyroidism, hypocalcemia and hyperphosphatemia is seen.

Hyperparathyroidism

Primary hyperparathyroidism is an endocrine disorder characterized by excessive uncontrolled release of parathyroid hormone (PTH) from adenomatous (single gland involvement, 80%), hyperplastic (multiple gland involvement, 20%) or malignant (<2%) parathyroid glands (104). Hyperparathyroidism associated with multiple endocrine neoplasia syndromes (MEN) is almost always due to disease of multiple glands. The hallmark of this disorder is hypercalcemia due to failure of the negative feedback cycle to suppress further PTH secretion. The etiology of this disorder is unknown although inheritance via an autosomal dominant trait has been described.

INCIDENCE

Earlier recognition of the disease through widespread use of routine serum calcium measurements has increased the detection of asymptomatic persons so that this disorder may be more common than previously thought. Various studies prior to 1969 indicate an incidence of 10 to 20 cases per 100,000 (105). In a careful population-based study, an incidence of 7.8 cases/100,000 jumped to 42 cases/100,000 after the introduction of routine calcium measurements. This increased prevalence of hyperparathyroidism is concentrated in persons greater than 40 years old and is 2 to 4 times more common in women than in men. The annual incidence is about 277 per million population (106).

Patient Characteristics		Incidence
	39 yr or less	10/100,000
Female	60 yr or greater	188/100,000
Male	60 yr or greater	92/100,000

PATHOGENESIS

Excessive release of PTH causes hypercalcemia and hypophosphatemia via the mechanisms previously described. Mild to moderate hyperchloremic acidosis may exist from PTH-induced bicarbonaturia. Hypercalciuria results when the renal threshold for reabsorbing calcium is exceeded, usually serum calcium elevations are greater than 12 mg/100 ml. Complications of nephrolithiasis are produced from the prolonged hypercalciuria in an alkaline medium (bicarbonaturia). Other extraskeletal metastatic calcifications may produce rheumatologic complaints of calcific tendinitis and chondrocalcinosis. Osteomalacia and osteitis fibrosa cystica are seen from depletion of vitamin D due to prolonged PTH renal conversion of 25-OH-D_3 to active 1-α-25 $(OH_2)D_3$.

DIAGNOSIS

Since the patient is frequently asymptomatic, the diagnosis is made in 80 to 90% of cases by finding an elevated serum calcium in conjunction with an elevated radioimmunoassay for PTH. Total serum calcium should be elevated on three separate measurements before hypercalcemia is established. The presence of nephrocalcinosis or other soft tissue calcifications deserves exclusion of primary hyperparathyroidism.

Other laboratory findings which may be present include hypophosphatemia, hypercalciuria, low serum bicarbonate, elevated serum chloride, and elevations in serum alkaline phosphatase if there is bone involvement. Radiographic manifestations of osteitis fibrosa cystica, nephrolithiasis, or other extra skeletal calcifications may be present. Other causes of hypercalcemia should be eliminated (see Table 26.12).

Table 26.12.
Causes of Hypercalcemia

1. Hyperparathyroidism
   a. Primary: parathyroid adenomas, hyperplasia or carcinoma
   b. Secondary: compensatory increase in PTH due to low calcium levels as in renal failure, osteomalacia, intestinal malabsorption
2. Granulomatous disease (sarcoidosis, tuberculosis)
3. Drugs
   a. Vitamin D, vitamin A, or calcium intoxification
   b. Milk-alkali syndrome
   c. Thiazide diuretics
   d. Lithium
4. Malignancies
   a. Nonhematologic (breast, bronchus)
   b. Hematologic (myeloma, leukemia, lymphoma)
5. Endocrine (Addison's, thyrotoxicosis)
6. Immobilization
7. Bone disorders (Paget's, osteoporosis)
8. Idiopathic hypercalcemia of infancy
9. Familial hypocalciuric hypercalcemia

CLINICAL PRESENTATION: SIGNS AND SYMPTOMS

Prior to the use of routine serum calcium measurements, patients classically presented with symptoms from severe hypercalcemia with bone and renal involvement (107). However, earlier detection of the disease has changed the clinical presentation so that most patients are relatively asymptomatic (108) or have nonspecific complaints of weakness and easy fatigability. In the high risk elderly female, the presenting picture may be one of confusion and dehydration (109).

The clinical spectrum and complications of primary hyperparathyroidism are presented in Table 26.13. The severity of the clinical manifestations, especially the degree of hypercalcemia, is generally proportional to the degree of hyperfunctioning tissue and level of PTH elevation.

Treatment of Hyperparathyroidism

SURGICAL MANAGEMENT

Surgical exploration of the neck and removal of adenomatous, hyperplastic, or malignant tissue is the definitive treatment of choice for symptomatic primary hyperparathyroid-

ism (110). Surgery is absolutely indicated in patients with: (a) serum calcium above 11 mg/100 ml, (b) evidence of bone involvement, (c) evidence of renal involvement, (d) complications from hyperparathyroidism, and (e) co-existing disease state which may be exacerbated by elevations in calcium such as in hypertension, arthritis.

In patients with mild asymptomatic rises in serum calcium the indications for surgery are less clear since the true progression of the disease is unknown (111, 112). In a 5-year prospective study of 134 patients with mild asymptomatic hyperparathyroidism, only 20% required surgical intervention due to progression of their disease while 58% had no deterioration in their clinical status (111). In this group it appears that the risks and costs of surgery must be weighed against presumed benefits. Such patients should probably be followed closely at 6- to 12-month intervals with serum calcium, phosphorus, renal function tests, and skeletal x-rays. If evidence for progression of the disease is found, surgical intervention should be considered (see section on "Medical Management").

The most critical consideration in the surgical treatment of primary hyperparathyroidism is the selection of an experienced and skilled surgeon. In competent hands the evidence of postoperative complications (i.e. vocal cord paralysis) is low while the cure rate is high.

Postoperatively, serum calcium levels may normalize or fall below normal within 24 to 48 hours. Hypocalcemia is usually mild and transient although tetany and permanent hypoparathyroidism may occur. Patients at high risk for the latter include those with evidence of bone demineralization, those with kidney involvement, those with steatorrhea, those undergoing total parathyroidectomy, and those undergoing multiple neck explorations (110).

Serum calcium levels should be monitored daily until levels stabilize about the 5th to 6th day. Symptoms of tetany or pretetany should be treated with 10 to 20 ml of 10% calcium gluconate given intravenously until symptoms are relieved. Modest degrees of hypocalcemia postoperatively need not be treated except by ensuring an adequate calcium intake. A small percentage of patients will develop permanent hypoparathyroidism requiring treatment with vitamin D (see section on "Hypoparathyroidism").

Table 26.13.
Signs and Symptoms of Hyperparathyroidism

System	Symptoms	Complications	Laboratory Tests
Gastrointestinal	Nausea, vomiting, anorexia, constipation, abdominal pain	Peptic ulcer disease 10–15%, chronic pancreatitis, fecal impaction/intestinal obstruction	↑ Amylase
Genitourinary	Polyuria, nocturia, polydipsia, symptoms of uremia, renal colic pain	Nephrocalcinosis 20–30%, renal failure, pyelonephritis	Hematuria, inability to concentrate urine, pyuria
Skeletal	Vague aches and pains, arthralgias, localized swellings	Osteitis fibrosa cystica, pathologic fractures, bone cysts; calcium depositions leading to gout, pseudogout	Radiologic → subperiosteal bone resorption
Neurologic	Emotional lability, slow mentation, poor memory, weakness, easy fatigability, drowsiness, coma	Depression, psychoses; headaches; myopathy (proximal)	Hyperactive deep tendon reflexes
Cardiovascular		Hypertension 20–60%	ECG: ↓ QT interval
Metabolic	Dehydration	Hyperchloremic acidosis	HCO_3 ↓ Cl ↑
Others	Pruritus due to ectopic calcifications in skin; ectopic calcifications in lungs, kidneys, etc.; red eyes	Anemia, band keratopathy, thrombosis	

MEDICAL MANAGEMENT

There is no pharmacological substitutes for the surgical management of hyperparathyroidism. However, medical management of hypercalcemia is necessary in patients who refuse surgery, in patients prior to surgery, in patients with life threatening hypercalcemia, in patients with resistant or recurrent hyperparathyroidism despite previous neck surgery, and in patients who are poor surgical candidates. Several modalities are available although not all are useful in the treatment of hypercalcemia from primary hyperparathyroidism (see Table 26.14). Hypercalcemia can be corrected by inhibiting bone resorption, increasing calcium excretion, or decreasing calcium absorption (113, 114).

General therapeutic measures should include adequate hydration, ambulation, restriction of dietary calcium and avoidance of thiazide diuretics which can decrease calcium urinary excretion.

In an emergency hypercalcemic situation, aggressive treatment with isotonic normal saline, furosemide, oral phosphates, as well as mithramycin may be required to prevent coma and death.

Several pharmacological agents have been investigated in hopes of finding a medical treatment for hyperparathyroidism. These have included the following:

Propranolol. Beta blockers have been recommended since beta-adrenergic catecholamines have been shown to stimulate PTH secretion. However, most studies with propranolol have been disappointing, suggesting that abnormal parathyroid glands may lose their normal responsiveness to catecholamines (115).

Cimetidine. The rationale that histamine stimulates release of PTH in vitro and in vivo has led to speculation that cimetidine may be effective. Although one study found cimetidine effective, most have found cimetidine ineffective (116).

Diphosphonates. These agents have great affinity for bone and appear to work by impairing the function of the osteoclast. The most promising agent is dichloromethylene diphosphonate (117).

Further investigations are required to find an effective medical treatment for primary hyperparathyroidism. Until such time surgery is still the treatment of choice.

Table 26.14.
Treatment of Hypercalcemia

Methods	Dose and Onset Treatment Characteristics	Effective in Primary Hyperparathyroidism	Comments
INHIBIT BONE RESORPTION			
Mobilization	Immobilization accelerates bone resorption	Yes	
Sodium Phosphates	May also inhibit calcium absorption through decreased production of 1,25-dihydroxy-vitamin D. IV up to 50 mmol (1.5 g phosphorus over 6–8 hr). PO elemental phosphorus 2–3 g/day given in 4 divided doses	Yes	Metastatic calcifications associated with hypotension, hypocalcemia, renal failure, death after IV can occur (Ref. 125). Oral causes diarrhea, nausea, vomiting
Mithramycin	Lowers serum calcium within 24–48 hr after a single 25–50 μg/kg injection. Maximum decline in 2–5 days	Yes	Toxicity of nausea, vomiting; hemorrhage, liver and renal damage most common with repeated doses in debilitated patients
Calcitonin	Doses of 4 MRC[a] units/kg induce falls of serum calcium of 1–2 mg/100 ml. Maximum effect in 6–9 hr, duration of 24 hr	No	Relatively free of toxicity; major benefit in Paget's disease
Estrogens	Option in postmenopausal women with hyperparathyroidism	Yes	Risks of estrogen therapy
INCREASE IN CALCIUM EXCRETION			
Hydration	Rehydration with normal saline can cause as much as 2–3 mg/100 ml drop in calcium	Yes	Watch for fluid overload and electrolyte disturbance, i.e., hypokalemia
Diuretics, i.e. furosemide	Use in conjunction with large doses of normal saline, as much as furosemide 100 mg every 2 hr may be required	Yes	Avoid thiazide diuretics which decrease calcium excretion. Replace electrolytes
DECREASE CALCIUM ABSORPTION			
Phosphates (see above)			
Cellulose phosphate	15 g/day		Watch for hypomagnesemia; Relatively free of toxic effects
Sodium phytate	6–9 mg/day	Yes	Diarrhea, nausea, vomiting, anorexia
OTHER MECHANISMS			
Steroids	Prednisone 30–100 mg/day or equivalent. Acts by decreasing calcium absorption, increasing calcium excretion and inhibits vitamin D effects	No	Most effective in malignant disorders, vitamin D intoxification, sarcoidosis
Diphosphonates	Appear to impair function of osteoclast	Yes	Investigational
Indomethacin	Dose 25 mg every 6 hr. May correct hypercalcemia caused by prostaglandin production	No	
Dialysis	Hemodialysis and peritoneal	Yes	Temporary effect; rebound with dialysis

[a] MRC = Medical Research Council.

PROGNOSIS

Surgical resection of benign parathyroid lesions is generally curative in primary hyperparathyroidism. Recurrences are common when multiple glands are involved but rare with single gland involvement.

Hypoparathyroidism

Hypoparathyroidism is an endocrine disorder characterized by a deficiency of parathyroid hormone, hypocalcemia, and hyperphosphatemia.

ETIOLOGY/INCIDENCE

The most common cause of hypoparathyroidism is related to surgical excision or exploration of the anterior neck. In experienced surgical hands the incidence of permanent hypoparathyroidism is less than 1% for all thyroid and parathyroid surgery (118). This risk is increased significantly after subtotal parathyroidectomy for parathyroid hyperplasia (multiple gland involvement) or after repeated neck surgery for recurrent disease.

Other rare causes include idiopathic hypoparathyroidism (unknown etiology), neonatal hypoparathyroidism, destruction of the parathyroid glands by radiation or metastatic disease, inactive parathyroid hormone, and target organ resistance to PTH (pseudohypoparathyroidism).

Functional hypoparathyroidism occurs with severe hypomagnesemia but is reversible with magnesium replacement. Magnesium is required for both PTH release from the gland and for the action of PTH peripherally. Some causes of hypomagnesemia include starvation, prolonged intravenous feeding, malabsorption, chronic alcoholism, diuretics, aminoglycoside, and cis-platinum therapy (114).

PATHOGENESIS

Deficiency of PTH hormone produces the following metabolic changes: (a) decreased bone resorption, (b) hyperphosphatemia and hypophosphaturia, (c) decreased intestinal absorption of calcium, (d) decreased levels of active $1-\alpha-25$-hydroxy-vitamin D_3, (e) hypocalcemia and hypercalciuria, and (f) metabolic alkalosis from decreased bicarbonate excretion.

DIAGNOSIS

The diagnosis of hypoparathyroidism should be suspected in the presence of hypocalcemia, hyperphosphatemia, undetectable levels of PTH, and a history of previous neck surgery. However, serum phosphates may not always be elevated because of dietary restriction; use of aluminum-containing phosphate binders, or increased mineral uptake by bone. The presence of normal or elevated PTH levels in the face of hypocalcemia excludes the diagnosis of hypoparathyroidism but strongly suggests end organ resistance to PTH (pseudohypoparathyroidism). Serum magnesium levels should be obtained to exclude the diagnosis of functional hypoparathyroidism. Other causes of hypocalcemia, including drug-induced, should be excluded (114) (see Table 26.15).

The long-term use of anticonvulsants such as phenytoin, phenobarbital, and structurally related compounds stimulate the hepatic conversion of vitamin D_3 and 25-hydroxy-D_3 to biologically inactive metabolites resulting in decreased concentrations of active 25-hydroxy-D_3, malabsorption of calcium, hypocalcemia and osteomalacia. This risk is higher in patients on long-term combination anticonvulsant therapy, patients with low dietary calcium intake, patients with little sunlight exposure, patients with diseases predisposing to vitamin D malabsorption, and blacks because of greater resistance to the irradiating effects

Table 26.15.
Causes of Hypocalcemia

1. Hypoparathyroidism
   a. Surgical: post-thyroidectomy, post-parathyroidectomy, post neck exploration
   b. Idiopathic (unknown)
   c. Neonatal
   d. Destruction of parathyroids, i.e. tumor, radiation
   e. Pseudohypoparathyroidism (end-organ resistance to PTH)
   f. Inactive PTH hormone
2. Magnesium deficiency (functional hypoparathyroidism)
3. Acute pancreatitis
4. Chronic renal failure
5. Osteomalacia
6. Drugs: phenytoin, phenobarbital, cholestyramine (see text); laxative abuse with phosphate enemas; aminoglycoside nephrotoxicity

of sunlight. Changes in serum calcium, alkaline phosphatase, and phosphate as well as the bony changes of osteomalacia should be closely monitored for in these patients. Fortunately, anticonvulsant-induced hypocalcemia and osteomalacia is responsive to vitamin D therapy (119, 120).

Another iatrogenic cause of hypocalcemia and osteomalacia is related to the long term administration of cholestyramine which binds the bile acids necessary for vitamin D absorption from the intestine. Therapy with higher doses of vitamin D is necessary to overcome the gut inhibitory effects of cholestyramine on vitamin D absorption (121, 22).

CLINICAL FINDINGS

The clinical manifestations of hypoparathyroidism is related to the severity of hypocalcemia as well as to the chronicity. Acute lowering of the calcium levels such as seen within the first 48 hours after parathyroidectomy are much more likely to produce hypocalcemic symptoms than slow depressions of calcium levels. Changes in acid-base status will also effect symptomatology. Alkalosis worsens hypocalcemia by decreasing ionized calcium through increased calcium binding by plasma proteins. The converse occurs in acidosis where ionized levels of calcium are increased.

The signs and symptoms of hypocalcemia and hypoparathyroidism are presented in Table 26.16.

Treatment of Hypoparathyroidism

Theoretically, the most appropriate therapy for hypoparathyroidism would be the administration of PTH although this is not very practical since no suitable oral preparation is available. However, an effective alternative to PTH is therapy with calcium supplementation and either vitamin D_2 or dihydrotachysterol (DHT) to increase intestinal calcium absorption.

Severe hypocalcemia complicated by tetany requires emergency treatment with intravenous calcium gluconate 10% until symptoms

Table 26.16.
Clinical Features of Hypocalcemia/Hypoparathyroidism

System	Signs/Symptoms	Complication/Sequelae	Comments
Musculoskeletal	Circumoral and distal numbness and tingling, muscle twitching; hyper-reflexia, positive Chvostek's and Trousseau's	Tetany: carpopedal spasm, laryngeal stridor, convulsions	Requires emergency treatment with intravenous calcium
Neurologic	Papilledema, increased CSF pressure; basal ganglia calcifications extra pyramidal symptoms; abnormal EEG	Epilepsy; parkinsonism: complication in 20% of patients with hypoparathyroidism	Improves with eucalcemia, increased sensitivity to dystonic reaction of phenothiazines
Psychiatric	Irritability	Depression, psychosis, mental retardation in 20% of children	May improve with eucalcemia
Integument	Dry scaly skin, coarse friable dry hair, longitudinal ridges on nails	Exfoliative dermatitis, atopic eczema, psoriasis, increase candida infection	May improve with eucalcemia
Ocular	Visual impairment and opacities of the lens	Lenticular cataracts: most common sequelae of hypoparathyroidism	Eucalcemia halts progression of cataracts
Others	Impaired dental development; intestinal malabsorption with steatorrhea; prolongation of QT interval; increased CPK, LDH		Improves with eucalcemia

Table 26.17.
Comparison of Vitamin Preparations

Vitamin D Preparations	Activity	Kinetics	Dose	Comments
Vitamin D$_2$ (ergocalciferol). Caps: 10,000, 25,000, and 50,000 units	Biologically inactive; require activation by hepatic 25-hydroxylation and by renal 1-α-hydroxylase; require bile salts for complete absorption in gut	Onset approximately 2 weeks (4–12 weeks range) long $t_{1/2}$ (half-life) highly protein bound, slow elimination: duration 3–6 mo	50–100,000 units/day	Least expensive; overdose may produce symptoms for up to 16–18 weeks after discontinuation
Dihydrotachysterol (DHT) (Hytakerol). Caps: 0.125 and 0.2 mg. Solution: 0.25 mg/ml	Requires only hepatic 25-hydroxylation for activation	Rapid onset within 2 hr, duration 7–15 days, short $t_{1/2}$	0.2–2.5 mg/day (average 0.5)	More expensive than vitamin D$_2$; useful when rapid effect desired, i.e. postoperative hypocalcemic tetany
1-α-25-dihydroxy vitamin D$_3$ (calcitriol) (Rocaltrol). Available as 0.25 and 0.5 μg	Active	Rapid onset, 1–3 days; $t_{1/2}$: 1–2 hr	Dose 0.25 μg initially, increase within 2–4 weeks; range 0.5–1 μg	Expensive; toxicity of decreased renal function. Useful in renal osteodystrophy or with defect in 1-α-hydroxylation
25-Hydroxy-vitamin D$_3$ (calcediol) (Calderol). Caps: 20 and 50 μg	Active	More rapid onset of action than vitamin D$_2$, but slower than DHT, metabolite has long $t_{1/2}$ of 16 days	50–100 μg/d; to be determined for each patient	Less expensive than DHT and 1-α 25-vitamin D$_3$; major disadvantage is long $t_{1/2}$ of metabolite (16 days)

are relieved or until serum calcium levels increase above 7.5 mg/100 ml. A continuous effect may be obtained by administering 100 ml of the 10% calcium gluconate in 1 liter of normal saline infused over 24 hours. Caution should be exercised in giving calcium to patients on digitalis and hypomagnesemia should be corrected if present. Oral supplements should be started immediately.

A daily intake of 1 to 2 g of elemental calcium and phosphate restriction via aluminum hydroxide binding gels may be all that is necessary to maintain calcium homeostasis in patients with mild hypoparathyroidism but in patients with serum calciums less than 7.5 mg/100 ml, concomitant therapy with vitamin D is often necessary to maintain eucalcemia.

If dietary intake is inadequate, calcium supplementation can be provided with any of the following salts although each has its own disadvantages. A large number of tablets are required when salts containing small amounts of calcium are given, i.e. gluconate although gastric irritation may be seen with salts containing large amounts of calcium, i.e. chloride.

The easiest and best tolerated calcium supplementation appears to be the use of Os-Cal-500 which contains 500 mg of calcium per tablet. Constipation is a potential problem with all calcium supplements. One gram of calcium is provided by the following salts:

Calcium carbonate	2.5 g	(40% calcium)
Calcium chloride	3.7 g	(27% calcium)
Calcium gluconate	12 g	(9% calcium)
Calcium lactate	9 g	(11% calcium)

A comparison of the available vitamin D preparations which differ mainly in cost, metabolism, and duration of toxicity is presented in Table 26.17 (123). Vitamin D_2 is commonly used since it is the least expensive of all the preparations. DHT is preferred over vitamin D_2 because of its more rapid onset of action as well as its more rapid dissipation in cases of inadvertent overdosage. The newer vitamin D_3 preparations are biologically active and superior to vitamin D_2 in terms of rapidity of onset and offset of action but are also more expensive. They appear to offer little advantage over DHT except in difficult to manage patients.

The main toxicity of all vitamin D preparations is hypercalcemia so that close monitoring of serum calcium, phosphorus, and alkaline phosphatase is indicated during dosage adjustment and on a regular basis thereafter. Calci-

triol may also be associated with deterioration of renal function in patients with previously stable renal function (124).

Therapy can be initiated with vitamin D_2 10,000 to 25,000 units/day and then gradually increased only after maximal effects are achieved in 4 to 6 weeks. Average doses range from 50,000 to 150,000 units daily. An alternative regimen is DHT 4 mg daily for 2 days, then 2 mg daily for 2 days, then 1 mg daily thereafter unless dosage adjustment is required. Serum calcium levels should ideally be maintained between 8.5 and 9 mg/100 ml leaving a margin for fluctuations. Serum calcium and phosphorus levels should be checked at least monthly till stable then every 3 to 6 months thereafter.

PROGNOSIS

The prognosis is excellent. Improvement in the majority of manifestations can be expected with restoration of serum calcium levels to normal.

References

1. Sterling K: Thyroid hormone action at the cell level part 1. N Engl J Med 300:117, 1979.
2. Sterling K: Thyroid hormone action at the cell level part 2. N Engl J Med 300:173, 1979.
3. Larsen PR: Thyroid-pituitary interaction: Feedback regulation of thyrotropin secretion by thyroid hormones. N Engl J Med 306:23, 1982.
4. Vagenakis AG, Braverman LE: Adverse effects of iodides on thyroid function. Med Clin North Am 59:1075, 1975.
5. Ingbar SH: Autoregulation of the thyroid: Response to iodide excess and depletion. Mayo Clin Proc 42:814, 1972.
6. Kaplan MM, Larsen PR, Crantz FR, et al: Prevalence of abnormal thyroid function test results in patients with acute medical illness. Am J Med 72:9, 1982.
7. Yamada T, Nobiuyuki N, Sato N, et al: Pituitary-thyroid feedback regulation in patients with Graves' disease during antithyroid drug therapy. J Clin Endocrinol Metab 54:83, 1982.
8. McFarland KF, Strickland AL, Metzger WT, et al: Thyrotropin-releasing hormone test. Arch Intern Med 142:132, 1982.
9. Jackson IMD: Thyrotropin releasing hormone. N Engl J Med 306:145, 1982.
10. Volpe R: The pathogenesis of Graves' disease: An overview. Clin Endocrinol Metab 7:3, 1978.
11. Zakarija M, McKenzie JM, Banovac K: Clinical significance of assay of thyroid-stimulating antibody in Graves' disease. Ann Intern Med 93:28, 1980.
12. Blum M: Thyroid function and disease in the elderly. Hosp Pract 16:105, 1981.
13. Okita N, Row VV, Volpe R: Suppressor T-lymphocyte deficiency in Graves' disease and

Hashimoto's thyroiditis. *J Clin Endocrinol Metab* 52:528, 1981.

14. Sridama V, Pacini F, DeGroot L: Decreased suppressor T-lymphocytes in autoimmune thyroid disease detected by monoclonal antibodies. *J Clin Endocrinol Metab* 54:316, 1982.

15. Bouzas A-G: Endocrine opthalmopathy. *Trans Ophthamol Soc U K* 100:511, 1980.

16. Gwinup G, Elias AN, Ascher MS: Effect on exopthalmos of various methods of treatment of Graves' disease. *JAMA* 247:2135, 1982.

17. McDougall IR, Kriss JP: Management of the eye manifestations of thyroid disease. *Pharmac Ther C* 2:95, 1977.

18. Miller JM: Hyperthyroidism from the thyroid follicle with autonomous function. *Clin Endocrinol Metab* 7:177, 1978.

19. Volpe R: Subacute (de Quervain's) thyroiditis. *Clin Endocrinol Metab* 8:81, 1979.

20. Hollander CS, Shenkman L, Mitsuma T, *et al.* Hypertriiodothyroninemia as a premonitory manifestation of thyrotoxicosis. *Lancet* 2:731, 1971.

21. Savoie JC, Massin JP, Thomopoulos P, et al: Iodine-induced thyrotoxicosis in apparently normal glands. *J Clin Endocrinol Metab* 41:685, 1975.

22. Blum M, Weinberg W, Shenkman L, et al: Hyperthyroidism after iodinated contrast medium. *N Engl J Med* 291:24, 1974.

23. Silas AM, White AG: Hyperthyroidism after use of contrast medium. *Br Med J* 4:162, 1975.

24. Kristensen O, Harrestrup-Anderson H, Pallisgaard G: Lithium carbonate in the treatment of thyrotoxicosis. *Lancet* 1:603, 1976.

25. McDougall IR: Treatment of hyper- and hypothyroidism. *J Clin Pharmacol* 21:365, 1981.

26. Amino N, Tanizawa O, Mori H, et al: Aggrevation of thyrotoxicosis in early pregnancy and after delivery in Graves' disease. *J Clin Endocrinol Metab* 55:108, 1982.

27. Wood LC, Ingbar SH: Hypothyroidism as a late sequela in patients with Graves' disease treated with antithyroid agents. *J Clin Invest* 64:1429, 1979.

28. Marchant B, Lees JFH, Alexander WD: Antithyroid drugs. *Pharmac Ther B* 3:305, 1978.

29. Greer MA, Kammer H, Bouma DJ: Short term antithyroid drug therapy for the thyrotoxicosis of Graves' disease. *N Engl J Med* 297:173, 1977.

30. Tamai H, Nakagawa T, Fukino O, et al: Thionamide therapy in Graves' disease: Relation of relapse rate to duration of therapy. *Ann Intern Med* 92:488, 1980.

31. Slingerland DW, Burrows BA: Long-term antithyroid treatment in hyperthyroidism. *JAMA* 242:2408, 1979.

32. Bouma DJ, Kammer H: Single dose methimazole treatment of hyperthyroidism. *West J Med* 132:13, 1980.

33. Kammer H, Srinivasan K: The use of antithyroid drugs in a single daily dose: Treatment of diffuse toxic goiter. *JAMA* 209:1325, 1969.

34. Greer MA, Meihoff WC, Studer H: Treatment of hyperthyroidism with a single daily dose of propylthiouracil. *N Engl J Med* 272:888, 1965.

35. Barnes HV, Bledsoe T: A simple test for select-

ing the thionamide schedule in thyrotoxicosis. *J Clin Endocrinol Metab* 35:250, 1972.

36. Totten MA, Wool MS: Medical treatment of hyperthyroidism. *Med Clin North Am* 63:321, 1979.

37. Reynolds LR, Kotchen TA: Antithyroid drugs and radioactive iodine: Fifteen years' experience with Graves' disease. *Arch Intern Med* 139:651, 1979.

38. Wartofsky L: Low remission after therapy for Graves' disease—Possible relation of dietary iodine with antithyroid therapy results. *JAMA* 226:1083, 1973.

39. Yamamoto M, Igarashi T, Kimura S, et al: Thyroid suppression test and outcome of hyperthyroidism treated with antithyroid drugs and triiodothyronine. *J Clin Endocrinol Metab* 48:72, 1979.

40. Davies TF, Evered DC, Rees Smith B, et al: Value of thyroid stimulating antibody determinations in predicting short term thyrotoxic relapse in Graves' disease. *Lancet* 1:1181, 1977.

41. McGregor AM, Rees Smith B, Hall R: Prediction of relapse in hyperthyroid Graves' disease. *Lancet* 1:1101, 1980.

42. Irvine WJ, Gray RS, Morris PJ, et al: Correlation of HLA and thyroid antibodies with clinical course of thyrotoxicosis treated with antithyroid drugs. *Lancet* 2:898, 1977.

43. Rosove MH: Agranulocytosis and antithyroid drugs. *West J Med* 126:339, 1977.

44. Wiberg JJ, Nutall FQ: Methimazole toxicity from high doses. *Ann Intern Med* 77:414, 1972.

44a. Cooper DS, Goldminz D, Levin AA, et al: Agranulocytosis associated with antithyroid drugs. Effects of patient age and drug dose. *Ann Int Med* 98:26, 1983.

45. Feek CM, Sawers JSA, Irvine WJ, et al: Combination of potassium iodide and propranolol in preparation of patients with Graves' disease for thyroid surgery. *N Engl J Med* 302:883, 1980.

46. Mazzaferri EL, Reynolds JC, Young RL, et al: Propranolol as primary therapy for thyrotoxicosis. *Arch Intern Med* 136:50, 1976.

47. Feely J, Forrest A, Gunn A, et al: Propranolol dosage in thyrotoxicosis. *J Clin Endocrinol Metab* 51:658, 1980.

48. Eriksson M, Rubenfeld S, Garber AJ, et al: Propranolol does not prevent thyroid storm. *N Engl J Med* 296:263, 1977.

49. Feely J, Crooks J, Forrest AL, et al: Propranolol in the surgical treatment of hyperthyroidism including severely thyrotoxic patients. *Br J Surg* 68:865, 1981.

50. Feely J, Stevenson IH, Crooks J: Increased clearance of propranolol in thyrotoxicosis. *Ann Intern Med* 94:472, 1981.

51. Riddell JG: Effect of thyroid dysfunction on propranolol kinetics. *Clin Pharmacol Ther* 28:565, 1980.

52. Safa AM, Schumacher OP, Rodriguez-Antunez A: Long-term follow-up of results in children and adolescents treated with radioactive iodine (I^{131}) for hyperthyroidism. *N Engl J Med* 292:167, 1975.

53. Freitas JE, Swanson DP, Gross MD, et al: Iodine-131: Optimal therapy for hyperthyroidism in

children and adolescents? *J Nucl Med* 20:847, 1979.

54. Dobyns BM, Sheline GE, Workman JB, et al: Malignant and benign neoplasms of the thyroid in patients treated for hyperthyroidism—A report of the cooperative thyrotoxicosis therapy follow-up study. *J Clin Endocrinol Metab* 38:976, 1974.

55. Robertson JS, Gorman CA: Gonadal radiation dose and its genetic significance in radioiodine therapy of hyperthyroidism. *J Nucl Med* 17:826, 1976.

56. Holm LE, Dahlqvist I, Israelsson A, et al: Malignant thyroid tumors after iodine-131 therapy: A retrospective cohort study. *N Engl J Med* 303:188, 1980.

57. Holm LE, Lundell G, Israelsson A, et al: Incidence of hypothyroidism occurring long after iodine-131 therapy for hyperthyroidism. *J Nucl Med* 23:103, 1982.

58. Holm LE: Changing annual incidence of hypothyroidism after iodine-131 therapy for hyperthyroidism: 1951–1975. *J Nucl Med* 23:108, 1982.

59. Wu SY, Chopra IJ, Solomon DH, et al: Change in circulating iodothyronine in euthyroid and hyperthyroid subjects given ipodate (Oragrafin), an agent for oral cholecystography. *J Clin Endocrinol Metab* 46:691, 1978.

60. Beng CG, Wellby ML, Symons RG, et al: The effects of ipodate on the serum iodothyronine pattern in normal subjects. *Acta Endocrinol* 93:175, 1980.

61. Sharp B, Reed AW, Tamagna EI, et al: Treatment of hyperthyroidism with sodium ipodate (Oragrafin) in addition to propylthiouracil and propranolol. *J Clin Endocrinol Metab* 53:622, 1981.

62. Wu S, Shyh T, Chopra J, et al: Comparison of sodium ipodate (Oragrafin) and propylthiouracil in early treatment of hyperthyroidism. *J Clin Endocrinol Metab* 54:630, 1982.

63. Beahrs OH, Sakulsky SB: Surgical thyroidectomy in the management of exopthalmic goiter. *Arch Surg* 96:512, 1968.

64. Bradley EL III, Digirolamo M, Tarcan Y: Modified subtotal thyroidectomy in the management of Graves' disease. *Surgery* 87:623, 1980.

65. Farnell MB, Van Heerdan JA, McConahey WM, et al: Hypothyroidism after thyroidectomy for Graves' disease. *Am J Surg* 142:535, 1981.

66. Burr WA: Thyroid disease. *Clin Obstet Gynecol* 8:341, 1981.

67. Fisher DA, Klein AH: Thyroid development and disorders of thyroid function in the newborn. *N Engl J Med* 304:702, 1981.

68. Galina MP, Avnet NL, Einhorn A: Iodide during pregnancy—An apparent cause of neonatal death. *N Engl J Med* 267:1124, 1962.

69. Prager EM, Gardner RE: Iatrogenic hypothyroidism from topical iodine-containing medications. *West J Med* 130:553, 1979.

70. Vorherr H, Vorherr UF, Pushpa M, et al: Vaginal absorption of povidone-iodine. *JAMA* 244:2628, 1980.

71. Postellon DC, Aronow R: Iodine in mother's milk: *JAMA* 247:463, 1982.

72. Cheron RG, Kaplan MM, Larsen PR, et al: Neonatal thyroid function after propylthiouracil therapy for maternal Graves' disease. *N Engl J Med* 304:525, 1981.

73. Mujtaba Q, Burrow GN: Treatment of hyperthyroidism in pregnancy with propylthiouracil and methimazole. *Obstet Gynecol* 46:282, 1975.

74. Kampmann JP, Hansen JM, Johansen K, et al: Propylthiouracil in human milk. *Lancet* 1:736, 1980.

75. Tegler L, Landstrom B: Antithyroid drugs in milk. *Lancet* 2:591, 1980.

76. Pruyn SC, Phelan JP, Buchanan JC: Long term propranolol therapy in pregnancy: Maternal and foetal outcome. *Am J Obstet Gynecol* 135:485, 1979.

77. Fischer DA: Pathogenesis and therapy of neonatal Graves' disease. *Am J Dis Child* 130:133, 1976.

78. Favus MJ, Schneider AB, Stachura ME, et al: Thyroid cancer occurring as a late consequence of head-and-neck irradiation. *N Engl J Med* 294:1019, 1976.

79. Hoffenberg R: Thyroid emergencies. *Clin Endocrinol Metab* 9:503, 1980.

80. Raber JH: The pharmacotherapy of thyroid storm. *Drug Intell Clin Pharm* 14:344, 1980.

81. Ibbertson HK: Endemic goiter and cretinism. *Clin Endocrinol Metab* 8:97, 1979.

82. Shopsin B: Effect of lithium on thyroid function. *Dis Nerv Syst* 31:237, 1970.

83. Bastenie PA, Bonnyns M, Vanhaelst L: Grades of subclinical hypothyroidism in asymptomatic autoimmune thyroiditis revealed by the thyrotropin-releasing hormone test. *J Clin Endocrinol Metab* 51:163, 1980.

84. Stock JM, Surks MI, Oppenheimer JH: Replacement dosage of L-thyroxine in hypothyroidism. *N Engl J Med* 290:529, 1974.

85. Rosenbaum RL, Barzel US: Levothyroxine replacement dose for primary hypothyroidism decreases with age. *Ann Intern Med* 96:53, 1982.

85a.Sawin CT, Herman T, Molitch ME, et al: Aging and the thyroid. Decreased requirement for thyroid hormone in older hypothyroid patients. *Am J Med* 75:206, 1983.

86. Levine HD: Compromise therapy in the patient with angina pectoris and hypothyroidism. *Am J Med* 69:411, 1980.

87. Mäenpää J: Congenital hypothyroidism—Aetiological and clinical aspects. *Arch Dis Child* 47:914, 1972.

88. Brennan MD: Clinical pharmacology series on pharmacology in practice 5 thyroid hormones. *Mayo Clin Proc* 55:33, 1980.

89. Rees-Jones RW, Rolla AR, Larsen PR: Hormonal content of thyroid replacement preparations. *JAMA* 243:549, 1980.

90. Sawin CT, Hershman JM, Fernandez-Garcia R, et al: A comparison of thyroxine and desiccated thyroid in patients with primary hypothyroidism. *Metabolism* 27:1518, 1978.

91. Stoffer SS, Szpunar WE: Potency of brand name and generic levothyroxine products. *JAMA* 244:1704, 1980.

92. Ingbar JC, Braverman LE, Ingbar SH: Equiva-

lence of thyroid preparations. *JAMA* 244:1095, 1980.

93. Montoro M, Collea JV, Frasier SD, et al: Successful outcome of pregnancy in women with hypothyroidism. *Ann Intern Med* 94:31, 1981.

94. Brown CL: Pathology of the cold nodule. *Clin Endocrinol Metab* 10:235, 1981.

95. Greenspan FS: Thyroid nodules and thyroid cancers. *West J Med* 121:359, 1974.

96. Hempelmann LH, Hall WJ, Phillips M, et al: Neoplasms in persons treated with x-rays in infancy: Fourth survey in 20 years. *J Natl Cancer Inst* 55:519, 1975.

97. Korff JM, DeGroot LJ: The management of radiation-induced tumors of the thyroid. *Clin Endocrinol Metab* 10:299, 1981.

98. Wenzel KW: Pharmacological interference with in vitro tests of thyroid function. *Metabolism* 30:717, 1981.

99. Cavalieri PR, Pitt-Rivers R: The effects of drugs on the distribution and metabolism of thyroid hormones. *Pharmacol Rev* 33:55, 1981.

100. Lawrence JR: Digoxin kinetics in patients with thyroid dysfunction. *Clin Pharmacol Ther* 22:7, 1977.

101. Bonelli J, Haydl H, Hruby K, et al: The pharmacokinetics of digoxin in patients with manifest hyperthyroidism and after normalization of thyroid function. *Int J Clin Pharmacol Bipharm* 16:302, 1978.

102. Hansten PD: Oral anticoagulants and drugs which alter thyroid function. *Drug Intell Clin Pharm* 14:331, 1980.

103. Vessell ES: The antipyrine test in clinical pharmacology: Conceptions and misconceptions. *Clin Pharm Ther* 25:275, 1979.

104. Arnaud CD: The parathyroid gland, in Wyngaarden JB, Smith LH Jr: *Cecil Textbook of Medicine*, ed 16. Philadelphia: W. B. Saunders, 1982, p 1286.

105. Boonstra CE, Jackson CE: Serum Ca: Survey for hyperparathyroidism results in 50,000 clinic patients. *Am J Clin Pathol* 55:523, 1971.

106. Heath H, Hodgson SF, Kennedy MD: Primary hyperparathyroidism. Incidence, morbidity and potential economic impact in a community. *N Engl J Med* 302:189, 1980.

107. Watson L: Primary hyperparathyroidism. *Clin Endocrinol Metab* 3:215, 1974.

108. Barzel US: The changing face of hyperparathyroidism. *Hosp Pract* 12:89, 1977.

109. Mundy GR, Cove DH, Fisken R: Primary hyperparathyroidism: Changes in the pattern of clinical presentation. *Lancet* 1:1317, 1980.

110. Davies DR: The surgery of primary hyperparathyroidism. *Clin Endocrinol Metab* 3:253, 1974.

111. Purnell DC, Scholz DA, Smith LH, et al: Treatment of primary hyperparathyroidism. *Am J Med* 56:800, 1974.

112. Coe FL, Favus MD: Does mild asymptomatic hyperparathyroidism require surgery? *N Engl J Med* 302:224, 1980.

113. Bilezikian JP: The medical management of primary hyperparathyroidism. *Ann Intern Med* 96:198, 1982.

114. Heath DA: The emergency management of disorders of calcium and magnesium. *Clin Endocrinol Metab* 9:487, 1980.

115. Vora NM, Kukreja SC, Williams GA, et al: Parathyroid hormone secretion: Effect of beta-adrenergic blockage before and after surgery for primary hyperparathyroidism. *J Clin Endocrinol Metab* 53:599, 1981.

116. Ljunghall S, Akerstrom G, Rudberg C, et al: Treatment with cimetidine in patients with primary hyperparathyroidism. *Acta Endocrinol* 99:546, 1982.

117. Shane E, Baquiran DC, Bilezikian JP: Effects of dichloromethylene diphosphonates on serum and urinary calcium in primary hyperparathyroidism. *Ann Intern Med* 95:23, 1981.

118. Witt TR, Meng RL, Economou SG, et al: The approach to the irradiated thyroid. *Surg Clin North Am* 59:45, 1979.

119. Hahn TA, Hendun BA, Scharp CR, et al: Effect of anticonvulsant therapy on 25-hydroxycalciferol. *N Engl J Med* 287:900, 1972.

120. Frame B: Hypocalcemia and osteomalacia associated with anticonvulsant therapy. *Ann Intern Med* 74:294, 1971.

121. Compston JE, Horton LWL: Oral 25-hydroxy vitamin D_3 in treatment of osteomalacia associated with ileal resection and cholestyramine therapy. *Gastroenterology* 74:900, 1978.

122. Heaton KW, Lever JV, Barnard D: Osteomalacia associated with cholestyramine for postileectomy diarrhea. *Gastroenterology* 62:642, 1972.

123. Kelly JF: New developments in the understanding of vitamin D and its metabolites. *Pharmacy and Therapeutics Forum*. Bulletin of the UC Hospital Pharmacy and Drug Information Analysis Service. UCSF. Vol 291, No. 1, 1981.

124. Massry SG, Goldstein DA: Is calcitriol [1,25-$(OH)_2D_3$] harmful? *JAMA* 242:1875, 1980.

125. Heath DA: Use of inorganic phosphate in the management of hypercalcemia. *Metab Bone Dis Relat Res* 2:213, 1980.

126. Ivey MF: Parathyroid disorders, in Herfindal ET, Hirschman JL: *Clinical Pharmacy and Therapeutics*, ed 2. Baltimore: Williams & Wilkins, 1979, p 470.

127. Stoffer SS, Szpunar WE: Potency of levothyroxine products. *JAMA* 251:635, 1984.

CHAPTER 27

Diabetes

R. KEITH CAMPBELL, B.Pharm., M.B.A.

Diabetes mellitus is a complex condition in that the effects of the disease touch on all areas of medicine. It is a condition in which there is still much to be learned; however, in recent years numerous changes have taken place in the understanding and treatment of diabetes mellitus. The effect of these changes on the diabetic patient has been dramatic. The process of self-blood glucose monitoring, in combination with better education programs and new treatment protocols, has been the most significant change in the treatment of diabetes since the discovery of insulin.

Some of the new developments in diabetes since 1980 include the following: a new classification system for diabetes; increased evidence to support "strict" control of blood glucose; new methods of monitoring control; greater emphasis on patient self-monitoring; more and better education programs; purer insulins; new treatment methods, including insulin infusion devices; a team approach to treatment including the pharmacist; numerous new products; the potential feasibility of transplantation of islet tissues; and a clearer but far from complete understanding of the many pathophysiological factors that can result in higher than normal blood glucose values.

A thorough, positive education program for the diabetic patient with respect to the disease, medication, blood and urine testing, and hygiene is a major component of diabetic management. Studies have demonstrated that poor control of diabetes is often the result of medication error, misinterpretation of test results, and ignorance of the disease (1). The diabetic needs a complete educational program that requires a total health team effort to be managed successfully. The physician must diagnose the condition accurately, clarify the type of diabetes, and stimulate the patient to learn to control and monitor the condition. The dietitian explains the importance of diet control and the food exchange system. The nurse helps the patient to develop a positive attitude, learn how to perform tests, monitor control, inject insulin and keep records of the factors that affect diabetic control. The pharmacist's easy access to the patient offers a unique opportunity to help the patient maintain a proper therapeutic regimen. The pharmacist can help answer patient questions about the disease, blood testing, urine testing, drug therapy, diet products and foot care, and can stress the information provided by other members of the team. The pharmacist also can monitor the course of diabetic patients. Since diabetic patients see pharmacists more often than any other health professional, the pharmacist is in a unique position to have a significant effect on the treatment of diabetic patients. Pharmacists who want to help their diabetic patients need to not only understand pharmacological facts but must also become competent in selecting, initiating and individualizing drug therapy for the various types of diabetic patients.

DEFINITION

Diabetes mellitus is a difficult condition to define because it is really a variety of conditions that have hyperglycemia as the common physiological problem that needs to be brought under control. Just a few years ago, everyone thought of diabetes as a single disease. It is clear now that diabetes is a heterogeneous group of disorders, almost all of which have a genetic basis, but in which the genetic types vary. Not only does the *insulin-dependent (type I)* form of diabetes differ from *non-insulin-dependent (type II)* diabetes, but within each of these two types there appears to be heterogeneity (2). Diabetes is a chronic disease characterized by disorders in carbohydrate (and associated fat and protein) metabolism due to an absolute or relative deficiency in the action of insulin and possibly abnormally high amounts of glucagon and other insulin-antagonizing substances such as growth hormone, sympathomimetic amines and corticosteroids. Insulin secretion in diabetes may progress from nearly normal capabilities to a totally deficient state.

Properly classifying the diabetic into one of several categories in which hyperglycemia is a clinical finding is critical in developing a treatment protocol to bring the patient under control. Diabetics in the past have been classified in numerous ways, including: degree of glucose tolerance; age of onset (juvenile or adult); body weight; degree of hyperglycemia or glucosuria, or both; susceptibility to ketoacidosis; insulin dependency; degree of severity and stability; treatment priority; and the presence or absence of large and small blood vessel lesions.

A classification of diabetes and other categories of glucose intolerance based on contemporary knowledge of this heterogeneous syndrome was developed by the National Diabetes Data Group in 1980 to assure consistency in treatment (3). Table 27.1 summarizes the new classification system and compares it to old methods as well as therapy recommended for each classification.

The two major clinical presentations of diabetes are maturity-onset and juvenile-onset types. Eighty percent of diabetics are identified after the age of 35 and are of the obese, maturity-onset type (4). They retain some pancreatic function and are relatively easily controlled on diet, or diet plus the use of oral hypoglycemic agents. Insulin may be required in 20 to 30% of cases although they rarely develop ketoacidosis (4). Many maturity-onset diabetics have normal or high levels of insulin, and it is possible that sluggish insulin secretion in response to glucose and a relative tissue resistance to insulin due to a low number of insulin receptors may be responsible for the symptomatology. Ten percent of type II diabetics are stable, nonobese, maturity-onset types; while 5% have brittle, adult-onset diabetes which more closely resembles the juvenile-onset presentation. Insulin-dependent (juvenile-onset) diabetes accounts for only 5% of diabetes (4). These patients have no pancreatic function and require insulin to control their symptoms. The blood glucose levels of juvenile-onset diabetics may fluctuate widely despite treatment, and these diabetics are more prone to ketosis than are the type II diabetics. Table 27.2 compares the distinguishing features of the two major clinical types of diabetes.

PREVALENCE

Diabetes mellitus and its complications are now the third leading cause of death in the United States, accounting for 300,000 lives each year (5). Almost 5% of Americans may have diabetes, and the incidence is increasing by 600,000 new cases yearly or at a rate of approximately 6%. If the present trend continues, by 1990 there will be over 20 million diabetics in the United States. Five to 6% of hospital admissions are due to diabetes. A new diabetic is diagnosed every 60 sec, and the chance of developing diabetes doubles with every 20% of excess weight and every decade of life (5).

Diabetes is the leading cause of new cases of blindness; diabetics are 25 times more prone to blindness than nondiabetics. Diabetics are 17 times more prone to kidney disease, and approximately half of insulin-dependent diabetics will succumb to chronic renal failure (5). Macroangiopathy occurs prematurely and progresses at an accelerated rate (killing 75% of non-insulin-dependent diabetics). Diabetics are twice as prone to heart disease and stroke as nondiabetics and are 5 times more prone to developing gangrene. Up to 50% of men with diabetes of long duration are sexually impotent, and as many as 25% of new renal transplant recipients are diabetic. The economic cost of diabetes is greater than 5 billion dollars annually and is growing. The average diabetic generated costs of $2,421 in 1979 (6). More than a billion dollars are expanded for diabetics with renal problems annually. The economic costs for insulin-dependent diabetics are approximately 13% higher than for type II diabetics.

Diabetics face the problem of being offered a bewildering selection of products that are not properly formulated, clearly labeled or safe to use. Thus the pharmacist has an excellent opportunity to act as a consultant to physician, nurse, dietitian and patient to disseminate useful information about diabetes care products and their proper use.

ETIOLOGY

Numerous factors have been associated with the development of diabetes. Table 27.3 summarizes some of the factors that have been linked to the development of diabetes. The understanding of diabetes is a continuous process and is far from complete and additional factors will undoubtedly be added in the

Table 27.1.
Classification and Therapy of Diabetes

Current Terminology	Others	Diet	Exercise	Insulin	Oral Hypoglycemic	Education
Type I Insulin dependent diabetes mellitus	Juvenile-onset Youth-onset Ketosis-prone Brittle	a) Regular meal schedule b) Restrict "simple sugars" c) No restriction of total carbohydrate (i.e., 50–60% of total calories) d) Limited fats (i.e., 30–50% of total calories) e) Avoid fad diets f) Increase fiber	Yes	Yes	No	Yes
Type II Noninsulin dependent diabetes mellitus a) Obese b) Normal weight	Adult-onset Maturity-onset Ketosis-resistant	*Obese:* a) Hypocaloric intake b) Limit fats *Nonobese:* a) Eucaloric intake b) Restrict "simple sugars" c) Limit fats d) Increase fiber e) Beware of "dietetic"	Yes	Not usually	Individualize	Yes
Diabetes associated with other conditions Secondary diabetes	Hyperglycemia secondary to: 1) Pancreatic disease 2) Endocrine disease 3) Drug or chemicals 4) Certain genetic syndromes	a) Change if underlying condition necessitates	Yes	Adjust to correct hyperglycemia	Individualize	Yes
Gestational diabetes	Gestational diabetes	a) Avoid simple sugars b) Avoid excessive weight	Yes	Use to tightly control diabetes	No	Yes
Impaired glucose tolerance	Asymptomatic diabetes Chemical diabetes Borderline diabetes Latent diabetes	Avoid extra calories; hypocaloric intake if overweight, or usual diabetic diet	Yes	Not usually	No	Yes

Table 27.2.
Distinguishing Features of Two Major Types of Diabetes Mellitus

	Insulin-Dependent Type I	Non-Insulin-Dependent Type II
Age of onset	Usually, but not always, during childhood or puberty	Frequently over 35
Type of onset	Abrupt	Usually gradual
Prevalence	0.5%	2–5%
Incidence	<10%	>75%
Family history of diabetes	Infrequently positive	Commonly positive
Primary cause	Pancreatic β-cell deficiency	End organ (insulin receptors) unresponsiveness to insulin action
Nutritional status at time of onset	Usually undernourished	Obesity usually present
Postglucose plasma or serum insulin (μU/ml)[a]	Absent	>100 at 2 hr
Symptoms	Polydipsia, polyphagia, and polyuria	May be none
Hepatomegaly	Rather common	Uncommon
Stability	Blood sugar fluctuates widely in response to small changes in insulin dose, exercise, and infection	Blood sugar fluctuations are less marked
Etiology	Unknown Possible factors include: *Inheritance:* associated with specific HLA tissue types, but only 40–50% concordance in twins *Autoimmune disease:* 50–80% circulating islet cell antibodies *Viral infections:* Coxsackie, mumps, influenza	Unknown Possible factors include: *Inheritance:* 95–100% concordance in twins, but not associated with specific HLA tissue types *Autoimmune disease:* negative; <10% circulating islet cell antibodies. No evidence for viral infections
Proneness to ketosis	Frequent, especially if treatment program is insufficient in food and/or insulin	Uncommon except in the presence of unusual stress or moderate to severe sepsis
Insulin defect	Defect in secretion; secretion is impaired early in disease; secretion may be totally absent late in disease	Insulin deficiency present in some patients; others are insulin resistant *Insulin deficiency:* in most patients, there is failure of insulin secretion to keep pace with inordinate demands engendered by the obese state; this defect may appear initially as a failure to respond to glucose alone, suggesting an impairment in the glucoreceptor of the pancreatic β-cell *Insulin resistance:* in some patients, there is a defect in tissue responsiveness to insulin and evidence of hyperinsulinemia; in such patients, insulin resistance may be mediated by decreased number of insulin receptors in target cells

Table 27.2—Continued

	Insulin-Dependent Type I	Non-Insulin-Dependent Type II
Plasma insulin (endogenous)	Negligible to zero	Plasma insulin response may be either adequate but delayed so that postprandial hypoglycemia may be present when diabetes is discovered or diminished but not absent
Vascular complications of diabetes and degenerative changes	Infrequent until diabetes has been present for ~5 years	Frequent
Usual causes of death	Degenerative complications in target organs; e.g., renal failure due to diabetic nephropathy	Accelerated atherosclerosis; e.g., myocardial infarction; to lesser extent, microangiopathic changes in target tissues; e.g., renal failure
Diet	Mandatory in all patients	If diet is utilized fully, hypoglycemic drug therapy may not be needed
Insulin	Necessary for all patients	Necessary for 20–30% of patients
Oral agents	Rarely efficacious	Efficacious

[a] Normal response is between 50 and 135 μU/ml at 60 min and less than 100 μU/ml at 120 min after 100 g of oral glucose.

near future. One factor that seems to be common to all of the types of diabetics is stress. It is also believed that, if a person lives long enough, he will develop an intolerance to glucose.

Type I diabetics have a defect in pancreatic β-cell function that could have numerous causes. Genetic defects in production of certain macromolecules may interfere with proper insulin synthesis, packaging, or release, or the β-cells may not recognize glucose signals or replicate normally. Extrinsic factors that affect β-cell function include damage caused by viruses such as mumps or coxsackie B4, by destructive cytotoxins and antibodies released by sensitized lymphocytes, or by autodigestion in the course of an inflammatory disorder involving the adjacent exocrine pancreas. Genetic susceptibility to insulin-dependent diabetes is conferred by two genes on chromosome 6, one associated with HLA-D/DR3, one with HLA-D/DR4 (7). The reaction of these predisposed individuals to certain environmental stimuli (β-cell-cytotoxic virus or chemicals?) is abnormal and leads to β-cell destruction directly, though "autoimmune mechanisms" or because of lack of regeneration of the β-cell after damage (7). The above hypothesis is being vigorously studied. It is possible that someday individuals susceptible to diabetes can be determined, and a preventive step

Table 27.3.
Etiology of Diabetes Mellitus

1. Obesity
2. Increasing age
3. Heredity
4. Emotional stress
5. Autoimmune β-cell damage
6. Endocrine diseases; i.e., Cushing's
7. Viral stress—decreasing β-cells
8. Vasculitis in tissue highly perfused with capillaries—eye, kidney, etc.
9. Insulin receptor defects
10. Drugs; i.e., cortisone, estrogen, thyroid, phenytoin, diazoxide, thiazide diuretics

taken. Refer to Table 27.2 for the various theories with reference to the etiology of the two major types of diabetes.

Many type II diabetics have excess insulin and are obese. The hyperinsulinism and insulin-resistance may be correlated with a decrease in insulin receptors. Studies have also shown that the tissues of type II patients exhibit reduced insulin binding. A reduced number of insulin receptors and the problem of insulin binding are major factors in the etiology of non-insulin-dependent diabetes (8).

Blood glucose levels can be elevated by a variety of mechanisms. Some diabetic patients may have elevated blood glucose due to an excess of glucagon. Others can have a defect in somatostatin or an excess of growth hormone, cortisol, epinephrine or other hormones that influence the regulation of blood glucose. Numerous drugs have also been indicated in increasing blood glucose levels, including: chlorothalidone, corticosteroids, diazoxide, phenytoin, epinephrine and other catcholamines, estrogens, ethacrynic acid, furosemide, lithium, nicotinic acid, thiazide diuretics, and thyroid preparations (9). Other drugs have been indicated in causing lower-than-normal blood glucose levels, and they include: anabolic steroids, ethanol, fenfluramine, monoamine oxidase inhibitors, propranolol, and large doses of salicylates (9).

In summary, an individual's blood glucose levels can be elevated via numerous mechanisms. There can be a decrease in the amount of insulin produced or released, a defect in an individual's ability to sense glucose and respond by releasing insulin, and a genetic mutation of the structure of insulin. Insulin antibodies can reduce the effectiveness of insulin. There can be decreased insulin receptor affinity, as well as a decrease in the actual number of receptors, and there are numerous hormones and chemicals that can affect blood glucose levels. It thus becomes highly critical that health care practitioners recognize the tremendous heterogenicity of diabetes mellitus and individualize each patient's treatment protocol by first trying to properly classify and determine the cause of the patient's diabetes.

PATHOPHYSIOLOGY AND SYMPTOMOLOGY

As with the etiology of diabetes, there is still a great deal that needs to be learned about the specific cellular biochemical mechanisms that are involved in the pathophysiology of diabetes. The consequences of a lack of insulin or a lack of the effect of insulin are well known. The consequences of high blood glucose levels should be reviewed in both the acute and chronic or long-term stages of hyperglycemia. Also note that, because we are dealing with a heterogeneous condition, the symptoms and consequences differ between type I and type II diabetics. The complex cellular effects of insulin provide numerous clues as to the type of intervention that should be made to improve the prognosis of a diabetic patient. The understanding of all of the cellular mechanisms involving insulin, glucagon, somatosta-

tin and the number and structure of insulin receptors is far from complete.

Normal Carbohydrate Metabolism

The important carbohydrate metabolism sites sensitive to insulin are the liver, where glycogen is formed, stored, and broken down; skeletal muscle, where glucose is oxidized to produce energy; and adipose tissue. where glucose may be converted to fatty acids, glyceryl phosphate, and triglycerides. Some important effects of insulin on carbohydrate metabolism in these tissues are increased glucose uptake by the tissues, increased glucose oxidation by all pathways, increased energy production from glucose, increased muscle and liver glycogen levels, decreased hepatic glucose output, increased synthesis of fatty acids and triglycerides, decreased lipolysis, decreased production of ketone bodies, and enhanced incorporation of amino acids into proteins (10).

In the nondiabetic, insulin—in concert with glucagon, somatostatin, growth hormone, corticosteroids, epinephrine, and parasympathetic intervention, plus other chemicals—maintains the blood glucose between 40 and 160 mg/100 ml (mg%) at all times. At least three types of cells have been identified in the islets of Langerhans of the normal human pancreas. The α-cells have been shown to produce glucagon, which has an opposite effect to insulin. The β-cell is responsible for producing, storing, and releasing insulin. The δ-cell produces a tetradecapeptide called somatostatin. These cells work in conjunction with each other to maintain control of glucose. Ingestion of a carbohydrate in a nondiabetic results in a prompt increase in the amount of insulin released into the blood. At the same time, there is a decrease in plasma glucagon. *Glucagon* is released in response to low blood glucose levels and the ingestion of protein. The release of glucagon stimulates insulin secretion, and insulin in turn inhibits the release of glucagon.

Somatostatin inhibits both insulin and glucagon secretion and suppresses growth hormone (10). Its primary effect is to suppress glucagon which thus results in a fall in blood glucose levels. Unfortunately, this effect persists for only 60 to 120 min.

A minimum blood glucose level of 40 mg/100 ml is required to provide adequate fuel for the brain, which is able to use only glucose as fuel and is not dependent upon the presence of insulin for its utilization. Glucose spills into the urine, resulting in energy and water loss, when blood glucose levels exceed the renal threshold of the kidneys (180 mg/100 ml). Muscle and fat also use glucose as a major source of energy but require the presence of insulin. If glucose is not available, the tissues respond by converting amino acids to carbohydrate (gluconeogenesis). This increases the blood glucose level all the more. If the muscle and fat cells continue to lack glucose because insulin is not available for the glucose to be transferred into these cells, eventually the cells metabolize stored fats. The end product of fat metabolism is the production of free fatty acids that are eventually oxidized to ketone bodies. Ketone bodies are then transferred into the blood, and the patient now has excess amounts of glucose and ketones in the blood, and both of these spill into the urine and help to establish a method by which patients can self-monitor the control of blood glucose levels. If insulin is not given to the patient, the patient will develop a process of ketoacidosis. The acidic ketones will cause the pH to drop, and the elimination of ketones and glucose will cause dehydration. The body's neutralizing factors will eventually be depleted and the patient will continue to deteriorate to the point of coma and eventually death. Figure 27.1 shows the clinical manifestations in an untreated type I diabetic who is insulinopenic.

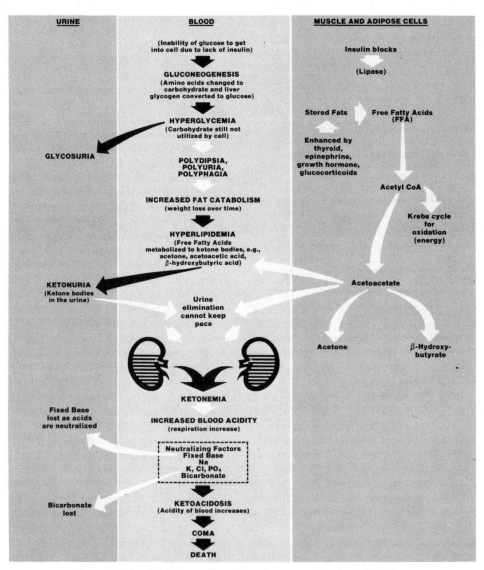

Figure 27.1. Clinical manifestations in untreated type I diabetics.

In type II diabetics the problem is not a lack of insulin but insulin that is not effective (11). Enough glucose gets into the muscle and adipose cells so that the process of fat metabolism to produce ketone bodies is not a factor. However, glucose does accumulate in the blood and can reach very high levels, resulting in a syndrome called diabetic nonketotic hyperosmolar coma. Both ketoacidosis and hyperosmolar coma are treated by first determining the cause of the problem, then giving fluids and electrolytes and low doses of insulin either intravenously or intramuscularly. Close monitoring of electrolytes to avoid complications is required.

Insulin is thus the major hormone related to glucose homeostasis. It is directly involved in carbohydrate, fat and amino acid metabolism; nucleic acid synthesis; glycerol formation; and growth regulation.

Insulin consists of 51 amino acids in two chains connected by two disulfide bonds. The initial protein is referred to as "proinsulin." The C-peptide is cleaved and stored along with the insulin chains and beta cell granules. The normal adult pancreas contains approximately 200 units of insulin at any point in time. Insulin is released from the β-cell constantly. Approximately 0.5 to 1.0 unit per hour is secreted. Insulin is also released as a response to an increase in blood glucose of 100 mg/100 ml or greater. The average daily insulin output in the adult is 25 to 50 units per day. Insulin is cleared metabolically by the liver, peripheral tissues, and the kidney. Insulin follows first order elimination kinetics in that the rate of elimination is proportional to the concentration.

In summary, in the "fed" state, a high insulin level is necessary for incorporation of glucose into liver and muscle glycogen; for muscle to consume glucose for energy needs; for both liver and adipose tissue to make fatty acid from glucose; for amino acids to be incorporated into muscle protein; for circulating chylomicrons to discharge their fatty acid into adipose tissue; and for these in turn to be reesterified and incorporated into the triglyceride storage droplet in the middle of the cell (10). Thus in patients who are insulinopenic (type I), the acute problems affect fat, protein and carbohydrate metabolism, resulting in high blood glucose and ketone levels. In patients who have ineffective insulin (type II), enough insulin gets into cells to meet the patient's energy requirements but glucose accumulates in

the blood causing hyperglycemia with relatively minor acute symptoms.

To complicate the picture even more, individuals diagnosing and treating diabetics should keep in mind that there are numerous other factors that cause an increase in blood glucose other than a lack of insulin. These factors include Cushing's disease, pheochromocytoma, aldosteronism, hyperthyroidism, pancreatitis, cirrhosis, pregnancy, emotional stress and miscellaneous drugs that have been mentioned earlier. One should also keep in mind that there are numerous factors that can decrease blood glucose levels, such as an exogenous insulin excess, nonfasting reactive hypoglycemia, fasting hypoglycemia, and several chemicals (12).

Symptoms

Whereas type I diabetes typically has a rapid onset with the usual signs of polyuria, polyphagia, polydipsia, weakness, weight loss and dry skin, type II diabetes frequently is unaccompanied by any symptoms. Type II diabetes is discovered most often when sugar is found in the urine or when elevated blood sugar is found in a routine examination. Careful study of these older, obese diabetics reveals glucosuria, proteinuria, postprandial hyperglycemia, microaneurysms, and even retinal exudates.

Other symptoms of hyperglycemia associated with diabetes include blurred vision, tingling, numbness in the feet, slow-healing skin infections, itching, drowsiness and irritability. Patients with the above symptoms, and also those patients who have a family history of diabetes or are overweight individuals in the 40-to 65-year-old age group, should be screened closely for hyperglycemia. Monilial infections of the vagina and anus and a history of complications during pregnancy also are warning signs to test for diabetes. The sooner diabetes is diagnosed, the more easily it can be brought under control and the better the chances of avoiding the complications of diabetes. Pharmacists should closely follow the medical literature for additional information concerning the relationship of insulin to the number and shape of insulin receptors, as well as the intracellular effects of insulin on cyclic AMP and various enzyme systems.

Long-Term Consequences of Hyperglycemia

Diabetics frequently develop kidney failure (*nephropathy*), lesions of the eye (*retinopathy*), and atrophy of the peripheral nerves (*neuropathy*). Generally, these processes occur because the walls of the capillaries that supply these tissues with blood and nutrients thicken. The molecular mechanisms leading to these late complications of diabetes have not been established conclusively (13, 14). Over the years there has been considerable debate on whether the lesions that develop within the diabetic's retina, kidneys, nerves and vascular system are due to a disorder in the structure and function of blood vessels or whether they are a consequence of prolonged hyperglycemia caused by inadequate metabolic control. Today few diabetologists believe that microvascular complications occur independently of hyperglycemia and insulin deficiency and that control of events is not a factor in their process. There is substantial evidence supporting the concept that the microvascular complications of diabetes are decreased by reduction of blood glucose concentrations (13, 14). Because of these findings there is a renewed emphasis on strict, but reasonable, control to prevent severe diabetic complications. Patients are being educated to normalize their blood glucose levels through multiple injections of insulins or the use of insulin infusion pumps in conjunction with self-blood-glucose monitoring and a strict diet and exercise program. The harmful effects of hyperglycemia are summarized in Table 27.4. Data proving that hyperglycemia is responsible for chronic complications are rapidly developing and causing significant changes in the attitude of physicians caring for diabetics with reference to the need for strict control. Table 27.5 summarizes the complications of diabetes mellitus and the treatment recommendations for each complication. At the present time, each of the complications promote the concept of strict control in both the prevention and treatment of each long-term diabetic disorder.

Table 27.4.
Harmful Effects of Hyperglycemia

1. Increased capillary basement membrane thickening
2. Glucose metabolized via polyol pathway → ↑ sorbitol
3. Faulty lipid metabolism → atherosclerosis
4. Abnormal minor (glycosylated) hemoglobins
5. Impairment of phagocytosis (ability to fight infection)
6. ↑ Platelet adhesiveness

Recently some major advances have been made in the treatment of some specific complications of diabetes. Retinopathy can be successfully treated by laser photocoagulation. If the patient has already suffered a retinal vitreous hemorrhage, surgical vitrectomy can be performed to help restore the patient's vision. Strict control before and during pregnancy has greatly reduced the incidence of perinatal mortality in infants of diabetic mothers (11). Neuropathies and diabetic cataracts improve with strict control and have also recently been treated experimentally with aldose reductase inhibitors. Furthermore, diabetic impotency can be treated surgically by inserting a penile prothesis (15). Training the diabetic to monitor foot care and vigorously treat any foot problems can reduce the incidence of gangrene in the extremities. Tight metabolic control can also reduce the thickness of basement membranes and improve the lipid blood levels in diabetic patients. Diabetics who are normalizing their blood glucose levels and their glycosylated hemoglobin levels have also been shown to have a decreased incidence in severity of infection (11).

Type I diabetic patients are predisposed to the development of diabetic nephropathy. The basement membrane of the capillaries in the glomerulus thickens and progresses to a nodular pattern (Kimmelstiel-Wilson syndrome). Nephropathy usually occurs in diabetics 10 to 15 years after diagnosis. Proteinuria is the first clinical manifestation with progression to hypertension, azotemia, hypoalbuminemia, and edema. Treatment is initiated to control the complications of nephropathy, and dialysis or transplantation may be necessary for patients who have progressive renal disease. Strict blood glucose control is necessary to reduce, or possibly prevent, pathological changes due to hyperglycemia.

Because of the high incidence of gangrene in diabetic patients, foot care is a major topic in the educational process of diabetics. This complication results from a combination of factors including atherosclerosis, decreased pain sensation due to neuropathy, and trauma. The reduced blood flow results in ischemic tissue changes. The diabetic, due to neuropathy, does not detect areas of injury or infection, and the progression to gangrene can be rapid. Diabetics should thus be instructed to monitor foot care on a daily basis, never go barefoot, strictly control their blood glucose, and avoid

Table 27.5.
Complications of Diabetes Mellitus and Their Treatment

Body Location	Description	Treatment
Eyes	Retinopathy, cataract formation, glaucoma, and periodic visual disturbances. Leading cause of new blindness	Strict control of blood glucose to prevent laser photocoagulation, vitrectomy
Mouth	Gingivitis, increased incidence of dental cavities and periodontal disease	Strict control and daily hygiene. See dentist often
Pregnancy	Increased incidence of large babies, stillbirths, miscarriages, neonatal deaths, and congenital defects	Strict control before and during pregnancy
Nervous system	Motor, sensory and autonomic neuropathy leading to impotency, neurogenic bladder, parathesias, gangrene	Strict control, daily foot care, surgery, and tricyclic antidepressants and phenothiazines
Vascular system	Large vessel disease and microangiopathy	Strict blood glucose control, artery bypass surgery
Skin	Numerous infections and specific lesions due to small vessel disease, increased lipids in blood, and pruritus	Strict control, daily hygiene
Kidneys	Diabetic glomerulosclerosis causing nephropathy	Strict control. Eventually diet low in proteins, prednisone, dialysis, and renal transplantation
Infections	Diabetics have a higher incidence of cystitis, tuberculosis, skin infections. They have a more difficult time overcoming infections. Moniliasis is very common in diabetic women	Strict control and aggressive antiinfection therapy

trauma to the feet by properly cutting toenails and selecting shoes that fit properly (12).

The pharmacist can have a significant role in monitoring the acute and chronic complications of hyperglycemia in diabetic patients. Patients who have abnormally high urine and blood glucose values should be encouraged to review their treatment protocol and bring their blood glucose levels down to more normal levels. The pharmacist can also monitor the patient for acute hypo- and hyperglycemic episodes and encourage the patient to self monitor for eye (16), kidney, nerve and foot complications.

DIAGNOSTIC TESTS

Most currently used diagnostic tests measure an individual's ability to handle a glucose load. Type I diabetics are usually easy to diagnose because they present with all of the classic symptoms of diabetes and high amounts of glucose in the urine and blood. Type II diabetics are more of a challenge because they often do not present with the classic symptoms. Furthermore, many of these patients are borderline, and the tests do not give a clear indication as to whether or not the patient is a diabetic. Table 27.6 summarizes the criteria that are now recommended for use in the diagnosis of diabetes and impaired glucose tolerance.

Oral Glucose Tolerance Test (OGTT)

This diagnostic test measures a person's ability to handle a glucose load over a period of time and, although controversial, is a quite reliable test for diabetes. Following an overnight fast, a morning fasting blood sugar is drawn and a 75-g glucose load is ingested by the patient, followed by blood samples drawn at ½-hour intervals for 2 hours, and at 3 hours. Urine samples are often taken at the same time and tested for glucose in order to estimate the renal threshold for glucose. In normal subjects the blood glucose returns to normal in less than 2 hours. In diabetics, the glucose peak is higher and occurs much later than in normal subjects; levels also decline at a slower rate. A normal OGTT occurs when the fasting plasma glucose is less than 115 mg/dl, the 2-hour

Table 27.6.
Criteria for Diagnosis of Diabetes and Impaired Glucose Tolerance

1. Diabetes—adult
   a. Unequivocal elevation of plasma glucose and classic symptoms (polyuria, polydipsia, weight loss)
   b. Fasting plasma glucose (FPG) $\geq$ 140 mg/dl on more than one occasion
   c. Oral glucose tolerance test (OGTT) with FPG < 140 mg/dl, 2-h PG $\geq$ 200 mg/dl, one intervening PG $\geq$ 200 mg/dl
2. Diabetes—children
   a. Plasma glucose $\geq$ 200 mg/dl with classic symptoms
   b. OGTT (1.75 g glucose/kg body weight up to maximum of 75 g) with FPG < 140 mg/dl, 2-hr PG $\geq$ 200 mg/dl, one intervening PG $\geq$ 200 mg/dl
3. Gestational diabetes
   Two or more of the following plasma glucose concentrations exceeded with a 100 g glucose dose: FPG 105/dl; 1-hr post dose 190 mg/dl; 2-hr post dose 165 mg/dl; 3-hr post dose 145 mg/dl
4. Impaired glucose tolerance
   OGTT with FPG < 140 mg/dl, 2-hr PG $\geq$ 140 mg/dl and < 200 mg/dl, one intervening value $\geq$ 200 mg/dl
5. Normal glucose values—nonpregnant adults
   OGTT with FPG $\leq$ 115 mg/dl, 2-hr PG < 140 mg/dl, intervening PG < 200 mg/dl

plasma glucose is less than 140 mg/dl, and the intervening glucose values are below 200 mg/dl.

Fasting Plasma Glucose (FPG)

Various blood or plasma tests for glucose are used in establishing the diagnosis of diabetes. The simplest test is the FPG, in which blood is drawn from the patient, usually after an overnight fast. A normal fasting plasma glucose depends upon the particular laboratory, but it is usually set between 65 and 110 mg/dl. Diabetes is suggested if two or more fasting plasma glucose tests are elevated above 140 mg/dl, but a normal fasting plasma glucose does not rule out diabetes. This test is used in nonpregnant adult patients who are neither receiving drugs nor have other diseases that could be responsible for the abnormal result.

2-Hour Postprandial (2HPP) Blood Glucose

The 2HPP is used as a screening test where a blood glucose level is drawn 2 hours following a 100-g glucose load. In nondiabetics, blood glucose levels return to normal in less than 2 hours following a glucose challenge, whereas hyperglycemia persists in a diabetic. Although this test is often used to evaluate diabetes control, it can easily be manipulated by the diabetic patient. All the patient needs to do is eat a small meal 2 hours before the test is determined.

Note that each of the blood glucose tests can be manipulated by the diabetic patient by improving his blood glucose control several days preceding the test. Furthermore, the blood glucose test can be elevated due to emotional stress, physical exertion and stimulants such as tobacco (17), coffee, and tea. Other causes of elevated blood glucose include acute stresses such as fever, trauma, major operations, myocardial infarctions, or cerebral vascular accidents (12). Chronic illnesses that cause prolonged physical inactivity, starvation and malnutrition can result in abnormally low fasting blood glucose levels. Potassium depletion from any cause can result in fasting hyperglycemia (12). Another cause of pseudohyperglycemia is chronic renal disease with uremia. Another factor to be considered in using diagnostic tests for diabetes is the caution of labeling a patient with the diagnosis of diabetes unless it is certain that the disease exists. To saddle a patient with a false diagnosis leads to personal frustrations, including insurance "riders," in some states driver's license limitations, and possible limitations in employment opportunities (12). Pharmacists monitoring elderly patients should be alert to the fact that, as an individual ages, tolerance to glucose decreases. This results in some elderly patients being labeled as diabetics and placed on medications that are probably unnecessary.

Glycosylated hemoglobin (Hemoglobin A$_{1c}$)

Glycosylated hemoglobin has recently been discovered to be abnormally high in diabetics with chronic hyperglycemia and reflects long-term metabolic control (18). Glycosylation of hemoglobin is a postsynthesis, nonenzymatic chemical reaction between glucose and phosphorylated sugar (glucose-6-phosphate) with the end-terminal valine of the B-chain of the hemoglobin molecule. Since hemoglobin is exposed to the ambient glucose concentration in the blood, a higher concentration will result in more glycohemoglobin formation. The result is that this hemoglobin becomes an important index of the long-term control of diabetes and may be a more reliable index than the degree of hyperglycemia or glucosuria. In the nondiabetic, glycosylated hemoglobin is between 3 and 8% of all hemoglobin, whereas in patients with poorly controlled diabetes it may range between 8 and 20%. The advantage of measuring glycohemoglobin as a parameter of diabetic control is that it indicates the level of control of the disorder for the previous 60 days when the red blood cells are about halfway through their 120-day cycle. The major form of the glycohemoglobins is termed hemoglobin A_{1c}. Some laboratories test specifically for hemoglobin A_{1c} and others test for all of the glycosylated hemoglobins. It thus becomes important to know which test a laboratory is using and what the normal range for the test is. Numerous recent studies have shown that when a relatively uncontrolled diabetic brings his blood glucose under strict control, there is a dramatic improvement in glycosylated hemoglobins (18). Studies are in progress to determine whether long-term hemoglobin A_1 values will correlate positively with diabetic microangiopathy. This test may be particularly useful for patients who have poor compliance in record-keeping or who make an extra effort to achieve acceptable plasma glucose levels only at a time of physician visits. Patients with changing renal functions and with changes in drug dosage may also benefit from monitoring with glycosylated hemoglobins. The test has an advantage also in that it can be taken at any time and is not affected by recent meals or physical activities.

The test is also used by some physicians to determine the appropriate time to prescribe insulin for type II patients who are not being adequately controlled on oral agents. Note that it is not a test done frequently, but rather 2 to 3 times a year.

Much work is also being done to develop additional tests to determine specific glycoproteins that will correlate well with diabetes control.

Self-monitoring of Blood Glucose

Since 1980, there has been a strong movement to educate diabetic patients to self-monitor blood glucose. This movement is continuing to gain momentum with the effect of having all types of diabetic patients involved in a daily process of checking their blood glucose levels to determine their degree of blood glucose control. The objective of diabetes treatment programs is to achieve blood glucose levels as close to normal as possible through a program of education, diet, exercise and medications. Achieving the objective requires active and routine patient involvement to determine whether or not blood glucose is being controlled. The trend to increasingly involve patients in the management of the disease has led to the development of blood glucose measuring devices which allow patients to measure their own blood glucose wherever they desire—at home, at work, during vacation, or while traveling.

Studies conducted over many years have accumulated a considerable body of evidence to suggest that tight, continuous control of blood glucose levels within normal limits appears to diminish the incidence and postpone the onset of diabetic complications. Besides the possibility of decreasing complications, strict blood glucose control can also decrease depression and avoid some of the problems inherent in urine testing. Urine tests are inconvenient, messy, affected by a wide variety of medications and do not reflect the prevailing blood glucose levels due to differences in patients' renal threshold and to residual urine left in the bladder (19).

Self-monitoring of blood glucose is feasible, practical, and acceptable to patients. It allows the patient to better understand the factors that affect blood glucose levels; gives an accurate reflection of the blood glucose after exercise, before and after meals and when the patient is placed on medications or is ill; helps the patient better understand diabetes and the objectives of therapy; assists in detecting and therefore avoiding hypoglycemia; helps the patient understand the symptoms of hypo- and hyperglycemia; improves the relationship between the health care professional and the patient; and helps the patient to become a more active, intelligent participant in managing diabetes.

The disadvantages of self-monitoring glucose, which include the increased expense and the annoyance of obtaining a drop of blood, are greatly outweighed by the many advantages. Several devices, i.e., the Autolet, are now available to assist the patient in obtaining a drop of blood easily and almost painlessly (20).

Several methods of determining blood glucose levels are available to diabetic patients.

Selection of a specific product should be made on the basis of cost, ability to perform the test accurately, accuracy of the method, convenience to the patient, and motivation of the patient to achieve strict control. Since maintenance of blood sugar control is impossible without measurement and since it is convenient and less costly for the patient to self-monitor, self-monitoring blood glucose is highly recommended for all types of diabetic patients. Pregnant diabetics, patients with altered or shifting renal threshold, labile patients who have difficulty bringing their diabetes under control, patients with frequent hypoglycemia, patients who have difficulty using a urine test, and patients who prefer monitoring their own blood glucose are all excellent candidates for self-monitoring blood glucose. It is a necessity for patients who are using continuous subcutaneous insulin infusion.

Each of the tests available for use by patients involves the glucose oxidase/peroxidase reaction to detect the glucose. Some of the tests use a reflectance photometer to read the strip and give a digital readout of the blood glucose values to the patient. Other methods have a color reaction on the strip which is compared to a chart on the side of the bottle that is visually read by the patient. Both types of tests require that capillary blood be placed on a semipermeable membrane that is impregnated with an appropriate test reagent.

Dextrostix can be read visually or can be read on a Dextrometer, a *Glucometer*, or a Glucoscan. The machines are calibrated to detect blood glucose levels from 0 to 399 mg/dl. A drop of blood is applied to the test strip for 60 sec, washed off with water, dried, and inserted in the Glucometer or other device for an immediate reading. Accurate timing is important. The use of self-monitoring of blood glucose is so great that there will be additional devices produced to read and display blood glucose levels for patients.

There are two products presently available that do not require a reflectance photometer and can be read visually by the patient. The first is the *Chemstrip bG*. It uses two reagent areas on a strip that are advocated to allow a more accurate determination of blood glucose. A drop of blood is placed on the reagent area for 60 sec, wiped off with cotton, and then compared 60 sec later with the manufacturer's color scale on the side of the bottle. The sensitivity of the Chemstrip bG is between 20 and 800. With a blood glucose above 240 it is dif-

ficult to read, but clinically this does not cause much of a problem because the patient recognizes that his blood sugar is too high and appropriate steps will need to be taken to bring it back to normal.

Another visually read strip is *Visidex II*. It also has two reagent areas on the strip that give a high-low scale for accurate visual reading. The top reagent area measures blood glucose between 20 and 110. The color changes go from yellow to dark-green. The second reagent area reads blood glucose levels between 140 and 800. The reagent area goes from yellow to a dark-orange. This strip requires that a drop of blood be placed on the reagent areas for 30 sec, wiped off, dried and compared with the color scale on the side of the bottle. It is unique in that the second reagent area does not change color unless the blood glucose is over 110.

The visually read strips have the advantage of being less expensive and very portable. The meter-read monitoring of blood glucose gives the patient a more accurate determination of blood glucose. Both systems, however, greatly improve the ability of the patient to understand the factors that affect blood glucose levels and therefore improve blood glucose control.

The trend of self-monitoring of blood glucose is considered by many to be one of the most significant advances in the treatment of diabetes since the discovery of insulin.

Urine Glucose Tests

Glucosuria is symptomatic of many conditions (e.g., pregnancy or impaired renal function), and is not a persistant finding in diabetes. It does occur when the mean blood glucose level is 180 mg/dl or more, but rarely when the level is less than 130 mg/dl. The major exception occurs when the renal threshold for glucose is increased with age; therefore older diabetics may "spill" no glucose at all despite a high blood glucose level. Thus one of the major disadvantages of urine testing to monitor diabetes is the fact that renal thresholds for glucose differ from patient to patient. There is also residual urine left in the bladder, even when the patient double-voids. This means that at any point at which the patient tests his urine, the test could be affected by his blood glucose levels for the previous 2 to 3 hours.

In spite of the fact that blood glucose monitoring by patients is gaining momentum, there is still a need for many relatively stable diabetics to continue to use urine tests to monitor their diabetes. The two types of tests available are the glucose oxidase method (*Tes-Tape, Clinistix,* and *Diastix*), which is specific for glucose, and the copper reduction method (*Clinitest*), which may be affected by reducing substances in the urine (20).

The glucose oxidase method is specific for glucose and the simplest to perform, but it is not the best method for monitoring insulin therapy because of its qualitative nature. Quantitative figures appear on many of the product labels, but glucose oxidase tests are quantitative only when the amount of glucose in the urine is less than 0.25%. Larger amounts (2, 3, and 4%) were misinterpreted as 0.5% or less in 502 out of 804 tests (21). Such a high rate of error makes the control of hyperglycemia difficult. Diastix is the only glucose oxidase method which makes quantitative claims; however, false low readings are common in the presence of high concentrations of glucose (greater than 1.5%) or moderate to large amounts of ketones. For this reason, difficult-to-control diabetics should be on a self-monitoring blood glucose program. The glucose oxidase tests are the tests of choice for type II diabetics who are treated with oral agents who are quite stable. Ascorbic acid in high doses (1 to 2 g) will interfere with the glucose oxidase test resulting in a false-negative reading.

When patients are using urine tests and are given medications, they should test their urine using both the glucose oxidase and the copper reduction methods. If the results are just the opposite, the only conclusion is that the urine tests are being interfered with by the drug.

Many hospitals and some physicians set up schedules for the dosing of regular insulin on the basis of urine glucose readings. These schedules are referred to as "the rainbow schedule" or "sliding scale." There is no standard schedule. However, generally 5 units of regular insulin are administered for each "plus" recorded by the copper reduction method, with supplemental insulin to be added should the patient spill acetone into the urine. These sliding scales have caused difficulty in that the various tests have previously used a plus type of system to indicate quantity of glucose, the trouble being that the plusses for each type of product indicated a different percent of glucose in the urine. Another problem with urine tests is the diabetic's lack of understanding of the disease and the errors

made in self-treatment or in performing tests. Labile patients should not use urine tests but instead should be encouraged to self-monitor for blood glucose. More stable patients can test their urine from 1 to 4 times per day. Some very stable patients test only 2 to 3 times a week.

At the first sign of stress, infection or change in control, the patient should be encouraged to test the urine or blood more often.

There are some cautionary notes with reference to using the copper reduction method. Most textbooks encourage the patient to use double-voided urine samples. However, there is now some controversy as to whether or not double voiding should be a requirement for urine testing (22). The Clinitest tablet generates its own heat and anaerobic environment with the production of foam. The test tube should not be agitated during the reaction. Also, the patient should observe the reaction while it is occurring since a very high glucose content results in the so-called "pass-through" phenomenon which is a fleeting bright-orange color which occurs during the "boiling" and fades to a greenish-brown once the reaction ceases. This color may then falsely be interpreted as 0.75 to 1% when there is actually more than 2% glucose in the urine. The "pass-through" phenomenon can be eliminated by using 2 drops of urine instead of 5 drops. Patients using Clinitest who spill more than 2% glucose should also test their urine for acetone. Many drugs are guilty of interfering with the copper reduction test to cause a false-positive reaction (23). These drugs are listed in Table 27.7 (23). Clinitest tablets disintegrate in the presence of moisture and light, therefore they

Table 27.7.
Substances Which May Cause False-Positive Glucosuria by Copper Reduction Method

Ascorbic acid (large quantities)
Cephalothin
Cephaloridine
Chloral hydrate
Isoniazid
L-Dopa
Metaxalone
Methyldopa
Nalidixic acid
p-Aminosalicylic acid
Penicillin (massive doses)
Probenecid
Salicylates
Streptomycin
Sugars (galactose, lactose, fructose)

should not be stored in the bathroom. The tablets change from a normal speckled robin's-egg blue to white with splotches of dark blue when exposed to moisture and light. Note that the Clinitest tablets are poisonous and caustic, the lid should be kept on tight, and the bottle kept out of the reach of small children. Should ingestion occur, it is important not to induce vomiting.

The pharmacist has a very special role with reference to assisting the diabetic patient in self-monitoring the control of his or her diabetes. There are numerous questions about how the specific urine and blood-testing products should be used. The pharmacist should be aware of the drugs that interfere with the laboratory tests and be able to explain to the patient how the various laboratory tests are interpreted with reference to levels of control. The pharmacist should also be aware of methods to assist visually impaired diabetics with self-monitoring (20) and should carry or be able to order a full line of diabetes care products that can assist the patient in achieving rigid control of blood glucose levels.

GENERAL PRINCIPLES IN THE TREATMENT OF DIABETES

The *treatment objectives* for diabetics are summarized in Table 27.8. In achieving the objectives, one must remember that diabetes is a heterogeneous condition and that there is tremendous variance among patients. The treatment protocol needs to be individualized and can be developed after first categorizing the type of diabetes the patient has. In general, glucose metabolism is normalized in diabetic patients who achieve excellent control. Current research has not definitely demonstrated that "excellent" control will prevent the occurrence of diabetic complications. However, there is very strong evidence to suggest that excellent control does decrease the severity of the complications and very possibly will postpone their onset. Excellent control will significantly improve the "quality" of life by producing a relative degree of healthiness. The most challenging of the diabetic patients is the type I insulin-dependent diabetic who has wide daily fluctuations of blood glucose.

The formula to achieve these objectives combines a program of weight loss and diet with an individualized exercise program and the use of medications, either insulin for the type I diabetic or possibly insulin or oral agents

Table 27.8.
Treatment Objectives for Diabetes Mellitus

1. Normalize glucose metabolism
   a. Normalize glycosylated hemoglobin
   b. Urine glucose and ketones negative
   c. Fasting blood glucose—70–150 mgm/dl
   d. 2-Hr postprandial < 180 mg/dl
   e. Urinary excretion of glucose < 5% over 24 hr
   f. Normal lipid blood levels
2. Avoid symptoms of diabetes mellitus
3. Avoid frequent hypoglycemia
4. Normalize nutrition and achieve ideal body weight
5. Achieve normal growth and development
6. Minimize or prevent complications
7. Acceptance of the diabetes state with a realistic but positive attitude
8. Normal and flexible life-style
9. Promotion of emotional well-being: have patient "take charge" of condition

for the type II diabetic. Diet, excercise and medications are glued together by a program of education and reeducation.

Education

In the *Guidelines for Diabetes Care* (24) that is published by the American Diabetes Association is a summary of specific guidelines for education of individuals with diabetes in both acute care and ambulatory care facilities. This document is worth reading because it specifically lists the steps that should be followed in training the diabetic patient to care for his own condition. The diabetic spends 365 days a year caring for his condition and monitoring the results of his efforts. It thus becomes essential that each diabetic be thoroughly trained in understanding diabetes and in following the specific steps necessary to care for the condition and to evaluate whether or not the treatment protocol is achieving its objectives.

The educational process requires a health team approach which includes a physician, a nurse, a dietitian, a pharmacist, and possibly a social worker and exercise physiologist. It is also important that the diabetic be continually educated and participate in understanding the condition along with other diabetic patients. This can be achieved by active involvement in the Juvenile Diabetes Foundation or the American Diabetes Association local affiliate. It is important that the educational process be well organized and assesses each individual patient's needs. It is also important that patients be periodically evaluated for their competence in performing urine or blood tests, mixing and injecting insulin, rotating injection sites, using the diet exchange system, and following an exercise prescription. Other topics include foot care and what to do during a sick day, and how to treat insulin reactions (hypoglycemia). Table 27.9 lists some of the statistics that show a strong need for diabetic patient education (5). It is not unusual to find a diabetic who has been diagnosed and told by a physician to take 24 units of NPH insulin and test the blood occasionally and try to limit the sweets that are eaten. There is also a problem in the initial announcement of the diabetes condition. If a physician has a negative attitude and the parents or other members of the diabetic's family respond in a negative way, it can cause long-term scars for the patient that are difficult to overcome even with a good educational program.

Basically the education prescription for a diabetic should be broken down into at least three areas:

1. Initial management of the diabetes which provides necessary information to bring the patient under control and gives the patient some time to adjust to the condition. This level of education is based upon the limitations of the individual and family to accept and/or assimilate all there is to know about diabetes at the time of diagnosis and the limitations of some settings to provide additional education.

2. Home management of diabetes places emphasis on increasing knowledge and flexibility as some experience is gained in living with diabetes. This level is perceived as essential for every individual but must be tailored to each person's needs and capacity. This type of educational experience is preferably offered in a nonhospital, as-close-to-home-as-possible environment.

3. Improvement in life-style is the third area in which educational guidelines should be developed. This form of education deals with advanced learning and is viewed as enriching the individual's life with flexibility, insight and self-determination. Many diabetics are forced to discover this information by trial and error. Although no educational program can or should entirely replace personal experience, the process need not be experienced by each individual. At each level of education there is information provided about nutrition,

Table 27.9.
Need for Patient Education

1. 3 out of 5 patients make errors in insulin measurement
2. 65–90% of patients have major deficits in selecting and using foods according to prescribed diet
3. Less than 10% of diabetics were following a "minimally adequate regimen"
4. 35% of patients lack any formal training
5. 17% placed on insulin without instruction
6. 50% who had been trained could not demonstrate skills in any of the major areas of self-care

medication, self-monitoring, what to do with hypoglycemia, how to handle hyperglycemic episodes and illness; what activities should be practiced on a daily basis, and specific steps in developing good hygiene and a routine schedule. Psychological adjustment is a method of assessing whether or not the patient is accepting the educational process.

Exercise

Although exercise is nearly always recommended by physicians as part of the treatment of diabetes, it is seldom prescribed. Recently more physicians undestand the improvement that exercise brings to the control of diabetes, and programs are being developed to specifically prescribe exercise treatment on a daily basis for diabetic patients (25, 26). Exercise lowers blood glucose by allowing glucose to penetrate the muscle cell and be metabolized without the assistance of insulin. Glucose may be utilized to varying degrees without insulin in all types of cells. Exercise also improves circulatory function, an important factor in diabetic management. Exercise also helps maintain normal body weight and aids in breathing, digestion and metabolism. An exercise log may help the patient maintain a regular daily schedule. Patients who monitor their own blood glucose become motivated to exercise because they easily see the beneficial effects of exercise on maintaining good blood sugar and control. An exercise program should be prescribed for both type I and type II diabetics. Diabetics should be evaluated before the exercise prescription is determined. The person's health, interests and motivation to exercise should be taken into consideration when developing a specific method of exercising. If blood glucose is greater than 300 mg/dl, exercise can result in an excessive rise in counter-regulatory hormones which, in the presence of inadequate insulin availability, can cause decreased muscle glucose uptake and an increase in liver glucose production that actually causes blood glucose to increase further (25). Thus type I diabetics should know their blood glucose level before beginning exercise. If the blood glucose is less than 300, injected insulin that has been absorbed subcutaneously can possibly be absorbed more rapidly, resulting in excessive insulin which, in combination with the exercise, can cause a serious drop in blood glucose. Diabetic patients over 40 years of age or who have had diabetes for greater than 25 years should have an exercise stress test and then have an individualized graded exercise program prescribed. Diabetics with peripheral sensory neuropathy and/or vascular insufficiency should avoid exercise that may cause trauma to the feet— for example, jogging. Diabetics with proliferative diabetic retinopathy should avoid strenous exercise which may induce hemorrhage. Another problem that needs to be considered in exercise programs is preventing hypoglycemia during exercise. Hypoglycemia can be prevented by ingesting additional carbohydrates before exercise begins (approximately 15 g 30 min before exercising). Patients should also inject insulin at a nonexercise site; i.e., in the abdomen if they are going to be running. The patient should log his exercise and monitor what effect it has on his blood glucose control. By doing this, a patient will be encouraged to exercise regularly. If hypoglycemia occurs repeatedly during regularly scheduled exercise, it may require a decrease in the insulin dose. Patients should also be warned to wear an identification bracelet or necklace when exercising in case they do become hypoglycemic. Diabetics should also carry a quick source of sugar with them when exercising in case of an insulin reaction.

Diet Treatment of Diabetes

Diet is the cornerstone of treatment of both type I and type II diabetics. It is the most critical treatment in type II diabetics and, in combination with exercise and insulin, is a necessary treatment for type I diabetics. Table 27.10 provides a quick overview of diabetes diet therapy. Pharmacists should make note of

Table 27.10.
Diabetes Diet Therapy

1. Diet compliance is critical
2. Avoid fad diets and prolonged fasting
3. Note that "dietetic" does not equal "diabetic"; read labels carefully
4. Avoid quick-acting (simple) sugars
5. Decrease consumption of animal (saturated) fats
6. Control calories—attempt to achieve an ideal body weight
7. Increase amount of fiber in the diet
8. Try to avoid alcohol
9. Avoid smoking
10. Take vitamin-mineral supplements
11. Understand and use the diabetic exchange diet system

the fact that they can offer much good advice to diabetic patients with reference to "sugarless" products and "dietetic" products that are often carried in pharmacies. Patients should be taught to read labels carefully because many sugarless and dietetic products actually contain a high number of calories and are not effective in helping the diabetic patient achieve or maintain an ideal body weight. Diabetics should also avoid quick-acting simple sugars because they cause a rapid rise in blood glucose levels. Animal (saturated) fats should be decreased because of the increased incidence of atherosclerotic disease in diabetic patients. The main factor in diabetes diet therapy is to control calories. Recently there have been some excellent studies done to show the importance of increasing the fiber in the diet of diabetics (27). However, each patient needs to see how he or she responds to the various types of fibers. Some of the fibers that have a high degree of pectin can cause constipation, where other fiber products, because of their bulk nature, can cause flatulence and diarrhea. To achieve the objectives of diet therapy, the patient must spend some time with a dietitian to specifically work out the number of calories to be ingested each day and the percent of those calories which should be carbohydrates, fat and protein. Patients also need to be educated in the relatively simple "diabetic diet exchange system." The diet exchange system allows patients to have a large variety of foods and, if the patient will follow the diet, weight can be lost and ideal body weight can be achieved. Remember, about 80% of diabetic patients are the obese, non-insulin-dependent type of diabetic. If weight loss can be achieved in this group, often the diabetes will disappear. Pharmacists who care for their diabetic patients should become familiar with the diabetes diet exchange system so that they can answer patients' questions and offer correct advice with reference to sugar-free and dietetic products.

Table 27.11 shows the dietary recommendations for type I and type II diabetics (28). Diet therapy in type II diabetics has a high degree of failure and often creates feelings of frustration, pessimism, failure and anger, which in turn result in poorly informed and inadequately motivated patients. The failure rate can also cause frustration and a negative attitude on the part of the physician who treats the patient. Successful diet programs require behavior modification on the part of the patient. Patients should be encouraged to join groups such as Weight Watchers and to keep a diet log similar to an exercise log. The patient should write down for a period of 4 to 10 days each time he eats, how much he eats and why he eats—whether food ingested was due to social pressure, loneliness, depression, nervousness or the time of day, or whether the patient truly needed nourishment. By having patients use smaller plates, take only one helping of food, and be conscious of why they eat,

it is possible to change dietary behavior. Diet support groups can be of assistance in modifying behavior (20).

One reason for diet therapy failure in diabetics is that physicians or dietitians prescribe changes in diet without first adjusting the dose of insulin or oral agents. The first step in diet therapy should be to prescribe an exercise program, lower the medication dose, and put the patient on a diet containing fewer calories. Insulin overtreatment is probably one of the most common causes of inadequrate diabetic control and weight gain. In one group of diabetic patients, 75% needed a reduction in insulin dose of at least 10%; 35% of the overtreated patients had large appetites; and 30% had hepatomegaly and headaches (29). Diabetic patients should be educated to determine whether or not they have involved themselves in a vicious cycle of taking too much insulin and then eating up to that level of insulin. Note also that type II diabetic patients have too much insulin to begin with, and even after eating a large meal still feel hungry, possibly due to their excess insulin levels. The pharmacist can play a supportive role in diet therapy by understanding some of the problems with it and encouraging diabetic patients to follow the prescribed diet and work with a well-trained dietitian.

Table 27.11.
Diet Recommendations for Type I and II Diabetics

Strategy	Obese Diabetics who Do Not Require Insulin	Nonobese, Insulin-dependent Diabetics
1. Decrease number of calories	Yes	No
2. Protect or improve pancreatic β-cell function	Very urgent priority	Seldom important because β-cells are usually extinct
3. Increase frequency and number of feedings	Usually no	Yes
4. Maintain day-to-day consistency of intake of calories	Not crucial if average caloric intake remains in low range	Desirable
5. Maintain day-to-day consistency of ratios of carbohydrate, protein, and fat for each of the feedings	Not crucial	Desirable
6. Time meals consistently	Not crucial	Desirable
7. Allow extra food for unusual exercise	Not usually appropriate	Usually appropriate
9. Use food to treat, abort, or prevent hypoglycemia	Not necessary	Important
9. During complicating illness, provide small frequent feedings or give carbohydrate intravenously to prevent starvation ketosis	Often not necessary because of resistance to ketosis	Important

Alcohol Use in the Diabetic

In general, alcohol use is discouraged in diabetic patients, but each individiaul diabetic should be assessed to see whether the advantages of alcohol (e.g., reducing emotional tension, relieving anxiety, and stimulating appetite) outweigh its potential effect on blood glucose control.

Either hyper- or hypoglycemia may develop in diabetics who ingest alcohol. Hypoglycemia is the most common effect. The hypoglycemic effect of alcohol is believed to be due to either increased early endogenous insulin response to glucose or to inhibition of hepatic gluconeogenesis. Relatively small quantities of alcohol (48 ml of 100-proof) may cause this effect. Thus, if a diabetic patient is fasting and consumes alcohol, hypoglycemia may be severe. If a diabetic has adequate amounts of glucose in the blood, then alcohol has a less clinically significant effect. Alcohol in combination with sugared mixture in a patient who is fed can add to the hyperglycemic state.

The additive hypoglycemic effects of alcohol with insulin have produced severe hypoglycemia resulting in coma, brain damage, and even death. Tolbutamide and chlorpropamide have been reported to interact with alcohol, resulting in a "disulfiram-like" reaction. Some diabetologists advocate the use of small amounts of dry wine for their diabetic patients. Diabetics on a diabetic diet alone or taking insulin or a sulfonylurea can consume up to 2 oz of dry wine without any significant alteration in blood glucose values. Diabetics taking other stronger forms of alcohol such as distilled liquor (gin) can run into problems from hyperglycemia and even ketosis. Diabetics should be well educated as to the type of alcohol-containing beverages and their sugar content.

MEDICATIONS IN THE TREATMENT OF DIABETES MELLITUS

The medications used to treat diabetes can be categorized into two broad areas: oral hypoglycemic agents and insulin. The oral agents are effective only in type II (non-insulin-dependent) diabetics. Insulin is used for all type I diabetics and in approximately 30% of type II diabetics. Insulin is also used in all diabetics during times of stress, such as infection, surgery, ketoacidosis or hyperosmolar coma.

Sulfonylureas

Drug therapy should never be considered in the mild, well-tolerated type II diabetic until the patient has been on a diet for an appropriate length of time (3 to 4 months). If diet therapy fails, then a trial of sulfonylureas is indicated. Before 1970, when the University Group Diabetes Program (UGDP) published its very controversial report, most non-insulin-dependent diabetics were placed on sulfonylureas. The UGDP (30) was a prospective study initiated in 1961 to evaluate the effectiveness of antidiabetic therapy in preventing vascular and late complications of diabetes. Eight hundred patients from 12 different diabetic clinics were included in the study. These newly diagnosed type II diabetics who could be treated by diet alone were assigned at random to one of five treatment programs: tolbutamide in fixed doses of 1.5 g, placebo or diet alone, insulin in a fixed dose, insulin in variable doses, and phenformin. The study was scheduled to continue, but an unexpected finding of a higher incidence of cardiovascular deaths in the tolbutamide- and phenformin-treated groups resulted in its early termination. Controversy surrounding the study is still not settled, and many emotional editorials have appeared in the literature about the faults of the study and the conclusions that were made. Many diabetologists feel that the sulfonylureas are effective and very safe medications to use in specific non-insulin-dependent diabetics. Nevertheless, the study made physicians more critical of drug therapy in type II diabetics, and a renewed emphasis on diet therapy has evolved. Because of the possibility that oral sulfonylureas can have an effect on increasing insulin receptors, the use of these agents is expected to increase in the future. Two new, more potent agents will become available in the United States, and the marketing of these products should also stimulate more prescriptions for oral antidiabetic agents.

Sulfonylureas stimulate insulin secretion by the pancreas and potentially increase the number of insulin receptors (31). Therefore, a minimum of pancreatic function is a prerequisite to sulfonylurea therapy. Since a normal pancreatized adult requires 40 to 60 units of insulin daily, an insulin requirement of less than 40 units would indicate that there is some pancreatic function remaining in the patient. Patients who seem to respond well to oral hypoglycemics have the following characteristics: they are not diagnosed as diabetics until after the age of 40, they are not overweight, and their insulin requirements are less than 40 units daily (preferably 10 to 20 units daily). Once a firm diagnosis of diabetes (by the oral glucose tolerance test) has been made, diet has been given an adequate trial, and the criteria for the use of oral hypoglycemics have been met, an appropriate drug can then be selected. The products that are or will soon be available in the United States are summarized in Table 27.12. Efficacy, potency and toxicity are major factors to consider in the selection of a drug. The differences in metabolism of each sulfonylurea account for clinical differences with reference to the onset and duration of action. Tolbutamide and chlorpropamide are the oldest drugs and are therefore best studied. Long-term studies of these agents indicate a primary failure rate of from 3 to 30%, an overall success rate of 20%, and the incidence of adverse effects less than 5%. In general, the incidence of adverse effects reported for chlorpropamide is higher than that for the other products—approximately 8% for chlorpropamide vs. 1 to 3% for tolbutamide. The severity of many of these side effects can be correlated with the differences in the half-life, metabolism and excretion of the drugs. Note that chlorpropamide has the longest half-life and also has the highest incidence of side effects of a serious nature. For this reason, some clinicians favor tolbutamide because of its short half-life and lesser toxicity. The sulfonylureas that are metabolized to inactive metabolites should also be safer for use in patients with kidney damage. The *side effects of sulfonylureas* (32) are summarized in Table 27.13. The most common side effect of the sulfonylureas is hypoglycemia. The pharmacist should thus tell the patient to be sure to carry some source of energy at all times. Other directions that the pharmacist should give to diabetic patients are summarized in Table 27.14. Frequent drug-drug interactions resulting in enhanced hypoglycemia can occur with alcohol, anabolic steroids, chloramphenicol, dicoumarol, monoamine oxidase inhibitors, phenylbutazone, propranolol, salicylates and sulfonamides (9). Drugs that may interfere with diabetes control by causing hyperglycemia include asparaginase, clonidine, corticosteroids, dextrothyroxine, diazoxide, estrogens, ethacrynic acid, furosemide, glucagon, levodopa, lithium, niacin (high doses), phenytoin, sympathomimetic amines, and thiazide diuretics (9).

Note also that chlorpropamide can cause an increased sensitivity to circulating levels of antidiuretic hormone which occurs in approximately 4% of patients. The chlorpropamide-induced inappropriate antidiuretic hormone activity is reversible. Improvement occurs within a week after the medication is discontinued.

Conditions in which the sulfonylureas are usually contraindicated include acidosis, severe infections accompanying diabetic onset, major surgery (during and after), sulfa sensitivity, and pregnancy. Sulfonylureas also are possible teratogens. They should not be used early in pregnancy, and are absolutely contraindicated late in gestation since they may cause prolonged and severe hypoglycemia. Pharmacists should be aware that approximately 40% of type II diabetics do not achieve satisfactory control with the oral agents. Secondary failures occur in patients who initially respond to oral agents but subsequently fail to be adequately controlled. The secondary failure rate ranges from 3 to 30%. The failure rate tends to increase year after year for patients experiencing initial satisfactory control.

Dosing of Sulfonylureas

The dose of sulfonylureas is increased weekly on the basis of blood glucose control, urine glucose and symptomatology. This is particularly important in the elderly because their poor eating habits and decreased renal function predispose them to hypoglycemic reactions. Lower doses are given once daily before breakfast, while higher doses are split and given two or more times throughout the day, depending upon the half-life of the drug.

In some patients the oral agents will not work, and the patient is labeled a "primary failure." In these patients insulin in combination with an oral agent or insulin by itself can be attempted. Doses of any given agent should be pushed to maximal levels before a decision to abandon therapy is made. Increasing the doses above maximum levels results in an increased incidence of adverse effects without producing any further decrease in blood glucose. The treatment with any given agent should continue for 1 month before a change in therapy is made.

In patients who suffer from "secondary fail-

Table 27.12.
Biopharmaceutics and Pharmacokinetics of the Oral Hypoglycemics[a]

Drug	Recommended Dose (g)	Maximum Dose (g)	Half-Life (hr)	Onset (hr)	Duration (hr)	Metabolism and Excretion	Comments
Tolbutamide (Orinase)	0.5–3.0 divided doses	2–3	5.6	1	6–12	Totally metabolized to inactive form; inactive metabolite excreted in kidney	Generally first drug of choice; most benign; least potent; short half-life; especially useful in kidney disease
Acetohexamide (Dymelor)	0.25–1.5 single or divided doses	1.5	5	1	10–14	Metabolite's activity equal to or greater than parent compound; metabolite excreted via kidney	Essentially no advantage over tolbutamide, although few patients who fail on tolbutamide are controlled; significant uricosuric effects
Tolazamide (Tolinase)	0.1–1.0 single or divided doses	0.75–1.0	7	4–6	10–14	Absorbed slowly; metabolite active but less potent than parent compound; excreted via kidney	Essentially no advantage over tolbutamide; said to be equipotent with less severe side effects
Chlorpropamide (Diabinese)	0.1–0.5 single dose	0.5	35	1	72	Previously thought not to be metabolized but recently found that metabolism may be quite extensive; significant percentage excreted unchanged	Most potent in use; caution in elderly patients and those with kidney disease; disulfiram-like reactions may occur with alcohol
Glyburide (Diabeta, Micronase)[b]	0.005–0.01 single or divided doses	.02	biphasic 3.2 + 10 hours	1.5	24	50% absorbed; completely metabolized in liver to nonactive derivatives; excreted in urine and bile 1:1	50–200 times more potent than other agents; good for kidney disease patients; no disulfiram reaction; low toxicity
Glipizide (Glucotrol)[b]	0.0025–0.005 single or divided doses	.045	3–7	1	24	Metabolized to inactive metabolite in liver; absorption ↓ by food	Potent; no disulfiram reaction; low toxicity; take on an empty stomach

[a] Adapted from M. A. Koda-Kimble (23).
[b] Approval by FDA expected soon.

Table 27.13.
Side Effects of Sulfonylureas

1. GI: less than 5%—take with meals
2. Skin: less than 2%
3. Antabuse effect: approximately 4%, especially with chlorpropamide
4. Hepatotoxicity: Rare, >500 mg Diabinese daily
5. Hematological: Very rare—cause and effect is questionable
6. SIADH: 4% with chlorpropamide yields hyponatremia (if on a diuretic, incidence increases)
7. Hypoglycemia: Especially in elderly and patients with renal insufficiency

Table 27.14.
What the Pharmacist Should Tell the Diabetic Taking Sulfonylureas

1. Name, purpose, directions for use
2. Can be taken with food
3. Take regularly, exactly as doctor prescribed
4. Contact M.D. if fever, sore throat or mouth lesions
5. Caution when using alcohol
6. Diet important—use drug in conjunction with diet
7. Use of other drugs should be doctor-approved and told to registered pharmacist
8. Carry sugar source for hypoglycemia

ure," once diabetogenic factors have been eliminated, the patient may be switched to a more potent sulfonylurea; i.e., from tolbutamide to chlorpropamide. If control is poor and symptoms are severe enough, the patient should be switched to insulin until control is achieved. Many patients can usually be successfully returned to oral therapy following control with insulin.

The role of the pharmacist in educating the diabetic patient to properly use oral sulfonylureas and in monitoring the compliance of the patient can be significant in achieving treatment objectives.

Insulin

Type I diabetics who have absolute insulin deficiency must be treated with exogenous insulin. Generally persons who require insulin initially tend to be younger than 30, lean, prone to developing ketoacidosis and markedly hyperglycemic even in the fasting state. Insulin also is indicated for type II diabetics who do not respond to diet therapy, either alone or combined with oral hypoglycemic drugs. Occasionally in type II diabetics doses of 10 to 20 units of intermediate-acting insulins are needed to bring hyperglycemia under control. Insulin therapy is also necessary in some type II diabetics who are subjected to the stress of infection, pregnancy or surgery. Thus, all classes of diabetics should be trained with reference to the use and injection of insulin.

Diabetic children should begin giving their own injections at around ages 8 to 9, although parents should administer one or two injections per week to stay in practice and should inject in areas difficult for the child to reach. By combining the appropriate modification of

diet, exercise, and variable mixtures of short- and longer-acting insulins, it has been possible to achieve acceptable but not excellent control of blood glucose. Patients using insulin should be strongly encouraged to self-monitor blood glucose levels.

INSULIN DOSING

A number of methods are used to determine the dose required by a type I patient. At some centers, insulin in the range of between 0.5 and 1.0 unit per kg is prescribed to take care of the needs of the diabetic patient. The total amount of insulin can either be given in one shot of intermediate-acting insulin or in two to three shots of short-acting insulin in combination with intermediate-acting insulin.

Other physicians will start with an "average" dose of insulin—i.e., 24 units of an intermediate-acting insulin—and have the patient try this amount and then through urine or blood glucose testing adjust the dose of the insulin up or down until the patient receives some degree of control. This trial and error method has many pitfalls.

A third method is to have the patient, in either an outpatient or inpatient setting, determine urine and/or blood glucose levels and take shots of regular (short-acting) insulin every 3 to 4 hours. The patient's objective is to bring the blood glucose under control at the time the tests are done. If accurate records are kept of the amount of regular insulin administered with each dose, a total of the regular insulin used over the 24-hour period is then determined. The doses of insulin are regulated by using the "sliding scale" for urine tests or by testing the blood and using approximately 1 to 2 units of insulin for each 50 mg/dl of desired fall in blood glucose levels. After the requirements for regular insulin is determined and the patient is under control, the multiple injections of regular insulin may be replaced by a single injection of intermediate-acting insulin (NPH or Lente). The dose of the intermediate-acting insulin is generally two thirds to three fourths of the 24-hour requirement of regular insulin and is supplemented with regular insulin as indicated by blood sugar levels. When the total requirement exceeds 40 units, the insulin may be given in two doses, two thirds in the morning and one third in the evening. Many physicians will order a blood sugar to be drawn at 4 P.M., the time at which intermediate-acting insulin exerts its peak activity, to assure that there is no mid-afternoon hypoglycemia. When the patient is discharged, the dose is decreased by 4 to 6 units to compensate for increased activity that is part of the outpatient process (4). Changes in diet and activity make further adjustments of dose on an outpatient basis almost inevitable, but fortunately the use of self-monitoring of blood glucose has greatly improved the ability of a patient to adjust insulin doses to achieve excellent control.

Another method to determine insulin requirements is to hospitalize the patient and attach him or her to a closed-loop insulin infusion device. The *Biostator* by Ames is such a machine. It automatically checks the blood glucose levels and administers the amount of insulin necessary to maintain the blood glucose at a predetermined level; i.e., 100 mg/dl. Over a 24-hour period, the amount of insulin used by the patient can be easily determined, and the change to rapid plus intermediate-acting insulins and the number of doses per day can be prescribed for the patient. Patients receiving a combination of regular and intermediate-acting insulins can experience mid-morning hyperglycemia secondary to the slow onset of the NPH or Lente insulins. Supplementation of the morning dose of the intermediate-acting insulins with small amounts of regular insulins will generally correct this problem. If mid-afternoon hypoglycemia with nighttime and early-morning hyperglycemia, is a problem the morning dose should be reduced and an additional evening dose given. This occurs in those patients who have a transient response to NPH insulin. Some patients experience a delayed onset of NPH insulin, leading to hyperglycemia throughout the day and hypoglycemia at night. This problem is managed by the addition of regular insulin to a lower dose of morning NPH. A snack before going to bed may also help alleviate nighttime hypoglycemia.

Several other problems can result in adjustments of insulin dose. The first is called the *"dawn phenomenon"* (33). This effect results from a rise in blood glucose levels which increases insulin need starting at about 5 A.M. and continuing until about 9 A.M. This condition has been detected in diabetics using insulin but not in nondiabetics. The early morning glucose rise can be caused by insufficient treatment; but in studies on patients with continuous subcutaneous insulin infusion, the dawn phenomenon still can occur. Food ingestion is another factor that could influence early morning rise. Yet in studies of fasting patients, blood glucose levels can increase in the early morning. Although the condition is not fully understood and the prevalence of the phenomenon is not totally known, it is a cause for concern in patients trying to achieve strict control. The most logical mechanism for the dawn phenomenon is an increased glucose production or decreased glucose utilization due to the morning rise of cortisol levels and/or other circadian factors.

Another problem requiring dosage adjustments is the "Somogyi phenomenon." This is a condition in which there is early morning hyperglycemia that is secondary to hypoglycemia. In simpler terms, a diabetic patient suffers an episode of hypoglycemia during sleep; this results in the release of hormones that increase blood glucose levels such as cortisol, glucagon and adrenalin; these hormones cause blood glucose levels to increase, and when the patient arises in the morning and tests his blood or urine glucose, it is elevated. Since the precipitating problem in the Somogyi phenomenon is hypoglycemia, the necessary step in treatment is to decrease the insulin dose.

The pharmacist can have a significant role in assisting the diabetic patient in understanding the onset and duration of insulin and insulin mixtures. Because there is increasing evidence that strict control of blood glucose can be achieved only through the use of continuous insulin infusion devices or through multiple injections of insulin, many new diabetic patients are being put on these types of regimens. By continuously receiving basal levels of insulin and then getting a bolus of insulin before meals, the patient's blood glucose levels can be much more easily normalized. By using a long-acting insulin (Ultralente) in combination with regular insulin, it is possible to achieve strict control of blood glucose levels. The Ultralente acts as a basal insulin because it has a slow, steady release over a long period of time. By combining regular and Ultralente insulin at breakfast, by giving regular insulin before lunch and combining regular and Ultralente insulin before dinner, the patient essentially has a basal level of insulin coming into the system with boluses before meals. These split regimens of insulin (two or more injections per day) can assist the patient in achieving strict control of hopefully prevent severe complications.

THE USE OF INSULINS

Table 27.15 summarizes the factors that are considered in comparing insulins. It is important that physicians, pharmacists and patients make special note of the species source and the purity of the insulins. There are two new manufacturers of insulin on the American market and over 30 different brand names of insulin from which to make a selection. Selecting insulins purely on the basis of cost has the possibility of causing adverse effects in some diabetic patients who require highly pure insulin. Table 27.16 summarizes the insulins available in the United States and compares their onset and duration of action as well as the species source, purity and strength. The short-acting insulins include semilente and neutral *regular insulins*. Intermediate-acting insulins include *NPH* and *Lente* insulins (globin zinc insulin is no longer manufactured or distributed in the United States). The long-acting insulins include *protamine zinc* and *Ultralente* insulins. Lente insulin is a combination of 70% Ultralente and 30% Semilente insulin. NPH insulin is a combination of 2 parts regular insulin and 1 part protamine zinc insulin.

In March 1980 the Food and Drug Administration decertified U-80 insulin. Thus at the present time there are two strengths of insulins available for diabetic patients: U-40 and U-100. U-500 insulin can be special-ordered and is available on prescription. In foreign countries patients are required to have a prescription from a physician to get insulin, and U-40 insulin is often the only strength available.

Table 27.15.
Factors Considered in Comparing Insulins

1. Onset and duration of action
2. Species source (human > pork > beef)
3. Strength—U-40 vs. U-100 vs. U-500
4. Methods of achieving long action; i.e., acetate buffers vs. protein, such as Protamine; Zn content
5. Purity
6. Mixability
7. Cost

Insulin vials and syringes from some manufacturers are color-coded to decrease errors and aid in the identification of the product. U-40 insulin vials and syringes designed to be used with U-40 insulins are color-coded red; U-100 insulin vials and syringes are color-coded orange with black lettering. All of the insulins are at a neutral pH of 7.4. All of the insulins are cloudy except regular insulin which is clear.

CLINICAL CONSIDERATIONS IN INSULIN USE

The *species source of insulin* can influence the effect of the insulin on blood glucose control and insulin resistance and sensitivity. Most commercially available insulins are derived from a mixture of beef and pork, although now pure pork or pure beef insulin is available and highly promoted. Human insulin is also currently available. High purification of pork insulin is possibly clinically important in reducing insulin dose, *lipoatrophy* (subcutaneous concavities caused by wasting of the lipid tissue), and insulin-binding capacity of serum. About 80% of the patients with persistent local allergy to mixed beef-pork insulin improve if treated with pure pork insulin (4). Beef insulin has greater antigenicity because it differs from human insulin by three amino acids, whereas pork differs by only one amino acid (4).

Another factor that affects insulin use in diabetic patients is purity. New analytical techniques using chromatography and electrophoresis to separate and isolate protein have made purer forms of insulin readily available. The average content of certain minor components of insulin, such as proinsulin, desamido insulin, arginine insulin, esterified insulin, and glucagon and somatostatin have been de-

Table 27.16.
Insulin Preparations[a]

Product (Manufacturer)	Species Source	Purity (ppm Proinsulin)	Strength
RAPID-ACTING (Onset ½–4 hr, duration 5–16 hr)			
Actrapid Regular Insulin (Squibb-Novo)	Pork, human	<1, <1	U-100
Insulin Quick, Velosulin (Nordisk)	Pork	<1	U-100
Humulin (Regular) (Lilly)	Human (re-combinant DNA)	0	U-100
Regular Iletin I (Lilly)	Beef and pork	<10	U-40, U-100
Regular Iletin II (Lilly)	Pork	<1	U-100, U-500
Regular Iletin II (Lilly)	Beef	<1	U-100
Regular Insulin (Squibb-Novo)	Pork	<25	U-100
Semilente Iletin I (Lilly)	Beef and pork	<10	U-40, U-100
Semilente Insulin (Squibb-Novo)	Beef	<25	U-100
Semitard Insulin Zinc Susp. (Squibb-Novo)	Pork	<1	U-100
INTERMEDIATE-ACTING (Onset 1–4 hr, duration 16–28 hr)			
Insulatard NPH (Nordisk)	Pork	<1	U-100
Lentard Insulin Zinc Susp. (Squibb-Novo)	Beef and pork	<1	U-100
Lente Iletin I (Lilly)	Beef and pork	<10	U-40, U-100
Lente Iletin II (Lilly)	Pork or beef	<1	U-100
Lente Insulin (Squibb-Novo)	Beef	<25	U-100
Mixtard, NPH + Regular Insulin (Nordisk)	Pork	<1	U-100
Monotard, Insulin Zinc Susp. (Squibb-Novo)	Pork, human	<1, <1	U-100
NPH Iletin I (Lilly)	Beef and pork	<10	U-40, U-100
NPH Iletin II (Lilly)	Pork or beef	<1	U-100
NPH (Isophane) Insulin (Squibb-Novo)	Beef	<25	U-100
Protaphane (NPH) Insulin (Squibb-Novo)	Pork	<1	U-100
LONG-ACTING (Onset 4–6 hr, duration 36+ hr)			
Protamine Zinc Iletin I (Lilly)	Beef and pork	<10	U-40, U-100
Protamine Zinc Iletin II (Lilly)	Pork or beef	<1	U-100
Ultralente Iletin (Lilly)	Beef and pork	<10	U-40, U-100
Ultralente Insulin (Squibb-Novo)	Beef	<25	U-100
Ultratard Zinc Susp. (Squibb-Novo)	Beef	<1	U-100

[a] Onset + duration of action may vary from patient to patient.

creased, resulting in fewer insulin-sensivity reactions. The very confusing terminology relating to purity of insulin as measured by proinsulin content is summarized in Table 27.17. The highly purified insulins have fewer than 10 parts per million of proinsulin. The recommendations for dosing insulin when changing from beef to pork or from conventional to purified insulin is summarized in Table 27.18 (34). Patients who should definitely use highly purified pork or human insulin are listed in Table 27.19. Note that patients who suffer from insulin allergy (local cutaneous reactions, rashes) should definitely be placed on a purified pork or human insulin. A few patients are allergic to pork insulin and can be put on purified beef insulin. If the local reactions continue, however, they may be treated by mixing an antihistamine such as diphenhydramine with the insulin before injection. Oftentimes if the patient will continue to use the insulin even though there is a local cutaneous reaction, the patient will become desensitized and the problem will disappear after several weeks. Desensitization kits can be obtained from Lilly.

Insulin resistance, a state requiring more than 200 units of insulin per day for more than 2 days in the absence of ketoacidosis or acute infection, occurs only in about 0.001% of diabetic patients. These patients almost invariably have high titers of insulin-neutralizing antibodies or are very obese. These patients should first be switched to a purified human insulin and if necessary placed on glucocorticoids (prednisone in a dose of 60 to 80 mg/

Table 27.17.
Proinsulin Contents of Insulins Available in the United States

Insulin	Proinsulin (parts per million)
Conventional USP	10,000–40,000
"Single Peak"	300–3,000
"Improved Single Peak"	50
"Improved (Low-PLI)"	20–25
"Purified"[a]	10[b]

[a] Novo pork and mixed insulins, Nordisk pork, Lilly pork (Iletin II pork) and beef (Iletin II beef), Squibb pork and beef.
[b] Internal specifications for manufacturers may vary.

Table 27.18.
Recommendations for Dosing Insulin When Changing from Beef to Pork or Conventional to Purified

1. Highly variable from patient to patient— MONITOR PATIENT CLOSELY
2. Decrease of 9–20% reported
3. Recommend 10% dose decrease if normal doses
4. Recommend 20% decrease if patient receiving >50 units/day

Table 27.19.
Patients Who Should Use Highly Purified Pork or Human Insulin

1. Patients with insulin resistance (using more than 100–200 units/day)
2. Patients with insulin allergy (local cutaneous reactions, rashes, etc.)
3. Patients with lipoatrophy or lipohypertrophy.
4. All type II diabetics using insulin for a short period of time (i.e., during surgery, infections)
5. Patients who are being treated for ketoacidosis?
6. Patients who have had a renal transplant?
7. Patients using insulin infusion pumps?
8. Patients who have been desensitized to pork insulin
9. Pregnant diabetics
10. All new diabetics?

Table 27.20.
Factors Affecting Formation of Insulin Antibodies

1. Species source:
   a. Beef most immunogenic
   b. Pork least immunogenic
2. Purity: greater the purity, lower the immunogenicity
3. Pharmaceutical form: regular (soluble) insulin is less immunogenic than Lente
4. Pattern of insulin treatment: episodic insulin therapy seems to accentuate antibody responses
5. Genetic factors

day) (4). Patients suffering from insulin lipodystrophy should be placed on purified human insulin. In the case of lipoatrophy, the purified human insulin should be injected in and around the scarred areas, and in a matter of 2 to 3 weeks cosmetically the appearance of the skin returns to normal. *Lipohypertrophy* is generally seen in patients who favor particular sites for insulin injection. This can be prevented by good rotation of injection sites and is an important factor because the hypertrophied areas can cause a decrease in insulin absorption.

The factors affecting formation of insulin antibodies (35) are summarized in Table 27.20. Other factors which affect the serum insulin concentration (36) are summarized in Table 27.21.

Determining the daily dose of insulin is challenging because of the many factors that can affect the optimal insulin level. Some of the factors known to cause changes in insulin requirements (36) include the following: age, endogenous insulin secretion, diet, duration of diabetes, antibodies, physical activities, degree of obesity, hormones, pregnancy, oral contraceptives, menstruation, intercurrent diseases, metabolic decompensation, drugs and anxiety. The hormones and drugs that are known to influence the requirements for insulin (9, 36) are summarized in Table 27.22.

MIXING AND STORING OF INSULIN

Because of improved purity, insulins are more stable and do not need to be refrigerated. Insulin should be injected at room temperature. If insulin is purchased in bulk, however, the vials that are not in use can be kept in the refrigerator.

For years the combination of regular plus NPH insulin or regular plus Lente insulin was assumed to be stable after mixing. Recent evidence has shown that the stability of these combinations lasts for only 5 min (34). New patients being put on regular plus NPH insulin or regular plus Lente insulin should be in-

Table 27.21.
Factors Affecting Serum Insulin Concentrations

1. Site of injection—abdominal > arm > leg > thigh
2. Exercise enhances absorption
3. Depth of injection
4. Concentration of insulin—in 40–100 U range—not significant
5. Increase in ambient temperature, increased absorption
6. Massage of site increases absorption
7. Insulin antibodies attract and hold insulin
8. Variance in degrading enzymes at site yields day-to-day variation
9. Insulins react with receptors

Table 27.22.
Hormones and Drugs Influencing the Requirements of Insulin

Increasing Requirement	Decreasing Requirement
Cortisol	Tetracycline
Prednisone	Salicylates
Glucagon	Alcohol
Growth hormone	Biguanides
Catecholamine	Sulfonylureas
Thyroxine	Propranolol
Oral contraceptives	
Diuretics	
L-Asparaginase	
Phenytoin	

Table 27.23.
Insulin Mixtures

1. Semi-Lente, Lente, Ultra-Lente
   a. May be mixed in any ratio
   b. Mixtures are stable for 18 months
2. Regular + Protamine Zinc Insulin (PZI)
   a. ≤1 to 1 mixture yields PZI
   b. 2 Regular to 1 PZI yields neutral protamine Hagedorn (NPH) type
   c. >2 Regular to 1 PZI yields regular + NPH type
   d. Stability of mixtures unpredictable
3. Regular + NPH
   a. Stable for only 5 min
   b. The lost regular yields more NPH
   c. After 30 min, reaches equilibrium
4. Regular + Lente
   a. Stable for only 5 min
   b. Continued state of flux for 24 hr
   c. Thought to yield Lente, but Semi-Lente produced
   d. Nordisk Regular + Lente is incompatible.

structed to use the insulin within 5 min of mixing. The Lente-type insulins can be mixed in any ratio, and the mixtures are stable for up to 18 months. Regular plus protamine zinc insulin causes a variety of problems, depending upon the ratio of the regular insulin to the protamine zinc insulin. Because of the very long action of the protamine zinc insulin, its low incidence of use, and the fact that few new diabetics are being put on the insulin, it will probably be removed from the market within the next 3 years. Table 27.23 summarizes the consequences of mixing various insulins. Because of the improvement in purity, most of the insulins are stable at room temperature for at least 18 months and for as long as 36 months. High temperatures may cause the suspensions of insulin (NPH, PZI and Lente) to clump (4). Potency is not necessarily lost, but there is a problem in drawing up the correct dose when clumping has occurred. Occasionally there can be a bad batch of insulin that results in the patient temporarily losing con-

trol. Patients should make special note of the control of their diabetes when they start on a new bottle of insulin in case their insulin has been exposed to high or low temperatures that could affect potency.

ADVERSE REACTIONS TO INSULIN

The major complications of insulin therapy (36) are summarized in Table 27.24. Other problems in insulin therapy are related to species source and insulin purity and hopefully will disappear with the availability of purified human insulins. Another major problem with reference to insulin use is the fact that patients do not achieve strict control and suffer the complications of diabetes that are secondary to inadequate control. Also, many diabetics are overtreated (inject too much insulin) (37).

A special effort should be made to educate the diabetic patient with reference to the symptoms and treatment of *hypoglycemia*. Factors predisposing the patient to insulin reactions (hypoglycemia) include insufficient food intake (skipping meals, vomiting, or diarrhea), excessive excerise, inaccurate measurement of insulin, concomitant intake of hypoglycemic drugs or termination of diabetogenic conditions. Symptoms include a parasympathetic response (nausa, hunger, or flatulence), diminished cerebral function (confusion, agitation, lethargy, or personality changes), sympathetic responses (tachycardia, sweating or tremor), coma, and convulsions. Ataxia and blurred vision are also common. In elderly patients with decreased nerve function, diabetes with advanced neuropathy, or patients receiving β-blockers, the symptoms of hypoglycemia are sometimes lacking, and the reaction may go undetected and untreated. All manifestations of hypoglycemia are relieved rapidly by glucose adminstration. In unconscious patients, injections of glucagon or IV glucose or dextrose may be required. Because of the potential danger of insulin reactions, the diabetic patient should always carry packets of table sugar or a candy role for use at the onset of hypoglycemic symptoms. Note also that if a hypoglycemic person is mistakenly thought to be hyperglycemic and given insulin, severe hypoglycemia and subsequent brain damage may result. Thus when there is doubt whether a diabetic is hypo- or hyperglycemic, sugar should be given initially until the condition can be evaluated accurately.

The pharmacist's role in insulin therapy can be significant. Pharmacists should monitor the type and strength of insulin the patient is using. The proper insulin syringe for use with the type and strength of insulin should also be monitored. Pharmacists should explain to the patient how insulin should be stored, mixed and injected. There should be a discussion of the rotation of injection sites with the patient. The pharmacist should also encourage the patient to self monitor blood glucose to make sure that the doses of insulin are appropriate. Because of the many recent changes in names, strengths and purity of insulins, the pharmacist should keep informed to help decrease the confusion among patients and health care practitioners.

INSULIN INFUSION DEVICES

A major frustration in treating type I diabetic patients with insulin was the fact that one or two shots of insulin per day do not simulate the normal relationship between insulin and the ingesting of food. A patient brings insulin on board in the morning, or in the morning and in the evening, and then eats up to the level of insulin injected. The insulin is not necessarily available in the right concentrations at the time the patient ingests food. In 1981 several manufacturers developed relatively small insulin infusion devices that provide the patient with a continuous subcutaneous basal injection of regular insulin. The basal rate takes care of the individual's blood glucose over a 24-hour period of time if no food is ingested (38). The rate of administration is approximately 1 unit of insulin per hour. This is approximately the amount of insulin that a nondiabetic secretes. Fifteen to 30 min before meals, the patient receives a bolus of regular insulin to handle the food that will be ingested. In the nondiabetic, upon eating, insulin is released from the pancreas to handle the rise in blood glucose levels. Diabetics on insulin pumps who receive insulin subcutaneously need to inject a bolus of insulin prior to eating. Table 27.25 summarizes the objectives of insulin pump therapy (38). Note that these objectives are not that different than the overall objectives in treating diabetics.

The insulin pump makes it much easier for the patient to have a more flexible life-style

---

Table 27.24.
Complications of Insulin Therapy

1. Related to insulin purity and/or species source:
   a. Insulin lipodystrophy (atrophic and hypertropic) 10%
   b. Insulin allergy (local, 5–10%; systemic <1%)
   c. Insulin antibody formation ~100% (including immunologic resistance
2. Unrelated to insulin purity and/or species source:
   a. Hypoglycemia ~100%
   b. Insulin edema
   c. Complications of diabetes secondary to inadequate control by conventional forms of insulin therapy

---

Table 27.25.
Insulin Pump Therapy Objectives

1. Normalize blood glucose values (70–140 mg/dl)
2. Keep blood glucose values under 200 mg/dl
3. Normalize glycosylated hemoglobin values
4. Prevent or reverse diabetic complications
5. Continue activities of daily living
6. Increase lifestyle flexibility (i.e., pump patients can more easily adjust eating, sleeping and exercise schedule)
7. Avoid weight gain by maintaining a well-planned diabetic diet
8. Avoid infections and problems with pump procedure
9. Achieve a sense of well being

and, in most patients, blood glucose values and glycosylated hemoglobins, as well as lipid values, are normalized within a 2- to 3-month period. A major problem is to properly educate the patient to not "cheat" when using the pump as this can result in a weight gain.

Table 27.26 summarizes the criteria used for selecting insulin pump patients (38). Numerous products are in the developmental stage. There are currently three companies that are marketing these devices. The pumps can be compared on the basis of insulin dilution requirements, size, ease of use, type and completeness of alarm system, supplemental dose features, whether or not they indicate the total amount of insulin given over a one-day period of time, and cost. The two most commonly used pumps are Model 9200—a CPI-Lilly Pump, and the Model AS-6C U-100 Auto-Syringe Pump. Numerous auxiliary items need to be purchased by pump patients. The pharmacist should keep abreast of these products so that they can special-order them for the diabetic patients using the pump.

All patients using pumps need to self monitor their blood glucose several times daily. The pharmacist should be aware of this and provide assistance to the patient in using the various methods available for self testing. Table 27.27 is a summary of the various *self-monitoring systems for blood glucose*. The pharmacist should carry the various blood testing products as well as explain to patients the proper use of the products. The pharmacist can also educate the patient in the simple and painless technique of obtaining a drop of blood and can have a significant effect in encouraging patients to self-monitor blood glucose.

PROGNOSIS

The outlook for the diabetic patient has never been more positive. More and more government funds are being allocated for diabetes research to better understand the condition and to develop systems of treatment that result in normalization of blood glucose levels and hopefully a decrease in the long-term complications. Many states have funds through the Center for Disease Control to develop diabetes control projects with the objective of reducing the morbidity and mortality of diabetes. Much research is also being done with reference to transplantation of pancreas or transplantation of islet tissues. Much work is also being done to develop a miniaturized closed-loop system that could be implanted in diabetic patients in

Table 27.26.
Criteria for Selecting Insulin Pump Patients

1. Pregnant diabetics
2. Diabetics with early complications
3. Diabetics who have had a renal transplant
4. Brittle (difficult-to-control) diabetics
5. Motivated type I diabetics
6. At present, type II and children are not being encouraged
7. All patients must be:
   a. Willing and highly motivated
   b. Capable of being educated
   c. Responsible for keeping records and following specific procedures
   d. Willing to perform and log blood tests daily
   e. Willing to be hospitalized for 2–4 days if necessary

Table 27.27.
Systems for Self-monitoring of Blood Glucose (BG)

System	Calibration Materials Needed	BG Range (mg/dl)	Reflectance Meter	Comments
Chemstrip bG (Bio-Dynamics)	Chemstrips, cotton swab	20–800	None required	Strips can be cut in half. Easy to use
Glucometer (Ames)	Dextrostix, water, tissue, calibration chips	0–399	Yes ~$150	Battery-operated, 60-sec timer, small, easy to carry. Holds calibration
AccuChek (Bio-Dynamics)	Chemstrip bG Strips, reagent standards	50–350	Yes ~$150	Relatively easy to use
Visidex II (Ames)	Visidex strip	20–800	None required	Visually read strip that has 2 reagent areas and allows patient to easily determine when BG is over 200

which their blood glucose could be determined and insulin would automatically be injected to maintain blood glucose at a preset level. With the massive amount of work being done in diabetes, it is expected that within 10 years there will either be a device that makes living with diabetes so easy that the patient is virtually unaware of being a diabetic, or there will be a surgical transplantation technique that will cure the condition. The new approach to educating patients and giving the patient the responsibility for self-monitoring should also produce positive results and decrease the complications while at the same time prolonging the diabetic's life span and improving the quality of his or her life.

CONCLUSION

Diabetes is a complex, heterogeneous disorder that requires a health team effort if treatment objectives are to be achieved. Through a combination of diet, exercise, medications and education that result in the patient "taking charge" of the condition, the outlook for the diabetic is continually improving. There is still much information needed if diabetes is to be conquered.

The role of the pharmacist in the treatment of diabetes has been overlooked too long. The pharmacist can have a significant effect in educating the patient and in monitoring the diabetic condition. Pharmacists have a unique opportunity, because of their position in the health care system, to impact upon the treatment of diabetes. The few pharmacists who have taken an active interest in the diabetic patient have achieved a great deal of positive professional feedback as well as increased income. One step that pharmacists can take to improve the care of the diabetic is to develop a diabetes care center within a community pharmacy. For the pharmacist to become involved in sincere effort is required. The pharmacist needs to communicate with other members of the health team and to reinforce the information they provide to the diabetic patient. It is also necessary for the pharmacist to actively participate in diabetes associations; to keep up on the various educational methods and programs relating to diabetes; pharmacists should become active in the American Association of Diabetes Educators. Last, the pharmacist must carry a complete line of diabetes care products that are sensitive to the needs of diabetic patients. The opportunity for pharmacists in the care of diabetes is great, and those who participate will find that the rewards are even greater.

References

1. Watkins JD, Roberts DE, Williams TF, et al: Observation of medication errors made by diabetic patients at home. *Diabetes* 16:883, 1967.
2. Salans LB: Diabetes mellitus, a disease that is coming into focus. *JAMA* 247:590, 1982.
3. National Diabetes Data Group: *Diabetes* 28:1039, 1979.
4. Waife SO (Ed): *Diabetes Mellitus*, ed 8. Indianapolis: Lilly Research Laboratories, 1980.
5. Podolsky S: *Clinical Diabetes: Modern Management.* New York: Appleton-Century-Crofts, 1980, p xvii.
6. Platt WG, Sudovar SG: *The Social and Economic Costs of Diabetes: An Estimate for 1979.* Washington, D.C.: Pracon, Inc., 1979, pp 3–4.
7. Nerup J: In Martin JM, Ehrlich RM, Holland FJ: *Etiology and Pathogenesis of Insulin-Dependent Diabetes.* New York: Raven Press, 1981, p 275.
8. Karam JH: In Krupp MA, Chatton WJ: *Diabetes Mellitus, Hypoglycemia, and Lipoprotein Disorders.* Los Gatos, Calif.: Lange Medical Publications, 1982, p 742.
9. Hansten PD: *Drug Interactions*, ed 4. Philadelphia: Lea & Febiger, 1979, pp 93–109.
10. Cahill GF Jr: Disorders of carbohydrate metabolism: diabetes mellitus. In Wyngaarden JB, Smith LH Jr: *Cecil Textbook of Medicine*, ed 16. Philadelphia: W. B. Saunders, 1982, vol 1, pp 1054–1056.
11. Kaplan SA: Diabetes mellitus, UCLA conference. *Ann Intern Med* 96:635–649, 1982.
12. Olson OC: *Diagnosis and Management of Diabetes Mellitus.* Philadelphia: Lea & Febiger, 1981, pp 10–17, 251–261.
13. Gerich JE: Diabetic control and the late complications of diabetes. *Am Fam Physician* 16:85, 1977.
14. Skyler JS: Complications of diabetes mellitus: relationship to metabolic dysfunction. *Diabetes Care* 2:499, 1979.
15. Bohannon NJ, Zilbergeld B, Bullard DG, et al: Treatable impotence in diabetic patients. *West J Med* 136:6–10, 1982.
16. Campbell RK, Klein OG: Eye care for the diabetic patient. *JAMA* 245:2087, 1981.
17. Hansten PD: Smoking interaction with drugs. *Drug Interaction Newslett* 2:14, 1982 (Applied Therapeutics, Inc., San Francisco).
18. Jovanovic L, Peterson CM: The clinical utility of glycosylated hemoglobin. *Am J Med* 70:331, 1981.
19. Skyler JS: Blood glucose monitoring. *Diabetes Outlook* 16:1, 1981.
20. Campbell RK: Diabetes care products. In *Handbook of Nonprescription Drugs*, ed 7. Washington, DC.: American Pharmaceutical Association, 1982.
21. Leonards JR: Evaluation of enzyme tests for urinary glucose. *JAMA* 163:260, 1957.
22. Guthrie DW, Hinnen D, Guthrie RA: Single-

voided vs. double-voided urine testing. *Diabetes Care* 2:269–271, 1979.

23. Koda-Kimble MA: Diabetes. In Herfindal ET, Hirschman JL: *Clinical Pharmacy and Therapeutics*, ed 2. Baltimore: Williams & Wilkins, 1979, p 381.

24. *Guidelines for Diabetes Care*: American Association of Diabetes Educators, Pitman, N. J./American Diabetes Association, New York, 1981.

25. Brownless M, Vlassara H: Exercise and the diabetic patient. *Drug Ther* p 66, 1982.

26. Richter EA, Ruderman NB, Schneider SH: Diabetes and exercise. *Am J Med* 70:201, 1981.

27. Kurtzman P: Role of food fiber in health. *U.S. Pharmacist* p 63, 1982.

28. West KM: Recent trends in dietary management. In Podolsky S: *Clinical Diabetes: Modern Management*. New York: Appleton-Century-Crofts, 1980, p 70.

29. Overtreatment of diabetics: *Diabetes Outlook* 6:2, 1976.

30. The University Group Diabetes Program: A study of the effects of hypoglycemic agents on vascular complications in patients with adult onset diabetes. *Diabetes* 19(Suppl 2), 1970.

31. Skillman TG, Feldman JM: The pharmacology of the sulfonylureas. *Am J Med* 70:361, 1981.

32. Pannelkoek JH: Side effects of drugs. In Meyler L, Herxheimer A: *Oral Antidiabetic Drugs*. Baltimore: Williams & Wilkins, 1968, vol 6, chap 28, p 422.

33. Schmidt MI: The dawn phenomenon. *Infusion* 1:1, 1982.

34. Galloway JW: Personal communication with author of studies done by Eli Lilly and Company on stability of insulin mixtures, 1981.

35. Galloway JA: When the patient is resistant or allergic to insulin. *Medical Times*, May 1980.

36. Galloway JA, DeShazo RD: The clinical use of insulin and the complications of insulin therapy. In Ellenberg M, Rifkin H: *Diabetes Mellitus: Theory and Practice*, ed 3. Garden City, N.Y.: Medical Exam Publishing Co., 1982.

37. Kromann H, Borch E, Gale EAM: Unnecessary insulin treatment for diabetes. *Br Med J* 283:1386, 1981.

38. Cambpell RK, Fredlund P: Insulin pumps: the state of the art today. *Practical Diabetology* 1:12, 1982.

CHAPTER 28

Adrenocortical Dysfunction

DONALD T. KISHI, Pharm.D.

Cushing's syndrome and Addison's disease result from disturbances in the regulation of cortisol synthesis-secretion. Cushing's syndrome is associated with chronic overproduction of cortisol. Addison's disease is the result of a chronic deficiency of cortisol and aldosterone. In its acute stage, this deficiency is known as Addisonian crisis.

PHYSIOLOGY

Cortisol is the major endogenous glucocorticoid produced in the body. In the normal individual, cortisol production and secretion are governed by the hypothalamic-anterior pituitary-adrenocortical (HPA) axis. It is the primary function of this axis to maintain and control the level of circulating cortisol (Fig. 28.1).

The adrenal cortex consists of three zones: the zona glomerulosa, reticularis and fasiculata. The zona reticularis and fasiculata comprise the inner zones responsible for cortisol production and secretion. The adrenal androgens are also produced and secreted from these inner zones. The zona glomerulosa is responsible for the production and secretion of aldosterone (1).

The production of cortisol is, in the normal individual, controlled by adrenocorticotropic hormone (ACTH) which is secreted from the anterior pituitary gland in response to low plasma cortisol levels. Conversely, high plasma cortisol levels result in an inhibition of pituitary ACTH secretion. This relationship between ACTH and cortisol manifests as a diurnal variation in their plasma levels (2).

The synthesis of cortisol is initiated by an ACTH stimulus to the conversion of cholesterol and its esters to form pregnenolone. Pregnenolone is converted by a series of enzymatic steps to form cortisol and some intermediary products such as the adrenal androgens. The final enzymatic step involves 11-hydroxylase, which will be discussed later in this chapter.

As mentioned previously, the secretion of ACTH follows a diurnal pattern; that is, there is a peak and valley effect of plasma ACTH each 24 hours. Consequently, it follows that cortisol production and secretion follow a diurnal pattern. Maximal ACTH levels occur between 2 A.M. and 6 A.M. During this time period, the stimulus to cortisol production is also at its maximum. After 8 A.M., ACTH and cortisol secretion gradually decline until the low point is reached—approximately 12 midnight. The low plasma cortisol level stimulates ACTH production and the diurnal pattern begins to repeat itself (Fig. 28.2).

The diurnal pattern of ACTH and cortisol secretion is a function of the sleep-wake or inactivity-activity pattern of an individual and not necessarily a function of daylight and night. For example, a person who works during the night and sleeps during the day will have an inverted diurnal pattern (3). Upon initiating this altered wake-sleep pattern, 1 to 3 weeks is required to completely invert the diurnal rhythm of ACTH and cortisol secretion (4). Individuals who have been comatose for any length of time lose the rhythmicity of ACTH and cortisol secretion (5).

The negative feedback relationship between the adrenal cortex and the anterior pituitary can be interrupted by the activation of the hypothalamic corticotropin-releasing center. ACTH secretion is stimulated by hypothalamic corticotropin releasing factor (CRF). CRF secretion is stimulated by a number of neurotransmitters including serotonin and dopamine (6). This activation is mediated by stressful stimuli which may be emotional, physical or chemical.

Stress activates the center and causes the CRF to enter the portal system of the pituitary. ACTH is then released from the anterior pituitary and, consequently, cortisol from the adrenal cortex. Sufficient cortisol, up to 300 mg in 24 hours, is secreted to deal with the stress. Normal cortisol production ranges from 5.0 to 27.9 mg/24 hours (7).

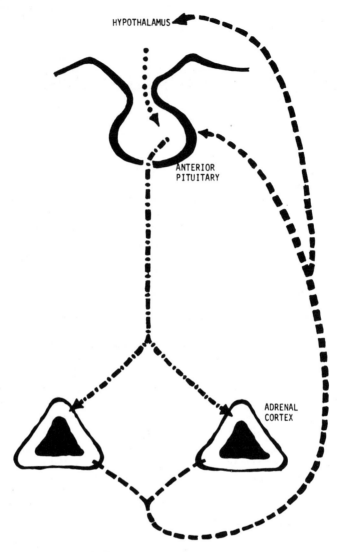

Figure 28.1. Normal hypothalamic-anterior pituitary-adrenal cortex axis. Note cortisol-negative feedback on hypothalamus and anterior pituitary. (····) corticotropin-releasing factor (CRF), (·−·−·) ACTH, (−−−) cortisol.

Once cortisol enters the circulation, it is bound primarily to an α_2-globulin known as corticosteroid-binding globulin (CBG) or transcortin and secondarily to albumin. In the normal individual, approximately 90% of the circulating cortisol is bound. The remaining unbound 10% is physiologically active and available for metabolism and excretion. It should be noted that pregnancy or estrogen therapy increases the amount of CBG available for cortisol binding. Conversely, CBG is decreased in conditions associated with decreased protein production or increased protein loss, e.g., cirrhosis and nephrosis (8).

Free cortisol is metabolized by the liver by conjugation with glucuronide. This glucuronidated form is physiologically inactive. The metabolism of cortisol can be enhanced by concurrent hyperthyroidism and by enzyme induction by phenytoin, phenobarbital and phenylbutazone (8, 9). Hypothyroidism and severe liver impairment inhibit the metabolism of cortisol (8). Free cortisol to the extent of approximately 1% is excreted unchanged in the urine (10).

CUSHING'S SYNDROME

In 1932, Cushing described the characteristic clinical manifestations found in a series of

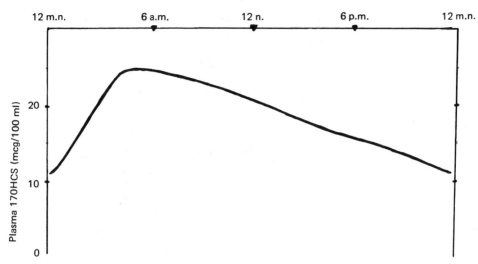

Figure 28.2.   Diurnal variation in plasma cortisol. (Reprinted with permission from Pincus et al. (5).)

12 patients with either documented or presumptive basophilic adenomas of the pituitary gland. The syndrome which he described and which was eventually to bear his name was most consistently characterized by the following features: adiposity of the face, neck and trunk; hypertrichosis of the face and trunk in females and preadolescent males; amenorrhea; cutaneous striae; hypertension; polycythemia; kyphosis and backaches; and fatigability and weakness (11). Cushing's work delineated one possible pathological abnormality which could account for the development of the syndrome. Cushing, however, could not elucidate the fundamental hormonal basis for the development of the syndrome. Subsequent work by endocrinologists revealed not only the basic hormonal disturbance, hypercortisolism, but also other pathological abnormalities which could lead to this hormonal disturbance and to the development of Cushing's syndrome. Consequently, this syndrome can now be defined as the group of clinical and metabolic abnormalities resulting from a chronic overproduction of cortisol (12).

Approximately 30 years ago, exogenous glucocorticoids were introduced into the physician's armamentarium of medical therapy. Consequently, an iatrogenic cause of Cushing's syndrome also exists. Aside from this iatrogenic hyperglucocorticoidism, Cushing's syndrome occurs in the general population at a rate of 1 per 1000. Females are afflicted 3 to 5 times more often than males. There is also a predominance in the age of onset; that is, over 50% of cases occur between 20 and 40 years of age (13).

Pathophysiology

The fundamental hormonal defect in Cushing's syndrome is the overproduction and secretion of cortisol (12). The overproduction of cortisol is the net result of pathological processes which relate primarily or secondarily to the adrenal cortex. Primary hypercortisolism relates to the overproduction of cortisol from an intrinsic disorder of the adrenal cortex. Secondary hypercortisolism relates to the excessive stimulation of normal adrenal cortices by an overproduction of ACTH (14).

Primary hypercortisolism is indicative of an adrenocortical tumor, usually an adenoma or carcinoma. The adenomas and carcinomas are usually unilateral and represent 15% and 10% of the cases of Cushing's syndrome, respectively (14, 15). The adrenocortical tumors are usually autonomous; that is, the production and secretion of cortisol by the adrenal cortex is independent of ACTH stimulation. In fact, the elevation of the cortisol levels results in a negative feedback on the normal pituitary. Plasma levels of ACTH in the presence of these autonomously functioning tumors are subnormal and may be undetectable (16, 17). The subnormal ACTH levels result in the atrophy of the contralateral adrenal cortex (15) (Fig. 28.3). However, even in patients with negligible ACTH, the conversion of cholesterol to pregnenolone and, eventually, to cortisol oc-

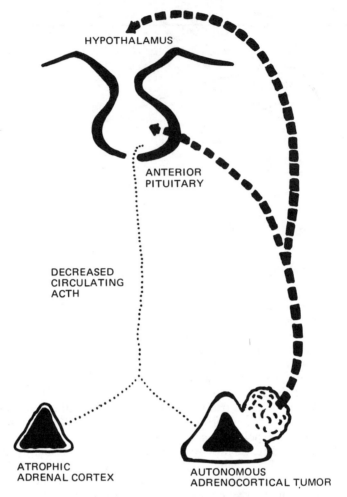

Figure 28.3. Autonomous adrenocortical tumor. Note negative feedback inhibition of ACTH and consequent atrophic contralateral adrenal cortex.

curs but at a very slow rate. The net result is the production of 0.5 mg per day of cortisol in these individuals (18).

Adrenocortical carcinomas occur in all age groups; however, the majority of cases occur in the 4th decade of life. There also appears to be a higher incidence in females—approximately 68% of the cases of adrenocortical carcinomas (19).

The adrenocortical carcinomas can metastasize to other tissues. The two most common sites of distant metastases are the lung and liver. Metastatic lesions have also been reported in bone, brain, skin, spleen, myocardium, ovary, bone marrow, thoracic duct and pelvis. The metastatic lesions usually manifest the same hormonal pattern as the primary tumor (19). Tissues adjacent to the primary tumor may also be involved.

Secondary hypercortisolism is related to the overproduction of ACTH. The excess ACTH can be from a pituitary origin or from an ectopic tumor. Although the adrenal cortex is fundamentally normal, the excess ACTH stimulation results in the hyperplasia of both adrenal cortices. Secondary hypercortisolism accounts for approximately 75% of the cases of Cushing's syndrome (15).

The pituitary origins of Cushing's syndrome are often referred to as Cushing's disease (14). The basophilic adenoma, carcinoma and the chromophobe adenoma represent primary anterior pituitary lesions which result in excess ACTH secretion (15). Secondary or nontumorous pituitary ACTH overproduction is the result of an overactive hypothalamus (20). The basophilic adenoma of the anterior pituitary and hypothalamic overactivity result in moderately elevated ACTH production. The chromophobe adenoma, in contrast, is associated with marked elevation of ACTH secretion. In the latter case, the minor melanocyte-stimulating properties of ACTH become significant. Consequently, the skin of patients with chromophobe adenomas is pigmented. Another contrasting feature which distinguishes the chromophobe adenoma from basophilic adenoma and hypothalamic overactivity is the size of the sella turcica. The chromophobe adenoma is associated with radiological evidence of sella turcica enlarge-

ment, whereas the hypothalamic overactivity and basophilic adenoma generally are not (15) (Fig. 28.4).

The ectopic nonendocrine tumors, which secrete an ACTH-like substance, result in mean cortisol secretion rates 3 times higher than that found in other forms of Cushing's syndrome (21). This is perhaps the most insidious cause of Cushing's syndrome since the clinical picture may not always suggest adrenocortical overactivity. The most common findings are progressive weakness, muscle wasting, edema and severe hypokalemic al-

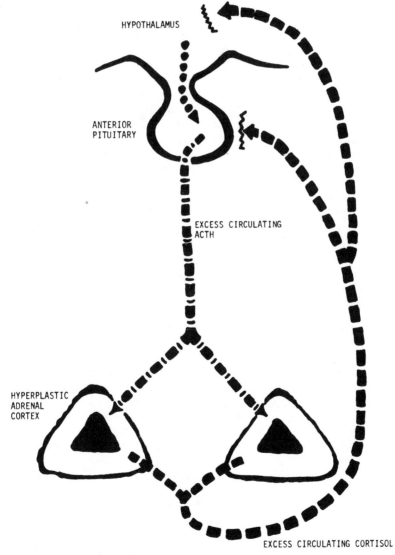

HYPOTHALAMUS

ANTERIOR
PITUITARY

EXCESS CIRCULATING
ACTH

HYPERPLASTIC
ADRENAL
CORTEX

EXCESS CIRCULATING CORTISOL

Figure 28.4. Bilateral adrenocortical hyperplasia due to excess anterior pituitary ACTH production. Note relative loss of negative feedback effect of excess cortisol.

kalosis. The severity of hypokalemic alkalosis appears to be a function of the degree of hypercortisolism and cortisol renal effect and may not relate to hyperaldosteronism. Death has been reported within days of the onset of these nonclassical findings (21).

The two most common ectopic ACTH-producing tumors are the oat cell carcinoma of the lung and pancreatic carcinomas. The former represents greater than 50%, and the latter 20%, of reported cases of ectopic ACTH-producing tumors. Other common sites of these ectopic tumors include the gall bladder, thymus and fibrosarcomas located retroperitoneally. Rarely reported sites include the breast, colon, ovaries, testes, prostate, kidney, thyroid, parotids, trachea and parathyroids. The metastatic lesions from these primary ectopic ACTH-producing tumors manifest the same hormonal patterns as the primary tumors (21).

The ectopic ACTH-producing tumors are usually autonomous. The tumors of the anterior pituitary and the hyperfunctioning hypothalamus lack this autonomous behavior and are responsive to high glucocorticoid plasma levels. It appears that the HPA axis negative feedback threshold for plasma glucocorticoid is abnormally elevated (21).

There is also evidence for ectopic tumors secreting CRF-like substances which result in the clinical picture associated with ectopic ACTH secreting tumors. Upton and Amatruda (22) reported two patients with the ectopic ACTH syndrome in whom CRF-like substances were isolated from a pancreatic tumor of one patient and the oat cell carcinoma and its metastases in the other.

It should be noted that the etiologies of Cushing's syndrome are not as clear-cut as defined in this section. There appears to be a definite intermediate form of adrenocortical hyperplasia and adenoma (23, 24). This rare intermediate form is termed "primary adrenocortical nodular dysplasia" (24). Gross pathological examination reveals adrenocortical hyperplasia with multiple small adenomas. Characteristically, this intermediate form is resistant to dexamethasone suppression, may show either a hyperactive or no response to exogenous ACTH stimulation and is associated with low plasma ACTH levels (24) (Fig. 28.5).

The manifestations of Cushing's syndrome can result from the therapeutic use of exogenous ACTH and/or glucocorticoids in the patient with an intact, normally functioning HPA axis or from the use of supraphysiological glucocorticoid replacement. The predictability or assignment of a minimal total daily dose of glucocorticoid or ACTH necessary to induce a given symptom, finding or the entire syndrome complex is not feasible. This lack of predictability is based on the individual variability of cortisol clearance. Although the total daily dose is a major factor in the development of some of the signs and symptoms of Cushing's syndrome, other factors also play a major role. Factors such as the dosage regimen, total dose and duration of therapy are also major factors in the rate of development of specific findings or manifestations of Cushing's syndrome. The picture of iatrogenic Cushing's syndrome is further complicated by the fact that a patient may have a predisposition for a given finding or manifestation.

"Pseudo-Cushing's syndrome" is a term which has been applied to a reversible condition in which the clinical manifestations of Cushing's syndrome, and hypercortisolemia are found in association with chronic alcoholism. The mechanism by which ethanol causes this syndrome has not been confirmed. Potential explanations include: decreased cortisol clearance secondary to alcoholic liver disease; compensatory hypersecretion of cortisol in response to decreased cortisol levels resulting from ethanol induction of hepatic enzymes; ethanol stimulation of CRF and/or ACTH secretion; and subacute withdrawal from alcohol and a resultant stress induced HPA axis stimulation (25).

Diagnosis

Patients with the manifestations of classic Cushing's syndrome can be easily recognized. Unfortunately, it is only the patient with long standing hypercortisolism who presents with these classic manifestations. Patients with a shorter history of hypercortisolism have variable signs and symptoms. This variability of presenting manifestations makes diagnosis of early Cushing's syndrome difficult. It is, therefore, recommended that patients even remotely suspected of hypercortisolism be tested (13).

The diagnosis of Cushing's syndrome involves two phases: documentation that hypercortisolism exists and the elucidation of the etiology of the hypercortisolism (26). In the normal adult, cortisol secretion rate varies from 5.0 to 27.9 mg/24 hours (7). In normal,

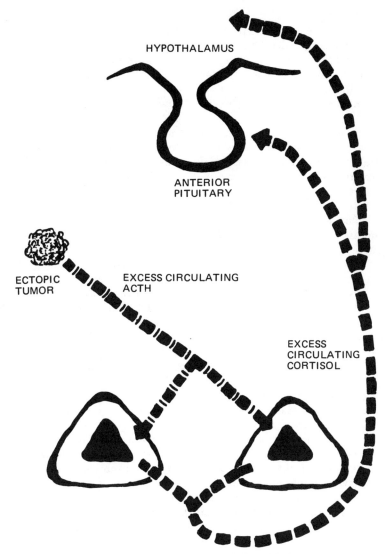

Figure 28.5. Ectopic ACTH-producing tumor with secondary adrenocortical hyperplasia. Note negative feedback inhibition of anterior pituitary ACTH secretion.

unstressed males' the mean secretion rate is 20.4 mg/24 hours. In normal, unstressed females' a mean secretion rate of 17.4 mg/24 hours has been reported (27). In infants less than 5 days old, the cortisol secretion rate is 18 mg/m²/day. By age 11 years, the secretion rate is 11 mg/m²/day, essentially the same as an adult (28). The diagnosis of Cushing's syndrome is based on direct or indirect evidence of hypercortisolism.

Screening Tests

It would seem logical that the demonstration of a single, elevated plasma cortisol level would be sufficient to document hypercortisolism. However, since cortisol secretion and production may be temporarily elevated by stress, a single plasma level may solely reflect such a temporary elevation and not sustained overproduction. It also should be noted that plasma levels of cortisol may be elevated by factors which elevate CBG, e.g., estrogens and pregnancy (29). If, on the other hand, two plasma cortisol levels are drawn, one in the early morning and the second in the later evening, loss of diurnal rhythm in plasma cortisol level owing to sustained overproduction of cortisol can be demonstrated. The presence of a diurnal rhythm in plasma cortisol levels, however, does not totally exclude the possibility that Cushing's syndrome exists (30). In general, it can be stated that, while the early morning plasma cortisol levels may be elevated or normal, the evening plasma cortisol level is abnormally elevated in Cushing's syndrome.

Medications can also affect plasma cortisol levels. Heparin and spironolactone have been noted to interfere with fluorometric assays of plasma corticosteroid levels. Carbenoxolone, nicotine, amphetamines, ethanol and vasopressin can elevate levels and lithium carbonate has been noted to decrease levels (31). Morphine administered acutely can result in elevated serum cortisol levels; however, chronic use of morphine blocks CRF release (32). Naloxone administered as intravenous bolus can cause serum levels of ACTH and cortisol to rise. This effect was not seen when the naloxone was administered as an infusion (33). Lysine vasopressin also is known to cause increases in serum ACTH and cortisol levels (34).

Based on animal models, the production and/or release of CRF may be influenced by a number of drugs. Dextroamphetamine, methamphetamine and Δ^9-tetrahydrocannabinol (marijuana) stimulate CRF release. Reserpine results in a transient increase in the basal secretion of CRF. The phenothiazines have been shown to have variable effects on CRF (35).

Indirect evidence of the overproduction of cortisol can be obtained by measurements of urinary 17-OHCS excretion. In the normal adult, 3 to 12 mg of 17-OHCS are excreted in the urine in 24 hours. In patients with a 17-OHCS urinary excretion which exceeds 12 mg/24 hours, Cushing's syndrome must be suspected (36, 37). Since obesity influences the rate of 17-OHCS excretion, a correction factor for body weight is made. This correction factor is based on urinary 17-OHCS excretion per g of urinary creatinine. In the normal adult, 3 to 7 mg of 17-OHCS is excreted per g of urinary creatinine. On the other hand, patients with Cushing's syndrome excrete greater than 10 mg of 17-OHCS per g of urinary creatinine (36, 37). Cortisol secretion rate can be measured by the radioisotope-dilution method. Unfortunately, although considered by some to be the definitive test for overproduction of cortisol, the limited availability of this test makes it an impractical method of testing.

Dexamethasone can be used as a diagnostic tool in the establishment of cortisol overproduction. The low dose dexamethasone-suppression test and the more simple dexamethasone-screening test are based on the negative feedback system of the HPA axis. Dexamethasone is used since it does not contribute significantly to the 17-OHCS levels, yet it has significant glucocorticoid activity. The dexamethasone-screening test is performed by administering 1 mg of the drug orally between 11 P.M. and 12 midnight with subsequent measurement of plasma 17-OHCS at 8 A.M. the following morning. In normal individuals, the level of plasma 17-OHCS is suppressed to less than 5 μg/100 ml when measured by the Porter-Silber method (38). If 17-OHCS is measured by the Eik-Nes method (39), normal individuals have a level of less than 11 μg/100 ml; plasma levels between 11 and 19 μg/100 ml are indeterminate and a level of 20 μg/100 ml or greater is considered evidence of the existence of Cushing's syndrome. Regardless of the method of measurement, it is recommended that sedation with flurazepam be given during the evening to eliminate the possibility of stress-induced activation of the HPA axis and resultant temporary increase in cortisol production (38).

The low dose dexamethasone-suppression test (12) consists of collecting two baseline 24-hour urine samples for 17-OHCS. Dexamethasone 0.5 mg is administered orally every 6 hours for eight doses. During the administration of the dexamethasone, 24-hour urine samples for 17-OHCS are collected. The normal patient will have 17-OHCS levels less than 2.5 μg and/or lower levels than the controls. Patients with Cushing's syndrome will show no suppression of 17-OHCS when compared to the baseline collections. However, there are reports which indicate that in some patients with Cushing's syndrome due to an adrenocortical neoplasm, dexamethasone suppression of urinary 17-OHCS during the low and high dose tests can occur (40).

Phenytoin has also been demonstrated to accelerate dexamethasone hepatic conjugation and biliary excretion. This results in lower dexamethasone levels which can result in a decrease in the negative feedback inhibition induced by the drug. There is evidence which suggests that the results of the low dose (0.5 mg every 6 hours) dexamethasone suppression tests are influenced by phenytoin. In the same study, the results of the high dose

(2.0 mg every 6 hours) dexamethasone test were not influenced (41). Since the dexamethasone screening test also uses a relatively small dose, the results of this test must be interpreted cautiously in patients receiving chronic phenytoin or other medications known to influence dexamethasone metabolism.

With the dexamethasone tests in particular, false positives and negatives may be due to the fixed doses used. That is, no consideration is given to the size of the patient. Similarly, it is now known that patients have different metabolic clearance rates—rapid metabolizers and slow metabolizers—for glucocorticoids (42).

Since there are several methods for assaying urinary 17-OHCS, the normal values will have to be verified with the laboratory doing the assay. Urinary assays are fraught with potential errors such as incomplete collection. Confounding these problems is that a number of drugs can interfere with the urinary 17-OHCS assays used. Drugs which may potentially interfere with these assays include: acetazolamide, ascorbic acid, colchicine, digitalis, TAO, erythromycin, hydralazine, hydroxyzine, menadione, methenamine, chloral hydrate, methprylon, phenazopyridine, phenothiazines, KI, quinine, quinidine, sulfamerazine, thiazides, meprobamate, reserpine, calcium, and carbamazepine. Drugs which have been noted to increase 17-OHCS excretion include: chlorthalidone, salicylates, and high doses of NaCl. Drugs which decrease 17-OHCS excretion include: oral contraceptives, propoxyphene, phenytoin, thiazides, glucocorticoids, aminoglutethemide and pentazocine (43).

In addition to medications which might interfere with testing for Cushing's syndrome, there are a number of conditions such as obesity, depression, hypertension, diabetes, and cancer, which have been reported to complicate the interpretation of the diagnostic tests (44). Elevated serum cortisol levels have been documented in patients with a variety of acute and chronic illnesses—cardiac, neurologic, hepatic, renal—but without lesions involving the HPA axis (45, 46).

It should be noted that in addition to false positive and false negative tests which occur with testing for Cushing's syndrome, there are reports of patients with documented Cushing's syndrome who have negative tests. These rare cases have intermittent periods in which cortisol production returns to normal (47).

It should be apparent that the diagnosis of Cushing's syndrome cannot be based on a single finding or test. Rather, by necessity, the diagnosis must be based on a number of findings and tests which must point toward the presence of chronic hypercortisolism.

Differential Diagnosis

Once chronic hypercortisolism has been established, localization of the underlying pathology to the adrenal cortex, hypothalamus-pituitary gland or ectopic ACTH producing tumor must be pursued. With the advent of plasma ACTH assays and technological improvements in visualizing the adrenal cortex, hypothalamus, and pituitary gland with tests such as computerized tomography, the necessity of using pharmacologic tests in the differential diagnosis of Cushing's syndrome has been minimized.

The plasma ACTH assay is the easiest and most reliable test available. In general, in the presence of elevated serum cortisol levels, an absent or low plasma ACTH level is diagnostic of an adrenal carcinoma or adenoma; a plasma ACTH level in the 100 to 200 pg/ml range is compatible with a pituitary lesion; and a plasma ACTH level of greater than 200 pg/ml is evidence of an ectopic ACTH producing tumor (48). For completeness, the pharmacologic tests are described below. The high dose dexamethasone test and the metyrapone test have been used to differentiate adrenal hyperplasia from adrenocortical tumors.

The high dose dexamethasone suppression test is an extension of the low dose test. If the low dose test indicates the presence of Cushing's syndrome, the high dose suppression test is initiated. In the high dose suppression test, 2 mg of dexamethasone are administered orally every 6 hours for eight doses. During this time period, two consecutive 24-hour urine samples for 17-OHCS are collected. If suppression of the production of cortisol occurs, as reflected by a comparison of the base-line 24-hour urinary 17-OHCS and the final 24-hour urinary 17-OHCS, the etiology of the hypercortisolism is hypothalamic-pituitary malfunction with secondary bilateral adrenal hyperplasia. If no suppression occurs, the diagnosis may be either adrenocortical tumor or ectopic ACTH-producing tumor.

Metyrapone has also been used in the differential diagnosis of adrenocortical hyperplasia and adrenocortical tumors. The basis of the metyrapone test is the responsiveness of hyperplastic adrenals and the autonomous behavior of tumors to ACTH stimulation. Metyrapone is administered orally in a dose of 750 mg every 4 hours until a maximum of 4.5 to 5.0 g is reached or an intravenous infusion of 30 mg per kg body weight in normal saline or 5% dextrose in water over a 2- 4- or 16-hour period (49, 50). At this dosage, metyrapone inhibits the 11-hydroxylation step of cortisol production. Consequently, plasma cortisol levels fall and initiate the stimulus for cortisol production via the HPA axis. In patients with normal or hyperplastic adrenal cortices, the response to the resultant increased ACTH production is a buildup of cortisol precursors which are measured as urinary 17-OHCS. Autonomously functioning adenomas and carcinomas of the adrenal cortex are not ACTH-dependent and do not respond to the ACTH stimulus. The metyrapone test is subject to interference by a number of drugs including phenytoin, meprobamate and chlorpromazine (51).

The differential diagnosis of adrenocortical tumor versus ectopic ACTH-producing tumor is based on the plasma ACTH levels. Ectopic ACTH-producing tumors result in elevated ACTH levels. Adrenocortical tumors are autonomous and, consequently, are independent of ACTH stimulation for cortisol production. Autonomous adrenocortical tumors producing excess cortisol result in the inhibition of pituitary ACTH release.

The differential diagnosis of adrenocortical adenomas versus adrenocortical carcinoma is not as clear. In general, it can be said that carcinomas are associated with an elevated urinary 17-ketosteroid (17-KS) and an elevated or normal 17-OHCS excretion, whereas adenomas may be associated with slightly elevated, normal or even low 17-KS urinary excretion levels (15, 19). Normal 17-KS urinary excretion approximates 10 ± 5 mg/24 hours in females, and 15 ± 5 mg/24 hours in males. Adrenocortical carcinomas have been associated with urinary 17-KS ranging from 40 to 100 mg/24 hours. Another potential distinguishing characteristic of the adrenocortical carcinoma is its lack of response to ACTH stimulation (15). Adrenocortical adenomas, on the other hand, may (rarely) respond to ACTH by increasing 24-hour urinary 17-OHCS excretion as compared to a control collection (52, 53).

The establishment of the diagnosis and the further delineation of the etiology of Cushing's syndrome is based primarily on the direct or indirect laboratory demonstration of hypercortisolism. The laboratory methods used in the determination of elevated cortisol levels are subject to interference by medications and chemicals. As a consequence, there must be an awareness by the diagnostician and his fellow clinicians of the possible interfering factors peculiar to their institution because variations in laboratory methods and facilities do exist. There are comprehensive tabulations available to assist in identifying potentially interfering substances (29) and physiological conditions.

Factors which alter the physiology and metabolism of cortisol should be sought out and corrected before evaluation begins. Drugs such as phenytoin and phenobarbital, which have been known to speed up the metabolism of cortisol, should be considered (29). Alteration of the protein binding of cortisol, such as pregnancy or estrogen-induced elevation of CBG, and consequently circulating plasma cortisol, should be noted (29). Patients who are acutely ill and/or under stress will also have an elevated plasma cortisol level.

Clinical Manifestations

The clinical manifestations and pathologies of Cushing's syndrome are primarily the result of the actions of a chronic excess of cortisol. However, since adrenal androgens are intermediary by-products of cortisol biosynthesis, manifestations of excess androgens can contribute to the clinical presentation of patients with Cushing's syndrome. Since secondary hypercortisolism is attributable to chronic excess ACTH production, extraadrenal manifestations as well as adrenal manifestations of ACTH can occur–transient aldosterone stimulation and melanocyte stimulation (2). Although ACTH is only $1/100$ as potent as melanocyte-stimulating hormone (MSH), ACTH in excess can cause pigmentation.

The patient with clinical manifestations of classic Cushing's syndrome is easily recognizable. However, since adrenocortical activity can be present in patients with few signs and symptoms suggestive of classical Cushing's syndrome, recognition of the existence of the syndrome may be difficult.

This difficulty may be attributable to the fact that cortisol possesses multiple actions which affect the metabolic processes of most tissues. These actions of cortisol on a given tissue can be augmented or counterbalanced by the actions of other hormones and other homeostatic mechanisms. Thus, the clinical manifestations and pathological findings due to excess cortisol are the net result of the interaction of cortisol and the counterbalancing hormone or other homeostatic mechanisms (54). However, the severity of a given cortisol-induced problem is not related to the plasma cortisol level (30), but certain signs, symptoms, effects or laboratory values may occur more frequently in relation to a higher cortisol level (15). Thus, there is considerable variability in the clinical manifestation in patients with Cushing's syndrome.

As the term "glucocorticoid" implies, cortisol and other compounds in this group have an effect on glucose. This involvement is primarily manifest in the intermediary metabolism of carbohydrates. In general, cortisol causes a glucose-sparing effect and increased glucose production through its influences on protein, lipid and carbohydrate metabolism. The net result is a tendency toward hyperglycemia (54).

The effect of cortisol on the metabolism of proteins, lipids and carbohydrates can be either catabolic or anabolic. The action of cortisol on muscle, lymphoid, connective, and adipose tissue is catabolic and results in the release of fatty acids, glycerol and glucose. In addition, cortisol may exert an antianabolic action on these tissues by inhibiting the passage of amino acids and glucose into these tissues (55, 56). Cortisol exerts an anabolic action on the liver which through the utilization of amino acids, fatty acids, and glycerol results in the increased production of protein, ribonucleic acid (RNA) and glucose (57). The clinical manifestations and frequency of appearance of these metabolic derangements in these and other tissues are noted in Table 28.1.

Hyperglycemia. The metabolic breakdown products—amino acids, glycerol and fatty acids—provide raw materials for hepatic gluconeogenesis. Cortisol also has a direct antiinsulin effect (58, 59). Consequently, hyperglycemia, decreased glucose tolerance, a relative resistance to insulin and glycosuria may occur (60). This hyperglycemic effect is dependent on the presence of excess cortisol for its persistence (61). Patients with latent diabetes will exhibit diabetes in the presence of hypercor-

Table 28.1.
Presenting Signs and/or Symptoms in Cushing's Syndrome

Sign or Symptom	(N = 601)[a] %	(N = 50)[b] %
Obesity	88	94
Generalized		60
Trunkal		40
Moonface	75	84
Menstrual irregularities	60	76[c]
Muscular weakness	61	58
Bruising	42	36
Psychological difficulties	42	
Acne	45	82
Hirsutism	65	
Backache	40	
Striae		52
Osteoporosis on x-ray		46
Hypertension		
BP 140/90		72
BP 100 diastolic		54
Renal calculi		16
Cholelithiasis		10

[a] Review of 601 patients (13).
[b] Report on 50 patients (23).
[c] Twenty-nine female patients (13).

tisolism. Patients with diabetes who develop Cushing's syndrome will experience exacerbation of the diabetes. In general, the diabetes of hypercortisolism is mild, reversible and not associated with ketosis.

Obesity, Moon Face, Buffalo Hump. Cortisol causes a redistribution of fat without a major alteration in total body fat (56). The manifestation of this redistribution of fat is the moon face, protuberant abdomen and buffalo hump of the classic Cushing's syndrome patient. The redistribution of fat results from the facilitation of lipolysis by cortisol and the lipogenic effect of insulin. The net result is deposition of fat in areas of the body where the lipogenic effect of insulin predominates—face, back, abdomen—and the loss of fat in tissues where the action of cortisol predominates (56).

Myopathy. The myopathy which results from excess cortisol is characteristically found in the proximal musculature of the extremities as seen on electromyography and tissue biopsy. The negative nitrogen balance—protein washing—which results from cortisol is the result of catabolism, as evidenced by a elevation of amino acids leaving the tissue, and an antianabolic effect, demonstrated as a decrease in amino acids entering the tissue (57). Additionally, inhibition of glucose uptake into muscle tissue may be a contributing factor (55).

The myopathy of Cushing's syndrome is usually moderate in severity, may not be progressive and clears upon correction of the endocrine defect. However, there are reports of persistent cases following the correction of hypercortisolism (62).

Osteoporosis, Compression Fractures of Vertebra, Low Back Pain, Nephrocalcinosis, Renal Stones. Cortisol-induced osteoporosis is generally accepted as being associated with prolonged elevations of cortisol. It can occur in all bones, but in primarily associated with vertebrae (2%), dorsal and lumbar vertebrae (54%), femoral neck (18%), ribs (12%), and other long bones (14%) (63).

The mechanisms responsible for cortisol-induced osteoporosis are several: inhibition of vitamin D and consequent reduction of intestinal calcium absorption (64), increased glomerular filtration and direct tubular action which increase urinary calcium clearance (65), and catabolism of the proteinaceous bone matrix with consequent decrease in surface area for calcium deposition (66).

Psychological Changes. There is no specific psychological picture associated with elevated cortisol levels. Rather, hypercortisolism amplifies preexistent psychological defects (67), which run the gamut from simple nervousness through hallucinations and paranoid ideation (68). Regestein et al. (67) reported such cases as Cushing's syndrome with associated mental aberrations. They noted the following correlations: Organic brain syndrome occurs more commonly in individuals 65 years of age or older; the same type psychological aberrations caused by excess cortisol may have been precipitated in the same individual previously by stress; and only nervousness was exhibited by an individual with no previous psychological problems and a secure background.

Hypertension, Edema. Cortisol exerts a permissive action on catecholamine effects (68). In the cardiovascular system, this permissive effect results in an increased heart rate, improvement in left ventricular efficiency and an increase in arterial pressure. Cortisol also enhances the hepatic production of angiotensinogen (68); this may result in an increase in angiotensin and consequent stimulus for vascular contraction and aldosterone production. The mineralocorticoid properties of cortisol and the ACTH stimulus to aldosterone production also provide other mechanisms for hypertension and edema in Cushing's syndrome.

Acne, Hirsutism, Amenorrhea. Adrenal androgens are produced in the zona fasciculata and reticularis of the adrenal cortex. The production of these androgens is initiated by ACTH. Thus the manifestations of excess androgen in Cushing's syndrome due to excess ACTH production are not unexpected. Adrenocortical tumors can secrete cortisol and androgens alone or in combination (19). Therefore, manifestations of excess androgens can also occur simultaneously with Cushing's syndrome secondary to adrenocortical tumors. Hirsutism, acne and amenorrhea are most commonly associated with increased androgens in Cushing's syndrome.

Impotence. Loss of libido, impotence and oligospermia occur in males with Cushing's syndrome. This has been related to a decrease in testosterone, luteinizing hormone and follicle stimulating hormone levels secondary to cortisol inhibition at the level of the testes and pituitary (69).

Short Stature. Short stature is found in all children with hypercortisolism (70). The mechanism of cortisol-induced growth suppression has not been fully defined; however, it is known that growth hormone secretion is not suppressed by elevated cortisol levels (71). This implies that there may be a block in the peripheral actions of growth hormone.

Ulcer. The incidence of peptic ulceration in Cushing's syndrome is no greater than that found in the general population—less than 10% (72, 73). This low incidence is contrary to the widely accepted belief that glucocorticoid therapy caused ulceration (74). The literature also does not support this belief. Nonarthritic patients receiving glucocorticoids for ulcerative colitis (75), asthma (76), other pulmonary diseases (77), and pemphigus (78) do not experience ulceration at a greater incidence rate than that found in the general population. A review of early reports of glucocorticoid-induced ulceration reveals that the patients under consideration were rheumatoid arthritics. No consideration was given to the concomitant gastric irritants—salicylates, phenylbutazone or indomethacin—which these patients commonly use. Thus, it appears that the significance of glucocorticoid-induced ulceration is questionable with the exception of patients known to have a predisposition to gastric ulceration. Therefore, it is not surprising that the incidence of peptic ulceration in patients with Cushing's syndrome approximates that in the general population.

Laboratory Manifestations

Erythrocytes. In his original report, Cushing noted a tendency toward erythemia in 5 of 9 patients studied. Cushing defined erythemia as a red blood cell count of greater than 5,000,000 per cu mm. However, based on their study and other reported cases, Ross et al. (75) concluded that polycythemia, if defined as a red cell count greater than 6,000,000, a hemoglobin concentration of 18 g/100 ml or a hematocrit of greater than 55%, is a rare occurrence in Cushing's syndrome.

White Blood Cells. Polymorphonuclear leukocytosis is often noted in Cushing's syndrome. In contrast, the lymphocytopenia and an eosinopenia are also noted in this syndrome. A lymphocytopenia of less than 25% was noted by Ross et al. (13) in 50% of their patients. Similarly, an eosinopenia of less than 100 eosinophils per mm^3 was noted in 37 of 42 patients studied. Of these 37 patients, the absolute eosinophil count was less than 10 eosinophils per $mm.^3$ The authors concluded that an eosinophil count of less than 10 per mm^3 favors the diagnosis of Cushing's syndrome, and that an eosinophil count in excess of 100 per mm^3 precludes the diagnosis of Cushing's syndrome.

Electrolytes. Cortisol and other glucocorticoids have varying degrees of mineralocorticoid properties. However, the serum sodium in Cushing's syndrome is usually normal (15, 13, 70). Exogenous glucocorticoid therapy is associated with a positive sodium balance. With continued therapy, however, an escape from the abnormal sodium retention occurs (79). The latter mechanism might also explain the normal serum sodium in Cushing's syndrome.

Hypokalemic alkalosis is associated primarily with Cushing's syndrome due to an ectopic ACTH-producing tumor or high dose glucocorticoid therapy (13, 70).

Calcium balance is negative owing to an inhibition of vitamin D and decreased calcium renal tubular reabsorption which result in increased fecal calcium and hypercalciuria. In spite of the negative calcium balance, serum calcium levels are normal. However, serum phosphate is reduced in 50% of Cushing's syndrome patients and is based on increased fecal and urinary phosphate clearance (13, 65, 66).

It is now recognized that a continued elevation of plasma glucocorticoid—loss of diurnal variation—is a basic characteristic of Cushing's syndrome. Consequently, iatrogenic Cushing's syndrome would occur more rapidly in the patient with a divided daily dose regimen than in the patient on a single morning dose, alternate day or intermittent dosing regimen. At the same time, the particular glucocorticoid preparation used is important since there is a difference in duration of tissue effects as exemplified by their variation in HPA axis suppression. With respect to this latter example, dexamethasone or betamethasone suppress the HPA for greater than 2.5 days; triamcinolone or paramethasone for 2.0 to 2.5 days; and cortisol or prednisolone for less than 1.5 days (74).

Systemic effects have also been reported during topical (80), ophthalmic (81), aerosol (82), and rectal (83) administration of glucocorticoids. Thus, the potential for development of iatrogenic Cushing's syndrome should not be thought of as being limited to systemic therapy. Rather, the possibility of iatrogenic Cushing's syndrome should be considered whenever a chronic course of glucocorticoid therapy by any route of administration is being considered.

When the incidence of clinical abnormalities of endogenous and iatrogenic Cushing's syndrome are compared, obesity, psychiatric symptoms, poor wound healing, and edema (cortisone) occurred with equal frequency. Benign intracranial hypertension, cataracts, pancreatitis, aseptic necrosis of bone and panniculitis were found to be unique to iatrogenic Cushing's syndrome. Hypertension, acne, menstrual disturbances and impotence (male), hirsutism or virilism, striae, purpura and plethora were found to be more common in endogenous Cushing's syndrome (84).

Therapy

Adrenocortical Adenoma and Adrenocortical Carcinoma. In Cushing's syndrome due to an adenoma or a nonmetastatic carcinoma of the adrenal cortex, the recommended mode of therapy is total unilateral adrenalectomy of the involved gland. This procedure is preferred over partial resection of the involved gland since the latter frequently is associated with recurrence of the tumor in the adrenal remnant (15).

In considering surgical intervention, it must be recalled that adrenocortical adenomas and carcinomas function autonomously. Consequently, the contralateral adrenal cortex is atrophic owing to the lack of ACTH stimulation. Since surgical excision of the adenomatous or carcinomatous gland results in removal of the only source of cortisol production in the body, supplemental exogenous glucocorticoid must be supplied to the patient until the atrophic contralateral adrenal cortex recovers.

If supplemental therapy with exogenous glucocorticoids is not provided during and after surgery, collapse due to acute adrenal insufficiency—addisonian crisis—can occur. A suggested regimen for providing exogenous glucocorticoids is noted in Table 28.2 (15).

Subsequent tapering of glucocorticoid replacement should be performed by eliminating the 4 P.M. dose. The morning dose should be tapered until there is no longer a need for exogenous glucocorticoid replacement owing to the recovery of the contralateral adrenal cortex. If tapering beyond that shown in Table

Table 28.2.
Pre-, Intra-, and Postoperative Management of Glucocorticoid Replacement for Cushing's Syndrome[a]

Relative Time	Medication	Dose (mg)	Route	Regimen
Evening prior to surgery	Cortisone acetate	100	IM	Single dose
Day of surgery	Cortisone acetate	100	IM	Single dose, preoperatively
	Hydrocortisone phosphate or sodium succinate	300	IV infusion	Intraoperatively, postoperatively, over the remainder of the operative day
	Cortisone acetate	50	IM	Single dose, evening of the operative day
Postoperative day:				
1	Cortisone acetate	50	IM	Morning and evening
	Hydrocortisone phosphate or sodium succinate	200	IV	Infusion, over the next 24 hr
2	Cortisone acetate	50	IM	Morning and evening
	Hydrocortisone phosphate or sodium succinate	150	IV	Infusion, over the next 24 hr
3	Cortisone acetate	50	IM	Morning and evening
	Hydrocortisone phosphate or sodium succinate	100	IV	Infusion, over the next 24 hr
4	Cortisone acetate	50/25	IM	Morning and evening
	Cortisone acetate	25	PO	q.i.d.
5	Cortisone acetate	50	IM	Morning
	Cortisone acetate	25	PO	q.i.d.
6	Cortisone acetate	50-25-25-25	PO	q.i.d.
7	Cortisone acetate	25	PO	q.i.d.
8	Cortisone acetate	25-12.5-25-12.5	PO	q.i.d.
9–14	Cortisone acetate	25-12.5-25	PO	t.i.d. (last daily dose 4 P.M.)
15–22	Cortisone acetate	25-12.5-12.5	PO	t.i.d. (last daily dose 4 P.M.)
22	Cortisone acetate	25		Morning
	Cortisone acetate	12.5		4 P.M.

[a] Adapted with permission from Lauler et al. (15).

28.2 is not possible owing to development of symptoms and signs of adrenal insufficiency, permanent glucocorticoid replacement therapy and concomitant ACTH stimulation therapy may be indicated. If at any time during the tapering procedure the patient is subjected to stress, the dose of replacement glucocorticoid may have to be temporarily increased to avoid acute adrenal insufficiency.

Inoperative Adrenocortical Carcinoma. Patients who are debilitated or who have metastatic lesions are considered to be inoperable. In these patients, chemotherapy is indicated to alleviate the overproduction of cortisol. Currently, two agents which can be used for the chemotherapy of Cushing's syndrome are mitotane (o.p.'-DDD) and aminoglutethimide.

Mitotane is a derivative of the insecticide, DDD. The latter chemical was noted to cause adrenocortical necrosis in the canine. However, it was also found to be too toxic in humans. Consequently, mitotane was developed. This compound is 20 times more potent as an adrenolytic agent and less toxic than its parent compound, DDD.

The mechanism of mitotane adrenolysis remains to be elucidated. The theoretical possibilities of suppression or inhibition of cortisol synthesis and/or the stimulation of conversion of cortisol to a more polar compound by this agent remain to be established (85). However, it has been demonstrated that the zona reticularis and the zona fasciculata of the canine adrenal cortex atrophy in response to mitotane. This atrophy, however, is not attributable to an inhibition of pituitary ACTH secretion (86). Consequently, the action of this drug is primarily directed toward the adrenal cortex.

The primary use of mitotane is in the treatment of adrenocortical carcinomas. When it is being considered for use, the following guidelines are applicable (87).

1. The use of mitotane in adrenocortical carcinomas should be reserved for those patients who are considered inoperable.

2. Metastatic lesions or local recurrences should be treated as early as possible to obtain remission.

3. Therapy should be pursued for 4 to 5 weeks following initiation of therapy, since 86% of patients require a minimum of 4 weeks to respond. If there is no response following a trial of 4 to 5 weeks of therapy, the prospect of obtaining response with continued therapy is poor (85).

4. If a response is obtained, therapy should be continued at a maximal tolerable dose for as long as possible.

5. The daily dose should approximate 10 g/day.

Tumor regression is the most reliable method of evaluating response to mitotane. Urinary 17-OHCS cannot be relied upon since the drug alters the ratio of cortisol metabolites (88). In the normal individual, tetrahydrocortisone and tetrahydrocortisol metabolites predominate over the more polar 6-p-hydroxy metabolite. In patients receiving mitotane therapy, the 6-p-hydroxy metabolite predominates. Since this latter metabolite is not extracted by the conventional methods for quantification of 17-hydroxycorticoids, values obtained are spuriously low and thus do not accurately reflect plasma cortisol levels.

Using objective evidence of tumor regression as criteria for response, Hutter and Kayhoe (85) noted a 34% response rate in a series of 138 patients treated with mitotane. A 35% response rate was noted when subjective symptomatic criteria were evaluated. The average dose required to obtain objective evidence of tumor regression was 8.1 g/day. Although the authors noted no correlation between age, sites or location of metastases and effectiveness of therapy, they did note that females responded to mitotane better than their male counterparts.

The adversities of mitotane therapy are most frequently associated with the gastrointestinal and neuromuscular systems. In the study by Hutter and Kayhoe (85) approximately 80% of 138 patients that were treated manifested anorexia, nausea, vomiting or diarrhea. Diarrhea occurred in 20% of the patients. Neuromuscular side effects appeared in 41% of the 138 patients. Lethargy and somnolence appeared in 26% and dizziness and vertigo in 14%. Muscle tremors, headache, confusion and weakness were also noted. The gastrointestinal and neuromuscular side effects are dose-related and are alleviated by discontinuance or reduction in the dose of the drug.

Dermatological reactions—skin rash—appeared in 14% of the patients. This reaction was not dose-related and may resolve itself spontaneously with continued therapy.

Other adverse reactions which were noted by Hutter and Kayhoe were: visual blurring, diplopia, reversible lens opacities, toxic actinopathy with papilledema and retinal hemorrhages, alopecia, erythema multiforme, hematuria, hemorrhagic cystitis, albuminuria, hypertension, orthostasis, aching pain and a decrease in protein-bound iodine (PBI) (85).

Aminoglutethimide was originally introduced as an anticonvulsant in the early 1950s. It was subsequently withdrawn from the market owing to the adverse reactions associated with the drug. The toxicities of aminoglutethimide include hypothyroidism and hypocortisolism which paradoxically may prove to be beneficial in Cushing's syndrome due to adrenocortical carcinoma.

Aminoglutethimide is a general adrenocortical poison as evidenced by vacuolization of the adrenal cortex in patients treated with the agent. There is also evidence for an inhibitory effect on cortisol synthesis which has been attributed to aminoglutethimide inhibition of the adrenocortical enzyme 20-hydroxylase (89). Thus, cholesterol is not converted to pregnenolone, the first step in adrenocortical cortisol synthesis (90).

The effectiveness of aminoglutethimide in alleviating the clinical and biochemical abnormalities of Cushing's syndrome varies with the etiology. Misbin et al. (91) reported that all 6 of their patients who had adrenal adenoma improved clinically and biochemically. Of the 21 patients with adrenocortical carcinoma, 13 improved clinically and biochemically and 3 demonstrated only biochemical improvement. Of the 6 patients with ectopic ACTH-secreting tumors, 4 improved clinically and biochemically. Of the 33 patients with bilateral adrenal hyperplasia, 14 improved clinically and biochemically and 5 improved only biochemically. Thus, the efficacy of aminoglutethimide is variable. The authors suggest that its use would be in inoperable patients; preoperative preparation to decrease morbidity; and in patients where other measures have failed.

Misbin et al. (91) reported side effects in 58% of the 66 patients they treated with aminoglutethimide. Thirty percent reported central nervous system (CNS) effects—lethargy, sedation, dizziness, blurred vision and/or depression; 18%—rash with fever; 12%—nausea, vomiting and/or anorexia; 5%—headache; and 6%—myalgia and malaise.

Aminoglutethimide is used in doses of 1 g/day in divided doses. Higher doses may be required to obtain control or recapture control if escape has occurred. Used in the appropriate doses, aminoglutethimide, in contrast to mitotane, is rapid acting. The onset of action occurs within days rather than weeks as in the case with the latter drug. Similarly to mitotane, tumor regression and not urinary 17-OHCS levels should be used to monitor the effectiveness of the compound. Unlike mitotane, aminoglutethimide only transiently affects the zona glomerulosa and, consequently, aldosterone production and secretion (92). Aminoglutethimide, therefore, would have the advantage of not requiring mineralocorticoid replacement therapy.

Ectopic ACTH-producing Tumors. The primary therapy for ectopic ACTH-producing tumors is surgical excision or radiotherapy. The majority of these tumors are malignant and nonresectable. Alternative therapy includes the adrenolytic agents, mitotane and aminoglutethimide, or in the early stages of the disease, bilateral total adrenalectomy. The alternative modes of therapy involve therapeutic maneuvers to correct the hypercortisolism and not the primary problem—the ectopic ACTH-producing tumor. The effectiveness of the adrenolytic agents in this type of Cushing's syndrome remains questionable (14, 21).

Trilostane inhibits cortisol, aldosterone and androstenedione production in the adrenal cortex. It has been tried in the treatment of Cushing's disease and appears to be effective in decreasing cortisol levels and reversing the metabolic and clinical manifestations of Cushing's syndrome. It has reputedly minor side effects—tiredness, paresthesias, increased salivation, and abdominal discomfort. It appears that its role will be for the treatment of Cushing's syndrome due to ectopic ACTH producing tumors (93).

Cushing's Disease. The primary therapy for Cushing's disease has been pituitary irradiation in doses of 4000 to 5000 rads over a 1-month period. Pituitary irradiation is effective in approximately 48% of the cases treated. Bilateral total adrenalectomy has been the alternative approach and was used in radiotherapy failures (14). However, newer forms of therapy are rapidly evolving.

If bilateral total adrenalectomy is to be performed, it should be emphasized that these patients will require permanent glucocorticoid- and mineralocorticoid-substitution therapy. The patient should be prepared preoperatively and intraoperatively as described in Table 28.1. Postoperative management is the same with the following exceptions: Or the 4th postoperative day, fludrocortisone 0.1 mg daily is initiated. Dosage of fludrocortisone must be titrated subsequently to provide adequate mineralocorticoid-replacement therapy permanently (15). It must be emphasized that the patient who is on permanent substitution therapy must be given an increased dose of cortisone acetate or other glucocorticoid during stress situations as they occur for the remainder of his life.

In patients who are not surgical candidates, mitotane therapy may be attempted. Mitotane therapy has only a minor effect on the zona glomerulosa of the adrenal cortex. Consequently, in contrast to surgical intervention, no mineralocorticoid replacement is required. The dose of mitotane required usually ranges from 3 to 6 g daily in divided doses. Therapy is usually continued for 4 to 6 months. If necessary, smaller maintenance doses may be continued for a longer period. In the 3- to 6-g/day dosage range, the primary side effects noted are nausea and ataxia (14).

Mitotane therapy alone and in combination with pituitary irradiation appears to be effective in the treatment of Cushing's disease. Luton et al. (94) in a study of 62 patients receiving mitotane alone or in conjunction with irradiation claim a 63% remission rate. It is interesting to note that the dose of mitotane ranged from 6 to 12 daily. the side effects included those listed previously in addition to a reversible gynecomastia in 50% of the males treated; a rise in serum alkaline phosphatase; and a reversible rise in serum cholesterol without concomitant triglyceride elevation.

Metyrapone has been used primarily diagnostically in Cushing's syndrome. The studies utilizing this 11-hydroxylase inhibitor as a therapeutic agent are few. Jeffcoat et al. (95) reported successful long term management (2 to 66 months) of Cushing's disease with metyrapone in 13 patients. In 8 of the 13, concomitant pituitary irradiation was given. The dose varied from 1.0 to 4.0 g daily in four divided doses. The patients' reponse was monitored by plasma cortisol levels. The clinical and biochemical improvement was rapid. The authors noted that metyrapone was used successfully in the ectopic ACTH syndrome and in adrenal tumors. The chronic metyrapone therapy was complicated by transient lightheadedness immediately following each dose in four patients. Hirsutism or aggravation of preexistent hirsutism was cited as the major complication.

Aminoglutethemide and metyrapone ther-

apy can be used in combination. This approach uses lower doses of both agents and consequently the dose related toxicities are decreased (96).

Cyproheptadine, a serotonin antagonist, was initially tried in the treatment of Cushing's disease by Krieger et al. (97) on the basis of experimental evidence that serotonin is involved in the ACTH release mechanism. They successfully managed 3 patients over a 3- to 6-month period by initiating cyproheptadine with 8 mg/day and increasing to 24 mg/day. All 3 patients demonstrated marked improvement on both a clinical and biochemical basis. Upon discontinuation of therapy 1 patient demonstrated biochemical signs of hypercortisolism. The major complaints or side effects of cyproheptadine related to increased appetite, weight gain and sluggishness. Of note is the fact that none of the above 3 patients recovered diurnal variation in plasma cortisol levels.

Since the above initial report on cyproheptadine, other reports have been published with varying degrees of success and failure (98–101). In a follow-up paper Krieger (102) reported a success rate of 60% in 40 patients treated.

Bromocriptine, a dopamine agonist, has been successfully used to reduce ACTH levels in patients with Cushing's disease; like cyproheptadine, this agent is thought to modify CRF stimulation of the anterior pituitary. The usual dose of bromocriptine is 10 mg/day. The drug is not without side effects and include: hallucinations, altered behavior, hypotension, dizziness and sluggishness (103).

Naloxone and valproate have been demonstrated to reduce the hypersecretion of ACTH in Nelson's syndrome and Addison's disease. It, however, has no effect on the hypersecretion of ACTH associated with Cushing's disease (33, 104).

Hypophysectomy is another method of treating Cushing's disease. The hypophysectomy can be performed by the frontal or transsphenoidal route. The frontal approach is usually reserved for the pituitary tumors with suprasellar extension, especially into the area of the optic chiasm. The advent of the operating microscope has made the transphenoidal route the preferred approach since it allows for selective isolation of tumors and microtumors. The procedure can be performed with minimal damage to adjacent anterior and posterior pituitary tissue. the transsphenoidal approach is 88% effective in treating Cushing's disease (105).

In contrast to the frontal approach, the selective nature of the transsphenoidal approach has minimized the necessity for replacement of anterior and posterior hormones. While all patients undergoing transsphenoidal surgery should be covered with glucocorticoid therapy during the operative and postoperative period, the patients should be evaluated for the need for continued glucocorticoid replacement in the following months. Similarly the need for thyroid hormone replacement must be evaluated periodically. During the immediate postoperative phase, patients should be monitored for diabetes insipidus. While this lack of vasopressin is usually transient, permanent diabetes insipidus has been reported. Cerebrospinal fluid rhinorrhea also complicates the transsphenoidal procedure. The significance of this occurrence is the potential development of a retrograde route for bacterial invasion and consequent meningitis. The mortality rate for this procedure at the Mayo Clinic was 1.1% of 250 patients (105).

Prognosis

Prior to the introduction of glucocorticoids as pharmacological agents, the prognosis for patients with Cushing's syndrome was poor. Indeed, the 5-year survival was reported to be less than 50%. Currently, the survival of patients with Cushing's syndrome due to adrenal adenoma and Cushing's disease has improved markedly owing to the introduction of glucocorticoid replacement therapy. In a recent report (14), a 100% cure was reported in 17 patients with adrenal adenoma following adrenalectomy. Patients with Cushing's disease were treated with pituitary irradiation (51 patients), adrenalectomy (28), mitotane (8), and hypophysectomy (3). The following results were obtained: pituitary irradiation—10 patients cured, 13 patients improved, 21 patients unimproved and 7 patients were followed less than 1 year; adrenalectomy—21 patients cured, 1 patient improved and the remaining patient did not improve; mitotane—8 patients cured; and hypophysectomy—1 patient cured and 2 patients did not improve. The basic factor for improved survival may be the development of an exogenous glucocorticoid source and, consequently, temporary or permanent replacement therapy

Patients with Cushing's syndrome due to adrenocortical carcinoma or the ectopic ACTH syndrome continue to have a poor prognosis. In the study previously noted in this section, 17 patients with the ectopic ACTH syndrome all died within 18 months of diagnosis in spite of surgery, radiation or chemotherapy. Of 12 patients with adrenocortical carcinoma, 9 were treated with adrenalectomy and 3 were treated with mitotane. The following results were obtained: adrenalectomy—3 patients cured, 2 patients improved, but with recurrent tumors and 4 died; mitotane—all 3 patients improved; however, 1 died after 10 months of therapy (14).

Summary

The basic hormonal defect in Cushing's syndrome is the overproduction of cortisol. The etiology of this hypercortisolism may be associated either primarily or secondarily with the adrenal cortex. Adrenocortical tumors comprise the primary lesion. Adrenocortical hyperplasias due to a defect in ACTH production of the anterior pituitary gland or from an ectopic nonendocrine tumor comprise the secondary lesions involved in the excess production of cortisol.

The clinical manifestations are primarily those of excess cortisol. The most frequently encountered manifestations include: hyperglycemia, osteoporosis, adiposity, stunted growth in children, menstrual irregularity, weakness, hirsutism, psychological difficulties and bruising.

The therapy of Cushing's syndrome is dependent on the etiology of the hypercortisolism and includes surgery, irradiation or chemotherapy. Adrenocortical neoplasms or ectopic nonendocrine tumors should be removed surgically if possible. Transsphenoidal hypophysectomy is favored in Cushing's disease. Adrenocorticolysis and adrenocortical inhibition generally are reserved for inoperable, refractory patients or those with metastatic lesions.

The prognosis is dependent on the etiology of the hypercortisolism. Cushing's disease and adrenocortical adenoma carry a favorable prognosis. On the other hand, adrenocortical carcinoma and the ectopic ACTH syndrome are related more closely to a poor prognosis.

ADDISON'S DISEASE

In 1855 Addison described the symptomatology of 11 patients afflicted with the disease which now bears his name—Addison's disease. These patients shared the following characteristics: anemia, lassitude weakness, gastrointestinal irritability, cardiac weakness, hyperpigmentation, and pathological changes in the adrenal cortex. While Addison could not elucidate the fundamental biochemical basis for this disease, it has, in subsequent years, been defined as a chronic insufficiency of cortisol and aldosterone.

The prevalence of Addison's disease, excluding the iatrogenic form, is 39 per 1,000,000 in the population between 25 and 69 years of age and 60 per 1,000,000 in the total population (106, 107). The disease occurs in all age groups but is less common early and late in life.

Women account for 55% and men for 45% of the cases of Addison's disease. However, this sex predilection varies with the etiology of the disease (108). The incidence of and predispositions to the iatrogenic form of the disease is not calculable.

Pathophysiology

The fundamental hormonal defect in Addison's disease is a chronic insufficiency in the production and secretion of cortisol and aldosterone from the adrenal cortices. The pathogenesis of this insufficiency relates to a progressive destruction or atrophy of the adrenal cortex. The destruction of these glands results from infections, and autoimmune and infiltrative processes (109). Hypocortisolism can also result from iatrogenic causes—surgical and medical.

Tuberculous Addison's Disease. Tuberculous infection has been a well known cause of Addison's disease for many years. In the 1920s involvement of the adrenal glands occurred in 2 to 5% of tuberculosis cases (107). With the advent of antitubercular therapy, tuberculosis as a cause of Addison's disease has been steadily declining. However, it still accounts for approximately 20% of the cases. Males appear to be slightly more susceptible to tuberculous Addison's disease as evidenced by a female to male incidence ratio of 1:1.2 (107).

The adrenal glands, although relatively resistant to the tuberculous organism, become infected via the hematogenous route. The adrenal cortices are slightly more resistant than the adrenal medullae (110). In patients with tuberculous Addison's disease, bilateral involvement occurs in 70% of the cases. Pathologically, the affected gland is enlarged owing

to the caseation which occurs. The caseous material is yellow-gray, confluent, and surrounded by a thin capsule. Within this material calcium deposits are found (107).

Idiopathic Addison's Disease. Idiopathic Addison's disease represents the largest pathological grouping for the disease and accounts for 79% of the cases (107). Within this 79% there is a definite sex predominance. Women appear to be predisposed as evidenced by a female to male incidence ratio of 2.5:1 (111). Overall the incidence of the idiopathic mechanism has been increasing relative to other causes of Addison's disease.

Until recently the idiopathic category included all cases for which no known cause for adrenocortical dysfunction was known. Currently, the pathologic mechanism is thought to have an autoimmune basis. Surgical specimens from patients with this form of the disease reveal a diffuse lymphocytic infiltration and atrophy of the glands. Adrenal antibodies have been isolated in 70% of patients. Adrenal antigen has also been identified in adrenal extracts and has been demonstrated to be organ-specific and species-nonspecific (112). It is also of note that idiopathic Addison's disease has often been found in association with other immunologic diseases (107).

Other Causes. The tuberculous and idiopathic mechanisms account for approximately 99% of Addison's disease. However, there exists another category of pathological conditions which have been implicated in causing adrenocortical destruction. This "other" group includes amyloidosis, sarcoidosis, Hodgkin's disease, systemic lupus erythematosus, periarteritis nodosa, infarction, hemochromatosis, giant cell granuloma, metastatic carcinoma, diastomycosis, coccidiomycosis, histoplasmosis, candidiasis and torulosis (107).

Iatrogenic Addison's Disease. Iatrogenic Addison's disease results from intentional and unintentional removal or destruction of adrenocortical tissue. In Cushing's syndrome or in the late stages of sex-hormone related carcinomas, bilateral adrenalectomy may be performed and permanent cortisol and aldosterone deficiency incurred.

Unilateral adrenalectomy for Cushing's syndrome owing to an autonomously cortisol-secreting tumor can result in a transient hypocortisol state (Fig. 28.3). These tumors are not reliant on ACTH stimulation for cortisol production. Rather, they produce excess cortisol autonomously. Consequently, the negative feedback system of the HPA axis becomes operative and results in a decreased secretion of ACTH. This ACTH deficiency, if prolonged, results in atrophy of the adrenal cortex of the contralateral, nontumorous gland. When unilateral adrenalectomy is performed, the only source of cortisol—the tumor—is removed. The atrophic adrenal is essentially nonfunctional and cannot secrete cortisol. The remaining gland will eventually recover function; however, exogenous glucocorticoid coverage is required during the operative and postoperative period until the gland regains its function.

Iatrogenic hypocortisolism can also result from destruction of the pituitary by irradiation, total hypophysectomy or cryohypophysectomy. These therapeutic measures used primarily in the treatment of pituitary tumors results in a deficiency of ACTH and consequently decreased levels of cortisol. The advent of operative microscope has allowed neurosurgeons to become more selective with respect to removal and/or destruction of pituitary tissue. The result of this selectivity is a transient rather than permanent decrease in ACTH and cortisol secretion (105).

Mitotane, a selective adrenocortical poison, is used in Cushing's syndrome to effect a chemical adrenalectomy. Mitotane irreversibly destroys the zonae reticularis and fasciculata. However, it has only a minor effect on the zona glomerulosa. Thus, cortisol insufficiency and, to a lesser degree, aldosterone insufficiency can result from the use of this agent (87).

Aminoglutethimide is used for selective destruction of the adrenal cortices in Cushing's syndrome and in inoperable metastatic breast carcinoma. Like mitotane, aminoglutethimide destroys the zonae reticularis and fasciculata which results in a hypocortisol state. Unlike mitotane, its effect on the zona glomerulosa and aldosterone is transient (91).

Hypocortisolism occurs following the withdrawal of chronic exogenous glucocorticoids owing to their suppressant action on the HPA axis. Axis suppression has been correlated with daily dose, total dose, duration and dosing regimen of glucocorticoid therapy (113, 114). Hydrocortisone 100 mg daily for 3 days, prednisone 30 mg daily for 5 days, and prednisone 20 mg daily for 7 days have been reported to induce HPA axis suppression based on adrenocortical unresponsiveness to exogenous ACTH stimulation (115, 116). Even physiologic doses—20 to 30 mg of hydrocortisone or equivalent—can cause suppression if administered in the afternoon, evening or night (117). This effect is related to the supplementation of the glucocorticoid level at a time when it is normally decreasing based on the circadian rhythm. Administration of physiologic doses in the morning or alternate day dosing with even higher doses can obviate or minimize suppression.

Metyrapone responsiveness of the HPA axis can be modified following 3 days of exogenous glucocorticoid therapy and is totally abolished following a total dose of prednisone ranging from 4.6 to 15 g (118, 119). Patients treated chronically for 16 months or less can retain metyrapone responsiveness; however, this responsiveness is totally abolished following 3 to 5 years of continuous therapy (118, 119). Consequently, during therapy the HPA axis is suppressed and the patient is at risk of cortisol deficiency during stress situations.

Following the withdrawal of chronic glucocorticoid therapy, 10 months may be required for full recovery of HPA axis function. This was described by Graber et al. (16) who monitored 6 patients after tapered withdrawal following 1 to 10 years of therapy. They described the recovery as having four phases.

Phase I. All patients had subnormal plasma 17-OHCS and ACTH levels and were unresponsive to exogenous ACTH. This period occurred during the 1st month following withdrawal.

Phase II. ACTH levels were normal or supranormal and 17-OHCS levels remained subnormal. The patients remained unresponsive to exogenous ACTH stimulation. This phase occurred between the 2nd and 5th month following withdrawal.

Phase III. ACTH and 17-OHCS levels were normal; however, response to exogenous ACTH stimulation remained subnormal. This phase occurred between the 6th and 9th month following withdrawal.

Phase IV. ACTH, 17-OHCS levels and response to exogenous ACTH stimulation were all normal. This phase occurred during the 10th month following withdrawal.

Acute Adrenal Insufficiency. During and following withdrawal from chronic exogenous glucocorticoid therapy the HPA axis is suppressed. These patients, if stressed, are at risk of developing acute adrenal insufficiency—

addisonian crisis. Sudden discontinuation of exogenous glucocorticoids can precipitate crisis owing to the inability of the suppressed adrenal gland to produce cortisol (120). This condition can also develop with rapid and complete adrenocortical destruction as occurs in the Waterhouse-Friedricksen syndrome, overwhelming meningococcal septicemia and associated massive bilateral adrenal hemorrhage. Similarly, anticoagulant therapy can cause bilateral adrenal hemorrhage and acute adrenal insufficiency (121).

Clinical Manifestations

Addison's Disease. The clinical manifestations of Addison's disease reflect a chronic insufficiency of cortisol and aldosterone. Subjectively, the patient complains of vague nonspecific symptoms of weakness, malaise, nausea, orthostatic dizziness and anorexia. Objectively, the patient is hypotensive in both the lying and standing positions; there is a history of weight loss; emesis and alternating episodes of diarrhea and constipation. As the disease progresses, diarrhea becomes the predominant finding.

Hyperpigmentation is the most characteristic finding. It is most noticeable in body creases such as those found on the palms, elbows, knuckles, waistline, perineal area, nipples and in newly formed scar tissue. In sun exposed and nonexposed areas there is a diffuse tanning of the skin. There can be multiple freckles on the skin and mucous membranes. This hyperpigmentation is the result of a chronically elevated ACTH levels owing to the cortisol insufficiency. Although ACTH possesses only $1/100$ the potency of melanocyte stimulating hormone (MSH), in excess it can cause sufficient stimulation of melanocytes to cause this pigmentation (2, 122).

Laboratory evidence compatible with Addison's disease involves abnormalities in the hematologic and electrolyte parameters of the patient. Pernicious anemia occurs in a small percentage of patients (123); however, since these patients can be hemoconcentrated owing to the aldosterone deficiency, the hematocrit can be falsely elevated. Leukocyte counts are usually depressed to a level of 5000/mm³ with an associated neutropenia, lymphocytosis, and eosinophilia (111).

Electrolyte abnormalities include hyponatremia and hyperkalemia due to aldosterone insufficiency. The sodium/potassium ratio is characteristically less than 30 (111). Calcium levels can be elevated owing to the loss of cortisol's antagonistic effect on vitamin D synthesis and gastrointestinal tract absorption of calcium, its negative effect on calcium renal tubular reabsorption and its hypophosphatemic effect (13, 65, 66).

Radiographic evidence consistent with Addison's disease includes a small heart and the presence of adrenal calcification. The latter finding occurs with tuberculous Addison's disease; however, calcification is present in only 50% of patients (108). Patients with evidence of pulmonary or other forms of tuberculosis and Addison's disease, with or without adrenal calcification, should be strongly suspected of the tuberculous form of the disease (107).

Addison's disease has been found in association with a number of other conditions including diabetes mellitus, thyrotoxicosis, myxedema, Hashimoto's thyroiditis, euthyroid goiter, pernicious anemia, gonadal insufficiency in both men and women, idiopathic hypoparathyroidism and diffuse cerebral sclerosis (107). Since these associations may exist, the clinical and laboratory evidence for Addison's disease may not be as easily discernible as described previously in this section.

Acute Adrenal Insufficiency. With the exception of pigmentation, the clinical manifestations of acute adrenal insufficiency are basically the same as those seen with chronic adrenocortical insufficiency. However, the onset of the manifestations is more abrupt and the acute insufficiency is usually associated or immediately preceded by some stressful event—surgery, infection or following acute adrenocortical damage—Waterhouse-Friedricksen syndrome or adrenocortical hemorrhage secondary to anticoagulant therapy. Acute adrenal insufficiency can also follow the inadvertent discontinuation of exogenous ACTH or glucocorticoid therapy without appropriate tapering. As such, the symptoms and findings can be complicated by the underlying cause. In the patient with undiagnosed Addison's disease, stress will also precipitate acute adrenal insufficiency (120). In this latter type of patient, pigmentation can be present.

Diagnosis

The onset of clinical manifestations of Addison's disease is usually insidious and may go unrecognized. If a patient is suspected of having Addison's disease, attempts to diagnose this condition are divided into two phases: (a) establishing that hypocortisolism exists and (b) establishing the source of the problem—adrenal or pituitary.

Screening Tests. In Addison's disease, diurnal periodicity of cortisol levels is lost. Consequently, demonstration of low plasma cortisol levels in the morning and evening is consistent with Addison's disease (109).

The cosyntropin (Cortrosyn) screening test is a rapid method of establishing adrenocortical insufficiency. Cosyntropin is a synthetic peptide unit of natural ACTH which is less allergenic and more potent than the exogenous ACTH preparations. One-tenth milligram (0.1 mg) is equivalent to 10 units of ACTH (124). This test is performed by obtaining a blood sample for a baseline plasma cortisol level. This is followed by the administration of 0.25 mg of cosyntropin intramuscularly. Thirty to 60 min following the injection a second blood sample for plasma cortisol is drawn. In patients with normal adrenocortical function the plasma cortisol level in the postinjection sample will be at least double the baseline level. The postinjection cortisol level in adrenally insufficient patients will be less than double the baseline value (125).

To differentiate primary from secondary adrenal insufficiency, a plasma ACTH level can be drawn. High levels are consistent with an adrenocortical lesion. Low levels are consistent with a pituitary lesion. However, since only a few institutions perform ACTH assays, alternative methods may be necessary to differentiate the location of the lesion. Similarly, antibodies to adrenal tissue can be tested for, if the test is available.

The ACTH infusion test will assist in the differentiation of primary and secondary adrenocortical insufficiency. However, this test requires 5 days to perform. On days 1 and 2 consecutive 24-hour urine collections for 17-OHCS are collected. On days 3, 4, and 5, ACTH, 40 units in normal saline, is administered intravenously over an 8-hour period—8 A.M. to 4 P.M. During these days, consecutive 24-hour urine collection for 17-OHCS are collected. In patients with primary adrenocortical insufficiency, the urinary 17-OHCS levels will not increase significantly beyond the baseline values from days 1 and 2. In patients with secondary adrenocortical insufficiency, the urinary 17-OHCS levels will progressively increase over days 3 through 5. This progressive increase reflects the gradual recovery of atrophic adrenal cortices when stimulated by ACTH (126). However, this is not conclusive evidence of secondary adrenocortical insufficiency since patients can have minimal pituitary ACTH production but are unable to secrete sufficient ACTH in response to stress. In these individuals the adrenal cortices are not atrophic and response to the serial ACTH infusions may be normal.

The final method utilized to distinguish between primary and secondary adrenocortical insufficiency is the metyrapone test. Metyrapone is an inhibitor of 11-hydroxylase which converts 11-deoxycortisol to cortisol. When metyrapone is administered, the production of cortisol is blocked and the circulating levels of cortisol decrease. This would, in a normal individual, result in an increased secretion of ACTH and resultant increase in cortisol production as measured by urinary 17-OHCS. In the patient with a pituitary lesion, neither increased ACTH secretion nor increased 17-OHCS excretion occurs.

The metyrapone test requires 4 days to perform. On days 1 and 2, consecutive 24-hour urine collections are made for baseline 17-OHCS levels. On day 3, the patient is given 750 mg of metyrapone every 4 hours for 6 doses. On days 3 and 4 consecutive 24-hour urine collections are made for 17-OHCS levels. If no pituitary lesion exists, then urinary 17-OHCS levels will be doubled on days 3 or 4. However, if a lesion exists, the 17-OHCS levels on days 3 and 4 will not vary significantly from the baseline values (127).

Two precautions must be taken with metyrapone: (a) It should not be given prior to the ACTH test since acute adrenal insufficiency can be produced when cortisol production is blocked in the patient with primary adrenal insufficiency. Also, with a test resulting in little or no change in urinary 17-OHCS levels compared to baseline, the level of the lesion—pituitary or adrenal—could not be differentiated. (b) Metyrapone should not be used in pregnancy since 11-hydroxylase is involved in the production of estrogen. This block can result in the abortion of the fetus.

The diagnosis of acute adrenal insufficiency is usually made on the basis of clinical manifestations. This is the result of the acute nature of the situation which prompts physicians to treat immediately. If the situation permits, a plasma cortisol level should be drawn prior to the implementation of therapy. This will provide documentation that adrenal insufficiency and not another condition is the precipitating problem.

Treatment

Specific therapy for Addison's disease is directed toward replacement of cortisol and aldosterone. Since cortisol is available commercially as hydrocortisone, replacement is readily achievable. Although the average adult male produces approximately 20.4 mg of cortisol daily and the average adult female produces 17.4 mg of cortisol daily, a slightly higher dose (20 to 30 mg) of hydrocortisone is recommended (126). Cortisone acetate can also be used and is recommended in a slightly higher daily dose of 25 to 37.5 mg per day owing to the 50 to 70% efficiency in biotransformation to hydrocortisone (128). The exact dose should be titrated to the individual.

The dosing regimen for replacement of cortisol should mimic the diurnal rhythm of cortisol secretion in a normal patient. This regimen can be accomplished by giving the patient two-thirds of the daily dose in the morning and one third in the late afternoon or early evening. For example, the patient is given hydrocortisone 20 mg in the morning on arising and 10 mg at 4 P.M. Another method is to give the hydrocortisone in three equally divided doses—10 mg in the morning, 10 mg at noon, and 10 mg at 4 P.M. Since hydrocortisone can cause stimulation, late evening or night dosing should be avoided to prevent insomnia (129).

Replacement of aldosterone can be accomplished by using fludrocortisone orally or desoxycorticosterone intramuscularly. Fludrocortisone is the 9α-fluoro derivative of hydrocortisone and possess 125 times the mineralocorticoid potency and 12 to 15 times the antiinflammatory potency of its parent compound. It is equipotent with aldosterone when given intravenously; however, no parenteral dosage form of fludrocortisone is available. The usual oral dosage ranges from 0.05 mg to 0.2 mg daily. The dose must be titrated for each patient. Too low of a dose is associated with hypovolemia and orthostatic symptoms. Too high a dose is associated with edema (130).

Desoxycorticosterone is a precursor to aldosterone. It possesses $1/30$ of the activity of aldosterone. The usual daily dose ranges from 1 to 4 mg. Like fludrocortisone, it must be titrated for each patient (131).

The best form of therapy for acute adrenal insufficency is prevention. Patients receiving chronic exogenous glucocorticoid therapy should be instructed not to discontinue therapy on their own volition. They should be educated regarding the signs and symptoms of impending acute insufficiency, situations which may precipitate them and how to handle the situation. Cards, bracelets or some other warning device should be worn or carried with information regarding the patient's condition. These latter suggestions should be especially emphasized to patients receiving replacement therapy. When a patient is tapered off chronic glucocorticoid therapy, both the patient and physician should be made to realize that acute insufficiency can be precipitated up to 10 months post-withdrawal. The patient should be instructed to inform all health care personnel involved in the care of his condition. Byyny (132) suggests giving a patient a preloaded syringe of dexamethasone and instructions on how and when to use it during and after tapering.

Patients on chronic exogenous glucocorticoids or replacement therapy should be premedicated with supplemental hydrocortisone if stressful situations such as surgery can be anticipated. Usually 100 mg of hydrocortisone can be given on call and another 200 to 300 mg in divided doses can be given daily during the operative and first postoperative day. The dosage can be tapered over the next few days to the level the patient was previously receiving (133). For a patient on replacement therapy a regimen similar to that displayed in Table 28.2 can be used.

Should acute adrenal insufficiency exist, therapy consists of administering hydrocortisone 100 mg intravenously immediately. This is followed by another 200 to 300 mg daily in divided doses until the precipitating cause is alleviated (120). This is then gradually tapered to the previous glucocorticoid dosage or to replacement doses.

At the high doses of hydrocortisone used for prophylaxis and/or treatment of acute adrenal insufficiency, mineralocorticoid replacement is unnecessary owing to the sodium retaining effects of the drug. However, since potassium wasting and fluid retention occur at these doses, patients should be monitored for hypokalemia and edema (120).

Interactions

As with Cushing's syndrome, the results of diagnostic tests can be altered by medications and other nonphysiologic states. Altered protein binding can lead to misinterpretation of tests for Addison's disease. The level of circulating endogenous cortisol can be elevated by pregnancy and estrogen therapy. Hypoproteinemic or dysproteinemic states can produce low levels of endogenous cortisol. Benzyl alcohol and spironolactone can interfere with the measurement of plasma cortisol by the fluorometric method. Calcium gluconate infusion, carbenoxolone, smoking, amphetamines and alcohol can cause elevation of cortisol levels on a pharmacologic basis. Lithium, on the other hand, has been associated with a lowering of cortisol levels (31). Urine tests for cortisol can be similarly altered by medications. Since there is considerable variability in the methods used for measurement of urinary 17-OHCS and in the medications which interfere with a specific test, a suitable reference source should be consulted once the test method used has been ascertained (45).

Consideration must also be given to drug-drug interactions. The metabolism of hydrocortisone and other glucocorticoids can be enhanced by hepatic enzyme induction. This is of particular significance in the patients receiving replacement hydrocortisone since this represents their only source of glucocorticoid. Enhancement of the metabolism can lead to a relative hypocortisol state in spite of full replacement dosing. Phenytoin and phenobarbital have been documented to cause this increased metabolic clearance of cortisol (8, 9).

Addisonian patients are particularly sensitive to narcotic analgesics. Use of these agents in these patients can result in an unexpected respiratory depression, coma and/or stupor (109).

Prognosis

The prognosis for Addison's disease prior to the advent of glucocorticoids in the late 1940s was poor. In excess of 80% of patients with Addison's disease died within a 2-year period following diagnosis. With the introduction of exogenous glucocorticoids, the feasibility of replacement therapy was realized. This, in conjunction with the introduction of antitubercular therapy, has resulted in a marked prolongation in the life expectancy of the addisonian patient (107).

Today, deaths related to Addison's disease are primarily due to the complications of an associated disease state or to acute adrenal insufficiency. In the latter instance, the inadvertent discontinuation of replacement of chronic glucocorticoid therapy, improper coverage for stressful situations and lack of patient understanding of his condition are the primary factors which contribute to an unnecessary and premature demise (120).

Summary

The basic hormonal defects in Addison's disease are chronic hypocortisolism and hypoaldosteronism. These deficits result from destruction of the adrenal cortices by tuberculous infection, organ-specific autoimmune reaction or other less common causes. Pituitary destruction can also cause hypocortisolism. Iatrogenic causes of Addison's disease include bilateral and, under special circumstances, unilateral adrenalectomy, hypophysectomy and chemotherapy. Acute adrenal insufficiency usually results from stress or unintentional acute discontinuation of chronic or replacement glucocorticoid therapy.

The clinical manifestations are primarily those of an insufficiency of cortisol and aldosterone. The most frequently encountered findings include nausea, vomiting, gastrointestinal irritability, dehydration, hypotension, pigmentation, hyponatremia, and hyperkalemia.

The treatment of Addison's disease is replacement glucocorticoid and aldosterone. Hydrocortisone and 9 α-fludrocortisone are the usual agents used chronically. For acute adrenal insufficiency, high dose intravenous hydrocortisone is the drug of choice.

The prognosis for Addison's disease is good; that is, if it is recognized. Prognosis is also dependent on the patient's compliance with therapy and his understanding of his condition. Patient education is critical to the patient's prognosis.

References

1. Thomas P: The structure and synthesis of steroids, in *Guide to Steroid Therapy*. Philadelphia: J. B. Lippincott, 1968, p 3.
2. Tucci JR, Espiner EA, Jagger PI, et al: ACTH stimulation of aldosterone secretion in normal subjects and in patients with chronic adrenocortical insufficiency. *J Clin Endocrinol Metab* 27:568, 1967.
3. Perkoff GT, Eik-nes K, Nugent CA, et al: Studies

of the diurnal variation of plasma 17-hydroxy-corticosteroids in man. *J Clin Endocrinol Metab* 19:432, 1959.

4. Orth DN, Island DP, Liddle, GW: Experimental alteration of the circadian rhythm in plasma cortisol (17-OHCS) concentrations in man. *J Clin Endocrinol Metab* 27:549, 1967.
5. Pincus G, Nakao T, Tait JF (eds): *Symposium on the Dynamics of Steroid Hormones.* New York: Academic Press, 1965, p 387.
6. Jones MT, Hillhouse EW, Burden J: Effect of various putative neurotransmitters on secretion of corticotrophin releasing hormone from rat hypothalamus in vitro. Model of neurotransmitters involved. *J Endocrinol* 69:1, 1976.
7. Cope CL, Black EG: The production rate of cortisol in man. *Br Med J* 1: 1020, 1958.
8. Beisel WR, DiRaimondo VC, Forsham PH: Cortisol transport and disappearance. *Am Intern Med* 60: 641, 1964.
9. Conney AH: Drug metabolism and therapeutics. *N Engl J Med* 280: 653, 1969.
10. Thomas P (ed): Measurement of steroids, in *Guide to Steroid Therapy.* Philadelphia: J. B. Lippincott, 1968, p. 12.
11. Cushing, HC: The basophil adenomas of the pituitary body and their clinical manifestations (pituitary basophilism). *Johns Hopkins Med J* 50:137, 1932.
12. Liddle, GW: Tests of pituitary-adrenal suppressibility in the diagnosis of Cushing's syndrome. *J Clin Endocrinol Metab* 20:1539, 1960.
13. Ross EJ, Marshall-Jones P, Friedman M: Cushing's syndrome: diagnostic criteria. *Q J Med* 35:149, 1966.
14. Orth DN, Liddle GW: Results of treatment in 108 patients with Cushing's syndrome. *N Engl J Med* 285:244, 1971.
15. Lauler DP, Williams GH, Thorn GW: Diseases of the adrenal cortex, in Thorn GW, Adams RD, Bennett IL et al: *Harrison's Principles of Internal Medicine,* ed 6. New York: McGraw-Hill, 1970, p 477.
16. Graber AL, Ney RL, Nicholson WE et al: The natural history of pituitary-adrenal recovery following long term suppression with corticosteroids. *J Clin Endocrinol Metab* 25:11, 1965.
17. Nelson DH, Sprunt JG, Mimms RB: Plasma ACTH determinations in 58 patients before or after adrenalectomy for Cushing's syndrome. *J Clin Endocrinol Metab* 26:722, 1966.
18. Bledsoe T, Island DP, Liddle GW: Studies of the mechanism through which sodium depletion increases aldosterone biosynthesis in man. *J Clin Invest* 45:524, 1964.
19. Hutter AM, Kayoe DE: Adrenal cortical carcinoma: clinical features of 138 patients. *Am J Med* 41:572, 1966.
20. Cope CL: Cushing's syndrome, in *Adrenal Steroids and Disease,* ed 2. Philadelphia: J. B. Lippincott, 1972, p 313.
21. Friedman M, Marshall-Jones P, Ros EJ: Cushing's syndrome: adrenocortical hyperactivity secondary to neoplasms arising outside the pituitary adrenal system. *Q J Med* 35:193, 1966.
22. Upton GV, Amatruda TT Jr: Evidence for the presence of tumor peptides with corticotrophin-releasing-factor-like activity in the ec-topic ACTH syndrome. *N Engl J Med* 285:419, 1971.
23. Choi Y, Werk EE, Sholiton LJ: Cushing's syndrome with dual pituitary adrenal control. *Arch Intern Med* 125:1045, 1970.
24. Meador CK, Owen WC, Farmer TA: Primary adrenocortical nodular dysplasia: a rare cause of Cushing's syndrome. *J Clin Endocrinol Metab* 27:1255, 1967.
25. Elias AN, Meshkin Pour H, Valenta LJ, et al: Pseudo-Cushing's syndrome: the role of alcohol. *J Clin Gastroenterol* 4:137, 1982.
26. Weiss ER, Rayyis SS, Nelson DH, et al: Evaluation of stimulation and suppression tests in the etiological diagnosis of Cushing's syndrome. *Ann Intern Med* 71:941, 1969.
27. Migeon CJ, Green OC, Eckert JP: Study of adrenocortical function in obesity. *Metabolism* 12:718, 1963.
28. Kenny FM, Janacyco GP, Heald FP, et al: Cortisol production rate in adolescent males in different stages of sexual maturation. *J Clin Endocrinol Metab* 26:1232, 1966.
29. Constatino NV, Kabat HF: Drug induced modifications of laboratory test values, revised 1973. *Am J Hosp Pharm* 30:24, 1973.
30. Ekman H, Hakansson B, McCarthy JD, et al: Plasma 17-hydroxycorticosteroids in Cushing's syndrome. J Clin Endocrinol Metab 21:684, 1961.
31. Hansten P: *Drug Interactions,* ed 4. Philadelphia: Lea & Febiger, 1979, p 336.
32. Briggs FN, Munson PL: Studies on the mechanism of stimulation of ACTH secretion with the aid of morphine as a blocking agent. *Endocrinology* 57:205, 1955.
33. Tolis G, Jukier L, Wiesen M, et al: Effects of naloxone on pituitary hypersecretory syndromes. *J Clin Endocrinol Metab* 54:780, 1982.
34. Del Pozo E, Martin PJ, Stadelmann A, et al: Inhibitory action of met-enkephalin on ACTH release in man. *J Clin Invest* 65:1531, 1980.
35. Frohman LA: Clinical neuropharmacology of hypothalamic releasing factors. *N Engl J Med* 286:1391, 1972.
36. Laidlow JC, Reddy WJ, Jenkins D, et al: Advances in the diagnosis of altered states of adrenocortical function. *N Engl J Med* 253:747, 1955.
37. Liddle GW: Cushing's syndrome, in Einstein AB: *The Adrenal Cortex,* Boston: Little, Brown, 1967, p 523.
38. Paveatos FC, Smilo, RP, Forsham, PH: A rapid screening test for Cushing's syndrome. *JAMA* 193:720, 1965.
39. Nugent CA, Nichols T, Tyler FH: Diagnosis of Cushing's syndrome: single dose dexamethasone suppression test. *Arch Intern Med* 116:172, 1965.
40. Rayfield EJ, Rose LI, Cain, JP, et al: ACTH responsive dexamethasone-suppressible adrenocortical carcinoma. *N Engl J Med* 284:591, 1971.
41. Jubiz W, Meikle AW, Levinson RA, et al: Effect of diphenylhydantoin on the metabolism of dexamethasone. Mechanism of the abnormal dexamethasone suppression in humans. *N Engl J Med* 283:11, 1970.

42. Gambertoglio JG, Amend WJC Jr, Benet LZ: Pharmacokinetics and bioavailability of prednisone and prednisolone in healthy volunteers and patients: a review. *J Pharmacokinet Biopharm* 8:1, 1980.

43. Hansten PD: *Drug Interactions*, ed 4. Philadelphia: Lea & Febiger, 1979, p 472.

44. Gold EM: The Cushing syndromes: Changing views of diagnosis and treatment. *Ann Intern Med* 90:829, 1979.

45. Sawin CT: Measurement of plasma cortisol in the diagnosis of Cushing's syndrome. *Ann Intern Med* 68:624, 1968.

46. Ramirez G, Etheridge P, Meikle W, et al: Evaluation of the pituitary adrenal axis in patients with chronic renal failure (abstract). *Clin Res* 26:148A, 1978.

47. Chajek T, Romanoff H: Cushing's syndrome with cyclical edema and periodic secretion of corticosteroids. *Arch Intern Med* 136:441, 1976.

48. Rees LH: ACTH, lipotrophin, and MSH in health and disease. *Endocrinol Metab* 6:137, 1977.

49. Liddle GW, Estep HL, Kendall JW, et al: Clinical application of a new test of pituitary reserve. *J Clin Endocrinol Metab* 19:875, 1959.

50. Gold EM, Kent JR, Forsham PH: Clinical use of a new diagnostic agent, metopirone (SU 4885), in pituitary and adrenocortical disorders. *Ann Intern Med* 54:175, 1961.

51. Kaplan HM: Methopyrapone test in primary hypothyroidism. *J Clin Endocrinol Metab* 25:146, 1961.

52. Sutter LJ, Geller J, Gabrilove JL: Response of the plasma 17-hydroxycorticosteroid level to gel ACTH in tumorous and nontumorous Cushing's syndrome. *J Clin Endocrinol Metab* 17:878, 1957.

53. Scott HW Jr, Foster JH, Liddle GW, et al: Cushing's syndrome due to adrenocortical tumor: an eleven-year review of 15 patients. *Ann Surg* 162:505, 1965.

54. Baxter JD, Forsham PH: Tissue effects of glucocorticoids. *Am J Med* 53:573, 1972.

55. Munck A: Glucocorticoid inhibition of glucose uptake by peripheral tissues; old and new evidence, molecular mechanism and physiologic significance. *Perspect Biol Med* 14:265, 1971.

56. Rudman D, Di Girolamo M: Effect of adrenal cortical steroids on lipid metabolism, in Christy NP: *The Human Adrenal Cortex* New York: Harper & Row, 1971, p 241.

57. Cahill GF: Action of adrenal cortical steroids on carbohydrate metabolism, in Christy NP: *The Human Adrenal Cortex* New York: Harper & Row, 1971, p 205.

58. Frawley TF, Kistler H, Shelley T: Effects of antiinflammatory steroids on carbohydrate metabolism with emphasis on hypoglycemia and diabetic states. *Ann NY Acad Sci* 82:868, 1959.

59. Valance-Owne J, Lilley M: An insulin antagonist associated with human albumin. *Biochem J* 74:18P, 1960.

60. Fajans SS: Some metabolic actions of corticosteroids. *Metabolism* 10:957, 1961

61. Thorn GW, Renold AE, Winegrad AI: Some effects of adrenal cortical steroids on intermediate metabolism. *Br Med J* 2:1009, 1957.

62. Muller R, Kugelberg E: Myopathy of Cushing's syndrome. *J Neurol Neurosurg Psychiatry* 22:314, 1959.

63. Rosenberg EF: Rheumatoid arthritis, osteoporosis and fractures related to steroid therapy. *Acta Med Scand* 162:Suppl. 341:211, 1958.

64. Kimberg DV: Effects of vitamin D and steroid hormones on the active transport of calcium by the intestines. *N Engl J Med* 280:1369, 1969.

65. Yrinis SL, Bercovitch DD, Stein RH, et al: Renal tubular effects of hydrocortisone and aldosterone in normal hydropenic man: comment on sites of action. *J Clin Invest* 43:1668, 1964.

66. Bernick S, Ershoff BH: Histochemical study of bone in cortisone-treated rats. *Endocrinology* 72:231, 1963.

67. Regestein QR, Rose LI, Williams GH: Psychopathology in Cushing's syndrome. *Arch Intern Med* 130:114, 1972.

68. David DS, Grieco MH, Cushman PJ: Adrenal glucocorticoids after twenty years: a review of their clinically relevant consequences. *J Chronic Dis* 22:637, 1970.

69. Luton JP, Thieblot P, Valck JC, et al: Reversible gonadotropin deficiency in male Cushing's disease. *J Clin Endocrinol Metab* 45:488, 1977.

70. McArthur TG, Cloutier MD, Hayles AB, et al: Cushing's syndrome in children. *Mayo Clin Proc* 47:318, 1972.

71. Anon: Cushing's syndrome in childhood (editorial). *Lancet* 2:267, 1972.

72. Kirsner JB, Kassreil RS, Palmer WL: Peptic ulcer, review of recent literature pertaining to etiology, pathogenesis and certain clinical aspects. *Adv Intern Med* 8:41, 1956.

73. Spiro HM, and Milles SS: Clinical and physiologic implications of steroid induced peptic ulcer. *N Engl J Med* 263:286, 1960.

74. Harter JG: Corticosteroids. Their use in allergic disease. *NY State J Med* 66:827, 1966.

75. Kirsner JB, Sklar M, Palmer WL: The use of ACTH, cortisone, hydrocortisone and related compounds in the management of ulcerative colitis; experience in 180 patients. *Am J Med* 22:264, 1951.

76. Schwartz D: Prolonged therapy with adrenocortical steroids in allergic diseases. *NY State J Med* 60:3973, 1960.

77. Smyllie HC, Connolly CK: Incidence of serious complications of corticosteroid therapy in respiratory disease. *Thorax* 23:571, 1968.

78. Sanders SL, Brodey M, Nelson CT: Corticosteroid pemphigus. *Arch Dermatol Syph* 82:717, 1960.

79. Relman AS, Schwartz WB: The metabolic effects of compound F. *J Clin Invest* 31:656, 1952.

80. Scoggins RB, Gliman B: Percutaneous absorption of corticosteroids, systemic effects. *N Engl J Med* 273:831, 1965.

81. Burch PG, Migeon CJ: Systemic absorption of topical steroids. *Arch Ophthalmol* 79:174, 1968.

82. Siegel SC, Heimlich EM, Richards W, et al: Adrenal function in allergy; IV. Effect of dexamethasone aerosols in asthmatic children. *Pediatrics* 33:245, 1964.

83. Farmer RG, Schumacher OP: Treatment of ulcerative colitis with hydrocortisone enemas: relationship of hydrocortisone absorption, ad-

renal suppression, and clinical response. *Dis Colon Rectum* 13:355, 1970.

84. Axelrod L: Glucocorticoid therapy. *Medicine* 55:39, 1976.
85. Hutter AM, Kayhoe DE: Adrenal cortical carcinoma: results of treatment with o,p'-DDD in 138 patients. *Am J Med* 41:581, 1966.
86. Brown JHU, Griffin JB, Smith RB, et al: Physiologic activity of an adrenocorticolytic drug in the adult dog. *Metabolism* 5:594, 1956.
87. Cope CL: Miscellaneous: o,p'-DDD the effects of triparanol, amino-glutethimide, in *Adrenal Steroids and Disease*. ed. 2. Philadelphia: J. B. Lippincott, 1972., p 697.
88. Bledsoe T, Island DP, Ney RL, et al: An effect of o,p'-DDD on the extra adrenal metabolism of cortisol in man. *J Clin Endocrinol Metab* 24:1303, 1964.
89. Cash R, Brough AJ, Cohen MNP, et al: Aminoglutethimide as an inhibitor of adrenal steroidogenesis; mechanism of action and therapeutic trial. *J Clin Endocrinol Metab* 27:1239, 1967.
90. Camacho AM, Cash R, Brough AJ, et al: Inhibition of adrenal steroidogenesis by aminoglutethimide and mechanism of action. *JAMA* 202:20, 1967.
91. Misbin RI, Canary J, Willard D: Aminoglutethimide in the treatment of Cushing's syndrome. *J Clin Pharmacol* 16:645, 1976.
92. Schteingart DE, Conn JW: Effects of aminoglutethimidine upon adrenal function and cortisol metabolism in Cushing's syndrome. *J Clin Endocrinol Metab* 27:1657, 1967.
93. Komanicky P, Spark RF, Melby JC: Treatment of Cushing's syndrome with Trilostane (WIN 24,540), an inhibitor of adrenal steroid biosynthesis. *J Clin Endocrinol Metab* 47:1042, 1978.
94. Luton JP, Mahoudeau JA, Bouchard PH, et al: Treatment of Cushing's disease by o,p-DDD. *N Engl J Med* 300:459, 1979.
95. Jeffcoate WJ, Rees LH, Tomlin S, et al: Metyrapone in the long term management of Cushing's disease. *Br Med J* 2:215, 1977.
96. Child DF, Burke CW, Burley DM, et al: Drug control of Cushing's syndrome. Combined aminoglutethemide and metyrapone therapy. *Acta Endocrinol* 82:330, 1976.
97. Krieger DT, Amorosa L, Linick F: Cyproheptadine induced remission of Cushing's disease. *N Engl J Med* 293:893, 1975.
98. Barnes P, Shaw K, Ross E: Cushing's disease; successful treatment with cyproheptadine (letter). *Lancet* 1:1148, 1977.
99. Ercole AJ, Morris, MA, Underwood LE, et al: Clinical note; treatment of Cushing's disease in childhood with cyproheptadine. *J Pediatr* 90:834, 1977.
100. Scott R, Espiner EA, Donald RA: Cyproheptadine for Cushing's disease (letter). *N Engl J Med* 296:57, 1977.
101. Hsu TH, Gann DS, Tsan KW, et al: Cyproheptadine in the control of Cushing's disease. *Johns Hopkins Medical J* 149:77, 1981.
102. Krieger DT: Cushing's disease and cyproheptadine (letter). *N Engl J Med* 295:394, 1976.
103. Benker G, Hackenberg K, Hamburger B, et al: Effects of growth hormone release-inhibiting hormone and bromocriptine in states of abnormal pituitary-adrenal function. *Clin Endocrinol* 5:187, 1976.
104. Allolio B, Winkelmann W, Kaulen D, et al: Valproate in Cushing's syndrome (letter). *Lancet* 1:171, 1982.
105. Salassa RM, Laws ER Jr, Carpenter PC et al: Northcutt, RC: Transsphenoidal removal of pituitary microadenoma in Cushing's disease. *Mayo Clin Proc* 53:24, 1978.
106. Stuart, MA, Meade TW, Lee JAH, et al: Epidemiological and clinical picture of Addison's disease. *Lancet* 2:744, 1968.
107. Nerup J: Addison's disease—a review of some clinical pathological and immunological features. *Dan Med Bull* 21:201, 1974.
108. Nerup J: Addison's disease—clinical studies. A report on 108 cases. *Acta Endocrinol* 76:76, 1974.
109. Irvine WJ, Toft AD: Diagnosing adrenocortical insufficiency. *Practitioner* 218:539, 1977.
110. Blalock JW, Rees EG: A study on the resistance of the adrenal cortex to tuberculous infection. *Br J Exp Pathol* 42:351, 1961.
111. Irvine WJ, Barnes EW: Adrenocortical insufficiency. *Clin Endocrinol Metab* 1:549, 1972.
112. Nerup J: Addison's disease—serologic studies. *Acta Endocrinol* 76:142, 1974.
113. Adams DA, Gold EM, Gonick HC, et al: Adrenocortical function during intermittent corticosteroid therapy. *Ann Intern Med* 64:542, 1966.
114. Jasani MK, Freeman PA, Boyle JA, et al: Studies of the rise of plasma 11-hydroxycorticoids in patients with rheumatoid arthritis during surgery. *Q J Med* 37:407, 1968.
115. Plager JE, Cushman P Jr: Suppression of the pituitary ACTH response in man by administration of ACTH or cortisol. *J Clin Endocrinol Metab* 22:147, 1962.
116. Christy NP, Wallace EZ, Jailer JW: Comparative effects of prednisone and of cortisone in suppressing the response of the adrenal cortex to exogenous adrenocorticotrophin. *J Clin Endocrinol Metab* 16:1059, 1956.
117. Nichols T, Nugent CA, Tyler FH: Diurnal variation in suppression of adrenal function by glucocorticoids. *J Clin Endocrinol Metab* 25:343, 1965.
118. Treadwell BLJ, Savage O, Sever ED, et al: Pituitary-adrenal function during corticosteroid therapy. *Lancet* 1:355, 1963.
119. Thomas P: Withdrawal of corticosteroid therapy in *Guide to Steroid Therapy*. Philadelphia: J. B. Lippincott, 1968, p 66.
120. Hubay CA, Weckesser EC, Levy RP: Occult adrenal insufficiency in surgical patients. *Ann Surg* 181:325, 1975.
121. Danese CA, Viola RM: Adrenal hemorrhage during anticoagulant therapy. *Ann Surg* 179:70, 1974.
122. Neelon FA: Adrenal physiology and pharmacology. *Urol Clin North Am* 4:197, 1971.
123. Turkington RW, Lebovitz HE: Extra adrenal endocrine deficiencies in Addison's disease. *Am J Med* 43:499, 1967.
124. Anon: Cosyntropin. *Med Lett* 13:33, 1971.
125. Maynard DE, Folk RL, Riley TR, et al: A rapid

test for adrenocortical insufficiency. *Ann Intern Med* 64:552, 1966.

126. Kenny FM, Preeyasombat C, Migcon CJ: Cortisol production rates; II. Normal infants, children and adults. *Pediatrics* 37:34, 1966.

127. Tyler FH: Laboratory evaluation of disorders of the adrenal cortex. *Am J Med* 53:664, 1972.

128. Jenkins JS, Sampson PA: Conversion of cortisone to cortisol and prednisone to prednisolone. *Br Med J* 2:205, 1967.

129. Cope, CL: Replacement corticosteroid therapy, in *Adrenal Steroids and Disease*, ed. 2. Philadelphia: J. B. Lippincott, 1972, p 558.

130. Cope CL: Replacement corticosteroid therapy, in *Adrenal Steroids and Disease*, ed 2. Philadelphia: J. B. Lippincott, 1972, p 561.

131. Haynes RC Jr., Larner J: Adrenocorticotrophic hormone, adrenocortical steroids and their synthetic analogues, inhibitors of adrenocortical biosynthesis, in Goodman LS, Gilman A: *Pharmacological Basis of Therapeutics*. New York: Macmillan, 1975, p 1484.

132. Byyny RI: Withdrawal from glucocorticoid therapy. *N Engl J Med* 295:30, 1976.

133. Plumpton FS, Besser GM, Cole PV: Corticosteroid treatment and surgery. *Anaesthesia* 24:12, 1969.

CHAPTER 29

Fluid and Electrolyte Therapy

PAUL M. JUST, B.Sc., Pharm.D.

Proper balance of fluid and electrolytes is essential for the rational management of most disease states. Paramount to the understanding of fluid and electrolyte therapy is the understanding of normal body composition. It is the purpose of this chapter to identify normal body composition and discuss the principles and therapy of fluid and electrolyte disorders.

WATER DISTRIBUTION (1–3)

Total body water (TBW) varies with age. It is highest at birth, about 75% of body weight, and diminishes to average 60% of body weight in men and 50% of body weight in women. TBW will vary with the quantity of adipose tissue present since this tissue contains negligible quantities of water. Therefore, when calculating TBW in obese individuals approximately 10% should be subtracted from the above TBW calculations.

TBW is divided into intracellular fluid (ICF) and extracellular fluid (ECF) volumes. The ICF contains approximately 60%, and the ECF, 40% of TBW. The ECF is subdivided into interstitial fluid (ISF), 80%, and intravascular fluid (IVF), 20%. Table 29.1 shows body fluid distribution.

Each of these volumes is uniquely composed of ionic and molecular particles. Homeostatic mechanisms maintain a general osmotic equilibrium between these volumes by regulating the passage of solute-free water through the selectively permeable membranes separating the different compartments.

Osmotic pressure is a major concept when considering fluid and electrolyte distribution in the body. Since the semipermeable membranes between each compartment allow free passage of water but not most solute, a pressure is established which is represented by serum osmolality. Normal serum osmolality is 270 to 300 milliosmoles per liter (mOsm/L), more than 90% of which is accounted for by serum sodium. A formula has been derived which allows for a rapid and easy estimation of serum osmolality (SO):

$$SO = 2\ Na^+_{serum} + \frac{glucose\ (mg/dl)}{18} + \frac{BUN\ (mg/dl)}{2.8}$$

However, because urea is freely permeable through most cell membranes it is so balanced in distribution that it can be omitted from the equation. Thus, effective serum osmolality is:

$$SO_{effective} = 2\ Na^+_{serum} + \frac{glucose\ (mg/dl)}{18}$$

Total water balance is regulated by the cardiac, renal, and central nervous systems. Peripheral baroreceptors, central osmoreceptors, the renin-angiotensin-aldosterone system, and antidiuretic hormone (ADH) from the posterior pituitary gland, are the effectors of this balance.

FLUID THERAPY

General Principles

In the healthy individual, water intake is equal to water output. Water is added to the system from three sources, body metabolism, in food, and as free water. Per day fluid losses are about 1500 ml as urine, and an "insensible loss" of 10 to 12 ml/kg from the lungs, gastrointestinal tract, and the integument (as perspiration). Thus, basic fluid requirements will increase during any condition which increases respiratory rate, causes vomiting and diarrhea, or fever.

To supply adequate fluid to the average person, 100 ml per kilogram body weight per day (ml/kg/day) should be supplied for the first 10 kg of body weight, 50 ml/kg/day for the second 10 kg, and 20 ml/kg/day for that weight greater than 20 kg. This works out to 2500 to 3000 ml/day for the average person. For each one degree centigrade the body temperature is above normal (37°) an additional 10% of daily fluid should be added to compensate for insensible loss.

Table 29.1.
Distribution of Body Water in a 70-kg Man (1–3)[a]

Compartment	Liter Quantity	Percent of Total Body Water
Total body water (TBW)	42	100
Intracellular fluid (ICF)	25.2	60
Extracellular fluid (ECF)	16.8	40
Interstitial fluid (ISF)	13.4	32
Intravascular fluid (IVF)	3.4	8

[a] For men, TBW is 60% of body weight; for women, TBW is 50% of body weight; in obese individuals, subtract 10% from these numbers.

When deciding what type of fluid replacement to use, a distinction should be made between loss of intracellular and extracellular volume. Although the terms overhydration and dehydration have commonly been used to refer to total body fluid balance, it is more accurate to use them to describe the state of intracellular water content. This differentiates ICF content from ECF content, specifically, intravascular volume.

By clinically evaluating these two distinct components, intravascular volume and intracellular volume, separately, a variety of general classifications can occur. One can have a normal, overloaded, or depleted intravascular volume combined with a normal, overhydrated or dehydrated cellular volume.

To monitor intravascular volume, heart rate, pulse force, blood pressure, urine output, mental status, and invasive techniques can be relied upon. With intravascular volume depletion, a reflex tachycardia will occur, pulse will be weak and thready in character, blood pressure will be low, possibly orthostatic, urine output will be decreased due to a reduction of renal blood flow and glomerular filtration rate and mental status will be decreased. Central venous pressure (CVP) and the more reliable pulmonary artery wedge pressure (PAWP) will be low. PAWP is a practical measure of left ventricular end diastolic pressure (LVEDP) or cardiac preload. For intravascular volume overload, heart rate will be normal or low, pulse will be strong and bounding in character, and blood pressure and urine output will be normal or high. CVP and PAWP will be high.

To monitor hydration status, assessment of thirst, mucous membranes, perspiration, skin turgor, and serum osmolality is useful. With dehydration, the patient will have notable thirst, dry mucous membranes, no perspiration, poor skin turgor (i.e. the skin when pinched will stay raised rather than flatten out immediately), and a high serum osmolality. A calculated effective serum osmolality greater than 300 mOsm/L represents dehydration. It should be noted that skin turgor in elderly patients is often poor and does not represent dehydration. Although it can be evaluated anywhere, the forehead may be the best spot to evaluate turgor since the skin is usually taut even in elderly individuals. With overhydration, the above would be normal except serum osmolality would be low. A calculated effective serum osmolality less than 270 mOsm/L represents overhydration.

As a practical and general guide to clinical assessment of water balance (in a 70-kg person), if the person is very thirsty this represents about a 2% loss of total body weight. If the person is thirsty, has no perspiration and a dry mouth, a loss of about 6%, or 4 liters, of total body weight can be estimated. If the above signs are present plus hypotension and mental status changes, a loss of about 10%, or 7 liters, of total body weight can be estimated.

In the last case, replacement of half the estimated loss could occur on the first day of therapy added to the normal daily requirements for fluid. On the second and successive days, reevaluate the fluid deficit.

Selection of Fluid Replacement

After determining the fluid abnormality one can decide on the necessary replacement solution. By considering the distribution characteristics of fluids through TBW it is possible to estimate how much of a given solution will be distributed to each body compartment. If free water is infused intravenously, because it passes readily through body membranes according to osmotic pressure gradients, it would equilibrate after a few hours such that distribution through all body compartments would be even, that is, 60% would go to the ICF and 40% to the ECF.

Intravenous infusion of a 0.9% solution of sodium chloride, however, is distributed only to the ECF. This "normal saline" solution, containing 154 milliequivalents (mEq) of both sodium and chloride ions, is slightly hypertonic and not "normal" in the true sense considering normal serum sodium and chloride are 136 to

145 mEq/L and 98 to 106 mEq/L, respectively. This restrictive distribution to the ECF occurs because sodium is the primary osmotically active particle holding water in the ECF spaces. Immediately after infusion, the saline solution remains in the intravascular volume, but later equilibrates evenly throughout the ECF volume, that is, 80% to the interstitial fluid and 20% remaining in the intravascular compartment.

Understanding this difference in total distribution helps in the selection of fluid for given disorders. When vascular volume is depleted, a 0.9% saline solution at equilibrium delivers more volume (as a percentage of the total volume infused) to the IVF compartment. When the ICF is depleted or a state of dehydration exists, a free water solution is necessary. However, water cannot be infused without osmotically active particles because the hypotonic fluid equilibrates rapidly with body cells, being drawn into them in excess and causing their destruction. Red blood cells are especially sensitive to this lysis. Free water then is given as 5% dextrose in water (D5W) which is basically isosmotic with blood. As the glucose is metabolized fairly rapidly, free water is provided and therefore distributed evenly through all body compartments, that is 60% to the ICF and 40% to the ECF.

Combination dextrose and saline fluids can be thought of in terms of how much free water is provided:

D50W	Dextrose 50% in water
D10W	Dextrose 10% in water

D5W	Dextrose 5% in water
D5/0.2S	Dextrose 5% with 0.2% saline
D5/0.45S	Dextrose 5% with 0.45% saline
D5/0.9S	Dextrose 5% with 0.9% saline
0.9S	0.9% saline (normal)
0.45S	0.45% saline (half-normal)
0.2S	0.2% saline (quarter-normal)

A liter of 0.45% saline (or half-normal saline) can then be thought of as delivering 500 ml of 0.9% saline and 500 ml of free water. Out of the whole liter, 300 ml end up in the ICF and 700 ml in the ECF. If this fluid is a combination of dextrose 5% with 0.45% saline, the distribution is essentially identical.

Table 29.2 lists the standard IV solutions used, their distribution to body compartments, osmolality, and pH. It should be noted that 0.2% saline is too hypotonic to infuse without other osmotically active particles added.

ELECTROLYTES

Disorders of electrolyte homeostasis can be mild and asymptomatic or severe with complications such as cardiac arrhythimias, seizures, hemolytic anemia, loss of energy stores or tetany. The major electrolytes found in the body are the cations sodium, potassium, calcium, and magnesium, and the anions chloride, phosphate, and bicarbonate (measured as total CO_2 content). Table 29.3 lists the normal laboratory values for these electrolytes (4). It is important to realize that there is no absolute number above or below which symptoms of an electrolyte disorder will be manifest. Even within an individual, tolerance to a single ab-

Table 29.2.
Osmolality, pH, and Distribution^a (ml) of 1 Liter of Common Intravenous Fluids

	D5W	D5/0.2S	D5/0.45S	D5/0.9S	0.9S	0.45S
Osmolality						
Calculated^b	278	353	432	586	308	154
Actual^c	252	321	406	560	308	154
pH (approx.)	4.7	4.4	4.4	4.4	5.3	5
Distribution						
Intracellular fluid	600	450	300	—	—	300
Extracellular fluid	400	550	700	1000	1000	700
Interstitial fluid	320	440	560	800	800	560
Intravascular fluid	80	110	140	200	200	140

^{a} After equilibration in a nonobese individual.
^{b} Calculated osmolality of a solution from formula:

$$mOsm/L = \frac{mg/L}{molecular\ weight} \times no.\ of\ particles$$

^{c} Commercially available solutions are based on the molecular weight of dextrose monohydrate rather than anhydrous dextrose.

Table 29.3.
Normal Electrolyte Concentrations (4)

Electrolyte	Serum Concentrations	(mEq/L)
Sodium	136–145	
Potassium	3.5–5.0	
Chloride	98–106	
CO_2	21–30	
Calcium	4.5–5.5	(9–11 mg/dl)
Phosphate	1–1.5	(3–4.5 mg/dl)

Table 29.4.
Total Body Electrolyte Composition (5–10)

Electrolyte	Sex	Concentration (per kg)
Sodium	M	45–46 mEq
	F	41–42 mEq
Potassium	M	41–46 mEq
	F	32–33 mEq
Chloride	M	26–28 mEq
	F	28 mEq
Calcium	M	173–188 mEq
	F	152–158 mEq
Phosphate		320–365 mmol

normal electrolyte value may change depending on total electrolyte balance or disease state.

The total quantity of electrolytes in the body remains fairly constant throughout adult life. The total body electrolyte content diminishes slightly with age beginning in the third to fourth decade of life. The most significant decrease occurs with calcium. Table 29.4 lists total body electrolyte content averaged over the adult life span of both men and women (5–7).

Sodium

Sodium (Na) is the major extracellular electrolyte although the total serum sodium is only approximately 11.2% of total body sodium (1). For clinical purposes, this number cannot be relied upon to calculate total body sodium since several variables, most significantly renal excretion, may change the total body to serum sodium ratio.

The main functions of sodium in the body are to maintain fluid volume and to participate in the activation and maintenance of membrane potentials.

The serum sodium concentration depends upon fluid status and is regulated primarily by renal excretion and ADH. Hyponatremia is more common than hypernatremia and will be reviewed first.

HYPONATREMIA

By definition, hyponatremia exists when serum sodium is below about 136 mEq/L, but practically, it is rarely significant until the level falls below 120 mEq/L. Symptoms of hyponatremia are listed in Table 29.5.

A widely accepted approach to hyponatremia is to classify it into dilutional, depletional or factitious hyponatremia. Dilutional hyponatremia is a manifestation of disorders such as congestive heart failure, hepatic cirrhosis, or the nephrotic syndrome. It is recognized by a

Table 29.5.
Signs and Symptoms of Hyponatremia (11, 12)

1. *Central nervous system:* Seizures, headaches, lethargy, confusion, delirium, lightheadedness, restlessness, psychosis, ataxia
2. *Neuromuscular:* Fasciculations, cramping, weakness, hypo- or hyperreflexia
3. *Cardiovascular:* Decreased cardiac output, blood pressure, left ventricular end diastolic pressure (LVEDP)
4. *Renal:* Decreased renal blood flow, glomerular filtration rate, urine volume
5. *Gastrointestinal:* Nausea, vomiting, anorexia

low serum sodium even though total body sodium and water are high. Patients are usually overhydrated, edematous, and have a normal pulse and blood pressure. Basic therapy is bed rest, restriction of fluid and sodium intake, and treatment of the primary disease. Diuretics alone are not helpful for chronic therapy because a common problem is decreased renal blood flow and thus delivery of sodium to the distal tubule. However, indications for diuretics would include respiratory or cardiac compromise secondary to fluid overload, physical discomfort, or a means of liberalizing sodium or fluid intake (1).

Depletional hyponatremia is caused by excessive loss of sodium from the body. Routes of loss are the gastrointestinal tract by vomiting, diarrhea, or nasogastric suction; excessive perspiration and replacement with free water; and, renal losses such as induced by chronic renal failure, adrenal disease, or excessive diuresis. Patients will show symptoms of dehydration, and, in more severe cases, volume depletion. If the patient exhibits severe symptoms of hyponatremia, therapy consists of intravenous replacement of sodium with a hypertonic saline solution (3% sodium chloride) (13).

An estimation of total body sodium deficit is helpful in calculating the quantity of this solution to be infused. Two assumptions are made in calculating this deficit. First, normal serum sodium is 140 mEq/L and second, sodium is equally distributed throughout TBW. The second assumption is a major source of error since sodium concentration in the extracellular fluid is 140 mEq/L and that in the ICF is much lower, about 5 to 40 mEq/L. The patient's current serum sodium is subtracted from 140 mEq/L and this value is multiplied by the liter quantity of TBW to provide the total body deficit in mEq of sodium. This calculated number is divided by 2 to give the quantity to infuse into the patient over the next 24 hours. This is conservative and done to correct for the incorrect assumption above. Sample Equation 1 gives an example of this calculation.

Sample Equation 1

The patient is a 70-kg woman with a serum sodium of 115 mEq/L. She is actively seizing. Calculate the amount of 3% saline solution needed to correct her sodium deficit over the next 24 hours.

$$3\% \text{ saline} = 513 \text{ mEq/L}$$
$$\text{TBW} = 50\% \text{ body weight} = 35 \text{ L}$$
$$\text{Normal Na}_{serum} = 140 \text{ mEq/L}$$
$$\text{Sodium deficit} = (140 \text{ mEq/L} - 115 \text{ mEq/L}) \times 35 \text{ L}$$
$$= 875 \text{ mEq}$$
$$\text{Sodium replacement} = 875 \text{ mEq} \div 2$$
$$= 437.5 \text{ mEq}$$
$$\text{Amount 3\% saline needed} = \frac{437.5 \text{ mEq/L}}{513 \text{ mEq/L}}$$
$$= 850 \text{ ml}$$

The serum sodium should be reevaluated after each such infusion and further doses based on new calculations of sodium deficit. Reevaluations need not wait 24 hours but should be done every 2 to 4 hours to follow the need for more rapid infusion. An important point is that the patient will probably become asymptomatic prior to normalizing serum sodium. If more rapid correction is necessary, furosemide may be injected IV (13) in a dose of 1 mg/kg (14).

For asymptomatic depletional hyponatremia, replacement with a 0.9% saline solution which contains 154 mEq/L sodium chloride will be adequate.

Factitious hyponatremia occurs when sodium is displaced from a unit volume of plasma by another substance. For each 100 mg/dl increase in plasma glucose concentration there is a 1.6 mEq/L decrease in plasma sodium concentration (15–17). Also, in hyperlipidemic or hyperproteinemic states where concentrations above 12 to 15 g/dl are reached plasma sodium is falsely decreased (18). To correct for the effect, plasma lipid (mg/dl) multiplied by 0.002, plus, the product of each g/dl of serum protein above 8 multiplied by 0.25, is added to measured serum sodium (8).

The most current classification of hyponatremic syndromes is by Narins et al. (8). They have defined three basic disorders, hypertonic, isotonic, or hypotonic hyponatremia with the hypotonic version further subdivided into hypovolemic, isovolemic, or hypervolemic forms based upon an assessment of ECF volume. This one scheme encompasses and expands on the previous scheme. For example, the factitious hyponatremias are separated with hyperglycemic being hypertonic hyponatremia and the hyperlipoproteinemic being isotonic hyponatremia. Dilutional forms fit into the hypervolemic hypotonic hyponatremia, and depletional forms into hypovolemic hypotonic hyponatremia. The isovolemic hypotonic form would include what previously were miscellaneous or combination syndromes such as water intoxication, reset osmostat, or the syndrome of inappropriate antidiuretic hormone secretion (SIADH).

HYPERNATREMIA (8, 11, 19, 20)

Hypernatremia in children and adults is associated with a high mortality rate. Although, by definition, it occurs when serum sodium rises above 145 mEq/L, it becomes most significant as levels exceed 160 mEq/L. At this level, mortality may range to a high of 45 to 75%. While thirst is normal it is rare to see hypernatremia as the body would respond to hyperosmolarity by increasing water intake. However, if a patient is unable to drink, has restricted access to fluid, or loses the sense of thirst for a prolonged period of time, hypernatremia may develop. Symptoms are listed in Table 29.6.

Hypernatremia can occur in patients with high, low, or normal levels of total body sodium. These are classified by Narins et al. (8) as hypervolemic, hypovolemic, and isovolemic hypernatremias based upon evaluation of the extracellular fluid volume. Contrary to hyponatremia, the serum is always hyperosmolar.

Table 29.6.
Signs and Symptoms of Hypernatremia (11, 12, 19)

1. *Central nervous system:* Lethargy, restlessness, fever, irritability, disorientation, ataxia, tremulousness, seizures, coma, cerebral hemorrhage, death
2. *Neuromuscular:* Weakness, myalgias, cramping, hyperreflexia, rhabdomyolysis
3. *Cardiovascular:* Decreased or increased (iatrogenic) blood volume
4. *Renal:* Prerenal azotemia

Once again, assessment of extracellular fluid volume is essential to proper diagnosis and therapy.

High total body sodium or hypervolemic hypernatremias are most commonly acute in origin and caused by excessive sodium loading. This is seen as the result of the administration of sodium bicarbonate in a cardiac arrest, inadvertent IV administration of hypertonic saline, or intentional overdose. Chronically this is seen in hyperadrenal or hyperpituitary states.

Therapy of hypervolemic hypernatremia is based on increasing the loss of sodium. This is accomplished by combining a potent natriuretic and diuretic agent, usually furosemide, with the IV infusion of some free water. Common solutions used to provide free water are D5W, D5/0.2S, D5/0.45S, and 0.45S. This causes a negative sodium balance since the administration of furosemide causes sodium to be lost in the urine in a concentration slightly exceeding that of half-normal saline (21). Reduction of serum sodium should not be rapid, rather it should be done over 48 to 72 hours. With more rapid correction of hypernatremia, the free water can distribute too quickly into brain cells causing cerebral edema and seizures. By using a solution containing some sodium it may be easier to control the rate of correction. A general guideline is to reduce serum sodium no faster than 1 mEq/hour. With severe renal disease, kidney or peritoneal dialysis may be used to decrease body water and sodium.

Low total body sodium, or hypovolemic hypernatremia occurs when there is loss of both water and sodium but proportionally more water. Loss from the gastrointestinal tract (vomiting, diarrhea), lungs, and integument can cause this state. Renal causes include kidney damage or obstruction, an osmotic diuresis (e.g. hyperglycemia), or diuretics.

In treating hypovolemic hypernatremia, diuretics should not be used since they may worsen the extracellular volume depletion. Therapy includes repletion of both water and sodium. Proper assessment of the extent of extracellular volume deficit is especially important here since the patient may be symptomatically volume depleted. In this case, replacement with 0.9S can be used to allow maximum distribution to the intravascular volume. Otherwise, initial therapy includes dextrose followed by a sodium-containing solution, usually D5/0.45S or 0.45S. Again, it is imperative that serum sodium be lowered gradually to prevent cerebral edema or seizures.

Normal total body sodium or isovolemic hypernatremia occurs with the virtually exclusive loss of free water. The most common nonrenal etiologies are central diabetes insipidus, a reset osmostat, increased respiratory loss of water, and loss from the integument. Nephrogenic diabetes insipidus is the most common renal etiology.

Treatment consists of replacing the lost free water slowly. Calculation of the free water deficit is useful, although not absolutely accurate. Once again, the deficiencies are that it is assumed that normal serum sodium is 140 mEq/L and that the distribution of sodium through TBW is equal. To calculate the deficit, determine the patient's total body water and multiply by the current serum sodium. This product is divided by normal serum sodium. From this value, subtract the calculated TBW. The answer is the amount of free water the patient is deficient.

Sample Equation 2

The patient is a 60-kg man with a serum sodium of 160 mEq/L. He is not currently seizing but is confused and has muscle fasciculations. Calculate the free water deficit.

$$TBW = 60\% \text{ body weight} = 36 \text{ L}$$
$$\text{Normal Na}_{serum} = 140 \text{ mEq/L}$$
$$\text{Water deficit} = 36 \text{ L} - \frac{36 \text{ L} \times 160 \text{ mEq/L}}{140 \text{ mEq/L}}$$
$$= -5 \text{ L}$$

The water deficit is added to the patient's normal daily fluid requirement and replaced over 48 to 72 hours.

Potassium (11, 19)

Potassium (K) is the major intracellular electrolyte with an intracellular concentration ranging from 140 to 160 mEq/L. Total plasma potassium accounts for only 0.4% of total body potassium (1). For this reason the reliability of serum potassium as an indicator of potassium balance can be questioned (22).

The major functions of potassium in the body include the maintenance of electrical transmission at neural and neuromuscular junctions, the regulation of aldosterone secretion, and a role in controlling the release of insulin (where increased potassium would increase release of insulin).

Although it would be convenient to think of disorders of potassium homestasis in terms of intake and excretion only, this is not possible because there are many internal factors which affect potassium balance. Prominent among these is acid-base balance.

It is generally accepted that blood pH significantly affects serum potassium concentration. The change in serum potassium is inversely proportional to pH. For each 0.1-unit decrease in pH, potassium is elevated by 0.6 mEq/L (as the ionized hydrogen replaces potassium intracellularly) and for each 0.1-unit increase in pH, potassium is lowered by 0.6 mEq/L. Adroque and Madias (23) agree with these qualitatively but not quantatively. Available data, they say, show that differences exist in the extent of change of potassium in each of the four primary acid-base disturbances. Not only do serum pH and bicarbonate affect the change, but also serum anions, osmolality, adrenergic activity, release of pancreatic hormones, and renal potassium excretion. Other important internal modifiers of potassium balance are adrenal (mineralocorticoid) activity and insulin secretion. Less important is body magnesium content. External factors are potassium intake, sodium intake, drugs, and renal function. Hypokalemia is far more common than hyperkalemia.

HYPOKALEMIA (8, 11, 19, 24)

Although by definition a patient is hypokalemic when serum potassium is less than 3.5 mEq/L, symptoms and significance are usually minimal until the level is less than 3.0 mEq/L. It is reported that when plasma potassium falls from 4 to 3 mEq/L total body stores are depleted 100 to 200 mEq. However, for each 1 mEq/L decrease below 3 mEq/L, there is a decrease of 200 to 400 mEq in total body potassium (19). Hypokalemia is of greatest significance in a person receiving a digitalis glycoside since digitalis toxicity is increased in the absence of potassium. Symptoms of hypokalemia are listed in Table 29.7.

Total body potassium can be low or normal in a patient with hypokalemia. In normal total body potassium hypokalemia there is a shift of potassium from extracellular to intracellular spaces. The most common etiology of this shift is alkalosis; others are excess insulin, hyperadrenal states (exogenous or endogenous), administration of cyanocobalamin (vitamin B_{12}) to severely depleted patients, and the rare disorder hypokalemic periodic paralysis (8, 24). This form of hypokalemia is occasionally seen in patients receiving diuretics due to the metabolic alkalosis that may be induced.

The treatment of normal total body potassium hypokalemia is to correct the basic abnormality. Administration of exogenous potassium as a routine therapy has little effect on reversing the apparently low concentration. It can be administered in an emergency situation where the person is symptomatic.

Low total body hypokalemia is usually caused by potassium-deficient diet or increased losses from the gastrointestinal tract (e.g. severe vomiting or diarrhea), or excessive kaliuresis occurring because the kidneys have no mechanism to conserve potassium. This can be seen during antibiotic therapy with carben-

---

Table 29.7.
Signs and Symptoms of Hypokalemia (11, 12, 24, 25)

1. *Central nervous system:* Confusion, drowsiness, decreased mental status, irritability, delirium, coma
2. *Cardiovascular:* ECG changes (flattening of the T wave, development U wave, increased P wave), occasional arrhythmias (especially with preexisting cardiac disease or digitalis), hypotension
3. *Muscular:* Weakness, muscle cramps, paralysis (all are usually first seen in the legs); atrophy, rhabdomyolysis, myalgias, fasciculations, areflexia
4. *Metabolic:* Abnormal glucose tolerance
5. *Renal:* Polyuria, polydipsia, nocturia, increased renin
6. *Gastrointestinal:* Nausea, vomiting, gastric atony, ileus

icillin, ticarcillin, and sodium penicillin G, or most commonly with diuretic therapy with thiazides, furosemide, or ethacrynic acid. For a complete list of etiologies the reader is referred elsewhere (8).

Treatment of this form of hypokalemia is directed at replacing the lost potassium although the underlying cause should be identified and corrected. Basic therapy of any hypokalemic disorder involves the decision of which of the many salts to use. This generally narrows down to using a salt which will or will not increase plasma bicarbonate.

In treating a hypokalemic alkalosis the chloride salt should be used. The bicarbonate, citrate, and gluconate salts should be avoided. These salts are ideal, however, if an acidosis is present (11). Another salt, potassium phosphate, is used in the presence of a combined phosphate deficiency as occurs in diabetic ketoacidosis or in patients receiving only parenteral nutrients.

When to treat is dependent upon symptoms, serum potassium, concurrent disease, and drug therapy. Unless the patient is symptomatic or has a serum potassium below 2.5 mEq/L (without symptoms) immediate potassium replacement is not warranted. The average patient who is asymptomatic with a stable serum potassium greater than 3 mEq/L does not require therapy. However, if there are only slight symptoms suggestive of deficiency or the patient has severe liver disease or congestive heart failure treated with digitalis and diuretics, oral supplementation with 20 to 60 mEq/day of potassium is recommended. Prophylactic therapy is often used in patients treated with digitalis and diuretics.

At any time severe symptoms (i.e. arrhythmias, respiratory paralysis) of potassium deficiency are evident, it may be replaced rapidly by the intravenous route. Where electrocardiographic monitoring is not available, the administration rate should be restricted to 10 mEq/hour due to the danger of precipitating cardiac arrhythmias. Where monitoring is available, potassium may be administered at rates up to 40 mEq/hour. This rate is limited by the distribution rate of potassium into the intracellular volume; if infused too quickly, symptoms of hyperkalemia may develop even in the presence of total body hypokalemia.

Another consideration is the concentration of the administered potassium, usually as chloride. Concentrations above 50 to 60 mEq/L are extremely irritating to peripheral veins. For a continuous infusion, the maximum concentration should be limited to 60 to 80 mEq/L. For acute administration, 10 mEq may be placed in each 100 ml of D5W or 0.9S and infused as above. Any concentration greater than this infused in a peripheral vein almost always causes the patient great discomfort. If pain occurs, either dilute the solution further, or decrease the rate of infusion.

HYPERKALEMIA (8, 11, 19, 26)

Hyperkalemia can be an insidious and especially dangerous electrolyte disorder since it may not be recognized clinically until life-threatening symptoms (e.g. cardiac arrhythmias) become evident. Symptoms of hyperkalemia are listed in Table 29.8.

The individual tolerance to an increased potassium concentration in the serum varies. Hyperkalemia occurs with either a normal or a high total body potassium content. Further complicating the assessment of hyperkalemia is the possibility of factitious, or pseudohyperkalemia. Because acid-base status affects serum potassium, the pH should always be considered when evaluating hyperkalemia.

Pseudohyperkalemia is most often caused by poor blood drawing technique which lyses red blood cells and releases potassium. This can occur when a tourniquet is either too tight or left on too long (greater than 5 min), the blood is drawn too fast through a small gauge needle, or it is refrigerated too long. It is also seen in extreme leukocytosis (above 50,000/mm^3) and thrombocytosis (above 1,000,000/mm^3) and may be identified by concurrent analysis of both serum and plasma potassium. Serum concentrations will be higher.

Other forms of normal total body potassium, or redistribution, hyperkalemia include aci-

Table 29.8.
Signs and Symptoms of Hyperkalemia (11, 12, 19, 27, 28)

1. *Cardiac:* Bradycardia, asystole, ventricular fibrillation, ECG abnormalities (in order of occurrence—peaked T waves, QRS widening, diminished amplitude of the P wave, depression of sinoatrial node)
2. *Neuromuscular:* Weakness, paralysis, fasciculations, myotonia, areflexia or hyperreflexia
3. *Central nervous system:* Fatigue, lassitude

dosis, high glucose, and drug therapy with β-blockers or digitalis glycosides.

High total body potassium hyperkalemia is caused by excess intake and/or decreased excretion. Most commonly hyperkalemia occurs with acute oliguric renal failure. It is much less common in chronic renal failure, unless the glomerular filtration rate is below 15 to 20 ml/min. This is because the remaining nephrons gain an increased ability to excrete potassium (called renal potassium adaptation) and excretion through the gastrointestinal tract is augmented (26). Excretion of potassium may also be diminished by drugs such as the potassium-sparing diuretics spironolactone, triamterene, and amiloride. Iatrogenic sources of exogenous potassium include oral potassium supplements, transfusion with stored blood, drugs (such as potassium penicillin G), salt substitutes, and hyperalimentation.

For a complete differential of hyperkalemia see Narins et al. (8) and DeFronzo et al. (26).

There are two major goals in the treatment of hyperkalemia, foremost is to protect the heart and then to lower serum potassium. When electrocardiographic abnormalities are seen, calcium, which acts as a myocardial protectant, should be the first drug administered. Calcium gluconate, 10 ml of a 10% solution supplying about 4.6 mEq of Ca^{2+}, may be injected intravenously over about 5 min. This is only a temporary measure since it does not decrease serum potassium. A constant infusion can be maintained to protect the heart until other measures lower serum potassium. If calcium chloride is used, it must be recognized that it provides about 13 mEq of Ca^{2+} per gram.

There are four standard methods for reducing serum potassium. Sodium bicarbonate ($NaHCO_3$) is used to raise the blood pH and cause a shift of potassium into cells. Acutely, 50 ml of 8.4% $NaHCO_3$ (1 ampule) is administered intravenously over 1 to 5 min followed by an infusion containing 2 to 3 ampules of $NaHCO_3$ in 1 liter of D5W or D10W at a rate adjusted to keep serum potassium low. This therapy is temporary, since it only shifts potassium within the body.

Dextrose with insulin is the next form of therapy. Insulin stimulates the cellular uptake of glucose with potassium following thus lowering its serum concentration. The minimum glucose to regular insulin ratio is 2 to 3 g of glucose for each unit of insulin. Both bolus and infusion methods are used to supply this combination. As a bolus 50 ml of D50W may be given with 10 units of regular insulin subcutaneously. Infusion techniques include combining 10 to 25 units of subcutaneously administered regular insulin with an infusion of D10W at a rate of 500 to 1000 ml/hour for the first hour and thereafter at 250 to 500 ml/hour. Alternatively, 25 to 50 units of regular insulin may be added directly to each liter of D10W and infused at 250 to 500 ml/hour. Sodium bicarbonate may also be added to each liter. This measure is also temporary as potassium is not removed from the body.

The final two standard measures are similar in that they both cause potassium to be removed from the body but act too slowly to be used in the acute treatment of hyperkalemia.

Administration of the cationic-exchange resin sodium polystyrene sulfonate (Kayexalate) either orally or rectally will cause the loss of potassium by exchanging it for sodium. One gram of sodium polystyrene sulfonate will remove approximately 1 mEq of potassium and supply 2 to 3 mEq of sodium. Since the resin is constipating it is combined with sorbitol (an osmotic laxative) and water prior to administration (see Chapter 31, "Renal Disease"). Complete exchange is dependent upon contact time in the gut, therefore the oral route is preferred since the retention time of enema is limtied. Initial doses of 25 to 50 g are used with continued therapy dependent upon serum potassium determinations.

Finally, in severely hyperkalemic patients, peritoneal dialysis or hemodialysis may be used.

Calcium

Calcium is one of the most vital minerals in the human body. It is regulated by the synchronous activity of several hormones, parathyroid (PTH), calcitonin, and 1,25-dihydroxycholecalciferol (the active form of vitamin D). It is also affected by serum concentration of phosphate and magnesium. The major role of the hormones is to regulate absorption, distribution, and excretion of calcium.

Only 50% of serum calcium is available for physiologic activity as ionized calcium. About 40% of serum calcium is bound to albumin and the remainder to various anions.

Calcium has multiple functions in the body. It is the major constituent of bone, with about 99% of total body calcium stored there. It is responsible for muscular contraction via activation of the actin-myosin complex. It causes the release of chemical transmitters in the nervous system and acts as a membrane stabilizer to decrease permeability and excitability. It also is active in the blood coagulation cascade as factor IV, inhibits enzymes of intermediary metabolism (phosphofructokinase, pyruvic kinase, and pyruvic carboxylase), stimulates gastrin which releases gastric acid, can cause a decrease in renal blood flow and glomerular filtration rate by renal vasoconstriction, and may inhibit renin release.

Disorders of calcium homestasis are rarely encountered in routine fluid and electrolyte therapy. Modifiers of serum calcium levels include albumin, globulin, and acid-base balance. For each 1 g/dl change in albumin, calcium changes 0.8 mg/dl in the opposite direction (29, 30). For each 1 g/dl change in globulin, calcium changes 0.2 mg/dl in the opposite direction (31). Finally for each 1 unit pH change serum ionized calcium changes 1.68 mg/dl in the opposite direction (30).

HYPERCALCEMIA (11, 30)

Although there are many causes of hypercalcemia there are three basic causes—increased intestinal absorption, increased bone resorption, and decreased renal excretion. The two most common etiologies are neoplasms and hyperparathyroidism. There are several mechanisms for the hypercalcemia of malignancy including ectopic production of: PTH, prostaglandins, osteoclast activating factor, a vitamin D-like sterol, a substance to stimulate prostaglandin synthesis within bone, and bone metastases causing direct lysis of bone. For a complete list of etiologies the reader is referred to Lee et al. (30). Symptoms of hypercalcemia are listed in Table 29.9.

The therapy of hypercalcemia is started with an infusion of normal saline IV to get a urine volume of about 100 ml/hour. Furosemide is then started at 1 mg/kg, maximum 100 mg, to maintain urine volume at 500 ml/hour. This is useful in all forms of hypercalcemia since it works by increasing the renal excretion of calcium. Thiazide diuretics should be avoided since they retain calcium.

Oral phosphate may be used in doses of 1 to 3 g/day in divided doses. Common preparations used are an oral Phospho-Soda solution containing approximately 800 mg phosphate per 5 ml and Neutraphos capsules or solution

Table 29.9.
Major Signs and Symptoms of Hypercalcemia (11, 12, 19, 30, 32, 33)

1. *Central nervous system:* Fatigue, lethargy, confusion, seizures, delirium, psychoses
2. *Cardiovascular:* Arrhythmias, ECG changes (decreased QT interval and sometimes increased PR interval)
3. *Renal:* Polyuria, calcium nephropathy
4. *Gastrointestinal:* Nausea, vomiting, anorexia, abdominal pain, constipation, diarrhea
5. *Skeletal:* Bone pain and fractures
6. *Neuromuscular:* Weakness, hyperreflexia

with 1 g of phosphate per 4 capsules or 300 ml solution, respectively. Intravenous phosphate as therapy for hypercalcemia should be avoided. It is absolutely the last resort because, although effective, it causes calcium phosphate to precipitate out in various body tissues (32).

Steroids are also useful in chronic management. The onset of action is 3 to 10 days and they work both at the bone to decrease resorption and in the liver to decrease the activation of vitamin D. Effective daily doses in 27 patients as described by Klein et al. (34) were 15 to 100 mg of prednisone daily. Steroids are useful in treating the hypercalcemia of a variety of neoplasms, tuberculosis, adrenal insufficiency, and vitamin D overdose. They are not effective in treating hyperparathyroidism (35).

Salmon calcitonin has been used frequently in the acute treatment of hypercalcemia due to its rapid onset of action and relatively short duration of 4 to 6 hours. Although relatively safe, a test dose of 1 unit should always be injected intradermally prior to use to test for an allergic reaction. Therepeutic doses are 2 to 8 Medical Research Units (MRC) per kilogram given intramuscularly every 4 to 6 hours or 3 to 6 MRC units/kg/day as a continuous infusion. The effect of calcitonin is usually brief, as "escape" occurs within 1 to 2 days of therapy. It is effective in most forms of hypercalcemia.

One of the most effective, but potentially toxic, therapies used is mithramycin. This drug acts directly to inhibit bone resorption by forming a complex with DNA in the presence of magnesium or another divalent cation to inhibit DNA-dependent RNA synthesis in the osteoclast. It is indicated when other drugs fail. It is dosed as 25 μg/kg up to a maximum weekly dose of 150 μg/kg. Its onset of action is

12 to 48 hours with a peak effect delayed sometimes up to 3 days and a duration of action of 3 to 7 days.

Combined therapy with calcitonin and phosphate or mithramycin have been used. Although effective, there is an increased risk of developing hypocalcemia.

Prostaglandin inhibitors have occasionally been used with some success in treating the hypercalcemia of malignancy. Indomethacin in doses of 50 to 150 mg a day in divided doses has been used. Possible indications would be a malignant solid tumor without bone metastases and with a low level of PTH detected in the serum; and when a high level of 7-α-hydroxy-5,11-diketotetraprostane-1,16-dioic acid (PGE-M) is detected in the urine (33, 36).

Finally, propranolol has been used in the mild form of hypercalcemia complicating hyperthyroidism. Doses of 80 to 100 mg/day have been used chronically (37, 38).

HYPOCALCEMIA (8, 11, 33, 39)

Most often hypocalcemia is seen as a subacute electrolyte disorder. Etiologies include hyperphosphatemia, pancreatitis, hypovitaminosis D, parathyroidectomy, and drugs. Cisplatin and gentamicin can cause a renal magnesium wasting which acts to decrease release of PTH. Phenytoin and barbiturates impair the activation of Vitamin D. Although PTH is the major regulator of calcium homeostasis, it is elevated in all the previous etiologies except parathyroidectomy. The chronic forms of hypocalcemia include primary hypoparathyroidism and diseases such as renal, liver, or neoplasia. A complete differential of hypocalcemia is available (8). Signs and symptoms are listed in Table 29.10.

In treating acute symptomatic hypocalcemia, calcium may be given intravenously as the gluconate or chloride salt. If necessary, 10 to 20 ml of a 10% calcium gluconate solution (4.6 to 9.2 mEq elemental calcium) may be given IV push or as a piggyback infusion over 30 min. This can be followed by the infusion of 0.75 to 1.0 mEq of calcium per kilogram of body weight over the next 4 to 8 hours in D5W. During the infusion blood pressure and ECG should be monitored. Serum concentration should be determined frequently and enough calcium should be supplied to keep the patient asymptomatic.

Following control of the acute episode, determination and treatment of the etiology usually make chronic maintenance therapy with

Table 29.10.
Signs and Symptoms of Hypocalcemia (11, 12, 39)

1. *Neuromuscular:* Tetany, fasciculations, cramping, carpopedal spasm, hyperreflexia, myalgias, laryngeal stridor, parasthesias
2. *Central nervous system:* Seizures, mental status changes, psychoses, increased intracranial pressure, choreoathetotic movements, calcification of the basal ganglia
3. *Cardiovascular:* ECG changes—prolonged QT interval, normal QRS; decreased contractility
4. *Skin:* Dry and scaly appearance, eczema-like dermatitis, impaired nail growth, decreased resistance to candida infection
5. *Other:* Cataract formation (irreversible), loss of body hair

calcium unnecessary. However, if the etiology will cause a chronic hypocalcemia, treatment with oral calcium and often vitamin D is required.

Oral calcium is available in several salts including calcium carbonate, the most concentrated form with 250 mg and 500 mg elemental calcium per tablet as well as calcium lactate (60 mg per 300 mg tablet) and gluconate (90 mg per 1000 mg as tablet or liquid). Typical doses range from 500 mg to 2000 mg elemental calcium per day in divided doses to decrease gastrointestinal discomfort.

When calcium supplementation alone is not adequate to maintain serum calcium in the normal range vitamin D must be added. Ergocalciferol, vitamin D_2, 50,000 to 200,000 units per day (1.25 to 5 mg) is the normal dose range. Due to an extremely long half-life it has a slow onset and long duration of action. The synthetic compound, dihydrotachysterol, has a quicker onset and shorter duration, is more potent with a dose range of 0.125 to 1.25 mg per day, but is much more expensive.

More active forms of vitamin D are available but their use is usually limited to patients with a vitamin D-resistant form of hypocalcemia. In these circumstances 1,25-dihydroxycholecalciferol, the most physiologically active form of vitamin D, is given in doses of 0.5 to 2 μg daily. Another highly active form, 25-hydroxycholecalciferol, is also used in doses of 300 to 350 μg administered in divided doses weekly.

Phosphate (10)

Phosphate, the most prevalent intracellular anion, has several essential roles within the body. Its most important function is providing the high energy phosphate bonds in adenosine triphosphate (ATP). It affects hemoglobin's oxygen carrying capacity as a component of 2,3-diphosphoglycerate (2, 3-DPG), cell membrane structure as phospholipid membranes, and cellular function as a constituent of cyclic nucleic acids and enzyme cofactors.

Phosphate metabolism is regulated by several factors including renal function, PTH, carbohydrate intake, quantity of total body phosphate, vitamin D, and acid-base status. The more common abnormality is hypophosphatemia since hyperphosphatemia is almost never seen in the presence of normal renal function.

HYPOPHOSPHATEMIA

There are three general causes for hypophosphatemia: decreased intake, increased excretion, and cellular redistribution of phosphate. Some causes of decreased intake are vomiting, diarrhea, the use of aluminum-containing antacids, and phosphate-poor hyperalimentation. Renal tubular damage, hypokalemia, and hypomagnesemia are included among causes of increased excretion of phosphate. Significant causes of internal shifts include alkalosis, glucose administration, and diabetic ketoacidosis. A more complete differential can be found elsewhere (8, 9, 40). Narins et al. (8) suggest that classifying hypophosphatemias by quantitating the amount in the urine is helpful in distinguishing nonrenal causes. If less than 100 mg daily it is nonrenal (8).

When assessing hypophosphatemia it must be considered that serum phosphate does not always represent total body phosphate. For example, when hypophosphatemia is secondary to cellular redistribution, total body content is usually normal.

The signs and symptoms (Table 29.11) of hypophosphatemia are most often absent until the serum level falls to or below 1 mg/dl. An exception is made in the case of chronic hypophosphatemia when symptoms may be seen at higher levels.

The treatment of hypophosphatemia depends on the symptoms seen. An asymptomatic patient with a low serum level requires identification and correction of the cause. With mild symptoms, dietary supplementation can be added, usually in the form of milk which contains 0.029 mmol phosphate per milliliter (41). Hypophosphatemia which is not

Table 29.11.
Signs and Symptoms of Hypophosphatemia (9, 10, 12, 40)

1. *Neuromuscular:* Extreme weakness, rhabdomyolysis, fasciculations, myalgias, paresthesias, anisocoria, intention tremor, malaise, paralysis
2. *Central nervous system:* Coma, seizures, decreased mental status, ataxia
3. *Cardiovascular:* Negative inotropy and reversible congestive heart failure
4. *Hematologic:* Decreased 2,3-diphosphoglycerate leads to tissue hypoxia, hemolysis, decreased platelet aggregation and survival, decreased white blood cell chemotaxis and phagocytosis
5. *Skeletal:* Osteopenia, osteomalacia, arthralgia, bone fracture
6. *Gastrointestinal:* Nausea, vomiting, anorexia, hepatic anoxia

life-threatening but is symptomatic or has a serum level less than 1 mg/dl can be treated by oral supplementation. A dose of 60 mmol/day in divided doses is all that is required (10). This can be conveniently given as 5 ml of an oral Phospho-Soda solution 3 times a day or as 500 mg oral capsules 4 times a day. A major problem with oral therapy is the high frequency of diarrhea it can cause. For long-term administration, calcium supplementation may be necessary since prolonged therapy with phosphate alone may induce hypocalcemia.

Intravenous phosphate therapy is generally reserved for the treatment of severe or life-threatening hypophosphatemia. The recommended dose is 0.08 mmol/kg for acute uncomplicated and 0.16 mmol/kg for chronic hypophosphatemia. Doses up to 50% higher should be used if the patient is symptomatic and a like amount lower in the presence of hypercalcemia (9, 10, 41). Each dose should be infused over a 6-hour period. Intravenous phosphate is also used prophylactically in hyperalimentation solutions to prevent the phosphate depletion that otherwise occurs. Phosphate at 15 mmol per liter is usually added.

Two forms of intravenous phosphate are available, potassium and sodium. Potassium phosphate contains 4.4 mEq of potassium per 3 mmol phosphate and the sodium form supplies 4.0 mEq for each 3 mmol phosphate.

HYPERPHOSPHATEMIA

Increased serum phosphate is rarely seen in a setting other than renal failure. Basic therapy is to reduce intake of exogenous phosphate as much as possible. Aluminum salts aid in this by binding phosphate in the gastrointestinal tract. Concentrated aluminum hydroxide gel, 600 mg/5 ml, given in a dose of 30 ml 4 times a day is the most potent binder. Other binders are aluminum carbonate and regular strength aluminum hydroxide.

Diuretics may be used to decrease phosphate acutely but are of little value in chronic therapy. Renal dialysis is an effective method of phosphate removal.

References

1. Edelman IS, Leibman J: Anatomy of body water and electrolytes. *Am J Med* 27:256, 1959.
2. Edelman IS, Olney JM, James AH, et al: Body composition: studies in the human being by the dilution principle. *Science* 115:447, 1952.
3. Moore FD, McMurrey JD, Parker V, et al: Total body water and electrolytes: intravascular and extravascular phase volumes. *Metabolism* 5:447, 1956.
4. Isselbacher KJ, Adams RD, et al. (eds): *Harrison's Principles of Internal Medicine*, ed 9. New York: McGraw-Hill, 1980.
5. Ellis KJ, Vaswani A, Zanzi I, et al. Total body sodium and chlorine in normal adults. *Metabolism* 25:645, 1976.
6. Cohn SH, Vaswani A, Zanzi I, et al: Changes in body chemical composition with age measured by total-body neutron activation. *Metabolism* 25:85, 1976.
7. Cohn SH, Abesamis C, Zanzi I, et al: Body elemental composition: comparison between black and white adults. *Am J Phys* 232:E419, 1977.
8. Narins RG, Jones ER, et al: Diagnostic strategies in disorders of fluid, electrolyte, and acid-base homeostasis. *Am J Med* 72:496, 1982.
9. Juan D: The causes and consequences of hypophosphatemia. *Surg Gynecol Obstet* 153:589, 1981.
10. Stoff JS: Phosphate Homeostasis and Hypophosphatemia. *Am J Med* 72:489, 1982.
11. Maxwell MH, Kleeman CR (eds): *Clinical Disorders of Fluid and Electrolyte Metabolism*, ed. 3. New York: McGraw-Hill, 1980.
12. Knochel JP: Neuromuscular manifestations of electrolyte disorders. *Am J Med* 72:521, 1982.
13. Ayus JC, Olivero JJ, Frommer JP: Rapid correction of severe hyponatremia with intravenous hypertonic saline solution. *Am J Med* 72:43, 1982.
14. Hantman D, Rossier B, et al: Rapid correction of hyponatremia in the syndrome of inappropriate secretion of antidiuretic hormone. *Ann Intern Med* 78:870, 1976.
15. Katz MA: Hyperglycemia-induced hyponatremia—calculation of expected serum sodium depression. *N Engl J Med* 289:843, 1973.
16. Crandall ED: Serum sodium response to hyperglycemia (letter). *N Engl J Med* 290:465, 1974.
17. Jenkins PG, Larmore C: Hyperglycemia-induced hyponatremia (letter). *N Engl J Med* 290:573, 1974.
18. DeFronzo RA, Thier SO: Pathophysiologic approach to hyponatremia. *Arch Intern Med* 140:897, 1980.
19. Schrier RW (ed): *Renal and Electrolyte Disorders*, ed 2. Boston: Little, Brown, 1980.
20. Ross EJ, Christie SBM: Hypernatremia. *Medicine* 48:441, 1969.
21. Wilson TW, Falk KJ, et al: Effect of dosage regimen on natriuretic response to furosemide. *Clin Pharm Ther* 18:165, 1975.
22. Dyckner T, Wester PO: The relation between extra- and intracellular electrolytes in patients with hypokalemia and/or diuretic treatment. *Acta Med Scand* 204:269, 1978.
23. Adroque HJ, Madias NE: Changes in plasma potassium concentration during acute acid-base disturbances. *Am J Med* 71:456, 1981.
24. Suki WN, Jackson D: Hypokalemia—cause and treatment. *Heart Lung* 7:854, 1978.
25. Jellett LB: Potassium therapy: when is it indicated. *Drugs* 16:88, 1978.
26. DeFronzo RA, Bia M, et al: Clinical disorders of hyperkalemia. *Annu Rev Med* 33:521, 1982.
27. Coniglione JC: Treatment of hypercalcemia and hyperkalemia. *Med Times* 106(7):69, 1978.
28. Newmark SR, Dluhy RG: Hyperkalemia and hypokalemia. *JAMA* 231:631, 1975.
29. Anon: Protein correction of serum calcium in mild primary hyperparathyroidism. *Acta Med Scand Suppl* 624:69, 1979.
30. Lee DBN, Zawada ET, Kleeman CR: The pathophysiology and clinical aspects of hypercalcemic disorders. *West J Med* 129:278, 1978.
31. Barreuthor AD: Calcium and phosphorus. *Hosp Pharm* 10(11):486, 1975.
32. Fulmer DH, Dimich AB, et al: Treatment of hypercalcemia. *Arch Intern Med* 129:923, 1972.
33. Bell NH: Hypercalcemic and hypocalcemic disorders: diagnosis and treatment. *Nephron* 23:147, 1979.
34. Klein RG, Arnaud SB, et al: Intestinal calcium absorption in exogenous hypercortisonism. *J Clin Invest* 60:253, 1977.
35. Austin LA, Heath H. III: Calcitonin. *N Engl J Med* 304:269, 1981.
36. Myers WP: Differential diagnosis of hypercalcemia and cancer. *CA* 27:258, 1977.
37. Rude RK, Oldham SB, et al: Treatment of thyrotoxic hypercalcemia with propranolol. *N Engl J Med* 294:431, 1976.
38. Shahshahani MN, Palmieri GMA: Oral propranolol in hypercalcemia associated with apathetic thyrotoxicosis. *Am J Med Sci* 275:199, 1978.
39. Schneider AB, Sherwood LM: Pathogenesis and management of hypoparathyroidism and other hypocalcemic disorders. *Metabolism* 24:871, 1975.
40. Fitzgerald F: Clinical hypophosphatemia. *Annu Rev Med* 29:177, 1978.
41. Lentz RD, Brown DM, Kjellstrand CM: Treatment of severe hypophosphatemia. *Ann Intern Med* 89:941, 1978.

CHAPTER 30

Obesity

MARTIN J. JINKS, Pharm.D.

"Leave gourmandizing, know that the grave doth gape for thee thrice wider than for other men."

William Shakespeare, 16th Century

Despite these perceptive words, Shakespeare and his contemporaries admired an ample form. Suppleness denoted a person graced by God, and was the hallmark of the opulent and idly rich. Rubens would certainly have scoffed at the idea of Twiggy as a model of beauty. It took the industrial revolution at the turn of this century to give obesity a bad reputation. Mechanization caused voluntary or forced reduction in average activity without a decrease in caloric intake and has caused obesity to become the single most prevalent metabolic disorder in the United States.

Obesity can be defined as a condition occurring from the sum total of the environmental, emotional and familial factors that have as the lowest common denominator an abnormal energy balance usually resulting from an excessive caloric intake and inadequate caloric loss. In simplest terms, obesity exists when there is excess body fat. In man, moderate obesity is present when adipose comprises more than 25% of ideal weight. The upper limit in females is 30%. Massive obesity is defined by adiposity in excess of 100% of ideal weight (1).

ETIOLOGY

Increasing body weight may be a reflection of fluid retention, adipose tissue accumulation or both. Weight gain in excess of 1 kg/day invariably implies fluid retention, and is frequently a signal of cardiovascular, renal or hepatic disorders (2). When medications produce weight gain, they usually do so by inducing fluid retention in susceptible individuals, either through direct (steroids and related drugs) or indirect mechanisms (medicinals high in sodium).

Obesity, an increased appetite with an accumulation of excess adipose tissue, is not a disease but a symptom. It has sometimes been viewed as a moral problem, namely gluttony, which represents "unrepressed hedonisitc tendencies or arrest of personality development at the oral stage" (3). These harsh attitudes are giving way to the appreciation that obesity is a complex interplay of life-styles, psychological influences, hereditary factors and metabolic changes which have, as their ultimate manifestation, chronic dietary indiscretion. Only rarely is obesity a symptom of a specific endocrinopathy, such as insulinoma or Cushing's disease. These uncommon disorders are easily differentiated by their peculiar fat distribution, attendant symptoms and a history of sudden appetite changes.

INCIDENCE

Obesity afflicts between 25 and 40% of adults in the United States. Between ages 30 and 39 years, 25% of men and women are moderately obese. Over 50 years, 34% of men and 49% of women are moderately obese. Of all adults, 5 to 7% are considered seriously overweight. Obesity is reported to be as high as 15% in children (1, 4). The condition touches every social, economic, racial and age group.

PATHOGENESIS

Research into the pathophysiology of obesity has branched into many related areas. The literature is replete with studies of the cause and effect of adipose tissue formation, structure and composition. In recent years, *Index Medicus* has contained several hundred citations per year relating to obesity research. The important findings can be summarized under the four following major topic areas.

Metabolic Abnormalities

Insulin refractoriness is the most significant metabolic deviation in obesity since insulin regulates the major pathways for fat accumulation and storage. It is thought that glucose intolerance results in a delayed response to blood sugar, triggering hyperinsulinemia and accelerated lipogenesis. This is an attractive hypothesis to explain the cause of obesity, but current evidence suggests that insulin refractoriness is a result, not a cause, of obesity.

Other endocrine changes are commonly associated with obesity and, like insulin refractoriness, are probably secondary to the physiological demands of obesity. Adrenal overactivity is a common finding in massively obese patients, as reflected by elevated urinary corticosteroids, mild hirsutism, borderline hypertension and glucose intolerance (5, 6). These abnormalities are probably a result of obesity rather than a cause. They develop in nonobese subjects following gorging, and they disappear as weight is returned to normal.

Metabolic enzyme deficiency resulting in abnormalities in thermogenic dissipation of calories in obese patients is currently receiving a great deal of attention. Cellular enzyme systems account for much of thermogenic calorie loss, and there is evidence that the obese may have inefficient catalytic rates (7–9). Impaired hormonal control by catecholamines and insulin (10) may be involved, but this hypothesis is controversial (11).

Genetic Factors

The role of heredity in obesity is a matter of great speculation and research. Inherited obesity has been proven in animals and is linked in humans. Statistically, when both parents are of normal weight, there is a 9% incidence of obesity in the offspring, while when one or both parents are obese, there is a 50% and 80% incidence of obese offspring, respectively. Obviously, cultural factors pertaining to food intake greatly confound research into this area, but evidence from adopted children and parents indicates that, in an affluent society, genetic factors more often dictate predisposition to obesity (3).

Dietary Indiscretion

Since the discovery over 65 years ago that obesity can be induced surgically in animals, a great deal of interest has developed in the relationship between abnormal appetite and possible aberrations within hypothalamic feeding centers. Lesions in the ventromedial nucleus of the hypothalamus result in hyperphagia, whereas lesions in the lateral hypothalamic areas result in cessation of eating (12, 13). Factors controlling these centers are unknown, but have been associated with endocrine and metabolic determinants. It is well appreciated that obese individuals exhibit behavior which might indicate a derangement in the satiety center. Research has demonstrated that when obese and nonobese individuals are allowed to ingest freely, the nonobese regulate food intake based on internal cues, such as hunger sensations and caloric density of the food, while obese individuals regulate food intake by external cues such as time and environment, regardless of the caloric density of the food (Fig. 30.1) (14).

It has been proposed that nutritional experiences in early life can produce changes in fat tissue and predispose individuals to obesity. Overfeeding in infancy has been linked to development of a hyperplastic adipose reserve (increased number of fixed adipose cells) which manifests as intractable obesity in later life. This contrasts with most forms of obesity which consist of hypertrophic obesity, the increase in the size of adipose cells. Since metabolic dysfunctions (e.g., insulin refractoriness, hyperglycemia, hypertriglyceridemia) are associated with the fat content per adipose cell, the therapeutic goal for hyperplastic-hypertrophic obesity may best be directed at correcting the metabolic abnormalities rather than aiming for the insurance-table weight norm (15). In hyperplastic-hypertrophic patients, the fat content per cell will be normalized long before insurance-table weight is achieved and attempts to reduce weight in these patients to norms for hypertrophic individuals can result in psychological and physical disability (16).

Since evidence favors the increased likelihood of chubby infants becoming obese adults (17), preventative measures are important. These measures include avoiding overfeeding of infants, encouraging the use of unsugared foods, keeping junk foods and snacks out of the house, and encouraging activity.

Psychological Factors

Familial and cultural eating habits are implanted in individuals at an early age. As a society, we place great emphasis on food—to most, one of life's enduring pleasures is a rich, hearty meal. The obese patient carries this gratification to an extreme level.

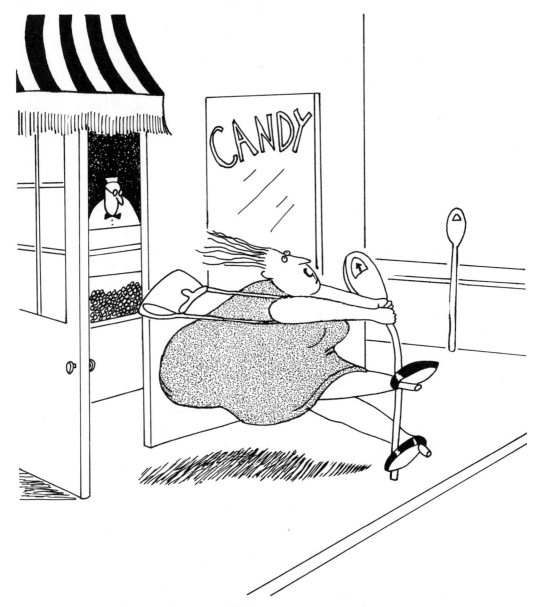

Figure 30.1. (From "Far Side" Chronicle Features, 1982.)

The obese often exhibit an immense appetite for psychological reasons. Overeating may be a manifestation of anxiety or depression, where the pleasures of food are substituted for the satisfactions missing from other sources. As a result, the obese characteristically dine until the food is gone or until they are overtly uncomfortable, while the nonobese usually stop eating when their hunger is gone.

Because obesity is often associated with neurotic traits, overeating is commonly considered to be a behavioral defect. In the pathologically obese, where no distinct underlying problem exists, psychological factors undoubtedly play a major role. However, obesity is most likely a complex interplay of psychological, genetic, and metabolic influences which manifest as abnormal appetite and resultant overweight.

DIAGNOSIS

The massively obese, the patient with peculiar fat distribution or the patient with sudden, rapid weight gain require extensive evaluation. However, common "idiopathic" obesity does not usually demand elaborate evaluation techniques.

Quantifying obesity is not difficult. The patient who is 136 kg (300 lb) overweight is readily recognized as obese. Moderately obese patients are easily diagnosed using standard height-weight charts. These charts have a 90% correlation with much more elaborate densiometry and radioisotope dilution techniques (1). However, height-weight charts are not without deficiencies, and the easiest and most accurate method is measurement of triceps, subscapular or suprailiac skinfold thickness with constant pressure calipers. Skinfold thickness measurements coupled with height-weight data give a convenient and accurate evaluation of the degree of obesity.

COMPLICATIONS

Many serious disorders are associated with severe obesity (Table 30.1). Significant excess weight is definitely detrimental to longevity and there is a definite statistical link between marginal and severe obesity and hypertension, diabetes, cardiovascular disease, and gastrointestinal disorders (Figs. 30.2 and 30.3). This link pertains primarily to moderate and severe obesity, since the marginally or slightly obese individual compares favorably in longevity to the nonobese.

Massive obesity during pregnancy is associated with a 7-fold increase in toxemia, a 10-fold increase in diabetes, and double the risk of maternal mortality (18). Substantial excess weight is also associated with altered pharmacokinetics of certain drugs (19).

Despite evidence of the detrimental effects of obesity on health, the prevalent factor motivating most individuals to lose weight is not health but cosmetic goals.

Table 30.1.
Disorders Associated with Obesity

Hypertension
Cerebrovascular disease
Congestive heart failure
Varicose veins
Diabetes
Hyperlipidemia
Respiratory distress syndrome (Pickwickian)
Gallbladder disease
Obstetric complications
Hiatus hernia
Osteoarthritis
Intertriginous dermatitis
Flat feet

TREATMENT

Except in the rare obese patient with severe psychological problems, weight reduction is uniformly desirable to avert complications and decrease mortality. There is no "standard treatment" that is effective in most or even a large fraction of obese patients, and each weight reduction program is designed to fit the personality, life-style and health status of the patient. Success depends on motivation and behavioral modification through the establishment of reasonable goals and expectations. Crash programs and demands for extreme alterations from established life-styles are uniformly unsuccessful in the long run, and potentially dangerous. Despite this simple and universally accepted approach, permanent weight reduction is a difficult achievement. To paraphrase Mark Twain, "... (dieting) is easy, having done it hundreds of times."

A comprehensive weight reduction program will incorporate components of diet restriction, exercise, counseling, and pharmacological approaches. The critical factor is that caloric expenditures must exceed caloric demands, and that permanent changes in patterns of caloric intake must be achieved to maintain the new weight at the desired level.

Regulation of Caloric Intake

Modest reduction of caloric intake through dieting and setting realistic goals and expectations is the most palatable and easily available method of treatment. A good diet prevents the patient from becoming too hungry and

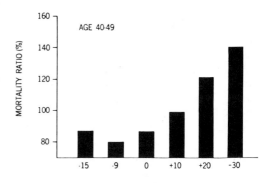

Figure 30.2. Effects of body weight on mortality. The death rate for variations of mean body weight are shown for persons aged 40 to 49 years. (Reprinted with permission from the Metropolitan Life Insurance Company.)

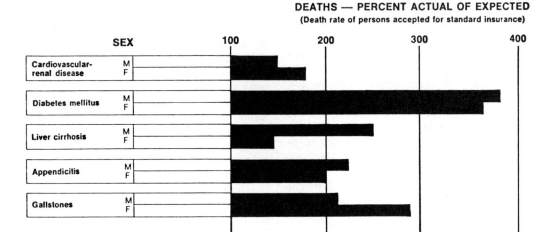

Figure 30.3. Relationship between obesity and serious medical disorders. (Reprinted with permission from the Metropolitan Life Insurance Company.)

noncompliant. Great emphasis should be placed on learning good eating habits and knowing caloric content of food varieties. Patient education is essential for subsequent maintenance of weight loss.

Weight loss should not accrue at a rate of more than 1 kg (2 lb) per week unless in an emergency or unless close medical supervision is involved (3). Any program resulting in weight loss of more than 0.3 kg (0.7 lb) per day is more fluid than tissue loss. During obesity, substantial fluid is sequestered in hydrated body tissues, and during initial caloric deficit an obligatory water loss occurs. This accounts for the accelerated weight loss during the first week or two of dieting. The use of diuretics for weight reduction will exploit this phenomenon, but is both illusory and hazardous (20).

In obese subjects, approximately a 3500-calorie deficit is required to lose 0.5 kg (1 lb) of tissue. To achieve this deficit, a bewildering array of diets have been advocated, each differing in ratios of carbohydrate, fat and protein, and each claiming superiority over all the others. Easy weight loss diets tend to exploit the obese individual who is not ready for a permanent level of change and discipline. Items like dietary drinks offer easy, short-term solutions, but their simplicity and convenience merely put off the essential need to learn about food and food values. Diet books appear with great regularity, and despite their guarantees and initial effectiveness, few effectively induce the permanent solutions of discipline and life-style changes.

All "crash diets" are dangerous in susceptible individuals when applied to extremes. Recent examples include the "Last Chance Diet," which resulted in dozens of fatalities despite medical supervision in many cases (21, 22), and the "Beverly Hills Diet," which promotes nutritional misinformation and can result in severe health problems (23, 24).

With all semistarvation diets, fluid and electrolyte abnormalities, arrhythmias, dehydration, ketoacidosis, hyperuricemia and teratogenesis are potential complications. Crash diets are contraindicated in patients with diabetes, cardiovascular disorders, kidney and liver disease and pregnancy. Total fasting is even more hazardous and is usually a hospital procedure.

Exercise

Dietary management of obesity alone has been called "the rhythm method of girth control." Unquestionably, exercise can be a valuable supplement to dieting. With dieting alone, a patient's basal metabolic rate (BMR) adapts by declining up to 40% in 6 months. On the other hand, exercising increases the BMR rapidly, and this elevation persists for up to 24 hours (25). Thus, regular exercise lessens the adaptive response of the BMR to dieting.

In order for exercise to be useful, it must be regular and of high quality. A regimen of thrice weekly exercise that expends in excess of 300 kcal over at least 30 min is recommended (26). The selection of an activity of moderate intensity and longer duration is important because a longer time-frame favors the utilization of fat stores. Unfortunately, quality exercise is not acceptable to many obese patients. They often turn to "effortless" weight reduction devices, such as mechanical vibrators, inflatable weight-reducing clothing or "spot reducers." As one author noted, these devices are little better than doing nothing, and the primary reduction often occurs in the exerciser's wallet (26).

Psychotherapy

Psychotherapy or behavior therapy can be a valuable adjunct to weight reduction, especially in the massively obese patient who requires help in accepting the seriousness of the problem. For the vast majority of obese individuals, weight reduction groups, such as TOPS and Weight Watchers, provide important psychological support and motivation to bring about permanent weight control measures. Weight Watchers alone claims nearly two million active members.

Appetite Suppressants

Obese patients who are instructed in dietary management and are treated with appetite suppressants lose more weight on the average than patients on diet alone. In a review of over 200 studies of appetite suppressants involving 10,000 patients, pooled data demonstrate an average loss of 0.25 kg (0.56 lb) per week more versus placebo (27). However, since these drugs are typically labeled for use for 2 to 4 weeks only, the average patient will lose only one additional kilogram when they are employed as recommended. When the decision is made to employ appetite suppressants, the patient must realize that improved dietary compliance is the goal of therapy and that diet, not the drug, is responsible for weight loss. Drug use is temporary, and restoration of drug-free dieting through behavior change is the desired outcome.

The routine use of appetite suppressants in the initial phases of a weight reduction program may detract from the importance of dietary/behavioral measures and provide a psychological escape from the need to change lifelong eating habits. A comparison of patients treated with either pharmacotherapy or behavioral therapy indicates that, while pharmacotherapy produces more weight loss, the benefits are short-lived and weight is rapidly regained when the drug is discontinued. At the end of a year of follow-up, patients treated with behavioral therapy alone weigh significantly less than patients treated with drugs alone. Also, combined pharmacotherapy and behavioral therapy produce long-term results which are poorer than if behavioral therapy alone is used (28).

Appetite suppressants are best reserved until after a reducing diet has been established and an unsatisfactory response observed. Their use is also appropriate in patients who reach plateaus after initial success with dieting alone or who relapse after a prolonged period of progress. Unfortunately, drugs are frequently prescribed as initial therapy. Many physicians seemingly cannot resist the pressures placed on them by patients who have invariably experienced failure with do-it-yourself dieting and present to the physician expecting more. Better long-term results could be realized if the physician would lend his esteem and credibility to dietary/behavioral approaches, including vigorous monitoring for compliance, rather than undermining the importance of self-motivated dieting by prescribing appetite suppressants in the initial stages.

Appetite suppressants are thought to exert their effect directly on the hypothalamic satiety center, which is under adrenergic control. Most augment brain catecholamine action except fenfluramine, which acts specifically on serotonin. Fenfluramine and mazindol also affect peripheral energy metabolism, such as triglyceride and glucose uptake and utilization, but the relationship of those effects to appetite suppression is unclear (29). These proposed mechanisms are not universally accepted, however, and many authorities feel the drugs act by inducing euphoria and suppressing appetite as a manifestation of a psychological defect.

Conventional wisdom holds that tolerance develops rapidly to the anorectic effects of these agents, as evidenced by the decelerating weight loss curves with continued use. This belief has led to recommendations that appetite suppressants be limited to short-term use. However, appetite suppressants appear to maintain weight loss as long as they are administered, and discontinuation following long-term use results in a rapid rebound in appetite and weight (30). Therefore, tolerance to the appetite suppressant effects may not be significant at the doses usually employed, and long-term treatment may be plausible for selected patients (31).

Because these agents are reinforcing (i.e., euphorigenic) central nervous system stimulants, their misuse potential is very high. However, misuse of these agents is not associated with anorectic use in motivated, obese patients. Misuse is more a result of indiscriminant prescribing with subsequent diversion for nonmedical, "recreational" use. Among the anorectic drugs, amphetamines account for most of the abuse episodes, and estimates are that over 10% of the legitimately manufactured amphetamines wind up in the hands of abusers (31). Much of the illegal diversion can be attributable to "fat doctors," some of whom prescribe sufficient quantities of amphetamines to initiate between 50 and 60 new patients per day for every day of the year (32). Under conditions of extreme misuse, amphetamines can produce intense psychological dependence and severe social dysfunction, and because there is no difference in efficacy over other anorectic agents in enhancing weight loss, attempts have been made to remove the obesity indication for amphetamines. This would reduce amphetamine production by 90% (31), but deletion of this indication continues to be met with resistance. Since much of the amphetamine abuse is due to indiscriminant prescribing, a ban on their use would most likely result in a compensatory increase in the misuse of the remaining drugs in this class, as has occurred in Canada.

In December 1978, the Advisory Review Panel on OTC Miscellaneous Internal Drug Products found the nonprescription ingredient, phenylpropanolamine (PPA), safe and effective for weight control. The widespread promotion of PPA as the "ultimate diet pill" and its close association with prescription ingredients (e.g., Dexatrim, Dex-A-Diet, etc.) have led to special problems of misuse. PPA is the most common ingredient in "look-alike" counterfeit drugs which are packaged in tablets and capsules to look virtually identical to amphetamines and sold as "legal stimulants."

No superiority has been shown for the appetite-suppressant effects of any of these agents. Thus, drug selection is best determined by side effects and duration of action. Side effects such as restlessness, insomnia, tremors, increased pulse, nausea, diarrhea, constipation, dry mouth and mydriasis are reported with all of these agents. In susceptible patients, elevated blood pressure and cardiac arrhythmias may occur. Recently, pulmonary hypertension has been reported in two patients receiving 120 mg and 160 mg of fenfluramine continuously for 8 months (33).

Product selection is determined by trial and error, using the entire spectrum of chemical classes (Table 30.2). Patients often tolerate an agent from one chemical class better than from another. Also, the duration of action can help determine the best anorectic agent for a given patient. If overeating occurs in the evening, little benefit is derived from morning doses. Likewise, long-acting agents are irrational when dietary indiscretion is limited to a particular time of day. In both instances, short-acting agents are preferred. Patients who overindulge in the evening, but suffer from drug-induced insomnia, may benefit from fenfluramine, which exhibits unique sedating properties (34). Combinations of anorectic agents with other ingredients, such as barbiturates or phenothiazines, probably possess no greater efficacy and exhibit an expanded array of side effects.

Pharmacist dispensing information includes advising the patient about stimulant side effects, dry mouth and possible insomnia. Dry mouth is minimized by sucking on sugarless hard candy. Insomnia from long-acting agents can be minimized by taking the dose early in the day. Patients receiving fenfluramine should be warned about possible drowsiness and additive depressant effects with ethanol or other sedatives. Drug interactions can occur with all of these agents, and the pharmacist should be alert to their concomitant use with monoamine oxidase inhibitors, antihypertensives, tricyclic antidepressants, and even caffeine. Lithium toxicity is reported to be precipitated by mazindol (35).

Appetite suppressants are to be dispensed with caution to pregnant patients. In studies involving amphetamines and morpholines, an increased incidence in oral clefts was noted when the drug was taken during the first 56 days of pregnancy (36).

Bulk Forming Agents

Bulk formers are indigestible hydrophilic colloids which swell when hydrated to give a sense of repletion. Clinical studies have been contradictory especially since use in recommended fashion can actually increase peristal-

Table 30.2.
Drugs Used to Treat Obesity

Drug	Usual Dose (mg)	Frequency of Administration per Day	Drug Enforcement Agency Schedule
I. Phenylethylamines			
A. Amphetamines			
1. Amphetamine sulfate	Tab: 5	1 or 2	II
	Cap: 15	1	
2. Dextroamphetamine sulfate	Tab: 5	1 or 2	II
	Cap: 15	1	
3. Dextroamphetamine HCl	Tab: 5	1 or 2	II
4. Dextroamphetamine tannate	Tab: 17.5	1 or 2	II
5. Amphetamine complex	Cap: 7.5, 12.5, 20	1	II
B. Amphetamine Congeners			
1. Methamphetamine HCl	Tab: 2.5, 5	1 to 3	II
	Long-acting: 5, 10, 15	1	
2. Benzphetamine HCl	Tab: 25, 50	1 to 3	III
3. Phentermine resin	Cap: 15, 30	1	IV
4. Phentermine HCl	Tab: 8	1 to 3	IV
5. Chlorphentermine HCl	Tab: 65	1	III
6. Chlortermine HCl	Tab: 50	1	III
7. Diethylpropion	Tab: 25	1 to 3	IV
	Tab: 75	1	
8. Fenfluramine	Tab: 20	1 to 3	IV
9. Phenylpropanolamine	Immediate release: ≾37.5	1 to 3	OTC
	Long-acting: ≾75		
II. Morpholines:			
A. Phenmetrazine	Tab: 25	1 to 3	II
	Tab: 50, 75	1	
B. Phendimetrazine tartrate	Tab: 35	1 to 3	III
	Cap: 105	1	III
III. Imidazoline: Mazindol	Tab: 1, 2	1	III

tic action (i.e., hunger pangs) (37). Bulk can be achieved through dietary means alone with the addition of high fiber fruits and vegetables. These are less expensive and more palatable means, and should become a part of the patient's lifelong diet anyway.

Gonadotropins

Nealy 30 years ago, it was noted that the distribution of excess fat in obesity resembled the syndrome characterized by human chorionic gonadotropin (HCG) deficiency. Based on this, a vigorous weight reduction scheme was proposed involving daily injections of 125 units of HCG 6 days a week for 40 treatments. The program also included daily consultation, psychological reinforcement and rigid diet restriction with monitoring. The total regimen works but critics feel that its success reflects the enthusiasm of its advocates and the daily patient monitoring. HCG is felt to be little more than a placebo.

Thyroid Hormones

Thyroid has been advocated for the treatment of obesity. Its early use was based on the incorrect observation that obesity was accompanied by an abnormally low basal metabolic rate (BMR). This observation was later shown to be an artifact due to the poor correlation between body surface area and BMR in grossly obese patients (2). Currently, advocates claim that caloric restriction causes a compensatory drop in BMR, and that thyroid hormone may prevent this phenomenon.

Critics argue that very substantial doses of thyroid are required (6 to 14 grains) to even slightly increase BMR, and these pharmacological doses can have deleterious effects in obese patients who are already predisposed to cardiovascular reactions. Long-term, high dose thyroid hormone use is associated with thyrotoxic cardiomyopathy. In addition, increased BMR would have the effect of appetite stimulation. In view of the risks, the consensus is to avoid thyroid in obesity without evidence of thyroid deficiency.

Surgery

Jejunoileal and gastric bypass surgery are employed for massively obese patients. The procedures involve bypassing a significant portion of the small intestine and stomach, respectively. Weight loss with either proceeds slower than with fasting and, unfortunately, may stop quite short of ideal weight. Jejunoileal bypass works by inducing a malabsorptive state and is associated with significant digestive discomfort, nutrient malabsorption, polyarthritis, fatty liver degeneration, oxalate nephrolithiasis, and tuberculosis (1, 4, 38). Gastric bypass surgery produces a decreased gastric reservoir which results in epigastric distress or vomiting when the capacity is exceeded. Gastric bypass may have fewer long-term complications but is technically more difficult and associated with a higher incidence of early postoperative complications. Nevertheless, despite these many complications, surgery remains the only viable solution in selected patients to avoid permanent disability or death.

CONCLUSION

In virtually all cases, obesity is preventable. When it occurs, the cure is uniquely simple and noninvasive. Despite this, a significant fraction of the population is suffering from what can be depicted as a "human energy crisis." This is due largely to the insensitivity of our society to the unfavorable health outcomes associated with sustained obesity and the unwillingness of obese individuals to undertake lifetime treatment (i.e., good dietary habits). Our acceptance of obesity as a benign condition leads to poor motivation and poor patient compliance.

Pharmacists can play an important role in the management of obesity. As has been emphasized, the use of drugs, though temporarily beneficial, can detract from the attainment of permanent solutions. The pharmacist is in a position to put the many components of treatment into perspective, and with educational and reinforcing techniques, assist the obese patient to achieve lasting results.

References

1. Bray GA, Davidson MD, Drenick EJ: Obesity; a serious symptom. *Ann Intern Med* 77:779, 1972.
2. Thorn GW, Cahill GF: Gain in weight; obesity. In *Harrison's Principles of Internal Medicine*, ed 7. New York: McGraw-Hill, 1974, p 232.
3. Mayer J: Some aspects of the problem of regulation of food intake and obesity. *N Engl J Med* 274 (3 parts): 610, 1966.
4. Van Itallie TB, Kral JG: The dilemma of morbid obesity. *JAMA* 246:999, 1981.
5. Danowski TS: The management of obesity. *Hosp Pract* pp 39–46 (April), 1976.
6. Angel A: Pathophysiology of obesity. *Can Med Assoc J* 110:540, 1974.
7. Galton DJ: An enzymatic defect in a group of obese patients. *Br Med J* 2:1498, 1966.
8. Miller DS, Mumford P, Stock MJ: Thermogenesis in overeating man. *Am J Clin Nutr* 20:1223, 1967.
9. Bondy PK: Metabolic obesity? *N Engl J Med* 303:1057, 1980.
10. Newsholme EA: A possible metabolic basis for the control of body weight. *N Engl J Med* 303:400, 1980.
11. Bray GA, Kral JG, Björntorp P: Hepatic sodium-potassium-dependent ATP-ase in obesity. *N Engl J Med* 304:1580, 1981.
12. Anand BK: Nervous regulation of food intake. *Physiol Rev* 41:667, 1961.
13. Celesia GG, Archer CR, Chung HD: Hyperphagia and obesity. Relationship to medial hypothalamic lesions. *JAMA* 246:151, 1981.
14. Schacter S: Obesity and eating: internal and external cues differentially affect the eating behavior of obese and normal subjects. *Science* 161:751, 1968.
15. Karam JH: Obesity: fat cells—not fat people. *West J Med* 130:128, 1979.
16. Stunkard A, Rush J: Dieting and depression reexamined—a critical review of reports of untoward responses during weight reduction for obesity. *Ann Intern Med* 81:526, 1975.
17. Charney E, Goodman HC, McBride M, et al: Childhood antecedents of adult obesity. *N Engl J Med* 295:6, 1976.
18. Edwards LE, Dickes WF, Alton IR, et al: Pregnancy in the massively obese: course, outcome, and obesity prognosis of the infant. *Am J Obstet Gynecol* 131:479, 1978.
19. Sketris I, Lesar T, Zaske DE, et al: Effect of obesity on gentamicin pharmacokinetics. *J Clin Pharmacol* 21:288, 1981.
20. Van Itallie TB, Yang M: Diet and weight loss. *N Engl J Med* 297:1158, 1977.
21. Linn R, Stuart SL: *The Last Chance Diet*. Secaucus, N.J.: Lyle Stuart, 1976.
22. Anon: Protein diets. *FDA Drug Bull* 8:2, 1978.
23. Mazel J: *The Beverly Hills Diet*. New York: Macmillan, 1981.
24. Mirkin GB, Shore RN: The Beverly Hills diet: dangers of the newest weight loss fad. *JAMA* 246:2235, 1981.
25. Straw WE, Sonne AC: The obese patient. *J Fam Pract* 9:317, 1979.
26. Franklin BA, Rubenfire M: Losing weight through exercise. *JAMA* 244:377, 1980.
27. Scoville BA: Review of amphetamine-like drugs by the Food and Drug Administration: clinical data and value judgments, in Bray GA: *Obesity in Perspective*. Washington, D. C.: U. S. Government Printing Office, 1976, pp 441–443.

28. Craighead LW, Stunkard AJ, O'Brien RM: Behavior therapy and pharmacotherapy for obesity. *Arch Gen Psychiatry* 38:763, 1981.
29. Sullivan AC, Comai K: Pharmacologic treatment of obesity. *Int J Obesity* 2:167, 1978.
30. Stunkard AJ: Anorectic agents: a theory of action and lack of tolerance in a clinical trial, in Garattini S: *Anorectic Agents: Mechanisms of Action and of Tolerance.* New York: Raven Press, 1981.
31. Anon: *The Green Sheet* Dec, 5, 1977.
32. Anon: *The Federal Register* 42:55374, October 14, 1977.
33. Douglas JG, Munro JF, Kitchin AH, et al: Pulmonary hypertension and fenfluramine. *Br Med J* 283:881, 1981.
34. Duhault J, Beregi L, deBoistesselin R: General and comparative pharmacology of fenfluramine. *Curr Med Res Opin* 6:3 (suppl 1), 1979.
35. Hendy MS, Dove AF, Arblaster PG: Mazindol-induced lithium toxicity. *Br Med J* 280:684, 1980.
36. Milkovich R, van den Berg BJ: Effects of antenatal exposure to anorectic drugs. *Am J Obstet Gynecol* 129:637, 1977.
37. Drenick EJ: Bulk producers (letter). *JAMA* 234:271, 1975.
38. Bruce RM, Wise L: Tuberculosis after jejunoileal bypass for obesity. *Ann Intern Med* 87:574, 1977.

SECTION 7
Renal Disease

CHAPTER 31

Renal Disease

DANIEL C. ROBINSON, Pharm.D.

The prognosis of patients with renal disease has increased dramatically during the last 2 decades due to numerous technologic advances in the areas of dialysis and transplantation. As of December 31, 1980, the Health Care Financing Administration Office of End Stage Renal Disease reported that 56,240 patients with chronic renal failure were undergoing maintenance dialysis in the United States. Coupled with the several million patients who have forms of renal disease not required dialysis, it can be seen that a thorough understanding of renal disease and its complications is essential to the management of any heterogeneous patient population.

Patients with renal failure frequently have other major medical problems requiring aggressive drug therapy. This chapter will emphasize the medical management of renal failure and its sequelae in addition to the pharmacokinetic adjustment of dosing in renal impairment.

ASSESSMENT OF RENAL FUNCTION

The laboratory parameters used to assess renal function do so through their ability to reflect glomerular filtration rate (GFR). An ideal substance should be freely filtered, not reabsorbed or secreted by the renal tubules, have no effect on filtration rate and be easily quantified in plasma and urine. Unfortunately the three parameters used clinically, blood urea nitrogen (BUN), creatinine, and creatinine clearance are less than ideal (1, 2).

Inulin, a fructose polysaccharide, is recognized as the substance whose clearance most accurately reflects GFR. Inulin clearance has had limited application in clinical medicine since it is an exogenous compound which must be given by continuous infusion and its measurement is not performed by most laboratories.

Hepatic deamination of amino acids liberates ammonia which combines with available CO₂ to form urea. Urea, which is primarily eliminated by the kidneys through glomerular filtration, undergoes reabsorption in the proximal tubule. The extent of reabsorption depends upon the urine flow rate so that 40% of the filtered urea is reabsorbed with diuresis and 60% is reabsorbed with antidiuresis. The normal values for BUN are 10 to 15 mg/dl and may increase to over 150 mg/dl with severe renal failure. The BUN is less accurate than serum creatinine and creatinine clearance in assessing renal function. Its major limitations are related to the number of factors which can alter BUN without changes in renal function (2). Urea production is dependent on protein catabolism and is, therefore, altered by changes in dietary intake, blood in the gastrointestinal tract, steroid induced catabolism, and by the antianabolic effect of tetracyclines—doxycycline being the only exception (3). Since urine flow rates are inversely proportional to the amount of urea reabsorbed, low flow states will elevate BUN disproportionately to changes in serum creatinine. Any factors which lower the absolute or effective blood volume and hence renal blood flow will increase BUN. Table 31.1 lists factors responsible for an elevation of BUN in the absence of renal impairment.

Creatinine production is a function of muscle metabolism which is relatively constant from day to day except in hypercatabolic states, myositis, muscle trauma, extreme exercise, and during prolonged gross motor seizures. Being a function of muscle mass, creatinine production is dependent on body size (surface area) and age. Because creatinine is filtered at the glomerulus and only slightly secreted by the renal tubule, its clearance closely approximates GFR. The normal values for serum creatinine are 0.8 to 1.3 mg/dl for men and 0.6 to 1.0 mg/dl for women.

Normal creatinine clearance is 97 to 140 ml/min for men and 85 to 125 ml/min for women

(4). Creatinine clearance is a derived term which requires a timed (usually 24 hours) and measured urine collection.

$$CL_{cr} = (U_{cr}/P_{cr}) \times V \qquad (1)$$

In the equation CL_{cr} = creatinine clearance in milliliters per minute, U_{cr} = urine creatinine concentration in milligrams per deciliter, P_{cr} = plasma creatinine concentration in milligrams per deciliter measured sometime during the collection period, and V = urine volume per unit time, i.e., total collection volume divided by time of collection express in milliliters per minute. It is important to note that the renal clearance of any measurable substance can be calculated in precisely the same way. A major disadvantage in determining creatinine clearance is the time and personnel required for its collection. A patient or nurse will, on occasion, accidentally omit or discard a voided sample without adding it to the total collection. Any such error, in addition to incomplete bladder emptying, results in underestimates of the patient's actual creatinine clearance. One method of estimating whether the creatinine clearance is valid is to use the creatinine index. If the patient's renal function is stable, creatinine production equals creatinine excretion. Based on data from 936 male and 219 female subjects, the rate of creatinine production (R_{cr}) can be calculated (4):

$$R_{cr} \text{ (mg/kg/24 hours)}$$
$$= 27 - (0.173 \times \text{age}), r^2 = 0.919 \text{ (male)} \qquad (2)$$

and

$$R_{cr} = 25 - (0.175 \times \text{age}),$$
$$r^2 = 0.966 \text{ (female)} \qquad (3)$$

If a 45-year-old 70-kg man with stable renal function produces 1345 mg of creatinine per day and the amount of measured creatinine collected in the urine is significantly less, the collection was probably incomplete and a repeat test should be performed.

Laboratory determination of serum creatinine is based on the alkaline picrate method of Jaffe, with minor modification to accommodate automation and increase specificity. Since this is a colorimetric test other noncreatinine chromogens can result in overestimation of creatinine (1). Some of these agents are reported in Table 31.2. A recent report of "cefoxitin-induced pseudo acute renal failure"

Table 31.1.
Factors Elevating BUN without Renal Impairment

1. High protein diet
2. Febrile illness with catabolism
3. Gastrointestinal bleeding
4. Hypovolemia
   a. Diuretic induced
   b. Hemorrhage
   c. Vomiting and diarrhea
5. Decreased cardiac output
   a. Congestive heart failure
   b. Mycocardial infarction
6. Peripheral vasodilation
   a. Antihypertensives
   b. Bacteremia
7. Steroids—catabolic effect
8. Tetracyclines—antianabolic effect

Table 31.2.
Agents Causing a False Elevation in Serum Creatinine by the Jaffe Method[a]

Acetoacetate	Levodopa
Acetone	Methyldopa
Aminohippuric acid	Phenolsulfonphthalein
Ascorbic acid	Pyruvate
Cefoxitin	Resorcinol
Fructose	Sulfobromophthalein
Glucose	

[a] From R. A. Sherman et al. (5) and D. S. Young et al. (6).

demonstrates that even with the use of more specific techniques new agents may be introduced which can cause gross overestimations of creatinine and lead to the implementation of inappropriate therapy (5). The observation of large elevations in creatinine without appreciable changes in BUN should preclude such overestimations.

A number of formulas are available for calculating the creatinine clearance from serum creatinine. A list of the commonly used methods appears in Table 31.3. An additional method utilizes the rate of creatinine production (R_{cr}) (equations 2 and 3) and the serum creatinine according to the relationship:

$$Cl_{cr} = (R_{cr} \times W \times 0.07)/S_{cr} \qquad (4)$$

Where Cl_{cr} = creatinine clearance in ml/min, R_{cr} = rate of creatinine production in mg/kg/24 hours, W = weight in kg, 0.07 for conversion of concentration units and S_{cr} = serum creatinine in mg/dl (4).

Table 31.3.
Methods of Creatinine Estimation[a]

1. Cockroft and Gault

$$CL_{cr} = \frac{(140 - age) \times weight}{72 \times S_{cr}}$$

CL_{cr} for women $\times$ 0.85

2. Jelliffe

$$CL_{cr} = \frac{98 - 0.8 \,(age - 20)}{S_{cr}}$$

CL_{cr} for women $\times$ 0.90
3. Siersbaek-Nielsen (per nomogram)

[a] From D. W. Cockroft and M. H. Gault (7), R. W. Jelliffe (8), and K. Siersbaek-Nielsen et al. (9).

URINALYSIS (10, 11)

A urinalysis is composed of the following major components.

Appearance. The urine should be clear, not turbid, and usually light yellow in color. Agents which may cause the urine to change color are shown in Table 31.4. Increasing amounts of bilirubin produce colors ranging from yellow-brown to deep olive green. Urine containing old blood, hemosiderin, or myoglobin is brown to black. Small amounts of red blood cells produce a characteristic smokey appearance. Patients with porphyria may void a normal colored urine but the sample may develop a deep purple or brownish color on standing.

pH. The pH of the urine varies between 4.5 and 8 in patients with healthy kidneys. The pooled daily specimen is usually acid (pH 6) leading some to erroneously call urine from 6 to 7 "alkaline." Decreased pulmonary ventilation during sleep causes respiratory acidosis and the development of a highly acid urine. Following meals the urine becomes alkaline for a few hours. Thus, urine pH varies widely depending on the time of collection. Highly concentrated urine is usually strongly acid and may be irritating. When urine stands, the urine becomes alkaline as urea is broken down to ammonia. Tests for pH should, therefore, always be done on freshly voided urine.

Urine which is persistently acid or alkaline may suggest the presence of systemic or urinary tract disease. Conditions associated with persistently acid urine and persistently alkaline urine are listed in Table 31.5.

Concentrating Ability. Specific gravity is the most convenient way of measuring the

Table 31.4.
Drugs Causing Changes in Urine Color Not Related to Disease[a]

Color	Drug
Darkening on standing	Chloroquine Levodopa Methocarbamol (Robaxin) Methyldopa Metronidazole Nitrofurantoin Phenytoin
Red-orange-brown	Anthraquinone laxatives Azulfidine Chlorzoxazone (Paraflex) Deferoxamine Phenazopyridine Phenothiazines Primaquine Rifampin
Blue-green	Amitriptylene Methylene blue Triamterene
Deep yellow	Atabrine Riboflavin

[a] From G. A. Porter and W. M. Bennett (12).

Table 31.5.
Conditions Associated with Persistent Changes in Urine pH

1. Persistently acid urine (pH < 7.0)
   a. Metabolic acidosis due to diabetic ketoacidosis, starvation, severe diarrhea, etc.
   b. Respiratory acidosis
   c. Pyrexia
   d. Phenylketonuria and alkaptonuria
2. Persistently alkaline urine (pH > 7.0)
   a. Urinary tract infections with urea splitting organisms such as *Proteus*
   b. Metabolic alkalosis due to the ingestion of alkali, vomiting, etc.
   c. Following the use of carbonic anhydrase inhibitors, e.g., acetazolamide
   d. Hyperaldosteronism

amount of dissolved solids in the urine; principally urea, sodium, and chloride. In health the specific gravity may range from 1.003 to 1.030. Concentration and dilution of the urine refer to specific gravities greater than or less than 1.010, respectively.

Although not a bedside procedure, the measurement of osmolality is more accurate and less influenced by large dense molecules such as protein and x-ray contrast media. To test concentrating ability the patient is either deprived of water for a number of hours or given vasopressin. Failure to concentrate urine to greater than 800 mOsm/kg water or 1.020 demonstrates decreased concentrating ability. When renal function approaches 20% of normal, the specific gravity and osmolality become fixed and stabilize at 1.010 and 300 mOsm/kg, respectively. The term isosthenuria is used to describe urine which is consistently at 1.010 or 300 mOsm/kg

Protein Content. Less than 150 mg of protein is normally excreted per day. The presence of proteinuria is an important indicator of renal disease. Its evaluation requires a knowledge of factors which cause proteinuria without renal pathology. Nonpathologic or functional proteinuria is transient in nature and usually occurs in young adults. Its occurrence may follow excessive exercise, cold exposure, or posturing such as a sustained lordotic position, or pregnancy which increases pressure within the renal vein. Proteinuria associated with renal disease occurs as a consequence of numerous disorders as listed in Table 31.6.

Nephrotic syndrome is the metabolic and clinical consequence of continued massive proteinuria (2 to 3 g of protein per day). In addition to proteinuria the other criteria for this syndrome include hypercholesterolemia, low serum albumin and edema.

Protein in the urine is measured by sulfosalicylic acid, heat and acetic acid, or dipstick methods. Because of its simplicity, the dipstick method is frequently used as a screening test for proteinuria. Drugs may cause false-positive results with the sulfosalicylic acid and heat and acetic method but not with the dipstick method (Table 31.7) (13).

Glucose and Ketones. Since these are of primary interest in diabetes mellitus the reader is referred to Chapter 27, "Diabetes." Causes of glucosuria other than diabetes may include patients who have undergone a gastrectomy, patients with familial renal glycosuria, preg-

nancy, those with Fanconi syndrome, nephrotic syndrome, Cushing's syndrome, following the injection of or endogenous liberation of epinephrine, and infection.

Cells and Casts. Normal urine contains a small number of red blood cells, white blood cells and hyaline casts. Casts are cylindrical elements with parallel sides which derive their shape and size from the tubular segment in which they were formed. They are formed from Tamm-Horsfall mucoprotein, a product of the renal tubules. Factors favoring cast formation are an acid pH, highly concentrated urine, proteinuria, and stasis within the tubules. The transparent hyaline casts are composed entirely of protein. Cellular casts represent red blood cells, white blood cells or renal epithelial cells trapped within the protein matrix. Granular casts represent degraded cellular casts and usually indicate renal parenchymal damage. Tables 31.8 and 31.9 list the cells and casts found in urine along with their significance.

CHRONIC RENAL FAILURE (14, 15)

Definition

Chronic renal failure is a progressive deterioration in renal function indicated by a rise in BUN and serum creatinine, a decline in creatinine clearance, and the development of uremic symptoms. Uremia refers to the symptom complex associated with severe renal impairment which may take from months to

Table 31.6.
Diseases Associated with Proteinuria

Amyloidosis
Systemic lupus erythematosus
Diabetic glomerulosclerosis
Multiple myeloma
Glomerulonephritis
Pyelonephritis

Table 31.7.
Causes of False Reactions in Some Protein Tests[a]

Conditions or Drugs	Methods		
	Heat and acetic acid	Sulfosalicylic acid	Albustix or Combistix
Highly buffered alkaline urine	−	−	−
p-Aminosalicylic acid in urine with preservatives	+	+	N
X-ray contrast media	+	+	N
Penicillin in high concentration	+	+	N
Sulfisoxazole metabolites	N	+	N
Tolbutamide metabolites	+	+	N

[a] False positive (+), false negative (−), not affected (N).

Table 31.8.
Cells Found in Urine

Cell	Normal Values	Clinical Importance
Red	0–2/HPF[a]	Genitourinary (GU) tract disorders; various systemic diseases; drugs—aspirin, anticoagulants
White	0–5/HPF	Urinary tract infections
Renal epithelial (nonsquamous)	0–2/HPF	Tubular damage; drugs—aspirin
Bacteria	Sterile	Urinary tract infection (10^5)
Oval fat bodies[b]	None	Nephrotic syndrome, diabetic glomerulosclerosis
Squamous epithelial	Occasional	Contamination from outer GU tract

[a] HPF, high power field.
[b] Renal tubular epithelial cell filled with fat.

Table 31.9.
Casts Found in Urine[a]

Cast	Clinical Importance
Hyaline	Few seen normally
Granular	Renal parenchymal disease, dehydration
Fatty	Nephrotic syndrome, diabetic glomerulosclerosis
Red cell	Glomerulonephritis, systemic lupus erythematosus, subacute bacterial endocarditis
White cell	Pyelonephritis
Epithelial cell	Tubular damage

[a] Casts originate from the distal tubules and therefore their presence indicates kidney involvement.

years to develop. A list of complications of chronic renal failure is provided in Table 31.10. Although the concentration of urea can be correlated with the degree of renal impairment, no specific uremic toxins have been identified as being responsible for all of the complications of the uremic syndrome. Other uremic toxins which have been identified include ammonia, guanidine, guanidinosuccinic acid, methylguanidine and myoinositol.

Etiology

The causes of chronic renal failure are multiple and can be divided into those originating in the kidney, those caused by systemic disease and those caused by drugs or chemicals. For a complete listing see Table 31.11.

Kidney damage which leads to chronic renal failure is generally irreversible; however, potentially reversible factors which further compromise kidney function can be identified and corrected. Some of these reversible factors are listed in Table 31.12.

Table 31.10.
Complications of Chronic Renal Failure

Sodium and water balance
Acid-base balance
Potassium balance
Anemia
Hemostatic defects
Calcium and phosphate abnormalities
Hyperuricemia
Carbohydrate abnormalities
Hypertension
Gastrointestinal problems
Neuromuscular disturbances

Table 31.11.
Etiology of Chronic Renal Failure

I. Those originating in the kidney
  A. Glomerulonephritis
    1. Acute
    2. Chronic
    3. Rapidly progressive
  B. Ischemic renal disease
    1. Bilateral renal artery stenosis
    2. Bilateral fibromuscular hyperplasia
  C. Urinary tract infection: Pyelonephritis
  D. Congenital anomalies
    1. Polycystic kidneys
    2. Medullary cystic disease
    3. Hypoplastic kidneys
II. Those caused by systemic diseases
  A. Diabetes
  B. Hypertension
  C. Systemic lupus erythematosus
  D. Polyarteritis nodosa
  E. Amyloidosis
  F. Chronic hypercalcemia
  G. Hyperuricemia
III. Those caused by drugs or chemicals
  A. Analgesic abuse
  B. Heavy metal poisoning
  C. Methysergide-retroperitoneal fibrosis
  D. Milk-alkali syndrome

Table 31.12.
Reversible Factors Causing Further Renal Function Impairment

1. Hypovolemia
2. Obstructive uropathy
3. Urinary tract infection
4. Congestive heart failure
5. Hypertension
6. Hypercalcemia
7. Hyperuricemia
8. Hypokalemia
9. Drugs
   a. Diuretics—volume depletion
   b. Antihypertensives—renal hypoperfusion
   c. Obstruction—sulfonamide crystalluria
   d. Nephrotoxins—methicillin, gentamicin, cephaloridine

Complications and Treatment

Of the numerous complications of chronic renal failure listed in Table 31.10 only the most common and clinically relevant factors will be discussed here. It is noteworthy that the majority of patients who have greater than 25% of normal renal function will have few if any symptoms due to the tremendous adaptive abilities of the failing kidneys.

Sodium and Water Balance

When creatinine clearance falls to less than 25 ml/min the kidney's ability to handle wide fluctuations in sodium and water intake is lost. If placed on a low sodium diet a majority of patients will be unable to reduce urine sodium excretion to match sodium intake resulting in hyponatremia. Some patients, usually with interstitial nephritis, medullary or polycystic kidney disease may require excessive sodium intake to maintain sodium balance.

Most patients with significant renal impairment will have an impaired ability to concentrate and dilute their urine. Nocturia is an early indicator of renal impairment since the kidney's ability to concentrate urine in response to the normal diurnal variation in antidiuretic hormone secretion is lost. A normal daily solute load of 600 mOsm can be excreted in 500 ml of urine if the urine can concentrate to 1200 mOsm per liter. The patient with renal impairment who is unable to concentrate urine greater than 300 mOsm per liter would require 2 liters of urine to excrete the same osmolar load. It can be seen that fluid restriction in such a patient would result in retention of normally excreted solutes such as urea and creatinine.

Acid-Base Balance

Metabolic acidosis is a common finding in advanced renal failure. Normal kidneys are responsible for excreting 60 to 70 mEq of hydrogen daily. The renal failure patient excretes 30 to 40 mEq per day resulting in a positive hydrogen ion balance, most of which is probably buffered by bone salts. Since hydrogen is a product of metabolism little can be done to control daily intake. When acidosis occurs, treatment consists of administering 20 to 30 mEq of sodium bicarbonate or sodium citrate daily.

Potassium Balance

Even though potassium is almost exclusively excreted in the urine, hyperkalemia rarely occurs in patients who have a GFR above 5 ml/min in the absence of acute changes in potassium load. This balance is maintained by increased potassium secretion in the distal renal tubule and increased fecal potassium losses. Factors which jeopardize this balance include the administration of potassium sparing diuretics such as spironolactone and triamterene, increased potassium intake, and acidosis which shifts potassium from the intracellular compartment.

Treatment of hyperkalemia depends on the serum potassium level and the absence or presence of electrocardiographic changes consistent with hyperkalemia. If peaked T waves, widened QRS complexes, prolonged P-R interval or absent P waves are noted therapy is begun with 5 to 10 ml of 10% calcium gluconate. This intravenous injection may be repeated in 5 to 10 min in order to provide 1 to 2 hours of protection from the electrical consequences of hyperkalemia. Since calcium does not effect serum potassium levels other measures must be instituted.

Sodium bicarbonate 50 mEq injected intravenously will increase serum pH which favors the intracellular movement of potassium. This may be repeated as needed to maintain a slightly alkaline serum pH.

A solution containing 2 g of glucose for every unit of regular insulin will also cause an intracellular shift of potassium. A typical solution might consist of 500 ml of 10% glucose with 25 units insulin to run over 4 hours. Sodium bicarbonate may also be added to this solution for continuous infusion. Careful monitoring is needed to avoid fluid and sodium overload with these regimens.

Since each of the above regimens have no effect on total body potassium and their effects are transient, a cation exchange resin (Kayexalate) given by retention enema is often needed to provide a sustained effect. Kayexalate, 50 g in 200 ml of 20% sorbital, retained for 30 to 60 min will lower serum potassium by approximately 1 mEq/liter. The enema is repeated as needed.

Calcium and Phosphorus Abnormalities (16)

At creatinine clearances below 25 ml/min urinary phosphorus excretion diminishes slightly. The modest elevation in serum phosphorus causes a reduction in ionized calcium which stimulates parathyroid hormone (PTH) production. An increase in PTH tends to normalize serum calcium by increasing calcium resorption from bone. In addition, PTH enhances renal tubular phosphorus excretion. The net effect is a relative normalization of phosphorus and calcium with a slight but significant increase in circulating PTH. As renal function further declines the kidney's ability to increase phosphorus excretion is impaired. A sustained elevation in serum phosphorus inhibits the renal conversion of 25-hydroxy-cholecalciferol (25-HCC) to 1,25-dihydroxy-cholecalciferol (1,25-DHCC) which results in impaired intestinal calcium absorption and bone resistance to PTH.

There are numerous skeletal abnormalities which result from disturbances in calcium and phosphorus metabolism secondary to chronic renal failure. These bone abnormalities can be collectively referred to as renal osteodystrophy. The management of renal osteodystrophy is aimed at keeping calcium and phosphorus near normal, suppression of PTH secretion, and improvement in skeletal metabolism. Early conservative management consists of restricting dietary phosphorus through reduction of high phosphorus-containing foods such as meat, milk, legumes and carbonated beverages or the use of phosphate-binding antacids. The phosphate binding capacity of antacids depends on their aluminum content. Those which are most often used are aluminum carbonate (Basaljel) and aluminum hydroxide (Amphojel or Alternajel). Given with or immediately following meals and at bedtime they complex dietary phosphorus or phosphorus contained in gastrointestinal secretions preventing absorption. Periodic measurement of phosphorus is necessary to titrate antacids and prevent hypophosphatemia.

Hypocalcemia, if present, may be treated with oral calcium supplements. A total daily calcium intake of 1 to 1.5 g may be provided in divided doses of calcium gluconate (9% Ca), calcium carbonate (40% Ca), or calcium lactate (13% Ca). Therapy should not be instituted unless serum phosphorus is less than 5.5 to 6 mg/dl. A calcium-phosphorus product (Ca × P) greater than 70 must be prevented in order to avoid soft tissue calcification.

In the event that serum calcium and PTH cannot be normalized with more conservative regimens a trial of vitamin D is warranted. Of the many vitamin D congeners available the newer potent form, 1,25-DHCC (Calcitriol), offers an advantage over ergocalciferol (Vit D_2) and cholecalciferol (Vit D_3) in that it has a shorter onset and duration of action. The potential for vitamin D intoxication and sustained hypercalcemia, which may require weeks for resolution, is a major hazard associated with pharmacologic doses of Vit D_2 and Vit D_3. If vitamin D intoxication occurs with the use of 1,25-DHCC it is rapidly corrected upon discontinuing therapy.

Platelet and Bleeding Abnormalities

Bleeding is a frequent complication of uremia manifested by ecchymosis, purpura, gastrointestinal bleeding and epistaxis. Capillary fragility and coagulation factor defects do not appear to play a major role. Quantitative and qualitative platelet abnormalities are presumed to be causative in the majority of patients. Although severe thrombocytopenia (less than 50,000/mm³) is rare, minor deficiencies (less than 150,000/mm³) have been noted in over half of those studied. Platelet factor 3 is reduced and platelet aggregation is inhibited in advanced renal failure, resulting in prolonged bleeding times and poor clot retraction. It is possible that uremic toxins are responsible for these abnormalities. Treatment for severe bleeding requires the administration of fresh platelet concentrates. Prevention depends on adequate treatment of the uremic state with hemo or peritoneal dialysis. Patients are told to avoid all drugs having anti-platelet activity and particularly aspirin.

Anemia (17)

Most patients with chronic renal failure will develop anemia. The anemia is normochromic and normocytic in nature and rarely does the hematocrit fall below 20%. In the absence of congestive heart failure and angina the anemia is usually well tolerated. The anemia is caused by a number of factors which are listed in Table 31.13. The earliest clinical signs are pallor and fatigue which occur when serum creatinine exceeds 3 mg/dl.

Treatment consists of replacing deficiencies such as folic acid with daily vitamin supplements and adequate oral nutrition. Iron deficiency should be treated with oral ferrous sulfate, 300 mg, 3 times daily, or parenteral iron in patients with gastrointestinal intolerance. A regular dialysis schedule will improve the anemia of uremia, often circumventing the need for blood transfusions.

Carbohydrate Abnormalities (18–20)

Most chronic renal failure patients (70%) have some degree of glucose intolerance as evidenced by elevated postprandial blood glucose even though fasting glucose levels are often normal. A major mechanism appears to be peripheral resistance to circulating insulin.

The kidney plays a major role in the metabolism and excretion of insulin. Thirty to forty percent of the insulin reaching the kidneys is cleared by this organ. In severe renal failure the insulin half-life is prolonged and the insulin requirements of uremic diabetes may be decreased. Insulin, however, remains the treatment of choice in the management of diabetes associated with chronic renal failure. In

Table 31.13.
Causes of the Anemia of Chronic Renal Failure

1. Decreased erythropoietin activity
2. Shortened red blood cell life span
3. Gastrointestinal blood loss
4. Due to dialysis:
   a. Iron deficiency from dialyzer blood loss
   b. Folic acid deficiency from dialyzer losses
   c. Red cell destruction from hemolysis
   d. Splenic sequestration

the rare event that oral hypoglycemic agents must be used, tolbutamide is the drug of choice. It has a relatively short half-life which is not increased with renal failure (see Chapter 27, "Diabetes").

Hyperuricemia (21, 22)

An elevated serum uric acid due to impaired renal excretion is commonly observed in chronic renal failure. The degree of hyperuricemia correlates with the severity of renal dysfunction. Serum urate levels are usually maintained within normal limits until the creatinine clearance falls below 30 ml/min. Urate levels may rise well above 20 mg/dl with severe renal failure. Complications which arise from hyperuricemia are gouty attacks and arthritis, uric acid stones, and urate disposition nephropathy. For unknown reasons chronic renal failure patients rarely develop gout unless they have a history of primary gout. The association between hyperuricemia and progressive renal disease due to urate deposition is also unclear. There is little evidence that deterioration of renal function occurs more rapidly in hyperuricemic patients than in nonhyperuricemia patients. Treatment is, therefore, aimed at those with a history of gouty attacks and those with evidence of urate stones.

In patients with adequate renal function management consists of liberal fluid intake to reduce renal urate concentration and the maintenance of a urinary pH between 6.0 and 6.5. Greater alkalinization favors calcium phosphate crystallization. In the absence of a response to the above measures or in patients unable to tolerate additional fluids, allopurinol is begun at 200 to 300 mg/day. Since allopurinol and its major metabolite oxypurinol accumulate in renal failure a fair number of patients will be controlled on smaller doses. Patients with essentially no renal function who require dialysis may be controlled sufficiently without allopurinol since uric acid is partially dialyzed.

Hypertension

The kidney plays a major role in the control of blood pressure through regulation of the extracellular fluid volume and the renin-angiotensin system. It is often difficult to determine whether the hypertension or the renal failure came first; however, the aggressive treatment of hypertension can improve long-term survival by limiting renal vascular injury.

Since extracellular volume expansion is a major cause of hypertension in those with impaired renal function, diuretics are used initially. Because thiazide diuretics are ineffective at creatinine clearances less than 20 to 30 ml/min, furosemide is the preferred agent. The dose can range from 40 to over 200 mg/day. In those with end stage renal failure, dialysis is an effective means of removing extracellular fluid and may obviate the need for diuretics.

Antihypertensive therapy at this point includes the use of methyldopa, propranolol, prazosin, or clonidine. Each of these drugs is capable of lowering renin release without compromising renal blood flow. Hydralazine may be combined with methyldopa, clonidine, or propranolol for further blood pressure control. In patients unresponsive to the above regimens, minoxidil is given with propranolol and furosemide. This combination has been effective in controlling blood pressure regardless of the degree of renal failure.

Gastrointestinal Disorders

Gastrointestinal complications such as anorexia, nausea and vomiting are common in patients with advanced renal failure. They frequently complain of a metallic or salty taste and their breath smells of ammonia or urine. They may develop stomatitis, parotitis, erosive gastritis, uremic colitis, and mucosal and submucosal ulcerations.

Uremics have salivary urea concentrations which undergo conversion to ammonia in the presence of bacterial ureases. Many symptoms are due to the irritative effects of ammonia on the GI tract.

Antacids are frequently administered to patients with GI irritation. When the creatinine clearance falls below 30 ml/min, magnesium-containing antacids should be restricted. If magnesium-containing antacids are given in chronic renal failure serum magnesium levels may rise above 6 mEq/liter causing depression of the central nervous system, lethargy, somnolence and depressed deep tendon reflexes. Dialysis effectively removes magnesium and may be indicated if severe toxicity develops.

ACUTE RENAL FAILURE (23–28)
Definition

The term acute renal failure is defined as a sudden decline in renal function accompanied by an accumulation of nitrogenous wastes normally excreted by the kidney. It is caused by a process within the kidney itself and is not reversed by correction of extrarenal factors. Urine volume may vary over a wide range. A urine volume less than 50 ml/day constitutes anuria. If the urine volume is less than 400 ml but greater than 50 ml/day, it is described as oliguria. Urine volumes which exceed 400 ml/day are referred to as nonoliguric or high output acute renal failure. It has been demonstrated that up to 50% of drug-induced acute renal failure is nonoliguric (28). Acute renal failure should be distinguished from acute tubular necrosis. Acute tubular necrosis is a histologic finding signifying necrotic damage to the renal tubules and not all patients developing acute renal failure exhibit tubular necrosis on renal biopsy. Unfortunately, these terms are often used interchangeably.

Etiology

Prerenal azotemia is caused by factors leading to decreased renal perfusion or intense renal vasoconstriction (Table 31.14). Postrenal azotemia is simply an accumulation of nitrogenous wastes secondary to obstruction of urine flow in the urinary tract (Table 31.15). Acute renal failure has been associated with numerous surgical and medical insults (Table 31.16).

Table 31.14.
Causes of Prerenal Azotemia

1. Hypovolemia
   a. Blood loss
   b. Vomiting, diarrhea
   c. Diuretic overuse
   d. Burns
2. Peripheral vasodilation
   a. Bacteremia
   b. Antihypertensive drugs
3. Decreased cardiac function
   a. Myocardial infarction
   b. Congestive heart failure
   c. Pulmonary embolism
4. Increased renal vascular resistance
   a. Anesthesia
   b. Surgery

Table 31.15.
Causes of Postrenal Azotemia

I. Bilateral ureteral obstruction
   A. Intraureteral
      1. Blood clots
      2. Stones
      3. Crystals (e.g., sulfonamides)
      4. Papillary necrosis (e.g., analgesics)
      5. Acute pyelonephritis
   B. Extraureteral
      1. Tumor
      2. Retroperitoneal fibrosis (e.g., methysergide)
II. Bladder neck obstruction
   A. Mechanical
      1. Bladder infection
      2. Prostatic hypertrophy
      3. Bladder carcinoma
   B. Functional
      1. Autonomic insufficiency (e.g., diabetes)
      2. Ganglionic blockers
      3. Anticholinergics
III. Urethral Obstruction

Table 31.16.
Causes of Acute Renal Failure

1. Sequelae of prolonged prerenal failure
2. Nephrotoxins
   a. Heavy metals
   b. Radiographic contrast media
   c. Antibiotics (e.g., aminoglycosides)
3. Ischemic disorders
   a. Massive hemorrhage
   b. Crush injury
   c. Transfusion reaction
   d. Septic shock
   e. Pregnancy
4. Glomeruli and small blood vessel diseases
   a. Acute poststreptococcal glomerulonephritis
   b. Subacute bacterial endocarditis
   c. Malignant hypertension
   d. Systemic lupus erythematosus
   e. Drug-induced vasculitis (e.g., allopurinol)
5. Other causes
   a. Hyperuricemia
   b. Hypercalcemia

Some specific drug-induced nephropathies will be discussed separately.

In a patient who suddenly develops oliguria and a rising BUN and serum creatinine, it is important to distinguish between (1) acute renal failure, (2) pre-renal azotemia, and (3) post-renal azotemia. Initial efforts should be directed toward ruling out urinary tract obstruction. Factors implicating obstruction include a normal urinalysis, rapid changes in urine output and residual urine on post-voiding catheterization. If renal calculi are present, a radiograph of the abdomen will detect the 90% that are radiopaque.

In the absence of obstruction the use of urinary indices provides the most reliable method of distinguishing pre-renal azotemia from acute renal failure. Table 31.17 will help in distinguishing pre-renal from acute renal failure but its usefulness would be limited following the administration of diuretics or in those with underlying chronic renal failure.

Treatment

The treatment of acute renal failure depends on the prevention of complications associated with acute renal failure. Infection and GI bleeding are complications which frequently plague the very ill patient in an acute care setting. Careful maintenance of intravenous lines, minimal use of indwelling bladder cath-

Table 31.17.
Urinary Findings in Pre-renal Azotemia and Acute Renal Failure [a]

	Pre-renal Azotemia	Acute Renal Failure
Urine sodium concentration (mEq/L)	<20	>40
Urine osmolality (mOsm/kg)	>500	<400
Urine/plasma creatinine (U/P creat.)	>40	<20
Renal failure index $\dfrac{U(Na)}{U/P(creat.)}$	<1	>2
Fractional excretion of sodium $\dfrac{U/P(Na) \times 100}{U/P(creat.)}$	<1	>1
Urine sediment	Normal	Granular casts Cellular debris

[a] Adapted from C. H. Espinel and A. W. Gregory (23), R. W. Schrier et al. (24), and R. W. Schrier (26).

eters and early recognition and treatment of wound and other infections is necessary. Surveillance for signs of blood loss such as testing stools for occult blood, monitoring of the hematocrit and control of gastric pH with H_2

blockers or antacids will minimize the morbidity associated with bleeding.

The early use of dialysis in the management of acute renal failure has been associated with increased survival. A small prospective study of Viet Nam casualties had demonstrated that patients whose BUN is maintained below 50 mg/dl and whose serum creatinine is maintained below 5 mg/dl have a mortality rate of 37%, whereas those given dialysis with a BUN greater than 120 mg/dl and serum creatinine greater than 10 mg/dl had a mortality rate of 80% (29). It is postulated that early dialysis provides a better biochemical environment for fighting infections and wound healing. It is for the same reason that maintenance of adequate nutrition during renal failure has been advocated (30).

Patients with nonoliguric renal failure have a better prognosis, with fewer complications, fewer patients requiring dialysis, and shorter hospital courses than those with oliguric renal failure. Although no carefully controlled studies exist, it is thought by some that the early conversion of oliguric to nonoliguric renal failure with furosemide will improve the patient's outcome (24, 31–33). Once acute renal failure has been established, furosemide administration will not alter the prognosis. Furosemide should not be administered if prerenal azotemia is suspected since it will promote volume depletion and further compromise renal blood flow.

Most patients developing acute renal failure have a complete clinical recovery if early supportive therapy is provided. Some, however, may regain only a fraction of their previous renal function and a few may go on to chronic end-stage renal failure.

DIALYSIS (20, 34, 35)

There are two types of dialysis, peritoneal dialysis and hemodialysis. In peritoneal dialysis a catheter is inserted into the peritoneal cavity. Dialysis fluid is then instilled and allowed to equilibrate and is then drained and replaced cyclically with fresh dialysate. In this type of dialysis the peritoneal membrane acts as the diffusion membrane. A significant complication of this form of dialysis is infection of the peritoneum; however, peritoneal dialysis can be initiated very rapidly in acute situations and is available in most hospitals. Hemodialysis requires the placement of an arteriovenous shunt (external) or fistula (internal)

for access to the systemic circulation. Arterial blood is routed to the artificial kidney (coil) where diffusion takes place through a thin Cuprophan membrane into the dialysate. The blood then returns through the venous blood line. Hemodialysis is more complicated than peritoneal dialysis and is available at hospitals where appropriate personnel and facilities are available. The complications of hemodialysis include infection at the access site, hepatitis, blood loss and air embolism. Anticoagulation with heparin is required during dialysis to prevent clotting in the membrane and tubing.

The length of the hemodialysis procedure is usually about 5 to 6 hours, 2 to 3 times per week. Peritoneal dialysis takes longer, usually 12 hours. In order to reduce the cost and inconvenience of dialysis, patients are being trained to dialyze themselves at home. This is not only easier for the patient, but is considerably less expensive. Chronic renal failure patients on hemodialysis experience considerable morbidity and mortality; the 5-year survival rate is 55 to 85%.

The principle of dialysis is the transfer of solute across a dialyzing membrane from an area of high concentration (patient's blood) to an area of low concentration (dialysate fluid). Waste products of metabolism such as urea and creatinine as well as a variety of other toxins are thus removed from the body. High molecular weight compounds which accumulate in uremic patients are not cleared well due to limitations in membrane permeability. Hemodialysis is considered more efficient than peritoneal dialysis, but the latter method is capable of removing larger molecules such as proteins.

The use of dialysis has significantly improved the prognosis for patients with end-stage renal disease who would otherwise die from uremia. Although it can sustain life, it is not a total substitute for a real kidney which performs a variety of endocrine functions in addition to its role of eliminating waste products and maintaining homeostasis.

TRANSPLANTATION (20)

Renal transplantation is a widely employed method of treatment for the patients with end-stage renal disease. Donors come from two groups, cadavers and live related (mother, father, brother or sister). Survival is generally greater in live-related transplants (70% 2-year graft survival) than in cadaver transplants

(50% 2-year graft survival), due to better antigen matching. Patients are given daily doses of the immunosuppressive drugs azathioprine and prednisone to suppress rejection. This regimen may result in leukopenia, cushingoid features, GI ulcers, pancreatitis, cataracts, aseptic necrosis of the hips and hyperglycemia. The patients are immunosuppressed and have a high susceptibility to develop infections caused by a wide spectrum of organisms. The infections are often caused by Gram-negative bacteria and the primary drugs useful against these are the aminoglycosides and/or cephalosporins which may cause nephrotoxicity. Fungal infections are also common and treatment with amphotericin B may endanger graft survival due to its nephrotoxic properties.

It is clear that transplantation is not ideal for all patients with end-stage renal disease and that chronic dialysis offers a more appropriate alternative to many patients.

DRUG-INDUCED NEPHROPATHIES (12, 14, 34–37)

In a survey of 11 major teaching institutions it was estimated that in 60% of the nephrology consultations, toxic or drug-induced nephropathy must be considered in the differential diagnosis. It is estimated that 24% of acute renal failure patients and 10% of all renal consultations are associated with nephrotoxins (12). The list of drugs capable of causing renal disease is extensive (Tables 31.18–31.23). Only a few of the drug-related syndromes will be considered in detail here.

Crush injuries have long been known to produce rhabdomyolysis, a destruction of muscle associated with myoglobinuria. Reports of nontraumatic rhabdomyolysis have appeared

implicating myopathies, seizures, strenuous exercise and in particular coma from drug overdose (38). Characteristic findings in these patients have included muscle pain and weakness, muscle swelling, pigmented granular casts and elevated muscle enzymes. Rapid rises in serum creatinine, potassium, uric acid and phosphate have also been observed. Limb ischemia appears to be of primary etiologic importance (39). Intramuscular pressures have been recorded in volunteers who were placed

Table 31.18.
Drugs Causing Glomerular Damage

Gold salts
Hydantoins
Hydralazine
Heavy metals
EDTA
Mercurial diuretics
Oxazolidine derivatives
Penicillamine
Procainamide
Quinidine
Sulfonamides
Allopurinol
Penicillin

Table 31.19.
Drugs Causing Direct Renal Tubular Damage

Aminoglycosides
Amphotericin B
Bacitracin
Capreomycin
Cephalosporins
Colistin/colistimethate
Methoxyflurane
Mercurial diuretics
Mithramycin
Pentamidine
Polymixin B
Radiocontrast Media
Streptozotocin
Tetracyclines
Platinum Compounds

Table 31.20.
Drugs Causing Functional Tubular Defects

1. Nephrogenic diabetes insipidus
   a. Lithium
   b. Demeclomycin
   c. Methoxyflurane
   d. Sulfonylureas
2. Fanconi syndrome: Out-dated tetracycline
3. Renal tubular acidosis
   a. Amphotericin B
   b. Streptozotocin

Table 31.21.
Drugs Causing Acute Interstitial Nephritis

Penicillin analogs (e.g., methicillin)
Azathioprine
Allopurinol
Cephalosporins
Furosemide
Thiazides
Phenytoin
Phenindione
p-Aminosalicylic acid
Rifampin
Sulfonamides

Table 31.22.
Drugs Causing Chronic Interstitial Nephritis

Phenacetin
Aspirin
Acetaminophen

Table 31.23.
Drugs Causing Obstructive Nephropathy

Acetazolamide
Allopurinol
ε-Aminocaproic acid
Calcium salts
Hydralazine
Methotrexate
Methoxyflurane
Methyldopa
Methysergide
Phenacetin
Phenazopyridine
Phenylbutazone
Radiopaque contrast media
Sulfonamides
Tetracyclines
Uricosuric drugs
Vitamin D

in positions common to overdose patients. Pressures were adequate to occlude or compromise muscle blood flow and presumably produce ischemic muscle injury. The result in a comatose patient would be sufficient muscle injury to simulate a crush syndrome with subsequent acute renal failure.

Among all classes of drugs none is more often associated with acute renal failure than the antibiotics. Among the antibiotics aminoglycosides and penicillins play a predominant role.

The study of aminoglycoside toxicity is complicated by the fact that patients requiring aggressive parenteral therapy also have diseases and concomitant drug therapy which can induce acute renal failure (36, 37). It is well established, however, that aminoglycosides are, in themselves, nephrotoxic. Toxicity generally occurs within the first 2 weeks of therapy. Early manifestations include proteinuria, pyuria, cylinduria and enzymuria. Renal concentrating ability may also be impaired. Abnormal urinary findings usually precede elevations in BUN and serum creatinine. Toxicity appears to be related to the extent of renal cortical tissue binding of the drug. Aminoglycosides are concentrated up to 20-fold in the renal cortex. The persistence of drug in the renal cortex probably explains the observation that acute renal failure can occur after the drug is discontinued. Factors which predispose to aminoglycoside nephrotoxicity include advanced age, volume depletion, preexisting renal dysfunction and prior administration of other nephrotoxins. Although the currently used cephalosporins rarely produce nephrotoxicity when administered by themselves the question of synergistic nephrotoxicity with aminoglycosides has been raised. One study which compared an aminoglycoside/cephalosporin combination with an aminoglycoside/methicillin regimen in a randomized fashion found evidence of nephrotoxicity in 12 of 47 (25.5%) of the former group and 3 of 43 (7.0%) of the latter group (40). Both groups were comparable in age, initial serum creatinine, duration of therapy and aminoglycoside

serum level. Caution is, therefore, advised when this combination is given.

Acute interstitial nephritis is characterized by interstitial infiltration and inflammation on renal biopsy. The penicillins as a class and methicillin in particular have been implicated in over 100 cases of acute interstitial nephritis. The lesions are immunologically mediated and may involve both humoral and cell mediated mechanisms (41, 42).

The diagnosis of methicillin-induced interstitial nephritis is based on urinary findings, white blood cell differential and clinical presentation. The onset of symptoms seldom occur prior to the 10th day of antibiotic administration and are heralded by microscopic hematuria (97%), proteinuria (94%), pyuria (93%), eosinophilia (79%), eosinophiluria (100%), fever (87%) and rash (24%). Impairment of renal function may be mild to severe requiring hemodialysis in some cases. Most patients regain full renal function with time. In one series of 14 patients, 8 received prednisone at an average daily dose of 60 mg and recovered baseline renal function within 9.3 days as compared to the non-prednisone-treated group who regained baseline function in 54 days. A trial of steroids appears warranted even though others have not experienced such beneficial results. A list of drugs which have been implicated in causing acute interstitial nephritis is provided in Table 31.21. Among the antistaphylococcal penicillins, nafcillin appears to be safer than methicillin. A recently published prospective analysis of 210 patients receiving nafcillin, including a 6-month follow-up reported no cases of interstitial nephritis (43).

An association between renal papillary necrosis, chronic interstitial nephritis and the ingestion of large amounts of analgesic drugs was first reported in 1953. There appears to be geographic differences in the extent of analgesic induced nephropathy. It has been reported that one third to one half of dialysis and transplant patients in Australia are the result of analgesic abuse. The incidence in the United States is somewhat less. Patients usually have a history of chronic pain such as headache or backpain, which require analgesics. Anemia and GI complaints are common especially in those ingesting aspirin containing products. Obtaining a history for analgesic abuse is difficult since patients typically understate their analgesic consumption or deny it all together. Any patient with a history of ingesting 1 g/day of an analgesic for more than 1 year or a cumulative intake of over 2 kg of analgesic should be considered at risk for developing analgesic nephropathy.

Phenacetin, acetaminophen and aspirin have all been implicated in causing renal disease. The majority of cases involve the use of combination products containing more than one of the above analgesics. Both phenacetin and acetaminophen concentrate in the renal papilla where they can cause oxidative breakdown of erythrocytes and lipid membranes, especially in the presence of inhibitors of the hexose monophosphate shunt such as aspirin.

Renal impairment is insidious in onset. An impaired concentrating ability is often the earliest sign of renal damage, followed by signs of renal tubular dysfunction. Progression to end stage renal failure is inevitable unless analgesic abuse is stopped. An abrupt change in renal function may be the result of sloughed papillary tissue which causes obstruction and acute renal failure.

PHARMACOKINETICS IN RENAL DISEASE

Drugs which are largely dependent on the kidney for elimination are expected to be greatly influenced by changes in renal function. The drugs in Table 31.24 have been divided into sections based on their extent of renal elimination. Drugs which are greater than 85% excreted unchanged by the kidneys will require a major dosing modification in the presence of renal impairment. Those drugs which are 40 to 85% excreted unchanged will require only minor modifications for severe renal impairment. Those drugs which are less than 40% excreted unchanged will generally require no modification regardless of the severity of renal impairment. The following scheme will allow dosing adjustments based on renal function.

A. Dosing in Renal Failure without Blood Levels
1. To calculate dosing weight (DW) (45, 46):
   Ideal body weight (IBW) = K + 2.3 [Ht (inches) − 60]
      where K = 45.5 for women, 50 for men
   If actual body weight (ABW) > IBW then
      DW = (ABW − IBW) 0.58 + IBW
   If ABW < IBW then
      DW = ABW
2. To calculate volume of distribution (V_d):
   $V_d = V_d^* \times DW$
   (*Average from literature expressed as liters/kg)
3. To calculate creatinine clearance (CL_{cr}) from serum creatinine

$$CL_{cr} = \frac{(140 - age)}{72 \times S_{cr}} \times DW \times K$$

   K = 1 for men, 0.85 for women
4. To calculate half-life ($t_{1/2}$)

$$t_{1/2}p = \frac{t_{1/2}}{f\left(\dfrac{CL_{cr}}{CL_{crn}} - 1\right) + 1}$$

   where $t_{1/2}$ = normal half-life
   $t_{1/2}p$ = patient's half-life
   CL_{crn} = creatinine clearance in normal subjects
   f = fraction excreted unchanged (from Table 31.24)
5. To calculate elimination rate constant (K_e)
   $K_e = 0.693/t_{1/2}$
6. To calculate loading dose (LD)
   $LD = C_{pmax} V_d$
   C_{pmax} = desired peak concentration
7. To calculate dosing interval (T)

$$T = \frac{\ln C_{pmax} - \ln C_{pmin}}{K_e}$$

Table 31.24.
Drugs Listed by Fraction Excreted Unchanged[a]

Excretion ≥0.85 (requires modification in renal failure):

Amikacin	0.98	Chlorothiazide	0.92	Methotrexate	0.94
Ampicillin	0.90	Gentamicin	0.95	Pyridostigmine	0.90
Atenolol	0.85	Hydrochlorothiazide	>0.95	Ticarcillin	0.86
Cefamandole	0.96	Kanamycin	0.90	Tobramycin	0.95
Cephalexin	0.96	Lithium	0.95	Vancomycin	>0.90
Cephradine	0.86	Methicillin	0.88		

Excretion 0.40–0.84 (requires minor modification in renal failure):

Acebutolol	0.40	Clonidine	0.62	Neostigmine	0.67
N-Acetylprocainamide	0.81	Dicloxicillin[b]	0.60	Oxacillin[b]	0.55
Amoxicillin	0.52	Digoxin	0.72	Pindolol	0.41
Carbenicillin	0.82	Disopyramide	0.55	Primidone	0.42
Cefazolin	0.80	Doxycycline	0.40	Procainamide	0.67
Cefoxitin	0.78	Ethambutol	0.79	Sulfisoxazole	0.53
Cephalothin	0.52	Flucytosine	0.84	Tetracycline	0.48
Cephapirin	0.49	Furosemide	0.74	Trimethoprim	0.53
Chlorthalidone	0.65	Methyldopa	0.63	Tubocurarine	0.43
Cimetidine	0.77	Nadolol	0.73		

Excretion <0.40 (requires no modification in renal failure):

Acetaminophen	0.03	Ethanol	<0.03	Nitrazepam	<0.01
Acetylsalicylic acid	0.01	Ethosuximide	0.19	Nitroglycerin	<0.01
Alprenolol	<0.01	Hexobarbital	<0.01	Nortryptyline	0.02
Amphotericin	0.03	Hydralazine	0.14	Phenobarbital	0.02
Carbemazepine	<0.01	Imipramine	0.01	Phenytoin	0.02
Chloramphenicol	0.05	Indomethacin	0.15	Prazosin	<0.01
Chlordiazepoxide	<0.01	Isoniazid	0.29	Propranolol	<0.01
Chlorpromazine	<0.01	Isosorbide dinitrate	0	Quinidine	0.18
Clindamycin	0.14	Lidocaine	0.02	Rifampin	0.16
Clofibrate	0.32	Lorazepam	<0.01	Sulfamethoxazole	0.30
Clonazepam	<0.01	Meperidine	0.22	Theophylline	0.08
Diazepam	<0.01	Metoprolol	0.10	Tolbutamide	0
Digitoxin	0.33	Minocycline	0.11	Triamterene	0.04
Doxepin	0	Morphine	0.10	Valproic acid	0.01
Erythromycin	0.15	Nafcillin	0.27	Warfarin	0

[a] Adapted from L. Z. Benet and L. B. Sheiner (44).
[b] These drugs require no modification since their hepatic clearance increases significantly in renal impairment.

C_{pmin} = desired minimum concentration (select a convenient dosing interval, usually every 4, 6, 8, 12 or 24 hours)

8. To calculate maintenance dose (MD)

$$MD = C_{pmax} V_d (1 - e^{-K_e T})$$

select a convenient dose

9. To calculate predicted C_{pmax} and C_{pmin}

$$C_{pmax} = \frac{MD}{V_d (1 - e^{-K_e T})}$$

$$C_{pmin} = C_{pmax} e^{-K_e T}$$

B. *Dosing in Renal Failure with Blood Levels*

10. To calculate K_e using predose and postdose levels (must be at steady state)

$$K_e = \frac{\ln C_{pmax} - \ln C_{pmin}}{T - (T_{post} - T_{pre})}$$

T_{post} = time post-dose level drawn
T_{pre} = time pre-dose level drawn

11. To calculate K_e using two post-dose levels (may be used in both steady state and non-steady state conditions)

$$K_e = \frac{\ln Cp^1 - \ln Cp^2}{TCp^2 - TCp^1}$$

Cp^1 = 1st post dose level
Cp^2 = 2nd post dose level
TCp^2 = time of Cp^2
TCp^1 = time of Cp^1

12. To calculate V_d

$$V_d = \frac{\text{dose } (1 - e^{-nK_eT})}{Cp^1 (1 - e^{-K_eT})} e^{-K_eT^1}$$

$T^1 = TCp^1$ minus time of dose (hours)
n = number of doses

Return to equations 7 to 9 to determine a new dosage regimen and accompanying plasma concentrations.

The above equations are based on intermittent bolus kinetics and are valid in patients with significant renal impairment since essentially no drug is being eliminated during the time of infusion. The dosing of patients who have good renal function should utilize intermittent infusion kinetics which are beyond the scope of this chapter.

References

1. Kampmann JP, Hansen JM: Glomerular filtration rate and creatinine clearance. Br J Clin Pharmacol 12:7–14, 1981.
2. Baum N, Dichoso CC, Carlton CE: Blood urea nitrogen and serum creatinine: physiology and interpretations. Urology 5:583–588, 1975.
3. Neu HC: A symposium on the tetracyclines: A major appraisal. Bull NY Acad Med 54:141–155, 1978.
4. Bjornsson TD: Use of serum creatinine concentrations to determine renal function. Clin Pharmacokinet 4:200–222, 1979.
5. Sherman RA, Eisinger RP, Weinstein MP, et al: Cefoxitin-induced pseudo acute renal failure. Clin Ther 4:114–117, 1981.
6. Young DS, Pestaner LC, Gibberman V: Effects of drugs on clinical laboratory tests. Clin Chem 1975; 21:1D–432D, 1975.
7. Cockroft DW, Gault MH: Prediction of creatinine clearance from serum creatinine. Nephron 16:31–41, 1976.
8. Jelliffe RW: Creatinine clearance: bedside estimate. Ann Intern Med 79:604–605, 1973.
9. Siersbaek-Nielsen K, Hansen JM, Kampmann J, et al: Rapid evaluation of creatinine clearance. Lancet 1:1133, 1971.
10. Kark RM, Lawrence JR, Pollak VE, et al: A Primer of Urinalysis, ed 2. New York: Harper & Row, 1963.
11. Kurtzman NA, Rogers PW: A Handbook of Urinalysis and Urinary Sediment. Springfield, Ill.: Charles C Thomas, 1974.
12. Porter GA, Bennett WM: Toxic nephropathies. In Brenner BM, Rector FC: The Kidney, ed 2. Philadelphia: W.B. Saunders, 1981.
13. Kory M, Waife SO: Kidney and Urinary Tract Infections. Indianapolis, Ind.: Lilly Research Laboratories, 1971.
14. Alfrey AC: Chronic renal failure: manifestations and pathogenesis. In Schrier RW: Renal and Electrolyte Disorders, ed 2. Boston: Little, Brown, 1980.
15. Valtin H: Chronic renal failure: adaptation of balances. In Renal Dysfunction: Mechanisms Involved in Fluid and Solute Imbalance, Boston: Little, Brown, 1979, p 257.
16. Coburn JW, Kurokawa K, Llach F: Altered divalent ion metabolism in renal disease and renal osteodystrophy. In M Maxwell, C Kleeman: Clinical Disorders of Fluid and Electrolyte Metabolism, ed 3. New York: McGraw-Hill, 1980, p 1209.
17. Fried W: Hematologic complications of chronic renal failure. Med Clin North Am 62:1363, 1978.
18. Bagdade JD: Disorders of carbohydrate and lipid metabolism in uremia. Nephron 14:153, 1975.
19. Rabkin R, Simon NM, Steiner S, et al: Effect of renal disease on renal uptake and excretion of insulin in man. N Engl J Med. 282:182, 1970.
20. Gambertoglio JG: Renal disease. In Herfindal ET, Hirschman JL: Clinical Pharmacy and Therapeutics, ed 2. Baltimore: Williams & Wilkins, 1979, pp 466–478.
21. Berger L: Renal function in gout: an analysis of 524 gouty subjects including long-term follow-up studies. Am J Med 59:605, 1975.
22. Lassiter WE: Uric acid and the kidney. In LE Early, CW Gottschalk: Strauss and Welt's Diseases of the Kidney, ed 3. Boston: Little, Brown, 1979, p 1217.
23. Espinel CH, Gregory AW: Differential diagnosis of acute renal failure. Clin Nephrol 13:73–77, 1980.
24. Schrier RW, Gardenswartz MH, Burke TJ: Acute renal failure: pathogenesis, diagnosis and treatment. Adv Nephrol 10:213–239, 1981.
25. Schrier RW, Conger JD: Acute renal failure: pathogenesis, diagnosis, and management. In RW Schrier: Renal and Electrolyte Disorders, ed 2. Boston: Little, Brown, 1980.
26. Schrier RW: Acute renal failure. Kidney Int 15:205–216, 1979.
27. Humphreys MH, Sheldon G: Acute renal failure in trauma patients. West J Med 123:148–153, 1975.
28. Anderson RJ, Linas SL, Berns AS, et al: Nonoliguric acute renal failure. N Engl J Med 296:1134–1138, 1977.
29. Conger JD: A controlled evaluation of prophylactic dialysis in post-traumatic acute renal failure. J Trauma 15:1056, 1975.
30. Blumenkrantz MJ, Kopple JD, Koffler A, et al: Total parenteral nutrition in the management of acute renal failure. Am J Clin Nutr 31:1831, 1978.
31. Brown CB, Ogg CS, Cameron JS: High dose frusemide in acute renal failure: a controlled trial. Clin Nephrol 15:90–96, 1981.
32. Powell HR, McCredie DA, Rotenberg E: Response to frusemide in acute renal failure: dissociation of renin and diuretic responses. Clin Nephrol 14:55–59, 1980.
33. Nierenberg DW: Furosemide and ethacrynic acid in acute tubular necrosis. West J Med 133:163–170, 1980.
34. Gordon A, Maxwell MH: Water, electrolyte, and acid-base disorders associated with acute and chronic dialysis. In MH Maxwell, CR Kleeman: Clinical Disorders of Fluid and Electrolyte Metabolism, ed 3. New York: McGraw-Hill, 1980, p 827.

35. Maher JF: Principles of dialysis and dialysis of drugs. *Am J Med* 62:475–481, 1977.

36. Appel GB, Neu HC: The nephrotoxicity of antimicrobial agents. *N Engl J Med* 296:663–670, 722–728, 784–787 (Parts I–III), 1977.

37. Bennett WM, Plamp C, Porter GA: Drug-related syndromes in clinical nephrology. *Ann Intern Med* 87:582–590, 1977.

38. Koffler A, Friedler RM, Massry SG: Acute renal failure due to nontraumatic rhabdomyolysis. *Ann Intern Med* 85:23–28, 1976.

39. Owen CA, Mubarak SJ, Hargens AR, et al: Intramuscular pressures with limb compression. *N Engl J Med* 300:1169, 1979.

40. Wade JC, Smith CR, Petty BG, et al: Cephalothin plus an aminoglycoside is more nephrotoxic than methicillin plus an aminoglycoside. *Lancet* 2:604, 1978.

41. Appel GB: A decade of penicillin related acute interstitial nephritis—more questions than answers. *Clin Nephrol* 13:151–154, 1980.

42. Galpin JE, Shinaberger JH, Stanley TM: Acute interstitial nephritis due to methicillin. *Am J Med* 65:756–765, 1978.

43. Barriere SL, Conte JE: Absence of nafcillin-associated nephritis. *West J Med* 133:472, 1980.

44. Benet LZ, Sheiner LB: Design and optimization of dosage regimens; pharmacokinetic data. In Gilman AG, Goodman LS, Gilman A: *The Pharmacological Basis of Therapeutics*, ed 6. New York: Macmillan, 1980.

45. Blouin RA, Mann HJ, Griffen WO, et al: Tobramycin pharmacokinetics in morbidly obese patients. *Clin Pharmacol Ther* 26:508–512, 1979.

46. Devine BJ: Gentamicin therapy. *Drug Intel Clin Pharm* 8:650–655, 1974.

SECTION 8
Rheumatic Diseases

CHAPTER 32

Rheumatoid Arthritis

ANDREW L. LEEDS, Pharm.D.

Patients often complain of "rheumatism," chronic pain, and deformity of the musculoskeletal system. Rheumatic diseases encompass those diseases which often share the common symptoms of "rheumatism" at some point in their course. Rheumatoid arthritis, the most prevalent of the rheumatic diseases (Table 32.1), has no known cause and no known cure. Though most prominently displayed in the structures of the joints, it can have profound systemic effects as well, such as weakness, fatigue, fever, and inflammation of other tissues. The goal of therapy is to minimize patient disability by decreasing the severity of symptoms and slowing, correcting or compensating for joint deformities. Therapy should be a coordinated, interdisciplinary effort of drug treatment and nondrug treatment, sometimes including rest, exercise, heat, and/or cooling therapy, and surgery.

EPIDEMIOLOGY

The prevalence of rheumatoid arthritis in the United States is about 1 to 3%. The disease may occur at any age, although its usual onset is between the ages of 20 and 40. It is 2 to 3 times more prevalent in women than men. The prevalence in men increases with age until, after age 50, it is about equal to that of women. There appears to be a genetic predispositon toward the disease, but no predisposition by race or geographic location.

PATHOGENESIS

Rheumatoid arthritis is an autoimmune disease. The antigen stimulating the initial autoimmune response and the genetic mechanism that promotes its development are unknown. Once underway, antigen-antibody complexes presumably activate complement and elicit the release of various mediators of inflammation in the synovial membrane. The inflammation and synovial-membrane destruction continues with the production of granulation tissue, called "pannus," which expands to destroy neighboring cartilage. Although this process is seen most often in joint structures, the same type of process may occur in many other parts of the body as well, such as the lungs, leading to pulmonary nodules, and the subcutaneous blood vessels, leading to cutaneous vasculitis and the occasional formation of rheumatoid nodules.

CLINICAL FEATURES

Inflammation, usually symmetrical, with tenderness, swelling, erythema, and warmth of the proximal interphalangeal joints of the hands and feet, is the most frequent clinical feature. Large joints, such as the knees, hips, and elbows, can also be involved. The arthritis, and the systemic effects of fever, anorexia, weight loss, and fatigue, are subject to spontaneous remissions and exacerbations. With progressing intensity come muscle weakness and atrophy, leading to decreasing grip strength and difficulty walking, depending on the joints involved. Symptoms are more intense upon rising, with complaints of persistent morning stiffness being a hallmark of the disease.

Several laboratory tests may be helpful in the diagnosis and monitoring of the disease. Though no laboratory test is specific for rheumatoid arthritis, erythrocyte sedimentation rate (ESR) is often elevated. Rheumatoid factor (RF), an antibody to γ-globulin, is present in up to 80% of patients with rheumatoid arthritis. Antinuclear antibodies (ANA) titers may also be elevated. A normocytic, normochromic anemia of chronic disease is found, usually in active cases of disease, and albumin levels are often reduced. Abnormal laboratory tests can indicate the presence of other rheumatic diseases and must be viewed in the context of physical signs and symptoms, possibly radiological studies, and patient history.

Table 32.1.
Rheumatic Diseases[a]

Rheumatoid arthritis
Ankylosing spondylitis
Psoriasis
Reiter's syndrome
Systemic lupus erythematosus
Polyarteritis nodosa
Rheumatic fever
Degenerative joint disease (osteoarthritis)
Arthritis associated with inflammatory intestinal disease
Acute bacterial arthritis
Gonococcal arthritis
Arthritis due to tuberculosis
Gout
Serum sickness and drug reactions

[a] From B. S. Katcher (19).

TREATMENT

The goal of treatment is to minimize patient disability. To reach that goal, pain and inflammation have to be reduced, the process of deformity has to be slowed, and patient activities have to be planned and supported to compensate for the disease.

The assessment methods for monitoring treatment range from objective measurement by an observer to subjective observation by the patient. The criteria measure joint inflammation and systemic disease and functional changes due to the ongoing disease. Joint circumference and the number of inflamed joints are useful criteria of articular inflammatory activity. Fatigue and duration of morning stiffness can be used to judge disease activity, as can ESR. Range of motion measurements are used to both identify inflamed joints (passive) and assess joint function. Grip strength and the time taken to walk a standard distance are commonly used to measure patient mobility and activity.

Physical therapy helps to preserve muscle strength and range of motion through a balanced program of joint rest, systemic rest, and exercise. Cooling or warming inflamed joints may increase patient comfort. Surgery, to remove synovial tissue, replace joints, and correct deformity, helps preserve function, as does the intermittent use of splints. Patient education about the disease and its treatment and, if necessary, specially designed appliances and occupational therapy to compensate for deformities and weakness are also very important in promoting patient activity.

DRUG THERAPY

Drug therapy of rheumatoid arthritis is primarily aimed at reducing inflammation. This decreases the pain and sometimes can slow the joint destruction due to chronic inflammation.

Because of the large numbers of people with this disabling and uncomfortable disease, the demand for effective drug treatment is enormous. In response to this demand, there are now several useful drugs available. The choice of drug, as with any treatment decision, should be made only after considering the anticipated risks and benefits of each drug as applied to the individual patient. In most cases of rheumatoid arthritis, drug treatment should be started with a single first-step nonsteroidal anti-inflammatory drug, appropriate for chronic use (usually aspirin), to provide initial relief and to reduce inflammation. Second-step drugs such as gold, penicillimine, and hydroxychloroquine, and steroids most often are added to the basic one-drug regimen, depending on the severity and progression of the disease, and as adjunctive therapy in the treatment of acute exacerbations and complications.

Nonsteroidal Anti-Inflammatory Drugs

The nonsteroidal anti-inflammatory drugs (NSAID) can be classified into two groups, according to their usual use in the treatment of rheumatoid arthritis. Members of one group are used for first-step chronic treatment (Table 32.2). Members of the other group, such as indomethacin and phenylbutazone, sometimes can be used for short-term adjunctive treatment of acute flares of the disease, but their long-term use is associated with a higher prevalence of adverse effects.

The mechanism of action of the NSAID is not completely understood. Their therapeutic effects and some adverse effects may be partially related to their common inhibition of prostaglandin synthesis, but there are other postulated mechanisms as well (1, 2). Benoxaprofen (withdrawn by the manufacturer in 1982), effective in treating rheumatoid arthritis, is a weak inhibitor of prostaglandin synthesis, which implies another mechanism for its theraputic effect (3). Asthmatic attacks, (especially in those patients with the syndrome of bronchial asthma, nasal polyps, and vasomotor rhinitis), and urticaria/angioedema are

Table 32.2.
Nonsteroidal Anti-inflammatory Drugs

Drug (Trade Name)	Approximate Serum Half-Life (hr)	Usual Dosing Interval (hr)	Usual Daily Dosage Range (mg)	Maximum Daily Dose (mg)[a]
Benoxaprofen (Oraflex)[b]	28	24	300–600	600
Fenoprofen (Nalfon)	3	8–12	900–2400	3200
Ibuprofen (Motrin)	2	6–8	900–2400[c]	2400
Naproxen (Naprosyn)	13	8–12	500–750	1000[d]
Piroxicam (Feldene)	50	12–24	20[e]	20
Sulindac (Clinoril)	16	12	300–400	400
Tolmetin (Tolectin)	1	8	600–1800	2000

[a] Manufacturer's recommendation.
[b] Benoxaprofen withdrawn by Eli Lilly & Co., current limited availability by special request. Dosing recommendations listed for information only and may not be currently recommended.
[c] Higher doses usually needed for rheumatoid arthritis.
[d] Maximum daily dose 1250 mg for pain relief.
[e] Long half-life implies that drug should be evaluated at least 2 weeks for therapeutic effect.

two severe types of adverse reactions associated with the NSAID. Asthma may be related to a decrease in certain prostaglandins which promote bronchodilation. Cross-sensitivity, especially of the asthmatic attack type, is a significant risk with other NSAID. They should be used cautiously in patients with bronchial asthma.

Renal function may be transiently decreased by NSAID, especially in patients with underlying renal disease (5).

SALICYLATES

Salicylates have analgesic, antipyretic, and anti-inflammatory properties, all of which are useful in treating rheumatoid arthritis. The most readily available, least expensive, and best known form of salicylate is aspirin, which, barring contraindication, is the drug of choice for the treatment of the disease. Other forms of salicylate, such as choline salicylate, can, in specific instances, have the advantage of causing fewer gastrointestinal problems, but in general aspirin should be the first drug to be tried for treatment.

It must be made clear to patients that the use of aspirin for their rheumatoid arthritis is for its anti-inflammatory effect, not its analgesic effect; and to achieve and maintain its anti-inflammatory effect, they must consume much higher doses than they use for headache, and must do it on a regular basis. Advising patients of ways to minimize gastrointestinal irritation, such as taking the aspirin with sufficient fluids to promote dissolution, is also important.

Therapeutic anti-inflammatory serum salicylate levels are between 15 and 30 mg/100 ml, with a wide interpatient range of levels produced by a given dose. Originally, this level was achieved without measuring salicylate levels, by dosing aspirin just to the point of tinnitus, a ringing or buzzing in the ears, then slightly reducing the dose. Unfortunately, tinnitus is neither always present nor the first sign of toxicity, especially in hearing-impaired patients. The total dose of aspirin needed to maintain a serum level by this method also may be greater than that needed for desired effects, increasing the risk of adverse effects. With the widespread availability and accuracy of serum salicylate determinations, the tinnitus method should not be used.

A reasonable conservative starting dose of aspirin is between 45 and 60 mg/kg daily, divided into 4- to 8-hour intervals. The patient is titrated to the maintenance dose, based on the drug's effects and steady state salicylate levels, measured in 5 to 7 days. Aspirin is rapidly and completely absorbed in 2 to 4 hours, depending on tablet formulation, and is rapidly hydrolyzed to salicylate. Salicylate is protein-bound, but the proportion of salicylate which is bound decreases with increasing salicylate concentration. Put another way, the amount of salicylate that is free to distribute into the tissues and to be renally excreted is greater at higher concentrations.

Salicylate is eliminated by renal excretion of the unchanged drug, and by four metabolic pathways (Fig. 32.1). Two of the four metabolic pathways are saturated at low salicylate concentrations. This can lead to unpredictably

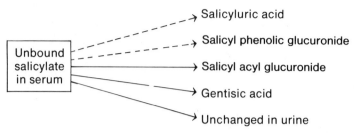

Figure 32.1. High dose salicylate kinetics. The *dotted lines* indicated capacity-limited processes. Protein binding is also capacity-limited and with higher doses the level of unbound salicylate increases, presenting more drug through the pathways depicted by the *solid lines*. (Reproduced from B. S. Katcher (19).)

large changes in concentration from small changes in dose. At therapeutic salicylate concentrations, protein (i.e., to albumin) becomes saturated, and the amount of salicylate free and available for renal excretion increases. Therefore, although the fraction of salicylate eliminated by metabolism decreases at higher concentrations, the fraction excreted by the kidney increases at the same time, and total salicylate clearance tends to remain constant (6). At lower concentrations, before protein saturation, increases in dose lead to greater than proportional increases in concentration. However, at therapeutic blood levels, after protein saturation, in the absence of renal failure, increases in dose tend instead to lead to roughly proportional increases in concentration. However, because of their proximity to toxic levels and interpatient variation, increasing the dose in patients already at higher concentrations still should be done very gradually.

Renal excretion of salicylate is pH-dependent; changes in urine pH may alter salicylate levels. Salicylate is filtered, actively secreted in the proximal tubule, and passively reabsorbed and secreted in the distal tubule. The passive processes are resistant to the passage of ionized molecules. Therefore, if the urine is more alkaline, a higher fraction of salicylate dissolved in it will be ionized and will not be readily reabsorbed, but will be excreted. The effect can be quite important in, for example, patients who are taking regular therapeutic doses of antacids while taking therapeutic doses of aspirin. It has been estimated that a fall in urine pH from 6.5 to 5.5 will cause serum salicylate levels to double (7). Occasional antacid use does not affect urinary pH, but the initiation or discontinuation of therapeutic antacid doses in patients who are also taking therapeutic doses of aspirin may lead to subtherapeutic or toxic salicylate levels.

In monitoring patients on chronic high dose salicylate therapy, a decrease in salicylate concentrations is sometimes observed over time. This decrease may be related to self-induction of metabolism rather than a decrease in compliance (8).

In addition to the adverse renal and antiplatelet effects shared with other NSAID, aspirin has been frequently associated with gastrointestinal blood loss. Aspirin hepatoxicity has been detected by abnormal liver-function tests and by biopsy (9).

Aspirin, and the other salicylates, increase the effect of oral anticoagulants. In addition to the reversible inhibition of platelet aggregation common to the NSAID, aspirin irreversibly acetylates platelets, to irreversibly decrease platelet adhesion. This may lead to elevated bleeding time for 7 to 10 days after a single dose. High doses of aspirin may also affect prothrombin time, especially in the presence of clotting factor deficiency (10). Aspirin should be used with extreme caution in patients with a coagulation disorder, or those who are at risk for bleeding episodes such as surgical patients on anticoagulation therapy (9).

In summary, salicylates, specifically aspirin, are the first choice for the drug treatment of rheumatoid arthritis. Salicylates are commonly associated with gastrointestinal intolerance, especially dyspepsia and nausea, and must be given in multiple doses per day. These problems, in addition to other adverse effects, may preclude its use and prompt the choice of another of the NSAID.

OTHER NONSTEROIDAL ANTI-INFLAMMATORY DRUGS

The other NSAID used for first-line, long-term treatment of rheumatoid arthritis are listed in Table 32.2. All of the drugs listed have been reported to be more effective than placebo, and to have less risk of gastrointestinal intolerance than aspirin. All are absorbed well, reaching peak plasma levels about 2 hours after a single dose.

The currently available propionic acid derivatives are fenoprofen, ibuprofen, and naproxen. Of this group, naproxen can be given twice daily.

Drugs chemically similar to indomethacin include sulindac and tolmetin. Sulindac is the sulfoxide prodrug. It is converted in the liver to two major metabolites, reversibly to the sulfide and irreversibly to the sulfone. The sulfide is the active form of the drug, in that it inhibits prostaglandin synthesis. Sulindac and its metabolites probably undergo enterohepatic recirculation, which contributes to the 16-hour half-life of the active metabolite and allows sulindac to to be given twice daily. It is reported to have fewer gastrointestinal effects, perhaps because the sulfoxide is inactive, and it has fewer central nervous system effects than indomethacin. Tolmetin is another drug that chemically resembles indomethacin, but is therapeutically more similar to the other first-line NSAID.

Piroxicam, at the present time, is the only member of the oxicam group to be approved for use in the United States. With a reported mean half-life of 50 hours, it can be administered once a day. It inhibits prostaglandin synthesis, and has been reported to be better tolerated than aspirin (11). Its safety in chronic use in laboratory animals has also been reported (12).

Indomethacin is effective in treating rheumatoid arthritis, but the doses needed for treatment produce adverse effects which preclude its use for chronic treatment. It sometimes can be useful in the treatment of some other rheumatic diseases. Side effects include headache, dizziness, and gastrointestinal pain and nausea, and sometimes blood dyscrasias.

Phenylbutazone and oxyphenbutazone should be used only for very short-term therapy. They are effective anti-inflammatory agents, but cause sodium and water retention, gastrointestinal intolerance, and can cause potentially lethal blood dyscrasias. They also interact with several other drugs, including oral anticoagulants. The risks involved relative to the other drugs available for treating rheumatoid arthritis preclude their use in other than extraordinary circumstances.

Once the decision has been made to try one of the NSAID listed in Table 32.2, the choice cannot be made on the basis of efficacy alone, since one drug has not been shown to be greatly more efficacious than the others. This does not mean that the use of each of the drugs will lead to identical patient response: there is wide variation in patient response. It has been reported that a drug requiring the fewest doses per day predicted patient and physician preference, with compliance being an important factor (13). It is further suggested that sequential trials of the NSAID are useful, since failure of one does not predict failure of another, due to the wide variation in patient response (13). This implies that the initial trial should be with a drug with a long enough half-life to allow once or twice-a-day administration and, in the event of treatment failure, not limited by adverse side effects, the other drugs could be tried sequentially.

ANTIMALARIALS

Antimalarial agents are a possible second step in treatment added to the NSAID. They have been used since the 1950s, but currently, hydroxychloroquine is the only member of the class approved for treating rheumatoid arthritis, since it may have less ocular toxicity associated with it. It is effective in treating rheumatoid arthritis, but is limited by its mild therapeutic efficacy and its sometimes severe ocular toxicity and minor adverse reactions, especially skin rash, gastrointestinal intolerance, and central nervous system effects.

The usual dose of hydroxychloroquine is 200 mg per day. Before treatment begins, a thorough ophthalmologic examination should be made and repeated every 3 months thereafter. The adverse ocular effects are of two types. The first, more common and less serious, is corneal deposits visible by slit lamp examination. They usually do not affect vision and usually disappear if the drug is discontinued. The corneal deposits may not be an indication to stop the drug, but may be one of the signs associated with the second and most severe toxicity of the drug: irreversible retinopathy.

Retinopathy occurs because hydroxychloroquine binds to melanin, found in high concentrations in pigmented tissue, including the retina. Melanin provides protection from light damage, however, the protection is removed by drug binding. The retinopathy may occur after the drug has been discontinued, since the drug may be bound to melanin for years. The condition is first manifested by retinal edema and can progress to macular degeneration and blindness. Fortunately, retinopathy is relatively rare. Its appearance seems to be associated with the daily dosage level and total cumulative dose given. It is more likely to occur at a cumulative dose greater than 600 g, but may occur at a lower total dose.

The mechanism of action of antimalarial agents in rheumatoid arthritis is unknown. Chloroquin, which preceded hydroxychloroquine in use, is known to suppress chemotaxis, stabilize lysosomal enzymes, and affect other processes involved with inflammation (14).

GOLD SALTS

Gold compounds have been used for treating rheumatoid arthritis for more than 50 years and can be quite useful in patients who tolerate them. Gold salts have been reported to slow progression of joint destruction. Gold therapy is usually best used for patients with active disease of less than 1 year's duration after failure of adequate trials of first-line NSAID.

The two gold salts currently available are gold thioglucose and gold thiomalate. They are given by intramuscular injection, usually starting with a test dose of 10 mg, then increasing the dose at weekly intervals by 10 to 15 mg to a dose of 50 mg per week. A dose of 50 mg is administered per week, up to a total cumulative dose of 1000 mg or until there is a favorable response, at which point the dosage interval is gradually lengthened to every 4 weeks. The onset of therapeutic effect is approximately 3 months; patients should be told not to expect an effect any sooner. If a cumulative dose of 1000 mg is reached without an adequate response, it is likely that gold will not be effective, and a retrial also would fail. The thioglucose salt is associated with fewer vasomotor reactions, such as flushing and dizziness, possibly because it is an oily suspension and is more slowly absorbed than the thiomalate salt. An orally active salt, auranofin, may soon be available in the United States. In addition to the convenience of oral administration, it is reported to have less risk of side effects.

Gold therapy should be discontinued at the first sign of any adverse reaction. It may be possible, based on the severity and type of reaction, to restart therapy, but with great caution. Discontinuance of intramuscular gold therapy due to adverse reactions has been estimated to be between 15 and 50%, usually in the cumulative dose range of 400 to 800 mg. Monitoring for adverse reactions, such as rash and stomatitis, blood dyscrasias, and proteinuria, should be done before each dose and sometimes more frequently, especially when lengthening the dosing interval. The cost of gold therapy is higher because of both the cost of injections and the need for close laboratory monitoring.

Cutaneous reactions are the commonest adverse effect of gold, manifested as oral ulcerations and stomatitis, and as pruritic rashes. These reactions can sometimes be managed by stopping the treatment and restarting it at a lower dose, then gradually increasing it. However, this form of reaction can also progress to exfoliative dermatitis, so rechallenge, though often successful, should be considered carefully.

Blood dyscrasias due to bone marrow suppression are the most serious form of adverse reaction to gold therapy. Aplastic anemia and pancytopenia are rare, but their risk calls for careful monitoring of hematologic values. Thrombocytopenia is much more common; fortunately, it is usually reversible, as is leukopenia associated with gold therapy, but both usually require permanent discontinuation of therapy.

Renal toxicity is another common form of adverse reaction to gold therapy. Transient trace proteinuria sometimes occurs, but proteinuria greater than 1000 mg/24 hours requires discontinuation of the drug (14). Nephrotic syndrome can occur, but is usually reversible when gold is discontinued. Proteinuria can continue for months after discontinuation.

Hepatitis, colitis, peripheral neuropathy, and pneumonitis have also been associated with gold therapy, but, fortunately, are very rare.

The mechanism of action of gold therapy in rheumatoid arthritis is unknown. It may be related to the action of gold on macrophages which are important in the development and maintenance of the immune response. Gold decreases the phagocytic activity and stabilizes the lysosomal enzyme of macrophages.

PENICILLAMINE

Penicillamine resembles the amino acid cysteine. Its first medicinal use was a chelating agent to promote the elimination and decrease the absorption of metals. Its efficacy in treating rheumatoid arthritis is approximately that of gold therapy, and, like gold, it may take months to see its maximum therapeutic effect.

The mechanism of action of penicillamine in rheumatoid arthritis is unknown. It is known that the drug causes a decrease in rheumatoid factor and interferes with several other processes in the immune system (14).

The initial dose of penicillamine is usually 250 mg/day. The dose can be increased at 1- to 3-month periods by 125 mg, to a daily dose of 750 mg. The dose can be increased thereafter by 125 mg every 2 or 3 months, usually to a maximum dose of 1000 mg. It is likely that, if there has not been a sufficient response at 1000 mg/day, the drug will be ineffective.

At higher doses, the chance of adverse reactions is much greater. Loss of taste can be transient. The two most serious adverse effects are blood dyscrasias and renal toxicity.

Thrombocytopenia is the most common adverse effect. The drug can be discontinued and restarted at half the dose, with careful monitoring for a month, then increased. If thrombocytopenia recurs, the drug should be discontinued. Leukopenia is less common, but can develop suddenly and be quite severe (15).

Proteinuria may occur early in therapy and can persist after the drug is discontinued. Hematuria may also occur. The proteinuria appears to be related to a glomerular lesion that has been detected by electron microscopy. At the present time, the significance of the renal toxicity is not really known and suggests discontinuing the drug.

Penicillamine is an effective drug to treat rheumatoid arthritis. It has major adverse effects, the extent of which are not really known. It has been associated with lupus-like syndrome, polymyositis, myasthenia gravis, and other rare diseases. Penicillamine, therefore, should be used cautiously, after adquate trials of other, older agents.

CORTICOSTEROIDS

Corticosteroids are very effective in the treatment of rheumatoid arthritis, but their use should be severely restricted. Their efficacy, prompt action, and sometimes drug-induced euphoria can lead to patient dependence (16) and overcompliance (17), with the increased risk of their numerous side effects and difficulty in tapering the dose of the drug.

Corticosteroids are used only after thorough consideration, if not trial, of more conservative therapy, including gold, hydroxychloroquine, and possibly penicillamine. They should be avoided in younger patients because, once begun, they are difficult to stop.

The goal of treatment in rheumatoid arthritis is to minimize patient disability. The corticosteroids are used to maintain the use of the most seriously involved joints. Large doses may be able to relieve most of the symptoms, but their risk precludes their use. The corticosteroid usually used is prednisone, starting at as low a dose as possible, generally between 2.5 and 5 mg/day. Once a maintenance dose is established, periodic attempts should be made to slowly taper the dose. In treating rheumatoid arthritis, the dose of prednisone should rarely need to exceed 10 mg/day. Alternate-day dosing, for example giving 10 mg every other day instead of 5 mg every day, may cause less adrenal suppression, but may also not provide enough effect on the "off" day.

The adverse effects of corticosteroids are well known, including increased susceptibility to infection, drug-induced cushingoid changes, sodium and water retention, euphoria or dysphoria, potassium depletion, cataracts, and osteoporosis. They may aggravate other concurrent diseases, such as diabetes mellitus, congestive heart failure, and peptic ulcer disease. They must be carefully tapered over time to avoid the effects of adrenal insufficiency and flares of arthritis.

Intra-articular injections of corticosteroids are sometimes used to treat chronic, severely inflamed joints. Relief in such a case is rapid and may last for weeks. There is a risk of infection from intra-articular injections, so they are reserved for those patients who have a few severely inflamed joints involved.

Corticosteroids are very useful in treating rheumatoid arthritis. Their significant adverse effects severely limit their use, as does their great patient acceptance and dependency. These potential hazards imply that they should be used for interim relief in severely debilitated patients, while waiting for the therapeutic effects of other agents with a slower onset of therapeutic effects.

IMMUNOSUPPRESSIVE AGENTS

Immunosuppressive agents, such as azathioprine and cyclophosphamide, which are most often used to treat neoplastic diseases and as adjuncts in organ transplantation are also useful in treating intractable rheumatoid arthritis. Azathioprine is the agent usually used, because of cyclophosphamide's greater risk of adverse effects. Azathioprine is a purine antagonist which interferes with actions of DNA and RNA, and has profound effects on the immune system. Its effectiveness is about that of gold or penicillamine. Among its side effects are gastrointestinal disturbances and hematologic complications, especially leukopenia and macrocytic anemia. The question also remains as to whether it causes cancer, since there may be a greater risk of neoplasia in transplant patients treated with the drug. Azathioprine is obviously not a drug for casual treatment and requires very careful monitoring. Its use is limited to intractable, severe, and progressive disease.

The feasibility of irradiation of the lymphoid tissues has been investigated as an alternative to the use of immunosuppressive drugs. The results associated a decreasing immune response with relief of joint inflammation. The patients in the study were candidates for treatment with azathioprine or cyclophosphamide or already had been treated with azathioprine without success (18). Further investigation is needed before radiation becomes an acceptable alternative to the immunosuppressive agents.

CONCLUSION

Rheumatoid arthritis is a disease of unknown cause and no known cure. It is an autoimmune disease which causes a chronic inflammation, which may lead to destruction of joint structures and decreasing joint function. It can also have serious systemic effects, involving multiple organ systems.

The treatment of rheumatoid arthritis is a coordinated multidisciplinary effort of drug and nondrug therapy aimed at minimizing patient disability. Drug treatment is generally started with an NSAID appropriate for chronic use, usually high dose aspirin. Other drugs generally are added to the NSAID, depending on the course of the disease. All of the drugs used can have serious adverse effects. These effects and the rationale behind their selection should be understood by pharmacists, who can

then become actively involved in promoting their appropriate use.

References

1. Kivilaakso E, Silen W: Pathogenesis of experimental gastric mucosal injury. N Engl J Med 301:364, 1979.
2. Simon LS, and Mills JA: Nonsteroidal anti-inflammatory drugs. N Engl J Med 302:1179, 1980.
3. Dawson W: The comparative pharmacology of benoxaprofen. J Rheum 7:5 (suppl 6), 1980.
4. Szczeklik A, Gryglewski RJ, Czerniawska-Mysik, G: Clinical patterns of hypersensitivity to nonsteroidal anti-inflammatory drugs and their pathogenesis. J Allergy Clin Immun 60:276, 1977.
5. Kimberly RP, Bowden RE, Keiser HR, et al: Reduction of renal function in newer NSAID. Am J Med 64:804, 1978.
6. Furst DE, Tozer TN, Melmon KL: Salicylate clearance, the resultant of protein binding and metabolism. Clin Pharmacol Ther 26:380, 1979.
7. Levy G, Leonards JR: Urine pH and salicyclate therapy. JAMA 217:81, 1971.
8. Dromgoole SH, Furst DE: Salicylates. In: Applied Pharmacokinetics. San Francisco: Applied Therapeutics, 1980, p 495.
9. Seaman WE, Plotz PH: Effects of aspirin on liver tests in patients with RA or SLE and in normal volunteers. Arthritis Rheum 19:155, 1976.
10. Rothschild BM: Hematologic perturbation associated with salicylates. Clin Pharmacol Ther 26:145, 1979.
11. Wilkens RF, Ward JR, Louie JS, et al: Double blind study comparing piroxicam and aspirin in the treatment of rheumatoid arthritis. Am J Med (suppl) February 16, 1982.
12. Wiseman EH: Pharmacologic studies with a new class of nonsteroidal anti-inflammatory agents—the oxicams—with special reference to piroxicam (Feldene®). Am J Med (suppl) February 16, 1981.
13. Wasner C, Britton M, Kraines G, et al: Nonsteroidal anti-inflammatory agents in rheumatoid arthritis and ankylosing spondylitis. JAMA 246:2168, 1981.
14. Bunch TW, O'Duffy JD: Disease modifying drugs for progressive rheumatoid arthritis. Mayo Clin Proc 55:161, 1980.
15. Mowat AG, Huskisson EC: D-Penicillamine in rheumatoid arthritis. Clin Rheum Dis 1:319, 1975.
16. Kimball CP: Psychological dependence on steroids? Ann Intern Med 75:111, 1971.
17. Nugant C, Ward J, MacDiarmid W, et al: Glucocorticoid toxicity. J Chronic Dis 18:323, 1965.
18. Kotzin BL, Strober S, Engleman EG, et al: Treatment of intractable rheumatoid arthritis with total lymphoid irradiation. N Engl J Med 305:969, 1981.
19. Katcher BS: Rheumatoid arthritis. In Herfindal ET, Hirschman JL: Clinical Pharmacy and Therapeutics, ed 2. Baltimore: Williams & Wilkins, 1979, pp 479–485.

CHAPTER 33

Gout and Hyperuricemia

RICHARD J. DE MEO, Pharm.D.

Gout was first referred to in the literature as podagra, meaning "foot seizure." The word gout was originated during the thirteenth century and was derived from the Latin word *gutta*, which translated into English means drop. It was believed that gout was due to a drop of poison entering the affected joint, drop by drop, and causing the joint to swell. During the nineteenth century, Sir Alfred Garrod demonstrated the presence of elevated uric acid concentrations in the blood of gout sufferers and postulated that gouty arthritis is an inflammatory reaction induced by crystals of sodium urate deposited in and around the joint. Recent progress in the research of gout has provided an extensive understanding of the disease and it is now known gout is a group of disease processes, either acquired or hereditary, characterized by hyperuricemia and acute inflammatory arthritis. The inflammatory response is induced by crystals of monosodium urate monohydrate and leukocytes in the synovial joint fluid. Deposits of urate crystals, called tophi, may occur in and around the joint sometimes causing severe debilitation to the affected joint. Extensive joint destruction is rare today due to effective pharmacological treatment. The term gout, therefore, refers to the presence of physical manifestations such as inflammatory arthritis and tophi deposition, induced by hyperuricemia. The term hyperuricemia does not imply gout is present, but only indicates the presence of elevated uric acid in the blood.

Hyperuricemia is defined by a serum uric acid level greater than 7 mg/100 ml. Concentrations greater than 7 mg/100 ml represent supersaturation and are associated with an increased risk of gout. Laboratory assay procedure and population variability accounts for some deviation of the "normal range." In the United States, the mean adult level in the men is 5.2 mg/100 ml and 4.9 mg/100 ml in the premenopausal women (1). Assay methodology, such as the Folin method adapted to an automated autoanalyzer, produces uric acid values 1 mg/100 ml higher than the true uric acid concentration. Interference caused by reducing substances such as caffeine, theophylline, ascorbic acid, acetaminophen, levodopa and glucose may falsely elevate uric acid test results. Serum uric acid values between 2 and 8 mg/100 ml are considered normal for men and a range of 2 to 6.5 mg/100 ml for women represents concentrations generally not associated with gout.

ETIOLOGY

Hyperuricemia is classified as primary or secondary. Primary implies that the major manifestation of the disease state is hyperuricemia. Secondary hyperuricemia is a condition that occurs along with some primary disorder, such as renal failure, in which the major manifestation is not hyperuricemia. Primary hyperuricemia is the most frequently occurring type of hyperuricemia and greater than 95% is of unknown etiology. The disorder may result from underexcretion of uric acid, overproduction of uric acid, or a combination of both. Overproduction is defined as a renal excretion of uric acid greater than 600 mg/day after a 5-day period of dietary purine restriction. This condition accounts for less than 10% of primary hyperuricemia. Normal 24-hour urinary excretion of uric acid is considered to be between 164 and 588 mg (2). The majority of primary hyperuricemia is due to underexcretion and occurs in the presence of normal glomerular filtration and creatinine clearance (Table 33.1). Elevation of uric acid in the presence of renal dysfunction is classified as secondary hyperuricemia. The mechanism of underexcretion is unknown, but has been postulated to result from either reduction of filtration of uric acid at the glomerulus, increased tubular reabsorption, diminished urate secretion per nephron, or increased postsecretory reabsorption.

Two rare, but identified, causes of primary

hyperuricemia involve enzymatic defects and account for less than 1% of primary hyperuricemia. Chemical mutants of phosphoribosyl-phyrophosphate (PP-ribose-P) synthetase results in a high rate of synthesis of PP-ribose-P and overproduction of uric acid. Partial deficiency of the enzyme hypoxanthine-guanine phosphoribosyl transferase (HGPRT) result in decreased consumption of PP-ribose-P and overproduction of uric acid. A complete lack of HGPRT results in secondary hyperuricemia (3).

Secondary hyperuricemia is associated with increased purine synthesis de novo, increased nucleic acid turnover, decreased renal function, or drug-induced decreased elimination of uric acid (Table 33.2). Glucose-6-phosphatase deficiency resulting in type 1 glycogen storage disease produces hypoglycemia and elevated serum concentrations of acetoacetic acid, β-

Table 33.1.
Classification of Hyperuricemia and Gout[a]

Type	Metabolic Disturbance	Inheritance
PRIMARY		
I. Undefined defects	Undefined (99% of primary)	
a. Overproduction (10%)	Not known	Polygenic
b. Underexcretion (90%)	Not known	Polygenic
II. Associated with enzyme defect	(1% of primary)	
a. Increased activity of PP-ribose-P synthetase	Overproduction of PP-ribose-P and uric acid	X-linked
b. Hypoxanthine-guanine phosphoribosyl-transferase deficiency (partial)	Overproduction of uric acid due to increased purine bio-synthesis	X-linked
SECONDARY		
I. Associated with increased purine biosynthesis de novo		
a. Glucose-6-phosphatase deficiency	Overproduction plus underexcretion of uric acid: type I glycogen storage disease	Autosomal recessive
b. Hypoxanthine-guanine phosphoribosyl-transferase deficiency (complete)	Overproduction of uric acid: Lesch-Nyhan syndrome	X-linked
II. Associated with increased nucleic acid turnover	Overproduction of uric acid	—
III. Associated with decreased renal clearance of uric acid	Reduced glomerular function; drug-induced retention of uric acid	—

[a] Adapted from *Harrison's Principles of Internal Medicine*, Ed. 9, p. 476.

Table 33.2.
Disease-induced Secondary Hyperuricemia

Hematopoietic-Lymphatic	Endocrine-Metabolic	Other
Acute myelogenous leukemia	Alcoholism (severe)	Acute renal failure
Chronic myelogenous leukemia	Diabetic ketoacidosis	Chondrocalcinosis
Hemolytic anemia	Hyperlipidemia	Chronic renal failure
Hemoglobinopathies	Hyperparathyroidism	Excessive purine intake
Hodgkin's disease	Hypoparathyroidism	(sweetbreads, liver)
Infectious mononucleosis	Myxedema	Psoriasis
Myeloid metaplasia	Obesity	Sarcoidosis
Multiple myeloma	Starvation	Paget's disease
Nontropical sprue	Toxemia	Lead poisoning
Pernicious anemia	Vasopressin-resistant diabetes insipidus	
Polycythemia vera		
Sickle cell anemia		
Thalassemia		
Waldenström's macroglobulinemia		

hydroxybutric acid and lactic acid. These organic acids inhibit tubular secretion of uric acid, thus producing secondary hyperuricemia. A complete lack of HGPRT is termed Lesch-Nyhan disease. This enzymatic defect not only results in severe secondary hyperuricemia, but is characterized by growth and mental retardation, choreoathetosis and self-mutilation by biting.

A common cause of secondary hyperuricemia is increased nucleic acid turnover. Neoplastic diseases, including the myeloproliferative and lymphoproliferative disorders, are the most common cause of excessive nucleoprotein turnover and secondary hyperuricemia. Psoriasis has an extremely high cellular turnover rate resulting in increased uric acid production. Paget's disease, sarcoidosis, and parathyroid dysfunction produce hyperuricemia for unknown reasons. Diabetes mellitus, when characterized by hypoglycemia, results in excessive formation of lactic acid and ketones, therefore preventing tubular secretion of uric acid. Fasting increases uric acid also by increasing ketones in the serum and decreasing tubular secretion (4). It is, therefore, advisable for the gouty patient to avoid "crash diets" as this may increase the frequency of gouty attacks. It is well known that acute alcohol ingestion increases uric acid levels by formation of lactic acid and decreased renal elimination. Secondary hyperuricemia can be caused by decreased renal excretion of uric acid as observed in intersitial renal disease, thiazide diuretics, and heavy metal toxicity such as lead poisoning. The thiazides increase tubular reabsorption and inhibit tubular secretion of uric acid. Furosemide induces hyperlactacidemia thus suppressing tubular secretion. The diuretics also deplete intravascular volume producing an increased uric acid retention. Extracellular volume replacement of sodium and water produces a normouricemia. Ethacrynic acid, chlorthalidone, and acetazolamide have also been identified to increase hyperuricemia. Other drugs known to increase uric acid levels include low dose aspirin (less than 2 g per day), ethambutol, nicotinic acid, methoxyflurane, levodopa and epinephrine. Drugs known to decrease uric acid levels are listed in Table 33.3. Serum uric acid levels have also been correlated to age, weight, sex, body surface area, social class, aptitude test scores, hemoglobin and plasma protein values (5). These parameters probably lead to more confusion than clarity and serve no useful purpose in identifying potential gout patients. The only useful parameter in determining possible gout patients is chronic elevation of uric acid.

Table 33.3.
Drugs and Chemicals That Increase or Decrease Serum Uric Acid

Increase	Decrease
Alcohol	Acetohexamide
Angiotensin	Adrenocorticotropic
Chemotherapeutic	hormone
agents	Allopurinol
Diuretics:	Chlorprothixen
Chlorothalidone	Glyceryl guaiacolate
Ethacrynic acid	Mannitol
Furosemide	Oxphenbutazone
Thiazides	Outdated tetracycline
Triamterene	Probenecid[a]
Ethambutol	Radiopaque dyes:
Levodopa	Iodipamide
Mecamylamine	Iodopyracet
Methoxyflurane	Iopanoic acid
Nicotinic acid (3–6 g/	Sodium diatrizoate
day)	Sodium ipodate
Pyrazinamide	Salicylates (>3 g/day)
Salicylates (<2 g/day)	Sulfinpyrazone[a]
Vasoconstrictors:	
Epinephrine	
Norepinephrine	

[a] Major uricosuric agent. May cause initial increase in serum uric acid when beginning therapy due to mobilization of tophi.

INCIDENCE

Gout occurs most frequently in the middle-aged hyperuricemic adult male patient. In the Heart Disease Epidemiology study conducted in Framingham, Massachusetts, 5127 subjects were evaluated and the incidence of gout was found to be 0.2%. Fourteen years later, the same subjects had an overall incidence of gout of 1.5% (6). The percent incidence of gout also increased with increasing uric acid concentrations. A serum uric acid level between 6 and 6.9 mg/100 ml corresponded with a 1.9% incidence in male subjects and increased to 25% when uric acid levels were between 8 and 8.9%. Of 212 men with uric acid levels greater than 7 mg/100 ml, 46 developed clinical gout representing a 20% incidence. The relationship of incidence of gout to serum urate levels is shown in Table 33.4.

PATHOGENESIS

Although the reason urate forms crystals in the joint fluid of gouty patients is still not

Table 33.4.
Relationship of Serum Uric Acid Levels to Incidence of Gout[a]

Serum Uric Acid Level (mg/100 ml)	Men			Women		
	Total No. examined	Gouty arthritis developed in		Total No. examined	Gouty arthritis developed in	
		No.	%		No.	%
6	1281	8	0.6	2665	2	0.08
6–6.9	790	15	1.9	151	5	3.3
7–7.9	162	27	16.7	23	4	17.4
8–8.9	40	10	25.0	4	0	0
9+	10	9	90.0	1	0	0
Totals	2283	65	2.8	2844	11	0.4

[a] Adapted from A. P. Hall et al. (6).

conclusively described, it is most likely a combination of factors such as hyperuricemia, rapidly changing urate levels, presence of certain protein polysaccharide substances, joint effusion of water and uric acid and the physical state of the joint. Acute gouty arthritic attacks develop from the deposition of urate crystals in the synovial fluid of the affected joint(s). The more distal the joint, the higher the incidence of occurrence. This effect may be explained by the fact the more distal joints are of lower body temperature than more proximal joints and uric acid is less soluble in lower temperatures. The solubility of urate in physiologic saline is 6.8 mg/100 ml at 37°C and decreases to 4.5 mg/100 ml at 30°C. The temperature of the ankle joint is approximately 30°C. Solubility of uric acid in the joint is also dependent on the concentration of substances such as chondroitin sulfate, hyaluronic acid and proteoglycans. Alterations or chemical mutants of these substances will decrease urate solubility and have been postulated as an explanation of why some patients develop gout and others do not at the same serum uric acid concentrations. Approximately 50% of first time gouty arthritic attacks are manifested in the great toe and about 84% will experience symptoms in their great toe during the course of gouty arthritis. A possible explanation for this clinical finding has been proposed by Simkin (7). He demonstrated that the diffusion of urate across the synovial membrane is slower than that of water. During the day, water will accumulate in the synovial joint due to walking and at night reabsorption of synovial fluid while the joint is at rest produces a transient increase in intra-articular urate concentration since water diffuses out more rapidly than urate. Acute gouty attacks have also been correlated with fluctuations in

serum uric acid concentrations. This has been demonstrated in the early treatment with uricosuric therapy, as rapidly lowering the serum uric acid concentration has been associated with an increased frequency of gouty arthritis attacks.

Once crystal formation of urate is formed in the synovial joint, an acute inflammatory response occurs. Although the precise mechanism is undefined, one possible process may involve activated Hageman factor resulting in high concentrations of kinin-like peptides producing vasodilation, increased vascular permeability, and leukocyte migration. Another factor involved in the acute inflammatory response is activation of the complement system. Regardless of the initial response to urate crystals, the major inflammatory response is dependent on the presence of polymorphonuclear leukocytes (PMN). Phagocytosis of urate crystals by the PMN leads to release of a chemotactic factor thereby increasing migration of more leukocytes. Urate crystals taken up within the phagosomes of the PMN result in lysis and release of enzymes which result in tissue injury and synovial inflammation. Within a few hours, the affected joint becomes hot, red, swollen, extremely tender and painful. The course of inflammation is self-limiting and may persist for several hours to months without treatment. The skin over the joint may desquamate as the attack subsides, and then the symptoms may completely resolve. Between attacks, recovery is complete and this inactive state is termed the intercritical period. In most patients, a second attack occurs within 6 months to 2 years. Subsequent attacks often are polyarticular, more severe, and longer in duration. Progressive development of gout leads to chronic symptoms such as visible tophaceous deposits. The extent and occurrence of tophi is dependent upon the degree of hyperuricemia and the duration. The crystalline deposits of urate form in the cartilage, synovial membranes, tendons, soft tissues and the helix of the ear. Progression of tophi deposits leads to increasing stiffness of the affected joints, persistent pain, and eventual destruction and deformity of the affected joint(s). The skin overlying the tophi becomes shiny and may ulcerate, exposing a white chalky exudate. Eventually erosion of the bone may occur resulting in fractures and deformity. Such deformity is rarely seen today due to effective drug therapy.

DIAGNOSIS AND CLINICAL FINDINGS

A definitive diagnosis of acute gouty arthritis requires the identification of sodium urate crystals in the synovial fluid of the joint. The American Rheumatism Association developed a criteria for the diagnosis of acute gout (Table 33.5) and a set of criteria necessary for a probable diagnosis. Diagnosis of acute gout is confirmed only when monosodium urate crystals are demonstrated in synovial fluid aspirated from the affected joint. A microscope using a first-order red compensator should be used for positive identification. A negative finding of the aspirated fluid does not rule out acute gouty arthritis as lack of urate crystals in synovial fluid in the acute gouty patient occasionally occurs (8). Due to the high incidence of gouty arthritis occurring in the great toe, aspiration of this joint may be beneficial in establishing a definitive diagnosis, even if the joint appears asymptomatic (9). A probable diagnosis can be made when six or more suggestive criteria are present (Table 33.5). These suggestive criteria are of value in establishing a diagnosis when aspiration of the joint cannot be performed prior to treatment. The clinical findings of pseudogout, hydroxyapatite calcific tendinitis, or sarcoid arthritis closely resemble the signs and symptoms of gout and therefore it is advisable to correctly establish the diagnosis of gout; otherwise, antihyperuricemic medications may be inappropriately prescribed.

Other clinical findings of acute gouty arthritis include hyperthermia, leukocytosis and elevation of the erythrocyte sedimentation rate. These findings may be also characteristic of inflammation of an infectious etiology.

Acute arthritic attacks frequently begin as monoarticular joint inflammation and prog-

Table 33.5.
Criteria for Diagnosis of Acute Gout[a]

Definite	Suggestive[b]
1. Demonstration of sodium urate crystals in affected joint	1. More than one attack of arthritis
	2. Development of maximum inflammation within 1 day
	3. Oligoarthritis attack
	4. Redness over joint
	5. Painful or swollen first metatarasophalangeal joint
	6. Unilateral attack on first metatarsophalangeal joint
	7. Unilateral attack on tarsal joint
	8. Tophus
	9. Hyperuricemia
	10. Asymptomatic swelling within a joint

[a] Criteria established by the American Rheumatism Association.
[b] A minimum of 6 criteria should be present to be suggestive of gout.

ress to polyarticular involvement. However, initial attacks that are polyarticular may occur in hyperuricemic patients as often as 39% of the time (10). Radiologic imaging has demonstrated in patients experiencing initial single joint attacks that actually many joints may be involved in the inflammatory process (11). The most frequently affected joint is the first metatarsophalangeal joint accounting for 50% of monoarticular attacks. Other joints frequently involved include the instep, ankles, heels, knees, wrists and fingers. The shoulder, hips, spine and sternoclavicular joint are rarely involved.

Physical stress induced by running, long walks or exercise involving use of the feet have been known to increase the frequency of subsequent attacks. The onset of the attack frequently occurs at night during sleep. The pathogenesis is probably related to the effusion of water out of the joint at night, causing a saturation of uric acid and ensuing inflammatory response (7). Laboratory diagnostic procedures should include a BUN and serum creatinine to assess renal function, a complete blood count (CBC), urinalysis, and a determination of serum uric acid concentration. A diagnosis of hyperuricemia cannot be made based on one serum uric acid concentration determination.

Spurious elevations of uric acid may be caused by many factors and diurnal variation in serum uric acid concentrations can produce misinterpreted results. Further evaluation of the hyperuricemic patient should include a 24-hour urinary uric acid excretion determination. Although such testing does not establish the etiology of hyperuricemia, a differentiation between underexcretors or overproducers can be helpful in deciding the appropriate antihyperuricemic medication. A 24-hour urinary uric acid excretion of less than 750 mg is generally considered an underexcretion and greater than 800 mg is consistent with findings of an overexcretion. Testing urinary samples for a 24-hour period is sometimes difficult to accurately perform due to patient cooperation and is subject to laboratory error. Another method, proposed by Simkin, involves an assessment from spot midmorning serum and urine samples. The test consists of a single 10 A.M. serum and urine analysis for creatinine and uric acid. The urine uric acid concentration (mg/100 ml) is divided by the urine creatinine concentration (mg/100 ml) and then multiplied by the serum creatinine concentration (mg/100 ml) which then yields a uric acid excretion ratio. A ratio greater than 0.8 indicates an overproducer, 0.6 to 0.8 is considered normal, and a ratio of less than 0.6 can also be normal or indicate an underexcretor (12). Although this method is easier to perform than obtaining a 24-hour sample, diurnal variation in uric acid excretion often leads to erroneous results (13).

Chronic tophaceous gout rarely occurs today. Previous to the discovery of antihyperuricemic agents, progressive hyperuricemia resulted in sodium urate crystal deposits in the joints, tendons, hands, ear and kidney. The incidence of visible tophi was 50 to 70% in the gouty patient when no medication was available.

A common physical finding associated with the hyperuricemic patient is renal disease. Both are common in many hypertensive patients and therefore gouty patients should be evaluated for blood pressure and renal function. Progressive renal failure is the cause of death in 17 to 25% of gouty patients. It was believed that hyperuricemia resulted in renal destruction and therefore asymptomatic hyperuricemia should be treated to prevent gouty nephropathy. This association of hyperuricemia and renal disease was noted to occur in patients also suffering from a primary nephropathy such as hypertension, glomerulonephritis, pyelonephritis or diabetes mellitus (14). Thus, the association between hyperuricemia and renal nephropathy is not clear and in fact it is now believed that asymptomatic hyperuricemia does not result in renal destruction (15, 16).

TREATMENT

Treatment of gout and hyperuricemia consists of first terminating the acute inflammatory arthritis, then gradual reduction of serum urate concentration in the hyperuricemic patient. Effective anti-inflammatory agents include colchicine, indomethacin, phenylbutazone, and nonsteroidal anti-inflammatory drugs such as naproxen and are prescribed for a period necessary to alleviate the acute gouty attack. Reduction of serum uric acid concentration should not be initiated until complete remission of the inflammatory process is accomplished as changes in serum urate concentration may precipitate further gouty attacks. Establishment of the etiology and severity of hyperuricemia should be made prior to initiating antihyperuricemic therapy. Asymptomatic hyperuricemia in patients experiencing infrequent mild joint pain does not warrant aggressive pharmacological therapy and may benefit from weight reduction programs and avoiding purine-rich foods. Unlike treatment of acute gouty arthritis which requires rapid and aggressive treatment, antihyperuricemic therapy is best approached through careful evaluation of the patient and gradual reduction of uric acid. Effective antihyperuricemic agents include allopurinol, a xanthine oxidase inhibitor, and the uricosuric drugs, probenecid and sulfinpryazone. The goal of antihyperuricemic therapy is to prevent recurrences of acute gouty arthritis by decreasing body stores of urate, and prevent or reverse complications due to urate deposition.

Acute Gouty Arthritis

The goal of therapy in treatment of acute inflammatory arthritis is to rapidly alleviate the pain and restore the affected joint to normal functioning capacity. Immobilization of the affected joint and administration of analgesic agents provide additional benefit to anti-inflammatory drug treatment in severe cases of gout. Anti-inflammatory treatment must be started within the first few hours of onset of pain.

Colchicine. Colchicine is effective in gout, pseudogout, calcific tendonitis and sarcoid arthritis. Unlike other anti-inflammatory agents, it is not effective in other inflammatory joint diseases. Therefore, when given in treatment of suspected gouty arthritis, colchicine's specificity aids in establishing a "probable" diagnosis of gouty arthritis following successful therapeutic results. Greater than 90% of patients with gouty arthritis respond adequately to colchicine therapy if treatment is initiated immediately; however, if treatment is delayed beyond 12 hours of presenting symptoms, the response is reduced to 75%. Colchicine is indicated in patients with previous history of successful treatment; however, it is not considered the drug of choice in patients with no prior medical history of gout. As one of the oldest therapeutic agents used in the treatment of gout, it is still used frequently.

Colchicine has been reported to exert anti-inflammatory activity through inhibition of PMN chemotaxis and lysosomal enzyme release. Recent evidence suggests the primary mechanism of colchicine action in ameliorating and preventing acute gouty attacks is by inhibiting the production or release of a cell derived glycoprotein chemotatic factor produced in urate-induced inflammation (17). Peripheral leukocyte migration is reduced in therapeutic doses. Pharmacological effects not related to therapeutic efficacy of colchicine include vasoconstriction, reduction of body temperature, respiratory depression, inhibition of release of histamine from mast cells, secretion of insulin from the pancreatic islets, and enhanced gastrointestinal activity by neurogenic stimulation.

Colchicine is rapidly absorbed from the gastrointestinal (GI) tract and reaches peak serum concentrations within 2 hours. The apparent volume of distribution is larger than total body water. The half-life in normal subjects is 60 min and is prolonged in liver disase. Hepatic metabolism and excretion in the feces accounts for the majority of drug elimination. Renal elimination of the unchanged drug is approximately 10 to 20% in normal subjects.

Colchicine, when given within the first few hours of an acute gouty attack, can reduce pain, swelling, and redness significantly in 95% of patients within 12 hours and provide complete remission in 48 to 72 hours. An initial dose of 1 mg followed by 0.5 mg every hour until symptoms subside or GI toxicity develops is the recommended regimen. Adverse effects of colchicine present most commonly as GI symptoms including nausea, vomiting, diarrhea, and abdominal pain. The incidence of GI toxicity is between 50 and 80% of all patients treated with a therapeutic dosage regimen of oral colchicine requiring some degree of dosage modification. Although paregoric or other drugs provide relief of abdominal discomfort, colchicine should be avoided in patients with preexisting GI disease (Crohns, diverticulitis), peptic ulcer disease, or history of internal bleeding. When colchicine is indicated in these specific disease states, it may be administered by the intravenous route, thus reducing the GI disturbances. An initial dose of 2 to 3 mg is followed, if needed, by an additional 0.5 to 1 mg every 6 hours up to a maximum dose of 5 mg. The colchicine should be diluted in 20 ml of normal saline and administered through a primary intravenous site cautiously to avoid any extravasation during the delivery. Small venous sites should be avoided as a route of administration as extravasation will lead to local necrosis and severe pain for the patient. As GI toxicity is minimized or negligible by this method of administration, doses greater than 5 mg could possibly be given if relief is not obtained. However, fatal doses have occurred with 10 mg and therefore the maximum safe dose is considered to be 5 mg during any one treatment (18). Serious adverse effects include bone marrow depression characterized by pancytopenia, and renal, hepatic and neurologic toxicity. These side effects are rare and generally occur in elderly patients, with preexisting renal or hepatic disease. Although colchicine is not considered the drug of choice in gouty arthritis by many rheumatologists, it is beneficial in patients with hypersensitivity to aspirin and the nonsteroidal anti-inflammatory drugs (NSAID). For example the patient with type 1 asthma will not be able to tolerate aspirin and the nonsteriodal agents. Consideration should be given to colchicine in patients receiving anticoagulant therapy as other agents used in the treatment of acute gout will effect the bleeding time, whereas colchicine does not present any problem in these patients. Patients with existing renal failure, congestive heart failure, and hypertension should also be considered for treatment with colchicine during acute gouty attacks as the NSAID indometha-cin and phenylbutazone will decrease renal blood flow and promote water and sodium retention. If colchicine cannot be used in these patients, the newer NSAID should be used versus indomethacin and phenylbutazone. Both indomethacin and phenylbutazone are both potent inhibitors of prostaglandin synthe-tase and will significantly reduce renal blood flow in the preexisting renally compromised patient and cause retention of sodium and water. Colchicine is also preferable in the al-coholic patient with cirrhosis (19). These pa-tients may present with preexisting GI disease, hepatic cirrhosis, renal insufficiency, and as-cites. Colchicine should be given by the intra-venous route to avoid GI distress and the dos-age should be reduced by one half in the presence of moderate to severe hepatic and renal dysfunction. As cochicine is metabolized by the liver, toxicity may result when full therapeutic dosage regimens are given in these patients.

Indomethacin. Indomethacin is very effec-tive in the treatment of acute gouty arthritis and is considered to be the drug of choice by most rheumatologists. Indomethacin is effec-tive as an anti-inflammatory agent in gout even when treatment is delayed several days from the onset of symptoms. Colchicine is rarely effective at this stage and should not be used unless treatment begins within the first few hours of the inflammatory reaction. Indo-methacin exerts its anti-inflammatory action through inhibition of prostaglandin synthesis and possibly inhibition of PMN migration. An initial dose of 75 mg followed by 50 mg every 6 hours with gradual dosage reduction as ad-equate response is achieved has been proven effective (20). Indomethacin should be avoided in patients with history of GI disease, espe-cially peptic or gastric ulcers. Indomethacin should be given with food or an antacid to reduce the incidence of gastric distress due to the acidity of the drug. Adverse effects include fluid and sodium retention, headache, depres-sion and allergic reactions. Severe hyperkale-mia and renal insufficiency may result from inhibition of prostaglandin synthesis and con-sequent hyporeninemic hypoaldosteronism in patients with preexisting renal disease and diabetes (21). Indomethacin should be used with caution in the elderly patient and pa-tients with compromised heart function. Hy-pertensive patients on furosemide present a

particular problem as indomethacin blocks the diuretic effect by inhibiting sodium excretion.

Phenylbutazone. Phenylbutazone and ox-phenbutazone, both potent anti-inflammatory agents, have been reported to be effective in 85 to 95% of patients suffering from an acute gouty arthritic attack (22). An effective dosage regimen of phenylbutazone consists of 200 mg, 4 times daily, then gradually reducing the dose as symptomatic relief is achieved. Phenylbu-tazone in doses of 200 mg can be given for the first 24 to 48 hours, then decreased to 200 mg, 3 times daily for another 24 to 48 hours. Ther-apy should not be required beyond a 4-day period. Due to enzyme induction, a higher dosage may result in lower serum concentra-tions and thereby compromising therapeutic efficacy. GI side effects are similar to that of indomethacin and therefore the same consid-erations and precautions are valid with phen-ylbutazone. Although hematological toxicities resulting in bone marrow suppression, aplastic anemia and agranulocytosis are well known adverse effects of phenylbutzone, their occur-rence is rare in patients receiving short-term therapy. As with indomethacin, phenylbuta-zone will cause sodium and water retention and therefore precaution should be used in the treatment of the patient with congestive heart failure and hypertension. Phenylbutazone will potentiate the pharmacological action of war-farin and the oral hypoglycemic agents. As phenylbutazone has some uricosuric proper-ties, a 24-hour urinary uric acid determination will be falsely elevated when this drug is given at the time of the test procedure.

Other Anti-inflammatory Agents. The new NSAID commonly used in rheumatoid arthri-tis such as ibuprofen, naproxen, tolmetin, su-lindac, and piroxicam are also effective agents in the treatment of acute gouty arthritis. These drugs exert their anti-inflammatory effect by inhibiting prostaglandin synthetase and may present a problem in the aspirin-sensitive pa-tient. Several cases of severe life-threatening bronchospasms in asthmatic patients have been reported in the literature (23). Therapeu-tic results can be achieved with the recom-mended doses of these agents for use in rheu-matoid arthritis. In one study, naproxen 750 mg as an initial dose, followed by 250 mg, 3 times daily, was as effective as phenylbuta-zone in treatment of acute gout (24). Daily doses and the recommended dosing intervals are listed in Table 33.6. As with indomethacin

Table 33.6.
Nonsteroidal Analgesic/Anti-inflammatory Drugs[a]

Drug (Trade Name)	Form (mg)	Daily Dose (mg)	Maximum Dose (Daily) (mg)	Dosing Interval
Ibuprofen (Motrin)	300	1,600–2,400	2,400	t.i.d.-q.i.d.
	600			
Fenoprofen (Nalfon)	200	800–2,400	3,600	t.i.d.–q.i.d.
	300			
	600			
Naproxen (Naprosyn)	250	500–750	1,500	b.i.d.
	375			
Piroxicam (Feldene)	10	10–20	40	Once daily
	20			
Tolmetin (Tolectin)	200	600–2,000	2,000	t.i.d.
Sulindac (Clinoril)	150	300–400	400	b.i.d.
	200			

[a] See also Table 42.4.

and phenylbutazone, the newer anti-inflammatory agents will cause GI disturbances and is the most frequently reported side effect (see Chapters 32 and 42.).

Hyperuricemia

The decision to treat hyperuricemia should be based on careful evaluation of the fact that the patient will have to take daily medication for a lifetime. Once antihyperuricemic therapy is initiated, therapy should be continued in order to maintain serum uric acid levels less than 6 mg/100 ml. The first step in evaluating the patient is identification of the etiological factors contributing to the hyperuricemia. In primary hyperuricemia pathologic metabolic disturbances may not be identifiable and therefore difficult to correct or reverse. The decision to treat is therefore based on the potential or present pathological consequences of not treating the patient. A mild or moderate hyperuricemia that is asymptomatic in an elderly patient is not likely to result in severely debilitating joint disease and therefore the benefits of treating may be outweighed by the side effects and cost of antihyperuricemic therapy. However, the decision to treat may be wise in the middle-aged adult presenting with tophi and frequent complaints of acute gouty arthritis. As the potential for gouty arthritis increases significantly in patients with serum uric acid concentrations greater than 10 mg/100 ml, therapy is reasonably justified in cases of this type. Once the decision is made to begin therapy, two methods of pharmacological management may be utilized. Uricosuric drugs

reduce the serum uric acid level by increasing renal elimination of uric acid whereas xanthine oxidase inhibitors, such as allopurinol, decrease the in vivo production of uric acid. Either method effectively reduces serum uric acid, therefore the choice of therapy is based on the pharmacological properties of the drug and the etiology of the hyperuricemia. Uricosuric agents are considered a logical choice in which hyperuricemia is due to underexcretion of uric acid, and allopurinol an appropriate choice in patients diagnosed as overproducers. Due to the increased propensity for crystallization of uric acid in the nephron of the kidney with the uricosuric drugs, and the fact that all types of hyperuricemia responds to the xanthine oxidase inhibitors, allopurinol is most commonly prescribed.

Probenecid. Probenecid is an effective uricosuric drug when prescribed in doses of 500 to 3000 mg, divided in 3 to 4 daily doses. Doses of 1 to 2 g daily result in a 4- to 6-fold increase of uric acid elimination. Initial therapy should begin gradually when possible to avoid uric acid saturation in the kidney. Therapy should begin with 250 mg every 12 hours for the first 3 to 4 days, and then increased to 500 mg twice daily for 1 to 2 weeks. At this point in therapy, the serum uric acid concentration should be determined. Adjustments in dosage can then be made to achieve and or maintain a serum uric acid target level of 6 mg/100 ml. Fluid intake of at least 2 liters/day is recommended to minimize the risk of urate crystals in the kidney. Alkalinization of the urine during the initial stages of therapy will increase the solubility of uric acid and therefore decrease the formation of crystals. Probenecid is rapidly and completely absorbed orally, and exhibits a half-life of 4 to 20 hours. The drug is metabolized by glucuronide conjugation and by oxidation of the alkyl side chains. As probenecid is characterized by dose-dependent kinetics, small dosage changes may result in significant fluctuation in the serum concentration and pharmacological effect. Renal excretion of the unchanged drug is minimal and is dependent on urinary pH (25). Clinical studies have documented drug-drug interactions with aspirin, penicillins, cephalosporins, nalidixic acid, rifampicin, sulfinpyrazone and the nonsteroidal anti-inflammatory agents. Concomitant low dose aspirin treatment is an absolute contraindication with probenecid as aspirin will significantly block the pharmacological therapeutic effect by preventing uric acid secretion. Probenecid will decrease excretion of indomethacin, penicillin, ampicillin, cefaclor, cefamandole, cefazolin, cefoxitin, cephaloridine, cephalothin, cephradine, nafcillin, indomethacin, naproxen and sulfinpyrazone and increase the renal elimination of allopurinol. Probenecid will also increase the levels of methotrexate when given concomitantly. When given to patients on low dose heparin, probenecid will increase the pharmacological effect and prolong the clotting time. In diabetic patients receiving chlorpropamide the blood glucose should be carefully monitored as probenecid prolongs the half-life. GI toxicity is the most frequently occurring side effect and is reported to be between 3.1% in short-term therapy and as high as 8.1% in chronic therapy. Uric acid stones have been reported in 9% of patients on chronic therapy. Variable incidences, usually less than 1%, have been documented for drug fever, skin rashes, and hypersensitivity reactions.

Sulfinpyrazone. Sulfinpyrazone, an analog of phenylbutazone, is a potent uricosuric agent when administered in maintenance doses of 200 to 400 mg daily. It is 3 to 6 times more potent than probenecid; however, as with probenecid, its efficacy is limited in the renally compromised patient. Fluid intake should be increased to assure minimum risk of nephrolithiasis. Therapy should begin with a 50-mg (½ tablet) dose administered twice daily. After 3 to 4 days the dose can be increased to 100 mg twice daily. Doses greater than 400 mg have a marginal dose/benefit ratio, and should be avoided. It is completely absorbed orally

and exhibits a half-life of 1 to 4 hours. Renal excretion of the unchanged drug is between 20 to 40% of the parent compound. Sulfinpyrazone lowers serum uric acid levels by inhibiting the tubular reabsorption of uric acid in the nephron. Adverse effects include dyspepsia, uric acid stones and hypersensitivity reactions. Recent case reports include rare, but serious nephrotoxicity characterized by acute oliguric renal failure. Renal biopsy in one study revealed acute tubular necrosis with no evidence of interstitial nephritis. The patient did not exhibit signs of a hypersensitivity reaction, but a direct chemical necrosis (26). Sulfinpyrazone significantly reduces platelet aggregation and has been demonstrated to reduce the risk of sudden death in the postmyocardial infarction patient (27).

Allopurinol. In patients with severe hyperuricemia, renal dysfunction characterized by a creatinine clearance less than 20 to 30 ml/min, or history of adverse effects with the uricosurics agents, allopurinol should be considered as a reasonable method of therapy to reduce serum uric acid. Many prescribers prefer allopurinol to any uricosuric drug as it is of equal efficacy in the underexcretor, the drug of choice in the overproducer, and presents less risk of uric acid nephrolithiasis. Therefore, allopurinol is the most commonly prescribed drug for treatment of hyperuricemia. Allopurinol is effective when given in a single daily dose of 300 mg. Doses of 400 to 600 mg/day may be required in severe hyperuricemia and can be given in divided doses. As with the uricosuric agents, allopurinol therapy should be initiated slowly to avoid rapid fluctuations in the serum uric acid level and possibly inducing acute gouty attacks. Allopurinol inhibits xanthine oxidase which is an enzyme that converts xanthine and hypoxanthine to uric acid. It also decreases intracellular phosphoribosyl pyrophosphate. Allopurinol has a half-life to 3 to 4 hours and is metabolized to an active metabolite, oxypurinol, which has a half-life of 28 to 44 hours. Oxypurinol is primarily renally excreted and therefore will accumulate in renal dysfunction, accounting for much of allopurinol's higher incidence of toxicity in the patient with poor renal elimination. Although no standard dosage adjustment is documented to reduce toxicity, allopurinol dosage should be reduced one third to one half in the presence of diminished renal function.

Allopurinol has an onset of action of 24 to

48 hours. The maximum therapeutic effect is obtained in 1 to 2 weeks and therefore serum uric acid determinations can be made after 2 weeks of therapy. Actual physical resolution of tophi requires 6 months to 1 year of daily therapy. When given concomitantly with the uricosuric agents a faster reduction in tophi can be achieved; however, uricosuric agents have been reported to increase the renal excretion of oxypurinol. The significance of this drug interaction is probably diminished by the fact that allopurinol will also increase the half-life of probenecid. Allopurinol is well tolerated provided the patient has adequate renal function or dosage adjustments are made in renal dysfunction. The most frequently reported adverse effects include GI upset and skin rashes. Epidermal toxic necrolysis, alopecia, bone marrow suppression manifested by leukopenia, thrombocytopenia and agranulocytosis, and hepatotoxicity have been rarely reported, but represent serious adverse effects (28–30). A significant increase in drug rashes has been documented when allopurinol is administered in the presence of concomitant ampicillin therapy (31). The reported incidence of drug rash with allopurinol alone is 2.1%, 7.5% with ampicillin alone, and 22.4% when both drugs are given together. The treatment of benign skin rashes is treated adequately with steroids or an antihistamine.

PROGNOSIS AND CONCLUSIONS

The disease gout is characterized by hyperuricemia and acute inflammatory joint disease. The progression of the disease state is dependent on physical and external factors characteristic of the individual and life-style. Fortunately, today the progression of hyperuricemia to physical discomfort and disability should not occur. Effective drug treatment to lower the serum uric acid level and eliminate crystal deposits in the joints and tissues should be instituted based on careful evaluation and consideration of patient factors. Not all hyperuricemia or gout requires treatment with drug therapy, as etiological factors may be reduced or eliminated.

References

1. Mikkelsen WM, Dodge HJ, Valkenburg H: The distribution of serum uric acid values in a population of unselected as to gout or hyperuricemia. Am J Med 39:242, 1965.
2. Seegmiller JE, Grayzel AI, Laster L: Uric acid production in gout. J Clin Invest 40:1304, 1961.
3. Wyngaarden JB: Metabolic defects of primary hyperuricemia and gout. Am J Med 56:651, 1974.
4. Maclachlan MJ, Rodnan GP: Effects of food, fast, and alcohol on serum uric acid and acute attacks of gout. Am J Med 42:38, 1967.
5. Munan L, Kelly A, Petitclerc C: Population serum urate levels and their correlates. Am J Epidemiol 103:369, 1976.
6. Hall AP, Barry PE, Dawber TR, et al: Epidemiology of gout and hyperuricemia. Am J Med 42:27, 1967.
7. Simkin PA: The pathogenesis of podagra. Ann Intern Med 86:230, 1977.
8. Romanoff NR: Gout without crystals on initial synovial fluid analysis. Postgrad Med J 54:95, 1978.
9. Weinberger A: Urate crystals in asymptomatic metatarsophalangeal joints. Ann Intern Med 91:56, 1979.
10. Halder NM, Franck WA, Bress NM, et al: Acute polyarticular gout. Am J Med 56:715, 1974.
11. Rosenthall L: Radionuclide joint imaging in the diagnosis of synovial disease. Semin Arthritis Rheum 7:49, 1977.
12. Simkin PA: Uric acid excretion: quantitative assessment from spot, midmorning, serum and urine samples. Ann Intern Med 91:44, 1977.
13. Wortmann RL: Limited value of uric acid concentration ratios in estimating uric acid excretion. Ann Intern Med 93:822, 1980.
14. Berger L: Renal function in gout. Am J Med 59:605, 1975.
15. Yu TF: Renal function in gout (Part V); factors influencing the renal hemodynamics. Am J Med 67:766, 1979.
16. Yu TF: Impaired renal function in gout; its association with hypertensive vascular disease and intrinsic renal disease. Am J Med 72:95, 1982.
17. Spilberg I: Mechanism of action of colchicine in acute urate induced arthritis. J Clin Invest 64:775, 1979.
18. Liu YK, Hymotwitz R, Carroll MG: Marrow aplasia induced by colchicine. A case report. Arthritis Rheum 6:21, 1978.
19. Nashel DJ, Chandra M: Acute gouty arthritis; special management considerations in alcoholic patients. JAMA 247:58, 1982.
20. Wortmann RL, Kelley WN: Gout and hyperuricemia; a rational approach to management. Clin Ther 1:159, 1977.
21. Findling JW, Beckstrom D, Rawsthorne L, et al: Indomethacin induced hyperkalemia in three patients with gouty arthritis. JAMA 244:1980.
22. Wallace SL: The treatment of the acute attack of gout. Clin Rheum Dis 3:133, 1977.
23. Salberg DJ, Simon MR: Severe asthma induced by naproxen—a case report and review of the literature. Ann Allergy 45:372, 1980.
24. Sturge RA: Multicenter trial of naproxen and phenylbutazone in acute gout. Ann Rheum Dis 36:80, 1977.
25. Cunningham RE, Israli ZH, Dayton PG: Clinical pharmacokinetics of probenecid. Clin Pharmacokinet 6:135, 1981.
26. Durham DS, Isbels LS: Sulphinpyrazone-in-

duced acute renal failure. *Br Med J* 282:609, 1981.

27. Anturane Reinfarction Trial Research Group: Sulfinpyrazone and the prevention of sudden death after myocardial infarction. *N Engl J Med* 302:250, 1980.

28. Fam AG, Paton T, Chaiton A: Reinstitution of allopurinol after cutaneous reactions. *Can Med Assoc J* 123:128, 1980.

29. Lang P: Severe hypersensitivity reactions to allopurinol. *South Med J* 72:1361, 1979.

30. Al-Kawas F, Seeff LB, Berendson RA, et al: Allopurinol hepatotoxicity. *Ann Intern Med* 95:588, 1981.

31. Boston Collaborative Drug Surveillance Program: Excess of ampicillin rashes associated with allopurinol in hyperuricemia. *N Engl J Med* 505:286, 1972.

SECTION 9
Diseases of the Blood

CHAPTER 34

Anemias

STANLEY G. KAILIS, Ph.D., F.P.S.
CONSTANTINE G. BERBATIS, M.Sc., F.P.S.

Anemia is a condition in which the erythrocytes are either reduced in number or deficient in the oxygen binding pigment hemoglobin and is said to be present when the blood hemoglobin concentration falls. The hemoglobin levels below which anemia is likely to manifest are: 11 g/100 ml for children 6 months to 6 years and 12 g/100 ml from 6 years to 14 years; 13 g/100 ml for men; 12 g/100 ml for women and 11 g/100 ml for pregnant women (1). There are approximately 100 different types of anemia and those relevant to the pharmacist will be reviewed. Anemias may result from chronic or acute blood loss, a decreased rate of erythrocyte production or an increased rate of erythrocyte destruction (Table 34.1).

GENERAL FEATURES

The severity of the clinical effects is determined by the degree of anemia and the ability of homeostatic mechanisms to compensate. Regardless of the cause of the anemia there are many signs and symptoms which are common to all severe cases. The overt signs of anemia are pallor of the skin, mucous membranes (particularly the conjunctiva) and nail beds. Symptoms relate to oxygen deficiency and are prominent in the cardiovascular and nervous systems. These include faintness, malaise, dizziness, fatigue, lack of concentration, shortness of breath particularly on exertion, intermittent claudication, irritability, headache, palpitations, ankle edema and angina. In severe cases cardiomegaly and high output heart failure develop.

Even though the symptoms accompanying anemia are distinctive, they can also be caused by a variety of other disorders. Therefore, for a definitive diagnosis of anemia and subsequent monitoring of its course, the use of laboratory tests is essential (2) (Tables 34.2 and 34.3).

A comprehensive history in addition to the physical examination is important in the assessment of the anemic patient. More specifically dietary habits, drug histories and occupation should be documented for the purpose of identifying any dietary deficiencies or drug induced causes. A family history is particularly useful in the identification of patients with hereditary disorders such as thalassemia, glucose-6-phosphate dehydrogenase deficiency and hereditary spherocytosis.

Laboratory tests used systemically are useful in establishing the cause of the anemia. The reticulocyte count is useful in determining whether a patient is failing to produce enough erythrocytes or their erythrocytes are undergoing abnormal destruction. A low reticulocyte count indicates decreased erythropoiesis. Reticulocytosis, an increase in the reticulocyte count, corresponds to the release of an increased number of immature erythrocytes from the bone marrow to the circulation and is indicative of bone marrow hyperactivity. Transient reticulocytosis often occurs in response to iron or vitamin B_{12} therapy following deficiency states.

A further dimension in the investigations of anemias is the use of erythrocyte indices. With the advent of automated and computerized blood cell counting technology these indices can be provided with relative ease. They include MCV (mean corpuscular volume), MCH (mean corpuscular hemoglobin) and MCHC (mean corpuscular hemoglobin concentration) and can be calculated from the erythrocyte count, hematocrit and hemoglobin concentration. For example in microcytic hypochromic anemias which occur in association with iron deficiency the MCV is lower than would be expected. In contrast, in the macrocytic anemias related to vitamin B_{12} deficiency, or folate deficiency, the MCV is elevated. Hypochromic anemias have a low MCHC value whereas hyperchromic anemias have an elevated MCHC.

A number of additional tests and investigations are available, including examination of blood smears and bone marrow, to identify the type of anemia and these are described in the subsequent sections.

Table 34.1.
Causes of Anemia and Corresponding State

Blood Loss	Chronic or Acute
Increased erythrocyte destruction	Hereditary cell defects, e.g. sickle cell anemia, hereditary spherocytosis, G6PD deficiency; exposure to hemolytic chemicals; development of antibodies against red cells, e.g. erythroblastosis fetalis
Reduced production of erythrocytes	Bone marrow disorders e.g. leukemia, aplastic anemia; deficiency of one or two nutrients e.g. iron, folic acid, vitamin B_{12}; deficiency of hormones, e.g. erythropoietin; drug induced; chronic diseases, e.g. chronic infection, widespread cancer, renal failure

GENERAL MANAGEMENT

As there are many different causes of anemia, treatment is either directed toward reducing the symptoms or where possible eliminating the cause. This may involve restoring missing nutrients in the deficiency anemias, identifying and removing toxic agents such as drugs in drug induced anemias, treating the primary causes with drug and nondrug measures or decreasing the extent of erythrocyte destruction by surgical methods such as splenectomy or restoring blood volume with transfusions.

IRON DEFICIENCY

Iron deficiency anemia results from decreased production of erythrocytes by the bone marrow due to a lack of available iron for hemoglobin synthesis. Iron deficiency has been classically defined as a hypochromic anemia because each erythrocyte contains less hemoglobin than normal. Hypochromia however is also a feature of other anemias such as those related to malignancies, chronic infection and genetically determined conditions such as thalassemia.

Table 34.2.
Selected Anemias and Their Laboratory Characteristics

Etiology	Reticulocyte No.[a]	Peripheral Smear	Additional Investigations
Iron deficiency	N↓	Hypochromic, microcytic	↓Fe ↑TIBC
Thalassemia	N↓	Hypochromic, microcytic	↑HbA$_2$, ↑HbF
Vitamin B_{12} deficiency	N↓	Macrocytic	↓B$_{12}$
Pernicious anemia	N↓	Macrocytic	↓B$_{12}$, achlorhydria
Folic acid deficiency	N↓	Macrocytic	↓Folate
Chronic inflammation	N↓	Normochromic, normocytic	↓Fe ↓TIBC
Uremia	N↓	Normochromic, normocytic	↑Creatinine
Liver disease	N↓	Normochromic, normocytic	Abnormal liver function tests
Myxedema	N↓	Normochromic, normocytic	↓T$_4$
Aplastic anemia	N↓	Normoblasts	Full blood count
Hemolytic—traumatic	↑	Polychromatophilia + schistocytes	
Immunohemolytic	↑	Normochromic, normocytic	Positive Coombs' test
Hereditary spherocytosis	↑	Spherocytes	Osmotic fragility
Sickle cell syndromes	↑	Sickle cells	
Glucose-6-phosphate dehydrogenase (G6PD) deficiency	↑	↓G6PD	Heinz bodies

[a] N↓ = normal or decreased.

Table 34.3.
Selected Hematologic and Biochemical Parameters (3, 4)

Component	Specimen[a]	Reference Range	
		Conventional	S.I.
Bilirubin (van der Bergh test)	S	1 min: 0.4 mg/100 ml	Up to 7 μmol/L
		Direct: 0.4 mg/100 ml	Up to 17 μmol/L
		Total: 1.0 mg/100 ml	
		Indirect is total minus direct	
Iron	S	50–150 μg/100 ml (higher in males).	9.0–26.9 μmol/L
		Shows diurnal variation higher in A.M.	
Total iron-binding capacity	S	250–410 μg/100 ml	44.8–73.4 μmol/L
Hematocrit	B	Male: 45–52%	Male: 0.42–0.52
		Female: 37–48%	Female: 0.37–0.48
Hemoglobin	B	Male: 13–18 g/100 ml	Male: 8.1–11.2 mmol/L
		Female: 12–16 g/100 ml	Female: 7.4–9.9 mmol/L
Erythrocyte count	B	4.2–5.9 million/mm^3	4.2–5.9 × 10^{12}/L
Mean corpuscular volume (MCV)	Ery	80–94 μm^3	80–94 fl
Mean corpuscular hemoglobin (MCH)	Ery	27–32 pg	1.7–2.0 fmol
Mean corpuscular hemoglobin concentration (MCHC)	Ery	32–36%	19–22.8 mmol/L
Ferritin			
Iron deficiency	S	0–20 ng/ml	0–20 μg/L
Iron excess	S	>400 ng/ml	>400 μg/L
Folic acid			
Normal	S	Greater than 1.9 ng/ml	>4.3 mmol/L
Borderline	S	1.0–1.9 ng/ml	2.3–4.3 mmol/L
Osmotic fragility of erythrocytes	B	Increased if hemolysis occurs in over 0.5% NaCl; decreased if hemolysis is incomplete in 0.3% NaCl	
Reticulocyte count	B	0.5–1.5% red cells	
Vitamin B$_{12}$	S	160–900 pg/ml	120–660 pg/ml

[a] S = serum; B = whole blood; Ery = erythrocyte.

Occurrence

Iron deficiency, estimated to occur in 500 million persons throughout the world and, perhaps 20 million persons in the United States, is the commonest cause of anemia (5). It is most frequently seen in male and female infants and menstruating women. In women it is prominent in pregnancy, being usually associated with folic acid deficiency.

In industrialized societies about 20% of all women and up to 50% of pregnant women are affected. In contrast, the prevalence of iron deficiency anemia in men is only about 3%. It occurs in approximately 30% of children peaking at approximately 1 year of age. In countries of the Orient, Africa and Central and South America, where hookworm infestation is endemic, iron deficiency anemia is common and can be severe.

Iron Absorption and Metabolism

Iron is an essential element for the body, being required for many physiologic processes including erythropoiesis, tissue respiration and as a cofactor of enzymic reactions (Table 34.4). It is generally obtained from a wide variety of foods, particularly meat and certain vegetables. Milk is a relatively poor source of iron as is a diet high in cereal content and low in animal protein. An average western diet contains approximately 10 to 20 mg of iron per day which is approximately the recommended dietary allowance (Table 34.5). The diet of the

Table 34.4.
Iron Distribution in the Body and Its Function

Site		Amount	Function
Functional			
Hemoglobin	Erythrocytes	2–2.5 g	Oxygen transport in blood
Myoglobin	Muscle	⎱ 140 mg	Oxygen transport in muscle
Cytochromes	Mitochondria	⎰	Electron transport system
Transferrin	Circulation	3 mg	Transport
Storage			
Ferritin and Hemosiderin	Reticuloendothelial cells of the liver and bone marrow	1 g (males), 100–400 mg (females)	Iron stores

Table 34.5.
Recommended Daily Dietary Allowances for Iron, Folic Acid and Vitamin B_{12} (8)[a]

Category	Age (yr)	Iron (mg)	Folacin[b] (μg)	Vitamin B_{12} (μg)
Infants	0–0.5	10	30	0.5
	0.5–1.0	15	45	1.5
Children	1–3	15	100	2.0
	4–6	10	200	2.5
	7–10	10	300	3.0
Men	11–18	18	400	3.0
	19–51+	10	400	3.0
Women	11–50	18	400	3.0
	51+	10	400	3.0
	Pregnant	30–60	+400	+1.0
	Lactating[c]	30–60	+400	+1.0

[a] For the maintenance of good nutrition for the majority of healthy persons in the United States.
[b] Folacin refers to dietary sources of folic acid as determined by *Lactobacillus casei* after treatment with enzymes.
[c] Continue for 2 to 3 months after parturition.

Table 34.6.
Factors Associated with Iron Absorption

Favoring absorption	
Inorganic iron	Ionic iron particularly in the ferrous form is better absorbed than ferric iron and organically bound iron
Ascorbic acid	Probably by assisting the conversion of ferric iron to ferrous iron
Acid	Gastric HCl promotes the release and conversion of dietary iron to the ferrous form
Chelates	Iron chelated to low molecular weight substances such as sugars (fructose and sucrose), amino acids and succinate faciliate binding of iron to the intestinal mucosa
Clinical states	Iron deficiency, increased erythropoiesis, pregnancy, anoxia, pyridoxine deficiency
Reducing absorption	
Alkaline	Alkaline pancreatic secretions containing phosphate probably convert iron to insoluble ferric hydroxide, antacids
Dietary	Dietary phosphates and phytates in cereals, tannins in tea (probably complex iron)
Clinical states	Chronic diarrhea, steatorrhea, iron overload, decreased erythropoiesis, acute or chronic inflammation

world's poorer populations today contains only a very low amount of iron.

Only a proportion of dietary iron is actually absorbed and utilized by the body. The amount absorbed depends on the iron status and rate of hematopoiesis of the individual, the nature of the foodstuff containing the iron and the ionic form of the iron (Table 34.6) (6). Dietary iron is closely linked to caloric intake with about 7 μg/1000 kcal intake with little variation among persons of different economic status. Adults with normal iron stores absorb approximately 5 to 10% of the dietary iron i.e. 1 to 2 mg/day. Absorption of iron may increase to 10 to 20% in patients with iron deficiency. In patients whose iron stores are severely depleted absorption may rise to as much as 50% of the total intake. For dietary iron to be absorbed, it must firstly be released by digestive enzymes from the organically bound form in the ingested foods. The availability of iron also varies according to the type of food (5). For example 10% of hemoglobin bound iron is absorbed compared to only 3% from eggs. Hemoglobin-bound iron and iron from other heme proteins such as myoglobin is absorbed as the intact heme molecule. Heme iron is highly available (20 to 40% in the iron-depleted subject), however it only represents a small fraction of dietary iron, particularly in the diet of poorer populations.

Furthermore dietary iron is converted to the ferrous form in the stomach and duodenum before it can be absorbed by the mucosal epithelial cells of the duodenum and ileum. Ferric iron is poorly absorbed, hence it is always desirable to administer iron in the ferrous salt form in the treatment of iron deficiency.

Ferrous iron is probably transported across the brush border of the intestinal mucosa bound to an intestinal gut protein, mucosal transferrin. The mechanism by which the intestinal epithelial cells respond to the body's iron requirements is not fully understood. After absorption the iron is either passed into the circulation where it is converted to the ferric form and combines with transferrin, a β_1-globulin plasma protein specific for iron transport or it remains within the epithelial cells combined with apoferritin to form ferritin. Iron bound to transferrin is transported to the bone marrow for hemoglobin synthesis and the liver for storage as well as to other tissues that require iron. At any one time the quantity of circulating iron (i.e. that bound to transferrin) is approximately 3 mg. Endogenous sources of iron include the breakdown of old erythrocytes by cells of the reticuloendothelial system (20 mg/day) and iron stores (10 to 15 mg/day).

Iron bound to ferritin remains in the mucosal epithelial cells if not required. This iron is excreted mainly in the feces when the epithelial cells slough off by the usual exfoliation process of the gut. Some iron is also lost by the continuous exfoliation of other epithelial cells such as of the skin and kidney. Adults lose approximately 0.6 mg of iron per day. The amount lost is higher in menstruating women and during pregnancy. Even though the concentration of serum iron is only 50 to 150 μg/100 ml, approximately 35 to 40 mg of iron is transported in the plasma each day, the major portion being taken for erythropoiesis. The erythrocyte mass accounts for approximately

2 to 2.5 g of iron. As the life span of the human erythrocyte is 120 days, and old cells are being continually replaced by new ones, 16 to 20 mg of iron is required daily for replacement.

Other factors which affect iron absorption in the small intestine are listed in Table 34.6. They include overt iron deficiency, pregnancy, anoxia and increased erythropoiesis due to hemorrhage, hemolytic states or high altitudes (7). The absorption of iron is usually lower when the body is overloaded with iron. In some clinical states such as primary hemochromatosis, thalassemia and sideroblastic anemia, iron absorption remains normal and even raised despite the presence of increased iron stores. Giving additional iron to these patients is therefore inappropriate and can be dangerous.

The quantity of iron lost by the body each day is similar to that absorbed. The daily iron requirements vary according to age and sex. It is high in menstruating women and during pregnancy, whereas normal men and postmenopausal women require only 1 mg each day (Table 34.7). The need for iron is high in the first year of life and subsequent childhood years because of rapid growth during this period. In women each menstruation can result in a loss of 30 mg or more of iron and the daily iron requirements increase to 2 to 3 mg a day. During pregnancy both the maternal and fetal iron requirements must be met by the mother and at least 3 to 4 mg of iron must be absorbed each day.

Etiology

Factors associated with iron deficiency include inadequate absorption of iron due to a dietary deficiency or an impairment of the iron absorbing process (e.g. gastrectomy) or mechanism (e.g. malabsorption); hemorrhage where

Table 34.7.
Daily Iron Requirements[a]

Infant	
0–4 months	0.5
5–12 months	1.0
Children	1.0
Adolescent male	1.8
Adolescent female	2.4
Menstruating female	2.8
Adult male	1.0
Post menopausal female	1.0
During pregnancy	3–4

[a] Values (mg) represent actual iron absorbed.

iron is being lost quicker than it can be replenished from the diet; and increased requirements such as in pregnancy (Table 34.8). Poor nutrition, defective intake or decreased assimilation of iron rarely causes iron deficiency in adults living in western countries. It may take many years for iron deficiency to manifest even if iron rich foods are excluded from the diet. In poor tropical countries, however, where large quantities of food of vegetable origin and little meat are consumed, women are more likely to suffer from nutritional iron deficiency anemia.

Blood lost through hemorrhaging is the commonest cause of iron deficiency in adults. In women of child-bearing age iron deficiency due to blood loss is most prevalent because of menstrual losses and the demands of pregnancy. Iron deficiency in men is usually a result of some underlying pathologic process e.g. malignancy or lesion of the gastrointestinal tract.

Iron supplementation during pregnancy is necessary because fetal demand is approximately 400 mg; loss at delivery, hemorrhaging, and iron in the placenta and uterus total another 325 mg. Iron-rich foods, iron-fortified food such as flour and bread or oral iron supplements are often given because the average diet is unable to meet the deficit.

During lactation, iron deficiency can be a risk for both mother and infant. Over a breast-feeding period of 6 months approximately 175 mg of iron may be lost by the mother. Care must be taken to supplement the infant's diet with more iron or iron-rich foods particularly if milk from either natural or artificial sources is the principal food.

Gastrointestinal bleeding associated with peptic ulceration or esophageal varices in alcoholics also results in iron deficiency. Bleeding may be occult or frank and manifested as hematemesis, darkening of the feces or melena. Other causes of blood loss are hemorrhoids, alimentary carcinoma, hookworm infestation and salicylate ingestion. Iron deficiency also arises in patients after partial or total gastrectomy where ability to absorb iron is reduced. Blood may also be lost from the gastric stump. These patients secrete reduced amounts or no gastric acid at all, so less ferric iron is converted to the better absorbed ferrous iron. Malabsorption conditions can also lead to iron deficiency. These, however, are rarely an important cause, unless the iron stores are low or there are other contributing factors such as blood loss or pregnancy.

Table 34.8.
Factors Associated with Iron Deficiency

Factor	Associations
Dietary	Starvation, poverty, vegetarians, religious practice, food faddism
Blood loss	
Females	Menorrhagia, postmenopausal bleeding, pregnancy
General	Esophageal varices, peptic ulcer, drug induced gastritis, carcinomas of stomach and colon, ulcerative colitis, hemorrhoids, renal or bladder lesions (hematuria), hookworm infestation, other organ bleeding (hemoptysis). Widespread bleeding disorders
Malabsorption	Celiac disease (gluten-induced enteropathy). Partial and total gastrectomy, chronic inflammation
Increased requirements	Rapid growth such as in childhood and adolescents, frequent pregnancies

Pathogenesis

Progressive depletion of iron in all tissues occurs if a state of negative iron balance exists. Iron is gradually mobilized from iron storage compounds such as hemosiderin and ferritin to meet the body's physiologic and metabolic needs. Mobilization occurs until stores are depleted. This is characterised by the absence of stainable iron in the bone marrow, increased iron absorption but no decrease in either the concentration of serum iron or whole blood hemoglobin. A second stage in the pathogenesis of iron deficiency anemia is when the iron depletion results in a fall of the serum iron concentration but with still no interference of erythropoiesis. In the final stage iron supply to tissues, particularly the bone marrow, is reduced and the features of iron deficiency begin to appear. Iron deficiency is readily reversed by giving iron. The initial response can be dramatic because iron deficient cells such as the erythroblasts of the bone marrow have an increased avidity for iron.

The number of nonerythroid tissue abnormalities described in iron deficient patients are assumed to result from the defective synthesis of tissue iron enzymes although biochemical and morphological correlates have yet to be established (9). The symptoms of the iron deficient patient may be related to metabolic changes including iron enzyme defects and mitochondrial abnormalities (9, 10). Such symptoms are described below.

Clinical Findings and Manifestations

Most individuals with iron deficiency have minimal anemia and are asymptomatic. Only patients with severe iron deficiency are likely to present with clinical manifestations typical of other chronic anemias (Table 34.9). These symptoms become evident when the hemoglobin concentration is less than 10 g/100 ml. Any significant degree of anemia is always associated with a decreased work capacity (10). People with sedentary life-styles may have a moderate degree of anemia and yet experience no symptoms. In poor countries severe iron deficiency anemia can reduce agricultural productivity. There is also conflicting evidence that increased infections are associated with iron deficiency particularly in infants and children. After reviewing the evidence, the U.S. Committee on Nutrition (1978) concluded that iron deficiency increased the risk of infection and that this was dependent upon the severity of the deficiency and whether it was nutritional in origin (10).

Laboratory Tests and Monitoring Parameters

Hematologic changes are evident in the more severe forms of iron deficiency. Blood hemoglobin concentrations fall if there is a depletion of iron stores and there is insufficient iron to maintain a normal erythrocyte mass. A fall is usually accompanied by erythrocyte changes reflected in decreased MCV and MCHC. In the early stages of iron deficiency anemia the amount of hemoglobin (MCH) in each erythrocyte falls as does the MCV. The MCHC remains within the normal range and the erythrocytes are classified as normochromic. When significant anemia accompanies the iron deficiency (e.g. blood hemoglobin of below 7 g/100 ml in women and 9 g/100 ml in men) the MCHC falls below normal and hypochromia is apparent. Hypochromic and microcytic cells, are seen in microscopic examination of the peripheral blood film along with small, pale and thin erythrocytes varying in size (anisocytes) and shape (elliptocytes), bizarre poikilocytes and some normally filled cells.

The erythrocyte count is usually near normal and the hematocrit is reduced. The proportion of reticulocytes is usually normal; however a transient reticulocytosis may follow acute hemorrhage or treatment with iron. The white cell count can be normal or reduced and the platelet count variable. Examination of the bone marrow shows moderate erythroid hyperplasia and many of the erythrocyte precursors such as the normoblasts have little cytoplasm.

Diagnosis

Diagnosis depends upon the finding of a blood picture of hypochromic anemia, depleted iron stores and in the case of suspected hemorrhage, the discovery of the source by clinical assessment, radiographic and/or endoscopic results.

An initial screen involving estimation of se-

Table 34.9.
Features of Patients with Iron Deficiency

Clinical manifestations	
Appearance	Tired, listless, lifeless appearance
Skin and hair	Pale skin, inelastic and often dry; dry and often scanty hair
Mouth	Papillary atrophy and erythema of the tongue, angular stomatitis
Eye	Pearly white sclerae
Nails	Flattened, longitudinally rigid, concave (koilonychia)
Cardiovascular system	Slight cardiomegaly, tachycardia, functional systolic murmur, cardiomegaly, ankle edema
Neurologic	Generally normal
Blood picture	
Hemoglobin	10–5 g/100 ml (moderate to severe)
MCV	Decreased
MCHC	Decreased
Marrow iron stores	Depleted
Serum iron	Reduced
TIBC	Increased

rum iron, total iron-binding capacity (TIBC) and transferrin saturation is useful (5). The first two parameters reflect iron availability to tissues, whereas the transferrin saturation, if below 16%, indicates that basal erythropoiesis cannot occur. Such a decrease can be due to either iron deficiency or inflammation. A decreased transferrin saturation and an increased TIBC is specific for iron deficiency and therefore differentiates between the two. Erythrocyte protoporphyrin is directly related to the iron needs of erythrocytes. Elevated circulatory levels indicate iron deficient erythropoiesis. Such elevated levels of protoporphyrin are also seen in lead toxicity and disorders of porphyrin metabolism. A relative deficiency occurs in hemolytic anemia and more specifically sickle-cell anemia.

As the iron stores must be depleted before significant anemia occurs in the presence of a relatively normal blood picture, serum iron and the TIBC are valuable monitoring tests. In iron deficiency the serum iron concentration is lower and the TIBC levels higher than normal which differentiates it from anemias of chronic illnesses where both serum iron concentrations and the TIBC levels are lower than normal.

The normal range of serum iron is 50 to 150 μg/100 ml, being higher in men than women. Serum iron concentrations are subject to diurnal variation with higher levels occurring in the morning (7). Larger variations occur in women particularly during menstruation. In a patient with iron deficiency anemia low blood hemoglobin concentrations (9 g/100 ml) are usually consistent with low serum iron concentrations. It is unlikely, however, that a patient with such low hemoglobin levels and a high serum iron concentration will have iron deficiency anemia.

Iron store status is inferred from bone marrow aspirates stained for iron, measuring serum transferrin saturation or serum ferritin levels. In iron deficiency anemia, in contrast to anemias of chronic disorders, no stainable iron is visible in the bone marrow. Transferrin saturations of less than 16% are generally consistent with lack of iron stores in patients with iron deficiency. Serum ferritin concentrations fall to one-tenth normal levels or lower. In adults 1 μg of ferritin per liter is equivalent to about 140 μg of storage iron per kilogram of body weight. A simple relationship between serum ferritin concentrations and iron stores cannot be assumed when ferritin concentrations exceed 4000 μg/liter or in patients who have received more than 100 units of transfused blood. Ferritin, a water-soluble protein-iron complex, is the major iron storage protein in the tissues (10). In normal persons, average serum ferritin concentrations vary with age and sex. It is about 30 μg/liter in children and in women remains at this level until menopause. In pregnancy during the first, second and third trimesters, it is 90, 30, and 15 μg/liter, respectively. In male subjects it increases from 30 μg/liter at 15 years to about 90 μg/liter from 30 years onward.

As indicated above serum ferritin concentrations are directly related to bone marrow iron stores within certain limits. The main clinical use of serum ferritin at the present time is in the evaluation of decreased iron stores (11). Low serum ferritin concentrations are a more sensitive indicator of iron deficiency than serum iron or TIBC, particularly in differentiating it from anemias of other causes. For example a patient with low serum iron and a high TIBC is probably iron deficient. A problem in the interpretation of serum ferritin concentrations is that the levels are inappropriately elevated particularly when associated with inflammation of ferritin-rich tissue, such as the liver. Increased serum ferritin concentrations are also associated with inflammatory conditions such as rheumatoid arthritis and in a variety of malignant states including carcinoma of the breast.

In the absence of a specialized hematology facility, a tentative diagnosis of iron deficiency can be made by giving a trial of oral iron therapy and monitoring hemoglobin concentrations and reticulocyte counts. Significant reticulocytosis occurs at 7 to 10 days after the commencement of treatment and the hemoglobin concentration increases at a rate of 0.2 g/100 ml per day over a period of 3 to 4 weeks.

Acute Hemorrhage

In the case of acute hemorrhage, a sudden loss of blood of 1 liter or more may result in shock due to a collapse of the peripheral circulation and a loss of 2 to 3 liters of blood over a very short period may prove fatal. A similar loss over 1 to 2 days allows the circulating blood volume to be maintained by transfer of tissue fluid into the blood. Following restoration of the circulating blood volume the symptoms of shock subside. If hemorrhage is severe than blood transfusions can be given.

Prophylaxis

In addition to ensuring a diet adequate in meat and vegetables, women with either heavy menstrual periods or those that have repeated pregnancies usually require iron supplementation. Such advice may be given by the pharmacist particularly during the prenatal period. Prophylactic measures for pregnant women include: routine estimation of hemoglobin at their first prenatal visit; iron therapy with ferrous sulfate 200 mg, 3 times a day, in combination with folic acid 300 μg per day (third trimester).

Symptoms of iron deficiency anemia are not as discernible in infants as they are in adults. To reduce the likelihood of iron deficiency in breast-fed babies or those on artificial milk supplementation (when essential), supplementary feeds of broth, ground meat, vegetable purees and other suitable food rich in iron can be given from the age of 4 to 6 months. Infants of a low birth weight may be given liquid iron supplements from 3 months onward.

TREATMENT OF IRON DEFICIENCY ANEMIA

A patient with iron deficiency anemia has lower circulating hemoglobin and inadequate iron stores. Treatment is therefore directed at these two problems. This is to increase the erythrocyte MCV and MCH to normal levels and replenish the depleted iron stores. Although restoration of erythrocyte parameters occurs within a few weeks, replenishing iron stores takes longer. As only a small percentage of the iron is absorbed (10 to 20%) it takes approximately 3 months and possibly up to 6 months for the iron stores to attain 1 g of elemental iron.

Iron deficiency anemia can be corrected by the administration of either oral or parenteral iron. But indiscriminate administration of iron may delay diagnosis. It is unwise to correct iron deficiency anemia by dietary means alone, a search for its cause is necessary.

Treatment failures with oral iron therapy are relatively high. In the absence of a response to oral iron therapy the following questions should be asked: 1) is the patient complying with the medication? 2) does the patient have a malabsorption problem? 3) is the patient bleeding so that iron loss is greater than intake? and 4) was the initial diagnosis correct?

Oral Iron Therapy

Since only a small and variable proportion of oral iron is absorbed, large oral doses of iron salts are necessary to reverse the deficiency state. The cheapest and safest method of treating a patient with confirmed iron deficiency anemia is the oral administration of ferrous sulfate ($FeSO_4$) 200 mg, 3 times a day (12). The effectiveness of therapy should be assessed 3 weeks after treatment is commenced. At the above dose a minimum response of an increased hemoglobin concentration of 2 g/100 ml should be expected provided sepsis, toxemia and hemorrhage are absent. In severe cases up to 1.8 g of ferrous sulfate can be administered daily in divided doses. The usual therapeutic dose of ferrous sulfate for children under 1 year is 180 mg daily; 1 to 5 years, 360 mg daily; and 6 to 12 years, 600 mg daily all in divided doses (12).

Maximum absorption of iron occurs if given before food. Large doses, which often produce gastrointestinal irritation and diarrhea, should be given after meals to avert these problems. Continued administration may sometimes produce constipation. Some patients may also complain of blackened or tarry stools during iron therapy which should not be confused with darkened stools or melena that can occur with gastrointestinal bleeding.

Treating anemias with a combination of iron with folic acid or vitamin B_{12} is undesirable because the effectiveness of each component may be difficult to assess. Such combinations may also be unnecessary and expensive. The claims of fewer side effects with sustained release preparations may be due to less ionic iron being presented to the gut at any one time.

Absorption of iron from ferrous sulfate is maximal in the fasting patient. The bioavailability of iron may be reduced by up to one half in patients fed various foods. However, taking ferrous sulfate on an empty stomach may increase the incidence of side effects such as nausea and vomiting. It is sometimes desirable to reduce the dose to alleviate such unpleasant effects and at the same time improve compliance. If side effects do occur then the patient should take the iron with or after meals. In patients with severe intolerance, parenteral iron may be necessary. Antacids also reduce the absorption of iron if taken at the same time, thus they should be separated by 1 to 2 hours.

Ferrous salts in the sulfate, lactate, succinate, glutamate and gluconate forms are absorbed to about the same degree. Care must be taken, however, when calculating the doses of these salts, as they each contain differing amounts of elemental iron (Table 34.10). Liquid iron preparations are also available without prescription over the counter for pediatric use.

Many strategies have been employed in the past to either improve iron absorption and/or reduce unpleasant side effects. Additives in iron preparations may enhance iron absorption. Of these, ascorbic acid (200 mg) is probably the most effective, increasing iron absorption by 30%. However, this may be associated with a greater incidence of side effects. To reduce side effects enteric-coated iron tablets have also been tried but are generally of no value. The use of sustained release formulations of ferrous sulfate has increased in recent years with claims of increased efficacy. Limited bioavailability data makes it difficult to compare them with other dosage forms.

Parenteral Iron Therapy

Iron is available in a colloidal (nonionic) form complexed to carbohydrate compounds. Two such preparations are iron dextran (50 mg Fe/ml) and iron sorbitex (50 mg Fe/ml) (12, 13). Iron dextran is the more commonly used and is administered preferably by the intramuscular route.

Iron dextran which consists of iron complexed to dextran is indicated only when iron deficiency anemia is refractory to oral iron treatment, or when oral medication is impractical or undesirable to administer; in some cases of rheumatoid arthritis; when serum iron and iron stores need to be rapidly achieved such as in emergency surgery in iron deficient patients; when iron deficiency is diagnosed in late pregnancy; and iron deficiency in premature infants. Parenteral iron is also useful in patients with gastrointestinal bleeding where oral iron therapy by darkening stools may mask melena.

The usual method of administration is by a deep intramuscular injection into the ventrolateral aspect of the upper and outer quadrant of the buttock. Care must be taken in using the correct technique for intramuscular injections. A recent study using computerized tomography scans suggested that in general injections intended for intramuscular use are often delivered into the subcutaneous region (intralipomatous) (14). In the case of iron dextran the injection technique must avoid leakage through the needle track or staining of the skin (z-track method). It is claimed that absorption of iron dextran from the injection site is virtually complete and maximum serum levels are reached within 1 or 2 days but

Table 34.10.
Common Iron Preparations

Proprietary Name	Active Ingredient	Elemental Iron	Iron (%)
Tablets			
Ferrous sulfate, USP (generic)	Ferrous sulfate heptahydrate	60 mg/300 mg	20
Feosol (initial formulation)	Ferrous sulfate dried	60 mg/200 mg	30
Fergon	Ferrous gluconate	39 mg/325 mg	11.5
Ircon	Ferrous fumarate	66 mg/200 mg	33
Chel-Iron	Ferrocholinate	39 mg/333 mg	12
Liquids			
Mol-Iron liquid	Ferrous sulfate	10 mg/ml	
Mol-Iron drops	Ferrous sulfate	25 mg/ml	
Feosol elixir	Ferrous sulfate	8 mg/ml	
Fer-In-Sol syrup	Ferrous sulfate	6 mg/ml	
Fer-In-Sol drops	Ferrous sulfate	25 mg/ml	
Fergon elixir	Ferrous gluconate	7 mg/ml	
Chel-Iron liquid	Ferrocholinate	10 mg/ml	
Chel-Iron drops	Ferrocholinate	25 mg/ml	
Ferrolip pediatric syrup	Ferrocholinate	4 mg/ml	
Ferrolip pediatric drops	Ferrocholinate	25 mg/ml	
Ferro drops	Ferrous lactate	25 mg/ml	

variable amounts bind locally for several months. The iron dextran is transported from the muscle by the lymphatic circulation to the blood, then to the liver, where it is taken up by reticuloendothelial cells. These cells are also known as mononuclear phagocytic cells. These cells release iron from the iron dextran complex which then enters the plasma compartment to combine with transferrin. Iron is utilized by the body or stored as ferritin or hemosiderin for later use. Some of the iron dextran remains trapped inside the reticuloendothelial cells but is gradually released. During the first week or so after injection the amount of iron in the plasma is largely due to the iron dextran present and is unrelated to transferrin bound iron.

The initial dose of iron dextran is usually 1 ml (50 mg Fe) on the first day and then 2 ml daily or at longer intervals, according to the hemoglobin response (12). The total volume of iron dextran injection required to restore hemoglobin levels to normal and replenish body iron stores can be calculated from the following formula:

Volume of iron dextran injection

$$= 0.66 \times W.D./50$$

W = body weight in kilograms

D = percentage hemoglobin deficiency

$$= 100 - \left(\frac{\text{patient's Hb (g/100 ml} \times 100)}{14.8} \right).$$

This formula does not take into account iron losses and iron bioavailability. Therefore higher doses of iron are probably required to give an increase in the whole blood hemoglobin by 0.2 g/100 ml/day.

An alternative method is to give periodic intramuscular injections until the hemoglobin level has returned to a desired level. Approximately 45 mg (approximately 1 ml) is needed for each 1% deficiency in the hemoglobin scale for a 70-kg adult. On this basis maximum doses for children are 0.5 ml for under 4 kg, 1 ml for 4 to 10 kg and 2 ml for children weighing more than 10 kg (12).

The intravenous route avoids deposition of iron into skeletal muscle and local reactions. The regimen involves several intravenous injections or the total dose is given as an infusion over a period of 6 to 8 hours diluted with 0.9% sodium chloride or 5% dextrose.

Arthralgias and myalgias occur with total dose infusions of iron dextran (15) and current practice is to administer them only by the intramuscular route at doses not exceeding 2 ml. Anaphylactoid reactions have also occurred after the administration of intravenous infusions of iron dextran. Allergic reactions and thrombophlebitis may arise at the injection site. Local phlebitis is less likely to occur if 0.9% sodium chloride is used as the diluent instead of 5% dextrose. Other adverse effects that have been reported include nausea, vomiting, flushing, sweating, fever, urticaria, leukocytosis, lymphadenopathy, dyspnea and circulatory collapse. In severe cases of dyspnea and circulatory collapse an injection of an antihistamine or adrenaline may be given subcutaneously.

Iron dextran injection should not be given to patients with severe liver disease or acute kidney infection. Patients with a history of allergy should be commenced in small doses followed by a graded series of injections. Large single doses should not be given to patients with rheumatoid arthritis because they may exacerbate the disease.

Iron Sorbitex

Intramuscular iron sorbitex injection is an alternative to intramuscular iron dextran injection (12, 13). It is unsuitable for intravenous administration. Each milliliter of the injection contains 50 mg of iron in the ferric form complexed to sorbitol and citric acid. After injection to an iron-deficient patient, half the dose enters the bloodstream within the first hour. Within 10 hours most of the iron is redistributed. Some of it is utilized for erythropoiesis by the bone marrow, the rest being stored in the liver. A darkening of the urine can occur after administration of iron sorbitex because part of the dose may be excreted by the kidneys.

Dosages of iron sorbitex for both adults and children are calculated on body weight. The initial dose is a volume equivalent to 1.5 mg of iron per kg body weight which for a 70-kg adult is about 2 ml. The total dose of iron sorbitex depends upon the hemoglobin level of the patient and is calculated on the basis that women require 200 mg of iron (4 ml) and that men require 250 mg (5 ml) to increase the blood hemoglobin concentration by 1 g/100 ml. To replenish iron stores an additional 0.5 to 1 g (10 to 20 ml) of iron is required. In pregnancy, five additional injections of 2 ml are administered after blood hemoglobin has returned to normal. For children the equivalent of 1.5 mg of iron/kg is administered on a daily or alternate day basis (12).

Iron sorbitex injection is rarely antigenic and the occurrence of urticaria is rare. Adverse reactions include nausea and vomiting. Some patients experience changes in taste sensation shortly after administration. A metallic taste is experienced if high doses of oral iron are inadvertently given after an injection of iron sorbitex. At least 24 hours should elapse before oral iron or a further injection of iron sorbitex is given. A week should pass if the patient has previously been given another parenteral iron preparation such as iron dextran beforehand. Iron sorbitex is contraindicated in hepatic disorders and renal diseases, particularly in pyelonephritis and untreated urinary tract infections.

IRON TOXICITY

Iron toxicity may be either acute, overdosage or accidental poisoning, or chronic as in iron overload.

Acute Toxicity

Oral ingestion of large amounts of iron salts are toxic (10, 12). Such ingestion has catastrophic effects partly because of the direct corrosive effects of iron salts on the gut and partly because of the toxic effects of the large quantities of ionic iron absorbed from the intestine (10). It has also been suggested that iron is toxic to mitochondria and the enzymes of the citric acid cycle because of marked lactic and citric acidosis prior to circulatory collapse, a major problem in acute iron toxicity. Death due to consumption of large amounts of iron salts in adults is rare and results from suicidal attempts. Fatal poisonings have occurred in young children (1 to 2 years old) after ingestion of ferrous sulfate. Doses of 1 g or more of ferrous sulfate should be considered toxic in children but 2 to 20 g are usually ingested in fatal cases. Signs and symptoms which may occur within the first hour after ingestion include abdominal pain, diarrhea and vomiting. The vomitus may be coffee brown in color and it may contain remains of the ingested tablets. The patient may be pale or cyanosed and lethargic. Hyperventilation due to acidosis and cardiovascular collapse are other serious prob-

lems. Death may occur within 6 hours or even 12 to 24 hours after ingestion. With earlier diagnosis of iron overdosage and subsequent implementation of treatment for shock, dehydration and acid base abnormalities mortality can be reduced from 45% to 1%.

If the victim is brought into the emergency room, deferoxamine mesylate (12, 13), a chelating agent with a specific affinity for iron can be administered for the removal of iron due to iron poisoning. It combines with any free iron in the tissues and the body fluids and is excreted through the kidneys. It is administered intramuscularly in 2-g doses dissolved in 8 to 12 ml of water for injections. Gastric lavage should then be performed promptly with 1% sodium bicarbonate solution. Oral administration of 5 g of deferoxamine mesylate in 50 ml of fluid is recommended to bind iron remaining in the stomach to prevent any further absorption. Intubation may be necessary in comatosed patients. Intramuscular injection may be repeated at intervals of 12 hours and if large amounts of iron have been taken it may have to be given to a maximum dose of 12 g (12).

Deferoxamine mesylate can also be administered by continuous intravenous infusion at a rate of not more than 15 mg/kg body weight per hour to a maximum dose of 80 mg/kg body weight in 24 hours; it may be added to sodium chloride injection or dextrose injection. The quantity of deferoxamine given by injection in poisoning should be related to the serum iron level. In suitable cases the above treatment may be given in the first instance and a decision whether to give injections is made after serum iron determinations. Infants or children with serum levels above 5 mg/liter or adults with serum levels of over 8 mg/liter require parenteral treatment.

If deferoxamine is not available, the patient should be made to vomit immediately followed by gastric lavage with a 5% sodium bicarbonate solution. About 300 ml of the solution should be left in the stomach. This procedure should only be undertaken within 1 hour of ingestion because of the danger of perforation. A saline cathartic should also be given to speed the elimination of the ferrous sulfate. Fluid loss should be replaced by administering compound sodium lactate injection or sodium chloride and dextrose injection. Exchange transfusions may be given in severe cases (12).

Chronic Toxicity

Parenchymal overload from chronic iron toxicity is more likely to be due to iron compounds in excess than free ionic iron. Iron overload exists when total iron stores exceed 4 g. It may be produced by three possible mechanisms: 1) inappropriately increased mucosal absorption of iron, 2) excessive intake of iron over a prolonged period, and 3) parenteral administration of iron either as blood transfusions or by injections of therapeutic iron preparations. With excessive iron intake, body iron stores gradually increase and excess iron is deposited as ferritin and hemosiderin in either parenchymal or reticuloendothelial cells (macrophages). The iron loading of parenchymal cells may be HLA-related, erythropoietic or associated with hepatic disease (5, 10, 16).

Hemachromatosis refers to a condition characterised by an increase in total body iron with predominately parenchymal cell deposition and iron induced damage. Inflammation and the continued trapping of iron by the macrophages leads to an increased iron absorption. Laboratory results include low to normal transferrin saturation and a progressive increase in serum ferritin and marrow hemosiderin with time. Most of the parenchymal iron is situated in the liver and the balance in other organs such as the heart and pancreas which can also be affected. Although an excess of iron in the parenchymal cells is usually due to excessive absorption it may also reflect enhanced internal redistribution of iron recycled from macrophages.

Idiopathic hemochromatosis refers to a genetic disorder of iron overload due to excessive iron absorption (5, 10, 16). It is associated with certain HLA types, HLA-H3 and HLA-B14, which are due to a somatic gene mutation. Its importance is that the hemochromatosis gene can be traced through a family without waiting for pathologic manifestations to occur (17). The homozygous form occurs in approximately 1 in 1000 persons with overt damage and symptomatic disease arising in 1 in 5000. The prevalence is lower in women, probably because of iron loss during menstruation. Alcohol consumption can increase the total iron overload up to 50%. Young homozygotes should be retested regularly to prevent severe overload and those patients considered to be heterozygous should be warned of the possible ill effects of alcohol and iron therapy.

Iron overload secondary to certain anemias can be divided into two classes: (a) those with a hypoplastic bone marrow where the main source of iron is blood transfusions used in the treatment of aplastic anemia and (b) those with hyperplastic marrow where the excess in iron results from increased iron absorption secondary to ineffective erythropoiesis. The latter usually arises in thalassemia major and sideroblastic anemia, but it has also been reported in thalassemia intermedia, congenital hemolytic anemia, sickle cell anemia, and other hemolytic anemias. Patients with aplastic anemia have little hepatic damage, whereas those with anemias and hyperplasia frequently have both heavy parenchymal iron overload and cirrhosis in the liver.

Iron overload occasionally develops in patients with liver disorders including cirrhosis and portacaval shunting. In these patients transferrin is saturated and serum ferritin elevated. This situation is distinguished from patients with idiopathic hemochromatosis by (a) the more abnormal liver function and (b) nearly normal urinary deferoxamine excretion and lack of evidence of iron overload in siblings of patients with liver disease.

Elevated serum ferritin is the most specific index of iron overload. Patients rarely present with serum ferritin concentrations in the reference range. Serum ferritin levels in excess of 70 μg/100 ml occur in patients with symptomatic hemochromatosis.

Clinical Manifestations

The clinical manifestations of iron overload correspond to the accumulation rate of iron. In thalassemia these develop most rapidly, progressing from hepatic fibrosis in early childhood; failure of the gonads in adolescence and if removal of iron is inadequate, possible cardiac death in early childhood. In HLA-related overload, the sequence of events is much slower. Clinical manifestations may not appear until the sixth decade. Their spectrum is variable and may include abdominal pain and hepatomegaly, diabetes, impotence and testicular atrophy, a bronze or gray pigmentation of the skin, and cardiac failure.

Treatment

Even if parenchymal iron overload is asymptomatic, treatment is desirable. Therapy for idiopathic hemochromatosis involves the removal of excess iron and treatment of complications such as diabetes, and cardiac and liver failure. Weekly venesection is used for patients with a hematocrit of above 30%. In young precirrhotic patients, iron stores should be reduced to normal within 1 to 2 years or less. After this, venesection is required only every 3 to 4 months to prevent reaccumulation of iron. The prognosis is excellent. In severely affected patients, venesection therapy results in 66% survival after five years and 32% survival after 10 years compared with 18 and 6%, respectively, for untreated patients. Regular phlebotomy is usually well tolerated, but occasionally hypovolemia may precipitate angina or cardiac arrhythmias.

Subcutaneous or intravenous deferoxamine is used in severely anemic patients. Liver failure, cardiac failure and diabetes mellitus are managed conventionally. Testosterone therapy (testosterone enanthate depot injection, 250 mg monthly) may partially relieve the loss of libido and changes in secondary sex characteristics.

In most patients with iron-loading anemias, venesection is not possible. Currently the treatment of transfusional iron overload must be directed to preventing the accumulation of iron in any way possible. Negative iron balance can be achieved by continuous infusions of deferoxamine regardless of the level of iron loading. Theoretically, reducing iron-rich foods in the diet such as meat and increasing the quantity of foods with a high phytate, phosphate or tannin content should be useful in the prevention or management of iron overload. However, dietary iron makes little contribution to the overloading.

A summary of recent developments in infusion iron chelator therapy with deferoxamine include (16):

1. Most patients require 1 to 4 g of deferoxamine over 12 to 24 hours to achieve negative iron balance.

2. Because of individual variation, dosage and duration of treatment should be individually adjusted for each patient by monitoring urinary iron excretion.

3. Patients should be ascorbate complete, because ascorbic acid deficiency has been shown to impair iron chelation. Concurrent administration of deferoxamine and ascorbic acid has been shown to improve iron excretion (see under "Thalassemias").

4. Treatment should be commenced early in life before gross iron overload develops.

5. The above regimen usually results in the urinary excretion of 1 to 4 mg of iron per kg body weight per day. Deferoxamine bound iron is also lost via the gastrointestinal tract. Elimination of 1 to 2 g of iron per month effectively maintains a negative iron balance in patients who receive 4 to 6 units of blood each month.

6. Iron absorption does not increase during deferoxamine treatment. Renal function is assessed because deferoxamine is cleared largely by the kidneys.

7. The following parameters should be monitored at 6 monthly intervals, or more often during treatment: urinary iron concentration; transferrin saturation; serum creatinine, iron, ferritin, albumin, bilirubin, aspartate aminotransferase and alkaline phosphatase levels; and hematologic measurements.

Contraindications of deferoxamine include pregnancy and severe renal disease. Transient cellulitis has occasionally been reported with subcutaneous infusions. Mild skin hypersensitivity reactions with pruritus, erythema and swelling sometimes arise at the injection site, but are readily controlled by an antihistamine given prior to administration of deferoxamine.

Prognosis

There is good evidence that deferoxamine therapy may arrest tissue damage in thalassemia. Using intravenous deferoxamine, normalization of iron balance occurs within months, even in patients with heavy loading. However, treatment is expensive and requires prolonged periods of infusions. Infusion over 12 hours is about as effective as 24 hours. This allows the infusion to be discontinued during the day. High dose continuous therapy offers the only hope currently to patients with cardiopathy due to iron overload. In patients with hereditary sideroblastic anemia prevention of tissue damage is preferable to treatment of impaired organs and tissues. Because of the expense and inconvenience of infusion therapy, effective oral chelators of iron are desirable.

The new drugs under investigation fall into three groups: (a) parenteral agents such as rhodotorulic acid, (b) oral iron chelators such as cholyhydroxamic acid and isoniazid pyridoxal hydrazone, and (c) depot preparations of deferoxamine or polymeric hydroxamic acids. None of the more experimental approaches of iron chelation using liposomes, combination therapy or drug entrapment into red cell ghosts has yet been found as a solution to the problem of iron overload.

MEGALOBLASTIC ANEMIAS

Megaloblastic anemias are characterized by impairment of DNA synthesis leading to disordered erythroid maturation. Microscopic examination of the bone marrow and peripheral blood reveals distinctive morphological changes. The main causes of megaloblastic anemia include either deficiency, malabsorption or impaired utilization of either vitamin B_{12} or folic acid or both. Malabsorption is the main cause of vitamin B_{12} deficiency, whereas a dietary lack is more likely to cause a folate deficiency. Next to dietary deficiency of folate, drug ingestion is the second most common cause of megaloblastic anemia.

Folic acid and vitamin B_{12} are required for the synthesis of purine and pyrimidine nucleotides, both precursors for DNA synthesis. During hematopoiesis, bone marrow cells differentiate and divide into the different cell lines including the erythrocyte series. If there is reduced availability of folic acid or vitamin B_{12} to the bone marrow for any reason, the rate of cell division decreases, the RNA:DNA ratio increases and larger erythrocyte precursor megaloblasts appear in the bone marrow. Why the megaloblast is large and how the characteristic chromatin pattern develops is not fully understood. The longer "s" phase in these cells probably allows greater RNA and protein synthesis to occur. When these cells mature and enter the circulation they are macrocytic and their MCV is in excess of 120 fl (see Table 34.3). It is useful to classify the hematologic changes as megaloblastic and macrocytic, because the presence of megaloblasts in the bone marrow and macrocytic cells in the circulation are features of vitamin B_{12} or folic acid deficiencies. All cell lines in the bone marrow are probably affected to some extent by the folate or B_{12} deficiency. These factors are also required for the formation and maintenance of other rapidly proliferating tissue particularly the mucosal epithelium of the gastrointestinal tract.

Malabsorption is the usual cause of B_{12} deficiency. The quantity of vitamin B_{12} in the diet and the level of B_{12} stores are usually sufficient to meet the body's needs. In strict vegetarians (i.e. absolutely no animal products are consumed) vitamin B_{12} deficiency sometimes occurs. In contrast, dietary folic acid intake is often marginal or inadequate and body stores relatively low. Deficiency therefore can develop quickly if there is a reduction in uptake or an increased utilization of folate. Malabsorption and possibly folate deficiency may occur either as the result of concomitant drug therapy, or if the patient has regional enteritis. Folate deficiency may result from these factors.

Vitamin B_{12}

Vitamin B_{12} is not a single substance. It comprises a group of closely related cobalt-containing compounds (cobalamins), which have similar physiologic activity. In humans the two metabolically active forms are adenosylcobalamin and methylcobalamin. Cyanocobalamin is the usual therapeutic form of vitamin B_{12} and has no known physiological activity and must be converted to a biologically active form such as adenosylcobalamin before it can be used by tissues. Little or no cyanocobalamin occurs in foods. Dietary vitamin B_{12} occurs in foodstuffs as a protein complex and is found predominantly in foods of animal origin such as liver, which is the richest source as well as kidney, meat and milk. It is also synthesized by many microorganisms including some of the intestinal flora. Foods such as fruits, vegetables and grains, however, are devoid of vitamin B_{12}. Most vegetarians will drink milk and so absorb modest amounts of vitamin B_{12}.

Vitamin B_{12} is relatively stable to heat and is therefore available in cooked food. The average diet in the United States supplies 5 to 15 μg/day, but diets vary from as low as 1 to 100 μg/day. It is well absorbed particularly at low dietary levels. The percentage of vitamin B_{12} absorbed decreases as the intestinal content increases. In man vitamin B_{12} is acquired exogenously from the diet and possibly from the intestinal flora. Absorption occurs by two processes. The principal mechanism involves intrinsic factor, calcium and the mucosal cells of the distal ileum. Intrinsic factor is a glycoprotein of molecular weight 50,000, secreted by the parietal cells of the gastric mucosa. The secretion of intrinsic factor generally parallels that of gastric hydrochloric acid. The absorption of vitamin B_{12} is a sequential process beginning with its release from foodstuffs, a complex formation with intrinsic factor, which passes into the intestinal lumen, followed by an association with specific binding sites in the mucosal cells of the distal ileum. The complex dissociates and the vitamin B_{12} is transferred through the mucosal cells to the capillary circulation.

The second mechanism, simple diffusion, provides small quantities and is only biologically significant when large amounts are ingested. There is now evidence that transcobalamin II has an active role in carrying vitamin B_{12} out of the ileal cell into the circulation.

In the circulation, vitamin B_{12} is transported by the serum globulin proteins transcobalamin I, II, and III (18). Of these, transcobalamin II is the most important because it binds newly absorbed vitamin B_{12} and is able to give it up to tissues such as the liver, bone marrow cells, placenta, brain and other tissues. Most circulating vitamin B_{12} is bound to transcobalamin I because that bound to transcobalamin II is rapidly cleared ($t_{1/2}$ = 1 hour), whereas from the former it takes a number of days. Because the daily cellular requirements of vitamin B_{12} are low, much of the ingested vitamin B_{12} is stored in the liver. The amount stored in the liver is about 1000 times the amount estimated to be necessary for daily uses and losses. The liver stores 40 to 90% of the total body content which is usually of the order of 2 to 5 mg. Vitamin B_{12} is conserved in the body by enterohepatic cycling whereby it is reabsorbed after combining with fresh intrinsic factor. If absorption of vitamin B_{12} was to cease abruptly in a normal individual with normal storage, a deficiency state would take 3 to 6 years to develop. Indeed the initial presence of a store of vitamin B_{12} accounts for the slow and insidious course of pernicious anemia.

Etiology

In Europe or North America vitamin B_{12} deficiency results from either a dietary lack which is rare, or much more commonly a defect in intestinal absorption. In contrast, in countries such as India, where poor nutrition is widespread, low dietary vitamin B_{12} is the major cause. Vitamin B_{12} deficiency manifests primarily as pernicious anemia, and is associated with a lack of intrinsic factor which will be described later. Other rare causes of vitamin B_{12} deficiency are a lack of its specific plasma protein transcobalamin II, a congenital absence of intrinsic factor or the genetically determined production of functionally abnormal intrinsic factor (Table 34.11).

Malabsorption can occur after either partial or complete gastrectomy. In the latter all patients will eventually develop megaloblastic anemia because with the removal of the stom-

Table 34.11.
Causes of Megaloblastic Anemias

Vitamin B_{12} deficiency	
Dietary	Inadequate intake
Malabsorption	Inadequate production of intrinsic factor, competition for vitamin B_{12}, disorders of terminal ileum, drug related
Impaired transport	Transcobalamin II deficiency
Folic acid deficiency	
Dietary	Inadequate intake, unbalanced diet, excessive cooking
Malabsorption	Intestinal mucosal changes
Increased requirements	Pregnancy, infancy, malignancy, increased hematopoiesis
Impaired metabolism	Drug related, enzyme deficiencies

ach there is an absolute absence of intrinsic factor. Similarly gastric erosion by corrosive chemicals reduces the ability of the mucosa to secrete adequate amounts of intrinsic factor and so a deficiency state is likely to develop.

In certain conditions, microorganisms such as bacteria, or parasites such as tapeworms, can compete for dietary vitamin B_{12} reducing its availability to the host. Microorganisms colonize intestinal strictures, diverticula and anastomoses. The tapeworm *Diphyllobothrium latum* infests many species of fresh water fish in northern European countries and in particular Finland. Infestations can occur when raw or inadequately cooked fish is eaten, resulting in B_{12} deficiency.

Abnormalities of the small intestine can also markedly reduce the absorption of vitamin B_{12} even in the presence of normal amounts of intrinsic factor. Such disorders include tropical sprue and other conditions which alter the absorptive capacity of the specific sites at the distal ilium (e.g. regional ileitis, Whipples disease and ileal resection). Drugs such as *p*-aminosalicylic acid, colchicine, neomycin, biguanides and slow release potassium interfere with the absorption of vitamin B_{12}.

Interesting observations of the effects of nitrous oxide gas on vitamin B_{12} metabolism have been made recently. First, persons exposed to nitrous oxide for prolonged periods of time show megaloblastic marrow changes which can be corrected by vitamin B_{12} administration. Second, peripheral neuropathy has occurred in dentists chronically exposed to nitrous oxide. Such changes are probably due to oxidation of the cobalt in methylcobalamin by nitrous oxide, and possibly a blocking of the homocysteine-methionine reaction in the bone marrow, brain and other tissues.

Clinical Manifestations

Certain clinical features are common to all forms of vitamin B_{12} deficiency. These include abnormalities of the blood, gastrointestinal tract and the nervous system (Table 34.12). The peripheral blood exhibits severe macrocytic anemia, leukopenia with hypersegmentation of the polymorphonuclear cells and thrombocytopenia. Symptoms include weakness, vertigo and tinnitus as well as palpitations, angina and other signs of congestive heart failure. The gastrointestinal problems occur because the normally rapidly proliferating epithelium is deprived of adequate amounts of vitamin B_{12}. Other consequences

Table 34.12.
Clinical Features of Pernicious Anemia

Symptoms and physical appearance[a]:
1. Pallor, slight jaundice and faint icterus of the sclera
2. Anorexia accompanied with a mild degree of weight loss; a flabby rather than a wasted appearance, diarrhea
3. Dyspnea, palpitations, sensation of extra heart beats, weakness, vertigo, tinnitus, precordial pain and heart murmurs
4. Paraesthesiae, difficulty in walking, loss of vibratory sense, incoordination of movements
5. Disturbed mentation, such as irritability, memory disturbances and mild depression, serious mental symptoms may develop
6. Mild pyrexia
7. Difficulty in urination

Organ involvement:
1. Atrophic glossitis
2. Mild hepatosplenomegaly
3. Enlarged heart
4. Nervous system-spinal cord and peripheral nerve degeneration
5. Achylia gastrica
6. Gastric cancer

[a] Similar features occur in all types of vitamin B_{12} deficiency.

include atrophic glossitis, anorexia, moderate weight loss and diarrhea.

A lack of vitamin B_{12} results in distinct neurologic changes beginning with demyelination of nerves. Neurologic abnormalities are common, particularly paresthesia of the toes and peripheral neuritis or subacute combined degeneration of the spinal cord. Reflexes may be diminished or increased. Mentation varies from mild irritability, memory disturbances and mild depression to severe dementia and psychosis (19).

Megaloblastosis and Neurologic Manifestations

Vitamin B_{12} is essential for hematopoiesis. In deficiency states abnormal erythroid maturation and megaloblastosis of the bone marrow results. Megaloblastosis occurs because of decreased DNA synthesis in the erythrocyte precursors. This results in a slower replication of cells, which have more nuclear chromatin than normal, but not enough for division, and larger cytoplasm than nucleus.

The proposed mechanism underlying the defect in DNA synthesis and megaloblastic maturation in patients with vitamin B_{12} deficiency is the impairment of the de novo formation of deoxythymidylic acid (dTMP) and deoxyuridylic acid (dUMP) in the developing erythrocyte (Fig. 34.1). dTMP is formed by

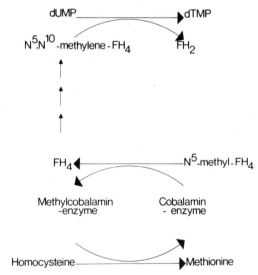

Figure 34.1. Vitamin B_{12} and folic acid metabolism in relation to the synthesis of thymidylate (dTMP) in the developing red cell.

methylation of dUMP with the participation of $N^{5,10}$-methylene tetrahydrofolate. This occurs during the methylation of homocysteine to methionine. In vitamin B_{12} deficiency states a significant proportion of N^5-methyltetrahydrofolate is trapped leading to a depletion of other folate forms including $N^{5,10}$-methylene tetrahydrofolate. The entry of N^5-methyltetrahydrofolate into erythrocytes also requires vitamin B_{12}, therefore in its absence erythrocyte folate levels are low even though serum folate is normal. The interrelationship between vitamin B_{12} and folate metabolism possibly explains why large doses of folic acid, given to patients with pernicious anemia, can result in a partial hematologic remission.

As mentioned earlier one of the late manifestations of vitamin B_{12} deficiency is neuropathy. Lack of this factor appears to interrupt the maintenance of myelin in the nervous system. At least two mechanisms have been suggested in the pathogenesis of the neuropathy. Firstly it may be related to the same block in the homocysteine-methionine reaction that results in megaloblastosis or secondly it may be related to a block in a vitamin B_{12} dependent but folate independent reaction in which methylmalonyl-CoA is converted to succinyl CoA. The latter defect is thought to result in the incorporation of abnormal fatty acids into the nervous system. Current evidence however does not favour the second mechanism as being the fundamental lesion.

PERNICIOUS ANEMIA

Pernicious anemia is a megaloblastic anemia caused by vitamin B_{12} deficiency specifically due to decreased or absent intrinsic factor secretion by the stomach. Deficiency may result from gastric atrophy or an inherited disorder. Pernicious anemia is particularly responsive to replacement therapy, but pharmacists should be careful not to confuse pernicious anemia with other anemias, as inappropriate treatment may complicate the disorder and delay its diagnosis.

Occurrence

Pernicious anemia is rare before the age of 30 years and between 45 and 60 years of age affects females more frequently than males. Juvenile pernicious anemia, an inherited condition is seen in children under 10 years of age. It has been generally accepted that there is a distinctive racial and geographic distribution of pernicious anemia, which is documented as being far more common in temperate regions such as North America, northern Europe (United Kingdom and Ireland) than in tropical countries. It occurs with a prevalence of 0.2 to 0.6%.

Etiology

In pernicious anemia there is a failure to absorb dietary vitamin B_{12} because the gastric mucosa does not produce the necessary intrinsic factor. Although the evidence is incomplete, pernicious anemia is considered to be an autoimmune disorder with a familial history. Antibodies against gastric mucosal cells can often be measured in the serum of persons with pernicious anemia and are implicated in the inactivation of intrinsic factor production, via a cellular immune mechanism. The majority of patients with pernicious anemia (90%) have measurable antiparietal cell antibodies and over half (60%) have anti-intrinsic factor antibodies. It should be noted however that half the patients with gastric atrophy with no evidence of pernicious anemia also have antiparietal cell antibodies. The case for an autoimmune pathogenesis is supported by its higher incidence in patients with other autoimmune diseases such as thyroiditis, Graves' disease and myxedema.

Diagnosis

Pernicious anemia can be differentiated from other forms of megaloblastic anemia by 1) the patient's age, 2) the finding of histamine-fast or pentagastrin-fast achlorhydria, 3) absence of pregnancy, and 4) no evidence of malnutrition, or structural or functional changes in the small intestine. Laboratory tests supportive of the diagnosis of pernicious anemia include plasma vitamin B_{12} and folate levels, the Schilling's test and an immunologic method for assaying intrinsic factor. In pernicious anemia plasma vitamin B_{12} is low (<160 ng/liter) and plasma folate is usually within the normal range. Schilling's test is used to demonstrate vitamin B_{12} malabsorption either due to a lack of intrinsic factor or an ileal defect. The tests consist of giving simultaneously 1 μg ^{57}Co-B_{12} orally and 1 mg of unlabeled vitamin B_{12} intramuscularly. The effect of the large intramuscular dose of vitamin B_{12} is to saturate the vitamin B_{12} binding proteins in the blood. Consequently there are less available binding sites for ^{57}Co-B$_{12}$ and so a substantial portion of this is excreted in the urine. Vitamin B$_{12}$ absorption is considered to be impaired if less than 10% of the labeled vitamin B$_{12}$ is excreted in the urine. If less than 5% of labeled vitamin B$_{12}$ is excreted then this is invariably consistent with a diagnosis of pernicious anemia. If the malabsorption was due to a deficiency in intrinsic factor then giving labeled vitamin B$_{12}$ and intrinsic factor simultaneously will return absorption to normal.

Clinical Findings

The onset of pernicious anemia is insidious and most patients present with signs and symptoms of anemia. Patients generally look well nourished although they may have lost weight. The skin and mucous membrane are usually pale and may even have a faint yellowish tint. The diagnostic triad of symptoms are weakness, painful tongue and numbness and a tingling in the extremities. In many instances at least two of these symptoms are encountered. The painful tongue often has a red raw appearance which eventually becomes smooth and atrophic. The numbness and tingling or paresthesia occurs in the fingers and toes in the majority of relapsed patients. Other neurologic manifestations involving the spinal cord rarely develop before the anemia.

Other symptoms may complicate the presenting clinical picture suggesting involvement of the gastrointestinal tract, the cardiovascular system or genitourinary system. In some cases the neural involvement is so advanced that a primary neurologic disease is suspected. The clinical features of pernicious anemia are presented in Table 34.12. Because pernicious anemia occurs in elderly persons it may be difficult to determine the extent that anemia, or degenerative changes of old age, contribute to the clinical findings. Finally psychiatric systems may occur when the serum vitamin B$_{12}$ levels are low even in the absence of hematologic abnormalities or signs of neuropathy. The laboratory findings in pernicious anemia are detailed in Table 34.13.

Management and Treatment

The aims of treatment for pernicious anemia are hematologic remission, reversal or retardation of the nervous system complications

Table 34.13.
Laboratory Findings in Pernicious Anemia

Parameter	Comments
Hematocrit	Normal to decreased
Peripheral smear	Macrocytic, occasional nucleated cells and a reticulocyte index well below the value of 1
Erythrocytes	Oval shaped, variations in size, some bizzare shaped (poikilocytes) mean corpuscular volume (MCV) is greater than normal (100–160 fl), mean corpuscular hemoglobin (MCH) is increased which results in a normal mean corpuscular hemoglobin concentration (MCHC)
Leukocytes	Hypersegmentation of polymorphonuclear cell nuclei is a consistent finding. If more than 3 cells have 5 lobes or a single cell has 6 lobes, this is presumptive diagnosis of a megaloblastic anemia; there can be mild to moderate neutropenia
Platelets	Reduced in number and bizarre in appearance on occasions
Serum B$_{12}$	Decreased
Serum folate	Normal, sometimes elevated due to folate metabolic trap
Gastric secretion	Achlorhydria (histamine-fast achlorhydria found in most patients), total volume of the gastric secretion and its enzyme content are markedly reduced
Antibodies	Antiparietal and anti-intrinsic factor antibodies present
Others	Methylmalonic acid excretion is enhanced; plasma unconjugated bilirubin and lactic acid dehydrogenase (type 1) increased because of enhanced intramedullary destruction of erythrocytes; iron kinetic data are abnormal

and the replenishment of the vitamin B_{12} body stores. The treatment of choice is IM therapy with either cyanocobalamin or hydroxocobalamin. Because the bioavailability of these agents by the oral route is poor and unreliable they are usually given by the IM route. The IV route can be used but there is no apparent advantage.

In severe cases of pernicious anemia the patient should be kept in bed until the hemoglobin has increased to about 7g/100 ml. Attention must be paid to the diet which should be light, easily digested and contain protein, iron and ascorbic acid. Blood transfusions are indicated in some patients including those dyspneic at rest who have not responded to vitamin B_{12} and have a low hemoglobin (3 to 4 g/100 ml). Packed cells should be infused slowly rather than whole blood to prevent any cardiovascular crisis.

VITAMIN B_{12}

Intramuscular injections of vitamin B_{12} can be given in any one of a variety of schedules (12, 20):

1. *Cyanocobalamin.* For pernicious anemia 5 intramuscular injections each of 1 to 2 mg are given within the first week, followed by 350 μg every 3 to 4 weeks. The dosage must be adjusted to the patient's response. For pernicious anemia patients with neurologic manifestations, the doses should be doubled. The initial dose in children is the same as that for adults. Subsequent dosage is determined after monitoring the appropriate hematologic parameters.

2. *Hydroxocobalamin.* In uncomplicated pernicious anemia and for patients with relapse, a weekly dose of 150 μg intramuscularly will usually produce a satisfactory response; however, 5 injections each containing 1 mg given within the first week will also restore depleted liver reserves. The usual maintenance dose is 250 μg every 3 to 4 weeks, but doses of 1 mg are often given at longer intervals. The dosage must be adjusted to the patient's response and in patients with neurologic manifestations the dose should be doubled. The dose for children is the same as the dose for adults.

Within 2 days of the first injection of vitamin B_{12}, the megaloblastic bone marrow becomes normoblastic. Reticulocytosis occurs with the maximum reticulocyte count occurring about the 4th to 7th day after commencement of treatment.

Factors such as infection, uremia, chloramphenicol consumption, concurrent iron use, folic acid deficiency or misdiagnosis can affect the therapeutic response. Cyanocobalamin or hydroxocobalamin should not be given except in the seriously ill patient, before a diagnosis of pernicious anemia has been fully established because of their ability to mask the clinical manifestations of subacute combined degeneration of the spinal cord. Folic acid should never be used alone because it does not halt the development of the irreversible neurologic damage although the megaloblastic anemia is improved. In some patients there is a pause in their response to vitamin B_{12} injections 2 to 3 weeks after the commencement of therapy and the hemoglobin fails to rise over 10 to 11 g/100 ml. This is probably due to a depletion of iron stores resulting from accelerated erythropoiesis after vitamin B_{12} replacement which responds to ferrous sulfate 200 mg, 3 times daily. The patient's progress should be followed by appropriate tests such as hemoglobin, hematocrit, erythrocyte and reticulocyte counts. In the seriously ill patient, it may be necessary to administer both vitamin B_{12} and folic acid while awaiting confirmation of the diagnosis.

Although cyanocobalamin should not generally be given orally because of its variable absorption, it may be justified for certain patients with bleeding disorders or who are allergic (very rare) to parenterally administered vitamin B_{12}. Only 1% of the oral dose is absorbed (by diffusion) and high doses are therefore needed to bypass the intrinsic factor defect in pernicious anemia. When oral formulations are used the tablet dosage is 50 to 150 μg daily, 1 hour before meals, and the liquid dosage is 35 to 20 μg daily, 1 hour before meals. The maintenance liquid dose for pernicious anemia is 140 μg/day. Such therapy is expensive and the results uncertain. Noncompliance is a problem and these patients require closer monitoring than those on parenteral treatment. "Shotgun" treatment, that is, combinations of a number of different hematinics should be discouraged as there is no rational basis for their use. An oral vitamin B_{12}-hog intrinsic factor combination has been used to expedite vitamin B_{12} absorption. If antibody formation to this heterologous agent occurs, patients become refractory to treatment.

Prognosis. If a case is properly treated with vitamin B_{12} the prognosis for pernicious anemia is excellent. The hematologic and other associated problems can be reversed. The nervous system manifestations can be stemmed and in situations where neurons are still viable, the neurologic lesions may be reversed. Both these responses depend on patient compliance with the treatment regimen. Gastric polyps, gastric cancer and other gastrointestinal problems occur in patients with pernicious anemia at three times the frequency of the general population. Other associated problems include diabetes, myxedema (with or without goiter), cardiac failure following fatty changes of the myocardium and intercurrent urinary tract infections due to lesions in the nerve supply of the urinary sphincter.

TRANSCOBALAMINS (18, 19)

Transcobalamin I and III, which are approximately 33% sugar, are closely related to the "R" vitamin B_{12} binding proteins present in body fluids such as saliva, gastric juice and milk. It is thought that these two proteins are synthesized by granulocytes, transcobalamin I by myelocytes and transcobalamin III by neutrophils.

There is a rare genetic condition in which transcobalamin I is absent, resulting in low serum vitamin B_{12} concentrations. In myeloproliferative disorders and certain tumors such as hepatoma and carcinoma of the breast, raised serum levels of transcobalamin I in association with high vitamin B_{12} levels have been observed. A benign increase in leukocytes such as in chronic inflammatory breast disease and also in polycythemia vera is often found with raised transcobalamin III with or without raised vitamin B_{12} levels. In contrast both transcobalamins I and III are increased in many patients with both benign and malignant increase in granulocytes.

The synthesis of transcobalamin II occurs in multiple organs including the liver and the ileum.

COBALAMINS

Large doses of either cyanocobalamin or hydroxocobalamin are irregularly absorbed when given orally or when absorption is impaired such as in intrinsic factor deficiency or when gastrointestinal disease is present. When cyanocobalamin is administered by intramuscular injection it is more rapidly excreted than hydroxocobalamin as it is less protein bound. Fifty percent of a dose is excreted in the urine in 48 hours along with significant amounts in the bile. Lower serum levels are obtained if equivalent doses of cyanocobalamin are used. The initial serum level after administration of cyanocobalamin is not as high or as sustained as that obtained after hydroxocobalamin administration. The biological half-life of cyanocobalamin is about 123 hours.

With impaired liver or renal function more frequent dosing is necessary. No adverse effects have been reported during pregnancy. The recommended daily maternal intake is 4 μg/day. Vitamin B_{12} crosses the placenta and at birth the neonate's level can be 2 to 5 times that of the mother's. It is excreted in breast milk and studies have shown that significant increases occur in breast milk after parenteral administration.

Cyanocobalamin is usually well tolerated and allergic reactions are rare. Mild diarrhea, polycythemia, peripheral vascular thrombosis, transitory exanthema, urticaria, pulmonary edema, congestive heart failure early in treatment, anaphylactic shock and death have been reported. An intradermal test dose of cyanocobalamin is recommended before it is administered to patients with a history of suspected allergic reactions to cobalamin.

Hypokalemia may occur upon the conversion of megaloblastic to normal erythropoiesis with vitamin B_{12} therapy as a result of the erythrocyte potassium requirements. Serum potassium concentrations need monitoring, particularly when potassium depleting diuretics are given concurrently. Most antibiotics, pyrimethamine and methotrexate invalidate microbiological vitamin B_{12} (and folic acid) assays. Colchicine, p-aminosalicylic acid, biguanides, heavy alcohol intake for greater than 2 weeks can cause malabsorption of the vitamin. Hydroxocobalamin is also used in conjunction with folic acid in the treatment of other macrocytic anemias associated with nutritional deficiencies and sprue. Cyanocobalamin is not acceptable for tobacco amblyopia, Leber's optic atrophy, transcobalamin II defect, methylmalonylhomocysteine aciduria and cyanide poisoning. In these instances hydroxocobalamin is used. It may also be necessary to give cobalamins in cases of vitamin B_{12} deficiency due, for example, to gastrectomy, disease or resection of the ileum or conditions in which there are abnormal intestinal flora.

FOLIC ACID DEFICIENCY

Folic acid is an important factor in cell division and without it division is stopped at metaphase. Adequate folic acid is required for normal erythropoiesis including the maturation of megaloblasts into normoblasts in the bone marrow.

Folic acid is present in many foods either as free folic acid or as polyglutamates, where folic acid is conjugated with several glutamic acid moieties. The best sources of folate are green leafy vegetables, meat, offal, yeast and cereals. Active absorption of folic acid occurs mainly in the proximal part of the small intestine. Conjugated folic acid is absorbed to a lesser degree than free folic acid, however, a conjugase enzyme in epithelial cells of the small intestine can convert the polyglutamates into absorbable monoglutamate forms. During absorption folic acid is reduced and methylated to N^5-methyltetrahydrofolic acid in the duodenal and jejunal cells. There is no specific plasma protein to transport the physiologic folates. The plasma folate concentration reaches a peak approximately 1 hour after ingestion. The principal circulating form of folate is N^5-methyltetrahydrofolic acid.

Serum folate loosely binds to albumin and possibly to α-macroglobulins. About one third is free. A number of specific folate binders have been found in body fluids and cells. However their main role may be to assist the excretion of oxidized folates and folate breakdown products. Intracellular folate binders may also help keep folate inside cells. The transport of reduced and nonreduced folates into cells occurs by separate mechanisms. For instance reduced forms are transported by an active, energy dependent and carrier mediated process.

The human requirements which depend on metabolic and cell turnover rates vary from 50 μg daily in infancy to about 100 μg daily in the adult. In normal persons the total body folic acid stores are 5 to 10 mg, half of which is in the liver. Liver folate is in the form of N^5-methyltetrahydrofolic acid. Upward of 2% is degraded daily and therefore a continuous dietary supply is essential. The rate of degradation increases in prolonged infection with pyrexia, hemolytic anemias and during pregnancy. The increased rate of degradation in these conditions is sufficient to cause folic acid deficiency. Small amounts are excreted in feces and urine. Additional amounts are probably metabolized and a small amount is lost by desquamation of cells from body surfaces.

Etiology

Folate deficiency is not uncommon. Causes include an inadequate intake of folates, malabsorption, increased requirements, enhanced metabolism and interference of its metabolism or clearance by drugs.

Folic acid intake may be reduced if insufficient attention is paid to the diet so that folic acid rich foods are excluded or food is poorly prepared and overcooked. Persons at risk include alcoholics, who may have poor diets, the elderly who often do not feel like eating, adolescents and teenagers who may skip meals and eat "junk" food, and some infants. Megaloblastic anemia due to a simple dietary deficiency of folic acid is common and sometimes severe among people in the tropics or developing countries; however, it is less common in more prosperous countries. Anemia develops within 5 to 6 months in a normal person on a folate-deficient diet. In comparison, patients who have undergone total gastrectomy do not develop the manifestations of vitamin B_{12} deficiency until after 2 years or more because of the long-term vitamin B_{12} stores.

Malabsorption of folate is frequently a problem in persons with gastrointestinal diseases such as tropical or nontropical sprue, inflammation of the gut such as regional ileitis or an anatomical lesion where resection of the small intestine has been undertaken. Signs of folate deficiency appear often among epileptics, but these are due primarily to their dietary habits rather than the effects of their drugs. Continuous use of phenytoin and primidone can lead to folate deficiency manifested by gingival hyperplasia, but megaloblastic anemia occurs only rarely. Oral contraceptives may impair folate absorption in some women.

An increased requirement for folic acid occurs during pregnancy, infancy, malignancy and during increased hematopoiesis such as in chronic hemolytic anemias. During pregnancy there is a large increase in the synthesis of nucleic acid associated with growth of the fetus, placenta and uterus and the increased maternal erythrocyte mass. Folate requirements may increase up to three fold and megaloblastic anemia due to folate deficiency may develop. Other problems during pregnancy affecting folate status in the mother include nausea, vomiting and urinary tract infections.

Impaired metabolism of folic acid either due to drugs or rare enzyme deficiencies, reduces the availability of the cofactor to rapidly dividing tissue such as the bone marrow. Drugs such as methotrexate, pyrimethamine, trimethoprim, triamterene and ethanol may cause megaloblastic anemia, particularly if the dietary intake of folic acid is inadequate or there is already some degree of megaloblastosis (alcoholics). Folinic acid can reverse the anemia if it is necessary to continue the offending drug. Anemia is more likely to occur if several contributing factors are present.

Drugs may cause megaloblastic anemia without interfering with folate or vitamin B_{12} metabolism usually by altering the supply of DNA precursors. For example 5-fluorouracil inhibits thymidylate synthesis, and hydroxyurea reduces the supply of dATP and dGTP by inhibiting ribonucleotide reductase. Cytosine arabinoside on the other hand competes with dGTP for binding sites on DNA polymerase resulting in an inhibition of DNA synthesis. Drugs which inhibit mitosis such as vincristine or alkylating agents such as chlorambucil, cyclophosphamide or busulfan do not cause megaloblastic anemia (18, 19).

Clinical Features and Course

Signs and symptoms include megaloblastosis, glossitis, diarrhea, weight loss and neurologic manifestations. The disease progresses slowly and the hemoglobin level may fall to an ominously low 2 to 4 g/100 ml. Plasma folate is less than 3 mg/ml and erythrocyte folate under 100 mg/ml.

Diagnosis

The laboratory evidence for folate deficiency include: 1) anemia and macrocytes in the peripheral blood, 2) megaloblasts in the bone marrow, 3) absence of folate stores, and 4) normal B_{12} stores.

Macrocytic cells are consistently found in severe forms of the anemia; however, an absence of macrocytes does not exclude folate deficiency. Additional evidence for megaloblastic anemia is that more than 3% of the polymorphonuclear cells have 5 or more lobes. Bone marrow biopsies provide evidence of megaloblastic erythrocyte precursors and this information must be interpreted in the light of vitamin B_{12} status because similar findings occur in vitamin B_{12} deficiency.

In practice a diagnosis is made on the finding of a macrocytic and megaloblastic anemia in a patient with normal B_{12} stores and low folate levels. The diagnosis is confirmed by giving the patient a therapeutic trial of folate and studying the response such as a transient reticulocytosis and increased blood hemoglobin concentration.

Folate store status is assessed by measuring serum folate concentrations or erythrocyte folate levels, the latter providing an indication of tissue stores. Most patients with megaloblastic changes due to folate deficiency have a low serum folate concentration and low erythrocyte folate level. Erythrocyte folate levels are a more reliable guide of folate stores because serum levels are sensitive to the dynamic state of folate metabolism. Even so measurements need to be interpreted in the light of the patient's B_{12} status. For instance patients with pernicious anemia often have low erythrocyte folate levels.

Folic Acid Therapy

Folic acid reverses the hematologic changes occurring in nutritional macrocytic anemia, megaloblastic anemia of infancy and pregnancy, celiac disease, steatorrhea, and postgastrectomy. It is therefore used in the management of the megaloblastic anemia in these conditions.

The daily dose of folic acid depends upon the cause of the deficiency. Daily doses of 5 to 10 mg or even less are effective. Seriously ill patients with hemoglobin levels of less than 5 g/100 ml need blood transfusions until folic acid therapy has increased erythropoiesis. Where possible the patient should be given a well balanced diet. Under some circumstances this may be impossible. Pregnant and lactating women have a greater need for folate than anyone else in the community. Here several regimens have been suggested which include 100 μg daily starting at the 20th week of pregnancy and 300 μg daily during the last trimester and during lactation.

Folic acid is of no value in the treatment of other types of anemia. It should never be given to persons suffering from pernicious anemia because it reverses the hematologic aberrations but not the neurologic manifestations such as irreversible degeneration of the spinal cord. Another danger is that indiscriminate self medication with preparations containing folic acid may mask hematologic manifestations in a person with undetected pernicious anemia to the point where neurologic changes have become essentially irreversible.

ANEMIA OF CHRONIC DISEASES

Anemia is often associated with chronic disorders such as chronic infections, renal failure, rheumatoid arthritis and neoplasms in hospitalized patients. The cause of the anemia is still poorly understood. However, at least three factors have been noted. First, erythrocyte production is reduced even though hemoglobin concentrations are low. Second, erythrocyte survival is reduced by extracorpuscular factors and third, the availability of iron from iron stores for erythropoiesis is reduced. The anemia is usually mild and erythrocyte function remains normal. The erythrocytes are usually normochromic but occasionally they are hypochromic and microcytic. Serum iron and TIBC are usually low and transferrin saturation is reduced. However, adequate iron stores are present in the bone marrow.

Anemias due to infections do not usually respond to either oral or parenteral iron therapy unless the primary cause is overcome. In uremia anemia is common and probably due to a deficiency of erythropoietin. The bone marrow however remains cellular until significant renal damage has occurred after which hypoplasia recurs. In hepatic cirrhosis the anemia is usually macrocytic or normocytic. Primary malnutrition is probably the cause of megaloblastic anemia in this condition, particularly in chronic alcoholics with primary cirrhosis. If iron deficiency anemia is also present, gastric or esophogeal bleeding which is more common in alcoholics is likely.

There are a number of causes of anemia in malignant disease. These include reduced appetite, malabsorption of nutritional factors, and blood loss from the alimentary tract. Occasionally hemolysis is also observed. Sideroblastic anemias result from abnormal utilisation of iron by the marrow.

APLASTIC ANEMIA

Aplastic anemia (AA) is a syndrome of bone marrow hypoplasia with pancytopenia. It may be characterized as severe or mild. Severe AA is defined as 1) a marrow of less than 25% normal cellularity or a marrow of less than 50% normal cellularity with less than 30% hematopoietic cells and 2) at least two of the following three peripheral blood values: granulocytes less than $500/mm^3$; platelets less than $20,000/mm^3$; anemia with reticulocytes less than 1% (corrected for hematocrit). Mild AA is marrow hypoplasia with pancytopenia not severe enough to meet the preceding criteria. While the above pictures may appear in patients receiving chemotherapy or radiotherapy for malignant disease, these patients usually recover and are not considered to have AA (21).

Etiology

About half the cases are of unknown etiology (idiopathic) and the rest are associated with synthetic agents or secondary to hepatitis (Table 34.14) (22).

Drugs and Chemicals. The association between drugs, or chemicals, and AA has followed the sequence of individual reports in the literature, leading to investigations into the causal relationship, then to resolution of the molecular mechanisms involved in the pathogenesis. The drugs and chemicals most frequently associated with AA are indicated in Table 34.14 and are described in two references (23, 24). Quinacrine, chloramphenicol, oxyphenbutazone and phenylbutazone have been studied for their causal relationship and

Table 34.14.
Etiologic Agents in Reported Series of Aplastic Anemia 1950–1977[a]

Agent	Adult (%)	Pediatric (%)
Total cases	100	100
Idiopathic	43	52
Chloramphenicol	26	29
Benzene	2	
Sulphonamides	2	1
Insecticides	3	1
Anticonvulsants	2	3
Phenylbutazone	4	
Infections	2	1
Solvents	1	2
Gold	1	
Hepatitis	1	4
Other	15	5

[a] Modified from Alter et al. (22) (for specific information, see references 23 and 24).

risk of use. Although quinacrine is rarely used worldwide, chloramphenicol is available in many countries. Phenylbutazone and oxyphenbutazone have been the drugs most frequently implicated in reports from countries which have controlled the use of chloramphenicol. This information provides a basis for pharmacists in advising on the appropriateness of prescribing drugs such as phenylbutazone where there is a considerably higher risk of aplastic anemia in the elderly, particularly females over 65 years old. This activity places pharmacists in a preventive role (25).

Pharmacists should critically examine reports collected retrospectively by national and international registries with respect to their method of classification (consideration: differing diagnostic criteria), incompleteness of collection (consideration: inaccurate numerator), the method of associating the drug and effect (consideration: variable criteria), against the background of drug usage, the denominator (consideration: different units) and the rational use of the drug (consideration: inappropriate indication and dosage regimen).

Two methods of evaluating the association between a drug or agent and adverse effect, are available. First is the individual case method which employs the criteria laid down by Irey (26) and applied by Pisciotta (27), to the relationship between drug therapy and blood disorders. These include: (a) a time relationship—the effect coincided with the administration of the drug and receded on suspension of treatment; (b) rechallenge—the effect recurred on reexposure to the drug; (c) pattern—the effect was consistent with previous pathological effects attributed to the drug; (d) detection and quantitation in tissue—this confirms the presence and level of drug in the body; and (e) singularity of drug—all other causes have been excluded. Many national registries and workers have adopted comparable guidelines. It should be noted that the individual case method is most applicable to adverse effects which are acute. The strength of association in each individual case is dependent on the number of criteria satisfied, some of which may be unethical (b), or difficult (d), to implement.

The second method of evaluating adverse effects to drugs is epidemiologic and applies criteria first reported by Bradford Hill (28) and modified by Jick and Vessey (29). These include: (a) the statistical significance of the association; (b) the strength of association—the stronger the association (i.e., the higher the relative risk), the more likely it is to hold and if there is a relationship between the rate of drug use and the incidence of adverse effects, this adds weight; (c) consistency—the results should be reproducible in other population studies, by different investigators; (d) biologic plausibility—other types of study, for example, biochemical, microbiologic or histopathologic, give results which support the epidemiologic data; and (e) epidemiologic plausibility—the association is consistent with other epidemiologic data, e.g., time trends, population or geographical clusters. Again, the strength of association is related to the number of criteria satisfied. The epidemiologic approach may be applied to adverse effects with a long latent period, which occur with a low frequency and/or which may be difficult to discern from disease processes arising naturally or from other causes.

Benzene and its derivatives, agents used in industry and the home, exemplify causes of aplastic anemia which occur with other hematologic abnormalities. For example, hemolytic anemia, refractory anemia associated with hypercellular marrow and myeloid metaplasia with leukemia may precede, follow or occur independently of AA. The molecular mechanisms involved in the production of the effects are unknown (23).

Other Etiologies. Ionizing radiation constitutes a potential hazard in persons occupationally or accidentally exposed to roentgen rays or radioactive isotopes. The severity of aplasia is dependent upon the dose and rate of the exposure to the bone marrow. An example of the congenital form of AA is that related to the inherited disorder, Fanconi's anemia. It manifests in children over the age of four years and is characterized by a variety of chromosomal aberrations, and may be associated with leukemia in later life. Over 200 cases have been described (23).

Occurrence

Data from Japan and other countries indicate incidences of fatal AA up to 10 per million per year (22, 25, 30).

Pathogenesis

The molecular and cellular mechanisms involved in AA have arisen from an understanding of normal hematopoiesis. Mature bone marrow cells are derived from stem cells committed specifically to producing granulocyte, erythrocyte and megakaryocyte progeny as well as the lymphocyte line of cells. Committed stem cells are in turn derived from pluripotent stem cells which have the dual capacity of self-replication and for differentiation into committed stem cells.

Amplification of the stem cell compartment occurs at the level of the committed cells. A number of factors are involved here including various hormones. For the erythroid cell lines the hormone erythropoietin is important in controlling erythropoiesis. Failure of committed stem cells would be expected to lead to a deficiency of a single cell line (21, 25). Aplastic anemia probably results from the defective function of stem cells or abnormal hormonal or cellular control of stem cell proliferation (21).

AA produced by drugs and chemicals may result from two types of actions: 1) a dose-dependent effect exemplified by the antineoplastic drugs, and 2) AA in the apparent absence of a dose-effect relationship. Factors involved in this susceptibility have not been elucidated.

Antineoplastic and immunosuppressive agents produce a bone marrow depression related to the dose or rate of administration of the drug. When combinations of these drugs are used their effects are both additive and cumulative. On their cessation, the bone marrow usually recovers quickly (21). Continued use results in gradual depletion of stem cell numbers, with consequent increased vulnerability to bone marrow depression from drug effects and a slower recovery.

Detailed studies of chloramphenicol have shown both types (types 1 and 2). Clinically it has exhibited a dose-related, reversible depression affecting mainly the formation of erythrocytes, and rarely the platelets and granulocytes. It occurred in most patients in whom blood chloramphenicol levels were above 25 μg/ml. The effect appeared to be mediated by inhibition of mitochondrial protein synthesis. Recovery occurred on suspension of the drug.

Aplastic anemia associated with chloramphenicol occurred rarely (1 in 20,000 to 40,000 treated patients) and was apparently unrelated to the dosage of the antibiotic. The effect may have been produced in individuals with abnormalities in (i) DNA synthesis in stem cells, (ii) elimination of chloramphenicol or (iii) in those with an already depleted bone marrow.

Diagnosis and Course

The diagnosis of AA is made largely by exclusion. Pancytopenia and hypoplastic bone marrow are also present in other blood disorders, therefore the careful investigation of exposure to environmental agents and the monitoring of clinical symptoms are essential. Patients may present with progressive weakness, bleeding and, less commonly, a bacterial infection (Table 34.15). The course of the disorder is variable, ranging from a short survival (months) to milder forms which may exhibit symptoms of anemia and linger for years. The severe form may be complicated by problems of hemorrhage or infection resulting from suppression of platelets or white cells, hemosiderosis from multiple transfusions, liver, kidney or other organ damage associated with therapy (23).

Laboratory Findings

Laboratory tests include examination of the blood and bone marrow and a study of iron utilization. The level of hemoglobin depends upon the severity of the conditions. It may be as low as 3 g/100 ml in the acute case, and usually varies between 7 g/100 ml and 10 g/100 ml in the chronic form. The white cell count is not depressed in every case and may vary at different times in the same individual. With an acute onset, the white cells may number less than 1000/mm³ with a marked reduction of neutrophils, and neutrophils may show toxic granulation. The degree of thrombocytopenia is variable, the platelet count usually being less than 140,000/mm³. Where there is severe hemorrhage and the onset is acute, a level below 40,000/mm³ is usually found.

Table 34.15.
Signs and Symptoms of Aplastic Anemia

Anemia	Pallor, mild progressive weakness, fatigue, exertional tachycardia
Thrombocytopenia	Ecchymoses, petechiae, purpura, epistaxis, gingival bleeding and retinal bleeding
Neutropenia	Infection; usual signs of inflammation may be absent
Others	Pyrexia; lymphadenopathy absent; hepatosplenomegaly absent

Bone marrow examination may reveal a hypocellular picture, but as the areas of activity and aplasia are often irregular, this can be deceptive. In this event a trephine biopsy of the iliac crest (for histologic sections as well as marrow smears) may be obtained. The replacement of hemopoietic marrow by fatty tissue and the irregular distribution of activity are usually evident on the section. Where doubt remains, confirmation may be forthcoming from ferrokinetic studies. A tracer dose of radioactive iron (^{59}Fe) will be cleared slowly from the plasma and the uptake by the red cells and marrow will be low.

Management and Treatment

The treatment of aplastic anemia involves consideration of supportive therapies and bone marrow transplantation. The severity of the aplasia and the resultant risks of hemorrhage and/or infection determine the supportive treatment. Recovery may take months or years and success is equated to the number surviving in the longer term. Treatment is considered under the headings: withdrawal of the causative agent, supportive care, restoration of adequate cell numbers, and marrow-stimulating agents. Bone marrow transplantation is discussed in the following section.

Withdrawal of the Causative Agent. The search for the removal of any drug or chemical is essential. Pharmacists should ensure that all items listed in Tables 34.14 and 34.16 have been investigated.

Supportive Care. Control of infection is central to the survival of the patient. Current practice includes good dental health, scrupulous aseptic technique, avoidance of direct contact with other individuals by the use of masks and isolation nursing and, where available, individual sterile units. Prophylaxis against endogenous infections from the nose, pharynx, mouth and gastrointestinal tract are undertaken. The use of antibiotics in this instance is not universal or standardized and may be complicated by the emergence of antibiotic-resistant organisms and other undesirable effects such as secondary infections by mycotic organisms. Antibacterial nasal sprays may be used. Other measures may include food with a low bacterial count and prophylactic bowel sterilization using a combination of nonabsorbable antibiotics such as neomycin, polymyxin, vancomycin, gentamicin and

Table 34.16.
History in a Patient with Aplastic Anemia

Occupation	Current and all previous occupations; inquire specifically about benzene, and solvents and radiation
Domestic activities	Ask about dry-cleaning fluids, insecticides, paint solvents and whether subject syphons gasoline (see references 23 and 24)
Prescribed and over-the-counter medicines	Take a drug history: ask patient or relative to produce any evidence of past and current medications or exposure to chemicals. If possible examine previous hospital records and contact local physician and pharmacists (see references 23 and 24)
Allergy	Ascertain any previous allergy or drug sensitivity

nystatin, or/and oral sulfamethoxazole and trimethoprim combination.

Specific anti-infective agents should be used early and vigorously in all patients showing signs of infections such as significant fever. Appropriate initial antibiotic therapy pending results of culture and sensitivity test may include the following:

1. For moderately ill patients, ampicillin and an aminoglycoside (e.g. gentamicin) are administered parenterally. These are effective against most Gram-positive and negative bacteria.

2. For the severely ill patient, ticarcillin, or cloxacillin and an aminoglycoside are given parenterally to provide cover against penicillin-resistant *Staphylococcus aureus* and *Pseudomonas aeruginosa*. The doses of aminoglycosides are determined by body weight or surface area and modified in patients with renal impairment. Their administration may be monitored by reviewing serum levels to ensure that the antibiotic is within the therapeutic range and that the peak level is below the toxic concentrations (e.g. 10 μg/ml for gentamicin). Nephrotoxicity associated with gentamicin usually occurs after 8 days of therapy, and renal function tests (e.g. serum creatinine)

should be closely followed at this stage (23, 31).

In addition, infection is hazardous in that it aggravates bleeding tendencies and may further deplete neutrophils and platelets. Other problems include 1) secondary infection (e.g. fungal), especially when antibiotics are given concurrently with corticosteroids; 2) phlebitis associated with administration of parenteral forms; and 3) adverse reactions including platelet dysfunction with high doses of carbenicillin or ticarcillin, hypokalemia following sodium introduced as the cation in antibiotic infusions, and organ damage outlined above.

Restoration of Cells. The decision to give transfusions depends on patients being candidates for bone marrow transplantation. Red cell transfusions are indicated when the hemoglobin level has fallen to 7 to 9 g/100 ml and may be increased in the event of certain cases such as menorrhagia in female patients. Suggested treatments for severe menorrhagia include anti-fibrinolytic agents such as oral contraceptives containing large doses of norethindrone. Each transfusion carries substantial risks, such as hepatitis, hemosiderosis and sensitization to erythrocyte and leukocyte (HLA) antigens. The type of blood used is important. The use of whole blood or packed cells even if carefully cross-matched often results in the appearance of white cell antibodies which cause severe clinical blood transfusion reactions. All blood transfusions should be white cell-free. The buffy coat may be removed by centrifugation or filtration but the best form of transfusion is frozen, reconstituted red cells.

Platelet transfusions are administered to maintain the platelet count at or above 20,000/mm³. Ideally the donor platelets should be HLA, ABO compatible and not from close relations who may be needed for bone marrow transplantation. The effectiveness of platelet transfusions is curtailed by fever and infection. Repeated transfusions may lead to antibody production which may impair or prevent successful marrow grafts. The best responses are obtained from HLA-identical siblings as there are other nonidentified minor tissue antigens which at the present time cannot be tested for. Agents, such as aspirin, ibuprofen, indomethacin, and mefenamic acid, impair platelet function and should therefore be avoided in the thrombocytopenic patient. Remissions of infections have been obtained with granulocyte infusions. Problems include febrile and immune reactions.

The hazards, logistic considerations, and expense outweigh the benefit of granulocyte transfusions for prophylaxis in most patients. Therapeutic granulocyte transfusions should be reserved for patients with granulocyte levels less than 500/mm³ and documented infections who fail to respond to a 48- to 72-hour trial of appropriate antibiotics (23, 31).

Marrow-stimulating Agents (23, 31). Androgenic steroid agents and adrenocorticosteroids have been used to improve the peripheral blood cell count and to regenerate the bone marrow with varying success. Usually a response is not seen in severe cases but where bone marrow transplantation is not feasible this modality of treatment may be tried. In milder cases and in the elderly it is worthwhile to attempt androgen therapy. The androgenic anabolic agent, oxymetholone (2 to 6 mg/kg daily) may be administered for 3 to 6 months to induce remission of the disorder. On evidence of a response, first revealed by erythropoiesis, the dose is reduced. Adverse effects of these agents include masculinization, fluid and salt retention. Oxymetholone, a 17-α-alkylated androgenic steroid, produces a hepatitis (cholestatic type) with a low frequency in these patients, and regular serum alkaline phosphatase tests are therefore often ordered. Normalization of liver function values usually occurs on withdrawal. Prednisone may also be used at doses of 40 to 60 mg daily for the purpose of prolonging the in vivo survival time of transfused cells. Adverse effects include capillary fragility, gastrointestinal bleeding and secondary infections in association with antibiotics. Therefore, it is advisable to avoid the use of this and similar agents at least in the acute stage of the asplastic anemia.

Immunologic Aspects

The possible role of abnormal immunologic reactions in the pathogenesis of aplastic anemia has led to the experimental use of immunosuppressive treatment such as antilymphocyte (ALG) or antithymocyte globulin (ATG) but the risks of adverse effects outweigh the benefits with ALG, while the efficacy of ATG in paients with severe aplastic anemia has not been established. Cyclophosphamide has also been used as immunosuppressive therapy in aplastic anemia but it is a dangerous drug to use in patients with bone marrow failure and should be considered only when there is unequivocal evidence of immune-mediated aplasia.

Bone Marrow Transplantation. Bone marrow transplantation involves the transference of stem cells from an immunologically compatible (histocompatible or HLA) donor to the patient. When the HLA identical sibling is available, then bone marrow transplantation offers the best prospects for recovery in a young patient with severe aplastic anemia. Overall, survival has been around 50% in reported series of bone marrow transplantation for aplastic anemia but where prior blood products have not been administered, then survival is of the order of 90% (32).

This is the basis for the different approach to the use of blood products in this situation. It is important that a young patient with aplastic anemia who has an HLA-identical sibling be referred to a bone marrow transplantation center as soon as the diagnosis is made. There, preparations are undertaken to immunosuppress the patient prior to bone marrow transplantation. Blood products are avoided unless absolutely vital to the welfare of the patient until immunosuppression is completed. Then all blood products are irradiated and closely HLA-matched preferably using a family member other than the marrow donor. Supportive care needs to be intense, as the immunosuppressive regimen is severely myelosuppressive (usually cyclophosphamide with total body irradiation being employed). After the transplant is performed, methotrexate is sometimes given intermittently in high doses to prevent graft-versus-host disease (GVHD) (31). The treatment of GVHD is neither satisfactory nor uniform. Encouraging results with the new immunosuppressive agent, cyclosporin A, holds promise as an acceptable treatment (31).

THALASSEMIAS

The thalassemias are a group of genetic disorders of hemoglobin synthesis characterized by a decreased rate of production of one or more of the globin chains of hemoglobin leading to imbalanced globin chain thesis (23, 32). In the β-thalassemias, the commonest form, β-chain production is deficient. Further differentiation of the thalassemias depends on 1) clinical presentation and 2) quantitation of HbA_2 (normally 1.4 to 3.2% of total adult hemoglobin) and fetal hemoglobin (HbF) levels.

The thalassemias, together with the sickle cell disorders, seem likely to be the first diseases amenable to the techniques of genetic engineering. Homozygous β (no β chains) and homozygous β (minimal β chain production) thalassemias are termed "thalassemia major" (or Cooley's anemia). In this condition, anemia manifests a few months after birth and, with inadequate treatment, there is stunting of growth and skeletal deformation caused by erythroid hyperplasia. These patients can be kept alive and well during childhood on high transfusion regimens, but usually succumb in the second or third decade of life from the effects of chronic iron overload. Most cases of heterozygous thalassemia or thalassemia minor are not associated with significant clinical manifestations. The mean hemoglobin level is about 15% lower than in normal persons of the same age and sex, the red blood cell count is usually elevated and the cells are microcytic. No treatment is indicated for such patients.

Management of the Major Thalassemias

The main lines of treatment are 1) regular blood transfusions to maintain hemoglobin above 7.5 g/100 ml, 2) the removal of excess iron with chelating agents, 3) the prevention and early treatment of infection, 4) splenectomy in selected cases, and 5) twice weekly supplements of folic acid because of the marrow requirements (erythroid hyperplasia). Technical difficulties with transfusions may be avoided using scalp vein or small butterfly needles throughout life to preserve veins and the use of disposable plastic donation sets to avert infections. Transfusion reactions may be averted with the use of washed red cells from which plasma and leukocytes have been removed.

The prevention and treatment of iron overload is based on the calculated transfusion of red cells, the use of chelating agents and avoidance of dietary iron. The chelating agent deferoxamine administered parenterally is now the established method of removing iron from thalassemics (23, 32, 33). Its effectiveness is limited by two factors: 1) at any time, only a small pool of iron is available for chelation even in patients with iron overload and 2) the plasma half-life of deferoxamine is short and much of it is excreted without iron. Progress in its use center on combinations of doses and methods used in its administration. Results from the United States and the United Kingdom have demonstrated the effectiveness and acceptability of administering deferoxamine by subcutaneous infusion overnight (12 hours) or by a portable infusion pump. Ascorbic acid enhances iron excretion but also increases the toxicity of tissue iron, therefore it should be confined to individuals who are not severely iron overloaded.

SICKLE CELL ANEMIAS

Sickle cell anemia is an inherited hemolytic disorder resulting from a single amino acid substitution in the β chain of adult hemoglobin. The resultant hemoglobin (HbS) is unstable under a variety of conditions leading to increased hemolysis and severe anemia. Life expectancy in sickle cell anemia is shortened although better medical management and improved social conditions have increased the lifespan of individuals into their 50s. The need for precise therapy and the promise of specific agents for the prevention of the sickling process makes this disease of increasing interest to pharmacists.

Pathogenesis

The molecular abnormality is caused by the substitution of glutamic acid, which is situated in the sixth position from the N terminus in the β chain, being replaced by valine. Although its heterozygous state (HbS trait) may occasionally give rise to clinical abnormality, its inheritance in homozygous form is associated with severe disease known as sickle cell anemia (SCA). Sickle cell diseases (SCD) refers to all the conditions in which the gene for HbS is associated with another abnormal hemoglobin gene, with accompanying clinical manifestations. The oxygenated form of HbS is similar in structure and behavior to HbA. However, when the concentration of deoxygenated HbS is sufficiently high, its properties differ markedly from those of deoxygenated HbA (normal adult hemoglobin) because of a polymerization of the molecules into filaments of high molecular weight. These polymers associate into filaments and bundles of filaments which distort cell into the characteristic sickle shape. A basis for this association may be the formation of intramolecular hydrophobic bonds between valine sites with a resultant structural complementarity between individual hemoglobins. The rigidity and distortion of the sickle cells lead to their premature destruction and to

anemia. The viscosity of the deoxygenated blood is increased, impeding capillary flow which leads to further deoxygenation and greater numbers of sickled cells. Blood vessels may become completely blocked causing the excruciating pain of the sickle cell crisis and the tissue damage typical of sickle cell disorders. HbS has a low oxygen affinity; thus, the relatively greater release of oxygen to the tissue compensates for the decreased access of blood to the tissues. It is the physical impedance to blood flow which is the most important factor. Effective antisickling action therefore requires an inhibition of the polymerization process itself.

Occurrence

Patients heterozygous for HbS are detected by simple laboratory tests, so it is convenient to discuss the distribution of HbS gene, or sickle cell trait. It occurs widely throughout tropical Africa, the eastern Mediterranean, Southern Arabia, India, and in countries with large numbers derived from these areas, e.g. North and South America and West Indies. The frequencies of the HbS gene in these areas are between 1 and 20% of the population. In the United States, the prevalence among blacks is about 8%, while approximately 0.16% have sickle cell anemia. In addition, the estimated frequency among U.S. blacks of sickle cell disease is about 0.17%.

Course of Sickle Cell Anemias

Fetal hemoglobin (HbF) is a good oxygen carrier and its presence masks the anemic effects of HbS up to the postnatal period. As the proportion of abnormal β chains increases, the pathophysiologic effects manifest in clinical symptoms. The acute manifestations of sickle cell disorders are best understood in terms of the vaso-occlusive and hematologic effects.

Vaso-occlusive Effects. 1) Cardiovascular abnormalities such as cardiac enlargement, systolic murmurs and ventricular gallops are common; 2) bone and joint changes are the results of ischemia in the marrow of the toes and fingers (dactylitis) and eventually other sites; 3) abdominal involvement includes abdominal pain, abdominal muscle tenderness, hepatic involvement and hyperbilirubinemia in the older age group; 4) pulmonary problems characterized by infarctions secondary to aggregated sickled cells and bacterial infections are common; 5) genitourinary signs such as priapism and eventual impotence occur and some renal impairment develops in the older age group; and 6) the eye and central nervous system may also be affected (34).

Hematologic Effects. The "splenic" sequestration syndrome" (hyperhemolysis) in young children results in an anemia. As well as anemia, aplastic episodes with changes in hematocrit and reticulocyte levels occur.

Treatment

The management of sickle cell disorders is divided into preventive and supportive measures which effectively prolong the intervals between acute hemolyses ("crises"), ameliorate symptoms and increase the life span. Treatment is directed at preventing or curtailing clinical crises, namely, the complications of vaso-occlusion and hemolysis. Controlled trials of treatment for sickle cell anemia have shown little effectiveness and the following measures reflect largely the impressions of experienced clinicians.

Preventive Measures. These are designed to avoid precipitating factors such as infection, cold, decreased blood flow, acidosis, dehydration and anesthesia. Prompt treatment of infections and even prophylactic antibiosis is advocated as these individuals are prone to salmonella osteomyelitis and pulmonary infections. Avoidance of cold conditions and constricting apparel is mandatory. The pharmacist should be aware of the possibility of associated glucose-6-phosphate dehydrogenase (G6PD) deficiency and the contraindication of oxidant drugs (Table 34.17). The need for sickle cell screening of patients prior to anesthesia and of pregnant women of Negro extraction is recognized as the risk of complications is higher in this group of patients. The risk of hypoxia in air flights should also be remembered. Daily folic acid of 0.25 mg is used to overcome the demand for folate, especially in pregnancy, alcoholism and patients on anticonvulsant therapy.

Supportive Measures. Bed rest, orally administered fluid and oral analgesics are first line measures in the advent of a crisis. If unsuccessful, hydration, either orally or parenterally (0.45% saline in 5% glucose at a rate of 5 ml/kg/hour) is recommended. Sodium bicarbonate, to correct acidosis, may be needed. Blood and urine osmolalities, cardiac and renal

Table 34.17.
Drugs and Agents Associated with Oxidant Hemolytic Anemias[a]

Antimalarials:
  Chloroquine[b, c]
  Hydroxychloroquine[b]
  Primaquine
  Pamaquine
  Pentaquine
  Quinacrine (mepacrine)
  Quinocide
  Quinine[d]
Antirheumatics/analgesics:
  Acetophenetidin (phenacetin)[b]
  Amidopyrine (aminopyrine)[d]
  Aspirin[b, c]
  Antipyrine[d]
  Probenecid[b]
Antibacterials:
  Chloramphenicol[b, d]
  Cotrimoxazole (sulfamethoxazole constituent)[b]
  Furazolidone
  Nalidixic acid
  Nitrofurantoin
  Nitrofurazone[d]
p-Aminosalicylic acid[b]
  Sulfonamides
  Sulfanilamide
  Sulfasoxazole[c]
  Sulfamethoxypyridazine
Miscellaneous agents:
  Chloramine[e]
  Dapsone
  Dimercaprol
  Fava beans
  Naphthalene
  Phenylhydrazine
  Toluidine blue
  Trinitrotoluene
  Vitamin K (aqueous preparations)

[a] Modified from WHO Technical Reports (39).
[b] Hemolytic anemia in those with G6PD deficiency, or/and other factors such as infection, ketoacidosis, renal failure, neonatal status but can occur in the absence of such factors in those with the Mediterranean variant of the enzyme.
[c] Reported to produce only mild hemolysis in healthy G6PD-deficient Negroes only when administered in high doses.
[d] Reported to produce significant hemolysis only in G6PD-deficient Caucasians but not in healthy primaquine-sensitive Negroes.
[e] Significant hemolysis in patients undergoing chronic hemodialysis.

status should be monitored during the procedure. Unremitting pain may be treated with parenteral morphine or meperidine (pethidine). In hospital infections (e.g. salmonella, pneumococcal and *Haemophilus influenzae*) are responsible for precipitating crises in the majority of children and in about 20% of adults. Oxygen (2 to 3 liters O_2/min by mask) is indicated if the PAO_2 level is below 80 mm Hg or there is evidence of pulmonary infection. Transfusion or partial exchange transfusion is vital for the restoration of hemoglobin levels and inhibition of erythropoiesis. Exchange transfusion is instituted only before general anesthesia or whenever an acute situation is deteriorating. After transfusion the proportion of sickle cells should be checked and additional red cells given if it is more than 50%.

Treatment of the vaso-occlusive effects (Table 34.18) in the cardiovascular system include a trial of digitalis therapy for pump failure. Treatment of the bone and joint problems includes appropriate analgesics and antibiotics (for salmonella osteomyelitis) and avoidance of weight bearing in cases of aseptic necrosis. A variety of orthopaedic procedures are available for aseptic necrosis of the femoral head. Total hip replacement is performed if patients are unable to remain ambulatory on crutches.

Liver dysfunction should be investigated to differentiate the vaso-occlusive effects from other possible causes such as viral hepatitis. Treatment is generally supportive. Surgery is recommended when complications such as cholelithiasis are evident. Pulmonary infarction is treated with full-dose sodium heparin. *Haemophilus* species are the most frequently isolated from sputum cultures. These infections are treated with ampicillin or a suitable antibiotic for the penicillin-allergic patient. If this therapy fails, *Mycoplasma pneumoniae*

should be suspected and, if confirmed, erythromycin is indicated.

Renal hematuria usually stops spontaneously within a few days. Lavage of the renal pelvis with silver nitrate, infusion of sodium bicarbonate or distilled water, and administration of diuretics are widely used, but none has been consistently effective. For prolonged hematuria, ϵ-aminocaproic acid, which inhibits urokinase may be given. This, however, may lead to formation of clots in the ureter rather than cessation of bleeding; in which case, fluids may need to be forced to prevent such clotting (35).

Priapism is alleviated with bed rest, sedation, in conjunction with hydration and a regimen of parenteral analgesics for severe pain along with transfusion of normal packed red blood cells to reduce HbS to less than 40% of the total hemoglobin level (35).

Optical integrity should be regularly assessed by an ophthalmologist. Vitreous hemorrhages and retinal detachment are serious complications which may respond to refined surgical methods. Leg ulcers are a distressing problem in many. They appear from the age of 10 years and are treated with saline soaks for 15 to 30 min, 3 times daily. The ulcers are covered with paraffin gauze between soaks. Debridement may be assisted by frequent dressings with Burrow's solution (35).

Developments

The value of oral urea or sodium cyanate as antisickling agents has not been validated in clinical trials.

Table 34.18.
Major Complications of Sickle Cell Disorders (23, 34, 35)

Site	Problem	Age (Where Applicable)	Treatment
Spleen	Sequestration, infarction		Oxidant drugs (!) contraindicated (Table 34.17)
Genitourinary	Kidney—hematuria		Diuretics, fluid lavage
Cardiovascular	Stroke	Children	Chronic transfusions
Bone and joint	Dactylitis	Children	Analgesics
	Aseptic necrosis	Older patient	Orthopaedic procedures, surgery
Eyes	Retinal, hemorrhages		Surgery
Leg	Ulcers	>10 yr	Saline soaks, debridement, bed rest
Liver	Variety		Supportive, surgery
Lung	Infarction		Heparin, full-dose
	Infection:		
	Bacterial		Penicillin (parenteral)
	Mycoplasma		Erythromycin

Genetic counseling and antenatal diagnosis as systematic preventive measures have been reported from many institutions (36). The most feasible future treatments seem to be either bone marrow transplantation or genetic engineering in the form of a drug or hormone which "switches" (derepresses) hemoglobin synthesis back to the production of fetal hemoglobin (HbF) in patients with sickle cell disorders (35). These latter developments are relevant, also, to the prevention and treatment of the thalassemias.

In recognition of the many complications arising from sickle cell diseases and the need to know more about their biological basis and rational treatment, a large multicenter study of more than 3000 cases is in progress (37).

Biological Significance

Sickle cell trait confers protection against infection with falciparum malaria. Much of the life cycle of malarial plasmodia is intracellular. The relative instability and shortened life of erythrocytes of individuals with sickle cell anemia is enhanced by the intracellular parasite which in turn impairs the viability of the plasmodia. The prevalence of sickle cell anemia and genetic hemolytic anemias (e.g. G6PD deficiency, thalassemic syndromes) among populations either residing or originating from endemic malarial areas provides strong evolutionary evidence for the persistence of these "abnormal" genes through history (38).

HEMOLYTIC ANEMIAS

Hemolytic anemia (HA) is an anemia resulting from an increased rate of destruction of red cells. It becomes clinically important when the excessive loss of cells is not adequately compensated by erythropoiesis. The life span of the normal erythrocyte is between 100 to 120 days, but in HA it is shortened by varying degrees and in severe cases may be only a few days. The development, structure and function of red cells is the best understood of all the blood cell lines. Developments in molecular biochemistry over the past 3 decades have laid a firm scientific foundation upon which clinical decisions can be made. This progress allows pharmacists to take precise and active monitoring and drug information roles.

Etiology

An etiologic classification of HA is presented in Table 34.19 (23). There are two broad categories, the first of which encompasses inherited disorders of the red blood cell which result in defects of the erythrocyte membrane, enzymes and of hemoglobin. The second includes those hemolytic disorders in which no evident inherited factor underlies the anemia, or, where an extrinsic agent has been identified as a cause. Many of the anemias in the second category have some immunologic involvement and future developments may reveal genetic components of these. Many reports of hemolytic anemia represent interactions between extrinsic agents (e.g. drugs), in the presence of a pathologic state (e.g. renal impairment), or an inherited disorder (e.g. G6PD deficiency).

Occurrence

Inherited Hemolytic Anemias. Sickle cell disorders are the most important of the inherited HA in the United States and the most prevalent form of HA due to an inherited defect of hemoglobin structure worldwide (see the preceding section). The thalassemias are the commonest inherited disorders of hemoglobin synthesis and occur with a high prevalence throughout the Mediterranean and the Middle and Far East. Of the inherited erythrocyte enzyme disorders, G6PD deficiency is the most common, with over 100,000 individuals throughout the world having a clinically significant enzyme deficiency (39). It has a similar distribution to the thalassemias, but in addition, occurs with a high frequency among black populations derived from certain areas in central and western Africa. Individuals from the specified regions have migrated to other countries and the frequency of the disorders in the host populations may be substantial. Many inherited HA comprise combinations of inherited defects (e.g. sickle cell and G6PD). Hereditary spherocytosis and hereditary elliptocytosis are disorders of the red cell membrane and occur with a frequency of 1 in 4000 to 5000 but are rarely clinically important. The molecular defects have not been identified, but these disorders are successfully managed by surgery (i.e. splenectomy).

Acquired Hemolytic Anemias. Swedish population studies showed about one third of

Table 34.19.
Classification of Hemolytic Anemias According to Etiology and Pathogenesis[a]

Inherited	Acquired
1. *Globin structure and synthesis defects:* Sickle cell anemia Doubly heterozygous disorders: hemoglo- bin SC disease, sickle-thalassemia Unstable hemoglobin disease Thalassemia syndromes	1. *Immunologic:* 1.1. *Transfusion reactions* 1.2. *Hemolytic disease of the new born* 1.3. *Warm antibody:* (1) Idiopathic (2) Secondary, e.g., virus, mycoplasma,
2.1. *Erythrocyte glycolytic enzymes deficiency:* Pyruvate kinase Hexokinase Glucose-phosphate isomerase Phosphofructokinase Aldolase Triosephosphate isomerase 2,3-Diphosphoglyceromutase Phosphoglycerate kinase Enolase	lymphoma, chronic lymphocytic leuke- mia, other malignant diseases, systemic lupus erythematosus (3) Drug-related (Table 34.21) 1.4. *Cold antibody:* (1) Cold agglutinin disease divided into *acute:* Mycoplasma infection, infectious mononucleosis; *chronic:* Idiopathic, lym- phoma
2.2. *Pentose phosphate pathway and glutathione* *metabolism enzyme deficiencies:* Glucose-6-phosphate dehydrogenase (G6PD) Glutathione reductase Glutathione peroxidase Glutathione synthetase	(2) Paroxysmal cold hemoglobinuria, syphi- litic and nonsyphilitic 2. *Traumatic and microangiopathic hemolytic* *anemias:* Prosthetic valves and other cardiac abnor- malities Hemolytic-uremic syndrome Thrombotic thrombocytopenic purpura Disseminated intravascular coagulation
2.3. *Miscellaneous erythrocyte enzyme* *deficiences:* Adenylate kinase Ribosephosphate pyrophosphokinase Adenosine triphosphatase Methemoglobin reductase	3. *Infectious agents:* *Protozoans:* malaria, toxoplasmosis, leish- maniasis *Bacteria:* bartonellosis, clostridial infection, cholera, typhoid fever and others
3. *Erythrocyte membrane defects:* Heteditary spherocytosis Hereditary elliptocytosis Abetalipoproteinemia Hereditary stomatocytosis Lecithin-cholesterol acyl transferase deficiency Defective phospholipid fatty acid transfer	4. (1) *Oxidant drugs and chemicals* (Table 34.17) (2) Nonoxidant chemicals, e.g., copper, ar- sine 5. *Others:* Thermal injury Ionizing radiation? Hypophosphatemia Spur cell anemia in liver disease Paroxysmal nocturnal hemoglobinuria

[a] Modified from Wintrobe et al. (23).

the cases to be idiopathic. The rest were associated with autoimmune, malignant and collagen diseases and uremia. Drugs were implicated in less than 10% of cases.

Course

After hemolysis, the course of HA is common to all types. Variation in details is dependent on the severity of the hemolytic process and the site of destruction of the red cell,
i.e. intravascular or extravascular.

After erythrocytes hemolyze, the freed hemoglobin breaks down to heme which is me-

tabolized to the pigment bilirubin. This is conjugated with glucuronic acid in the liver and
passes into the bile duct to the intestine. Here
the bilirubin is mainly metabolized by bacteria
to urobilinogen and excreted in the feces.
When erythrocyte destruction is excessive,
however, the serum bilirubin level rises because the liver is incapable of clearing it. In
intravascular hemolysis red cells release their
contents directly into the blood and unconjugated hyperbilirubinemia may result. This is a
feature of severe episodes of oxidant hemolysis
(see below).

Patients with hemolysis have decreased levels of haptoglobin and hemopexin. These plasma constituents bind free hemoglobin and the resulting complexes are taken up by the mononuclear phagocytic system and metabolized. The heme iron is incorporated into the iron storage proteins, ferritin and hemosiderin and the heme is catabolized to bilirubin.

Once the plasma hemoglobin binding capacity is exceeded, free hemoglobin passes through the renal glomeruli and is normally reabsorbed by the proximal tubules. In hemolysis, this capacity may be exceeded and hemoglobinuria results. This indicates severe intravascular hemolysis. The presence of hemosiderin in the urine is indicative of chronic hemolysis.

Diagnosis of Hemolytic Anemia

Reticulocytosis and hyperbilirubinemia often, with visible jaundice, are the main clinical criteria suggesting an active hemolytic process. The severity of HA is indicated by the decrease in hematocrit, the presence of unconjugated serum bilirubin and elevations of the reticulocyte count and total serum bilirubin. Table 34.20 indicates the laboratory data required for a diagnosis of HA with specific procedures necessary for the differential diagnosis of inherited and acquired hemolytic disorders.

INHERITED ENZYME DISORDERS

Glucose-6-phosphate dehydrogenase is one of the enzymes of the pentose phosphate pathway which is crucial to the generation of chemically reduced substances in the red cell and its deficiency leads to a marked decrease in the reducing capacity of the red cell. This state renders the red cell susceptible to oxidant stresses arising from within the cell and exogenously from oxidant agents (Table 34.17). It is the most frequently occurring and clini-

Table 34.20.
General Evidence of Hemolysis

1. *Evidence of increased hemoglobin breakdown:*
   a. Jaundice and hyperbilirubinemia
   b. Increased fecal and urinary urobilinogen
   c. Reduced plasma haptoglobins
   d. Hemoglobinemia
   e. Hemoglobinuria
   f. Hemosiderinuria ⎫ Evidence of intravascular hemolysis
   g. Methemalbuminemia ⎭
2. *Evidence of compensatory erythropoietic hyperplasia:*
   a. Reticulocytosis and erythroblastemia
   b. Macrocytosis
   c. Erythroid hyperplasia of the bone marrow
   d. Skeletal x-ray: radiologic changes in the skull and tubular bones (inherited anemias only)
3. *Evidence of damage to the red cells:*
   a. Spherocytosis and increased osmotic fragility
   b. Fragmentation and contraction of red cells
4. *Demonstration of shortened red Cell life span:*
   a. Radioactive chromium method (method used in clinical practice)
   b. Ashby (differential agglutination) method
5. *Specific procedures and type of hemolysis:*
   a. Antiglobulin (Coombs) tests—immunologic
   b. Heinz bodies—oxidant hemolysis
   c. Red cell methemoglobin—oxidant hemolysis
   d. Hemoglobin electrophoresis—sickle cell, thalassemias, other inherited hemoglobin disorders
   e. Detection of abnormal hemoglobin and thalassemia—inherited hemoglobin disorder
   f. Red cell enzyme studies—inherited enzyme disorder
   g. Warm and cold agglutinins—warm and cold antibody hemolytic anemias
   h. Acid serum (Ham's) test and sucrose lysis test—paroxysmal nocturnal hemoglobinuria
   i. Donath-Landsteiner test—differentiate cold antibody anemias—paroxysmal cold hemoglobinuria
   j. VDRL or Wassermann test—paroxysmal cold hemoglobinuria
   k. Family studies in hereditary hemolytic anemias
   l. Investigations to demonstrate an underlying disease such as disseminated lupus erythematosus, lymphoma, lead poisoning, etc.

cally important inherited enzyme disorder of red cells. The African (A-) and Mediterranean varieties have been characterized most thoroughly. Different types of G6PD deficiency may often coexist in the same populations. G6PD deficiency is an X-linked trait, affecting males having a single enzyme-deficient red cell population. Homozygous females also have a single enzyme-deficient red cell population whereas the more frequent heterozygous females have two red cell populations, one normal and one deficient. The ratio of abnormal cells varies from 1% to 99% with a mean of 50%. Only abnormal cells are drug-sensitive and in most heterozygous females the drug-related hemolysis is mild. About one third of heterozygous females have enough abnormal cells to predispose them to clinically significant hemolysis.

The African type (A-) is characterized by enzyme activity 8 to 20% of normal and high electrophoretic mobility. The youngest red cells have normal or almost normal enzyme activity and red cells younger than 50 days have sufficient enzyme levels to protect against damage by oxidant drugs. The older cells are susceptible to destruction and even during drug administration hemolysis is self-limited. The Mediterranean type of G6PD deficiency is marked by severe enzyme deficiency (0 to 4% of normal). Even younger cells are affected and hemolytic episodes are therefore not self-limited. Hemolysis is more severe, even life-threatening and cells are sensitive to a wide range of drugs. The East and Southeast Asian variants differ from the above two types. Some may be as severe as the Mediterranean type and characterization has identified many variants (23).

The molecular and cellular basis of drug-induced hemolysis of G6PD-deficient red cells is described in a following section. The common clinical manifestation of G6PD deficiency is an acute hemolytic episode precipitated by drugs, food or infections. Neonatal hyperbilirubinemia leading to kernicterus may occur in G6PD-deficient infants of Mediterranean, Chinese and African origin after the exposure of the child or mother to certain agents.

The pharmacokinetics of oxidant drugs may be influenced by renal impairment or acetylator status, thereby aggravating the toxicity. Additionally, diabetic acidosis, electrolyte disturbances and concurrent infections may alter the hemolytic sensitivity of the red cells.

Prevention of Oxidant Drug Hemolysis

Awareness of the distribution and frequency of G6PD deficiency in populations is a prerequisite to preventing drug-induced oxidant hemolytic anemia. Table 34.17 lists contraindicated drugs. The decision to use or cease potentially hemolytic drugs should be guided by: 1) the disease and its severity; 2) availability of alternative, safer drugs; 3) the type of G6PD deficiency; 4) sex of the patient; 5) concurrent patient factors which may precipitate an acute episode, e.g. renal impairment, infection (see "Acquired Hemolytic Anemias" in Table 34.19); and 6) the presence of deformed cells (with or without Heinz bodies) in laboratory preparations, contraindicates the use of oxidant drugs.

ACQUIRED HEMOLYTIC ANEMIAS

Acquired HA (Table 34.19) are not attributable to hereditary defects. This section includes certain immunologic HA with emphasis on factors associated with drug-related HA.

Autoimmune Hemolytic Anemias

Autoimmune HA are caused by antibodies that are produced by the patient's own immune system. These anemias are classified according to the thermal properties of the anti-red cell antibody: warm-reactive antibodies bind to red cells most avidly at 37°C, whereas cold-reactive antibodies seldom interact with red cell antigens at 37°C but display progressively greater affinity as the temperature is lowered to 0°C (23, 40).

WARM ANTIBODY TYPE

The warm antibody immunologic HA (Table 34.19) are characterized by the following features: the anti-red cell antibodies are either IgG or IgM, or a combination of these and the antibodies have mainly Rh specificity. There is evidence that genetic factors (HLA association) and selective T-cells (e.g. suppressor activity) occur principally in the 40- to 70-year-old segment of the population with a predilection for women. The most common associated features are neoplastic disease and infections. The usual diagnostic procedure is the direct (Coombs) antiglobulin test which is positive for IgG and occasionally IgA, but not for C3 (complement) while the indirect antiglobulin test is negative. Associated findings include hyperbilirubinemia, decreased haptoglobin levels and splenomegaly. In its most severe form, patients present with overt hemolysis, together with hemoglobinemia, hemoglobinuria, and shock. Without adequate treatment facilities patients may expire (23).

COLD AGGLUTININ DISORDERS

Cold agglutinins are usually IgM antibodies which interact with red blood cells at temperatures below 37°C. Cold agglutinin disease is most frequently associated with *Mycoplasma pneumoniae* and infectious mononucleosis infections. Paroxysmal cold hemoglobinuria which was the first of the autoimmune HA to be recognized, is divided into the syphilitic and nonsyphilitic types. It is now a rare problem and is most commonly associated with viral infections. Its definitive laboratory diagnosis is the Donath-Landsteiner test which demonstrates cold agglutination with a special antibody preparation.

MANAGEMENT OF AUTOIMMUNE HEMOLYTIC ANEMIAS (23, 40)

Drugs and agents which have been associated with autoimmune HA (Table 34.21) should be excluded before the following procedures are instituted. Mild forms of these warm antibody autoimmune HA are initially treated with corticosteroids (prednisone, 1 mg/kg/day). More than 75% improve, but half of these will relapse due to eventual reduction of steroid therapy. Splenectomy, the second line of management, is indicated for patients for whom steroid and immunosuppressive therapy was inadequate or if they were unable to tolerate these drugs. A favorable response is evident in the majority of patients but splenectomy has a substantial mortality in those patients with an underlying disorder of the lymphoid system. The immunosuppressive agents azathioprine and cyclophosphamide are being evaluated as adjuncts to the above treatments. The severity of the disease and the evaluation of the treatment procedures are assessed by monitoring of hematocrit, regular antiglobulin testing and examination of the blood film for the presence of spherocytes. Transfusions may be necessary in patients with severe anemia. Cold agglutinin disorders invariably respond to the avoidance of cold environments and the administration of chlorambucil.

Pathogenesis of Hemolytic Anemias Associated with Drugs

Hemolytic anemias associated with drugs may be categorized into two types: (a) intracorpuscular, e.g. oxidant HA and (b) extracorpuscular, e.g. immunologic HA.

INTRACORPUSCULAR

The intracorpuscular type includes those drugs or their metabolites, which, by their physicochemical nature, enter the red blood cell and stress the membrane directly or indirectly (Fig. 34.2). Into this latter category fall oxidant substances including drugs, which increase the oxidizing forces within the red blood cell. Oxidant hemolysis refers to the lysis of red cells accompanied by Heinz body deposition and/or methemoglobinemia. The survival of erythrocytes relies largely on their capacity to counter oxidant stresses. These stresses may arise exogenously from oxidizing chemicals including drugs available over-the-counter or on prescription only (Table 34.17). The oxidant effect of these substances is dependent mainly on their concentration in the serum, their permeability into erythrocytes and the reducing ability of erythrocytes. The most important reducing agents in erythrocytes are the reduced form of cofactors including NADH, NADPH, and glutathione which arise from electron transfer reactions normally occurring. The sources of these reduced cofactors are the metabolic pathways including, in priority, the pentose phosphate shunt and glycolysis, which are coupled to the reduction of methemoglobin (Fig. 34.2) to oxyhemoglobin (41).

Oxidant hemolysis may result from one, or a combination of two mechanisms. The first mechanism involves the oxidation of hemoglobin (Fe^{2+} to methemoglobin (Fe^{3+}). If there is inadequate NADH, NADPH, or reduced glutathione, or, if methemoglobin reductase activity is decreased, methemoglobin is sequentially oxidized to hemichromes, which are denatured to Heinz bodies. Heinz bodies are precipitated denatured globin chains, with or without the heme groups of hemoglobin. There are some substances (e.g. nitrites) which may produce methemoglobinemia without Heinz bodies or hemolysis because they inhibit further oxidation of methemoglobin. The red cells with denatured protein on their mem-

Table 34.21.
Drugs and Agents Associated with Hemolysis due to Antibodies[a]

Mechanism	Features of Drug-induced Immunologic Hemolytic Anemias			
	Red cell complex with	Ig class	Detection test	Drug examples[b]
Red cell autoantibodies ("autoimmune")	IgG	IgG (warm type)	Antiglobulin (red cells, no drug needed)	Methyldopa, levodopa, mefenamic acid
Drug adsorption (Type II)	Drug or hapten	IgG	Antiglobulin (drug-treated red cells)	Penicillins (high dose), cephalosporins (high dose), carbromal? methadone?
Immune complex adsorption (Type III allergic)	Drug or hapten and Ig complex with complement activation	Often IgM, and IgG	Hemolysis, agglutination antiglobulin (drug plus red blood cell plus serum)	Stibophen, quinidine, p-aminosalicylic acid, quinine, phenacetin, antihistamines, isoniazid, sulfonamides, aminopyrine, dipyrone, sulfonylureas, insulin, rifampicin, acetaminophen, hydrochlorothiazide, tetracycline
Membrane modified—nonspecific adsorption of protein	Drug or hapten and non-Ig protein	—	Direct non-Ig-protein antiglobulin	Cephalosporins (high dose)

[a] Compiled from Petz and Garratty (40).
[b] Hydralazine and chlorinated hydrocarbon-containing insecticides (toxaphene, dieldrin and heptachlor) have been substantiated as causes of immunologic hemolytic anemias, but the mechanism was not clear from the reports.

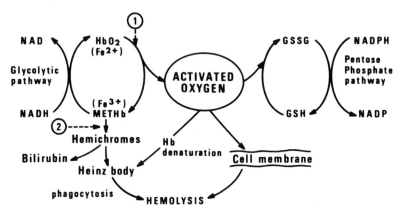

Figure 34.2. Mechanisms of oxidant hemolysis (modified from Carrell et al. (41)): *1, 2,* sites of oxidant drug and agent action; Hb, hemoglobin; METHb, methemoglobin; NAD, nicotinamide adenine dinucleotide; NADP, nicotinamide adenine dinucleotide phosphate; GSH, glutathione; GSSG, oxidized glutathione.

branes are phagocytosed as they pass through the spleen and other sites of the mononuclear phagocytic system. Deformed erythrocytes called "bite" or "pitted" cells result, which may be seen under the microscope. These are more susceptible to hemolysis and are removed from circulation more rapidly than normal cells.

The second mechanism depends on the presence of higher concentrations of activated oxygen. The term "activated oxygen" includes the molecules peroxide, hydroxyl free radical and singlet oxygen which are generated by a number of reactions, including the oxidation of hemoglobin (Fe^{2+}) to methemoglobin (Fe^{3+}). If levels of activated oxygen increase, as in situations of decreased reducing factors, it may exert a damaging oxidant effect on hemoglobin and/or on the red cell membrane. The direction of the pathogenic effect depends on factors described fully by Carrell and associates (41). The fate of the red cell is identical to that described for the other oxidant mechanism. Reports indicate that the most common circumstances involved in cases of drug-induced oxidant hemolytic anemia are the administration of oxidant agents (e.g. sulfonamides) to patients with renal impairment, or G6PD deficiency (e.g. antimalarial drugs to blacks). The significance of these reactions to the pharmacist is that, when signs of oxidant hemolysis are present, the prescriber should be informed that oxidant drugs (Table 34.17) are contraindicated, because of the hazard of hemolysis (Fig. 34.2).

EXTRACORPUSCULAR

In the extracorpuscular type, drugs or their metabolites act directly or indirectly (i.e. immunologically) on erythrocytes. There are no substantiated clinical examples of drugs which act directly on the erythrocyte membranes, although a group of compounds the holothurin derivatives contained in sea cucumber, have been shown to elicit hemolytic crises by this mechanism. Drugs may act indirectly through immunologic processes to produce hemolytic anemia. The first reports of drugs and an associated immunologic HA were those of a patient with Coombs positive hemolytic anemia and pancytopenia secondary to mephenytoin in 1953 and another in 1954, of a patient with stibophen in whom acute intravascular hemolysis developed. In vitro studies in the latter case showed that the patient's serum agglutinated his own or normal erythrocytes or sensitized them to agglutination with antiglobin serum only in the presence of the drug. In both cases, there was a return of hemoglobin concentrations to normal values on cessation of drug treatment. Since that time, many other drugs have been implicated in immunologic HA (Table 34.21) (40).

The features of immunologically mediated HA, tests for their detection and causative drugs are summarized (Table 34.21). The types of drug-related immunologic HA are as follows.

Erythrocyte Autoantibody ("Autoimmune")

Type. Since the first reports of methyldopa-associated autoimmune HA, a number of mechanisms have been proposed for the genesis of the antibody reacting against red cells. One of the important clinical questions that remains unsolved is the reason for 15% of patients administered methyldopa eliciting Coombs positive reactions while only a small percentage (0.01 to 0.8%) exhibit anemia. A genetic factor may underly this susceptibility as a significant HLA association was found in patients given this drug and who formed anti-erythrocyte antibodies (23).

Drug Adsorption (Type II Allergic Reaction). The immunogenicity of penicillin is due to its ability to react chemically with tissue proteins to form haptenic groups. Hemolysis becomes evident only when sufficient penicillin has coated the red cells for the anti-penicillin antibody to react. Complement is activated and lysis follows (40).

Immune Complex Adsorption (Type III Allergic Reaction). The drug or metabolite combines with antibody in the serum of patients previously sensitized to the drug (or metabolite). The complex of hapten and immunoglobulin (usually IgM) adsorbs to erythrocytes, stimulates the complement system and lysis results (40).

Membrane Modified and Nonimmunologic Protein Adsorption. In high doses cephalothin has been shown to alter the erythrocyte membrane. Proteins may adsorb to these cephalothin-modified membrane sites. Cephalothin antibodies in previously sensitized patients attach to these sites, with subsequent lysis (40).

CONCLUSIONS AND ROLES OF PHARMACISTS

Drug information and monitoring roles of pharmacists in individual cases and surveys of aplastic (42) and hemolytic anemias of the inherited (43) and acquired (44) categories have been reported. The role of pharmacists in the monitoring of adverse reactions has been generally accepted, but the analysis and feedback of the data emanating from such surveys to prescribers, has not been carried out methodically and continuously as the WHO recommends (45). A further specific role which should be exploited is that of providing technical information and participating in the laboratory investigation of drug-associated blood disorders and their mechanisms (46).

Drug information may be divided into two categories: prevention and treatment. In this context prevention encompasses (a) careful selection of therapeutic agents, (b) careful selection of patients treated with such drugs, (c) the detection of early manifestations of drug effects, (d) the need for regular blood examinations with certain therapy and in certain patients, (e) the systematic avoidance of re-exposure to agents which have been associated with blood disorders, and (f) procedures to prevent exposure of relatives to agents in cases of blood disorder with a suspected inherited component. The treatment of the blood disorders included in this chapter has progressed markedly: there is an increasing number of drugs, more precise dosage regimens and better methods of administration of therapy. As the molecular mechanisms of pathogenesis become defined and the evaluation of management procedures more refined, it is imperative that the pharmacist has a good knowledge base and is aware of developments in this area. Without these requirements and sound professional judgment, it will be difficult for pharmacists to contribute substantially to patient care without clashing with other health professionals.

References

1. WHO: Technical Report Series No. 563: Nutritional anemias. Geneva: WHO, 1975.
2. Kailis SG, Jellett LB, Chisnal W, et al: A rational approach to the interpretation of blood and urine pathology tests. Part 1—Principles. *Aust J Pharm* 61:221–230, 1980.
3. Scully ER, McNelly BU, Galdabini JJ: Case records of the Massachusetts General Hospital, weekly clinicopathological exercises—normal reference laboratory values. *N Engl J Med* 30:37–48, 1980.
4. Kailis SG, Jellett LB, Chisnal W, et al: A rational approach to the interpretation of blood andurine pathology tests. Part 2—Reference ranges. *Aust J Pharm* 61:303–307, 1980.
5. Finch CA, Huebers H: Perspectives in iron metabolism. *N Engl J Med* 306:1520–1528, 1982.
6. Hallberg L: Bioavailability of dietary iron in man. *Annu Rev Nutr* 1:123–147, 1981.
7. Hoffbrand AV: Iron. In Hoffbrand AV, Lewis SM: *Postgraduate Haematology*, ed 2. London: William Heinemann, 1981, ch 2, pp. 35–71.
8. Food and Nutrition Board: *Recommended Daily Allowances*, ed 9. Washington, D.C.: National Academy of Sciences, 1980, p 187.
9. Beutler E, Fairbanks VF: The effects of iron deficiency. In Worwood M: *Iron in Biochemistry and Medicine II*. London: Academic Press, 1980.
10. Jacobs A: Disorders of iron metabolism. *Recent Adv Haematol* 3:1–23, 1982.

11. Wheby MS: Effect of iron therapy on serum ferritin levels in iron deficiency anemia. *Blood* 56:138–140, 1980.

12. *Pharmaceutical Codex*, ed 11. London: Pharmaceutical Press, 1979.

13. *United States Pharmacopeia*, ed 20. Washington, D.C.: United States Pharmacopeial Convention, Inc., 1980.

14. Cockshott PW, Thompson GT, Seeley ET: Intramuscular or intralipomatous injections. *N Engl J Med* 307:356–358, 1982.

15. Hamstra RD, Block MH, Schocket AL: Intravenous iron dextran in clinical medicine. *JAMA* 243:1726–1731, 1980.

16. Halliday JW, Bassett ML: Treatment of iron storage disorders. *Curr Ther* 11:71–82, 1981.

17. Simon M, Fauchet R, Hespel JP, et al: Idiopathic hemachromatosis: a study of biochemical expression in 247 heterozygous members of 63 families: evidence for a single major HLA-linked gene. *Gastroenterology* 78:703–708, 1980.

18. Hoffbrand AV, Wickremasinghe RG: Megaloblastic anaemia. *Recent Adv Haematol* 3:25–44, 1982.

19. Isselbacher KJ, Adams RD, Petersdorf RG et al: Megaloblastic anemias. In *Harrison's Principles of Internal Medicine*, ed 9. New York: McGraw-Hill, 1980, ch 311, pp 1518–1525.

20. Australian National Drug Information Service: Profile on cyanocobalamin, Canberra, 1980.

21. Appelbaum FR, Fefer A: The pathogenesis of aplastic anemia. *Hematology* 18:241–257, 1981.

22. Alter BP, Potter NU, Li FP: Classification and etiology of the aplastic anemias. *Clin Haematol* 7:431–65, 1978.

23. Wintrobe MM, Lee GR, Boggs DR, et al: *Clinical Hematology*, ed 8. Philadelphia: Lea & Febiger, 1981.

24. Swanson M, Cook R: *Drugs, Chemicals and Blood Dyscrasias*. Hamilton, Ill.: Drug Intelligence Publications, 1977.

25. Berbatis CG, Herrman RP, Kailis SG: Aplastic anaemia associated with phenylbutazone: evaluation of treatment. *Aust J Pharm* 60:797–801, 1979.

26. Irey NS: Tissue reactions to drugs. *Am J Pathol* 82:617–629, 1976.

27. Pisciotta V: Drug-induced agranulocytosis. *Drugs* 15:132–142, 1978.

28. Bradford Hill A: *Principles of Medical Statistics*, ed 7. London: Lancet, 1971.

29. Jick H, Vessey MP: Case-control studies in the evaluation of drug-induced illness. *Am J Epidemiol* 107:1–8, 1978.

30. Aoki K: Aplastic anaemia and chloramphenicol. In Gent M, Shigematsu I: *Epidemiological Issues in Reported Drug Induced Illnesses*. Hamilton, Ont.: McMaster University Library, 1978.

31. Gale RP, Champlin RE, Feig SA, et al: Aplastic anemia: biology and treatment. *Ann Intern Med* 95:477–494, 1981.

32. Weatherall DJ, Clegg JB: *The Thalassaemia Syndromes*, ed 3. London: Blackwell, 1981.

33. Propper R, Nathan D: Clinical removal of iron. *Annu Rev Med* 33:509–19, 1982.

34. Sears DA: The morbidity of sickle cell trait: a review of the literature. *Am J Med* 64:1021–36, 1978.

35. Charache S: Treatment of sickle cell anemia. *Annu Rev Med* 32:195–206, 1981.

36. Alter BP: Prenatal diagnosis of haemoglobinopathies: a status report. *Lancet* 2:1152–5, 1981.

37. Gaston M, Rosse WF: The cooperative group. The cooperative study of sickle cell disease: a review of study design and objectives. *Am J Pediatr Hematol Oncol* 4:197–201, 1982.

38. Friedman MJ, Trager W: The biochemistry of resistance to malaria. *Sci Am* 244:112–124, 1981.

39. WHO: Technical Report Series No. 524: Pharmacogenetics. Geneva: WHO, 1973.

40. Petz LD, Garratty G: *Acquired Immune Hemolytic Anemias*. London: Churchill Livingstone, 1980.

41. Carrell RW, Winterbourn CC, Rachmilewitz EA: Activated oxygen and hemolysis. *Br J Haematol* 30:259–266, 1975.

42. Swanson M, Cook R: Detection of drug induced blood dyscrasias. *Am J Hosp Pharm* 30:534–536, 1973.

43. Berbatis CG, Diekman J, Eckert GM, et al: Oxidant type hemolytic anemia in a glucose-6-phosphate dehydrogenase deficient individual—a problem in patient compliance. *Aust J Hosp Pharm* 7:44–47, 1977.

44. Berbatis CG, Eckert GM, Savdie E: Oxidant hemolysis associated with sulfamethizole toxicity. *Aust J Pharm* 58:397–400, 1977.

45. WHO: Technical Report Series No. 563: Evaluation of Drugs for Use in Man. Geneva: WHO, 1975.

46. Hemmaplardh D, Kailis SG, Morgan EH: The effects of inhibitors of microtubule and microfilament function on transferrin and iron uptake by rabbit reticulocytes and bone marrow. *Br J Haematol* 28:53, 1974.

SECTION 10
Neurological and Psychological Disorders

CHAPTER 35

Insomnia and Anxiety

MARTIN J. JINKS, Pharm.D.

Insomnia and anxiety are important health problems in our society, as reflected by recent drug-use statistics published by the National Institute on Drug Abuse. In 1981, nearly 92 million prescriptions for hypnotics and antianxiety agents were filled in the United States, with hypnotics accounting for about 21 million prescriptions (1, 3). It is estimated that 10 million Americans use a benzodiazepine antianxiety agent in any given year (2), and their widespread use has probably reached the proportions of a mass cultural phenomenon. Diazepam, which accounts for over half of benzodiazepine prescriptions, has routinely occupied first place as the most frequently prescribed drug, including new and refill prescriptions.

This considerable amount of prescribing may or may not reflect the usefulness or effectiveness of these agents. Insomnia and anxiety are largely unquantifiable disorders with subjectively derived therapeutic indications and endpoints. Unlike with hypertension or diabetes, no laboratory value will divulge adequate drug response. The abundant literature on anxiety and sleep disorders has fallen short in providing prescribers with quantifiable and scientific parameters for diagnosis and prescribing. Thus, therapy of these disorders is apt to be more art than science, and the decision to use these agents based more on philosophical bent than measurable indication.

INSOMNIA

Occasional insomnia is universal in any patient population, and chronic insomnia is a relatively common complaint. About one third of adults report some sleeping difficulty during a given year, and one half of these consider the problem serious (4). About 3 to 4% of the adult population use prescription hypnotics, and an estimated 1% of adults report taking these drugs continuously for 2 months or more (5, 6). In institutionalized patients, insomnia is

the second most common indication for drug therapy (7).

Evaluation of Sleep Disorders

The Insomniac. Sleeping time in individuals varies significantly. Most humans require 7 to 8 hours sleep, but this can range 2 to 3 hours more or less in individuals. The usual lower limit of normal is 5 hours (8).

Sleep patterns and requirements undergo subtle changes with aging. The usual 7 to 8 hours of uninterrupted sleep are replaced by a pattern of increased sleep latency and a subsequently more fitful sleep during which the older adult is more easily disturbed. Complaints of difficulty in staying asleep may be as high as 48% in adults over 50 years of age (9). However, the popularly held belief that the aged sleep less may not actually be the case, and instead with normal aging there is a reappearance of more natural polycyclic patterns of sleep with daytime naps as occurs in infancy. The total daily sleep time may not change significantly. These normal age-related changes are important to recognize to avert unnecessary prescribing of hypnotics in older adults. Thirty-nine percent of hypnotics prescribed in one report were for persons over the age of 60 (6), and in another survey nearly half of the persons over 65 years of age reported the use of prescription and nonprescription hypnotics "every night" or "frequently" (9).

Since insomnia is often a symptom of an underlying physical or emotional disorder, the physician is obliged to consider a number of possible etiologies before resorting to pharmacological control. Some type of sleep disorder occurs in all emotional disturbances, and delineation of the pattern of insomnia is important. For example, insomnia characterized by early morning awakening indicates depression and, in severe depression, hypnotics will not help the sleep disorder and may actually aggravate the depression. Based on incidence figures for depression, it has been speculated that inappropriate hypnotic use in this group of patients probably accounts for a large percentage of the 21 million hypnotic prescriptions per year in the United States (10). In one literature review, psychiatric disorders were the most common cause of insomnia, accounting for 35% of the cases (11).

In addition to emotional etiologies for insomnia, physical disorders may cause insomnia and may be overlooked. Often the physical disorders are subtle in nature and/or the patient is unable to articulate them well or associate them with sleeping difficulties. Underlying pathology, such as dyspnea from angina or congestive heart failure, or hyperthyroidism, may be manifested early as insomnia. Consideration of the patient's age is extremely important since the incidence of sleep apnea and nocturnal myoclonus (periodic leg movements) is greatly increased in the aged. The physician with a low index of suspicion may prescribe a hypnotic agent, which can aggravate these disorders or delay diagnosis, instead of treating the underlying condition.

A careful drug history is always an important part of the workup of the insomniac patient. A number of drugs such as appetite suppressants, antiasthmatic agents, and prescription and nonprescription sympathomimetic agents (both systemic and topical) can produce central nervous system (CNS) stimulation and wakefulness. Other drugs such as narcotics, reserpine, phenothiazines and tricyclic antidepressants can produce disturbances in normal sleep patterns.

A history of social drug habits also is important, since caffeine ingestion (especially in middle-aged patients) and heavy alcohol ingestion can produce inability to fall asleep and early morning wakefulness, respectively. Drug and alcohol misuse is a leading cause of insomnia, accounting for over 12% in one study (11).

Evaluating Hypnotic Efficacy

Objective methods to evaluate hypnotic efficacy were unknown 10 years ago. Now, through the development and sophistication of sleep laboratory techniques, certain basic criteria measuring duration and quality of sleep have been identified, and these criteria have some usefulness in the study of drugs that affect sleep and relieve insomnia. The major problem with sleep laboratory techniques is that expense and limited facilities preclude the accumulation of a large patient data base relating to hypnotic therapy.

It has been shown that sleep is composed of a succession of two main functional states, rapid eye movement (REM or dream sleep) and non-rapid eye movement (NREM) sleep. NREM sleep is further divided into four distinct stages. In the normal, young adult, electroencephalograph (EEG) monitoring demonstrates cyclical progressions in and out of REM sleep so that the normal REM duration is about 20 to 25% of the total sleep time. The aged normally show altered sleep patterns in which the initial awake period is prolonged, REM periods are quantitatively different and awakenings are more frequent. Therefore, older adults generally have reduced total sleep time at night, which is entirely normal.

Patients with insomnia who have been studied in the sleep laboratory in the absence of hypnotic therapy not only have prolonged initial awake periods but show suppression of REM and stage 4 NREM sleep. This has important implications for pharmacological management because hypnotic agents, while beneficial in initiating sleep, suppress REM and NREM sleep with chronic use, and therefore can aggravate the underlying EEG abnormalities. REM and NREM suppression is believed to be related to the development of tolerance, dependence and hypnotic-withdrawal insomnia, although these relationships are not proven. It is known, however, that there is significant reduction in REM sleep time in insomniacs taking hypnotics compared to insomniacs not taking these drugs.

Complete REM deprivation over prolonged periods by physically awakening the subject has been shown to cause irritability, anxiety and, rarely, psychotic episodes. However, partially suppressed REM sleep in humans by hypnotic agents can continue for months without severe adverse psychological effects. In certain circumstances, REM deprivation with drugs has theoretically beneficial possibilities. Nocturnal anginal attacks most often occur during REM sleep, and REM suppression may reduce the frequency of such attacks. It also has been suggested that hypnotic-induced REM deprivation may be beneficial following eye surgery when avoidance of rapid eye movement is desirable.

A number of drugs have been evaluated using sleep laboratory parameters. Results indicate that all drugs promoted for hypnotic use are equally effective in inducing and maintaining sleep initially. However, with the exception of the benzodiazepine hypnotics, all show marked decrease in these indices in 2 weeks or less. Several, including pentobarbital, glutethimide, methyprylon and methaqualone, produce symptoms of REM rebound in as little as 3 days. The benzodiazepine hypnotics affect sleep stages in a manner similar to the barbiturates, but their sleep-inducing and sleep-maintenance effects persist much longer.

Kales and Kales (12) have cited a number of shortcomings in the sleep laboratory evaluation of hypnotic drugs and offer them as guidelines for assessing hypnotic drug literature. Two major types of shortcomings exist.

General Methodological Inadequacies of the Trials. Ten weeks is the longest period of time any hypnotic has been studied under sleep laboratory conditions. The majority of published sleep laboratory trials involve a single night's administration, or 3 nights' administration at the most. Short-term studies of efficacy and side effects are often not applicable to intermediate and long-term use and often do not replicate the usual pattern of prescribing. In one study of hypnotic utilization, 40% of patients received sleep medication in excess of 3 months (13).

A second methodological inadequacy is the evaluation of several drugs in a crossover design without allowing adequate wash-out time between drugs. The wash-out period assures that the previously administered drug does not interfere with the drug currently being evaluated. Since the effects of most hypnotic drugs persist 24 hours or longer, the wash-out factor is crucial. For example, drug-induced REM changes one night can cause worsening of sleep by placebo or active drug the following night from REM rebound, and the evaluation of the second drug is adversely affected.

Promotional Claims Based on Sleep Laboratory Studies. There are a number of instances where sleep laboratory data have been misused in the promotion of hypnotic agents. First, studies in normal subjects may not be relevant to those in patients with disturbed sleep even though studies in normal subjects are frequently promoted as proof of efficacy. Secondly, although most trials are relatively brief, this information is not disclosed in the manufacturer's literature. Statements of effi-

cacy without specifying the duration of the trial mislead the prescriber into assuming that the hypnotic agent is effective for both short- and long-term use. Third, there is a clear lack of knowledge regarding the specific importance of any sleep stage. In fact, it has even been suggested that the effects of hypnotics on eye movement may not represent a primary effect on sleep mechanisms, but rather a depression of occulomotor activity that simply becomes apparent during sleep (14).

The Hypnotic Drugs

Hollister (8) has outlined the criteria for an ideal hypnotic drug: (a) rapid onset; (b) no disturbance of normal sleep patterns; (c) sufficient duration of action to maintain sleep throughout the night; (d) little residual sedation; (e) no tolerance, habituation or withdrawal; and (f) safety from accidental or intentional suicide. Unfortunately, no hypnotic drug currently available meets all of these basic criteria.

Sedatives, antianxiety agents and hypnotics cannot be separated pharmacologically since all depress the CNS. Promotion by the drug manufacturer and dosing determine the therapeutic use. Both long-acting agents (e.g., flurazepam versus diazepam) and short-acting agents (e.g., temazepam versus lorazepam) are divided in their use as either hypnotics or antianxiety agents, but this is with little pharmacological or pharmacokinetic basis.

Upon initiation, hypnotics decrease sleep latency, awake time and number of awakenings, and they increase total sleep time. With continued use, these favorable effects are superceded by reduction in REM sleep and certain NREM stages. This occurs with even small doses nightly for only a few days. With nonbenzodiazepine hypnotics, tolerance develops rapidly, and with both non-benzodiazepine and short-acting benzodiazepine hypnotics, "REM rebound" occurs, resulting in restlessness, nightmares and worsening insomnia. Thus, both tolerance and hypnotic-withdrawal insomnia have been linked to continuous REM deprivation, and the degree to which a hypnotic reduces REM and certain NREM stages of sleep has become a criterion for evaluation.

The effects of benzodiazepine hypnotics on sleep stages are qualitatively similar to non-benzodiazepine hypnotics, but their beneficial effects on sleep induction and sleep maintenance persist longer. Exactly how long the beneficial effects last is unknown. The longest reported administration of flurazepam and temazepam under sleep laboratory conditions is 30 and 35 days, respectively. Nitrazepam, a benzodiazepine available in Great Britain, has been studied in the sleep laboratory for up to 10 weeks, and triazolam has been studied in clnical trial for 6 months. In each instance, the benzodiazepine hypnotic was shown to retain effectiveness for the duration of the study. However, hypnotic-withdrawal insomnia occurs with the short- and intermediate-acting benzodiazepines, such as triazolam, nitrazepam, temazepam, and lorazepam (15, 16). Long-acting benzodiazepines, such as flurazepam and diazepam, have not been implicated as yet.

For the non-benzodiazepine hypnotics, the development of tolerance and ineffectiveness can lead to multiple dosing, hypnotic misuse and withdrawal phenomena. With short- and intermediate-acting benzodiazepines, the patient may continue to use the drug to avoid the unpleasant consequences of withdrawal. The syndrome of hypnotic-withdrawal insomnia is a compelling reason to avoid uninterrupted use patterns. Because of this hazard, the American Medical Association Council on Scientific Affairs has determined that the long-term, nightly use of hypnotic agents (i.e., no more than 2 weeks for barbiturates and no more than 6 weeks for benzodiazepines) is unjustified (5).

Adverse publicity and the concern of health professionals about overprescribing and misuse of hypnotic agents has resulted in an appreciable decline in hypnotic prescribing during the past decade. Between 1971 and 1977, the number of hypnotic prescriptions decreased by 39%, and a major shift from barbiturates to benzodiazepine hypnotics occurred (6). These changes in utilization most likely reflect the prescribers' greater appreciation of the limitations of hypnotic agents, as well as the restriction of barbiturates to schedule II status.

For patients caught in a cycle of insomnia, hypnotic tolerance and hypnotic withdrawal phenomena, a protocol for discontinuing hypnotic drugs with a minimum of withdrawal symptoms has been suggested (17): (a) withdraw the hypnotic drug very gradually at the rate of one therapeutic dose every 5 or 6 days;

(b) inform the patient that severe changes may occur, including increased dreaming, vivid dreams and even nightmares, and that these symptoms are reflections of transient physiological changes; and (c) where total withdrawal of the drug is difficult, replace the drug with a hypnotic which has been demonstrated in sleep laboratory studies to retain effectiveness for relatively longer periods (e.g., long-acting benzodiazepines) and limit the hypnotic drug use to the lowest adequate dose.

THE BARBITURATES (PENTOBARBITAL, SECOBARBITAL, ETC.)

A number of chemical entities and products in this class are marketed, but there is little pharmacological distinction among them. Those commonly used for sleep are called "short-acting" barbiturates, but the term "short-acting" is a misnomer because all barbiturates used commonly for sleep induction have half-lives in excess of 24 hours. The property which makes "short-acting" barbiturates more suitable as hypnotic agents is their rapid onset of action.

Low cost is the primary advantage of the barbiturate hypnotics. Disadvantages include: (a) rapid onset of sleep stage abnormalities, tolerance and withdrawal phenomena; (b) low safety index, as indicated by the large number of successful suicides involving barbiturates; (c) induction of liver drug metabolizing enzymes, resulting in numerous drug interactions; and (d) class II Drug Enforcement Agency (DEA) scheduling, making them less convenient to prescribe and dispense.

Barbiturate hypnotic prescribing has declined by nearly 80% during the past decade until they now account for only 17% of all hypnotics prescribed. Barbiturate-related deaths have decreased by over 50% during this same period. Interestingly, general and family practitioners prescribe barbiturates most frequently, while psychiatrists have virtually abandoned the barbiturates in favor of benzodiazepines (5, 6).

THE GLUTARIMIDES (GLUTETHIMIDE AND METHYPRYLON) AND METHAQUALONE

Despite wide promotion as nonbarbiturate hypnotics, these drugs are very similar to the barbiturates chemically and pharmacologically. The glutarimides and methaqualone do not share the advantage of low cost with the barbiturates. They do, however, share most of the disadvantages. A particular problem with all these agents is that they are highly lipid soluble and in overdose produce an exceedingly troublesome intoxication to treat. Also, methaqualone (i.e., Quaalude, Parest) is the leading illicit drug used next to marijuana, and in terms of abuse morbidity, it outstrips even heroin and cocaine in urban areas (18).

HALOGENATED HYDROCARBONS (CHLORAL HYDRATE, ETHCHLORVYNOL)

Chloral hydrate is an old drug which is enjoying a resurgence in popularity. The reasons for its resurgence are multiple: (a) low cost; (b) in low doses, sleep abnormalities and appearance of tolerance are insignificant with short term use (at higher doses, i.e., 1 g daily or more, efficacy declines within 2 weeks); and (c) DEA schedule IV classification makes it simpler to prescribe, purchase and dispense.

Ethchlorvynol is a chemically related hypnotic but has properties similar to the barbiturates and glutarimides with regard to tolerance and overdose.

THE BENZODIAZEPINES

Within the benzodiazepine class of drugs there are little qualitative differences in pharmacological effects that would make some uniquely suitable as hypnotics (see tables, next section). Nevertheless, only flurazepam, temazepam and triazolam have emerged, through promotion, for insomnia. Wide acceptance by prescribers of the perceived benefits of benzodiazepines for sleep-induction is reflected by the fact that flurazepam is ranked 15th in *American Druggist's* survey of top 200 in 1982 and first among all hypnotic agents (68) (Table 35.1).

Flurazepam. Because of early favorable results in sleep laboratory studies, flurazepam has been heralded as a solution to the hypnotic problem. Flurazepam does have unique properties that give the drug advantages when prolonged (i.e., more than 1 to 2 weeks) therapy is required. In usual doses, a delayed onset of REM deprivation of 1 to 3 weeks is characteristic (19). This delay contrasts with most other hypnotics which suppress REM sleep immediately. The delayed REM deprivation explains earlier reports of flurazepam's lack of

Table 35.1.
Commonly Prescribed Hypnotic Agents

Drug	Trade Name	Strength (mg)
Flurazepam	Dalmane	15, 30
Lorazepam	Ativan	1, 2
Temazepam	Restoril	15, 30
Triazolam	Halcion	0.25, 0.5
Nitrazepam	Mogadon	—[a]
Chloral hydrate	Noctec	250, 500
Pentobarbital	Nembutal	30, 50, 100
Secobarbital	Seconal	50, 100
Amobarbital/ secobarbital	Tuinal	50, 100, 200
Glutethimide	Doriden	250, 500
Methyprylon	Noludar	50, 200, 300
Ethchlorvynol	Placidyl	100, 200, 500, 750
Ethinamate	Valmid	500
Methaqualone	Quaalude or Parest	150, 200, 300, 400

[a] Not marketed in the United States.

REM disruption, since earlier studies were short term. Besides the REM abnormalities, stage 4 NREM sleep is virtually absent with flurazepam use after 3 days and takes up to 2 weeks to return after withdrawal from extended use. A compensatory increase in other NREM sleep stages appears to occur, however.

REM and stage 4 NREM suppression is associated with the production of tolerance and hypnotic-withdrawal symptoms with the non-benzodiazepine hypnotics, but with flurazepam significant tolerance to the sleep induction and sleep maintenance effects has not yet been reported. Also, discontinuation of flurazepam after short or intermediate term therapy produces very slight rebound REM, but there are usually little or no withdrawal symptoms. Indeed, with flurazepam discontinuation, a continued pattern of improved sleep may persist up to 3 days. Withdrawal from most other hypnotics, even after only a few days, results in immediate return to predrug sleep difficulties or even worsening insomnia. The "carry over" effect of flurazepam is perhaps related to the slow elimination of an active metabolite over several days.

With long-term use (i.e., up to 1 month) a slight diminution of effectiveness appears with flurazepam, and minor withdrawal symptoms often appear, causing a slight reduction of insomnia parameters over baselines during the 2-week period following discontinuation. The carry over effect is still present up to the third night after discontinuation, and thus, up to 1 month, withdrawal insomnia is relatively insignificant. Thus, flurazepam demonstrates advantageous characteristics with extended use over other hypnotics in that tolerance and withdrawal symptoms are insignificant. Fortunately, hypnotic agents are rarely indicated for extended periods and, in fact, flurazepam promotional literature states that "since insomnia is often transient and intermittent, prolonged administration is generally not necessary or recommended."

Flurazepam is rapidly absorbed and produces a peak effect from a single oral dose in ½ to 1 hour. This rapid action contributes to its specific usefulness as a hypnotic. However, flurazepam is converted to an active metabolite with a half-life of 47 to 100 hours. Therefore, multiple dosing with flurazepam may result in cumulative effects. In one study of flurazepam in nursing home patients, 25% of patients were found to have symptoms of oversedation after a few weeks of continuous therapy (20). It is recommended that patients be started on 15 mg of flurazepam and held at this dose for at least 1 to 2 weeks to assure maximal effect before increasing the dose. The use of conservative doses is particularly important in geriatric patients.

Temazepam. Temazepam is a recently marketed benzodiazepine hypnotic agent which can be considered intermediate-acting. It has an average half-life of 14.7 hours with a range of 8 to 38 hours (16). Its major route of elimination is conversion to the inactive glucuronide. Its metabolism is not significantly changed in older adults.

Temazepam alters sleep stages in sleep laboratory studies, although its effect on REM sleep appears small in the doses employed. No reduction in sleep benefits is seen after 35 consecutive nights of administration, but a mild form of rebound insomnia occurs following discontinuation. A clinical disadvantage of temazepam is its delayed peak effect of 2½ to 3 hours. Patients with disturbances of sleep onset may not benefit from temazepam unless the drug is administered 2 hours before bedtime.

Triazolam. Triazolam, a new benzodiazepine hypnotic, has a short half-life of 3 hours and a rapid onset of less than 30 min. In long-term clinical trials, triazolam maintains a shortened sleep latency and increased sleep duration in most patients, although some tolerance is apparent in 25% of the cases after 6 months (21). Rebound insomnia is reported in 14 days with triazolam which is attributed to its rapid elimination and lack of active metabolites (22).

There are important clinical implications associated with the differences between benzodiazepine hypnotics. Patients requiring short-term hypnotic drug use (e.g., during a brief hospitalization) would benefit from any of the rapid-acting agents, including the non-benzodiazepines. If long-term use (i.e., more than 1 to 2 weeks) is anticipated, the benzodiazepines are preferred. Benzodiazepines with a rapid onset make better hypnotics, particularly in patients with sleep latency disorders. Rapid acting benzodiazepines include flurazepam and triazolam.

The use of agents with long-acting metabolites can be both beneficial and detrimental. Flurazepam is the only benzodiazepine promoted for sleep that is long-acting. It is converted to an active metabolite with a half-life of 47 to 100 hours, and a carry-over daytime sedative effect is commonly seen. In patients who have an anxiety component to their sleep disturbance, the carry-over effect can reduce daytime anxiety. Diazepam, although not promoted for sleep induction, has a rapid onset and long duration, and can be used very effectively in these patients. An important advantage of long-acting benzodiazepines is they produce minimal rebound insomnia upon discontinuation.

A major disadvantage of long-acting benzodiazepines is that they may seriously impair coordination due to hangover effects and may present a potential hazard for the patient who, thinking that the effects of the sleeping pill taken the night before have worn off, drinks alcohol or takes other sedating medication. Geriatric patients are especially vulnerable to the carry-over effects since they do not generally metabolize the long-acting benzodiazepines as efficiently as younger adults. Accumulation and daytime oversedation commonly occur. Alternative hypnotics to use in geriatric patients are the short- and intermediate-acting benzodiazepines which do not accumulate with multiple dosing. These include temazepam and triazolam. Lorazepam and oxazepam are also short-acting benzodiazepines which are useful in geriatric patients, although not promoted for sleep induction. Temazepam, lorazepam and oxazepam all share the disadvantage of a slow onset, taking 2 to 4 hours to exert their peak effects. The short-acting benzodiazepines have all been associated with REM rebound and hypnotic-withdrawal insomnia, and thus extended use (i.e., more than 1 to 2 weeks) requires that discontinuation be achieved by a careful tapering process.

A distinct advantage of the benzodiazepine hypnotics over other hypnotics is that they are relatively "suicide-proof" in massive doses in the absence of other drugs, and no fatalities have been reported from them. However, this reassuring knowledge must be tempered by the fact that morbidity—that is, illnesses and/or hospital admissions from suicide attempts with the benzodiazepines (often combined with alcohol and other drugs)—is significant so that the suicide-proof characteristic does not preclude patient suffering from an overdose. Therefore, the admonition regarding the dangers of indiscriminantly prescribed hypnotic drugs applies equally to benzodiazepine hypnotics.

Tricyclic Antidepressants

Because insomnia is a common complaint in depression, depression must always be ruled out. The use of hypnotics in depression is dangerous because these drugs may aggravate the condition and may also provide a means for attempting suicide.

Certain tricyclics have significant sedative properties. Twenty-five milligrams of amitriptyline has hypnotic properties equivalent to 100 mg of secobarbital. If depression is a cause of insomnia, the tricyclic antidepressants are appropriate. Unfortunately, tricyclic antidepressants often are used unknowingly but successfully for insomnia in the absence of depression because of their sedative properties. This, according to one author, is "like using a sledgehammer to drive a tack."

Recommendations and Conclusions

Lennard et al. (23) point out that "as more and more facets of ordinary human conduct are considered to be medical problems ... intervention through the medium of psychoactive drugs (has become) desirable or required (for conditions) which in the past have been viewed as falling in the bounds of the normal trials and tribulations of human existence." To avoid hypnotic drug use for insomnia falling "within the bounds of the normal trials and tribulations of human existence," the prescriber must be discreet in selecting patients for hypnotic therapy. The importance of losing a night's sleep should not be exaggerated. Older adults, in particular, often respond to reassurance and education regarding reduced sleep requirements in later years. Minor changes in life-style or social drug habits may be all that is required. Physicians quick to write a prescription for hypnotics tend to reinforce the patient's notion that pathological insomnia exists, even when it does not, and may overlook a correctable underlying pathology or condition. A noninvasive strategy for improving nightly sleep is illustrated by the patient information sheet in Table 35.2. Initial educational approaches such as this are best exhausted before imposing the risks of hypnotic drugs on any patient.

Until a more precise method of evaluating and classifying pathological insomnia is developed, the decision to use hypnotics will remain empirical, based on physician attitudes and social pressures. Once the decision is made to employ a hypnotic agent, the following therapeutic guidelines are offered:

1. Instruct the patient that the ultimate therapeutic goal of treatment is to *restore* normal sleep without the use of drugs. Educate the patient that an occasional imperfect sleep is both normal and harmless.

2. If hypnotic agents are indicated, educate the patient regarding their limited usefulness. Patients encouraged to keep hypnotic drug use at a minimum are significantly more likely to do so than those not given instructions.

3. Begin theapy with the smallest dose possible and allow an adequate therapeutic trial before assuming ineffectiveness and increasing the dose.

4. In all possible cases, prescribe hypnotic agents for short periods of time or with frequent interruptions or "holidays." Intermittent therapy will tend to delay the onset of tolerance, habituation and hypnotic-withdrawal insomnia.

5. Prescribe hypnotic agents in sublethal quantities.

6. For patients in whom episodic therapy of not more than a few days at a time is adequate, most hypnotic agents will be equally effective. Avoid prescribing these agents for more than a few days at a time because of rapid appearance of withdrawal phenomena.

7. If, upon initial workup, or after an unsuc-

Table 35.2.
Patient Information Sheet for Insomnia

TO THE PATIENT: Suggestions for improving your nightly sleep

1. Increase your level of physical activity *gradually*. A sudden violent attempt to increase levels may actually make sleep worse; however, a steady program of adequate exercise will improve sleep
2. Exercise several hours before bedtime. This usually has a mild sedating effect; but again, avoid strenuous exercise right before bedtime
3. Try to regulate your daily schedule and set up a regular time to go to bed
4. Go to bed when you are sleepy; don't stay in bed when you're not
5. Try to do something relaxing before bedtime such as watching TV or reading, as opposed to an anxiety-producing activity such as balancing your checkbook
6. Coffee is a common sleep disturber; as you get older, coffee may tend to disrupt your sleep more than it did in younger years
7. Alcohol may actually cause poor sleep. A drink in the evening may improve sleep early in the night, but since alcohol is rapidly metabolized, minor withdrawal symptoms may occur in the early morning hours making later sleep more restless. It is better to have warm milk or cereal at bedtime instead of a snack that includes an alcoholic beverage
8. Your doctor is your best source of information about sleep disorders and proper treatment for them. Despite claims made on TV and in magazines, modern sleep laboratory studies have demonstrated that nonprescription sleep aids are ineffective in treating most insomnia. Moreover, these drugs may have unpleasant or dangerous side effects. Don't use them without the knowledge and approval of your physician

---

cessful short-term trial with a non-benzodiazepine hypnotic, it is determined that long-term, daily therapy is needed, the benzodiazepines are the drugs of choice.

8. If flurazepam is selected, begin with 15-mg doses and increase only after an adequate trial of 1 to 2 weeks. Inform the patient that maximal results are expected only after a few days and that daytime sedation may appear. Once adequate sleep is attained, the drug will be discontinued as soon as possible. A 1- to 2-month course should not be exceeded. If discontinuation within this time frame is not possible, institute "drug holidays" to prepare the patient for ultimately discontinuing the hypnotic and to minimize tolerance.

9. If a shorter-acting benzodiazepine is selected (e.g., temazepam or triazolam), caution the patient against abruptly discontinuing the drug without medical supervision.

10. For patients who consume hypnotics chronically and who display symptoms of tolerance, habituation and hypnotic-induced insomnia, attempt to withdraw the hypnotic (or at least minimize its use) according to Kales' protocol described earlier in the text.

In conclusion, little evidence exists that normal, physiological sleep can be achieved with the use of any hypnotic drug. However, using the basic principles outlined, hypnotic therapy can be optimized with regard to effectiveness and safety.

ANXIETY

Clinical anxiety consists of a kaleidoscope of symptoms which, to some degree, are experiences common to everyone. Pathological anxiety is anxiety severe enough to produce dysfunction, discomfort and inability to maintain work or social activities. Obscure and inconsistent psychic and somatic symptoms are present, ranging from a subjective sense of fear, tension, apprehension and depersonalization to bodily symptoms of autonomic hyperactivity, nervousness, dizziness, lightheadedness, paresthesias of hands and feet, perioral numbness, weakness, irritability, shortness of breath, palpitations, tachycardia, chest pain, tachypnea, diaphoresis, jitteriness and hyperactive reflexes.

In the differential diagnosis of anxiety, three etiologies must be considered and evaluated in order to select the most appropriate therapy: (a) an underlying medical illness, (b) a primary anxiety disorder, or (c) a situational anxiety reaction. These three etiologies and their medical treatments are outlined in Table 35.3.

Underlying Medical Illness. The initial presentation of anxiety should always be viewed as a symptom with a possible underlying cause rather than a simple diagnosis with prognostic implications. The association of anxiety with medical illness is substantial. Prominent anxiety symptoms are associated

Table 35.3.
Treatment of Anxiety by Diagnosis[a]

Disorder	Therapy	Medication[b]
1. Underlying medical illness	Specific medical/surgical approaches	Adjunctive benzodiazepines
2. Primary anxiety disorder (e.g., agoraphobia, social phobia, panic attacks)	Behavior therapy (e.g., desensitization, forced immersion, etc.)	MAOI; TCA; β-blockers; clonidine; adjunctive benzodiazepines
3. Situational anxiety	Counseling; relaxation techniques	Benzodiazepines; β-blockers

[a] Adapted from M. A. Schuckit (25).
[b] MAOI = monoamine oxidase inhibitor; TCA = tricyclic antidepressant.

with paroxysmal tachycardia, thyrotoxicosis, pheochromocytoma, acute and chronic pain, and hypoxic states. Psychiatric disorders, such as schizophrenia and depression, often present with anxiety complaints. Other examples include encephalopathies, seizure disorders, senile dementia, angina pectoris and premenstrual tension.

Intolerance to drugs may be an important cause of anxiety symptoms. Prescription drugs are common culprits. The stimulant side effects of bronchodilators in asthmatic patients or the akathesia secondary to antipsychotic medication are two examples. Excessive use of caffeine, ethanol or sedative-hypnotics produce anxiety symptoms. Long-term or high dose use of antianxiety agents can result in "rebound anxiety" when discontinuation is attempted.

Whenever an underlying medical illness exists, treatment is directed at the specific medical cause. Antianxiety agents are adjunctive therapy at best.

Primary Anxiety Disorders. These disorders are major psychiatric diseases which are currently classified by the *Diagnostic and Statistical Manual of Mental Disorders* of the American Psychiatric Association (24). They consist of acute panic disorders or chronic phobias, such as agoraphobia (fear of being away from a familiar environment) and social phobias (fear of humiliation or public scrutiny). Each disorder is characterized by an intense avoidance reaction in the absence of a preexisting affective illness or coexisting alcohol or drug abuse, and each entails some degree of restricted activity (25).

Panic disorders and phobias are the most common of the primary anxiety disorders, and they are often part of the same syndrome. The natural history of acute panic disorder with phobia begins with the sudden onset of a panic attack characterized by an intense apprehension, fear, terror and a feeling of impending doom. The acute attack typically lasts for seconds to minutes with severe autonomic symptoms, such as tachycardia, dyspnea, tremulousness, dizziness, diaphoresis and a desire to escape. If random panic attacks periodically recur, the patient's overall anxiety level becomes elevated and a severe and persistent anticipatory anxiety component develops, leading to avoidant behavior (i.e., phobias).

Treatment consists of a combination of drug therapy and behavioral modification. Drug therapy is used to specifically interrupt the acute panic attacks, while behavior therapy attempts to resolve phobias and anticipatory anxiety. Drugs used successfully for primary anxiety disorders are tricyclic antidepressants, monoamine oxidase inhibitors, β-blocking agents and clonidine.

Tricyclic antidepressants (TCAs), particularly imipramine, are 80 to 90% effective in treating acute panic attacks (26). Doses used are the same as those used to treat endogenous depression and range from 150 to 300 mg daily. As in depression, doses must be titrated carefully up to therapeutic levels. The onset of action may be delayed 3 weeks or longer after therapeutic doses are reached.

Monoamine oxidase inhibitors (MAOIs) appear to be similar in effectiveness to TCAs. MAOIs may be more effective than TCAs for the psychic symptoms of acute panic and chronic phobias (27), but proof of this requires more study. The MAOI agent most commonly used is phenelzine in doses of 45 to 90 mg daily. A maximum response is seen in 6 to 8 weeks.

The β-blockers and clonidine are reported to have limited usefulness in the primary anxiety states. Propranolol reduces somatic autonomic symptoms (e.g., tachycardia, dyspnea, etc.), but is still considered a second-line drug to the TCAs and MAOIs. Clonidine is a centrally acting α_2-agonist which theoretically inhibits central anxiety modulation by the locus ceruleus (28). Clonidine is effective in acute panic attacks, especially for the psychic component, but due to troublesome side effects, clonidine will not likely supplant TCAs and MAOIs for primary anxiety disorders.

Benzodiazepine antianxiety agents should not be used alone in the treatment of primary anxiety disorders. These drugs decrease the anticipatory anxiety between panic attacks but do nothing to abort the attack. As the level of anticipatory anxiety increases from uncontrolled panic attacks, the patient may continue to increase the benzodiazepine dose to a level at which dependence becomes a problem. It has been suggested that the mistaken diagnosis of situational anxiety for anticipatory anxiety secondary to panic attacks is a common cause of benzodiazepine misuse by patients (29).

Once the acute panic attack has been controlled with a TCA or MAOI, behavior therapy is initiated to resolve the avoidance component of the panic-phobia complex. Techniques such as relaxation therapy, desensitization, forced immersion into the threatening situation, and several other approaches have all been employed.

Situational Anxiety. After careful screening to rule out an underlying medical illness or a primary anxiety disorder, many patients are found to suffer from anxiety related to a situational state or cause. The anxiety may have a clear-cut focus or may be free-floating, i.e., not clearly related to an internal or external stimulus. The natural history of situational anxiety is usually short-term when a precipitating cause is identified, or episodic in the free-floating form, with acute anxiety typically lasting 1 to 3 weeks (25, 30).

If the patient is not overwhelmed by anxiety and can function, counseling is the simplest and least hazardous treatment. In anxiety reactions severe enough to produce dysfunction or discomfort, temporary use of an antianxiety agent is indicated. What exactly constitutes dysfunction or discomfort depends on the combined and negotiated perceptions of both the patient and physician. The optimal choice between pharmacological management and psychotherapy is not "either/or," but "both."

Antianxiety agents are frequently used as adjunctive treatment in medical conditions where stress is a factor. Anxiolytics for presurgical induction, endoscopy procedures, cardioversion and for somatic symptoms of hypertension, coronary artery disease, or gastrointestinal disorders represent common situational uses. Recent data indicate that two thirds of diazepam prescriptions are for adjunctive therapy of anxiety associated with serious organic or functional disorders (31). Temporary, symptomatic and judicious use of antianxiety agents in conjunction with medical illnesses is rational as long as specific treatment is concurrently undertaken, but long-term, uninterrupted therapy is inappropriate due to the risk of dependence and abstinence syndromes.

Certain forms of acute situational anxiety are characterized by a predominance of somatic symptoms and minimal cognitive symptoms. Common examples are public speaking jitters, final exam jitters, and stage fright. Doses of propranolol averaging 60 mg daily or more have improved performance in acute situational anxiety states manifested mainly by somatic complaints (35, 36). Since β-adrenergic blockers do not affect cognitive symptoms of anxiety, and because they have numerous undesirable side effects, their general application in anxiety is limited.

The therapeutic benefits derived from antianxiety agents, weighed against the risks and perceived disadvantages, have been a matter of considerable controversy. The popularity of these drugs in medical practice has led to public allegations that ours is an overmedicated society. Extensive discussion in lay publications has criticized the current "Valiumania" and indicted liberal benzodiazepine prescribing as a public health problem leading to adverse reactions and physical dependence. Even "Valium Anonymous" groups have sprung up (32, 33).

Critics of widespread use argue that the increasing reliance of large numbers of patients on antianxiety agents to treat symptoms usually related to common life experiences denies the patient the benefits and reduced risks of non-pharmacological solutions and reinforces the notion that the patient is indeed sick rather than confronted with normal stresses. In most cases, anxiety is a normal prerequisite to coping with problems, and pharmacological intervention is rarely indicated. In the best interests of most patients, drugs are to be avoided whenever possible and reassurance and counseling substituted.

The opposing point of view holds that antianxiety agents, particularly the benzodiazepines, can do no harm in therapeutic doses. Patients cannot—and should not have to—cope with problems causing or resulting in anxiety without chemical support. It is pointed out that patients have extremely conservative attitudes toward these drugs and are not apt to use them on a daily basis. It has even been suggested that the evolutionary development of man has not kept pace with the rapid advances of a technocratic civilization and that an artificial means to alleviate stress is natural and logical (34). With the discovery of endogenous benzodiazepine receptors in the brain, could it be that anxious patients are born with a 10-mg Valium deficiency?

Prescriptions for benzodiazepine have slipped 32% from 1973 to 1981, and the bulk of the loss was recorded by Valium, down by one third (55). Much of this decline can be attributed to adverse publicity about overuse and dependence. The rising popularity of alternative therapies for relaxation, such as jogging, has also played a role. Certainly the FDA has affected use by making benzodiazepines schedule IV drugs. The FDA has also deleted the "stress and stressful situation" indication in package labeling, prohibited claims that benzodiazepines do not cause physical dependence, and required manufacturers to warn health professionals against prolonged (i.e., >4 months) prescribing of antianxiety agents.

The Antianxiety Agents

Prior to 1950, treatment of anxiety was limited to barbiturates, opiates, chloral hydrate and bromides. In 1955, the glycerol derivative, meprobamate, was marketed for anxiety and was favorably received. Although many prescribers continue to regard the barbiturates and meprobamate as reliable and effective, their use has declined substantially since the introduction of the first benzodiazepine in 1960. It is now generally accepted that benzodiazepines are more effective than barbiturates and meprobamate, and that their reduced sedation and dependence liability and increased safety have made them the drugs of choice in anxiety. Thus, the majority of the discussion on antianxiety drugs will focus on benzodiazepines.

THE BENZODIAZEPINES

Benzodiazepines are the most commercially successful drugs ever marketed. Throughout the decade of the 1970s, counting new and refilled prescriptions per year, Valium has continually ranked first in frequency of prescribing. In 1973, Valium and Librium ranked first and second, respectively, of all prescription drugs. Surveys during this time showed that, during any 3-month period, 10% of the adult population consumed Valium. However, as mentioned earlier, the most recent surveys indicate an overall tendency for decreased consumption over the past 4 years.

The success of the benzodiazepines, compared to other antianxiety agents, can be attributed to several factors: (a) they are more selectively anxiolytic, (b) they produce less drowsiness and sedation at the therapeutic doses, (c) they produce less disruption in sleep, (d) they are associated with a marked decrease in mortality and morbidity in overdoses, (e) tolerance develops more slowly and physical dependence is less likely to occur, and (f) they do not significantly induce drug-metabolizing enzymes and thus are not subject to the drug interactions of other antianxiety agents. On the basis of these advantages, the benzodiazepines have become the mainstay in the treatment of anxiety.

Mechanism. Although not well understood, the benzodiazepines are thought to exert their effects indirectly by facilitating the inhibitory neurotransmitter, γ-aminobutyric acid (GABA). The discovery of specific benzodiazepine receptors in human brain tissue and the observation that their distribution parallels the distribution described for GABA receptors led to this theory (37). Furthermore, the high density of these receptors in the cerebral cortex and limbic forebrain and low density in the brainstem may account for the greater anxiolytic specificity of the benzodiazepines and their reduced toxicity in overdose, particularly their lack of fatal respiratory depressant effects (38).

Pharmacology and Kinetics. Benzodiazepines have more similarities than differences. However, they can be divided into two broad categories with respect to pharmacological and kinetic differences, and these differences can determine their clinical application: (a) long-acting benzodiazepines and (b) short-acting benzodiazepines (see Table 35.4).

Long-acting benzodiazepines have an extended effective duration of action due to the slow elimination half-life $(t_{1/2\ \beta})$ of the parent compound and/or the production of a major active metabolite with a slow $t_{1/2\ \beta}$. Most long-acting benzodiazepines are metabolized in the liver through a common pathway, undergoing N-dealkylation to desmethyldiazepam (nordiazepam) or its halogenated homologues. This major active metabolite has a half-life of about 50 hours. Most of the long-acting benzodiazepines are considered pronordiazepams since much of their pharmacologic effect can be attributed to desmethyldiazepam (DMD). Clorazepate and prazepam are two agents which are specific DMD prodrugs. Clorazepate undergoes hydrolysis and decarboxylation to DMD in the stomach before absorption, and prazepam requires first-pass liver transformation to DMD for activation. Diazepam, flurazepam, and halazepam also have DMD or its halogenated homologue as a major metabolite, but each parent drug also has anxiolytic activity. Chlordiazepoxide is active and has a number of active metabolites, of which DMD is a minor one. Once formed, DMD is hydroxylated to oxazepam and then glucuronidated and excreted.

The short-acting benzodiazepines include oxazepam, lorazepam, temazepam, triazolam and alprazolam. These drugs have shorter half-lives and are rapidly inactivated and eliminated without the production of active metabolites. Alprazolam and temazepam have been called intermediate-acting benzodiazepines because their half-lives are slightly longer, but neither accumulate with multiple dosing. Alprazolam and triazolam appear to have a minor active metabolite, but their effects are

Table 35.4.
The Benzodiazepines

Drug	Indication: A = anxiety H = hypnotic	Usual Daily Dose (mg)	Peak Plasma Level (hr)	Elimination $t_{1/2}$ (hr)	Metabolites	Intramuscular Bioavailability	Protein Binding (%)
LONG-ACTING AGENTS							
Chlordiazepoxide (Librium)	A	15–100	1–4	6–30	Active	Poor	96
Clorazepate (Tranxene)	A	15–60	—	See DMD	Active	N/A	97 (DMD)
Desmethydiazepam (DMD or nordiazepam)	See Figure 35.1			50–100	Active	N/A	97
Diazepam (Valium)	A	6–40	0.5–2	20–80	Active	Poor	98
Flurazepam (Dalmane)	H	15 or 30	0.5–1	Short but active metabolite, 47–100	Active	N/A	—
Halazepam (Paxipam)	A	80–160	1–3	14	Active	N/A	97 (DMD)
Prazepam (Centrax)	A	20–60	6	See DMD	Active	N/A	97 (DMD)
SHORT-ACTING AGENTS							
Alprazolam (Xanax)	A	0.75–4	1–2	12–15	Inactive	N/A	80
Lorazepam (Ativan)	A H	1–10 2 or 4	2–4	10–15	Inactive	Good	85
Oxazepam (Serax)	A	30–120	2–4	5–20	Inactive	N/A	87
Temazepam (Restoril)	H	15 or 30	2–4	15	Inactive	N/A	96
Triazolam (Halcion)	H	0.25 or 0.5	0.5–1	3	Inactive	N/A	80

generally insignificant (39). The metabolic relationships between the long- and short-acting benzodiazepines are illustrated in Figure 35.1.

The differences between the long- and short-acting benzodiazepines can be clinically important. With repeated doses, long-acting agents may take 1 to 2 weeks to reach steady-state levels. Therefore, the full therapeutic effects may be delayed and oversedation can result. This effect may be exaggerated in older patients due to age-related changes in volume of distribution and reduced metabolic efficiency, making older patients at higher risk for accumulation and oversedation. Conservative dosing and careful titration of long-acting agents is necessary in the aged. Accumulation is also a major concern in patients with cirrhosis or acute viral hepatitis. Hepatic disorders result in 2- to 5-fold increases in half-lives of the long-acting benzodiazepines. Finally, long-acting benzodiazepines can produce residual sedative effects and impaired motor performance for a substantial period of time following discontinuation. For example, alcohol use may result in additive sedation up to 10 hours after the last dose of a long-acting agent (40).

Long-acting benzodiazepines have certain advantages. They usually need to be administered only once or twice daily. Anxious patients with sleep disorders can be given a long-acting agent with a rapid onset (e.g., diazepam, flurazepam) at bedtime, and this will serve as both hypnotic and daytime sedative. With long-acting agents, a missed dose is of little consequence, and abrupt discontinuation after prolonged use generally does not result in a severe rebound syndrome. Abstinence syndromes do occur, however.

Short-acting benzodiazepines may be particularly useful in older patients and in patients with hepatic disorders. They do not accumulate with multiple dosing and they attain plasma steady state levels in 1 to 3 days. Their major disadvantage is that they must be taken 2 to 4 times a day and that abrupt discontinuation from prolonged use can result in the rapid emergence of a rebound anxiety syndrome (15). Alprazolam, a recently marketed triazolo-benzodiazepine agent, has structural similarities to the antidepressant trazodone. It is reported to be effective in anxiety with depression. This broadened indication may or

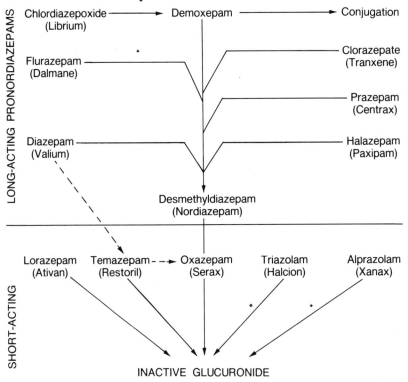

Figure 35.1. Metabolic relationships of benzodiazepines. * = more steps; – – – – = minor pathway. (Adapted from C. Bellantuono et al. (40).)

may not be deserved since preliminary evidence concerning its antidepressant effectiveness is difficult to evaluate (39).

Benzodiazepines differ in their onset of action with single doses. A benzodiazepine with a slow onset would be less effective when used intermittently for quick relief of anxiety-provoking stimuli or settings. This is a major advantage of diazepam which has a rapid onset. However, before steady state levels are reached, diazepam loses effectiveness quickly due to rapid tissue redistribution. Therefore, if daily therapy is to be employed, diazepam might best be given in divided doses during the first week. None of the other benzodiazepines promoted for anxiety, including the short-acting agents, are as rapid in onset as diazepam. Flurazepam and triazolam have rapid onsets, but both are promoted for sleep-induction (see Table 35.4).

Most of the benzodiazepines are highly protein bound, and in conditions associated with hypoalbuminemia, increased sensitivity may be seen (41). Benzodiazepines with lower protein binding, such as oxazepam or alprazolam, may be less effected.

Lorazepam is the intramuscular product of choice. Intramuscular injection of lorazepam produces little discomfort and is rapidly and reliably absorbed. By contrast, intramuscular chlordiazepoxide or diazepam produce considerable pain and are slowly and erratically absorbed (42).

Acute Toxicity and Side Effects. Benzodiazepines are considered very safe drugs. It has been said that "the only way to kill an animal (with benzodiazepines) ... is to smother it under a mound of tablets" (43). When taken alone, even in massive doses, benzodiazepines rarely cause life-threatening symptoms, and clinical manifestations mainly include drowsiness or stupor. However, it should be stressed that despite (or perhaps because of) the low mortality associated with benzodiazepine overdose, morbidity, in the form of emergency room visits and hospitalizations, is high. Next to alcohol, diazepam is the most commonly mentioned drug in emergency room admissions, and it is the most common single agent ingested (44). In combination with alcohol or other drugs, diazepam has been implicated in a substantial number of drug-related deaths (45).

Most common side effects of benzodiazepines are an extension of their desired pharmacological effects. Age- and dose-related sedation occurs most frequently and can impair cognitive performance and motor reflexes. Based on these sedating properties, a 5-fold increase risk of automobile accidents has been suggested in anxiolytic drug users (46), but two more recent studies have disputed this (47, 48).

Benzodiazepines can produce a number of adverse behavioral effects, including confusion, sleep disturbances and depression, especially in older adults. Triazolam has recently been associated with a psychosis syndrome (22, 49). Suicidal thoughts and impulses have been associated with therapeutic doses of diazepam (50). On rare occasions, benzodiazepines produce paradoxical reactions characterized by agitation and hostility. Benzodiazepines, with the possible exception of oxazepam, should be prescribed with care in patients experiencing interpersonal frustrations (e.g., marital discord) who have a history of acting out their frustrations or anger, or in whom impulse control is tenuous (51). Oxazepam may lack paradoxical hostility reactions (52).

Benzodiazepines must be used with caution during early pregnancy and during the perinatal period. Chlordiazepoxide, diazepam and clorazepate have all been associated with fetal abnormalities, primarily cleft lip or palate (40, 53, 54). Long-acting benzodiazepines accumulate in the fetal compartment with multiple dosing, and newborn hypothermia, respiratory depression and lethargy can occur if given during the perinatal period. A neonatal withdrawal syndrome has also been described with maternal use of high dose chlordiazepoxide or diazepam during the perinatal period (40). The use of benzodiazepines in women of childbearing age is of special concern in light of the fact that the majority of recipients of antianxiety agents are women.

Rare side effects reported with the benzodiazepines include skin rashes, occulomucotaneous reactions, hepatitis, ovulation suppression, galactorrhea and blood dyscrasias (40).

Dependence and Withdrawal. True physical dependence due to benzodiazepines is rare considering their overall rate of use and has been estimated as infrequently as 1 in every 50 million patient-months of use (25). Nevertheless, much concern has been expressed over the increasing reports of dependence and severe benzodiazepine abstinence syndromes. Much of the concern focuses on long-term, uninterrupted prescribing patterns. In a recent report from the National Academy of Sciences, 15% of third-party recipients received uninterrupted therapy for more than 4 months, and 8% used higher doses than prescribed (55). Long-term use and high doses are the two main predisposing factors for dependence.

The benzodiazepine withdrawal syndrome typically occurs after prolonged administration (i.e., > 4 months) of high doses (60 to 160 mg/day of diazepam or equivalent). Diazepam dose equivalents of 30 mg daily or less for three months or less is not associated with dependence. Much higher doses for shorter periods (e.g., 100 to 600 mg/day of diazepam for 7 days), or lower doses for prolonged periods (e.g., 15 mg/day of diazepam for 4 to 6 months; 30 to 45 mg/day of diazepam for 20 months; 15 to 25 mg/day of diazepam for 6 years; 45 mg/day of oxazepam for 3 years; 8 to 12 mg/day of lorazepam for 6 months) have produced abstinence syndromes (56–59).

The abstinence syndrome can be mild and resemble a "rebound anxiety." Failure to recognize mild withdrawal symptoms may perpetuate unnecessary drug use. Severe withdrawal symptoms resembling ethanol or barbiturate withdrawal can occur. Acute withdrawal from long-acting benzodiazepines begins in 2 to 9 days following abrupt discontinuance, with symptoms of tremors, nervousness, agitation, nausea, vomiting, cramps and diaphoresis. Severe psychosis has also been reported (60), and seizures, if they occur, usually appear between the 7th and 9th days. The abstinence syndrome following abrupt discontinuation of short-acting benzodiazepines is similar except that the time course is accelerated. For example, withdrawal seizures associated with oxazepam and lorazepam occur 25 hours (61) and 60 hours (59), respectively, following discontinuation. A chronic withdrawal state has been reported with long-acting agents and may appear between the 9th and 20th days and persist from 15 to 45 days (57, 62). This phase is characterized by depression, insomnia and exaggerated symptoms of anxiety.

Prevention of the benzodiazepine withdrawal syndrome involves tapering of the drug in any patient taking doses greater than 30 mg of diazepam equivalent per day and/or taking the drug continuously for longer than 3 months. In general, discontinuation is accomplished by a gradual tapering of the dose, not exceeding a 10% reduction of the first day's dose each day (51). If abstinence symptoms appear, temporary reinstitution of the drug will reverse the symptoms, and a more gradual tapering schedule will be required.

Benzodiazepine Drug Interactions. Benzodiazepines are likely to have additive CNS depressant activity with any sedative drug, including ethanol. There is evidence that ethanol may increase the absorption of diazepam (63). Diazepam interference with the antiparkinson effect of levodopa has been reported (64). Drugs which inhibit or compete with the mixed-function hepatic oxidative enzyme system can substantially impair the metabolism of long-acting benzodiazepines. Rapid and significant increases in half-life occur when combined with cimetidine (65) and low-dose estrogen-containing oral contraceptive steroids (66).

Principles of Benzodiazepine Therapy. One of the most difficult decisions facing the conscientious physician is whom to treat with benzodiazepines. In a world filled with anxiety, the decision is as much a philosophical matter as it is a medical one. The main concern is that anxiolytic use will delay confrontation with, and solution of, anxiety-producing problems. Nevertheless, when simple measures fail—such as counseling, reassurance and support—benzodiazepines effectively treat the symptoms of disabling situational anxiety.

Situational anxiety typically has an acute onset followed by a gradual decrease in symptoms over 1 to 3 weeks. Therefore, benzodiazepines are most appropriately used episodically within this timetable. Episodic use not only provides symptom relief consistent with the natural course of anxiety but also minimizes the potential for physical and psychological dependence. Even in patients who complain of persistent anxiety, it is best to use the benzodiazepine only during exacerbations. If indefinite treatment is judged necessary, the patient should be given the lowest possible dose and reevaluated regularly. Homeopathic doses often suffice (e.g., one fourth of one 2-mg Valium tablet) in patients "needing" chemical support (67). Continuous therapy is justified only when coping and problem solving are enhanced and avoidant behavior is diminished.

Patients vary widely in their individual dose requirements, and each patient must be titrated carefully to relieve symptoms without producing oversedation. When the long-acting agents are used, an initial dose of 2 mg of diazepam or its equivalent can be given at bedtime and doubled each night until a good night's sleep is obtained with a slight hangover effect the next day. After the initial response is achieved, further dose adjustment should not not be made more often than weekly. This applies to all pronordiazepam drugs which take 1 to 2 weeks to reach steady state levels.

Some patients may prefer the ritualistic procedure of taking divided doses throughout the day, and in this case short-acting agents may be better. Other situations in which the short-acting agents may be preferred are in geriatric patients and in patients with hepatic disorders. Oxazepam may have unique application in patients who exhibit paradoxical reactions to the other benzodiazepines.

The clinician should be prepared to use the full range of therapeutic options offered by the benzodiazepines. The individualization of therapy with regard to dosing and drug selection is important for the successful treatment of situational anxiety.

References

1. Anon: *National Prescription Audit, Therapeutic Category Report*, Ambler, Pa.: IMS America, 1982.
2. Anon: *FDA Drug Bull* 10:2, 1980.
3. Anon: *Am Drug* 185:20, 1982.
4. Bixler EO, Kales A, Soldatus CR, et al: Prevalence of sleep disorders in the Los Angeles metropolitan area. *Am J Psychiatry* 136:1257, 1979.
5. Anon: Council on Scientific Affairs: hypnotic drugs and treatment of insomnia. *JAMA* 245:749, 1981.
6. Solomon F, White CC, Parron DL, et al: Sleeping pills, insomnia and medical practice. *N Engl J Med* 300:803, 1979.
7. Miller RR; Drug surveillance utilizing epidemiologic methods; a report from the Boston Collaborative Drug Surveillance Program. *Am J Hosp Pharm* 30:584, 1973.
8. Hollister LE: Psychiatric and neurological disorders, in Melmon KL, Morrelli HF: *Clinical Pharmacology*. New York: Macmillan, 1972, p 482.
9. Bonnett MH, Kramer M: Interactions of age, performance and hypnotics in the sleep of insomniacs. *J Am Geriatr Soc* 29:508, 1981.
10. Brumback RA: Use of hypnotics (letter). *N Engl J Med* 292:217, 1975.
11. Coleman RM, Roffwarg HP, Kennedy SJ, et al: Sleep-wake disorders based on a polysomnographic diagnosis. *JAMA* 247:997, 1982.
12. Kales A, Kales JD: Shortcomings in the evaluation and promotion of hypnotic drugs. *N Engl J Med* 243:826, 1975.
13. Kales A, Kales JD, Bixler EO, et al: Effectiveness of hypnotic drugs with prolonged use; fluraze-

pam and pentobarbital. *Clin Pharmacol Ther* 18:356, 1975.
14. Feinberg I, Fein G, Walker JM, et al: Flurazepam effects on sleep EEG. *Arch Gen Psychistry* 36:95, 1979.
15. Kales A, Scharf MB, Kales JD, et al: Rebound insomnia. *JAMA* 241:1692, 1979.
16. Milter MM: Evaluation of temazepam. *Pharmacotherapy* 1:3, 1981.
17. Kales A, Bixler EO, Tan T, et al: Chronic hypnotic-drug use. *JAMA* 227:513, 1974.
18. Anon: Methaqualone abuse. *JAMA* 246:813, 1981.
19. Kales A, Bixler EO, Scharf M, et al: Sleep laboratory studies of flurazepam: a model for evaluating hypnotic drugs. *Clin Pharmacol Ther* 19:576, 1976.
20. Marttila JK, Hammel RJ, Alexander B, et al: Potential untoward effects of long-term use of flurazepam in geriatric patients. *J Am Pharm Assoc* NS17:692, 1977.
21. Deberdt R: Long-term triazolam. *Curr Ther Res* 26:1005, 1979.
22. Einarson TR: Hallucinations from triazolam. *Drug Intell Clin Pharm* 14:714, 1980.
23. Lennard HH, Epstein LJ, Bernstein A, et al: Hazards implicit in prescribing psychoactive drugs. *Science* 169:438, 1970.
24. *Diagnostic and Statistical Manual of Mental Disorders*, ed 3. Washington, D.C.: The American Psychiatric Association, 1980.
25. Schuckit MA: Current therapeutic options in the management of typical anxiety. *J Clin Psychiatry* 42:11, 1981.
26. Anon: Treating panic attacks. *Biol Therap Psychiatry* 5:1, 1982.
27. Gonzales ER: New studies confirm MAO inhibitors' efficacy in treating severe anxiety. *JAMA* 245:1799, 1981.
28. Hoehn-Saric R, Merchant AF, Keyser ML, et al; Effects of clonidine on anxiety disorders. *Arch Gen Psychiatry* 38:1278, 1981.
29. Muskin PR, Fyer AJ: Treatment of panic disorder. *J Clin Psychopharmacol* 1:81, 1981.
30. Hollister LE: *Clinical Use of Psychotropic Drugs*. Springfield, Ill.: Charles C Thomas, 1973, p 133.
31. Anon: *FDC Reports* 42:T&G8, 1980.
32. Cant G: Valiumania. *New York Times Magazine*, Feb. 1, 1976, p 34.
33. Anon: Overcoping with Valium. *FDA Consumer*, Dec. 1979–Jan. 1980, p 21.
34. Sachs SB: Chronic anxiety or tranquilizers—the doctor's dilemma. *S Afr Med J* 60:1260, 1981.
35. Brewer C: Beneficial effect of β-adrenergic blockade on "exam nerves." *Lancet* 2:435, 1972.
36. Bonn JA, Turner P, Hicks DC: β-Adrenergic-receptor blockade with practolol in treatment of anxiety. *Lancet* 1:814, 1972.
37. Richter JJ: Current theories about the mechanisms of benzodiazepines and neuroleptic drugs. *Anesthesiology* 54:66, 1981.
38. Study RE, Barker JL: Cellular mechanisms of benzodiazepine action. *JAMA* 247:2147, 1982.
39. Evans RL: Alprazolam. *Drug Intell Clin Pharm* 15:633, 1981.
40. Bellantuono C, Reggi Y, Tognoni G, et al: Ben-

zodiazepines: clinical pharmacology and therapeutic use. *Drugs* 19:195, 1980.

41. Greenblatt DJ: Clinical toxicity of chlordiazepoxide and diazepam in relation to serum albumin concentration. *Eur J Clin Pharmacol* 7:259, 1974.

42. Greenblatt DJ, Shader RI, Franke K, et al: Pharmacokinetics and bioavailability of intravenous, intramuscular, and oral lorazepam in humans. *J Pharm Sci* 68:57, 1979.

43. Mathew H: Are there safer hypnotics than barbiturates? *Lancet* 1:224, 1974.

44. Ungerleider JT, Lundberg GD, Sunshine I, et al: The drug abuse warning network (DAWN) program. *Arch Gen Psychiatry* 37:106, 1980.

45. Khantzian EJ, McKenna GJ: Acute toxic and withdrawal reactions associated with drug use and abuse. *Ann Intern Med* 90:361, 1979.

46. Skegg DCG, Richards SM, Doll R: Minor tranquilizers and road accidents. *Br Med J* 1:917, 1979.

47. Jick H, Hunter JR, Dinan BJ, et al: *Am J Public Health* 71:1399, 1981.

48. Landauer A: Diazepam and driving ability. *Med J Aust* 1:624, 1981.

49. Einarson RR, Yoder ES: Triazolam psychosis—a syndrome? *Drug Intell Clin Pharm* 16:330, 1982.

50. Zisook S, DeVaul RA: Adverse behavioral effects of benzodiazepines. *J Fam Pract* 5:963, 1977.

51. Rosenbaum JF: The drug treatment of anxiety. *N Engl J Med* 306:401, 1982.

52. Salzman C, Kochansky GE, Shader RI, et al: Is oxazepam associated with hostility? *Dis Nerv Syst* 36:30, 1975.

53. Anon: Teratogenicity of minor tranquilizers. *FDA Drug Bull* 5:14, 1975.

54. Patel DA, Patel AR: Clorazepate and congenital malformations. *JAMA* 244:135, 1980.

55. Anon: *FDC Reports* 44:T&G3, 1982.

56. Haskell D: Withdrawal of diazepam. *JAMA* 233:135, 1979.

57. Winokur A, Rickels K, Greenblatt DJ, et al: Withdrawal reaction from long-term low-dosage administration of diazepam. *Arch Gen Psychiatry* 37:101, 1980.

58. Pevnick JS, Jasinski DR, Haertzen CA: Abrupt withdrawal from therapeutically administered diazepam. *Arch Gen Psychiatry* 35:995, 1978.

59. de la Fuente JR, Rosenbaum AH, Martin HR, et al: Lorazepam-related withdrawal seizures. *Mayo Clin Proc* 55:190, 1980.

60. Preskorn SH: Benzodiazepines and withdrawal psychosis. *JAMA* 237:36, 1977.

61. Einarson TR: Oxazepam withdrawal convulsions. *Drug Intell Clin Pharm* 15:487, 1981.

62. Hall RCW, Kirkpatrick B: The benzodiazepines. *Am Fam Physician* 17:131, 1978.

63. Hayes SL, Pablo G, Radomski T, et al: Ethanol and oral diazepam absorption. *N Engl J Med* 296:186, 1977.

64. Hansten PD: *Drug Interactions*, ed 4. Philadelphia: Lea & Febiger, 1979, p 275.

65. Klotz U, Reimann I: Delayed clearance of diazepam due to cimetidine. *N Engl J Med* 302:1012, 1980.

66. Abernethy DR, Greenblatt DJ, Divoll M, et al: Impairment of diazepam metabolism by low-dose estrogen-containing oral-contraceptive steroids. *N Engl J Med* 306:791, 1982.

67. Macpherson ELR: To tranquillize, or not to tranquillize,—that is the question. *Practitioner* 225:1275, 1981.

68. Anon: *Am Drug* 187:13, 1983.

CHAPTER 36

Affective Disorders

GLEN L. STIMMEL, Pharm.D.

Disturbances of mood, which include mania and depressions, represent the most common psychiatric condition. Studies in the United States and Europe indicate that approximately 18 to 23% of adult females and 8 to 11% of adult males have had at least one major depressive episode. Bipolar, or manic-depressive illness, is much less common with a prevalence of 0.4 to 1.2% of the adult population, with an equal distribution in women and men (1, 2).

DIAGNOSTIC CLASSIFICATION

There are four major categories of affective disorders (Table 36.1) (1). Bipolar patients are those with mania, whether or not they have also had depression. A growing body of evidence suggests significant genetic, biochemical, pharmacological, clinical and physiological differences between unipolar and bipolar patients (3). Bipolar patients are further divided into type I and type II, depending on the natural course of their illness. Bipolar type I ptients have both acute manic and depressive episodes. Bipolar type II patients have only hypomanic (slightly manic) episodes as well as depressive episodes. The interval between episodes can vary from months to years, and there is no predictable pattern in the sequence of manic and depressive episodes.

Major depressive disorders include single and recurrent episodes. Single episodes constitute 30 to 50% of all unipolar patients, while 50 to 70% will suffer a recurrence of depression sometime in their lives. Depressive episodes are subclassified based upon accompanying symptoms such as psychotic features and melancholia. Typical psychotic features include delusions and hallucinations. When present their content is usually clearly consistent with the predominant mood (mood-congruent). Common examples include persecutory delusions, nihilistic delusions of world or personal destruction, somatic delusions of cancer or other serious illness, delusions of poverty and auditory hallucinations that involve voices which berate the individual for sins or shortcomings. Melancholia is added to the diagnosis when the following symptoms are present: loss of pleasure in most all activities, lack of reactivity to pleasureable stimuli, excessive or inappropriate guilt, depressive mood is regularly worse in the morning and marked psychomotor retardation or agitation (1).

Cyclothymic disorder is a chronic mood disturbance involving numerous periods of depression and hypomania. Symptoms are of shorter duration and less severity than bipolar disorder. Intervals of normal mood may last months at a time. Prevalence is unknown, but it is no longer believed to be rare (1). Cyclothymic disorder is frequently found in relatives of bipolar patients, and may in fact represent a subaffective or "abortive" form of bipolar disorder (4). These patients do not develop psychotic symptoms and rarely require hospitalization. Substance abuse is particularly common as a self-treatment for these mood disturbances.

Dysthymic disorder is a chronic disturbance of mood involving either depressed mood or loss of interest or pleasure in almost all activities, but not of sufficient severity and duration to meet the criteria for a major depressive episode. For adults, dysthymic disorder can be diagnosed only after a duration of 2 years. There may be periods of normal mood lasting a few days to a few weeks, but no more than a few months (1).

NATURAL COURSE

The episodic nature of affective disorders distinguishes it from most other major psychiatric disorders. Onset of depressive disorders may begin at any age, and age of onset is fairly evenly distributed throughout adult life. The first manic episode of bipolar patients typically

Table 36.1.
Affective Disorders Classification

1. Bipolar disorder
    Mixed
    Manic
    Depressed
2. Major depression
    Single episode
    Recurrent
3. Cyclothymic disorder
4. Dysthymic disorder (depressive neurosis)
5. Both manic and depressive episodes are further subclassified as
    A. Manic episode:
        In remission
        With psychotic features
        Without psychotic features
    B. Depressive episode
        In remission
        With psychotic features
        With melancholia
        Without melancholia

Table 36.2.
Stages of Mania

Stage I (euphoria)
    Increased psychomotor activity
    Euphoria mood
    Grandiose, overconfident
    Coherent, but tangential thinking
    Increased sexual preoccupation
    Insight generally intact
Stage II (irritability, anger)
    Increased pressure of speech
    Open hostility and anger
    Explosive and assaultive behavior
    Definite flight of ideas
    Increasing cognitive disorganization
    Overt paranoid and grandiose delusions
Stage III (severe panic)
    Desperate, panic stricken state
    Frenzied bizarre psychomotor activity
    Incoherent and loose associations
    May see disorientation, hallucinations, ideas of reference

occurs before age 30 (1). One third of bipolar patients are hospitalized before their 25th birthday, and at least 20% show evidence of illness as adolescents (5). For most untreated depressive episodes, their expected duration is 3 to 6 months. Depression in bipolar patients tend to be shorter than in unipolar patients. The expected duration of an untreated manic episode is about 3 months. Between episodes, patients with primary affective disorder usually function well, though there may be occasional residual symptoms. With increasing age, both unipolar and bipolar patients have diminishing symptom-free intervals between episodes (3). Because affective disorders will spontaneously remit without treatment, the goal of pharmacotherapy is to shorten the episode by eliminating manic or depressive symptomatology.

CLINICAL FEATURES

Mania

The three cardinal features of mania are euphoria, hyperactivity and flight of ideas. Euphoria may be replaced by irritability in some patients. Three stages, or degrees of severity, have been described for mania (Table 36.2) (6). The three stages are defined primarily by the predominant mood. Stage I, corresponding to hypomania, is when euphoria predominates. These patients are perceived as happy, hyper-

active, somewhat tangential in thinking, impulsive, distractable, hyperverbal, but not out of control. Stage II, often called acute mania, is when the euphoria is replaced by irritability and anger. The racing thoughts of stage I lead to definite flight of ideas, or skipping rapidly from one thought to another. The grandiose or paranoid suspicions of stage I become more intense and appear as well-developed fixed false beliefs (delusions). Stage III, often called delirious mania, can be indistinguishable from acute schizophrenia (7, 8). Although differential diagnosis may be difficult in stage III mania, patients will appear more classically manic both earlier in the course and later as the episode resolves. The rate of progression of mania may be very rapid, but the sequence of stages is often consistent and predictable. Use of longitudinal sequential analysis of changing symptom patterns rather than simple cross-sectional enumeration of symptoms yields increased diagnostic clarity for mania.

Depression

Depression is characterized by a persistent dysphoric mood accompanied by a variety of physiologic symptoms (Table 36.3). A diagnosis of major depression can be made if symptoms are present nearly every day for at least 2 weeks. Most depressed patients will describe their mood as depressed, sad, hopeless or blue. Others will deny depressed mood but will describe loss of interest and caring, or an inability to experience pleasure. Sleep and appetite are typically decreased, but occasionally both may be increased. Psychomotor agitation may be manifest as pacing, wringing of hands, pulling or rubbing hair, skin, clothing and outbursts of shouting. Psychomotor retardation may be manifest as slowed speech, increased pauses in speech, slowed body movements and muteness (1).

ETIOLOGY

Although a biochemical model for affective disorders has been rather well defined, deficiencies of neurotransmitters alone does not account for the clinical syndromes of affective disorders. For example, depression depends not only upon biogenic amine changes, but also on genetic background, cognitive state of the individual, and the ability to cope with the altered mood state (9). The biochemistry of affective disorders will be discussed later only in terms of its relationship to drug effects.

TREATMENT

Mania

The value of lithium for treating affective disorders is evidenced by its rapid acceptance shortly after its introduction in the United States. This quick acceptance is even more noteworthy considering lithium's reputation as a toxic and lethal agent when used as a salt substitute in the late 1940s (10). Lithium has been described as one brake on rising medical expenses (11). A conservative estimate suggests that in ten years, from 1969 to 1979, the United States saved at least $2.88 million in medical costs and gained $1.28 billion in production as a consequence of the use of lithium to treat bipolar affective disorder.

Acute Mania

Lithium is the treatment of choice for acute mania. Compared to neuroleptic drugs, lithium is more specific in ameliorating core symptoms of mania and does so without sluggishness and sedation. Because lithium has a lag time of effect of 7 to 10 days, neuroleptic drugs may need to be given with lithium for the first 1 to 2 weeks. Chlorpromazine is useful for initial control of increased psychomotor activity, although haloperidol is probably equally effective yet lacks chlorpromazine's sedative and hypotensive effects (12, 13). Once

Table 36.3.
Clinical Features of Depression

Psychological
  Dysphoric mood (sad, despondent, discouraged)
  Excessive guilt
  Pessimism, hopelessness, self-pity
  Loss of interest in usual activities
  Social withdrawal
Physiological
  Sleep disturbances
  Anorexia, weight loss
  Loss of energy, fatigue
  Psychomotor agitation or retardation
  Decreased libido
  Menstrual irregularities
  Palpitations, constipation, headaches
  Varied non-specific bodily complaints
Thinking
  Decreased concentration and attention span
  Confusion, poor memory
  Slowed thought processes
  Persecutory, somatic, or religious delusions
  Suicidal ideation

lithium levels are within therapeutic range, the neuroleptic drug should be tapered and discontinued to assess lithium's efficacy alone. Electroconvulsive therapy (ECT) should be used cautiously in a patient receiving lithium since memory loss and confusion are increased and ECT efficacy decreased (14). Early studies of lithium efficacy for acute mania were overly optimistic, reporting 90 to 100% efficacy, but later controlled studies suggest lithium treatment results in remission or marked improvement of mania in 70 to 80% of patients after 1 to 2 weeks (12, 15). Indicators of favorable lithium response include a definite diagnosis of primary affective disorder, occurrence of less than four episodes of mania and depression in 1 year, psychotic features present in both manic and depressive episodes, the more typical euphoric-grandiose symptomatology, a family history of bipolar illness, and response of family members to lithium. Patients with retarded depression, severe anxiety and thought disorder are poor lithium responders. Each of these factors alone are not reliable indicators, but should be considered together (16, 17). Advanced age has no effect on lithium efficacy, but any evidence of chronic dementia or extrapyramidal movements disorder results in poorer response and more frequent and severe neurotoxicity (18). Another report challenges the concept that there are nonresponders and responders to lithium (19). The 20 to 30% nonresponse to lithium is felt to be episode related rather than a permanent characteristic of individual patients. Thus lithium nonresponse once does not necessarily mean the patient will be nonresponsive to lithium in the future.

PROPHYLAXIS

Lithium has been clearly established as effective in preventing future manic episodes, and to a lesser degree, useful in preventing future depressive episodes in both bipolar and unipolar patients. The overall relapse rate of all controlled studies including both manic and depressive relapses is 34% on lithium compared to 79% on placebo (20). Regardless of the indication, the decision to initiate lithium prophylaxis in an individual patient should depend upon the chances of further episodes in the near future and what would be the impact of another episode on the patient, his job and his family. Because bipolar patients cycle much more frequently than unipolar patients, lithium prophylaxis for bipolar patients is more common (21). Patients with good insight regarding their illness and a good family support system who have episodes less frequently than once every 1 to 2 years may not need prophylactic lithium. Others may need prophylaxis who experience a minimum of 2 episodes in 7 years (16).

More recently, lithium has been suggested as an effective treatment for depressive episodes for some bipolar patients. Most all studies, however, have methodological problems and more investigation is needed before lithium can seriously be considered an antidepressant. Current evidence suggests that lithium may be considered a second or third choice treatment for bipolar patients unresponsive to tricyclic antidepressants (TCAs) (22).

Lithium has also been tried in a variety of other psychiatric and nonpsychiatric conditions, but all such studies suffer from inadequate sample size or lack of adequate controls (23). The most interesting is its use in schizophrenia, which directly challenges earlier notions that lithium can worsen schizophrenia (24). It is too early to recommend use of lithium for schizophrenic patients either as an adjunct to neuroleptics or when neuroleptic drugs fail. Lithium can be used for children and adolescents (25). Lithium can successfully treat affec-tive disorder in the presence of epilepsy, mental retardation, previous encephalitis and positive EEGs. The small subgroup of children who can be expected to favorably respond to lithium are those with classic bipolar symptoms or major periodic disruptions of mood and a family history of bipolar illness.

Lithium Kinetics

Lithium carbonate is virtually totally absorbed from the gastrointestinal tract within 8 hours of oral administration with peak blood levels occurring in 2 to 4 hours. Distribution is throughout body water but tissue uptake is not uniform. Liver and CSF levels are about 50% of plasma levels, brain levels are about equal to plasma levels, and muscle, kidney, bone and thyroid levels are 2 to 4 times the plasma level. Lithium is not bound to proteins or metabolized, but excreted unchanged in the urine. Lithium is freely filtered through the glomerulus, about 80% is reabsorbed in the proximal tubule, competing with sodium (26, 27). Diuretics such as thiazides, furosemide and ethacrynic acid do not increase lithium excretion, but their naturesis can cause total body lithium to increase. Average plasma half-life is 18 to 20 hours, but can reach 36 hours in the elderly.

Several slow release lithium preparations have recently been released in the United States. The potential advantages of a slow release lithium formulation include a decreased amplitude of post absorptive plasma lithium levels, thus decreasing the fluctuations experienced during a single dose interval; decreased frequency of lithium administration per day, thus increasing patient compliance; and decreased incidence and intensity of side effects including decreased risk of renal damage. A variety of such preparations have been studied in Europe, Canada and the United States using ion exchange resins, imbedding lithium in a gel, and decreasing lithium solubility. The results have been mixed, the major problem being decreased bioavailability. Lithobid shows equal total availability with peak height and time-to-peak-height significantly different from the standard formulation (28). Steady state lithium level is slightly higher, and fluctuations in levels during a single dosage interval is one half that observed with the standard release formulation. These findings suggest this slow release formulation can be used interchangably with the standard formulations, and the twice daily dosing offers a significant advantage in terms of patient acceptance and compliance. Eskalith-CR is a recently marketed drug which differs in that it releases 150 mg immediately with 300 mg as a slow release.

BLOOD LEVELS

For acute manic episodes, a plasma level of 0.8 to 1.5 mEq/liter is recommended, and for prophylaxis, a level of 0.6 to 1.2 mEq/liter. Levels above 1.5 mEq/liter are regularly associated with some signs of toxicity, and levels above 2.0 mEq/liter result in serious toxicity. The narrow range between therapeutic and toxic levels makes plasma level determinations an important part of monitoring lithium therapy. Standardization of lithium levels requires consistency of sampling time. A 12-hour interval between the last dose and drawing the blood sample in a patient receiving the same divided daily dosage for at least 1 week will yield a standardized lithium value which is reproducible (29).

Several attempts have been made to predict the dosage needed to achieve therapeutic lithium levels. The most convenient method is one in which the individual dosage requirement can be predicted from a single blood sample drawn 24 hours after administration of 600 mg of lithium carbonate. The method has been shown to be accurate and reproducible, and also valid for a slow release formulation (29, 30).

The erythrocyte-lithium to plasma-lithium ratio has received considerble attention in the last several years. It was thought that the RBC lithium level more accurately reflected CNS lithium levels than plasma levels, and thus there should be better correlation with clinical response and toxicity. More recently, mechanisms of lithium transport in human RBCs have been identified with genetic and racial aspects of lithium transport described (31). So far the RBC lithium level or ratio does not aid in the clinical management of an individual lithium patient. There is considerable inter-subject variation in the extent of lithium accumulation by erythrocytes. The most consistent finding is that bipolar patients have a higher mean lithium ratio than unipolar patients or normals (32). One potential clinical use of ratios are in assessment of lithium compliance. The noncompliant patient who skips several days of lithium but takes it the day before the blood sample is drawn will have an apparent therapeutic plasma level, but the ratio will be low. Similarly, the patient with relatively stable plasma levels but significant swings in the ratio over repeated visits is probably not being compliant (32).

Finally, saliva lithium concentrations have been proposed as capable of providing all the information necessary to formulate rational lithium dosage regimens once the plasma: saliva ratio is determined for the patient. Because plasma:saliva ratios vary much more between individuals than within an individual, the saliva lithium determination may be a useful method to approximate plasma levels and thus adjust lithium dosage. Clinical use of saliva lithium levels is minimal even though studies have now been available for over 5 years. Some clinicians question the predictive values of saliva levels (33), while others suggest its value only in clinically stabilized patients (34).

INITIATING LITHIUM THERAPY

Before lithium is begun, a physical examination and history should focus on detection of cardiovascular, endocrine and renal disease. Laboratory tests useful as baseline values before lithium begins include serum creatinine, blood urea nitrogen, complete blood count, urinalysis, thyroid function tests, electrolytes and an ECG if the patient is over 40 or has cardiovascular disease. In acute manic episodes, a daily dose of 1500 to 2400 mg is usually necessary to achieve a blood level of 0.8 to 1.5 mEq/liter. The initial dose, however, should be small and divided to assess tolerance of side effects. A starting lithium dose of 300 mg, 4 times daily, is conservative, and can be increased by 300 mg increments every 2 or 3 days if necessary. More aggressive therapy may be necessary for inpatients whose mania is severe or whose past history suggests the need for larger doses. For these patients, 600 mg, 3 times daily, may be used initially. Dosage titration is then dependent upon side effects, plasma levels during the first week, and clinical response after the first week. Blood level determinations preferably should be done after 1 week at a given dose to reflect steady state levels, but may need to be done more quickly for inpatients who may only be in the hospital 2 or 3 weeks. Blood should be drawn 10 to 12 hours after the last dose, the most convenient time is before the first dose in the morning. Initiation of lithium between episodes for prophylaxis should be conservative. Since desired blood levels are 0.6 to 1.2 mEq/liter, an oral daily dose of 900 to 1500 mg is usually adequate. Dosage initiation and titration must be conservative since these patients will be outpatients. A starting dose for prophylaxis might be 300 mg twice daily with weekly increments of 300 mg following steady state plasma level determinations. Once the desired level is reached, monthly blood levels are sufficient.

SIDE EFFECTS AND TOXICITY

Side effects and their relationship with therapeutic lithium levels as well as those unrelated to plasma level are found in Table 36.4. Although the list is long and the symptoms dramatically worsen with lithium levels above 1.5 mEq/liter, a majority of patients on therapeutic levels experience no side effects. Gastrointestinal effects are most apparent during initiation of lithium and usually disappear

Table 36.4.
Lithium Side Effects and Toxicity

Plasma Level (mEq/L)	Effects
Therapeutic (less than 1.5)	Nausea, diarrhea Polyuria, polydipsia Muscle weakness Fine hand tremor ECG T-wave alteration
1.5–2.0	Coarse hand tremor Persistent nausea, diarrhea Slurred speech Confusion
2.0–5.0	Stupor Seizures Increased deep tendon reflexes Irregular pulse, hypotension Coma Death
Non-dose-related and chronic effects	Leukocytosis Nephrogenic diabetes insipidus Nontoxic goiter Cogwheel rigidity Weight gain Maculopapular or acneiform reactions ? renal damage

after the dose is stabilized. For the patient who continues to complain of GI effects, the daily dose should be divided further since the steeper the rise in lithium levels the more severe and frequent are the GI effects (35). Such a patient is an ideal candidate for a slow release lithium preparation. More than 50% of lithium patients will experience polyuria and polydipsia, and almost 25% will continue to experience it after 1 to 2 years of lithium treatment. Fortunately, for most patients, it is of little concern and does not interfere with continued treatment. Muscle weakness is present in about 30% of patients initially, but disappears quickly. Fine hand tremor is noticeable in over 50% of patients initially decreasing with time, but may persist (36). Again, for most patients, the tremor is of no concern and does not interfere with functioning. Most patients are unaware of the tremor until they are asked to extend their arms and fingers, or may notice it when holding a full cup of coffee.

Lithium toxicity usually develops when plasma levels exceed 1.5 mEq/liter (35). Patients should be instructed to temporarily discontinue lithium and contact their physician if any symptoms in the second or third group in Table 36.4 appear.

Lithium also causes several effects not directly related to dosage. Leukocytosis during lithium therapy is secondary to neutrophilia and is accompanied by lymphocytopenia. The white count may reach 14,000/cu mm, may persist throughout therapy, and is reversible when lithium is discontinued (35). Although a benign effect, it is useful to obtain a baseline complete blood count before lithium therapy begins.

A more serious effect is the diabetes insipidus-like syndrome. The polyuria and polydipsia seen in many patients progress in a few to include 3 or more liters of urine output per day and a urine specific gravity falling as low as 1.002 to 1.005 following a 12-hour water deprivation test. This syndrome is unresponsive to vasopressin, but usually fully reversible upon discontinuation of lithium. A few cases have been reported in which the diabetes insipidus persisted for up to 20 months after lithium was discontinued (37). Thiazides have been suggested to treat this syndrome, although lowering the lithium dosage may be of benefit without adding another drug (35, 38).

Lithium can induce a diffuse nontender goiter, and some patients may become hypothyroid. The most consistent laboratory abnormality is an elevated serum TSH level. Incidence of thyroid pathology in lithium patients ranges from 3 to 20%. A benign reversible exopthalmos has also been reported. In most cases, no treatment is needed, or if so, thyroid supplementation is sufficient and lithium need not be discontinued. Use of thyroxine 0.05 to 0.2 mg daily will correct the hypothyroidism within 3 months (35, 39).

Although of unknown etiology, cogwheel rigidity has been reported in patients receiving long-term lithium therapy, 27.8% with mild cogwheel rigidity and 7.6% with moderate cogwheel rigidity. Mild cases occur in up to 25% of patients, are typically unnoticed by the patient, and are of doubtful clinical significance. Moderate severity is found to occur in 8% of patients on long-term lithium therapy. Increasing age and presence of tremor either predispose or are associated with moderate cogwheel rigidity. Anticholinergic drug treatment is ineffective, suggesting lithium cogwheeling may not be at the extrapyramidal level (40, 41).

Cardiovascular effects of lithium are few and of concern only in patients with preexisting cardiovascular disease. In normal patients, ECG changes are confined to lowering of T-wave amplitude. Lithium may aggravate preexisting ventricular arrhythmias. Abnormalities of the sinus node consisting of bradycardia and sinoatrial block have also been described (42).

Dermatological reactions to lithium include folliculitis, acneiform eruptions, pruritic maculopapular rash, psoriasis and exfoliative dermatitis (43). The incidence of any dermatological effect is unknown since all evidence so far is case reports. Although two cases of lithium-induced psoriasis have been reported, lithium should be cautiously used in a patient with psoriasis since exacerbation is likely.

The issue of most concern regarding lithium effects is the possibility of renal damage with long-term lithium therapy (44). The most comprehensive report documents 14 cases of tubular atrophy and/or interstitial fibrosis in patients receiving lithium for 1.8 to 15 years. The lithium patients, on renal biopsy, had twice the amount of interstitial connective tissue, three times the degree of tubular atrophy, and five times the number of sclerotic glomeruli compared to age matched controls (45). A unique specific tubular lesion caused by lith-

ium has also been described (46). The lesion is found in the cortical and medullary collecting ducts and distal convoluted tubules, develops soon after lithium is started and is absent 1 year after lithium has been stopped. The site of the lesion is where the vasopressin receptors are thought to be, suggesting this lesion may be the pathological basis of the vasopressin-resistant diabetes-insipidus-like syndrome caused by lithium. A comparison of renal-biopsy material from patients taking lithium for 5.5 years, patients about to start lithium, and a group of age-matched donor kidneys used for transplantation raised some question as to lithium's role in observed renal changes. Significant histological changes were found in both the pre-lithium and lithium groups compared to the control group, but no differences were found between pre-lithium and lithium material. Thus other drugs used to treat affective disorders may be suspect as well as lithium in being nephrotoxic.

It is premature to suggest a direct causal effect of lithium. Furthermore, there has been no correlation of the findings to actual occurrence of chronic renal failure. The role and significance of risk factors, such as lithium blood levels, number of acute intoxications and duration of treatment, remain unknown. In the meantime, caution is very important. Pre-lithium baseline should include urinalysis, serum creatinine and BUN. Serum creatinine should be obtained several times a year and compared to the baseline value. Increases in serum creatinine would indicate obtaining a creatinine clearance. Concern over nephrotoxicity should result in lithium being used only when it is appropriately indicated.

TREATMENT OF DEPRESSION

Treatment options for depression include antidepressant drugs (tricyclics, monoamine oxidase inhibitors and new nontricyclic drugs), ECT and psychotherapy. Drugs and ECT are primarily indicated for major depressive disorders and depressions in bipolar patients. Drugs are often ineffective in treating dysthymic disorder. The comparative value of psychotherapy for depression has not been adequately evaluated. For ambulatory depressed patients, once weekly interpersonal psychotherapy can be equal to tricyclic antidepressant therapy, and the combination superior to each treatment alone (47). For maintenance therapy, drugs will reduce relapse rates and prevent symptom return, while psychotherapy will improve social function. These two effects should be viewed as complimentary (48).

Electroconvulsive Therapy

ECT remains the most effective treatment for major depressions. Compared to drugs, ECT is more effective (95% versus 60 to 80%), more rapidly ameliorates symptoms, and is safer in patients with cardiovascular disease. The major disadvantage is frequent relapse within several months of treatment. Many patients will require antidepressant drug maintenance after a successful series of ECT to maintain response. The past abuse and overuse of ECT has caused a very negative social stigma and even legislation restricting its use. For these reasons, ECT is primarily indicated for acutely suicidal patients needing rapid response, and for patients who are unresponsive or for whom drug therapy is contraindicated (49, 50). Drug modification of ECT by use of anesthetic and neuromuscular blocking drugs have increased patient acceptance and decreased ECT morbidity. Methohexital and succinylcholine are the respective drugs of choice (51, 52).

Monoamine Oxidase Inhibitors

Until recently, MAO inhibitors (MAOI) were viewed as less effective and more toxic than tricyclic antidepressants. They were either never used or used only after all other treatments failed. During the last several years, however, there has been renewed interest in MAOI as being very effective in selected depressions, and their dangers put in proper perspective.

Whereas TCAs are indicated for major depressions, MAOIs have been shown to be most useful in atypical depressions and some phobic disorders (53–55). Table 36.5 indicates predictors of positive response to TCAs and MAOIs (56). TCAs remain the drugs of first choice for most depressed patients, and MAOIs should be reserved for atypical depressions and phobias as well as secondary drugs for TCA drug failures (53).

Phenelzine and tranylcypromine are the two more commonly used MAOIs. Although earlier studies suggested tranylcypromine to be more effective and safe, phenelzine is now the preferred MAOI since it has been more thoroughly studied recently in terms of indi-

Table 36.5.
Predictors of Antidepressant Response

Imipramine > Placebo	Amitriptyline > Placebo
Insidious onset	Anorexia
Weight loss	Middle, late insomnia
Middle, late insomnia	Psychomotor retardation
Psychomotor retardation	Psychomotor agitation
Upper socioeconomic class	Upper socioeconomic class
Low urinary MHPG[a]	High urinary MHPG

Imipramine = Placebo	Amitriptyline = Placebo
Neurotic, hypochondriacal, hysterical traits	Neurotic, hypochondriacal, hysterical traits
Multiple prior episodes	Multiple prior episodes
Delusions	Delusions

MAO Inhibitors > Placebo

Hypochondriacal, hysterical traits
Initial insomnia or hypersomnolence
Phobic anxiety
Psychomotor agitation
Increased appetite, weight gain

[a] 3-Methoxy-4-hydroxyphenethylene glycol.

cations, efficacy, dosage and safety (53). An effective dosage for phenelzine is 1 mg/kg/day (60 to 90 mg daily). MAO inhibition reaches its peak within 2 to 4 weeks, which corresponds to clinical improvement. Sixty to eighty percent inhibition of platelet MAO correlates with clinical response (56, 57). Sixty percent of ultimate improvement occurs by the end of 14 days, and maximum improvement is attainable at the end of the 4th week. Another correlate with clinical response is that clinical improvement usually coincides with the onset of REM suppression (53). Although phenelzine is a hydrazine MAOI, acetylator status has shown no definite relationship with clinical response (55).

Side effects do not correlate well with phenelzine dosage. Common side effects are autonomic—dry mouth, orthostatic hypotension, constipation, delayed ejaculation (53, 55, 56). Of particular concern, primarily with tranylcypromine, is hypertensive crisis. The patient on MAOIs should avoid foods and drugs with indirect acting sympathomimetic amines. Tryamine is found in significant concentration in well ripened cheeses (Camembert, Edam, cheddar), yeast extract, red wines, chicken livers and beer. Similarly, pressor effects can be potentiated by drugs such as ephedrine, cocaine, amphetamines and other sympatho-mimetic amines. Common prodromal symptoms of hypertensive crisis include severe occipital headache, stiff neck, sweating, nausea and vomiting, and sharply elevated blood pressure. Although the α-blocking agent phentol-amine is a specific treatment, a more readily available drug in most psychiatric settings that can abort a hypertensive reaction is chlorpromazine.

Drug therapy compliance is a recognized problem in general, but dietary compliance is of additional concern if MAOIs are to be used. Patients often report that they occasionally cheat on their MAOI diet without ill effects. In a study of 98 tranylcypromine patients, 32% reported a high degree of compliance and 40% admitted to extensive non-adherence to dietary restrictions (58). The remaining 28% admitted accidental or occasional indiscretions. The most common items eaten were chocolate, cheeses, sour cream and various alcoholic beverages. Only 11 patients experienced hypertensive reactions, 5 serious enough for brief emergency room and drug treatment. The most common precipitants of these reactions were cheeses and liqueurs (Drambuie, Kahlua and creme de cacao).

Antidepressant Drugs

Seven tricyclic and three newer nontricyclic antidepressant drugs are currently available for use in the United States. Early studies with imipramine and amitriptyline showed that they were equal in antidepressant efficacy, that about 70% depressed patients would show favorable response to either one compared to 40% response rate to placebo. More recent evidence concerning the biochemistry of affective disorders and the different biochemical effects among these drugs suggests that drug selection must be tailored to the individual patient, and if done, a response rate of 80 to 90% is possible (59). The one exception to major depressions being highly responsive to antidepressant drugs is delusional depression. Presence of delusions negatively correlates with drug response (Table 36.5), and ECT has been suggested to be the treatment of choice (60). The concept that TCAs are ineffective in primary depressive disorders if delusions or other evidence of psychosis is present has been challenged however (61). Poor response in past studies is attributed to inadequate dosage and

duration of TCA therapy. Imipramine proved to be effective for delusional depressions when the dose reached 300 mg daily for 5 weeks. A comparison of five treatment regimens for psychotic depression found antipsychotics alone, antipsychotic-antidepressant combinations, ECT, and ECT-antipsychotic combinations to be effective, but antidepressants alone to be ineffective when paranoid delusions are present (62). There are also reports of MAOIs being effective for delusional depressions (63).

DRUG SELECTION

Once the decision is made that an antidepressant will be used, two factors should influence drug selection: past history of drug response and side effect differences. An evaluation of both factors will maximize therapeutic success and will allow tailoring of the drug to the patient.

A complete drug history is essential when selecting an antidepressant. History of positive response to a particular drug for a previous depressive episode would obviously suggest the same drug to be used for the current episode. A history of nonresponse to a drug should prompt several questions. Was the patient compliant? Was the dose at adequate levels for at least 4 weeks? Finally, the patient's attitude toward individual drugs should be assessed. A strong postitive or negative attitude toward a particular drug should weigh heavily in the selection decision since compliance will be affected. A drug history which includes these factors is much more useful than a mere list of drugs taken in the past.

The other major factor to consider in drug selection is differences in side effects. Among the many possible side effects, the incidence or degree of sedation and anticholinergic activity varies among antidepressants enough to be of clinical significance (Table 36.6). Sedation is greatest with amitriptyline and doxepin, least with protriptyline and desipramine, and moderate with imipramine and nortriptyline. Sedation is often a desirable effect since most depressed patients sleep poorly. Choice of a sedating drug dosed at bedtime also eliminates the need for a hypnotic drug. On the other hand, the patient with psychomotor retardation does not need additional sedation from the drug, so choice of a less sedating drug is most appropriate. The other side effect category of clinical importance is anticholinergic effect. Dry mouth or blurry vision are usually

Table 36.6.
Antidepressant Drug Side Effect Profile

Drug	Sedation	Anticholinergic Effect
Tricyclics		
Amitriptyline	High	High
Nortriptyline	Moderate	Moderate
Protriptyline	Low	Moderate
Imipramine	Moderate	Moderate
Trimipramine	Moderate	Moderate
Desipramine	Low	Low
Doxepin	High	Moderate
Tetracyclic		
Maprotiline	Moderate	Low
Dibenzoxazepine		
Amoxapine	Low	Low
Triazolopyridine		
Trazodone	Moderate	Very low

only bothersome effects, and can be minimized by once daily dosing of the drug. For some patients, however, anticholinergic effects represent a serious problem particularly the elderly. Preexisting benign prostatic hypertrophy, dementia, glaucoma and constipation may be aggravated. For these patients, a drug with very low anticholinergic effect should be used (Table 36.6) (64, 65).

Based on the above information, selection of an antidepressant can be precise and tailored to the individual patient. A drug history which includes specific information on past response, adverse effects, current medical problems and patient attitude can form the basis for most appropriate drug therapy decisions.

NEW ANTIDEPRESSANTS

After nearly a 10-year gap during the 1970s, several new antidepressants were introduced in the early 1980s. These drugs are being called second generation antidepressants since they are chemically and pharmacologically unique and are not merely chemical cousins of existing TCAs. Maprotiline, amoxapine and trazodone are the first three drugs to become available, and several more are close to being marketed. Also, one "chemical cousin" type drug, trimipramine, is new to the United States (66).

Maprotiline is the first tetracyclic compound. While it shares similar types of side effects, maprotiline causes fewer and less severe anticholinergic and orthostatic hypotensive effects compared to amitriptyline and imipramine. Maprotiline is moderately sedating.

Toxicity in overdose is different but no less serious than seen with the TCAs. Cardiac arrhythmias are less frequent, but seizures and delirium are more common with maprotiline in overdose (67, 68).

Amoxapine is a dibenzoxazepine and a metabolite of loxapine. Side effects are similar but less frequent and severe compared to TCAs. Extrapyramidal effects have been rarely reported, likely due to a minor metabolite which has dopamine blocking activity. Although still a controversial issue, amoxapine has the best evidence for a more rapid onset of effect. A majority of controlled studies show some items on depressive rating scales to have an earlier onset of response with amoxapine compared to standard antidepressants. It is too early to judge amoxapine's relative safety in overdose (69, 70).

Trazodone has the least anticholinergic effects of the currently available antidepressants. Too little is known at present to evaluate its relative safety in overdose (71, 72).

Trimipramine, although relatively new in the United States, has been used for many years in other countries. It possesses significant sedative orthostatic hypotensive and anticholinergic effects. Frequency and severity of these effects appears to be less than amitriptyline but more than imipramine (73).

BIOGENIC AMINES AND RECEPTOR SENSITIVITY

A prominent neurochemical effect of antidepressants is their enhancement of monoamine effect via blockade of reuptake in presynaptic neurons. From this emerged the hypothesis that depression is the result of monoamine deficiency, and antidepressant drugs are effective in treatment because they increase these monoamines. Later it was found that antidepressant drugs differ greatly in their relative effect on serotonin and norepinephrine activity (59). Amitriptyline and trazodone selectively enhance serotonin activity, while desipramine and maprotiline selectively enhance norepinephrine activity. Nortriptyline, imipramine and amoxapine enhance the activity of both neurotransmitters. Further, it was suggested that there may be two subtypes of depression representing deficiency of each neurotransmitter. Measurement of urinary 3-methoxy-4-hydroxyphenethylene glycol (MHPG), a major metabolite of brain norepinephrine, could suggest which type of drug should be selected for a patient. A low MHPG level would indicate the need for a drug specific in affecting norepinephrine, while a normal MHPG level would indicate the need for a serotonergic drug (74). Most recently, however, attention has shifted away from effect on neurotransmitters to amine receptor sensitivity (75). Discovery of new antidepressants which do not significantly inhibit uptake of either neurotransmitter as well as in explainable differences in time course of drug effect have caused this shift in focus. Of some concern is the dilemma that monoamine reuptake blockade occurs within minutes to hours after one dose of antidepressant, but onset of clinical response is seen only after several weeks. For these reasons, the slower adaptive changes in amine receptor systems induced by long-term antidepressant use must be considered as at least part of these drugs' mechanism of action. Although this hypothesis is in preliminary stages, TCAs, newer nontricyclic drugs, MAOIs and even electroshock therapy all produce consistent changes in postsynaptic receptor sensitivity. Long-term treatment reduces β-adrenergic sensitivity while responses to α-adrenergic and serotonergic stimulation are enhanced. Presynaptic autoreceptors are also included in this modification of the original monoamine hypothesis. The major mechanism regulating release of norepinephrine is the feedback inhibition, which is mediated by stimulation of a presynaptic α_2-inhibitory adrenergic receptor (76, 77). Long-term antidepressant administration decreases the sensitivity of these receptors resulting in an increased release of neurotransmitter.

Attempts have also been made to identify with a biochemical marker those depressed patients who might be most likely to respond to antidepressant drugs. The interaction of thyroid function, catecholamines and β-adrenergic receptor response has been described (78). Of most clinical relevance thus far has been the identification of dysfunction of the hypothalamic-pituitary-adrenal axis in up to 50% of depressed patients. A relatively safe and easy test is the dexamethasone suppression test (DST) (79). A 1 mg dose of dexamethasone at 11 P.M. will normally suppress plasma cortisol levels for up to 24 hours. The DST will not suppress cortisol levels in up to 50% of depressed patients, and for these patients antidepressant drugs are indicated. The DST is now commonly used to help determine if drug treatment is indicated.

PHARMACOKINETICS

All antidepressants are virtually 100% absorbed. Peak plasma levels occur within 2 to 6 hours for all drugs except protriptyline, which peaks in 6 to 12 hours (80). Volumes of distribution have been reported from 10 to 20 liters/kg (81). The tertiary amine drugs are demethylated to their corresponding secondary amines which are active metabolites. The major inactivation route for both the tertiary and secondary amines is hydroxylation, which then undergo glucuronidation and urinary excretion. The hydroxy metabolites were once thought to be inactive, but recent studies with imipramine and desipramine suggest these metabolites must be considered in evaluation of efficacy and adverse effects (82). Two aspects of metabolism influence dosage requirements for individual patients as well as among drugs. First pass metabolism varies greatly. Only 15% of protriptyline is metabolized on first pass, while nortriptyline is 46 to 59%, imipramine is 53%, amitriptyline 60%, and doxepin highest at 73%. The rate of hydroxylation can also vary greatly among individuals, resulting in variation of steady state plasma levels as high as 30-fold in individuals ingesting the same oral dose (83, 84). This individual variation was found to be far more important in determining adequate dosage than factors such as age, sex, weight and smoking history. All antidepressant drugs have elimination half-lives within a range of 12 to 30 hours except protriptyline's 74 hours. Nomifensine, a new antidepressant close to marketing, is of interest since it virtually lacks anticholinergic and cardiac effects, and is unique with an elimination half-life of only 2 hours (85).

TCA BLOOD LEVELS

Tricyclic antidepressant blood levels have finally emerged from research status to enter the clinical arena. Table 36.7 lists the current therapeutic TCA plasma levels. Nortriptyline's therapeutic plasma levels can be regarded as well-established, levels for imipramine and amitriptyline will probably not change much with further research, but the other drugs are very tentative in regard to correlation with clinical response. Routine use of TCA levels is not recommended at this time, but rather reserved for patients failing to respond to determine if their level is at the lower or upper end of the therapeutic range, patients with sus-

Table 36.7.
Therapeutic Plasma Levels for Tricyclic Antidepressants

Drug	Therapeutic Range (ng/ml)
Nortriptyline	50–150
Amitriptyline (plus nortriptyline)	125–250
Desipramine	—[a]
Imipramine (plus desipramine)	>180
Doxepin (plus desmethyldoxepin)	>110
Protriptyline	>70
Trimipramine	—
Maprotiline	200–300
Amoxapine	200–400
Trazodone	—

[a] Not established.

Table 36.8.
Effective Dosage Ranges

Drug	Dose (mg/day)
Amitriptyline	150–300
Nortriptyline	50–150
Protriptyline	30–60
Imipramine	150–300
Desipramine	150–250
Doxepin	150–300
Trimipramine	150–300
Maprotiline	150–300
Amoxapine	200–600
Trazodone	200–600
Phenelzine	60–90
Tranylcypromine	20–40
Isocarboxazid	20–60

pected toxicity, patients on maintenance therapy to determine how far the dosage might be tapered, and suspected noncompliant patients. Blood level information should still be viewed as only one aspect of a total assessment of a patient's TCA therapy (86, 87).

A most interesting finding with TCA blood level research is the concept of a therapeutic window, or curvilinear response pattern for nortriptyline. Maximum therapeutic efficacy with nortriptyline correlates with plasma levels of 50 to 150 ng/ml, and poor therapeutic response correlates with levels lower than 50 or higher than 150. The evidence of imipramine supports a linear relationship between plasma levels and clinical response (87). The remaining TCA drugs have not been adequately studied to determine whether a linear or curvilinear relationship exists. The upper limits of levels in Table 36.7 for drugs other than nortriptyline reflect levels at which side effects occur without further therapeutic gain.

INITIATION OF TREATMENT

Drug therapy should begin with a small divided dose to assess how the patient will tolerate side effects particularly sedation and orthostatic hypotension. A reasonable starting dose for a healthy adult would be 25 mg, 3 times daily for amitriptyline or imipramine. If the patient tolerates that dose well, the dose can be quickly titrated up to a dose of 150 mg daily by the end of the first week. Table 36.8 lists the generally effective dosage ranges for antidepressants (56). Geriatric patients and those with cardiovascular disease require more conservative initial dosing and titration. Once the lower end of the therapeutic dosage range is reached, further dosage increases should be done on a weekly basis. The expectable pattern of response is that the physiological symptoms of depression will show improvement within the first week to 10 days, while the psychological symptoms typically improve after 2 to 4 weeks (Table 36.3) (30). So, the patient on amitriptyline 150 mg for 1 week should show improvement in sleep, an increased appetite and energy level. There is usually no change in mood, guilt or pessimism. If physiological symptoms do not significantly improve after 1 week of 150 mg daily, the dosage should be raised to 50-mg increments per week. When the physiological symptoms improve, the dose should be maintained at that level as the psychological symptoms should respond in a week or 2. A trial of 4 weeks at doses of 250 mg per day or more constitute an adequate trial, after which an alternative drug should be considered for the nonresponsive patient. Blood levels, if available, should be obtained for nonresponders.

Patient education about their antidepressant is critical. Side effects may start the first day, but improvement in mood may take up to 3 or 4 weeks. Add to this the pessimistic nature of a depressed patient, and noncompliance within the first 2 weeks of TCA therapy becomes a seemingly reasonable option to the patient. Patients should be counseled on expectable side effects, what to do if they occur, and understand that there is a lag time in onset of effect. A useful fact in patient education during the first week is an explanation that the improved sleep and energy is a good predictor that the drug is working and a beneficial effect on mood can be expected.

MAINTENANCE THERAPY

After a depressive episode successfully responds to drug therapy, the next decision becomes how long the treatment should be maintained. Drug maintenance is divided into continuation therapy and prophylactic therapy. Remembering that the natural duration of an untreated major depressive episode is approximately 6 months, continuation therapy is defined as the time period that the underlying pathophysiology presumably continues to run its course. Prophylactic therapy is the time period when the patient would normally be between episodes of depression and the drug is used to prevent future episodes. Although it is often impossible to determine the natural untreated duration of a depressive episode for an individual patient, continuation therapy has been arbitrarily determined to be 6 months after remission of depression. The evidence is convincing that all major depression disorder patients should receive continuation therapy. Continuation therapy reduces the risk of relapse in these patients by 20 to 50%. Although this means 50 to 80% of patients will receive continuation therapy unnecessarily for 6 months, the likelihood of serious drug side effects during 6 months is very small compared to the damaging effects of a depressive recurrence shortly after recovery (88).

The value of antidepressant prophylaxis is much less clear. Adding imipramine to lithium in bipolar patients does not decrease depressive episodes and increases the risk of mania (89). In major depressive disorder, imipramine is equal to lithium in prophylactic effect, although lithium is often not effective in preventing depressive episodes (88, 90, 91). In spite of conflicting evidence, many clinicians continue to use antidepressants prophylactically. A reasonable guide to such use is that prophylaxis be used only in patients with an established history of frequent relapse, and for patients who have infrequent severe depressions with dangerous suicide attempts (88). For bipolar patients, lithium is the preferred prophylactic drug since it can also prevent future manic episodes while TCAs cannot (90).

Another factor in antidepressant maintenance therapy is the recognition that acute depressive episodes can be superimposed on chronic depressive disorders. Less than total response to antidepressant therapy, or continuing depressive symptoms after the drug is discontinued, does not necessarily indicate resumption of drug treatment. Up to 25% of patients with a major depressive disorder may have an underlying chronic depressive disorder (92). Response to drug treatment must be defined as either response to the acute episode or of both disorders.

A final factor contributing to the question of prophylaxis is the recent finding that antidepressants can induce more rapid cycling between mania and depression in bipolar patients (93, 94). The question is raised whether "antidepressant" is a misnomer, and actually these drugs act to accelerate the natural evolution of affective disorders, thus acting synergistically with the cyclic manic-depressive process in all of its phases (93). Clearly this evidence speaks against the use of TCA maintenance therapy for bipolar patients, and lithium alone may be the preferred drug.

SWITCH PROCESS

Approximately 10% of depressed patients who receive a tricyclic or MAOI will experience a switch to hypomania or mania (95). The switch is usually dramatic—a patient may switch from a nonverbal, psychomotor retarded depression to a hyperactive psychotic manic state within one hour. The switch typically occurs during the first week of antidepressant therapy. Bipolar patients are more vulnerable to switches to mania. Major depression disorder patients are less vulnerable and are more likely to experience hypomania rather than mania. Hypomania can be of 1 or 2 days duration, while a switch to mania often lasts a number of weeks. One implication of this phenomenon is that bipolar patients on lithium who become depressed should have their lithium continued while the antidepressant drug is added.

SIDE EFFECTS AND TOXICITY

Side effects of concern include sedation, anticholinergic effects and cardiovascular effects. Sedation is rarely a problem since it can be adjusted by drug selection and once daily bedtime dosing. Anticholinergic effects differ significantly among the antidepressants (Table 36.6). Constipation is usually easily treated. Because anticholinergic-induced constipation results from slowed gut motility and results in hard dry stools, optimal treatment is a stool softener or a bulk laxative when diet is inadequate. Stimulant laxatives should be avoided except for occasional use. Prompt treatment of constipation is necessary since it may lead to impaction, paralytic ileus and even death. Dry mouth and blurred near vision cannot be treated except by lowering the dose or switching the dose to bedtime. These effects should be a definite part of patient education since some dry mouth or blurred vision may have to be tolerated to gain the therapeutic benefit of the drug.

Abrupt withdrawal of antidepressants can cause a variety of symptoms which are primarily associated with cholinergic rebound. Typically seen are symptoms such as nausea, vomiting, diarrhea, abdominal cramps, malaise, headaches, dizziness, sleep disturbance, restlessness and anxiety (96, 97). Two cases with imipramine occurred after only one dose was missed with symptoms consisting of nausea and dizziness. Withdrawal reactions can easily be misinterpreted by patients or therapists as depressive relapse. Thus all patients treated with antidepressants who complain of increased sleep disturbance and anxiety should be questioned regarding compliance, and patients should be advised of the possibility of withdrawal symptoms with abrupt noncompliance.

Cardiovascular effects of antidepressants are by far the most common serious effect (42, 98). While cardiotoxicity is an obvious concern with overdose, cardiovascular effects at therapeutic doses are more subtle. Orthostatic hypotension is the most common serious effect of these drugs. So far, the safest drug is nortriptyline which very rarely causes orthostatic hypotension (98). The newer antidepressants may also offer this advantage but more data is needed to validate such a claim. The symptoms of orthostatic hypotension, e.g. dizziness upon arising, typically improve with time, but the hypotension itself does not. All patients begun on an antidepressant should be warned of the possibility of orthostatic hypotension, and instructed how to rise slowly to prevent dizziness and syncope.

Antidepressants at therapeutic plasma levels frequently prolong the P-R interval and QRS complex, which reflect action in both the ventricular specialized conducting system and ventricular muscle. The only patients in danger of A-V or H-V block are those with preexisting bundle-branch block. Antidepressants may also aggravate sinus node dysfunction, even though they show a preferential effect on bundle of His-ventricular conduction over atrial-bundle of His conduction. This is in contrast to lithium which shows a preferential effect on the sinus node (98). Interestingly, imipramine has an antiarrhythmic effect markedly suppressing spontaneous atrial and ventricular premature contractions. The similarity of effect of quinidine and procainamide suggests the two drugs should be used very cautiously together, and the dose of antiarrhythmic drug may need to be decreased in the presence of an antidepressant (98).

Antidepressant toxicity in overdose is manifest as CNS effects (toxic psychosis; seizures; coma with respiratory depression), cardiovascular effects (sinus and supraventricular tachycardias; impaired conduction leading to A-V block, intraventricular block, ventricular arrhythmias or fibrillation and asystole; and depressed myocardial contractility), and peripheral anticholinergic effects (urinary retention, decreased bowel sounds and paralytic ileus). Treatment consists of first preventing absorption and interfering with enterohepatic recirculation by gastric lavage and activated charcoal. Physostigmine is not an "antidepressant antidote," and should be reversed for treating supraventricular tachycardias causing significant problems. Fluids require careful monitoring since too vigorous hydration may result in pulmonary edema. Intensive cardiac monitoring can be discontinued when the plasma level falls below 500 ng/ml or when the ECG has been normal for more than 2 days (99). An ingestion of a 1-week supply of a TCA can cause a serious intoxication. Generally, 1.5 g of amitriptyline or its equivalent is considered a serious toxicity. This suggests more care be taken in evaluating the amount of drug given patients in one prescription, and patients with children should be particularly cautioned regarding this danger.

References

1. American Psychiatric Association: *Diagnostic and Statistical Manual*, ed 3. Washington, D.C.: American Psychiatric Association, 1980, pp 205–224.
2. Hirschfeld RMA, Cross CK: Epidemiology of affective disorders. *Arch Gen Psychiatry* 29:35–46, 1982.
3. Goodwin FK: Diagnosis of affective disorders, in Jarvik ME: *Psychopharmacology in the Practice of Medicine*. New York: Appleton-Century-Crofts, 1977, pp 219–228.
4. Akiskal HS, Djenderejian AH, Rosenthal RH, et al: Cyclothymic thymic disorder: validating cri-

teria for inclusion in the bipolar affective group. *Am J Psychiatry* 134:1227–1233, 1977.

5. Loranger AW, Levine PM: Age at onset of bipolar affective illness. *Arch Gen Psychiatry* 35:1345–1348, 1978.

6. Carlson GA, Goodwin FK: The stages of mania. *Arch Gen Psychiatry* 28:221–228, 1973.

7. Bond, TC: Recognition of acute delirious mania. *Arch Gen Psychiatry* 37:553–554, 1980.

8. Garvey MJ, Tuason VB: Mania misdiagnosed as schizophrenia. *J Clin Psychiatry* 41:75–78, 1980.

9. Akiskal HS, McKinney WT Jr: Overview of recent research in depression. *Arch Gen Psychiatry* 32:285–305, 1975.

10. Talbott JH: Use of lithium salts as a substitute for sodium chloride. *Arch Intern Med* 85:1–10, 1950.

11. Reifman A, Wyatt RJ: Lithium: a brake in the rising cost of mental illness. *Arch Gen Psychiatry* 37:385–388, 1980.

12. Goodwin FK, Zis AP: Lithium in the treatment of mania. *Arch Gen Psychiatry* 36:840–844, 1979.

13. Shopsin B, Gershon S, Thompson H, et al: Psychoactive drugs in mania, a controlled comparison of lithium, chlorpromazine, and haloperidol. *Arch Gen Psychiatry* 32:34–42, 1975.

14. Small JG, Kellams JJ, Milstein V, et al: Complications with electroconvulsive treatment combined with lithium. *Biol Psychiatry* 15:103–112, 1980.

15. Goodwin FK, Murphy DL, Bunney WE Jr: Lithium carbonate treatment in depression and mania: a longitudinal double-blind study. *Arch Gen Psychiatry* 21:486–496, 1969.

16. Ananth J, Pecknold JC: Prediction of lithium response in affective disorders. *J Clin Psychiatry* 39:95–100, 1978.

17. Ananth J, Engelsmann F, Kiriakos R, et al: Prediction of lithium response. *Acta Psychiatr Scand* 60:279–286, 1979.

18. Himmelhoch JM, Neil JF, May SJ, et al: Age, dementia, dyskinesias, and lithium response. *Am J Psychiatry* 137:941–945, 1980.

19. Carroll BJ: Prediction of treatment outcome with lithium. *Arch Gen Psychiatry* 36:870–878, 1979.

20. Klerman GL: Long term treatment of affective disorders, in Lipton MA, DiMascio A, Killam KF: *Psychopharmacology: A Generation of Progress.* New York: Raven Press, 1978, pp 1303–1311.

21. Zis AP, Goodwin FK: Major affective disorder as a recurrent illness. *Arch Gen Psychiatry* 36:835–839, 1979.

22. Donnelly EF, Goodwin FK, Walkman IN, et al: Prediction of antidepressant responses to lithium. *Am J Psychiatry* 135:856–859, 1978.

23. Schou M: Lithium in the treatment of other psychiatric and non-psychiatric disorders. *Arch Gen Psychiatry* 36:856–859, 1979.

24. Miller FT, Libman H: Lithium carbonate in the treatment of schizophrenia and schizo-affective disorder: review and hypothesis. *Biol Psychiatry* 14:705–710, 1979.

25. Youngerman J, Canino IA: Lithium carbonate use in children and adolescents. *Arch Gen Psychiatry* 35:216–224, 1978.

26. Schou M: Lithium in psychiatric therapy and prophylaxis. *J. Psychiatr Res* 6:67–95, 1968.

27. Amdisen A: Serum level monitoring and clinical pharmacokinetics of lithium. *Clin Pharmacokinet* 2:73–92, 1977.

28. Cooper TB, Simpson GM, Lee JH, et al: Evaluation of a slow release lithium carbonate formulation. *Am J Psychiatry* 135:917–922, 1978.

29. Grof P: Some practical aspects of lithium treatment. *Arch Gen Psychiatry* 36:891–893, 1979.

30. Cooper TB, Simpson GM: The 24 hour lithium level as a prognosticator of dosage requirements: a two year follow-up study. *Am J Psychiatry* 133:440–443, 1976.

31. Pandey GN, Dorus E, David JM, et al: Lithium transport in human red blood cells: genetic and clinical aspects. *Arch Gen Psychiatry* 36:902–908, 1979.

32. Frazer A, Mendels J, Brunswick D, et al: Erythrocyte concentrations of the lithium ion: clinical correlates and mechanisms of action. *Am J Psychiatry* 135:1065–1069, 1978.

33. Vlaar, H, Bleeker JAC, Schalken HFA: Comparison between saliva and serum lithium concentrations in patients treated with lithium carbonate. *Acta Psychiatr Scand* 60:423–426, 1979.

34. Rosman AW, Sczupak CA, Pakes GE: Correlation between saliva and serum lithium levels in manic-depressive patients. *Am J Hosp Pharm* 37:514–518, 1980.

35. Reisberg B, Gershon S: Side effects associated with lithium therapy. *Arch Gen Psychiatry* 36:879–887, 1979.

36. Schou M, Baastrup PC, Gros P, et al: Pharmacological and clinical problems of lithium prophylaxis. *Br J Psychiatry* 116:615–619, 1970.

37. Simon NM, Garber E, Arieff AJ: Persistent nephrogenic diabetes insipidus after lithium carbonate. *Ann Intern Med* 86:446–447, 1977.

38. Singer I, Forrest JN: Drug induced states of nephrogenic diabetes insipidus. *Kidney Int* 10:82–95, 1976.

39. Lindstedt G, Nilsson LA, Walinder J, et al: On the prevalence, diagnosis and management of lithium induced hypothyroidism in psychiatric patients. *Br J Psychiatry* 130:452–458, 1977.

40. Asnis GM, Asnis D, Dunner DL, et al: Cogwheel rigidity during chronic lithium therapy. *Am J Psychiatry* 136:1225–1226, 1979.

41. Tyrer P, Alexander MS, Regan A, et al: An extrapyramidal syndrome after lithium therapy. *Br J Psychiatry* 136:191–194, 1980.

42. Stimmel B: *Cardiovascular Effects of Mood Altering Drugs.* New York: Raven Press, 1979, pp 133–166.

43. Deandrea DM, Walker NR, Mehlmauer M, et al: Dermatological reactions to lithium: a critical review of the literature. *J Clin Psychopharmacol* 2:199–204, 1982.

44. Ramsey TA, Cox M: Lithium and the kidney: a review. *Am J Psychiatry* 139:443–449, 1982.

45. Hestbech J, Hansen HE, Andisen A, et al: Chronic renal lesions following long term treatment with lithium. *Kidney Int* 12:205–213, 1977.

46. Kincaid-Smith P, Burrows GD, Davies BM, et al: Renal biopsy findings in lithium and prelithium patients. *Lancet* 2:700–701, 1979.

47. Weissman MM, Prusoff BA, DiMascio A, et al: The efficacy of drugs and psychotherapy in the

treatment of acute depressive episodes. *Am J Psychiatry* 136:555–558, 1979.

48. DiMascio A, Weissman MM, Prusoff BA, et al: Differential symptom reduction by drugs and psychotherapy in acute depression. *Arch Gen Psychiatry* 36:1450–1456, 1979.

49. Greensblatt M: Efficacy of ECT in affective and schizophrenic illness. *Am J Psychiatry* 134:1001–1005, 1977.

50. Fink M: Myths of shock therapy. *Am J Psychiatry* 134:991–996, 1977.

51. Allen RE, Pitts FN, Summers WK: Drug modification of ECT: methohexital and diazepam. *Biol Psychiatry* 15:257–264, 1980.

52. Marco LA, Randels PM: Succinylcholine drug interactions during electroconvulsive therapy. *Biol Psychiatry* 14:433–445, 1979.

53. Robinson DS, Nies A, Ravaris L, et al: Clinical pharmacology of phenlzine. *Arch Gen Psychiatry* 34:629–635, 1978.

54. Davison JRT, Miller RD, Turnbull CD, et al: Atypical depression. *Arch Gen Psychiatry* 39:527–534, 1982.

55. Tyrer P, Gardner M, Lambourn J, et al: Clinical and pharmacokinetic factors affecting response to phenelzine. *Br J Psychiatry* 136:359–365, 1980.

56. Gelenberg AJ: Prescribing antidepressants. *Drug Ther* 9:95–112, 1979.

57. Stern SL, Rush AJ, Mendels J: Toward a rational pharmacotherapy of depression. *Am J Psychiatry* 137:545–552, 1980.

58. Neil JF, Licata SM, May SJ, et al: Dietary non-compliance during treatment with tranylcypromine. *J Clin Psychiatry* 40:33–37, 1979.

59. Maas JW: Biogenic amines and depression. *Arch Gen Psychiatry* 32:1357–1361, 1975.

60. Glassman A, Kantor S, Shostak M: Depression, delusions and drug response. *Am J Psychiatry* 132:716–719, 1975.

61. Quitkin F, Rifkin A, Klein DF: Imipramine response in deluded depressive patients. *Am J Psychiatry* 135:806–811, 1978.

62. Minter RE, Mandel MR: A prospective study of the treatment of psychotic depression. *Am J Psychiatry* 136:1470–1472, 1979.

63. Lieb J, Collins C: Treatment of delusional depression with tranylcypromine. *J Nerv Ment Dis* 166:805–808, 1978.

64. Snyder SH, Yamamura HI: Antidepressants and the muscarinic acetylcholine receptor. *Arch Gen Psychiatry* 34:236–239, 1977.

65. Shein K, Smith SE: Structure-activity relationships for the anticholinoreceptor action of tricyclic antidepressants. *Br J Pharmacol* 62:567–571, 1978.

66. Stimmel GL: Antidepressants old and new. *Clin Pharm* 1:462–463, 1982.

67. Stimmel GL: Maprotiline. *Drug Intell Clin Pharm* 14:585–590, 1980.

68. Pinder RM, Brogden RN, Speight TM, et al: Maprotiline: a review of its pharmacological properties and therapeutic efficacy in mental depressive states. *Drugs* 13:321–352, 1977.

69. Lydiard RB, Gelenberg AJ: Amoxapine—an antidepressant with some neuroleptic properties? *Pharmacotherapy* 1:163–78, 1981.

70. Stimmel GL: Amoxapine commentary. *Pharmacotherapy* 1:177–8, 1981.

71. Rawls WN: Trazodone. *Drug Intell Clin Pharm* 16:7–13, 1982.

72. Bryant SG, Ereshefsky L: Trazodone: review and evaluation of its antidepressant properties. *Clin Pharm* 1: 1982 (in press).

73. Settle EC, Ayd FJ: Trimipramine: twenty year's worldwide clinical experience. *J Clin Psychiatry* 41:266–274, 1980.

74. Cobbin DM, Requin-Blow B, Williams LR, et al: Urinary MHPG levels and TCA drug selection. *Arch Gen Psychiatry* 36:1111–1115, 1979.

75. Charney DS, Menkes DB, Heninger GR: Receptor sensitivity and the mechanism of action of antidepressant treatment. *Arch Gen Psychiatry* 38:1160–1180, 1981.

76. Garcia-Sevilla JA, Zis AP, Hollingsworth PJ, et al: Platelet α_2-adrenergic receptors in major depressive disorder. *Arch Gen Psychiatry* 38:1327–1333, 1981.

77. Charney DS, Heninger GR, Sternberg DE, et al: Presynaptic adrenergic receptor sensitivity in depression. *Arch Gen Psychiatry* 38:1334–1340, 1981.

78. Targum SD, Sullivan AC, Byrnes SM: Neuroendocrine interrelationships in major depressive disorders. *Am J Psychiatry* 139:282–286, 1982.

79. Kalin NH, Risch SC, Janowsky DS, et al: Use of the dexamethasone suppression test in clinical psychiatry. *J Clin Psychopharmacol* 1:64–69, 1981.

80. Ziegler VE, Biggs JT, Wylie LT, et al: Protriptyline kinetics. *Clin Pharmacol Ther* 23:580–584, 1978.

81. Gram LF: Plasma level monitoring of tricyclic antidepressant therapy. *Clin Pharmacokinet* 2:237–241, 1977.

82. Potler WZ, Calil HM, Stutfin TA, et al: Active metabolites of imipramine and desipramine in man. *Clin Pharmacol Ther* 31:393–401, 1982.

83. Taska RJ: Clinical laboratory aids in the treatment of depression. *Curr Concepts Psychiatry* 2:12–20, 1977.

84. Ziegler VE, Biggs JT, Rosen SH, et al: Imipramine and desipramine plasma levels: relationship to dosage schedule and sampling time. *J Clin Psychiatry* 39:660–663, 1978.

85. Fields ED: Nomifensine evaluation. *Drug Intell Clin Pharm* 16:547–552, 1982.

86. Hollister LE: Plasma concentrations of tricyclic antidepressants in clinical practice. *J Clin Psychiatry* 43:66–69, 1982.

87. Risch SC, Huey LY, Janowsky DS: Plasma levels of tricyclic antidepressants and clinical efficiency: review of the literature, Parts I and II. *J Clin Psychiatry* 40:4–16 and 58–69, 1979.

88. Quitkin FM, Rifkin A, Klein DF: Prophylaxis of affective disorders: current status of knowledge. *Arch Gen Psychiatry* 33:337–341, 1976.

89. Quitkin FM, Kane J, Rifkin A, et al: Prophylactic lithium carbonate with and without imipramine for bipolar I patients. *Arch Gen Psychiatry* 38:902–907, 1981.

90. Prien RF, Klett CJ, Caffey EM Jr: Lithium carbonate and imipramine in prevention of affective episodes. *Arch Gen Psychiatry* 29:420–425, 1973.

91. Peselow ED, Dunner DL, Fieve RR, et al: Lithium prophylaxis of depression in unipolar II, and

cyclothymic patients. *Am J Psychiatry* 139:747–752, 1982.

92. Keller MB, Shapiro RW: Double depression: superimposition of acute depressive episodes on chronic depressive disorders. *Am J Psychiatry* 139:438–442, 1982.

93. Wehr TA, Goodwin FK: Rapid cycling in manic-depressives induced by tricyclic antidepressants. *Arch Gen Psychiatry* 36:555–559, 1979.

94. Pickar D, Murphy DL, Cohen RM, et al: Selective and nonselective monoamine oxidase inhibitors. *Arch Gen Psychiatry* 39:535–540, 1982.

95. Bunney WE Jr: Psychopharmacology of the switch process in affective illness, in Lipton MA, DiMascia A, Killam KF: *Psychopharmacology: A Generation of Progress.* New York: Raven Press, 1978, pp 1249–1259.

96. Santos AB, McCurdy L: Delirium after abrupt withdrawal from doxepin: case report. *Am J Psychiatry* 137:239–240, 1980.

97. Stern SL, Mendels J: Withdrawal symptoms during the course of imipramine therapy. *J Clin Psychiatry* 41:66–67, 1980.

98. Glassman AH, Bigger TJ Jr: Cardiovascular effects of therapeutic doses of tricyclic antidepressants. *Arch Gen Psychiatry* 38:815–820, 1981.

99. Preskorn SH, Irwin HA: Toxicity of tricyclic antidepressants—kinetics, mechanism, intervention: a review. *J Clin Psychiatry* 43:151–156, 1982.

CHAPTER 37

Schizophrenia

GLEN L. STIMMEL, Pharm.D.

Schizophrenia is no longer the concern of only state mental hospitals, since the emphasis on community treatment engages virtually all health professionals in a variety of practice settings. Residential care facilities, or board and care homes, are becoming an important part of many community pharmacy services. Community hospitals are also providing more care to schizophrenic patients, requiring the hospital pharmacist to update and maintain knowledge of psychiatric disorders and their treatment. The knowledgeable pharmacist in either setting can significantly influence appropriate and rational drug treatment of psychiatric disorders.

Before describing what schizophrenia is, it is necessary to describe what it is not. Schizophrenia is not a split personality. Portrayal of schizophrenia as a Dr. Jekyll-Mr. Hyde syndrome or as multiple personalities is inaccurate. Multiple personalities do exist, although rarely, and they more appropriately fit under personality disorders rather than psychotic disorders. Schizophrenia also is not directly associated with mental retardation. Although television and movie productions tend to portray schizophrenic patients as intellectually impaired, schizophrenia is not a cause or result of mental retardation. Schizophrenic patients may at times be floridly psychotic and bizarre, yet between psychotic episodes they may be in total control of their behavior, feelings and thoughts.

PREVALENCE

The prevalence of schizophrenia admitted to psychiatric hospitals is generally quoted as 24 to 40%, but use of modern diagnostic criteria has revealed admission prevalence of schizophrenia of 7%. In the same study, 26% were manic, 9% were depressed, 45% were diagnosed as organic brain syndromes, alcoholism, drug abuse, personality disorder, neurosis, stress reaction, or no illness, with the remaining 13% undiagnosed (1). This study and others challenge the commonly accepted belief that the morbidity risk for schizophrenia in the general population is 1 to 2%, but may be as low as 0.4 to 0.6% (1). The importance of this challenge is that schizophrenia may be too liberally used as a diagnostic label when in fact patients have other disorders such as affective disorder. Such an error results in a patient not receiving specific treatment with lithium and the patient is subjected to serious adverse affects from unnecessary chronic neuroleptic therapy.

ETIOLOGY

There is no clear etiologic explanation for the schizophrenias. A schizophrenic illness represents a complex interaction of biologic and social factors. There seems to be a definite genetic basis for schizophrenia, but of equal importance are the family and social experiences and stresses during the many phases of development. Although the mechanism by which neuroleptic drugs exert their antipsychotic effect is beginning to be understood, suggestions regarding a biochemical basis for schizophrenia are still indirect and tentative (2).

DIAGNOSIS AND CLINICAL FINDINGS

The essential features of schizophrenic disorders are the presence of certain psychotic features during the active phase of the illness, characteristic symptoms involving multiple psychological processes, deterioration from a previous level of functioning, onset before age 45, and a duration of at least 6 months (3). Schizophrenia is most easily understood as a thought disorder. Disturbances characteristically involve content and form of thought, perception, affect, sense of self, volition, relationship to the external world, and psychomotor behavior. The major disturbance in content of thought involves delusions (fixed false belief). Delusions may involve the belief that others are spying on, spreading false rumors about, or planning harm, that one's thoughts are being broadcast aloud or have been inserted or withdrawn by some external force, or that one's impulses, thoughts, or actions are controlled. Less commonly delusions involve somatic, grandiose, or religious concerns. Form of thought disturbances are manifest as "loose associations" in which the patient may shift from one thought to another without any awareness that the topics are unrelated. Thinking and speech may be tangential, circumstantial, or in the most severe cases, derailment of thought processes may be observed. Perception disturbance primarily involves hallucinations, in which there is a sensory awareness without a sensory stimulus. The most common hallucination in schizophrenic disorders is auditory (hearing voices) which are perceived usually as coming from outside the head. Disturbances of affect involves blunting, flattening, or inappropriateness of the expression of mood. The frequency of common schizophrenic symptoms is listed in Table 37.1 (4). No single feature is invariably present or seen only in schizophrenia.

TYPES

The lack of diagnostic precision for schizophrenic disorders that characterized the 1960s and 1970s has been addressed with the introduction of the American Psychiatric Association's new diagnostic criteria (DSM-III) (3). Five types of schizophrenic disorders are recognized—disorganized, catatonic, paranoid, undifferentiated, and residual (Table 37.2). In addition to these five types of schizophrenic disorders, there are two similar disorders which are now classified separately.

Table 37.1.
Frequency of Schizophrenic Symptoms

Symptom	Frequency (%)
Lack of insight	97
Auditory hallucinations	74
Ideas of reference	67
Suspiciousness	66
Flatness of affect	66
Voices speaking to patient	65
Delusions	64
Thoughts spoken aloud	50

Schizophreniform Disorder

Schizophreniform disorder shares identical features with schizophrenic disorders except that the duration is less than 6 months but more than 2 weeks. It is classified separately because there is a greater tendency toward acute onset and resolution, recovery to premorbid levels of functioning is more likely, and there is no increased incidence among family members as there is with schizophrenic disorders. A majority of acute schizophrenic episode diagnoses of the past will now be called schizophreniform disorder.

Schizoaffective Disorder

There continues to be no consensus regarding the definition of schizoaffective disorder. Distinguishing mania from schizophrenia can be very difficult. Many patients present with symptoms common to both diagnoses. Schizoaffective disorder is too convenient as a diagnosis, and unfortunately is too often used in place of an adequate diagnostic assessment. This diagnostic category was retained in DSM-III without diagnostic criteria but is defined such that it should become an uncommon diagnosis. The need for such a category is

Table 37.2.
Types of Schizophrenic Disorders

Disorganized
  Frequent incoherence
  Absence of systematized delusions
  Blunted, inappropriate or silly affect
Catatonic
  Dominated by any of the following: stupor,
    rigidity, negativism, excitement, posturing
Paranoid
  Dominated by one or more of the following:
    persecutory delusions, grandiose delusions,
    delusional jealousy, hallucinations with persecutory or grandiose content
Undifferentiated
  Prominent delusions, hallucinations, incoherence or grossly disorganized behavior but
    does not meet the criteria for any of the
    previously listed types or meets the criteria
    for more than one
Residual
  Subchronic (duration < 2 years)
  Chronic (duration > 2 years)
  Subchronic with acute exacerbation
  Chronic with acute exacerbation
  In remission

uncertain, and if needed, its relationship to schizophrenia and affective disorders must be determined. Previously diagnosed schizoaffective disorder patients would likely now be diagnosed as schizophreniform disorder, major depression or bipolar disorder, or schizophrenia with a superimposed atypical affective disorder.

TREATMENT

Drugs, psychotherapy, and psychosocial treatments should play supplemental roles rather than competing roles for schizophrenic disorders. Neuroleptic drugs are effective in relieving psychotic symptoms and preventing their return. Reality-based supportive psychotherapy, occupational rehabilitation and social skills training are most effective in facilitating day-to-day coping (5).

Drug of Choice

Once a decision is made to treat a patient with a neuroleptic drug, a particular drug must be selected. An examination of factors important in the drug selection process provides a useful way to present the clinically significant differences among neuroleptic drugs. There are 16 neuroleptic drugs available for use in the United States, although only about 6 or 8 are commonly used (Table 37.3). Among a

Table 37.3.
Available Neuroleptic Drugs

Phenothiazines
  Aliphatics
    Chlorpromazine (Thorazine)
    Triflupromazine (Vesprin)
  Piperidines
    Thioridazine (Mellaril)
    Mesoridazine (Serentil)
    Piperacetazine (Quide)
  Piperazines
    Trifluoperazine (Stelazine)
    Fluphenazine (Prolixin; Permitil)
    Perphenazine (Trilafon)
    Butaperazine (Repoise)
    Acetophenazine (Tindal)
    Prochlorperazine (Compazine)
Thioxanthenes
  Thiothixene (Navane)
  Chlorprothixene (Taractan)
Butyrophenones
  Haloperidol (Haldol)
Dibenzoxazepines
  Loxapine (Loxitane; Daxolin)
Dihydroindolones
  Molindone (Moban; Lidone)

group of available drugs, the selected drug should ideally be the most effective, have the least side effects for the particular patient, and the patient should have had a positive response to it when given in the past. For compliance reasons, the patient should also have a positive or at least a neutral attitude toward the drug selected. For neuroleptic drugs, each of the above factors are important for selection except the first one. There is no evidence suggesting any one neuroleptic drug has a greater antipsychotic efficacy than another (6), and it is also not possible to select a more efficacious drug for certain symptoms or subtypes of schizophrenia (7). This does not suggest, however, that all patients will respond equally to all neuroleptic drugs. It is not possible to predict which neuroleptic drug to use for a patient based upon efficacy studies and psychotic symptoms or diagnosis, but individual patients often show better response to a particular neuroleptic drug. The explanation for this finding most likely is that efficacy differences among neuroleptics are so small that they cannot be detected in a series of patients and studies. Of the many attempts to correlate a particular neuroleptic with specific symptoms, the best evidence, although still a minority opinion, is that paranoid patients may show better response to loxapine (8). Otherwise, efficacy differences do not seem to be of value in drug selection.

A major difference among neuroleptic drugs of great clinical significance is comparison of side effect incidence and severity. The incidence of four side effects differ enough among neuroleptic drugs to play a major role in drug selection (Table 37.4). Unfortunately, choice of any drug means dealing with some side effects. The large differences in the incidence of side effects makes it possible to tailor the drug to the individual patients. Sedation may be a

Table 37.4.
Neuroleptic Side Effect Profiles[a]

Drug	Sedation	Extrapyramidal	Anticholinergic	Hypotension
Haloperidol	1	4	1	1
Fluphenazine	1	4	2	1
Thiothixene	2	3	2	1
Trifluoperazine	2	3	2	2
Loxapine	2	3	2	2
Molindone	2	3	2	2
Chlorpromazine	4	2	3	4
Thioridazine	4	1	4	4

[a] 1 = low, 4 = high.

desirable side effect in a patient with agitation or insomnia. A past history of problems with extrapyramidal symptoms (EPS) or noncompliance due to EPS might suggest use of thioridazine. For the patient with glaucoma, prostatic hypertrophy, or chronic constipation, a drug low in anticholinergic effects is most desirable. For the patient already taking another drug with orthostatic hypotensive effects, or elderly patients in whom hypotension can decrease cerebral perfusion causing increased organic symptoms, a drug low in hypotensive effects would be most desirable. One drug selection issue of some interest is whether thioridazine or haloperidol is preferred for patients with a psychosis associated with organic brain syndrome. Thioridazine is frequently chosen for this patient population, but haloperidol has more recently been suggested to be advantageous since it is much less likely to cause cardiovascular changes, sedation and anticholinergic effects. These potential advantages are not supported by comparative studies, however. The cardiovascular effects of thioridazine are generally of no consequence for most geriatric patients, sedation may be a desirable effect, and the anticholinergic effect advantage quickly disappears when benztropine must be added to halperidol for extrapyramidal effects. Comparative studies of these two drugs for patients with organic brain syndrome and psychosis yield a conclusion that either drug may be used safely and effectively (9, 10). As can be seen, information from the drug history, medical history and current symptoms can suggest the most appropriate drug choice for a particular patient. For the physically healthy patient, the choice usually is between sedation and extrapyramidal effects. Differences in anticholinergic activity usually disappear since the haloperidol patient often requires an anticholinergic agent for treatment of EPS. Table 37.4 is also useful in patient counseling since it identifies the expectable side effects for a particular drug.

In addition to differences in side effects, a patient's past history of response and present attitude toward neuroleptics must be considered in drug selection. Questions during the drug history such as "Which drug helped you the most in the past?" and "What side effects have you had the most difficulty with?" can help identify which neuroleptic should be chosen for the current episode. Most schizophrenic patients have been treated with several or many different neuroleptic drugs in the past, and often have definite opinions about individual neuroleptics. If a negative attitude is elicited about a particular drug, it makes no sense to choose that drug since drug compliance will likely be poor. Some chronic patients have very negative attitudes about many neuroleptic drugs, and will refuse to take them if prescribed. In this case, drug selection becomes a matter of finding a neuroleptic untried by the patient. Other patients are firmly committed to one drug, refusing to try anything else in spite of other considerations such as side effects. These two types of patients make a strong case for a very liberal formulary of neuroleptic drugs. Based on efficacy studies alone, there is need for only one neuroleptic. Based on side effect profile, maybe three neuroleptics could be justified. But based upon patient attitude and resultant compliance, virtually all neuroleptic drugs should be included in drug formularies. It has been shown that a patient's subjective response to a neuroleptic can be used as a predictor of symptomatic outcome (11). Response to questions such as "How does the medication agree with you?" "Did it make you feel calmer?" "Did it affect your thinking?" and "Do you think this would be the right medicine for you?" were rated based on euphoric or dysphoric responses after a test dose of chlorpromazine. Patients with an early euphoric response improved more than patients with an early dysphoric response during the subsequent hospital stay. The early dysphoric response seemed to persist, since 88% of the dysphoric responders eventually refused to continue taking chlorpromazine because of persisting dysphoria against only 23% of the early euphoric responders. Therefore, in addition to seeking a patient's past history of drug response and attitude, it seems worthwhile to assess a patient's early subjective response to a neuroleptic drug.

Treatment of Acute Psychosis

Once a particular drug has been chosen for a patient, the lower end of the daily dosage range is given in a divided schedule initially (Table 37.5), for example chlorpromazine 100 mg q.i.d. or thiothixene 5 mg q.i.d. A divided schedule initially allows evaluation of tolerance of adverse effects with low doses. The dosage can then be titrated upward by 25 or 33% increments of the initial dose on a weekly basis. No change in target symptoms over 1 week suggests an increased dose is necessary,

Table 37.5
Oral Dosage and Potency

Neuroleptic	Acute Dosage (mg/day)	Potency[a]
Chlorpromazine	400–1000	100
Thioridazine	400–800	100
Loxapine	40–120	10
Molindone	40–120	10
Trifluorperazine	20–60	5
Thiothixene	20–60	5
Fluphenazine	10–40	2
Haloperidol	10–40	2

[a] Chlorpromazine, 100 mg, has equal antipsychotic activity to haloperidol, 2 mg.

while partial reduction of some psychotic symptoms after 1 week suggests no increase in dosage is necessary. Full therapeutic effect from a given dose is seen at 6 to 8 weeks, but at least slight efficacy should be seen within one week to justify maintaining the current dosage. This titration schedule must be slowed in geriatric patients or patients experiencing adverse effects, and can be accelerated in patients whose psychotic symptoms and psychotic agitation is severe. If no response is seen at the top end of the dosage range, the diagnosis should be reevaluated, drug compliance should be questioned, and an alternative neuroleptic drug considered. If partial response is seen at the top end of the dosage range, the dose should be increased further. Some acute patients will require very high doses for response, such as haloperidol 100 mg daily. These patients, however, should constitute a minority rather than majority of patients in a treatment facility. The best candidate for high dose therapy is the patient whose psychosis is acute, past history of episodes brief, and physical examination and medical history unremarkable.

RAPID TRANQUILIZATION

Occasionally, an acutely psychotic patient will require rapid control of symptoms for the protection of self or others. A technique of rapid intramuscular neuroleptic drug treatment has been described as useful for these patients (12). While an appealing concept, the indications are few. Rapid tranquilization is most effective for quick control of psychotic agitation, bizarre acting-out of psychotic ideation and insomnia. It is not more rapid than conventional oral dosage titration previously discussed for the core psychotic symptoms,

such as loose associations, thought broadcasting or insertion, delusions and hallucinations. Rapid tranquilization should be considered only on inpatient wards with nursing staff adequately trained and available to recognize and treat adverse effects. Acute dystonic reactions are most common, and laryngospasm can be life-threatening.

Fluphenazine, thiothixene and haloperidol are the most commonly used drugs for rapid tranquilization, primarily because of their virtual lack of sedative and cardiovascular effects. Other advantages in using one of these drugs includes their availability in concentrated form, allowing large doses to be given intramuscularly without significant muscle trauma, coupled with their low incidence of local irritation on injection.

Various methods for rapid tranquilization have been described, but a basic technique has been proposed as a safe, effective, and quick method to manage acutely decompensated psychotic patients (12). Using fluphenazine hydrochloride as an example, a 5-mg intramuscular dose is given every hour until the symptoms abate, the patient sleeps, or significant adverse effects develop. Usually 20 to 60 mg will be needed during the first 24 hours, although some patients may respond after only 5 to 10 mg. Most patients can be switched to an oral dosage form on the 2nd day, using the conversion of 1:1 or 1:1.5 parenteral to oral. Dystonic reactions are common, but usually respond extremely well to diphenhydramine, 50 mg IM or IV, or to benztropine mesylate, 2 mg IM or IV, and do not modify the rapid tranquilization procedure.

DOSAGE SCHEDULE

Once an effective dosage is found, the drug can be shifted to a once daily bedtime schedule. Once daily dosing is equally efficacious, enhances compliance, reduces anticholinergic side effects, reduces cost, often eliminates the need for a hypnotic drug, and does not cause significant behavioral disruptions compared to divided dosing schedules. The few disadvantages include patients who require or desire daytime sedative effect, and patients who experience frightening dreams (pavor nocturnus) (13).

Maintenance Therapy

Until recently, it was generally assumed that a schizophrenic patient should remain on neuroleptic drugs indefinitely to prevent psychotic exacerbations. Many patients have been told they need neuroleptics like diabetic patients need insulin. A common clinical practice was to give neuroleptic drugs for 1 year after the first psychotic episode, for 2 years after the second episode, and indefinitely for 3 or more episodes. Placebo controlled drug withdrawal studies as well as longitudinal studies have clearly demonstrated neuroleptic drugs can reduce the incidence of relapse compared to placebo. Analysis of comparable studies shows that maintenance neuroleptic therapy in 2153 patients resulted in a relapse rate of 30%, while in 1077 placebo patients the relapse rate was 65% over several years. Drug-placebo differences in relapse rate range from 12 to 59% with a median value of 40% (14). Thus neuroleptic drug maintenance is essential for 40% of schizophrenic patients for survival in the community. This number potentially could be higher if all patients on maintenance therapy were receiving optimal drug therapy. Even allowing a significant increase for theoretical optimal drug maintenance, there remain a large percentage of chronic schizophrenic patients who can do well without neuroleptic drug maintenance.

Because it is impossible to predict which patients do and do not need maintenance neuroleptic drugs, every chronic schizophrenic outpatient maintained on neuroleptic medication should have the benefit of an adequate trial without drugs. If a patient's drug history reveals that drug withdrawal or dosage reduction in the past was followed by clinical relapse, it can be assumed that a new attempt at withdrawal is likely to fail. Without such a history, every chronic outpatient should be gradually withdrawn from their neuroleptic.

No criteria exist for selecting the time for drug withdrawal, but criteria developed and used by this author require drug and dosage stabilization for at least 6 months, absence of psychotic symptoms for at least 6 months, lack of prior history of relapse with drug withdrawal, reliability of the patient to keep appointments once drugs are discontinued, and willingness of the patient to be without medication. Patients withdrawn from neuroleptic drugs should be closely monitored for at least one year since clinical relapse may occur at any time during the first 12 months.

DEPOT FLUPHENAZINE

One specific aspect of maintenance neuroleptic therapy is the use of either fluphenazine enanthate or fluphenazine decanoate. The unique advantage of these preparations is that a patient can be given an injection every 1 to 4 weeks rather than ingesting daily capsules or tablets. These long-acting drugs are given intramuscularly for patients who respond well to neuroleptics but consistently refuse to take neuroleptics as outpatients. Although several studies suggest the depot fluphenazine be used for acute psychosis, use of a depot drug with variable onset and duration cannot be justified. The flexibility of dosage titration from oral or IM hydrochloride preparations is not available with the depot form.

Although both fluphenazine enanthate and fluphenazine decanoate are available for use, only the decanoate form should be used. Fluphenazine decanoate has a significantly longer duration of effect, causes a slightly lower incidence of extrapyramidal effects, yet is equally effective compared to the enanthate (15, 16).

The contribution of depot fluphenazine to maintenance neuroleptic therapy is substantial considering the magnitude of noncompliance with drug therapy. There are several danger areas, however, that should be monitored for and prevented. The convenience and success of depot fluphenazine can result in some sloppiness of drug prescribing. Routine doses and schedules can lead to lack of individualization of dosage, dosage titration and adjustment. Continuous monitoring is needed to ensure that the convenience of staff remains secondary to actual patient needs. A final caution is that use of depot fluphenazine for outpatients contradicts the basic philosophy of community treatment, which is to allow patients to assume as much responsibility as possible for their own care. A clinic with 15 to 25% of neuroleptic treated patients being given depot fluphenazine is probably appropriate, but when the number reaches 50% or more, the number of valid indications for its use should be questioned.

The techniques of conversion from an oral neuroleptic used to treat the acute episode to fluphenazine decanoate are many, though most are based upon clinical experience rather than validated by clinical trial. If it is known early that the patient will be converted to the depot form, oral fluphenazine should be used for treatment of the acute phase of psychosis. If a patient happens to be on another neuroleptic, it is preferable but not mandatory to convert to oral fluphenazine before instituting the fluphenazine decanoate. The average dose of fluphenazine decanoate is 25 to 75 mg every 1 to 2 weeks, which can be lengthened to 25 mg every 3 to 4 weeks for chronic maintenance.

Two techniques of conversion from oral to depot fluphenazine are compared in Table 37.6. The first method is to use 25 mg of fluphenazine decanoate every 2 weeks for up to 20 mg of oral fluphenazine. For each 5 mg above 20 mg, add 12.5 mg of decanoate to the biweekly schedule (12). This formula is useful for low and moderate neuroleptic doses, but quickly over estimates decanoate dosage when oral dose is high. A practical useful conversion this author developed is based upon literature information plus extensive clinical experience with fluphenazine decanoate. It is well established that the dose of oral fluphenazine used to treat an acute psychotic episode ranges from 10 to 40 mg daily with some patients requiring 60 mg or more. The usual dose of fluphenazine decanoate is 12.5 to 75 mg every 1 to 2 weeks (6, 15). To maintain this relationship, a simple conversion is to take the daily oral fluphenazine dose or its equivalent (Table 37.6), increase it to the nearest 0.5 ml amount of decanoate (25 mg/ml), and give that amount every 1 to 2 weeks depending on the acuteness and severity of the psychotic episode. Once pharmacokinetic parameters are better defined for fluphenazine and the decanoate, dosage conversion can become much more precise.

Because of the delayed onset of effect with fluphenazine decanoate, conversion from oral to depot is not simply a matter of stopping one and starting the other. A reasonable conversion would be to give the depot injection, taper the oral neuroleptic over 1 to 2 weeks and discontinue the oral when the second depot injection is given. The depot may need to be given weekly for the first two or three injections, then lengthened to every 2 weeks. Some chronic maintenance patients do well with

Table 37.6.
Conversion Formulas for Fluphenazine Decanoate (FD)

Mason and Granacher (12):	25 mg FD for first 20 mg PO, plus 12.5 mg FD for each additional 5 mg PO
Stimmel:	Increase daily PO fluphenazine dose to nearest 0.5 ml amount of FD (e.g. 20 mg PO converts to 25 mg FD; 50 mg PO to 62.5 mg FD)

fluphenazine decanoate given once every 3 to 4 weeks (15).

Pharmacokinetics

The pharmacokinetics of neuroleptic drugs make them very difficult to analyze since low dosage and ease of tissue distribution yields low blood levels. Analysis is made more difficult when the metabolites of varying pharmacodynamic profiles and different kinetic behaviors are considered. Chlorpromazine, being the first available neuroleptic drug, has undergone two decades of clinical use and studies, and as yet no correlation has been shown between blood levels and clinical response. Biotransformations of chlorpromazine result in more than 100 metabolites and involve very complex metabolic pathways. There is some suggestion that pharmacogenetic differences may help explain clinical findings of why the effective dosage range of chlorpromazine is so large or why some patients are responders and others are nonresponders. Higher levels of the active 7-hydroxy metabolites have been correlated with good clinical response, while patients with higher levels of the inactive sulfoxide metabolite showed poor response. Such differences in relative percentage of active versus inactive metabolites has been suggested as an explanation for the wide therapeutic dosage range for chlorpromazine. Another finding of clinical interest is that calculations of overall accumulation of chlorpromazine and metabolites in various animal and human autopsy tissues make it probable that no more than a total of 1 to 2 days' chronic chlorpromazine doses are stored in body tissues (17).

Piperazine phenothiazines yield higher blood concentrations than chlorpromazine, and may be the best candidates for demonstration of clinical correlation. Piperazine phenothiazines are well absorbed in the gastrointestinal tract, with peak blood levels occurring between 2 and 4 hours.

Plasma Levels

Neuroleptic plasma levels are not yet useful for clinical management of patients. Chlorpromazine has been studied most, and a level of 30 to 300 ng/ml has been associated with improvement of psychotic symptoms. Toxicity, in the form of tremors and convulsions have been reported with levels above 750 ng/ml, and psychotic exacerbation presumably caused by chlorpromazine can be improved when levels are reduced from the 700 ng/ml range down to 300 ng/ml. Although tempting, such data must be regarded as preliminary and tentative since it is based upon small, heterogeneous sample sizes, and interpretation of data in studies is inadequate or biased (18).

One of the few more carefully controlled studies with thiothixene suggested that a correlation of plasma level to clinical response exists. Plasma levels of 10 to 22.5 ng/ml were necessary for therapeutic effects of thiothixene in 15 patients. Daily oral doses necessary to achieve the desired plasma level ranged from 15 to 60 mg (19). One study of haloperidol in acute schizophrenics showed therapeutic response with a plasma level of 10 ng/ml (20). A study of fluphenazine decanoate found fluphenazine serum levels to be substantially lower than levels observed by oral administration (21). Explanation of its efficacy in spite of very low serum levels is either due to the transient rise in levels seen within the first 3 days after injection, or that chronic patients need only these very low levels for maintenance.

Adverse Effects

Neuroleptic drugs can affect many systems in the body (Table 37.7). Discussion will focus primarily upon their relative clinical significance, differential incidence among neuroleptic drugs and management.

Extrapyramidal Effects. Extrapyramidal symptoms (EPS) are the most significant neuroleptic side effects in terms of frequency and reason for noncompliance with drug therapy.

Table 37.7.
Neuroleptic Adverse Effects

Extrapyramidal	*Cardiovascular*
Pseudoparkin-	Orthostatic hypo-
sonism	tension
Dystonic reactions	ECG changes
Akathisia	*Endocrine*
Tardive dyskinesia	Amenorrhea
Autonomic	Galactorrhea
Dry mouth	Gynecomastia
Constipation, ileus	Weight change
Blurred near vision	*Pigmentation*
Urinary retention	Corneal, lenticular
Delayed ejaculation	Retinopathy
Central	Skin
Sedation	*Allergic*
Toxic psychosis	Skin
Seizures	Hepatic
	Hematologic

EPS are divided into three major groups—pseudoparkinsonism, dystonic reactions and akathisia. A fourth, tardive dyskinesia, is technically an extrapyramidal effect, although its cause, mechanism and treatment are actually opposite that of the first three. Table 37.8 describes these effects (22, 23). Pseudoparkinsonism manifests itself in a similar way as does Parkinson's disease. Early signs or more mild forms consist of a reduction of facial movements and arm movements. Akinesia, characterized by lessening of spotaneity, paucity of gestures, diminished conversation and apathy can be easily confused with depression, demoralization and residual schizophrenic symptoms. Onset of pseudoparkinsonism

Table 37.8.
Extrapyramidal Side Effects

Pseudoparkinson
Akinesia:
    Rigidity and immobility
    Stiffness and slowness of voluntary movement
    Masklike facial expression, drooling (sialorrhea)
    Stooped posture
    Shuffling, festinating gait
    Slow, monotonous speech
Tremor:
    Regular rhythmic oscillations of extremities, especially hands and fingers; pill-rolling movement of fingers
Dystonic Reactions
Oculogyric crisis: Fixed upward gaze
Torticollis: Neck twisting
Opisthotonus: Arching of back
Trismus: Clenched jaw
Others: Spasm of muscles resulting in facial grimaces, exaggerated posturing of head or jaw, and difficulty in speech and swallowing.
Akathisia
Inability to sit still, constant pacing
Continuous agitation and restless movements
Rocking or shifting of weight while standing
Shifting of legs, tapping of feet while sitting
Tardive Dyskinesia
Mouth: Rhythmical involuntary movements of tongue, lips or jaw; protrusion of tongue, puckering of mouth, chewing movements (bucco-linguo-masticatory triad)
Choreiform: Irregular purposeless involuntary quick movements of the extremities; flailing movements
Athetoid: Continuous arrhythmic worm-like slow movements of the extremities
Axial hyperkinesis: To and fro clonic movement of spine

symptoms is usually at least several weeks after the neuroleptic drug is begun, and sometimes may be delayed as much as 3 months. Dystonic reactions are characterized as an acute tonic contraction of a muscle group. About 90% of all dystonic reactions occur within the first 72 hours of neuroleptic therapy, and can occur after only one dose. While pseudoparkinsonism tends to be more common in older females, dystonic reactions occur more often in younger males. Dystonic reactions can be an extremely terrifying experience and can affect future drug compliance. Fortunately, most reactions are brief and easily treated. The only potentially life-threatening dystonia is laryngospasm which may interfere with respiration. Whereas chlorpromazine and thioridazine are more likely to cause pseudoparkinsonism if they produce an EPS, the piperazine phenothiazines, thiothixene, loxapine, molindone and haloperidol are more likely to cause dystonic reactions and akathisia. Akathisia is the most common and troublesome of all EPS. It is often difficult to differentiate from psychotic agitation and is least likely of all EPS to respond to treatment. Akathisia misdiagnosed as psychotic agitation may result in the neuroleptic drug dosage being increased, resulting in a worsening of akathisia. Akathisia has no preference for an age group, and has its typical onset several weeks after neuroleptic drug therapy is begun. Akathisia is also noteworthy in that it is the primary cause for neuroleptic drug noncompliance (22–24). The difference in incidence of EPS among neuroleptic drugs is presented in Table 37.4. The approximate incidence of a neuroleptic causing any type of EPS is 10 to 15% for thioridazine, 20 to 25% for chlorpromazine, and up to 40 to 50% for piperazine phenothiazines and haloperidol. Fluphenazine enanthate causes a greater incidence of EPS than fluphenazine decanoate, especially akathisia. One study reported on EPS incidence with fluphenazine enanthate of 69% and fluphenazine decanoate of 57%. Significant akathisia developed in 26% of enanthate patients and in only 4% of decanoate patients (25). The incidence of EPS with the depot fluphenazines is usually considered to be greater than with oral fluphenazine, but a more recent study showed the incidence to be the same (26). This 7-week study showed oral fluphenazine to fluphenazine decanoate akathisia to be 25 to 27%, and pseudoparkinsonism to be 32 to 35% at the end of week 7.

Neuroleptic-induced EPS result from neuroleptic postsynaptic blockade of dopaminergic receptors in the corpus striatum. Normal motor function depends upon a balance of dopaminergic and cholinergic activity in the striatum. Neuroleptic dopaminergic blockade produces a relative striatal dopaminergic deficiency, resulting in the clinical signs and symptoms of pseudoparkinsonism. This imbalance is mechanistically the same as seen in Parkinson's disease, where dopamine neurons degenerate and die, also producing a relative dopaminergic deficiency in the striatum (27).

In contrast to the simplified striatal dopaminergic-cholinergic balance model, it has also been suggested that neuroleptics differ in their ability to cause EPS due to differences in their effect on dopaminergic receptors (28). Two different dopamine receptors may exist which are not strictly localized in distinct anatomical regions. Neuroleptic drugs with a high incidence of EPS (e.g. haloperidol) seem to affect one type of receptor while neuroleptic drugs like thioridazine with a low incidence of EPS affect the other type of dopaminergic receptor. This pharmacologic distinction could have important implications for screening new neuroleptic drugs.

Even though EPS are common, can interfere with compliance, and can be severe, they are generally very easily treated with centrally active anticholinergic agents. Acute dystonic reactions are most responsive to treatment, typically responding to one parenteral injection of either benztropine or diphenhydramine. Pseudoparkinson symptoms show a variable response to antiparkinson drugs, but typically show moderate improvement at least. The muscle rigidity usually is more responsive than akinesia. Akathisia is the least responsive EPS of the three (22). The available antiparkinson drugs and usual doses are in Table 37.9. Measurement of anticholinergic drug levels has verified efficacy of these drugs by showing an inverse relationship between serum levels and severity of acute extrapyramidal effects from neuroleptic drugs (29). As expected, a few patients receiving normal therapeutic doses of benztropine experienced either nonresponse or anticholinergic toxicity. The nonresponders were found to have very low serum levels, and an increase in dose up to 12 mg daily was necessary to achieve response and therapeutic levels. The patient experiencing toxicity was found to have an extremely high serum level, which was resolved with dosage reduction while maintaining control of EPS. A serum level near 0.7 pmol of atropine equivalents will yield therapeutic efficacy. The two more commonly used drugs are trihexyphenidyl and benztropine. They are equal in antiparkinson efficacy and side effects, but three differences should be noted. Both are available as 2-mg tablets, but benztropine is twice as potent as trihexyphenidyl. Although it is too frequently done, these two drugs are not interchangable on a milligram-for-milligram basis. This potency difference has resulted in the incorrect clinical impression that benztropine causes more side effects. The other two differences between these drugs form the basis for benztropine to be recommended as the drug of choice for treating EPS. First, the duration of effect of benztropine is longer, allowing once daily dosing for most patients, and twice daily dosing at most. Trihexyphenidyl, as well as procyclidine and biperiden, have shorter half-lives and must be dosed 3 to 4 times daily for best efficacy. In addition to once daily dosing increasing compliance and decreasing costs, it makes no sense to use trihexyphenidyl on a 3 times daily basis when the neuroleptic drug is being used once daily. Trihexyphenidyl is sometimes given once daily, but the need for the drug should be questioned if the patient is having no EPS. The second advantage of benztropine is that it does not have the abuse problem and street value that trihexyphenidyl has among patients. Procyclidine and biperiden are less commonly prescribed drugs, but can be viewed as virtually identical to trihexyphenidyl. Diphenhydramine is a less effective oral antiparkinson drug alone, and is best used as an adjunct to benztropine or trihexyphenidyl for EPS particularly akathisia. As a treatment for acute dystonic reactions, parenteral diphenhydramine is equal in efficacy to parenteral benztropine.

Amantadine, a dopaminergic agonist, is an approved drug for treating neuroleptic-induced EPS. It should still be viewed as a second choice drug, or as a good alternative when a patient cannot tolerate the peripheral anticholinergic effects of drugs like benztropine. Rather than decreasing cholinergic activity to restore balance in the striatum, amantadine works by increasing dopaminergic activity to help restore the striatal cholinergic-dopaminergic balance. A dose of 200 mg daily of amantadine equals the efficacy of 8 mg daily of trihexyphenidyl (30, 31). It is still unclear why amantadine may be useful while levo-

Table 37.9.
Drugs for Neuroleptic-induced Extrapyramidal Side Effects

Drug (Trade Name)	Daily PO Dose (mg)	Daily Dosing Frequency	IM/IV Dose (mg)
Benztropine (Cogentin)	2–6	1–2	2
Trihexyphenidyl (Artane, Tremin)	4–15	3–4	—
Procyclidine (Kemadrin)	5–15	3–4	—
Biperidin (Akineton)	4–12	3–4	—
Diphenhydramine (Benadryl)	100–300	3–4	25–50
Amantadine (Symmetrel)	200–400	2	—

dopa is not effective in treating neuroleptic-induced EPS. Levodopa is believed to be ineffective since its effect is blocked by the postsynaptic receptor blockade of the neuroleptic. Another concern with levodopa is that it may exacerbate the psychosis, but this concern has not been raised with amantadine except indirectly (22, 32).

In addition to the use of antiparkinson agents, other considerations are necessary in the management of EPS. Before an additional drug is added, a slight reduction of neuroleptic dose or change in scheduling to bedtime dosing may eliminate the EPS. When treating akathisia, there may only be partial response to maximal doses of antiparkinson drugs which are accompanied by their own anticholinergic side effects. A better solution often is to switch from fluphenazine or haloperidol to thioridazine, which is very unlikely to cause akathisia (Table 37.4).

A final consideration in the use of antiparkinson drugs is their prophylactic use when neuroleptic drugs are begun. Most authors agree that use of antiparkinson agents beyond 3 months should be justified by a drug withdrawal and demonstration of reemergence of EPS. The real decision, then, is if the first 3 months of low dose antiparkinson drug therapy is justifiable even though it may be unnecessary. The majority of patients begun of neuroleptics should not receive prophylaxis. Certainly patients given very low doses or given thioridazine or chlorpromazine do not need prophylaxis since the likelihood of EPS is low. Antiparkinson prophylaxis is justified however when factors are present such as history of noncompliance due to EPS, or paranoid young patients given moderate to high doses of neuroleptics with a high EPS incidence. For these patients, benztropine 2 mg daily for 2 to 3 months will be of benefit yet will contribute very little additional anticholinergic side effects.

A remaining controversy is whether anticholinergic drugs antagonize the therapeutic effect of neuroleptic drugs. It has been found that, when anticholinergic drugs are added to a neuroleptic drug regimen, therapeutic effect is diminished (33). One explanation of this finding is that anticholinergic drugs lower neuroleptic blood levels, which has been shown in several studies (34, 35). The first placebo controlled study with a crossover design and adequate sample size, however, refutes the idea that anticholinergic drugs decrease plasma levels of neuroleptics (36). What now remains to be explained is how anticholinergic drugs can antagonize the therapeutic effect of neuroleptic drugs.

Tardive Dyskinesia. Tardive dyskinesia is a late appearing effect which looks like an EPS but in most aspects is exactly opposite in terms of etiology and responsiveness to treatment. The typical clinical features of tardive dyskinesia are the bucco-linguo-masticatory triad (Table 37.8). These mouth movements are usually mild, and many patients are unaware of the movements until someone brings it to their attention. Tardive dyskinesia often appears as if patients are chewing gum or have ill fitting dentures. The more severe cases may include choreoathetoid movements of the extremities. Although unusual, severe axial dystonia, respiratory dyskinesias and intense facial grimacing can produce marked discomfort as well as social and physical disability (37, 38). The jerky choreiform movements are often made to look like purposeful movements, such that a patient with choreiform movements will be constantly readjusting clothing or glasses, or smoothing hair or scratching their head. Observation of fingers and toes at rest may reveal constant involuntary dyskinetic movement. In elderly subjects, dyskinesias can spontaneously develop. A comparison of spontaneous dyskinesias to neuroleptic-induced dyskinesias conducted in a French retirement home found 18% of patients who never received neuroleptics had dyskinesias, while 42% of those who received neuroleptics had dyskinesias, establishing the primary etiologic role of neuroleptic drugs (39). Before tardive dys-

kinesia was well recognized, clinicians would attempt to deal with it as another type of EPS. Several major differences were noted, however, in that tardive dyskinesia: (a) often appears upon neuroleptic dose reduction or withdrawal, (b) improves when neuroleptic dosage is increased, (c) worsens when anticholinergic drugs are given, and (d) may persist for months or years after neuroleptic drugs are discontinued. Because most patients have been on several different neuroleptic drugs, it is not yet possible to distinguish relative incidence among individual neuroleptic drugs. Major differences in reported incidence are probably due to nonstandardized rating scales and varied patient populations. One estimate suggests that 3 to 6% of patients in a mixed psychiatric population receiving neuroleptics will exhibit some aspect of tardive dyskinesia (23). A review of 44 epidemiologic studies concludes the prevalence of tardine dyskinesia to be 24 to 56% in chronic neuroleptic users (40). Tardive dyskinesia is not restricted to schizophrenic patients since it has been seen in medical patients receiving prochlorperazine for chronic gastritis and anxiety (41). Duration of neuroleptic therapy seems to be the most important variable in the development of tardive dyskinesia. Neuroleptic dose and the particular neuroleptic drug used are not significant risk factors (42). The most consistent suggestion, however, has been that drugs with a stronger dopamine-receptor blocking effect (haloperidol) are more likely to induce tardive dyskinesia than neuroleptics with a weaker dopamine-receptor blocking effect (thioridazine). Long-term administration of anticholinergic drugs with neuroleptic drugs has been identified as a significant increased risk factor (43, 44). Tardive dyskinesia may be irreversible. A syndrome resembling tardive dyskinesia is withdrawal dyskinesia (45). Withdrawal dyskinesias appear within 6 weeks, and usually within 1 week of neuroleptic drug withdrawal, are self-limited and slowly decrease and disappear over 1 to 12 weeks. Withdrawal dyskinesia is thought to be due to a temporary hyperdopaminergic state in the basal ganglia following the discontinuation of the dopamine blocking neuroleptic drug. Withdrawal dyskinesias may represent the mild end of a continuum with irreversible tardive dyskinesia at the other end. Emergence of tardive dyskinesia after neuroleptic withdrawal is differentiated from withdrawal dyskinesia by the persistence of symptoms beyond 6 to 12 weeks. Covert dyskinesia has been introduced as a third category, which refers to tardive dyskinesia which remains masked by neuroleptic drugs and is manifest clinically only when neuroleptics are withdrawn.

The pathophysiology of tardive dyskinesia can be deduced from the clinical observations of changes induced by various drugs. Improvement with increasing neuroleptics and worsening associated with use of antiparkinson drugs or decreased neuroleptic dosage suggests a relative striatal hyperdopaminergic activity. The best accepted suggestion is that dopaminergic receptors subjected to prolonged blockade become hypersensitive. Thus, while the other EPS are caused by a relative striatal dopaminergic activity deficiency, tardive dyskinesia is caused by a relative striatal dopaminergic hyperactivity. Tardive dyskinesia remains reversible if only hypersensitivity develops, but may become irreversible if dopamine receptors undergo permanent structural change and/or an increased number of dopamine receptors develop (46, 47). This model has been supported by studies of the influence of various cholinergic and dopaminergic agonists and antagonists on tardive dyskinesia. If striatal dopaminergic receptors can become hypersensitive, then mesolimbic dopaminergic receptors should be able to become hypersensitive. Since blocking dopaminergic activity in the mesolimbic area with neuroleptic drugs results in diminished psychotic symptoms, mesolimbic dopaminergic receptor hypersensitivity should result in increased psychotic symptoms. Such a supersensitivity psychosis has been described, although it is rarely seen even in patients with tardive dyskinesia (48, 49).

Treatment of tardive dyskinesia has followed two logical courses based upon the proposed pathophysiology. Since there is dopaminergic predominance in the striatum, either decreasing dopaminergic activity or increasing cholinergic activity will restore balance and eliminate symptoms. More recently, GABA agonists have been shown to be useful in the treatment of tardive dyskinesia (50, 51). Studies of the effect of a variety of drugs have helped define the pathophysiology of tardive dyskinesia, but their value in the long-term management of tardive dyskinesia is uncertain. The first step in management is to discontinue any anticholinergic drug and neuroleptic drug, if possible, or if needed for psychosis taper the neuroleptic dosage down to the least amount possible (52). Because the dyskinesia is not sufficiently bothersome for most patients, attempts to treat it with other drugs, cannot be justified. Only when the dyskinesia seriously interferes with functioning, causes significant social difficulties or threatens relationships with a spouse should drug treatment be tried. If neuroleptic therapy is required in the presence of tardive dyskinesia, thioridazine is the preferred drug choice (47).

Because treatment of tardive dyskinesia is still disappointing, attention to preventive measures becomes most important. The first step in prevention is to restrict neuroleptic use to treatment of psychoses, and avoid long-term use for anxiety states, personality disorders, insomnia, gastrointestinal disorders or mania. Each of these conditions can usually be equally or more effectively treated by other drug classes or non-drug treatment. Patients who receive maintenance neuroleptics should be assessed for presence of early signs of tardive dyskinesia-vermicular tongue movements, facial tics such as frequent eye blinking, and choreoathetoid finger or toe movements. Early detection is crucial since reversibility seems to decrease the longer neuroleptic drugs are continued. In addition to regular evaluation of patients for early signs of dyskinesia, drug holidays can detect covert dyskinesia. There is an unknown number of patients on neuroleptic therapy who have developed dopaminergic receptor hypersensitivity, but clinical evidence is masked by the neuroleptic drug. To detect covert dyskinesia, a drug holiday of 4 to 6 weeks will uncover these receptors and allow assessment of any hypersensitivity that has developed (45, 47). A period of 3 drug-free months has been suggested as sufficient to judge the reversibility of dyskinesia (53).

Anticholinergic Effects. Peripheral anticholinergic effects may commonly accompany thioridazine and chlorpromazine therapy (Table 37.4). Additionally, patients on the other neuroleptic drugs often require anticholinergic agents for EPS so they too are bothered by dry mouth, blurred near vision or constipation. These effects are directly dose-related and are additive. Usually these symptoms are bothersome but not significant unless there is preexisting prostatic hypertrophy, glaucoma or constipation. These effects can usually be minimized by switching to bedtime dosing or by decreasing neuroleptic or antiparkinson drug dosage. The dry mouth and blurred vision are worse during initiation of therapy and some tolerance usually develops. There is no treatment of proven value except alteration of drug or dosage. Constipation is the more serious peripheral effect. The reduction in gut motility and secretions typically results in constipation characterized by hard dry stools. Response is best achieved with use of a stool softener such as dioctyl sodium sulfosuxinate (DOSS) 100 to 500 mg daily accompanied by increased fluid intake. DOSS need not be given continuously but on an interrupted basis for 4 to 7 days at a time. Patients often require some education regarding normal physiology and role of exercise and diet. Constipation is one side effect which should be specifically inquired about during a medication assessment since many patients attempt self-treatment and the consequences of untreated chronic constipation can be severe (54). Reported cases of megacolon, ileus and even death all were preceded by a period of chronic constipation left untreated.

Temperature Regulation. Neuroleptic drugs may also interfere with normal temperature regulation. The most common effect is neuroleptic-induced relative poikilothermia, in which the environmental temperature can produce either hypothermia or hyperthermia. Hyperthermia is more frequently reported in patients receiving phenothiazines in hot humid weather. Hyperthermia results from an inhibition of the hypothalamic temperature control area, an increase in peripheral vasodilation and diminished heat loss due to decreased sweating. Patients on high doses of chlorpromazine and thioridazine should be warned to avoid sustained outdoor activity in hot humid weather.

Sexual Dysfunction. The most frequently reported side effect relating to sexual function is disorders of ejaculation. The major problem is an absence of ejaculation on masturbation or sexual intercourse, with a few patients reporting suprapubic pain on orgasm. In addition to the effect on α-adrenergic receptors in the pelvic plexus to interfere with the ejaculatory mechanism, neuroleptics with high anticholinergic effect can also relax the internal sphincter muscle of the bladder resulting in "retrograde ejaculation" by means of reflux of semen into the bladder. Patients may complain of white urine. Patients should be reassured that these effects are reversible upon discontinuation of the drug, or can be eliminated by switching to a neuroleptic with lower anticholinergic activity. A complaint of impotence or ejaculation disorder should not be routinely assumed to be drug-induced since sexual dysfunction due to the psychotic disorder is common.

Cardiovascular Effects. Orthostatic hypotension is the most frequent cardiovascular effect of neuroleptic drugs. It is more common with the aliphatic and piperidine phenothiazines and unusual with the other neuroleptic drugs except when given intramuscularly (55). This effect is most prominent during the first hours or days of treatment, and most patients develop a compensatory tolerance during the first week (6). The consequences of a fall due to this effect can be serious, and prevention through patient education is simple. Patients begun on an aliphatic or piperidine phenothiazine, or when dosage is increased, should be warned to rise slowly from a sitting or reclining position. Elderly patients and those on other drugs with hypotensive effects should be particularly cautioned. Treatment of a hypotensive episode usually only requires elevating the feet of the patient in a prone position. Nonresponse, which is unusual, will then require administration of fluids, and if necessary, vasopressors. Because of the α-adrenergic blockade of neuroleptic drugs, α-agonists are preferred. Thioridazine, and to a lessor extent chlorpromazine, may induce ECG changes, T-wave abnormalities in particular. Doses above 300 mg daily are necessary to see this effect in most patients. This change is thought to represent a benign disturbance of myocardial repolarization.

Controversy still remains whether there is a syndrome of phenothiazine sudden death (55). Sudden death in young healthy patients receiving phenothiazines, usually chlorpromazine or thioridazine, has been reported, but no direct causal effect of phenothiazines has been demonstrated. Three possible mechanisms for these deaths have been suggested: cardiac arrhythmias and arrest, sudden catastrophic hypotension, and asphyxia due to aspiration. The sudden deaths are described as unpredictable and unpreventable, and autopsies are not generally helpful in fixing an anatomic cause of death. The only possible predictive information from the many reported cases is that a majority of cases involved patients with psychomotor agitation, given large oral or intra-muscular chlorpromazine, and often were in physical restraint. Perhaps when this set of circumstances develops, use of a drug like haloperidol might be preferable. Other cases of sudden death seem totally unpredictable, sometimes patients are found dead in bed with no signs of agonal struggle.

Endocrine Effects. Common endocrine effects of neuroleptic drugs include galactorrhea (lactation) and amenorrhea in women and gynecomastia (breast enlargement) in males. Galactorrhea results from the suppression of prolactin inhibitory factor in the median eminence of the hypothalamus by neuroleptic drugs, allowing secretion of prolactin from the anterior pituitary. No specific treatment is indicated, and lowering the dosage may lessen or eliminate this effect. The patient should be assured it is a reversible effect. Amenorrhea and irregular menses are common findings in psychiatric patients. A 1942 study (pre-drug era) of schizophrenic women of child-bearing age showed an 18% incidence of amenorrhea and 31% had delayed or prolonged menstrual cycles (56). With the introduction of neuroleptic drugs, the incidence seems not to have increased, although there is recognition that neuroleptics can pharmacologically interfere with the menstrual cycle. All women of child-bearing age should have a menstrual history taken to use as a baseline before drug therapy is initiated. Gynecomastia is a relatively rare side effect with few cases reported. Typical onset is several months after neuroleptic therapy is begun.

Neuroleptic drugs can also influence body weight. Phenothiazines, thiothixene and haloperidol have been associated with weight gain, while loxapine and molindone have been reported to cause weight loss. This difference can be a significant factor in drug selection for an individual patient. The mechanism of neuroleptic drug-induced weight change is unknown, but an alteration of hypothalamic monitoring of plasma glucose, pathological glucose tolerance and carbohydrate craving have been postulated (57).

Pigmentary Effects. Pigmentary effects in the skin and eye occur with high dose long-term phenothiazine therapy. Chlorpromazine and thioridazine are most likely to cause pigmentation since they are given in hundreds of milligrams daily while piperazine phenothiazines are given in tens of milligrams daily.

Thioxanthene drugs can also cause pigmentation, but haloperidol does not. Based upon chemical structural differences, molindone and loxapine should not cause pigmentation changes either, although it is still too early to know. Ocular pigmentation is described as a light dusty pigment on the lens capsule which eventually may take the form of a stellate cataract. Skin pigmentation may range from a slate gray to a metallic purple color and is confined to skin exposed to sunlight. The color changes are often so gradual that the patient may not notice, while other patients may suddenly adopt wearing high-necked long-sleeved clothes and heavy makeup to cover the pigmentation. Any patient with skin pigmentation should be referred for ophthalmologic examination since there is close correlation of skin and eye changes. One author found a 30% incidence of significant ocular pigmentation in patients taking chlorpromazine who had either received a total of 600 g or had a total of 200 g in 1 year (58). A specific problem with thioridazine in doses over 1200 mg daily for 4 to 8 weeks is pigmentary retinopathy. This is a serious effect since it can interfere with visual acuity. There are no cases reported of any pigmentary retinopathy at 800 mg daily or less. Once any pigmentation is observed, the neuroleptic should be switched to a drug unable to contribute to it. Piperazine phenothiazines and thiothixene have both been associated with pigmentation, so haloperidol, molindone or loxapine is the best choice. Most evidence suggests that pigmentary changes are slowly reversible over a period of months once the phenothiazine is discontinued.

Allergic Reactions. Skin eruptions take a variety of forms, but the most common neuroleptic reaction is a macropapular rash on the face, neck, upper chest and extremities which occurs between 14 and 60 days after the start of medication. Often allergic skin reactions are mild and transitory and can be treated with antihistamines without discontinuing the neuroleptic drug. Allergic skin manifestations must be differentiated from photosensitivity reactions which are characterized by erythematous lesions in sun-exposed areas of the body.

Hepatic toxicity is now rare with the neuroleptic drugs. Cholestatic jaundice with chlorpromazine typically occurs within the first 4 weeks of therapy, and most cases have classic prodromal symptoms which precede the jaundice by about 1 week. Laboratory findings are consistent with that seen in other types of obstructive jaundice. Onset of prodromal symptoms is usually abrupt. Chlorpromazine-induced hepatitis is usually short-lived and self-limiting.

Hematological effects of neuroleptic drugs are varied but generally rare. A review of outpatient phenothiazine use and bone marrow depression studied 1,048 patients admitted to a psychiatric hospital and found no evidence of subclinical depression of white cell count attributed to neuroleptic drugs. Of 18,587 patients admitted to a medical ward, 34 had bone marrow depression, only one of which had a questionable chlorpromazine etiology. Of 24,795 medical, surgical and gynecological patients, four had bone marrow depression, one of which was a reversible leukopenia due to trifluperazine (59). Agranulocytosis, the most significant hematological effect, had an abrupt onset in which the leukocyte count drops rapidly at the beginning of the illness and reaches a low point in 2 to 5 days. Ninety percent of cases occur within the first 8 weeks of therapy. Agranulocytosis begins with symptoms of localized infection, usually in the pharynx, such as fever, pharyngeal erythema and adenopathy. Mortality due to phenothiazine-induced agranulocytosis is 10 to 40%, usually secondary to infection. Virtually all neuroleptics have been reported as causative agents, but chlorpromazine has the highest incidence. Prevention centers on careful clinical monitoring for signs of infection during the first 8 weeks of therapy.

Teratogenicity. There is no definite proof of teratogenicity of neuroleptic drugs, but the possibility exists. Obviously phenothiazines should be used in the pregnant patient only when absolutely necessary and then at the lowest possible dose, but current evidence supports their use when the benefits outweigh these risks.

Neuroleptic Malignant Syndrome. Neuroleptic malignant syndrome (NMS) is a recently recognized, potentially lethal complication of neuroleptic drug therapy (60). It is characterized by muscular rigidity, hyperthermia, altered consciousness and autonomic dysfunction. Over 60 cases have been reported in the world literature since 1960. NMS can occur from hours to months after initial neuroleptic drug exposure. Once initiated, NMS signs develop explosively over 24 to 72 hours. Muscular rigidity is commonly described as "lead

pipe" or "plastic" rigidity. Rigidity and akinesia develop simultaneously or shortly before temperature elevations as high as 41°C. Consciousness fluctuates from an alert but dazed mutism through stupor and coma. Sialorrhea, dyskinesias and dysphagia are common. Autonomic symptoms include severe tachycardia, labile blood pressure, profuse diaphoresis, dyspnea and incontinence.

Neuroleptic drugs seem necessary but not totally sufficient to trigger the onset of NMS. In some cases neuroleptics have been restarted without recurrence of symptoms after the acute syndrome has resolved. A common factor in many cases is presence of physical exhaustion and dehydration prior to the onset of the syndrome, suggesting that the physiologic state of the patient at the time of drug exposure may be an important variable. All but one case of NMS resulted from the use of high potency neuroleptics. While the majority of cases reported in the United States involve depot fluphenazine, depot fluphenazine preparation account for 16 of 60 cases. Of these 60 cases, 12 were fatal. Of 44 patients treated with oral neuroleptics, only 6 (14%) had a fatal outcome while 6 of 16 (38%) of patients with NMS from depot fluphenazine had a fatal outcome. There are no proven specific treatments for NMS. Management of this syndrome consists of early recognition, immediate discontinuation of psychotropic drugs, and prompt institution of intensive supportive medical and nursing care focusing on respiratory, renal and cardiovascular function. Anticholinergic drugs and antibiotics did not affect the mortality rate or expected duration of symptoms. With oral neuroleptics, NMS lasts 5 to 10 days, while with depot fluphenazine the duration is 2 to 3 times longer. NMS can be described as disorders or crises of hypothalamic, basal ganglia and brainstem function, but the etiology and pathogenesis is unknown. NMS seems to be clinically distinct from neuroleptic heat stroke and temperature regulation dysfunction.

References

1. Taylor MA, Abrams R: The prevalence of schizophrenia: a reassessment using modern diagnostic criteria. *Am J Psychiatry* 135:945–948, 1978.
2. Freedman AM, Kaplan HI, Sadock BJ: *Modern Synopsis of Comprehensive Textbook of Psychiatry II*, ed 2. Baltimore: Williams & Wilkins, 1976, p 418.
3. American Psychiatric Association: *Diagnostic and Statistical Manual of Mental Disorders*, ed 3.

Washington D.C.: American Psychiatric Association, 1980, pp 181–203.

4. Keith SJ, Gunderson JG, Reifman A, et al: Special report. *Schizophr Bull* 2:509–565, 1976.

5. May PRA: Rational treatment for an irrational disorder: what does the schizophrenic patient need? *Am J Psychiatry* 133:1008–1012, 1976.

6. Davis JM, Casper R: Antipsychotic drugs: clinical pharmacology and therapeutic use. *Drugs* 14:260–282, 1977.

7. Hollister LE, Overall JE, Kimbell I Jr, et al: Specific indications for different classes of phenothiazines. *Arch Gen Psychiatry* 30:94–99, 1974.

8. Bishop MP, Simpson GM, Dunnett CW, et al: Efficacy of loxapine in the treatment of paranoid schizophrenia. *Psychopharmcology* 51:107–115, 1977.

9. Cowley LM, Glen RS: Double blind study of thioridazine and haloperidol in geriatric patients with a psychosis associated with organic brain syndrome. *J Clin Psychiatry* 40:411–419, 1979.

10. Smith GR, Taylor CW, Linkous P: Haloperidol versus thioridazine for the treatment of psychogeriatric patients: a double blind clinical trial. *Psychosomatics* 15:134–138, 1974.

11. Van Putten T, May PRA: Subjective responses as a predictor of outcome in pharmacotherapy. *Arch Gen Psychiatry* 35:477–480, 1978.

12. Mason AS, Granacher RP: Basic principles of rapid neuroleptization. *Dis Nerv Syst* 37:547, 1976.

13. Strayhorn JM, Nash JL: Frightening dreams and dosage schedule tricyclics and neuroleptic drugs. *J Nerv Ment Dis* 166:878–880, 1978.

14. Gardos G, Cole JO: Maintenance antipsychotic therapy; is the cure worse than the disease? *Am J Psychiatry* 133:32, 1976.

15. Groves JE, Mandel MR: The long acting phenothiazines. *Arch Gen Psychiatry* 32:893, 1975.

16. Kane J, Quitkin F, Rifkin A, et al: Comparison of the incidence and severity of EPS with fluphenazine decanoate. *Am J Psychiatry* 135:1539, 1978.

17. Usdin E, Forrest IS (Eds): *Psychotherapeutic Drugs; Part II. Applications.* New York: Marcel Dekker, 1977.

18. May PRA, Van Putten T: Plasma levels of chlorpromazine in schizophrenia: a critical review of the literature. *Arch Gen Psychiatry* 35:1981–1087, 1978.

19. Hobbs DC, Welch WM, Short MJ, et al: Pharmacokinetics of thiothixene in man. *Clin Pharmacol Ther* 16:473–478, 1974.

20. Ericksen SE, Hurt SW, Change S: Haloperidol dose, plasma levels, and clinical response: a double blind study. *Psychopharmacol Bull* 14:15–16, 1978.

21. Tune LE, Creese I, Coyle JT, et al: Low neuroleptic serum levels in patients receiving fluphenazine decanoate. *Am J Psychiatry* 137:80–82, 1980.

22. Donlon PT, Stenson RL: Neuroleptic induced extrapyramidal symptoms. *Dis Nerv Syst* 37:629–635, 1976.

23. American Psychiatric Association Task Force: Neurological syndromes associated with antipsychotic drug use. *Arch Gen Psychiatry* 28:463–467, 1973.

24. Matbie AA, Cavenar JO Jr: Akathisia diagnosis: an objective test. *Psychosomatics* 18:36–39, 1977.

25. Kane J, Quikin F, Rifkin A, et al: Comparison of the incidence and severity of extrapyramidal side effects with fluphenozine enanthate and fluphenazine decanoate. *Am J Psychiatry* 135:1539–1542, 1978.

26. Gelenberg AJ, Doller JC, Schooler NR, et al: Acute extrapyramidal reactions with flupheazine hydrochloride and fluphenazine decanoate. *Am J Psychiatry* 136:217–219, 1979.

27. Klawans HL: The pharmacology of tardive dyskinesia. *Am J Psychiatry* 130:82–86, 1973.

28. Ljundberg T, Ungerstedt U: Classification of neuroleptic drugs according to their ability to inhibit apomorphine-induced locomotion and gnawing: evidence for two different mechanisms of action. *Psychopharmacology* 56:239–247, 1978.

29. Tune L, Coyle JT: Serum levels of anticholinergic drugs in treatment of acute extrapyramidal side effects. *Arch Gen Psychiatry* 37:293–297, 1980.

30. Fann WE, Lake CR: Amantadine versus trihexyphenidyl in the treatment of neuroleptic-induced parkinsonism. *Am J Psychiatry* 133:940–943, 1976.

31. Stenson RL, Donlon PT, Meyer JE: Comparison of benztropine mesylate and amantadine hydrochloride in neuroleptic-induced extrapyramidal symptoms. *Compr Psychiatry* 17:763–768, 1976.

32. Hausner RS: Amantadine-associated recurrence of psychosis. *Am J Psychiatry* 137:240–241, 1980.

33. Singh MM, Kay SR: Therapeutic antagonism between anticholinergic antiparkinsonism agents and neuroleptics in schizophrenia. *Neuropsychobiology* 5:74–86, 1979.

34. Gautier J, Jus A, Villeneuve A, et al: Influence of the antiparkinsonian drugs on the plasma level of neuroleptics. *Biol Psychiatry* 12:389–399, 1977.

35. Rivera-Calimlin L, Nasrallah H, Strauss J, et al: Clinical response and plasma levels: effect of dose, dosage schedules and drug interactions on plasma chlorpromazine levels. *Am J Psychiatry* 133:646–652, 1976.

36. Simpson GM, Cooper TB, Bark N, et al: Effect of antiparkinson medication on plasma levels of chlorpromazine. *Arch Gen Psychiatry* 37:205–208, 1980.

37. Tarsy D, Granacher R, Bralower M: Tardive dyskinesia in young adults. *Am J Psychiatry* 134:1032–1034, 1977.

38. Jackson IV, Volavka J, James B, et al: The respiratory components of tardive dyskinesia. *Biol Psychiatry* 15:485–487, 1980.

39. Bourgeois M, Bouilh P, Tignol J, et al: Spontaneous dyskinesia vs. neuroleptic induced dyskinesias in 270 elderly subjects. *J Nerv Ment Dis* 168:177–178, 1980.

40. Tepper SJ, Hass JF: Prevalence of tardive dyskinesia. *J Clin Psychiatry* 40:508–516, 1979.

41. Klawans HL, Bergen D, Bruyn GW, et al: Neuroleptic-induced tardive dyskinesias in non-psychotic patients. *Arch Neurol* 30:338–339, 1974.

42. Jus A, Pineau R, Lachance R, et al: Epidemiology

of tardive dyskinesia; Part I and II. *Dis Nerv Syst* 37:210–214, and 257–261, 1976.

43. Gerlach J, Simmelsgaard H: Tardive dyskinesia during and following treatment with haloperidol, haloperidol and biperiden, thioridazine, and clozapine. *Psychopharmacology* 59:105–112, 1978.

44. Mallya A, Jose C, Baig M, et al: Antiparkinsonics, neuroleptics, and tardive dyskinesia. *Biol Psychiatry* 14:645–649, 1979.

45. Gardos G, Cole JO, Tarsy D: Withdrawal syndromes associated with antipsychotic drugs. *Am J Psychiatry* 135:1321–1324, 1978.

46. Tarsy D, Baldessarini RJ: The pathophysiology of tardive dyskinesia. *Biol Psychiatry* 12:431–450, 1977.

47. Klawans HL, Goetz CG, Perlik S: Tardive dyskinesia: review and update. *Am J Psychiatry* 137:900–908, 1980.

48. Chouinard G, Jones BD: Neuroleptic induced supersensitivity psychosis: clinical and pharmacological characteristics. *Am J Psychiatry* 137:16–21, 1980.

49. Davis KL, Rosenberg GS: Is there a limbic system equivalent of tardive dyskinesia? *Biol Psychiatry* 14:699–703, 1979.

50. Chien CP, Jung K, Ross-Townsend A: Efficacies of agents related to GABA, dopamine and acetylcholine in tardive dyskinesia. *Psychopharmacol Bull* 14:20–22, 1978.

51. Mackay AVP, Sheppard GP: Pharmacotherapeutic trials in tardive dyskinesia. *Br J Psychiatry* 135:489–499, 1979.

52. Jus A, Jus K, Fontaine P: Long term treatment of tardive dyskinesia. *J Clin Psychiatry* 40:72–77, 1979.

53. Jeste DV, Potkin SG, Sinha S, et al: Tardive dyskinesia—reversible and persistent. *Arch Gen Psychiatry* 36:585–590, 1979.

54. Evans DL, Rogers JF, Peiper SC: Intestinal dilatation associated with phenothiazine therapy: a case report and literature review. *Am J Psychiatry* 136:970–972, 1979.

55. Stimmel B: *Cardiovascular Effects of Mood Altering Drugs.* New York: Raven Press, 1979, pp 117–131.

56. Ripley HS, Papanicolaou GN: The menstrual cycle with vaginal smear studies in schizophrenia, depression and elation. *Am J Psychiatry* 98:567–573, 1942.

57. Doss FW: The effect of antipsychotic drugs on body weight: a retrospective review. *J Clin Psychiatry* 40:528–530, 1979.

58. Wheeler RH, Bhalerao UR, Gilkes MJ: Ocular pigmentation extrapyramidal symptoms and phenothiazine dosage. *Br J Psychiatry* 115:687–690, 1968.

59. Swett C: Outpatient phenothiazine use and bone marrow depression. *Arch Gen Psychiatry* 32:1416–1418, 1975.

60. Caroff SN: The neuroleptic malignant syndrome. *J Clin Psychiatry* 41:79–83, 1980.

CHAPTER 38

Epilepsy

WILLIAM A. PARKER, Pharm.D., M.B.A.

Epilepsy has plagued mankind for centuries. It was probably first described in ancient Egyptian writings about 2000 B.C. and was a popular topic of the Greek and Roman scholars. The "sacred disease" or "falling sickness," as it was frequently called by the ancients, was closely identified with supernatural forces and was considered a manifestation of the gods and spirits.

The modern era of epilepsy began with the writings of Jackson in the late 1850s. His extensive treatise and the later publications of Gowers established the neuroanatomical basis for epileptic phenomena. The introduction of bromides in the late 19th century and phenobarbital in the early 20th century finally afforded the physician a means of treating this disabling disorder. Since the introduction of electroencephalography by Berger in the 1930s, our understanding of the basic neurophysiology of the disorder has greatly expanded. Improved understanding has resulted in the development of a large number of potent and specific drugs for various seizure types, and the basis for rational therapeutics and patient monitoring.

Unfortunately, the lay public still nurtures many false notions about epilepsy. For example, it is not true that epilepsy causes insanity, nor is it disfiguring or painful. Electroencephalograms do not reveal the patient's intelligence, nor do they apply electrical current to the brain. Provided epilepsy is not secondary to birth or head trauma, the intelligence of an epileptic is equal to the intelligence of the general public. While the disorder itself probably does not directly shorten one's life span, patients with epilepsy tend to die earlier secondary to other causes, such as drug side effects or seizure-induced trauma like drowning.

A seizure usually, but not always, denotes an alteration of environmental consciousness that might be accompanied by a change in behavior, motor, autonomic, or sensory activity. Patients may, however, remain fully conscious during some seizure variants. A convulsion specifically denotes motor involvement. "Epilepsy" is a term used to define a disorder characterized by recurrent, usually transient seizures having a sudden onset and a spontaneous resolution. It excludes extracerebral causes such as syncope and episodic psychiatric syndromes. It is not a disease, but rather a condition in which a patient suffers from a complex set of symptoms.

Pharmacists should educate the patient and family, the public, and colleagues about epilepsy and its rational therapeutic management. We must also expand our knowledge of the disorder and become familiar with the new advances in therapy, thereby affording more epileptics improved seizure control with fewer complications. Other responsibilities include careful anticonvulsant product selection (since differences in bioavailability between some generic products may affect seizure control), selective monitoring of drug effectiveness and toxicity/side effects and promotion of drug compliance by the patient.

ETIOLOGY/CLASSIFICATION

Epilepsy consists of a complex set of symptoms, including altered states of consciousness and changes in behavioral, perceptual and/or motor functions, and is due to the activation or inactivation of neurons which exhibit an abnormal degree of electrical discharge [1].

Epilepsies are classically divided into two main groups: primary, idiopathic or cryptogenic in which no identifiable cause can be determined (comprises the largest group), and secondary or organic in which seizures exist in conjunction with an identifiable precipitating factor (comprises the smallest group [1, 2]. There are also several different types of epileptic seizures which are classified on the basis of the affected cerebral area and the subsequent clinical symptomatology. An example of the International Classification of Epileptic Seizures is presented in Table 38.1; older, more

Table 38.1.
International Classification of Epileptic Seizures[a]

Partial seizures (local onset)
1. Partial seizures with elementary symptomatology
   [Generally without impaired consciousness]
   Motor symptoms (includes Jacksonian seizures)
   Sensory/somatosensory symptoms
   Autonomic symptoms
   Compound forms
2. Partial seizures with complex symptomatology (temporal lobe/psychomotor seizures)
   [Generally with impaired consciousness]
   Cognitive symptoms
   Affective symptoms
   Psychosensory symptoms
   Psychomotor symptoms
   Compound forms
3. Partial seizures secondarily generalized
Generalized seizures (bilaterally symmetrical without local onset)
   Simple absences (petit mal)
   Bilateral massive epileptic myoclonus
   Infantile spasms
   Clonic seizures
   Tonic seizures
   Tonic-clonic seizures (grand mal)
   Atonic seizures (drop attacks)
   Akinetic seizures
Unilateral seizures
Unclassified epileptic seizures

[a] From H. Gastaut (2).

Table 38.2.
Examples of Causative Factors in Seizures

Nearly all cerebral (brain) and neurological (nervous system) disorders are known to have produced seizures. In addition to specific disease factors, there are numerous other known precipitants. Representative examples of disease and non-disease precipitants of seizures are listed.

1. Congenital and hereditary diseases (e.g., trisomy D (Down's) syndrome, rubella infections *in utero*)
2. Antenatal and perinatal causes (e.g., birth trauma, anoxia)
3. Metabolic disorders (e.g., alkalosis, hypocalcemia, hyponatremia, hypomagnesemia, hypoglycemia, pyridoxine deficiency, porphyria)
4. Head injury (e.g., trauma, increased intracranial pressure)
5. CNS infections (e.g., meningitis, encephalitis, syphilis)
6. Cerebrovascular incidents (e.g., hemorrhage, thrombosis, hypertension, tumors, cysts, aneurysms)
7. Degenerative diseases (e.g., Alzheimer's disease, multiple sclerosis)
8. Drugs and chemicals[a] (e.g., amphetamines, phenothiazines, tricyclic antidepressants, abrupt alcohol, barbiturate, benzodiazepine and anticonvulsant withdrawal, pentylenetetrazol, IV penicillin, IV lidocaine, lithium, theophylline, metoclopramide, epinephrine, insulin, lead, carbon monoxide, DDT, α-benzene hexachloride (Kwell), iron)

[a] Most drug effects are the result of high dose therapy or overdose, long-term therapy, and/or abrupt drug withdrawal.

common names for some of the seizure states are included. The seizures are subdivided on the basis of generalized/nongeneralized (partial) activity, convulsive/nonconvulsive activity, or their pattern of physiologic expression (1–3).

A number of factors are known to precipitate seizures (Table 38.2), although these factors are responsible for only a small proportion of seizures. Most epilepsies are classified as primary or idiopathic in origin. There are many precipitating factors which do not directly cause but which can trigger abnormal electrical discharges in susceptible individuals. These factors include edema, hyperventilation, flickering lights, emotional stress, fatigue, and febrile illnesses. At the present time, febrile convulsions remain one of the most common pediatric problems, accounting for half of all seizures in children under the age of 5 years. The risk of developing epilepsy by age

20 has been reported to be about 6% for all children who have experienced febrile convulsions (4). However, this risk figure consisted of a combination of 2.5% of children without prior neurologic disorder or atypical or prolonged seizures, and 17% of those children with such complications. Overall, the most prevalent identifiable cause of seizures is the patient's own irregular intake of anticonvulsant medication. Pharmacists should take an active role in educating the patient about proper drug intake and ensuring his drug compliance.

PATHOPHYSIOLOGY

Propagation of nerve impulses in the brain is largely asynchronous; electrical charges fire sporadically and the electrical potential is close to zero. Any process which damages, irritates or otherwise compromises the gray matter of the brain may result in the activation or inactivation of neurons by an unknown mechanism. This leads to a sudden, excessive, synchronous electrical discharge. The result of synchronous firing is a summation of activity resulting in an electrical potential. This area of aberrant tissue is called the focal lesion, or focus. This primary discharge will either remain localized, resulting in partial seizures, or it will spread and involve the entire cerebrum, resulting in generalized seizures.

The seizure threshold is a function of the excitability of the neurons as well as the electrical instability of surrounding tissue. With hyperexcitable cell membranes there is modified cation transport intracellularly. This increases post-tetanic potentiation (the augmentation of postsynaptic compound action potentials elicited by repetitive presynaptic stimulation) at synapses and the spread of discharges to adjacent areas, although the focus may continue to discharge locally. The location of the primary discharge and the pattern of spread from the site of initiation determine the seizure's clinical expression (Fig. 38.1) (5). Synaptic transmission refers to the transmission of electrical energy by chemical means. Excitatory and inhibitory changes in the brain are associated with, and perhaps directly caused by, significant changes in electrolytes and amino acid metabolism within the brain. Al-

though these findings offer no conclusive evidence as to the extent of chemical involvement in the pathophysiology of epilepsy, imbalance in excitatory transmitters such as acetylcholine and inhibitory transmitters such as γ-aminobutyric acid (GABA) provide new insights into the pathogenesis and treatment of seizure disorders (6, 7).

Once the seizure activity has peaked, there is a decrease in the frequency of neuronal discharge and an increase in the refractory period of the neurons, processes resulting in a cessation of hypersynchronous discharge and seizure activity (3). Factors contributing to this termination probably include a loss of cerebral energy reserves, local tissue anoxia, accumulation of toxic metabolites of neuronal metabolism, and inhibitory neuronal feedback mechanisms (1–3).

INCIDENCE

The incidence rate (number of new cases of epilepsy occurring within a given population within a given time period) is usually given as 0.5%, although the Epilepsy Foundation of America reports a rate of approximately 4%. The prevalence rate (number of epileptics in a given population at a specific point in time) is reported at 2%. These figures vary considerably depending on the populations sampled, the definition of epilepsy, and the cause of the seizures. Over 90% of epileptics suffer from

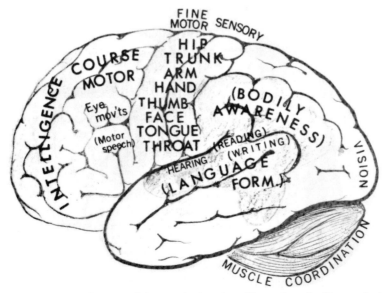

Figure 38.1.   Main functional areas of the cerebral cortex. (Reproduced with permission from A. B. Baker: *An Outline of Applied Neurology*, Kendall/Hunt, Dubuque, Iowa, 1970 (5).)

generalized tonic-clonic seizures, and many suffer from multiple forms of the disorder. There is a higher incidence in males than females, but the ratio varies according to age at onset. The incidence rate for primary generalized tonic-clonic and absence seizures is highest in infants and children and decreased after adolescence. Secondary seizures of these two types more commonly have their onset at the extremes of age. Birth defects, anoxia, trauma, and central nervous system (CNS) infection explain the high incidence in children, whereas vascular disease and toxic encephalopathy, such as from alcoholism and tumor, are causative in the older age group. Partial seizures commonly have their onset during adolescence and the older age groups. Between 80 and 90% of epileptics experience their first seizure by the age of 20 years. In general, onset of seizure activity for the first time after 25 years of age is indicative of either vascular or neoplastic destructive CNS lesions (1).

There is evidence to indicate that there is a genetic trait in primary generalized tonic-clonic and possibly absence epilepsy. When one parent is an epileptic, there is an 8% chance that offspring will also be epileptic. The incidence increases to as high as 25% when both parents are epileptic (1, 8).

DIAGNOSIS

Drug usage implies that a specific diagnosis has been made. However, the difficulty encountered in attempting to make a correct and definitive diagnosis, to differentiate in effect between a "fit or faint" or other causes of passing unconsciousness, is often greater than the problems encountered concerning treatment. This differentiation is very important. Once medication is instituted, one is committed to a prolonged period of therapy. The costs may be great in terms of prescription costs, hazards arising from therapy, and emotional problems resulting from the social stigma directed against the diagnostic label. It should be remembered that one seizure does not an epileptic make. Epilepsy is by definition a *recurrent* seizure disorder. An individual, for example, with a low seizure threshold may have a seizure brought on by various presumably innocuous events, such as relative sleep deprivation, or abstinence from food or consumption of alcohol. This individual should be considered as having suffered a seizure episode and should not be designated as an epileptic individual.

All epilepsies are diagnosed on the basis of tests. However, the most useful information is the description of the attack by an observer. This description, coupled with a history of any recent or past head trauma, drug or alcohol abuse, and a detailed neurological examination prove invaluable.

Routine tests include a complete blood count (CBC), serum electrolytes, liver function tests, urinalysis (UA), cerebrospinal fluid (CSF), and test for syphilis (VDRL). The physician will usually pay special attention to the serum sodium, calcium and glucose as these tests may be indicative of chemically induced seizures. Of importance to the pharmacist is the possibility of ingestion of various chemicals and drugs, such as antidepressants and amphetamines (Table 38.2). A general seizure workup also includes x-rays of the patient's skull (skull series) and a computerized axial tomography (CAT) scan which together may reveal etiological evidence of skull fracture, brain calcifications or intracranial masses. The brain scan and arteriography (radiocontrast studies of the cerebral circulation) may also be performed.

Perhaps the most important diagnostic tool is the electroencephalogram (EEG). It measures the electrical activity of the brain with the aid of harmless scalp electrodes. The electrical impulses (measured in cycles per second; cps), which are classified according to frequency, amplitude and wave form, present specific diagnostic patterns from the different lobes of the brain. Thus, the EEG may confirm a clinical suspicion or it may provide assistance in a situation that defies correct interpretation of the clinical data. However, a fairly high percentage of false positive and negative results may occur, and one should not institute therapeutic decisions on the basis of the EEG alone.

Various ways exist in which a more accurate reading of the EEG may be obtained. One method especially useful in absence attacks is to have the patient hyperventilate, creating a respiratory alkalosis which can activate abnormal activity not usually seen at rest in a susceptible individual. Other techniques include sleep deprivation or induction, photostimulation, and the administration of small amounts of analeptic drugs, such as pentylenetetrazol, all of which help to precipitate a seizure and reveal focal brain lesions. Intensive monitoring by video recording of seizures and EEG telemetry may also be necessary.

CLINICAL MANIFESTATIONS (1–3, 9)

Generalized Seizures

Generalized tonic-clonic (grand mal or major motor) epilepsy occurs in about 90% of epileptics, making it one of the most common seizure disorders. In actuality, many of the attacks may represent partial seizures which have secondarily generalized.

In about half the patients there is an altered sensory perception (aura), a brief moment before the attack begins. Auras differ from patient to patient but are relatively consistent within an individual, and may consist of strange visions, smells, or sensations. Auras generally indicate the site of a focal lesion. The aura quickly proceeds to the tonic or muscular contraction phase. Intense muscular contractions cause the patient to fall to the ground where he loses consciousness and lies rigid. There may be arching of the back, flexion of the arms, extension of the legs, and clenching of the teeth. Air is forced up the larynx, extruding saliva as foam and producing an audible crylike sound which is not, however, an indication of pain. Respirations stop and the patient may become cyanotic. The tonic phase usually lasts 20 to 60 sec before a diffuse trembling, then jerks alternating with relaxation of extremities, begins; this is the clonic phase, which is bilaterally symmetrical. Slight at first, it gradually becomes more violent and involves the whole body musculature. Patients often bite their tongues and become incontinent of urine or feces. Usually within 60 sec this phase proceeds to a resting, recovery phase of flaccid paralysis and sleep lasting 2 to 3 hours (postictal depression). When the patient awakens, he has no recollection of the preceding events. The severity, frequency and duration of attacks are highly variable. They may be from 1 to 30 min long and occur as frequently as daily or as infrequently as once every several years.

The generalized tonic-clonic attack may be centrocephalic in origin or the result of an abnormal impulse arising from some cortical region. The abnormal discharges generally arise from the thalamic and putaminal areas of the brain. EEG patterns associated with attacks may not always be aberrant, but often show high frequency abnormalities during the interseizure period, and 8 to 14 cps spiking during the seizure. Approximately 90% or more of patients may be rendered seizure-free or show an improvement in seizure frequency and severity with appropriate anticonvulsant therapy.

Other types of generalized convulsive seizure disorders include the following (1–3, 9): (a) *tonic seizures*, which are characterized by sustained tonic extension of voluntary muscles; (b) *clonic seizures*, which are characterized by sustained body clonus; and (c) *focal onset generalized seizures*, which are characterized by an initial selective, focal symptom before proceeding to a generalized tonic-clonic seizure.

First Aid

Pharmacists should be familiar with the following first-aid measures for a generalized tonic-clonic attack (3). If the patient is standing or sitting at the beginning of an attack, ease him to the floor so that he will not fall. If he is on his back, put him in the coma position: on his side with his head turned to the side so that his tongue will not fall posteriorly and obstruct his airway, and to help prevent any aspiration of secretions. Loosen restrictive clothing, such as ties, to facilitate breathing, and check for emergency medical information (necklace, bracelet, wallet card). *If his mouth is already open*, you might place a *soft object* such as a handerchief between the *sides of his teeth* to minimize tongue-biting, *taking care not to obstruct his airway.* If his mouth is closed, do not try to open it. *Never put your fingers or anything hard or sharp into his mouth.* To prevent him from banging his head, kneel and cradle it in your lap or on a pillow. Remove any hard or sharp objects which may injure the person, but *do not hold him down* to prevent him from thrashing around, as you may easily cause dislocations or fractures secondary to the powerful contractions during the seizure. You cannot stop a seizure (without drugs) once it has started, so do not try. If the attack persists beyond a few minutes, or if the person seems to experience two or more seizures without regaining consciousness between attacks, call a doctor immediately. This constitutes a medical emergency—status epilepticus—discussed below. Finally, carefully observe what happens before, during, and after the attack so that you may inform the patient's doctor.

Simple absence (petit mal) epilepsy is a nonconvulsive seizure disorder of childhood, and although it may occasionally continue into adult life, it does not arise de novo in adults. There is an association with generalized tonic-clonic epilepsy in about 50% of cases. Occasionally, as these patients reach adulthood, they are maintained on therapy for the generalized tonic-clonic component but that for the absence attacks is discontinued since this expression of the seizure predisposition may well have lessened considerably or completely with increasing age.

Absence epilepsy most commonly begins between 4 and 8 years of age and rarely before 3 or after 15 years of age. The attacks recur frequently, with some patients experiencing 50 to 100 daily. They occur most frequently during the first few hours after awakening.

Attacks consist of paroxysmal episodes of altered environmental consciousness lasting for 5 to 20 sec. There is an absence of prodromal and postictal phenomena, and many attacks may pass unnoticed. Attacks begin suddenly and end abruptly, and the patient is almost always able to immediately continue the interrupted activity. Simple attacks consist of a sudden, vacant stare into space, with or without a flickering of the eyelids or faltering in speech. There may also be associated automatisms, such as chewing or swallowing movements, lip smacking, or mumbling. Because of their nonconvulsive nature, attacks do not extensively affect the voluntary motor system as in the previously discussed seizure types.

Patients with absence attacks exhibit characteristic 3 cps spike and wave activity on EEG, with discharges commonly occurring in the putaminal area. Approximately 80% of patients may be rendered seizure-free with appropriate anticonvulsant therapy.

Other types of generalized nonconvulsive seizures include the following (1–3, 9):

1. *Infantile spasm* (hypsarrhythmia) is a childhood disorder characterized by frequent flexor spasms of musculature resulting in massive myoclonic seizures in the recumbent position and head-dropping attacks in the sitting position. Extensor spasms are less frequent. There is often a high incidence of concomitant mental retardation.

2. *Atypical absence* (petit mal variant, Lennox-Gastaut syndrome) epilepsy is similar to infantile spasms but with a brief period of unresponsiveness and occasionally a precipitous forward fall (astatic or akinetic seizure).

3. *Myoclonus/myoclonic* epilepsy involves lightning-like repetitive contractions of the voluntary muscles of the extremities, trunk and head. It is not uncommon for patients to lose their balance and fall to the floor in an akinetic state. These attacks occur most frequently at night as the patient enters the sleep threshold.

Unilateral and Partial Seizures

The most common types of nongeneralized seizures are unilateral seizures and partial seizures (1–3).

Unilateral seizures involve seizure activity confined to one side of the brain. The seizures, which may last minutes to several hours, are characterized by marked hemiclonus with or without loss of consciousness. Although the seizure activity is limited to one side of the brain at a time, it may alternate between sides of the brain during the same seizure episode or between episodes. Following an attack, the patient's affected side is generally left with a postictal paralysis which clears over time. The most common cause of unilateral seizures in adults is an underlying brain tumor or vascular lesion (1, 3).

Partial seizures (those beginning locally) are subdivided into two main categories: those with elementary symptomatology, namely partial motor (focal cortical) seizures and partial somatosensory seizures, and those with complex symptomatology (psychomotor or temporal lobe seizures) (1–3, 9).

Partial motor seizures involve localized convulsions of voluntary muscles, usually clonic in nature. They are indicative of a structural cortical or subcortical lesion. Generally lasting only a few minutes, the partial motor seizure activity may spread in an orderly fashion to adjacent muscle groups, enlisting further motor clonus ("Jacksonian march" or Jacksonian seizures), or it may eventually spread across the entire cerebral cortex, resulting in a generalized tonic-clonic seizure.

Partial somatosensory seizures are characterized by local sensory abnormalities, such as paresthesias (abnormal spontaneous sensations, like burning or tingling), numbness, or altered proprioception (position-sense) resulting in abnormal posture. Although these seizures usually involve the fingers, hands or face, they may spread in a pattern similar to the partial motor seizures.

Partial seizures with complex symptomatology arise predominantly from eliptogenic foci in the temporal lobes of the brain. The temporal lobe stores memory and complex events which may be relived in the patient's mind during seizure activity. Purposeful but irrelevant motor activity, hallucinations, illusions, sudden feelings of fear, amnestic episodes, bizarre visceral sensations, distortions of spatial or body perception, and a vast panorama of other psychic or motor activity can occur as a result of seizures arising in the temporal lobe or its immediate anatomical connections, which include the limbic system. The limbic system exerts an important influence upon the endocrine and autonomic motor systems, as well as affecting motivational and mood states. Although the patient's outward appearance may be normal and he is conscious throughout, he is in a type of dream state. The attacks, which may occur several times daily and last several minutes, commonly end in sleep or with a clouded sensorium with no recollection of the events of the attack.

The protean clinical expression of this large group of seizures obligates the physician to investigate thoroughly every patient with recurrent, stereotyped aberrations of behavior that cannot be easily relegated to a specific psychiatric syndrome. Besides psychiatric conditions, partial complex seizures are also frequently confused with absence attacks in children. Partial complex seizures are also compounded by the occurrence of supervening generalized tonic-clonic seizures. However, the EEG often proves helpful in locating the focus, showing spiking, slow wave or sharp wave activity localized to the anterior temporal lobe.

Partial complex seizures are difficult to control, yielding results less favorable than with either generalized tonic-clonic or absence seizures. Better results are often obtained with combination therapy.

A more detailed description of all of the aforementioned seizure types may be found elsewhere (1–3).

Status Epilepticus

Status epilepticus is a serious medical emergency requiring immediate medical intervention and treatment to prevent permanent brain damage or death. Status is usually defined as either repetitive seizure activity in which the patient does not regain consciousness between seizures, or a continuous, single seizure episode lasting 30 min or more, with or without alteration of consciousness (10). Although status may involve any one of several seizure entities, such as generalized tonic-clonic, absence, partial complex, and focal motor seizures, the most frequent and most serious form is associated with generalized tonic-clonic epilepsy. It is estimated that 8000 patients are hospitalized each year with generalized tonic-clonic status epilepticus, with mortality rates beween 6 and 18% (10). Morbidity may include irreversible cortical, cerebellar, frontal, and temporal lobe damage, probably secondary to anoxia. While mortality is less of a concern with the other types of status, there may still be associated chronic memory or psychological impairments.

A common precipitant of status is noncompliance with anticonvulsant medication. Rapid cessation of therapy, as for example when changing from one medication to another, may precipitate rebound seizure activity which may manifest itself as status. Should medication alteration be required, then, if at all possible, withdrawal should be performed slowly (days to weeks). Pharmacists should encourage all epileptics to get their anticonvulsant prescriptions refilled before running out. Should an anticonvulsant prescription expire before authorization to refill can be obtained, the pharmacist should provide the patient with enough medication to cover the period. Status may also occur secondary to any of the factors that are listed in Table 38.2 which upset the CNS homeostasis. Although status may present as the initial symptom, most cases occur in patients with chronic seizure disorders, the frequency being much higher in secondary epilepsy than from an idiopathic cause. As a general rule, status in an idiopathic epileptic is much easier to bring under control than when it arises as a manifestation of a recently acquired organic CNS lesion. In either case, an adequate airway and adequate ventilation are mandatory, as the patient will continue with seizure activity if hypoxia is superadded despite the concomitant administration of anticonvulsants. A more detailed discussion of status epilepticus and its treatment may be found elsewhere (9–13).

DRUG THERAPY

The prime objective of anticonvulsant drug therapy is to reduce seizure frequency and severity within a framework of an acceptable level of side effects. This goal may be realized by removing the underlying cause, increasing the seizure threshold to seizure activity, or preventing the synchronous spread of impulses once the threshold is exceeded. Efficacy depends on many factors, such as the type of seizure and the patient's age at onset, the choice of drug agent, and the clinical pharmacology and pharmacokinetics of the drug. Complete seizure control may not always be possible. Generally, the severity of epilepsy will partly determine the drug response. The patient who has had only a few isolated seizures before initiating therapy usually has a better prognosis for drug control than does the patient who is having many seizures a day. Until all indicated anticonvulsants have been tried and proven ineffective (in conjunction with serum drug level determinations), there is no accepted rationale for not using drug therapy. When the correct seizure diagnosis is made and the correct drug is administered in the correct amount, many seizures considered to be drug resistant can be brought under control (9, 14, 15). The chief causes for treatment failure are patient noncompliance, administration of inappropriate dosages, and selection of inappropriate drugs.

Practical Considerations

Several general therapeutic principles exist for managing the epileptic (3, 9, 14, 16):

1. Factors known to lower the patient's seizure threshold, such as fever, edema, hypoglycemia, or specific drugs, should be recognized and corrected by specific means whenever possible.

2. An appropriate drug should be selected for a particular seizure type. Indications for the most commonly prescribed anticonvulsants are presented in Table 38.3. Rational selection based on seizure type is essential. In general, drugs that are effective in the management of generalized convulsive seizures involving tonic-clonic expression may be useful in the management of partial complex seizures, and vice versa, but they have little value in the management of absence, akinetic or myoclonic seizures, and may even exacerbate their control. Drugs which are effective in absence attacks may be of some value in akinetic and myoclonic seizures but generally are not useful in generalized tonic-clonic or partial complex seizures. The patient's history, age, sex, and socioeconomic character should all be taken into consideration when choosing alternate agents.

3. The initial treatment should be started with one drug only. Single drug therapy permits lower costs and easier patient titration and assessment of drug effect and toxicity, should adverse effects develop. When there is little urgency for completely protecting the patient from recurrent seizures, one may minimize side effects by gradually increasing the drug to a dosage that will maintain effective

Table 38.3.
Primary and Secondary Anticonvulsant Drugs and Therapies

	Generalized Tonic-Clonic	Absence	Partial Complex	Status[a]
First choice(s)	Phenobarbital or Phenytoin	Ethosuximide or Valproic acid	Carbamazepine or Phenytoin or Primidone	Diazepam[b] or Lorazepam[b]
Alternatives Primary	Combination[c] Carbamazepine Primidone Valproic acid	Combination[c] Clonazepam	Combination[c]	Phenobarbital Phenytoin[b]
Secondary	Clonazepam Ethotoin Mephenytoin Mephobarbital	Acetazolamide Methsuximide Trimethadione	Clonazepam Ethotoin Mephenytoin Methsuximide Valproic acid	Lidocaine Paraldehyde[b] Pentobarbital Thiopental

[a] Intravenous administration.
[b] Effective in alcohol withdrawal seizures.
[c] Many clinicians recommend combination therapy with first choice drugs before adding alternative agents.

serum concentrations. Phenytoin, phenobarbital and ethosuximide may be started at the maintenance level or by means of a loading dose, whereas the dosage of carbamazepine, valproic acid and primidone should be gradually increased (14).

4. The decision to add a second drug should be supported by analysis of serum concentrations of the first drug. Additional drugs should be added one at a time and increased gradually. Rational combinations might include the concomitant use of anticonvulsants with different mechanisms of action or side effects, such as phenobarbital and phenytoin. If seizure control is obtained following the necessary addition of a second drug, one should attempt to gradually remove or reduce the first drug.

5. Any changes in the therapeutic regimen should be done slowly so that the effect can be properly evaluated over time. Basic pharmacokinetic parameters (Table 38.4) have been reviewed elsewhere (9, 14, 16–20) and must be followed to ensure attainment of therapeutic steady state concentrations before discounting the value of a particular agent. Increasing doses too quickly may lead to toxicity while decreasing too quickly may lead to drug withdrawal seizures.

6. The daily drug regimen should be adjusted to the known pharmacological and pharmacokinetic features of each drug. Dosages vary greatly from patient to patient and often within the same patient. Differences exist with regard to drug absorption, distribution, metabolism, excretion, product formulation, and disease state. Therapy must, therefore, be highly individualized and closely monitored (see below). Several agents usually having long half-lives, such as phenytoin and phenobarbital, may often be administered once daily in adults, thus minimizing certain side effects and enhancing patient drug compliance. However, an anticonvulsant drug should not be administered in intervals greater than one serum half-life because it is undesirable to have fluctuations greater than 50% of the serum drug concentration. Sensitivity to the degree of fluctuation varies with the anticonvulsant. Children may require twice daily dosing of the above agents because of their higher metabolic rates. As well, children's medication regimens should be reviewed frequently, especially during puberty, in order to keep pace with changing utilization patterns related to weight, metabolism, and seizure type.

7. Medication must be taken on a regular, daily basis, and should never be stopped without professional advice. Patient noncompliance is the primary factor behind poor seizure control. Reduction or withdrawal of anticonvulsants should always be done slowly. As mentioned previously, abrupt discontinuation may result in the precipitation of status, an increased seizure frequency and severity, or a relative refractoriness to the agent abruptly withdrawn.

DRUGS

Barbiturates

All barbiturates are useful in the management of epilepsy; however, only phenobarbital, mephobarbital, metharbital, and primidone are used prophylactically because they are effective anticonvulsants in subhypnotic doses. Other barbiturates, such as pentobarbital and thiopental, are occasionally used parenterally to terminate status epilepticus (see below).

Anticonvulsant effects are multiple and rather nonselective. The primary action is believed to be reduction of mono- and polysynaptic transmission resulting in decreased excitability of the entire nerve cell, as well as increasing the threshold for electrical stimulation of the motor cortex. Although this pharmacologic action is associated with a protective effect in generalized tonic-clonic, focal cortical, and febrile-induced seizures, phenobarbital is not a broad-spectrum anticonvulsant and is of little use in the treatment of absence or partial complex seizures.

When indicated, phenobarbital is usually considered the initial drug of choice, particularly in infants, young children, and pregnant females. It is considered by many clinicians to be the least expensive and the least toxic agent, two important considerations for a chronic maintenance drug. Mephobarbital and metharbital are metabolized in vivo to phenobarbital and barbital, respectively. Although barbital has less anticonvulsant activity and greater sedative properties than phenobarbital, it may be tolerated by patients who react adversely to phenobarbital (excluding hypersensitivity). Other features appear similar to those described for phenobarbital.

Phenobarbital is nearly completely absorbed following oral doses of 2 to 3 mg/kg, with peak levels reached within 12 to 18 hours. Unlike phenytoin, it is well absorbed following IM injection. Following IV dosing, it rapidly

Table 38.4.
Clinical Pharmacokinetic Parameters of Major Anticonvulsant Prototypes.[a]

Property	Phenytoin	Phenobarbital	Primidone	Ethosuximide	Carbamazepine	Valproic Acid	Clonazepam	IV Diazepam
Daily dose adult (mg/kg)[b]	4–7	1–3	5–20	20–40	5–20	15–60	0.01–0.02	5–10 mg/dose
Absorption rate (T_{max}) (hr)	5–8	4–5	4–6	1–4	3–8	3–7	1–3	—
Volume of distribution (V_d) (L/kg)	0.6	0.7–1.0	0.6	0.7	0.8–1.4	0.15–0.4	2–3	1–2
Protein binding (%)	>90, lower in uremia	40–50	0–20	0	70–80	>90, lower in uremia	40–50	>90
Elimination Biotransformation (%)	>95	75	60–80	80	99	>95	>95	>95
Unchanged (%)	<5	25	20–40	20	1	<5	<5	<5
Metabolites	Inactive	Inactive	Active, PEMA, Phenobarbital	Inactive	Active, carbamazepine-10,11-epoxide	Active, 3-hydroxy-2-propylpentanoic acid	Inactive	Active, n-desmethyl-diazepam, oxazepam
Plasma half-life ($t_{1/2}$) (average value) (hr)	12–36 (24)[d]	48–144 (96)	6–18 (12)	48–72 (30 children) (60 adults)	6–20 (12)	6–18 (12)	24–36 (29)	24–48
Plasma clearance (L/kg/hr)	0.02[d] at linear kinetics	0.004	0.02–0.07	0.01–0.02	0.02	0.04–0.07	0.05–0.1	0.03
Elimination kinetics	Linear → nonlinear[d]	Linear	Linear	Linear	Linear	Linear	Linear	Linear
Therapeutic plasma range (mg/L)	10–20	15–40	4–12	40–100	5–12	40–100	0.02–0.08	—
Time to reach steady-state plasma concentrations (days)	5–7	14–28	2–4	10–15	2–4	2–4	5–7	—

reaches high concentrations in most vascular organs except the brain which requires a distribution time of 20 to 60 min because of a low fat/water partition coefficient. Therefore, status epilepticus will respond to phenobarbital more slowly than to certain other medications, such as diazepam or phenytoin. The half-life of phenobarbital ranges from 53 to 140 hours, depending on the age of the patient, urine flow and pH, and the presence of certain other drugs. Therefore, 10 to 30 days are required to achieve steady state concentrations. If it is desired to achieve steady state levels rapidly, a loading dose (LD) of phenobarbital can be given. Assuming a volume of distribution (V_d) of 0.7 liter/kg, bioavailability (F) of 1, and a desired plasma concentration ($Cp_{desired}$) of 20 mg/liter, the equation

$$LD = \frac{(V_d)\ (Cp_{desired})\ (\text{body weight in kg})}{(F)} \tag{1}$$

yields a loading dose of about 15 mg/kg. The loading dose is generally divided into 3 or more portions and administered over several hours by the oral, IM or IV route. It should then be followed by initiation of regular maintenance therapy in order to maintain steady state concentrations. Because of its long half-life, phenobarbital may usually be administered in a once daily dosing regimen in adults.

Although the therapeutic uses of primidone are similar to those of phenobarbital, it is used primarily in the management of partial complex and generalized tonic-clonic seizures. Primidone is unique among the commonly used anticonvulsants; the parent compound is a potent anticonvulsant agent with two active metabolites, phenylethylmalonamide (PEMA) and phenobarbital. The relative amounts of primidone, PEMA and phenobarbital vary according to the dose of primidone and concurrent drug therapy. Because of the generation of phenobarbital, caution and close attention to serum phenobarbital monitoring must prevail when using primidone and phenobarbital concurrently if phenobarbital toxicity is to be avoided.

Primidone is rapidly and nearly completely absorbed following oral doses of 4 to 5 mg/kg, with peak levels reached within 3 hours, although there is wide interindividual variability. In order to minimize CNS toxicity, primidone should be started in small doses (250 mg/day) and increased gradually in 125 to 250 mg/day increments every 3 to 4 days, espe-

a Adapted from References 9, 14, and 16–20. Many values are subject to significant inter- and intra-individual variation dependent upon age, dose, duration of therapy, route of administration, and concomitant drug therapy.

b Higher mg/kg doses are generally required for children because of their higher rates of metabolism.

c Based on chronic, single-drug regimens, half-lives are subject to significant inter- and intra-individual variations. Half-lives are generally less in children because of their higher rates of metabolism. Most of the drugs used in the treatment of tonic-clonic and partial seizures are potent inducers of hepatic microsomal drug-metabolizing enzymes, thus resulting in a progressive decline of the half-life and steady-state plasma concentration during the first 4–6 weeks of therapy. Carbamazepine undergoes significant autoinduction.

d Dependent on plasma concentration; Michaelis-Menten capacity-limited metabolism. The most useful parameters are $V = (V_m \times C)/(K_m + C)$, where V = rate of reaction; V_m = maximum rate of metabolism (~7 mg/kg/day); K_m = constant equal to plasma concentration at which the rate of metabolism is one-half the maximum (~4 mg/L); C = plasma concentration.

cially when primidone is being initiated as the first anticonvulsant. Because of its short half-life (3 to 12 hours), primidone needs to be given in a multiple dose regimen.

The most frequently occurring side effects (9, 14, 21) common to all chronically administered anticonvulsants, and especially the barbiturates, are related to the CNS: drowsiness, sedation, dizziness, ataxia (muscular incoordination), diplopia (double vision), nystagmus (rhythmical oscillation of the eyeballs), and loss of concentration. These side effects are usually dose-related. The drowsiness, sedation and loss of concentration may or may not be dose-related, as they are most noticeable during initial therapy, frequently decrease or disappear during continued therapy, and can be minimized by starting with low doses and gradually increasing dosage. Patients should be cautioned that these drugs may impair their ability to perform hazardous activities requiring mental alertness or physical coordination. Side effects that may not be dose-related include paradoxical excitement and hyperactivity in children, excitement, confusion or depression in the elderly, rash (including severe exfoliative forms and Stevens-Johnson syndrome), nonspecific hepatic changes, and rarely, teratogenic effects (notably cleft lip and cleft palate) and blood dyscrasias (including the coagulation defects of neonates of mothers given the drug during pregnancy). However, since uncontrolled seizures may also be associated with fetal malformations, phenobarbital is not contraindicated during pregnancy (9, 22, 23). Studies have also shown an increased incidence of hypocalcemia and osteomalacia with the barbiturates, as well as other anticonvulsants. Although some clinicians recommend that patients be prophylactically treated with vitamin D and calcium supplements, this is probably not necessary if patients are maintaining adequate, balanced nutrition.

Barbiturates are also potent inducers of metabolizing enzymes. Pharmacists must, therefore, closely monitor these patients for possible drug interactions (see below). As well, it should be remembered that the excretion rate of the long-acting barbiturates (30 to 50% unchanged) is dramatically affected by urinary pH—the more acidic the urine, the more unionized the drug and the greater the reabsorption from the renal tubules (resultant toxicity), while the more alkaline the urine, the more ionized the drug and the greater the excretion rate (resultant loss of seizure control). Also, if a patient's urine output is significantly impaired (creatinine clearance of 10 to 20 ml/min/1.73 m^2), the excretion rate will be decreased and serum concentrations will be increased.

Hydantoins

The hydantoin derivatives are useful agents for the treatment of many seizure types, including generalized tonic-clonic, partial elementary and complex seizures. They are not effective against absence attacks or febrile-induced convulsions. Their primary action is believed to be the limitation of seizure propagation by reduction of post-tetanic potentiation of synaptic transmission, as well as stabilizing excitable membranes and preventing cortical seizure foci from detonating adjacent cortical areas.

Three derivatives are used clinically: phenytoin, mephenytoin, and ethotoin. Phenytoin is considered the drug of choice. Mephenytoin is usually reserved for patients refractory to less toxic agents. Ethotoin is the least toxic and least effective agent.

The absorption of phenytoin varies considerably depending on its site of administration, the pH at this site, the dose, the solubility of the preparation based on formulation characteristics, and the presence of food in the stomach. Phenytoin is slowly absorbed following oral doses, with peak levels reached in 4 to 8 hours. The absorption may be slower following large doses or concomitant administration of food and antacids, which may also decrease total absorption. Because of insolubility at the pH of muscle and crystallization of phenytoin in the muscle tissue, the IM route of administration is not recommended. Although absorption is nearly complete, it is very slow, and the injection painful. If the IM route is unavoidable, when switching from oral to IM phenytoin increase the IM dose by 50% of the oral. When switching back to the oral from IM, a dose equal to one half the original oral dose should be administered for the same period of time that the patient received the IM phenytoin (24). The preferred parenteral route is IV. Because of solubility problems, it is generally recommended that phenytoin be administered by direct IV infusion. Since cardiovascular toxicity (hypotension and asystole) may result from too rapid an administration of phenytoin and its propylene glycol diluent, the rate of administration should not exceed 50 mg/min. However, direct IV push of moderate to large doses of phenytoin (as are necessary during status epilepticus or loading a patient) is slow and difficult to administer, as well as being extremely painful secondary to the alcohol-propylene glycol diluents. For this reason, several authors have shown that phenytoin can be safely mixed in concentrations of 1 to 10 mg/ml in 0.9% sodium chloride without precipitation (25, 26). These admixtures result in colloidal solutions which remain crystal-free over the time period necessary for infusion, usually less than 30 min. Since crystals will form over longer periods of time, phenytoin infusions should be prepared fresh and administered immediately.

The half-life of phenytoin, which is dependent on the mode of administration, the age of the patient, the size of the dose, and the presence of certain other drugs which stimulate its metabolism, is approximately 24 hours in adults following standard oral doses. This long half-life permits once daily dosing schedules in many adults. Children, because of their higher metabolic rates, generally require at least twice daily dosing. Because of the long half-life in adults, initiation of usual maintenance doses will not result in steady state concentrations for 5 to 7 days. If it is desired to achieve steady state levels more rapidly, a loading dose can be given. Using equation 1 with a V_d of 0.75 liter/kg, an F of 1, and a $Cp_{desired}$ of 20 mg/liter, one gets about 15 mg/kg. This may be given orally in 3 divided doses over a 4-hour period or by IV infusion, followed by initiation of regular maintenance therapy at 4 to 7 mg/kg/day to maintain steady state concentrations. Large interindividual differences exist with regard to daily dosage requirements. Similarly, differences in bioavailability have been noted between different generic phenytoin products, as well as between different phenytoin oral dosage forms. The capsules and tablets contain the sodium salt in a macroparticle form while the liquid suspensions contain phenytoin acid in a microsuspension, which is absorbed more rapidly than the macroparticle form. Because of phenytoin's narrow therapeutic index, switching from one dosage form or brand to another should be discouraged and closely monitored.

Phenytoin exhibits saturation kinetics within its therapeutic range. This means that when phenytoin dosage is incrementally increased at lower dosages, the serum concentration rises proportionately. However, when the amount of phenytoin present exceeds the metabolizing capacity of the enzyme system responsible for its metabolism, a standard dosage increment will result in a rapid and disproportionate rise in the serum concentration. Therefore, dosage adjustments of phenytoin should be made carefully and in small increments within the therapeutic range, and should be monitored by means of serum drug concentration determinations.

Chronic uremia influences both the hepatic metabolism of phenytoin and the renal excretion of its metabolites. Uremia results in reduced protein binding and higher free fractions of phenytoin in the serum, and the drug's biological half-life is decreased as a result of enhanced hepatic metabolism. Although alkalinization of the urine enhances the excretion of phenytoin, it is much less prominent than with phenobarbital, probably because of phenytoin's high degree of protein binding.

Frequently occurring dose-related side effects (9, 14, 21) of phenytoin are related to the CNS: drowsiness, nystagmus, diplopia, dizziness and ataxia, and at higher concentrations, clouding of the sensorium, abnormal extrapyramidal movements, and exacerbation of the seizure disorder.

The most common side effect not dose-related is gingival hyperplasia (overgrowth of gum tissue), which may occur in over 20% of all patients. Most common in children, it may be minimized by good oral hygiene (regular brushing of the teeth and gumline, flossing). If hyperplasia persists, alternate anticonvulsant therapy and surgical resection may be necessary. Another common complaint is gastrointestinal (GI) distress, particularly when phenytoin is used in a once daily dosing regimen. The GI distress may be minimized by administering the drug with a full glass of water or with food. Antacids should be avoided because of drug interaction and reduced absorption.

Other less common side effects, not necessarily related to dose, include hypersensitivity reactions, such as rashes. Generally morbilliform (measles-like), the rash may be accompanied by fever, lymphadenopathy, eosinophilia, and acute systemic lupus erythematosus (SLE)-like symptoms. Because these skin reactions can precede potentially fatal reactions, such as exfoliative dermatitis and Stevens-Johnson syndrome, the drug should be discontinued immediately if they occur. Phenytoin also produces hypertrichosis (hirsutism or excessive body and facial hair) which is frequently irreversible in some patients. Because of its androgenic effect on hair follicles, it has also been implicated in the production and aggrevation of acne. Studies show an increased incidence of megaloblastic anemia, hypocalcemia, and osteomalacia in some patients receiving long-term phenytoin therapy. The effect appears to be mediated through both intestinal malabsorption of vitamins and minerals and altered folic acid and vitamin D metabolism. Some clinicians recommend that all patients receiving phenytoin be prophylactically treated with folic acid, cyanocobalamin, and vitamin D therapy. However, as in the case with phenobarbital, this is probably not necessary if the patient is maintaining adequate, balanced nutrition. Long-term therapy has also been associated with pyridoxine deficiency and peripheral neuropathy in some individuals. Once again pyridoxine replacement is probably not necessary if the patient is well nourished, unless other drugs known to interfere with pyridoxine, such as isoniazid or oral contraceptives, are being used concurrently.

Although blood dyscrasias rarely occur following the administration of hydantoins, pharmacists should be alert to patient complaints of sore throats, fever, easy bruising, petechiae (pinpoint skin hemorrhages), epistaxis (nose bleeds), or other signs of infection or bleeding tendency which may indicate hematologic toxicity. Severe liver disease also occurs rarely in association with the hydantoins, and pharmacists should be alert to patient complaints about jaundice (such as scleral icterus or yellowing of the whites of the eyes), dark urine, anorexia, abdominal discomfort, or pruritus. Phenytoin has also been infrequently associated with hyperglycemia, occasionally of significant clinical importance. Finally, phenytoin has been the anticonvulsant most frequently implicated in the production of birth defects, notably cleft lip, cleft palate, and the "fetal hydantoin syndrome" (9, 22, 23). However, like phenobarbital, phenytoin is not contraindicated during pregnancy.

In conclusion, although the above list of phenytoin-induced complications is large, most of those not related to dose are rare considering the great frequency of phenytoin use.

Valproic Acid

Valproic acid or valproate, a relatively new agent, is useful in many seizure types, including absence, generalized tonic-clonic, myoclonic, and partial complex seizures, and probably has the widest range of activity among the currently marketed anticonvulsants. It appears to inhibit the spread of abnormal discharges through inhibition of an enzyme responsible for the catabolism of GABA, an inhibitory neurotransmitter. In this way, higher concentrations of GABA are built up, resulting in a presumed stabilization of focal areas.

Valproic acid is rapidly and nearly completely absorbed following oral doses, with peak levels reached within 4 hours. Therapy should not be started at typical maintenance doses because of intolerable side effects, such as nausea. Instead, therapy should be started at dosages below 15 mg/kg/day, with weekly increases of 5 mg/kg/day. About 25% of patients with uncontrolled seizure disorders will need daily dosage of valproic acid greater than 30 mg/kg/day. Valproic acid is usually given in a divided regimen because of its relatively short half-life (8 to 12 hours), but less frequent dosing schedules have been reported effective. The relationship between daily dose and corresponding serum level is variable, possibly due to differences in absorption or elimination; enzyme saturation does not occur. Therefore, dosage adjustments should be made in small incremental doses monitored by means of serum drug concentration determinations.

Common side effects (9, 14, 21) include nausea, vomiting, diarrhea, abdominal cramps and indigestion. These effects occur early in treatment and usually respond to a temporary reduction of the drug, or giving the drug with food. Neurologic side effects, such as sedation and ataxia, have occurred, but may be secondary to protein-binding displacement of other anticonvulsants due to valproic acid's high affinity for binding. Other side effects occur less often, but include increased weight gain, transient alopecia (hair loss), and rarely, hepatotoxicity, pancreatitis, and altered platelet function.

Carbamazepine

Carbamazepine, chemically related to the tricyclic antidepressants and pharmacologically related to phenytoin, is useful in the management of generalized tonic-clonic, simple and complex partial seizures, particularly those which are refractive to the primary agents. Carbamazepine may be preferred in children who often experience hyperactivity, irritability and alterations in sleep patterns with phenobarbital and primidone and gingival hyperplasia, acne, and hirsutism with phenytoin. The drug's precise mechanism of action is unknown, but several effects are similar to those of phenytoin, such as depression of synaptic transmission which helps to reduce the generalization and spread of seizure discharge, and some depression of post-tetanic potentiation at high concentrations.

Carbamazepine is slowly and incompletely absorbed following oral doses, with peak levels reached in 6 to 12 hours. Absorption and attainment of peak levels occur more rapidly with long-term therapy, and when the drug is taken with meals. The initial dose should be 100 to 200 mg in 2 daily doses for adults to minimize GI and other side effects. This dosage can then be increased by 200 mg daily every 3 to 5 days until seizure control or therapeutic serum concentrations are achieved. Drug administration should be in 2 to 3 divided daily doses, taken with meals, to relieve GI discomfort.

The half-life of carbamazepine is quite variable and is dependent on the age of the patient, the size of the dose, the presence of certain other drugs that might stimulate its metabolism, and the chronicity of treatment. Carbamazepine undergoes clinically significant autostimulation of its own metabolism with chronic therapy.

Frequently occurring dose-related side effects (9, 14, 21) of carbamazepine are similar to those of phenytoin and are related to the CNS: drowsiness, sedation, dizziness, ataxia, diplopia and blurring of vision, headache, and vertigo. The drowsiness, sedation, and headache may or may not be dose-related, as they are most noticeable during initial therapy, frequently decrease or disappear during continued therapy, and can be minimized by starting with low doses and gradually increasing dosage. Nystagmus is not a good indicator of toxicity because it can occur with low carbamazepine concentrations. Other side effects possibly related to dose include anticholinergic side effects such as urinary frequency and retention and, uncommonly, an antidiuretic effect resulting in hyponatremia and water intoxication.

Other side effects, not necessarily dose-related, include GI disturbances such as nausea, vomiting and anorexia, transient elevations of liver enzymes with rare hepatotoxicity, rash (including severe exfoliative forms and Stevens-Johnson syndrome), and blood dyscrasias (including bone marrow suppression and aplastic anemia). Although use of carbamazepine was initially restricted because of early reports of aplastic anemia, the incidence of hematological toxicity is rare. A transient decrease in the white blood cell count is commonly seen during initiation of therapy, but it does not require withdrawal of the drug. The monitoring parameters for blood dyscrasias and hepatotoxicity discussed above for phenytoin should be followed.

Because of its chemical structure, carbamazepine should not be coadministered with monoamine oxidase inhibitors, nor should it be used in patients with known sensitivity to tricyclic compounds. It should also be used with caution in patients with cardiac irregularities or coronary artery disease (9).

Succinimides

Succinimide derivatives elevate the seizure threshold in the cortex and basal ganglia and reduce synaptic response to low frequency repetitive stimulation. They successfully suppress the paraoxysmal spike and wave pattern of discharge common in absence seizures. Succinimide anticonvulsants are used chiefly in the management of absence seizures, with ethosuximide considered to be the drug of choice. Some clinicians have also reported good results with ethosuximide in the treatment of myoclonic seizures. Methsuximide and phensuximide have similar pharmacological properties, but are generally less effective and are prescribed for patients refractive to ethosuximide.

Ethosuximide is rapidly and nearly completely absorbed following oral doses, with peak levels reached within one to 4 hours. Like phenobarbital and phenytoin, the typical maintenance dose, 20 to 40 mg/kg/day, may be given at the beginning of therapy. Protein binding and enzyme induction are insignificant factors. However, the rate of metabolism and half-life vary with patient age, with an average half-life of 30 and 60 hours in children and adults, respectively.

Generally, adverse reactions to ethosuximide are rare and of minor consequences and usually clear with continued treatment (9, 14,

21). Dose-related side effects include nausea, vomiting, anorexia, headache, fatigue, lethargy, dizziness, and hiccups. More serious but less common side effects unrelated to dosage include rashes, blood dyscrasias (leukopenia, eosinophilia, agranulocytosis), periorbital edema, renal and liver dysfunction. The monitoring parameters for those conditions discussed above under phenytoin may be followed here as well.

Benzodiazepines

Direct intravenously administered diazepam, having the most rapid onset and shortest duration of all anticonvulsants, is generally considered the drug of first choice for terminating most forms of status epilepticus. The usual adult dose of diazepam is 0.15 to 0.3 mg/kg by IV injection at a rate of 2 mg/min, up to a maximum of 10 to 20 mg. Due to rapid and extensive redistribution out of the intravascular space, repeat dosage may be necessary, and therapeutic supplementation should be provided with parenteral phenobarbital or phenytoin to provide long-lasting control. Diazepam should not be given IM because of slow and erratic absorption. Diazepam may also occasionally be given by IV infusion in at least a 1:10 dilution in dextrose 5% in water or 0.9% sodium chloride. Because the drug interacts with plastic IV bags and tubings, glass containers should be used (27). Severe central depression of cardiovascular and respiratory functions may occur, especially if diazepam is coadministered with other CNS depressants, such as barbiturates or paraldehyde, or if the rate of administration exceeds 5 mg/min.

Four milligrams of lorazepam diluted with 1 ml of 0.9% sodium chloride and administered IV over a 2-min period is also very effective in controlling various types of status. It may also be administered by IM injection with good absorption. Lorazepam is a potent anticonvulsant as equally effective as diazepam but without significant cardiorespiratory depression or prolonged somnolence. It often works in cases where diazepam has failed. It also has a longer duration of action than diazepam (approximately 12 hours versus 30 to 90 min), thus not usually requiring repeat dosage (10). Lorazepam does not appear to interact with plastic administration set tubings.

Chronic oral diazepam has probably been most effective for the control of infantile spasms and in controlling certain anxiety states which may be contributing to the breakthrough of seizures in patients who would otherwise be well controlled.

Clonazepam has been most effective for the treatment of typical and atypical absence, myoclonic, akinetic seizures and infantile spasms. As adjunctive therapy, it has also been found effective in patients with generalized tonic-clonic, complex partial, and mixed seizures. Clonazepam is rapidly absorbed following oral doses, with approximately 80% bioavailability and peak levels reached within 3 to 4 hours. Therapy should not be started at typical maintenance doses because of intolerable side effects. Instead, therapy should be started at doses of 0.01 to 0.03 mg/kg/day in children and one to 1.5 mg/day for adults, increasing dosage weekly by 0.25 mg/day in children and 0.5 mg/day in adults up to daily doses of 0.1 to 0.2 mg/kg. Administration in divided doses minimizes side effects.

Common side effects (9, 14, 21) of clonazepam include drowsiness, sedation, ataxia, behavioral changes (hyperactivity and irritability with an aggressive component), and the development of tolerance to its anticonvulsant effect. Hypersalivation and increased bronchosecretion may also be seen. Using low doses initially and slowly increasing the dose significantly reduces the incidence of side effects, although the problem of tolerance remains. When tolerance does develop, increasing the dose of clonazepam will allow a reinitiation of anticonvulsant response in about two thirds of tolerant patients (3).

Paraldehyde

Paraldehyde is an effective alternative agent for treating status epilepticus when diazepam, phenytoin, or phenobarbital cannot be used or fail. It is also effective for controlling seizures secondary to alcohol withdrawal reactions. Paraldehyde can cause corrosion of local mucosa when given orally or rectally, and it can cause painful tissue necrosis when given IM. The recommended dosage for status is 0.1 to 0.15 ml/kg by the IV route, repeated every 2 to 4 hours, if needed. It should preferably be diluted at least 20-fold in 0.9% sodium chloride and injected slowly, 0.5 ml/min paraldehyde, since IV administration has the potential for causing pulmonary edema and cardiorespiratory collapse. Because paraldehyde deteriorates in the presence of air to acetaldehyde and acetic acid (which have been implicated in the toxic reactions), only freshly opened vials of paraldehyde should be used. Since paraldehyde is incompatible with many types of plastics, only glass syringes and containers should be used.

Miscellaneous Agents

Other agents found effective in refractory cases of status epilepticus include IV lidocaine, rectally administered valproic acid, and general anesthesia by means of IV short-acting barbiturates such as thiopental and pentobarbital. These drugs' doses, regimens, and special considerations have been reviewed in greater detail elsewhere (9–13).

Acetazolamide, a carbonic anhydrase inhibitor, has also been shown to have anticonvulsant properties. Inhibition of carbonic anhydrase results in systemic acidosis and a concomitant increase in the concentration ratio of extracellular/intracellular sodium, a shift which appears to stabilize neuronal tissues. It may be useful in the management of refractory absence and generalized tonic-clonic seizures, and as an adjunct to regular therapy in cases of seizures triggered by premenstrual edema in females. However, tolerance to the anticonvulsant effect usually develops within 6 to 12 months when it is used alone. Other side effects include anorexia, polyuria, lassitude, and drug interactions through its effect on urine pH.

Corticotropin and corticosteroids are often used in the management of infantile spasms and myoclonic seizures in infants. Generalized tonic-clonic and refractory absence seizures have also been favorably affected, but only in children. Since the beneficial effects of these agents correlate with the relative maturation of the CNS, their value as anticonvulsants declines with the age of the patient.

Although magnesium sulfate injection (50%) is used primarily for the prevention and control of seizures in severe preeclampsia or in eclampsia (a condition marked by hypertension, edema and/or proteinuria during pregnancy), parenterally administered magnesium sulfate may also be useful in controlling epileptic seizures associated with low magnesium serum levels, as is frequently seen in alcoholics.

Other drugs used in the past, such as bromides, the oxazolidinedione derivatives trimethadione and paramethadione, and phenacemide, are rarely used today. Their relative ineffectiveness and high degrees of toxicity have relegated them to use in cases refractive to safer therapy.

The clinical pharmacology, therapeutics, and pharmacokinetics of all of the above described anticonvulsants have been reviewed and referenced in much greater detail elsewhere (9, 14, 16–20).

MONITORING THERAPY

Laboratory studies should be performed frequently at the beginning of therapy with any new anticonvulsant. The laboratory examination should be designed to include any unique toxicity of the drug in question. Urinalysis, CBC, liver function tests, and assessment of cerebellar function, such as tandem walk, ataxia, finger-to-nose movements, slurred speech patterns and nystagmus, should be routinely performed regardless of the duration of therapy.

Anticonvulsant serum levels (and less commonly performed, saliva levels) have revolutionized drug management of the epileptic. Because of large inter- and intraindividual variability of anticonvulsant drug concentrations in relation to dose, drug level monitoring is essential in the treatment of epilepsy. Procedures for performing the anticonvulsant assays may be found in the literature (9, 28, 29). Drug levels are indicated in patients with poorly controlled and recurrent seizures, suspected toxicity, suspected noncompliance, liver or renal disease, and for establishing a baseline for monitoring long-term therapy (9). Numerous studies have reported good correlations between serum, CSF, and brain concentrations of anticonvulsants as they relate to therapeutic control and developing toxicity. For example, the therapeutic serum range for phenytoin is 10 to 20 mg/liter, which is extremely close to its toxic level. In general, nystagmus occurs with a serum level above 20 mg/liter, ataxia, slurred speech and a cerebellar syndrome develops at about 30 mg/liter, with obtundation and confusion at levels of 40 mg/liter or more. Many patients may tolerate higher concentrations, or some signs and symptoms may develop before others, but the general step-wise progression holds true. Similar patterns may be seen with other anticonvulsants, such as phenobarbital. Therapeutic serum concentration ranges are shown in Table 38.4.

Because of progressively changing maternal physiology during pregnancy and the rather more rapid return to the normal state after parturition, monitoring serum drug levels needs to be carried out at frequent intervals during pregnancy, and even more frequently in the puerperium (the 6 weeks following termination of labor). There is good evidence that serum phenytoin levels fall during pregnancy and rise again during the puerperium. There is reasonable evidence that similar changes occur in serum phenobarbital levels, and a suspicion that such changes also occur with other anticonvulsants, such as ethosuximide and carbamazepine, although possibly due to different mechanisms (23, 30). Since serum anticonvulsant levels fall early during pregnancy (first trimester), and may be associated with increased seizure frequency, one should measure drug levels every 4 weeks from the outset of pregnancy, adjusting dosage accordingly. Because anticonvulsant requirements may change within a few days of parturition, or not for several weeks, one should monitor drug levels weekly after birth for 2 to 3 weeks, and then every 2 weeks, making dosage adjustments as necessary until drug levels stabilize at pre-pregnancy levels (30).

Suggested therapeutic serum levels are merely ranges; they do not represent "all-or-none" phenomena. Some patients will be adequately controlled with levels below "normal" while other patients may require levels in the "toxic" range for adequate control. The most common cause of suboptimal anticonvulsant serum levels and subsequent failure to control seizures is patient noncompliance with their drugs. Up to 75% of patients designated "refractory" to phenytoin have been shown to have an unreliable drug intake (15). This is followed in frequency by administration of homeopathic doses. Rapid metabolism, drug interactions, and/or inadequate bioavailability should also be considered when confronted with lower than expected serum levels. In uremia, serum phenytoin and valproic acid levels (total) are often lower than expected, possibly because of alterations in plasma protein binding. However, the free (active) concentration of the drugs increases. Attempts to bring the serum drug concentrations (usually measured and reported as "total drug") back into the usual therapeutic range may result in drug toxicity. Elevated serum levels may be the result of patient overcompliance (from fear of experiencing a seizure), liver or renal disease, inappropriate dosage regimens, slow metabolism, drug interactions, and/or differential bioavailability.

DRUG INTERACTIONS

Concurrent administration of numerous drugs with anticonvulsants has been reported to affect either the patient's response to the anticonvulsant or to the other drug. Most of the reported drug interactions relate to phenobarbital, phenytoin, or valproic acid, but the possibility of similar interactions with other drugs of the same chemical class should be considered. Extensive reviews on anticonvulsant drug interactions, their mechanisms of action, and clinical significance and management have been reported elsewhere (31, 32).

Drug interactions involving phenytoin are numerous. Drugs that frequently prolong the half-life of phenytoin, and thus produce a higher steady state serum level, include dicumarol, disulfiram, isoniazid, and phenylbutazone. Phenytoin's half-life is occasionally prolonged by trimethadione, mephenytoin, diazepam, methylphenidate, chlorpromazine, prochlorperazine, chlordiazepoxide, estrogens, chloramphenicol, and halothane. The prolongation of half-life is probably secondary to competition for sites on the liver microsomes. Drugs that have lowered steady state phenytoin levels include carbamazepine, ethanol, and sedative-hypnotics through microsomal enzyme induction and increased biotransformation; aluminum and magnesium hydroxide and calcium-containing antacids through decreased absorption; and valproic acid and other highly protein-bound drugs through changes in protein binding and increased excretion. Phenytoin may also displace other highly protein-bound drugs, such as the oral hypoglycemics, oral anticoagulants, sulfonamides, and valproic acid, thereby affecting their actions. Although phenytoin appears to have weak, clinically insignificant enzyme-inducing properties, it does have an important effect on the metabolism of carbamazepine and primidone (causing considerably more phenobarbital to accumulate at steady state).

Phenobarbital, primidone, and carbamazepine drug interactions are primarily concerned with their induction of drug metabolizing enzymes. Phenobarbital and primidone may cause either increased or decreased phenytoin levels. Initiation of therapy may increase the levels through competition for microsome sites, whereas chronic therapy lowers the levels through enzyme induction. Because phenobarbital may compete for protein binding sites, it may temporarily increase the effect of other drugs bound to protein, such as warfarin. Isoniazid has been shown to inhibit primidone metabolism, increasing the half-life nearly 2-fold. Carbamazepine undergoes clinical autoinduction of its own metabolism with chronic therapy, and may decrease serum levels of phenytoin and other drugs as well. In addition, phenytoin, phenobarbital, and primidone may all increase the metabolism of carbamazepine, thereby decreasing its serum level and effectiveness.

Valproic acid is highly protein-bound and interacts with other protein-bound drugs similar to phenytoin. It may increase phenobarbital serum levels from 35 to 200% and may reduce total serum phenytoin while increasing free phenytoin. Phenytoin, phenobarbital, or primidone may decrease the half-life of valproic acid, but the mechanism is unclear. Because of the potential for significant and often unpredictable interaction over time between 2 or more anticonvulsants, it is desirable to monitor serum levels of each drug during initial therapy, making dosage adjustments as necessary.

SURGERY

Surgery is frequently the only treatment for epilepsy secondary to brain tumors or other acute brain pathology. It has been recommended most often in treatment of partial complex seizures. Proponents of epileptic surgery emphasize that surgery is limited to patients who could not be satisfactorily controlled by any anticonvulsant after diligent trials of at least one year. In addition, they must have a clear focus: a consistent, limited, single area of abnormally discharging neurons, and the focal area must be accessible to surgery, in an area of the brain that can be removed without creating a neurological deficiency. An aura, if present, usually indicates the site of the focal lesion.

One complication of such surgery is hemiplegia (paralysis of one side of the body), occurring in about 5% of patients. Recently, a new surgical procedure, implantation of cerebellar electrical stimulators to prevent seizures, has been successfully performed. Following surgery, patients should continue to take anticonvulsant medication. If there are

no seizures in the month following surgery, the dose of the drug may be gradually reduced.

DIET

The ketogenic diet, which supplies 80% or more of daily calories in the form of fats or medium-chain triglycerides, is infrequently used in patients with refractory, intractable absence seizures. The mechanism by which this regimen controls seizures is unknown, but it may be due to a shift in the acid-base balance to the acidotic side, or it may relate to changes in electrolyte balance, possibly increasing excretion of sodium and potassium. The diet is more effective in children between 2 and 5 years of age. Older children do not respond as well as they fail to maintain an adequate degree of ketosis. Compliance is poor, and the diet is rarely considered as a part of today's therapeutic regimen.

PROGNOSIS

How long treatment should be continued after the last seizure depends upon a number of factors, including the age of the patient, seizure frequency, type of seizure, etiologic factors, and neurologic and EEG findings.

The threshold to seizures is lowest, and the withdrawal of therapy particularly hazardous, at 7 to 10 years of age and at puberty. The following criteria should be satisfied before a gradual reduction of the dose is attempted: (a) the patient should have been seizure-free for at least 2 to 3 years (with some clinicians recommending at least 5 years); (b) the EEG should be free of seizure discharges; and (c) signs of structural cerebral defects should be absent. Focal seizures and persistence of a focal abnormality on the EEG are indications for the continued use of anticonvulsants for much longer periods of time than is necessary in the case of generalized tonic-clonic or absence seizures.

Attempted withdrawal of medication should be initiated gradually. Anticonvulsants should be discontinued one at a time, withdrawing the least effective first. The dosage should be slowly decreased over 6 to 8 weeks until the drug is completely withdrawn. If the patient then remains free of seizures for 1 month, the second drug is discontinued in the same manner, and so on (9). Very close contact with and monitoring of the patient should be maintained during this period of time, and stressful events known to precipitate seizures should be avoided. If seizures should recur, drug therapy should be restarted. If all anticonvulsants have been withdrawn, monotherapy should be restarted adhering to the general principles described previously.

Anticonvulsants provide only a therapeutic cure for as long as they are taken. Complete remission in epilepsy is dependent upon many factors elucidated above. Absence seizures show the best prognosis of idiopathic epilepsy, with remission rates as high as 75%; partial complex seizures have among the worst prognosis, as do those with an identifiable focal lesion. Seizures themselves, apart from trauma secondary to head-banging or prolonged anoxia seen with status epilepticus, are relatively free of complications. Often the most hazardous complications are those inflicted through treatment, as well as people's attitudes arising from misunderstanding of the disorder.

CONCLUSION

The judicious and rational use of anticonvulsants can provide most epileptics a normal, seizure-free life. Adjunctive measures, which include adequate nutrition, rest, and emotional support, are also important. As pharmacists, it is our responsibility, through education of the patient and his family and the monitoring of his total drug therapy, to see that we do not substitute drug intoxication for seizure control. Pharmacists desiring additional information about epilepsy and its treatment, either for themselves or their patients, should write the Epilepsy Foundation of America (1828 L Street, NW, Washington, DC 20036).

References

1. Gilroy J, Meyer JS: *Medical Neurology*, ed 2. New York: Macmillan, 1975, pp 201–226.
2. Gastaut H: Clinical and electroencephalographical classification of the epileptic seizures. *Epilepsia* 11:102, 1970.
3. Piepho RW, Lorenzo AS: Therapeutic management of seizure disorders. *US Pharm* 4(9):36, 1979.
4. Annegers JF, Hauser WA, Elveback LR, et al: Risk of epilepsy following febrile convulsions. *Neurology* 29:297, 1979.
5. Baker AB: *An Outline of Applied Neurology*. Dubuque, Ia.: Kendall/Hunt, 1970, p 3.
6. Deupree JD: Mode of action of anticonvulsant drugs: membrane effects, in Tyrer JH: *Treatment of Epilepsy*. Philadelphia: J. B. Lippincott, 1980, pp 1–28.
7. Meldrum BS: Mode of action of anticonvulsant drugs: biochemical effects, in Tyrer JH: *Treatment of Epilepsy*. Philadelphia: J. B. Lippincott, 1980, pp 29–59.
8. Parsonage M: Epilepsy in adults, in Tyrer JH: *Treatment of Epilepsy*. Philadelphia: J. B. Lippincott, 1980, pp 275–321.
9. Wilder BJ, Bruni J: *Seizure Disorders: A Pharmacological Approach to Treatment*. New York: Raven Press, 1981.
10. Peck MG: Status epilepticus in adults. *US Pharm* 6(11/12):81, 1981.
11. Treiman DM, Delgado-Escueta J: Status epilepticus, in Thompson RA, Green JR: *Critical Care of Neurologic and Neurological Emergencies*. New York: Raven Press, 1980, pp 53–97.
12. Browne TR: Drug therapy reviews: drug therapy of status epilepticus. *Am J Hosp Pharm* 35:915, 1978.
13. Whitty CWM: Status epilepticus, in Tyrer JH: *Treatment of Epilepsy*. Philadelphia: J. B. Lippincott, 1980, pp 349–376.
14. Penry JK, Newmark ME: The use of antiepileptic drugs. *Ann Intern Med* 90:207, 1979.
15. Porter RJ, Penry JK, Lacy JR: Diagnostic and therapeutic reevaluation of patients with intractable epilepsy. *Neurology* 27:1006, 1977.
16. Woodbury DM, Penry JK, Schmidt RP (Eds): *Antiepileptic Drugs*. New York: Raven Press, 1972.
17. Hvidberg EF, Dam M: Clinical pharmacokinetics of anticonvulsants. *Clin Pharmacokinet* 1:161, 1976.
18. van der Kleijn E, Schobben F, Vree TB: Clinical pharmacokinetics of antiepileptic drugs. *Drug Intell Clin Pharm* 14:674, 1980.
19. Eadie MJ: Pharmacokinetics of the anticonvulsant drugs, in Tyrer JH: *Treatment of Epilepsy*. Philadelphia: J. B. Lippincott, 1980, pp 61–93.
20. Winter ME, Katcher BS, Koda-Kimble MA: *Basic Clinical Pharmacokinetics*. San Francisco: Applied Therapeutics, 1980, pp 175–199.
21. Eadie MJ: Unwanted effects of anticonvulsant drugs, in Tyrer JH: *Treatment of Epilepsy*. Philadelphia: J. B. Lippincott, 1980, pp. 129–160.
22. Bodendorfer TW: Fetal effects of anticonvulsant drugs. *Drug Intell Clin Pharm* 12:14, 1978.
23. Dam M, Dam AM: Epilepsy in pregnancy, in Tyrer JH: *Treatment of Epilepsy*. Philadelphia: J. B. Lippincott, 1980, pp 323–347.
24. Wilder BJ, Serrano EE, Ramsey E, et al: A method for shifting from oral to intramuscular diphenylhydantoin administration. *Clin Pharmacol Ther* 16:507, 1974.
25. Salem RB, Yost RL, Torosian G, et al: Investigation of the crystallization of phenytoin in normal saline. *Drug Intell Clin Pharm* 14:605, 1980.
26. Salem RB, Wilder BJ, Yost RL, et al: Rapid infusion of phenytoin sodium loading doses. *Am J Hosp Pharm* 38:354, 1981.
27. Parker WA, MacCara ME: Compatibility of diazepam with intravenous fluid containers and administration sets. *Am J Hosp Pharm* 37:496, 1980.
28. Riedmann M, Rambeck B, Meijer JWA: Quantitative simultaneous determination of 8 common antiepileptic drugs and metabolites by liquid chromatography. *Ther Drug Monit* 3:397, 1981.
29. Rambeck B, Meijer JWA: Gas chromatographic

methods for determination of antiepileptic drugs: a systematic review. *Ther Drug Monit* 2:385, 1980.

30. Eadie MJ, Lander CM, Tyrer JH: Plasma drug level monitoring in pregnancy. *Clin Pharmacokinet* 2:427, 1977.

31. Perucca E, Richens A: Anticonvulsant drug interactions, in Tyrer JH: *Treatment of Epilepsy.* Philadelphia: J. B. Lippincott, 1980, pp 95–128.

32. Perucca E: Pharmacokinetic interactions with antiepileptic drugs. *Clin Pharmacokinet* 7:57, 1982.

CHAPTER 39

Parkinsonism

SAM K. SHIMOMURA, Pharm.D.

In 1817, a general practitioner in London, Dr. James Parkinson, first described a disease he called the "shaking palsy" or "paralysis agitans." It has since become known as Parkinson's disease, parkinsonism or Parkinson's syndrome. Even today very little can be added to his description of the symptomatology of this disease. A brief excerpt from "An Essay on the Shaking Palsy" characterizes this disease as follows:

> Involuntary tremulous motion, with lessened muscular power, in parts not in action and even when supported; with a propensity to bend the trunk forward, and to pass from a walking to a running pace; the senses and the intellects being uninjured....

Historically, anticholinergics have been the mainstay of treatment for Parkinson's disease. Surgical treatment has benefited a few patients, but it has not been proven to ameliorate the symptoms of the vast majority of patients. The introduction of levodopa has been hailed by an editorial in the *New England Journal of Medicine* as "... the most important contribution to medical therapy of a neurological disease in the past 50 years because of its usefulness in one of the more prevalent and disabling neurologic illnesses of man." By understanding the rationale for the use of levodopa in parkinsonism, the pharmacist can contribute significantly to the medical treatment of this neurological disease by monitoring patients for adverse reactions, drug interactions and laboratory test interferences. The pharmacist also can contribute to the education of the patient regarding his drug therapy and its relationship to his disease.

BIOCHEMICAL BASIS OF PARKINSONISM

In recent years, much has been elucidated about the biochemical basis of parkinsonism,

but, as yet, not all the information is in. A cholinergic component appears to be involved, since anticholinergics have been found to be useful in the treatment of Parkinson's disease for over 100 years. This cholinergic overactivity has been confirmed by studies that show that centrally acting cholinesterase inhibitors, such as physostigmine, aggravate parkinsonian tremor, while centrally acting anticholinergics, such as benztropine, will reverse the effect.

Acetylcholine has predominantly excitatory effects on the central nervous system and is responsible for the positive signs of parkinsonism such as tremor. However, the primary defect in Parkinson's disease appears to be a state of dopamine deficiency. In the normal state, there is a balance between the effects of excitatory acetylcholine and the inhibitory effects of dopamine. While the concentration of acetylcholine seems to be unchanged in parkinsonism, the deficiency of dopamine disturbs this balance, and cholinergic activity predominates. Other neurotransmitters, such as serotonin, norepinephrine, and γ-aminobutyric acid, may also be involved in producing the manifestations of parkinsonism. Parkinsonism may be caused by any degenerative, toxic, infective, traumatic, or neoplastic pathology altering the balance between acetylcholine and dopamine in favor of cholinergic overactivity. Therefore, based on this hypothesis, anticholinergics are given to decrease central cholinergic activity, and dopamine, as its precursor, levodopa, is given to increase dopaminergic activity (1).

INCIDENCE

Approximately 200,000 to 300,000 patients in the United States are estimated to suffer from the manifestations of parkinsonism. Each year there are another 20 new cases per 100,000 population. The risk of developing parkinsonism sometime during one's lifetime is 2 to 3%. At least 66% of all those afflicted have onset of symptoms between 50 and 69 years of age. The age of onset is the same in men and women. It is slightly more common in males (55 to 60%) than in females.

ETIOLOGY

The signs and symptoms of parkinsonism are produced by many different causes. Before a diagnosis of primary parkinsonism is established, secondary causes of parkinsonism must be ruled out. Unlike idiopathic parkinsonism, many of the secondary-like states can be cured.

Idiopathic Parkinsonism

The term "idiopathic" denotes a disease of unknown cause. Many theories have been proposed, and each in succession has been refuted or abandoned owing to lack of supporting evidence. This chapter will focus on idiopathic parkinsonism, since secondary causes make up only a small percentage of cases.

Trauma-induced Parkinsonism

Severe injuries to the head very rarely produce tremor and extrapyramidal rigidity similar to that seen in primary parkinsonism. Usually this occurs soon after injury, and recovery is the general rule.

Chemical-induced Parkinsonism

Many chemicals produce parkinsonism-like symptoms upon acute ingestion of large amounts or occasionally upon chronic exposure. Acute carbon monoxide poisoning can be a cause of secondary parkinsonism. It is not a common sequela of carbon monoxide intoxication, but when it does occur, recovery may be slow. Chronic exposure to heavy metals, such as lead, manganese and mercury, may cause symptoms of parkinsonism. Other chemicals which have been reported to produce some or all of the signs of parkinsonism are carbon disulfide, cyanide, methylchloride and some photographic dyes. In most cases of chemical-induced parkinsonism, recovery is complete if the patient survives the acute exposure to the chemical.

Drug-induced Parkinsonism

Phenothiazines (e.g., chlorpromazine) commonly produce extrapyramidal side effects which ultimately may manifest themselves as a parkinsonism-like syndrome (Table 39.1). Early in the treatment with phenothiazine derivatives, a dystonic syndrome may develop. This side effect consists of torsional movements involving most muscles of the body, especially those of the tongue and face. Stiff neck (torticollis), facial grimacing and retrocollis are often seen. Dystonic reactions occur twice as frequently in males and most often between 5 and 45 years of age. The parenteral administration of diphenydramine 50 mg or benztropine 2 mg will produce dramatic response within 10 to 30 min. Akathisia may occur after a few weeks of phenothiazine therapy. Patients with akathisia appear jittery and very anxious. They may pace the floor, tap their fingers and generally give the impression of restlessness. This occurs twice as often in females as in males and usually in patients between 12 and 65 years of age. The true parkinsonism-like syndrome usually becomes apparent 2 to 3 months after initiation of drug therapy. It consists of the usual symptoms associated with idiopathic parkinsonism, namely rigidity, tremor, bradykinesia, drooling, slurred speech, masklike face, festinating gait and seborrhea; and it occurs most frequently in patients over 50 years of age.

Even phenothiazines that are thought to have little extrapyramidal side effects, such as thioridazine, may cause or unmask parkinsonism-like signs and symptoms in low doses. Parkinsonism caused by phenothiazines may persist for a considerable time (up to 2 years in some cases). Therefore, all newly diagnosed parkinsonism patients should be questioned carefully about their prior use of neuroleptic agents. If there is any suspicion that the patient may have taken a phenothiazine in the past, a "drug holiday" every 6 months would reveal

Table 39.1.
Examples of Phenothiazines That Produce Extrapyramidal Effects

Drug	Relative Degree
Trifluoroperazine	High
Perphenazine	High
Fluphenazine	High
Prochlorperazine	High
Promazine	Moderate
Chlorpromazine	Moderate
Thioridazine	Low

if the condition was entirely or partly drug induced (2).

Other drugs besides the phenothiazines have the potential for producing a parkinsonism-like syndrome (Table 39.2). Haloperidol and other butyrophenones produce pharmacological effects similar to those of the phenothiazines, and the same precautions should be observed. Reserpine depletes the brain of dopamine and in high doses can produce a parkinsonism-like syndrome. Methyldopa is a decarboxylase inhibitor which can also produce parkinsonism-like symptoms when given in large doses.

Other drugs which have been reported to produce extrapyramidal symptoms are carbamazepine, thiothixene, and chlorprothixene.

Postencephalic Parkinsonism (Encephalitis Lethargica)

Between 1917 and 1925 there was an epidemic of encephalitis lethargica (von Economo's disease). A sequela of this viral infection was an onset of symptoms similar to parkinsonism which include seborrhea of the face, sialorrhea, occulogyric crisis and a respiratory tic. Although new cases are rare, it is currently one of the major causes of secondary parkinsonism. Because of its viral origin, investigators have been trying to establish a viral basis for primary parkinsonism. At present, there is no evidence to support this hypothesis.

Infection-induced Parkinsonism

Besides the viral etiology of postencephalic parkinsonism, a number of other infectious diseases mimic parkinsonism as an occasional complication. A few examples are syphilis, poliomyelitis, malaria, typhoid, herpes zoster and coxsackievirus.

Tumor-induced Parkinsonism

Another rare cause of parkinsonism-like symptoms is intracranial tumor. The symptoms are usually unilateral and very rarely produce a masklike facies.

DIAGNOSIS AND CLINICAL FINDINGS

The symptoms of advanced parkinsonism are so striking and unique that it hardly ever poses a diagnostic challenge. The patient presents with rigidity, bradykinesia, seborrhea,

Table 39.2.
Drugs Which May Produce a Parkinson-like Syndrome

Amitriptyline and other tricyclic antidepressants
Carbamazepine
Chlorpromazine and other phenothiazines
Chlorprothixene
Haloperidol and other butyrophenones
Reserpine
Thiothixene

festinating gait, flexed posture, drooling, and a characteristic "pill rolling" tremor. With further observation, the clinician notices a "reptilian stare" consisting of frozen, masklike facies, infrequent blinking of the eyes, and the tendency to sit for long periods of time in a stationary position. The voice initially may be hoarse and harsh which, with time, decreases in volume and resonance into a low monotone.

Most of the clinical features of parkinsonism fall into three general categories: bradykinesia, rigidity and tremor. Bradykinesia and akinesia are a slowing down of voluntary actions with apparent difficulty in initiating movement. This is often severe enough to cause the patient to "freeze" into immobility. This can be tested for by assessing the inability of the patient to perform rapid, alternating movements. Rigidity is the tendency to move "en bloc." There is an increased hypertonicity with resistance to passive and active movements of muscles. Muscle control and normal associated movements are hampered. Cogwheel rigidity is seen upon applying force to bend the limbs; the muscles yield jerkily giving the impression of cogwheels moving one upon another. It has a higher frequency and may not be related to resting tremor. The tremor of parkinsonism is generally coarser, slower and of wider amplitude than that associated with alcoholism, hyperthyroidism or nervousness. Resting tremor is seen in a relaxed patient and is a slow, rhythmical tremor.

Although moderately advanced to advanced parkinsonism is easily diagnosed, early features and findings of the disease frequently can be confused with many other diseases. The early presenting signs and symptoms vary from patient to patient.

The masking of facial expression is often an early feature of parkinsonism appearing long before more overt symptoms such as the festinating gait. A friendly, outgoing and smiling individual may slowly appear to become more restrained, emotionless and depressed. There is a subtle restraint of smile, a drawing down of the lips and lower face into an unchanging and worried expression. A slight bulging of the eyes and the barely noticeable tremulousness of early parkinsonism can easily mislead the physician into a diagnosis of anxiety, nervousness or depression. Not only can this diagnosis destroy the confidence and self-esteem of the patient, but it sets in motion a self-fulfilling prophecy wherein the patient actually becomes depressed, anxious and nervous. The patient may be referred to a psychiatric clinic where treatment with a phenothiazine may exacerbate the extrapyramidal symptoms of the disease.

Another patient may present with weakness and stiffness of one hand. There may be no tremor or other symptoms of parkinsonism. He also may complain of "stiff joints" and difficulty in turning over in bed or getting up out of a chair. His wife may complain of his slowness of movement and inability to button the top button of his shirt or to put on his cuff links. These presenting symptoms can often be misdiagnosed as arthritis or, when unilateral involvement is apparent, the possibility of a stroke may be raised.

Early symptoms of parkinsonism frequently involve only one of the three cardinal symptoms of rigidity, bradykinesia, and tremor. Symptoms often are unilateral and almost imperceptible at first and slowly progress in severity and spread from one area of involvement such as one finger, hand, or shoulder to the whole body. The upper part of the body is usually affected first with involvement of the lower part of the body, e.g., shuffling gait, a later finding.

Dementia and impairment of intellectual capacity are encountered in some parkinsonism patients. Advancing age and senility may account for part of these findings, and the amount of intellectual loss is usually not of major proportions.

TREATMENT

Treatment is aimed primarily at providing maximal symptomatic relief of symptoms and maintaining the independence and movement of the patient. At present, there is no cure for this disease, but dramatic improvement in drug therapy in the form of levodopa has greatly improved the prognosis of parkinsonism. Successful treatment involves a total program consisting of drug therapy, physical therapy, psychological support and, occasionally, surgical intervention.

Drug Treatment

ANTICHOLINERGICS

Drugs with anticholinergic properties have been the mainstay of parkinsonism therapy for over a century. The mechanism of action involves the suppression of cholinergic overactivity in the brain. Anticholinergics that do not cross the blood-brain barrier, e.g., quarternary ammonium compounds such as propantheline, are ineffective. Centrally acting anticholinergics produce moderate symptomatic improvement in tremor and rigidity with some improvement in akinesia in one half to one third of the patients.

The belladonna alkaloids such as atropine and scopolamine have been replaced in therapy by the synthetic anticholinergics. Although the synthetic agents are not more effective, they produce somewhat fewer side effects.

Of the synthetic anticholinergics, trihexyphenidyl is currently the most popular. A number of congeners such as procyclidine, cycrimine, and biperiden are also available. There is no clinically apparent difference among these agents. Any one of this group is suitable for initial therapy. One should begin with low doses and gradually increase the dose, weighing satisfactory response against undesirable side effects.

Benztropine is used widely because of its long duration of action. One to 2 mg at bedtime will allow most patients mobility upon arising during the night or getting up out of bed in the morning.

All of the anticholinergics share these common side effects: blurred vision, dry mouth, drowsiness, mild confusion, constipation, and urinary retention. In toxic doses, they may produce hallucinations, agitation and elevation of body temperature.

ANTIHISTAMINES

Diphenhydramine is the most popular agent in this group and provides mild anticholinergic and antiparkinsonism effects. The other drugs in this class, orphenadrine and chlorphenoxamine, are similar in action. Diphenhydramine is also useful as a hypnotic in parkinsonism patients who have difficulty going to sleep or staying asleep.

AMANTADINE

Amantadine is an antiviral agent that produces moderate improvement in parkinsonism. Currently, the mechanism of action is unknown, although it is postulated that amantadine may inhibit the reuptake of dopamine and other catecholamines from neuronal storage sites. Side effects include slurred speech, ataxia, depression, hyperexcitability, insomnia, dizziness, livedo reticularis, and, in extremely large doses, convulsions and hallucinations. The usual dose is 100 mg/day with breakfast for the first week and then 100 mg with breakfast and lunch thereafter. Approximately 90% of amantadine is excreted unchanged in the urine, and therefore, the dose must be reduced in patients with renal impairment (3). Tachyphylaxis occurs after 4 to 8 weeks in about one half of patients. Amantadine is not a first-line drug, but it may be useful as an adjunct to therapy with anticholinergics and levodopa.

LEVODOPA

Cotzias first demonstrated the efficacy of levodopa in parkinsonism in 1967. Although small doses of dopa were tried as early as 1961 in parkinsonism, most investigators reported transient or no improvement. By switching to the levo isomer of dopa and gradually increasing the dose of the drug, Cotzias and associates were able to push the dose high enough to achieve therapeutic results while keeping the gastrointestinal (GI) side effects at a tolerable level.

The next major breakthrough in the use of levodopa was the addition of carbidopa, a decarboxylase inhibitor, to levodopa therapy. High doses of levodopa, 4 to 8 g per day, are generally needed, because much of the levodopa is wasted through extracerebral metabolism. Decarboxylase inhibitors which do not cross the blood-brain barrier are useful in preventing the conversion of levodopa to dopamine outside the brain. This enables the dose of levodopa to be reduced to one fourth of the original dose with concomitant decrease in nausea, vomiting and cardiac arrhythmias (4).

Akinesia is generally the first symptom to improve, followed by improvements in rigidity and tremors. Overall, therapy with levodopa can be expected to produce 50% or greater improvement in about two thirds of patients. Levodopa is approximately 3½ times more effective in treating parkinsonism when compared to anticholinergic therapy.

The rationale for the use of levodopa is based on the findings that parkinsonism may be caused by the depletion of dopamine in the basal ganglia. Dopamine seems to act as a specific transmitter at certain dopaminergic synapses. Dopamine itself was tried in the treatment of parkinsonism, but it does not cross the blood-brain barrier to any appreciable extent. However, the immediate precursor of dopamine, levodopa, does so easily, and it is therefore effective in restoring dopamine levels in the brain.

Dosage and Administration

The careful titration of dosage for each individual patient is of the utmost importance in achieving successful therapy. The usual effective dose of levodopa is 2 to 8 g/day in divided doses given with meals or food. Therapy begins with low doses of 300 to 500 mg and then is increased by 100 to 500 mg every 3 to 4 days as tolerated by the patient. The doses are divided into four and sometimes more doses to decrease side effects and to produce a more even response. Full dosage is usually achieved in 5 to 7 weeks. If patients have difficulty swallowing the tablet or capsules, the tasteless powder can be removed from the capsule and sprinkled on food.

When the levodopa/carbidopa combination is used, the dose of levodopa can be reduced by 75%. The patient may be started on 1 tablet of 100 mg levodopa and 25 mg carbidopa 3 times a day. The dose may be rapidly increased to effective levels, since the necessity to develop tolerance to the peripheral effects of dopamine is minimized. As the dose is increased, the patient may be switched to tablets containing 250 mg levodopa and 25 mg carbidopa. The maximum recommended dose of levodopa in such a combination is 2.0 g/day. When switching a patient from levodopa to the combination, wait at least 8 hours after the last dose of levodopa to prevent toxic effects.

Absorption, Metabolism and Excretion

Approximately 80% of orally administered levodopa is absorbed, primarily in the small intestine. Peak levels occur ½ to 2 hours after an oral dose is given in a fasting state. Although food delays absorption, generally it is administered with meals to decrease nausea and vomiting. Even before absorption begins, some levodopa is metabolized in the gut. Once it reaches the general circulation, metabolism is fairly rapid, with detectable levels present for only 4 to 6 hours. Levodopa is converted to dopamine in the stomach, liver, and kidneys, as well as in the brain. The metabolic transformation is shown in Figure 39.1. Initially, it is decarboxylated to dopamine and then it is further metabolized to norepinephrine, epinephrine and a host of other metabolites. Most of these metabolites are excreted in the urine within 6 hours, with very little excreted unchanged.

Side Effects

Gastrointestinal. Nausea and vomiting are seen at one time or another in almost all patients taking levodopa. Anorexia may also occur in conjunction with the nausea and vomiting but occasionally may occur alone. The nausea and vomiting are probably a result of both the local and central effects of levodopa.

In order to prevent the GI side effects, levodopa should be initiated with low doses and then slowly increased as tolerated by the patient. Administering the drug with food or antacid will decrease the nausea. If nausea and vomiting become severe enough to limit the dosage despite slow increases in dose and administration with food, symptomatic treatment may be required. Phenothiazine derivatives, such as prochlorperazine, should be avoided, since they may counteract the therapeutic effects of levodopa.

Nausea and vomiting are significantly decreased when carbidopa is used in conjunction with levodopa. Other GI side effects include abdominal pain, diarrhea, constipation, peptic ulcer and GI bleeding.

Cardiovascular. Cardiac arrhythmias, most commonly sinus tachycardia, and premature ventricular contractions occur in a small number of patients. This side effect can be attributed to the stimulation of β-adrenergic receptors in the heart by dopamine and its metabolites, such as norepinephrine. Treatment consists of discontinuing the levodopa and starting an antiarrhythmic agent. Propranolol is the

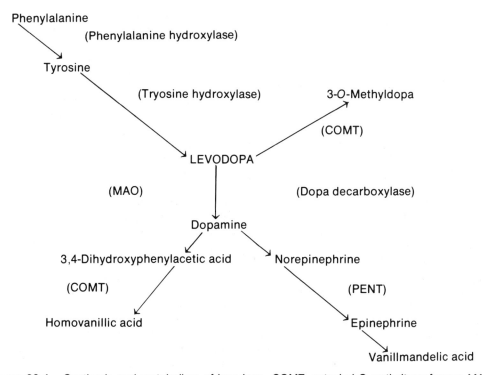

Figure 39.1. Synthesis and metabolism of levodopa. *COMT,* catechol-*O*-methyltransferase; *MAO,* monoamine oxidase; *PENT,* phenylethanolamine-*N*-methyltransferase.

logical agent since it has primarily β-blocking actions. Decarboxylase inhibitors such as carbidopa may decrease the prevalence of cardiac arrhythmias.

The orthostatic hypotension frequency found in patients with parkinsonism can be aggravated by levodopa. Several different mechanisms have been proposed including direct β-effects of dopamine on blood vessels producing vasodilation, α-blockade of the peripheral vascular system, and depletion of norepinephrine from adrenergic nerve endings by dopamine. Whatever the mechanism, it occurs in excess of 25 to 35% of patients early in treatment, but, fortunately, the blood pressure usually returns to normal within 2 to 3 months after initiation of therapy. If symptoms are severe, treatment with elastic stockings, increased salt intake or sympathomimetic drugs, such as ephedrine, is indicated.

Central Nervous System. Levodopa causes behavioral changes manifested as hallucinations, depression, paranoia, agitation, delusions and loss of judgment. The magnitude of these behavioral changes is difficult to determine, since parkinsonism occurs primarily in older patients who may develop impairment of memory, dementia and other personality changes independent of levodopa therapy.

Abnormal involuntary movements are related to high doses and prolonged therapy with levodopa. After 6 months or more of therapy, over half the patients show symptoms of grimacing, chewing, active tongue movement, bobbing of the head and neck, and rocking movements of the trunk. When the carbidopa/levodopa combination is used, the onset of abnormal involuntary movements and other central nervous system reactions may be shortened to a few weeks, since more levodopa is available to enter the brain.

The "on-off" effect is a complication of levodopa therapy that often occurs after 2 to 3 years of treatment. There is an abrupt fluctuation in the patient's response to levodopa from being symptom-free "on" to experiencing full-blown parkinsonism signs and symptoms "off." It may occur at any time and persist in either phase for minutes to hours. In about half of the cases of the "on-off" effect, the "off" phase occurs 3 to 4 hours after the last dose of levodopa and is called "end-of-dose deterioration." Improvement "on" begins about an hour after the next dose. The exact mechanism for the "on-off" effect is unknown but may be due to

factors which cause fluctuation in the blood level of levodopa or alter the sensitivity of dopamine receptors.

The treatment of the "on-off" effect includes more frequent administration of levodopa, the use of the levodopa/carbidopa combination, and the substitution of a direct-acting dopamine agonist such as bromocriptine.

Drug Interactions

A number of drugs have a potential for interacting with levodopa. The clinical significance of these interactions is largely unknown, because most reports of the interactions are either theoretical in nature or only anecdotal.

Pyridoxine (Vitamin B₆). Even small amounts of pyridoxine can antagonize the beneficial effects of levodopa due to an enhancement of the peripheral metabolism of levodopa. A pyridoxine-dependent enzyme catalyzes the conversion of levodopa to dopamine. For this reason, pyridoxine was initially administered to potentiate the effect of levodopa but instead completely reversed it. By enhancing the conversion of levodopa to dopamine in the gut, liver and kidneys, pyridoxine decreases the amount of levodopa available to cross the blood-brain barrier. Although even 5 to 10 mg may antagonize the therapeutic effects of levodopa, in some patients such doses may be given to overcome the torsion dystonia produced by levodopa. However, reducing the dose slowly usually will produce the same effects and is the preferred method for treating this side effect. Small doses of pyridoxine may be given to overcome pyridoxine deficiency resulting from the large amount utilized in levodopa metabolism or to prevent the peripheral neuropathy associated with isoniazid or hydralazine therapy. Since most parkinsonism patients now receive carbidopa, a decarboxylase inhibitor, with their levodopa, even large doses of pyridoxine will not counteract the beneficial effects of levodopa. Therefore, pyridoxine restriction is unnecessary in patients receiving this combination.

Phenothiazines and Butyrophenones. It is well known that phenothiazines in large doses cause extrapyramidal side effects. Phenothiazines apparently produce extrapyramidal symptoms by their ability to block dopamine receptors in the brain. Although low doses of phenothiazines for short periods of time do not significantly reverse levodopa effects, it is best to avoid this combination if possible. An additive hypotensive effect may also complicate therapy with this combination. Clinicians unaware of this interaction may try to treat the nausea produced by levodopa with prochlorperazine or one of the other phenothiazine antiemetics. Haloperidol, a butyrophenone, has actions similar to those of the phenothiazines and produces considerable extrapyramidal side effects.

Reserpine. Reserpine can also antagonize the "dopa effect." In fact, the discovery that it depletes the brain of dopamine and produces a parkinsonism-like syndrome was an important clue in determining the biochemical defect in parkinsonism. Reserpine should be avoided in parkinsonism patients whether or not they are on levodopa.

Food. Early reports suggested that certain foods, such as Chianti wine, old cheese, and chocolate, antagonize the effects of levodopa, but subsequent reports indicate there is no antagonism from these foods. High protein intake also has been implicated as a factor in decreasing the beneficial effects of levodopa. Since levodopa is absorbed and transported like other amino acids, it has been suggested that high protein diets may interfere with the absorption of levodopa or other common pathways. In addition, there was initial concern that dietary pyridoxine might antagonize the effects of levodopa. However, this has not been a problem, since the average American diet is estimated to contain less than 1 mg/day, much less than the 5 to 10 mg needed to nullify levodopa effects. In summary, foods do not significantly interfere with the action of levodopa.

Monoamine Oxidase Inhibitors. Monoamine oxidase inhibitors (MAOI) prevent the inactivation of catecholamines such as dopamine and norepinephrine, and they may interact with many other drugs. MAOI have been tried in combination with levodopa to decrease the metabolism of dopamine and thereby potentiate its action. Although they appear to increase the effectiveness of levodopa, they also can produce a hypertensive reaction. This is due to a buildup of dopa metabolites, such as norepinephrine, which have vasopressor activity. The combination of levodopa and MAOI is potentially dangerous and should be avoided.

Benzodiazepines. The benzodiazepines, chlordiazepoxide and diazepam, occasionally may antagonize the beneficial effect of levodopa. Only a handful of cases has been reported thus far, and the reversal of levodopa effects may have been just coincidental. Many patients take benzodiazepine derivatives and levodopa without apparent untoward reaction. The mechanism and clinical significance are unknown. Drugs of this class are not contraindicated in parkinsonism, but if patients do not respond as expected to levodopa while on benzodiazepines, it may be prudent to discontinue the benzodiazepine and observe the results (5).

Papaverine. The beneficial effects of levodopa may be reversed over a period of several weeks when papaverine in doses of 100 mg/day is added to the treatment regimen. Once the papaverine is discontinued, the expected response to levodopa returns to 5 to 7 days. While the mechanism is unknown, there is some evidence to suggest that papaverine may block dopamine receptors in the striatum.

Phenytoin. Therapeutic doses of phenytoin (300 to 500 mg/day) have been reported to produce a return of hypokinesia, rigidity and postural instability in five patients previously well controlled on levodopa or levodopa/carbidopa. When the phenytoin was discontinued, the patients slowly returned to their previous level of control over a 2-week period. While the mechanism for this interaction is unknown, it has been postulated that phenytoin may interfere with either the binding of dopamine or the reactivity of the brain to the dopamine.

Laboratory Test Interference

Very few laboratory abnormalities have been noted thus far with levodopa therapy. There is no significant interference with the hematological system, renal function, endocrine function or liver function. There have been reports of slight, transient elevations of serum glutamic oxaloacetic transaminase (SGOT) and serum glutamic pyruvic transaminase (SGPT), and interference with determination of serum uric acid by the colorimetric method, but not by the more specific uricase test. Levodopa also produces an excess excretion of catecholamine metabolites in the urine. Certain metabolites of levodopa cause false positive reactions for ketoacidosis by the dipstick method. The urine, saliva and sweat may turn reddish and then black owing to levodopa metabolites. Positive Coombs' test without frank hemolysis may also be noted. Phenistix, used to test for phenylketonuria, is relatively sensitive to levodopa. In fact, it can be used as a screening test for consumption of levodopa in patients who may not respond to levodopa therapy as expected.

BROMOCRIPTINE

While levodopa has helped the large majority of patients with Parkinson's disease, there is an increasing number of patients who fail to maintain this beneficial response as their disease progresses. In order for levodopa to be active in the brain, it must be converted to dopamine by pigmented neurons in the substantia nigra. As parkinsonism progresses, the brain loses this ability to convert levodopa to its active metabolite, and the patient becomes more and more refractory to the beneficial effects of this agent. Drugs which will stimulate intact postsynaptic receptors directly would be the ideal solution to this problem.

Bromocriptine (Parlodel) is a direct-acting dopamine agonist that originally was approved by the FDA for endocrine disorders such as amenorrhea/galactorrhea associated with hyperprolactinemia. Since late 1981, it has also been approved for the treatment of parkinsonism. While levodopa requires conversion in the brain to its active form, dopamine, bromocriptine acts directly to stimulate intact postsynaptic receptors. Bromocriptine appears to be about as effective as levodopa and is predominantly reserved for severely disabled Parkinson patients who no longer respond adequately to levodopa alone. It has the advantages of a longer half-life (6 to 8 hours versus about 3 hours for levodopa), greater efficacy against tremors, and a reduction of the "on-off" effect caused by levodopa. Adverse reactions to bromocriptine are qualitatively similar to those of levodopa. Orthostatic hypotension and mental changes are more frequent with bromocriptine, and involuntary abnormal movements and the "on-off" effect are decreased as compared to levodopa (6).

While most studies indicate that the optimum dose for parkinsonism patients not taking levodopa is 30 to 90 mg in three divided doses, a recent study gives hope that low-dose therapy (average dose 15 mg) may be just as effective. Teychenne and associates (7) started their patients on 1 mg of bromocriptine daily and slowly increased by not more than 1 mg daily at intervals of one week or more. At four "dose-stage points" (4, 7.5, 10 and 12.5 mg/day), the dose was not increased for 2 weeks to determine the status of the patients. In their study of 25 patients (14 levodopa-treated patients and 11 not on levodopa), there was a significant improvement (39%) in the combined scores of tremor, rigidity and bradykinesia while on bromocriptine therapy. Because optimum response to low dose bromocriptine is delayed for several weeks, rapid increase in drug dosage may place the patient on a larger dose than is necessary. The dosage recommendation in Table 39.3 is the FDA-approved dose from the package insert. Bromocriptine is very expensive and should therefore be used in the lowest possible dose. Currently, most neurologists use bromocriptine only in those parkinsonism patients who no longer respond to levodopa, or who experience severe "on-off" phenomena or other intolerable adverse effects from levodopa.

General Comfort Medications

Many of the minor symptoms of parkinsonism can be corrected easily with simple over-the-counter medications. For example, constipation is a common symptom of parkinsonism. It is frequently aggravated by the anticholinergic drugs and levodopa. A stool softener such as docusate sodium or a mild laxative like milk of magnesia is usually effective. Another common complaint of parkinsonism is blurred vision, especially while watching television or movies. This can be attributed to the infrequent blinking of the eyes in parkinsonism. The lubricating action of "artificial tears" eye drops often gives relief. The blurred vision may also be due to therapy with anticholinergic drugs and a reduction of dosage may be beneficial in this case. Parkinsonism patients often have difficulty falling asleep and staying asleep. After initiation of therapy with levodopa, more patients may begin to complain about insomnia even though studies indicate that levodopa neither improved nor worsened sleeping difficulties. This may be explained by the observation that prior to levodopa therapy, daytime symptomatology may be so severe that sleeping difficulties at night are overlooked. As their condition improves, patients may become more aware of their sleeping difficulties and report them to the physician. The drug of choice in this situation is diphenhydramine, because not only is it an effective

Table 39.3.
Antiparkinsonism Drugs

Drug	Dose	Side Effects
ANTICHOLINERGICS		
Trihexyphenidyl (Artane) (2- and 5-mg tablets; 5-mg time-released capsules; 2 mg/5 ml elixir)	1 to 5 mg t.i.d., start with low doses. Doses over 20 mg/day are rarely tolerated	Blurred vision, dry mouth, vertigo, drowsiness, muscle weakness, mild confusion. In toxic doses tachycardia, hallucinations, agitation, elevation of body temperature. Contraindicated in narrow-angle glaucoma
Biperiden (Akineton) (2-mg tablets)	2 mg 3 to 4 times/day	See above
Cycrimine (Pagitane) (1.25- and 2.5-mg tablets)	Initially 1.25 mg, 2 to 3 times/day. Usual range 3.75 to 15 mg daily in divided doses	See above
Procyclidine (Kemadrin) (2- and 5-mg tablets)	Initially 2.5 mg, 2 or 3 times/day. Usual dosage range 10 to 20 mg daily in 3 or 4 doses	See above
Benztropine (Cogentin) (0.5-, 1.0- and 2.0-mg tablets)	Initially 0.5 to 1 mg daily with slow increase to 1 to 2 mg/day. Maximum dose 6 mg in divided doses	See above
Diphenhydramine (Benadryl) (25- and 50-mg capsules; 12.5 mg/5 ml elixir)	Initially 25 mg at bedtime and 75 mg daily in divided doses. Usual range 75–150 mg daily with 300 mg/day maximum	Drowsiness, confusion, dizziness, atropine-like effects
Chlorphenoxamine (Phenoxene) (50-mg tablets)	Initially 50 mg t.i.d. May increase to 100 mg q.i.d.	See above
DOPAMINERGIC DRUGS		
Levodopa (Larodopa, Dopar, Levopa, Bendopa) (100, 250, and 500 mg)	Initially 300–500 mg/day with slow increase to 2–8 g/day.	Nausea, vomiting, anorexia, hypotension, abnormal movements, behavioral changes, cardiac arrhythmias
Levodopa/Carbidopa (Sinemet) (100 mg/10 mg, 100 mg/25 mg and 250 mg/25 mg tablets)	300/75 to 1500/150 mg/day in 3–4 divided doses. Maximum dose 2000/200 mg/day	Same as above, except less nausea, vomiting, and cardiac arrhythmias
Amantadine (Symmetrel) (100 mg capsules; syrup containing 50 mg/5 ml)	100 mg with breakfast for 5–7 days and then 100 mg with breakfast and lunch	Hyperexcitability, tremor, slurred speech, ataxia, depression, hallucinations, insomnia, livedo reticularis
Bromocriptine (Parlodel) (2.5-mg tablet and 5-mg capsule)	Start with 1.25 mg twice a day with meals. If necessary, the dosage may be increased every 14–28 days by 2.5 mg/day with meals. The usual dosage range is 30–90 mg/day in 3 divided doses. The safety of bromocriptine has not been demonstrated in doses exceeding 100 mg/day	Similar to levodopa. Nausea, abnormal involuntary movements, hallucinations, confusion, etc.

hypnotic, but it possesses significant antiparkinsonism effects as well. Flurazepam and diazepam have been recommended for insomnia in parkinsonism, but benzodiazepine derivatives have been reported occasionally to antagonize the beneficial actions of levodopa.

Supportive Psychotherapy

The symptoms of parkinsonism frequently can be aggravated by psychic factors. The patient usually has suffered much humiliation from the readily obvious symptoms of his disease and often becomes defensive, uncommunicative, and introverted. Since the patient's outlook and motivation can seriously influence his disease, it is important for all members of the health care team to provide reassurance, sympathetic understanding and encouragement. To add to the problem, many drugs used in the treatment of parkinsonism produce hallucinations, paranoid delusions and changes in mood and behavior.

Physical Therapy

The purely neurological symptoms, such as tremor and rigidity, do not respond to physical therapy. However, certain secondary disabling manifestations, such as bradykinesia, festinating gait and freezing of motion, can be lessened, although sometimes only temporarily. The goal is to turn a normally unconscious, automatic, voluntary movement, such as walking, into a conscious, voluntary movement where the patient attempts to place undivided attention on the performance of a series of small sequential acts. Activities such as getting up from a chair and walking are broken down into prearranged units so that the patient can practice performing these acts in a flowing, coordinated motion.

Heat and massage are also helpful in alleviating painful muscle cramps, and exercise can be useful in preventing flexion contractions. A program of physical therapy may slow down the progression of the disabling symptoms of parkinsonism and allow these patients many added years of independence.

Surgical Treatment

In carefully selected patients, surgery may relieve the tremor and rigidity of parkinsonism in over 70% of cases for periods up to 5 years or longer. Surgical intervention is primarily directed to the interruption of one or more neural pathways in the globus pallidus or the ventrolateral nucleus of the thalamus. While tremor and rigidity may be effectively reduced, the akinesia and disturbances in gait, posture and voice are not significantly improved. For this reason, surgery has not been a wholly satisfactory treatment, since the akinesia rather than the rigidity or the tremor is the disabling factor in parkinsonism.

Those patients most likely to benefit from surgery are those with primarily unilateral tremor and rigidity rather than akinesia; reasonably good health, i.e., no hypertension, mental deterioration or extreme old age; sufficient motivation to carry out the postoperative physical rehabilitation program; and inadequate response to medical treatment.

Postoperative neurological complications occur in 5 to 20% of patients and are generally transient. Permanent neurological complications occur with a frequency of 2 to 6%. The most common cause of postoperative death is hemorrhage and edema of the brain. Nonfatal complications include hemiplegia, hyperkinetic movements, transient inability to open the eyes, and changes in mentation.

At present, thalamotomy appears to be beneficial only in a few well-selected patients with primarily unilateral rigidity and tremor. Probably less than 10% of parkinsonism patients will derive any significant improvement with this form of therapy.

PROGNOSIS

Parkinsonism is a slow, progressive disease. Surgery has decreased the tremor and rigidity in some cases, but very few patients are suitable surgical candidates. Drugs may relieve many of the signs and symptoms of parkinsonism but do not cure the disease.

Before the introduction of levodopa, a study found that parkinsonism significantly shortened life, with mortality being 2.9 times that of the general population of the same age, sex and race. The average patient died about 9.4 years after onset of symptoms, but some have survived for 30 years or more. The most common cause of death was cardiovascular complications, bronchopneumonia and cancer.

Several studies indicate that the introduction of levodopa may have decreased the mortality rate of parkinsonism patients almost to that of the general population. A multicenter study of 1,625 parkinsonism patients followed for 4,358 patient-years found a mortality rate of 1.03. When their data were adjusted for the mortality rate of the drop-outs, the adjusted mortality rate was 1.33 (8). Marttila et al. (9) investigated 349 patients treated with either levodopa or levodopa combined with a decarboxylase inhibitor during 1969 to 1975 inclusive and found the ratio of actual to expected deaths of 1.85. The excess mortality was accounted for by patients with severe disease at entry in the study.

CONCLUSION

The parkinsonism patient must be closely monitored to achieve maximum benefit from drug therapy. The complex combination of drugs often used in these patients must be frequently adjusted, because they have a high potential for adverse reactions, drug-drug interactions, and drug-laboratory interferences. With proper therapy, the signs and symptoms of parkinsonism may be controlled for many years, and the life span of these patients may approach that of the general population.

References

1. Hoehn MM: Recent advances in the treatment of parkinsonism. *Drug Ther Hosp* 7:81, 1982.
2. Murdoch PS, Williamson J: A danger in making the diagnosis of Parkinson's disease. *Lancet* 1:1212, 1982.
3. Horadam VW, Sharp JG, Smilack JD, et al: Pharmacokinetics of amantadine hydrochloride in subjects with normal and impaired renal function. *Ann Intern Med* 94:454, 1981.
4. Boshes B: Sinemet and the treatment of parkinsonism. *Ann Intern Med* 94:364, 1981.
5. Yosselson-Superstine S, Lipman AG: Chlordiazepoxide interaction with levodopa. *Ann Intern Med* 96:259, 1982.
6. Parkes JD: Bromocriptine in the treatment of parkinsonism. *Drugs* 17:365, 1979.
7. Teychenne PF, et al: Bromocriptine: low-dose therapy in parkinson's disease. *Neurology* 32:577, 1982.
8. Joseph C, et al: Levodopa in Parkinson's disease; a long-term appraisal of mortality. *Ann Neurol* 3:116, 1978.
9. Marttila RJ, et al: Mortality of patients with Parkinson's disease treated with levodopa. *J Neurol* 216:14, 1977.

CHAPTER 40

Headache

RICHARD GRANT CLOSSON, Pharm.D.

Headache is said to be the most frequent symptom reported to the general physician as well as to most specialists. Scandinavian studies show that as many as 73% of women and 58% of men may experience headache during a year (overall prevalence = 66%) (1). In a homogeneous population of almost 10,000 young men, 4.4% had recurrent headache: 1.7% had migraine, 0.09% had cluster headaches and 2.6% had nonmigrainous headaches (2).

Pharmacists also see patients with pain complaints. In a study of community pharmacists as providers of primary care, 183 "primary care contacts" were recorded during two survey days at five pharmacies (3). Twenty-five of those contacts were regarding pain other than stomach and abdominal pain. This frequency was surpassed only by contacts for upper respiratory tract problems (36 contacts) and stomach and bowel problems (32 contacts). In 72% of the complaints of pain, the pharmacist was able to recommend a nonprescription item for relief (only 12% required referral to medical care, while 16% received some other recommendation). It is reasonable to assume that a substantial portion of these patients with pain had headache, even though the type of pain was not recorded.

Because of mass media promotion of nonprescription pain relievers, it is extremely rare for a patient to seek medical care for headaches without first having sought informal advice from a health professional and having tried self-medication. Pharmacists must rank high in this role as informal health advisors due to their availability and education (4). For this reason, it is important to be familiar with the recognition and management of common problems, such as headache.

It is well known that simple questions from patients for advice may really require a great deal of background information for an adequate response. Even for neurologists, diagnostic information is largely historical; therapy monitoring is entirely by patient report. Physical examination of the head is not usually helpful (5) and sophisticated diagnostic procedures (e.g., brain scan, computerized tomography, cerebral angiography) are expensive and usually reserved for the patients with headaches unresponsive to treatment or suggestive of organic disease (Table 40.1) (6).

A short, informal history should be obtained from any patient with headaches before recommending any course of action. A baseline description of the headaches must be established from which we can tell subsequently if recommended therapy has been successful. An important part of the history of any particular complaint is the establishment of its *onset* or first occurrence of symptoms. Most of us see patients who have had headaches in the past and who have treated them before. Often it is only in the situation of incomplete success that a patient will seek the opinion of a pharmacist or physician. Rarely, these chronic pains are due to brain tumors or other serious organic diseases about which patients worry most. It is the onset of new head pain, previously unknown to the patient, which should be of greatest concern. Frequent headache of recent onset or new head pain unusual to the patient probably all require medical evaluation.

Included in the characterization of any headache should be descriptions of its *quality, duration, intensity, location,* the factors which *produce* it, make it *worse* or make it *better,* and the response to previous therapy. With this information, one might better understand what causes a patient's headaches and might feel more confident about recommending a medication for analgesia or sedation, or recommending a trial of physical measures or routines, or recommending that the patient seek medical care.

The *quality* of the headaches might be described as constricting, dull, aching, boring, burning, pulsating, steady, sharp, intermittent, or many other terms. The *duration* might be

Table 40.1.
Serious Disorders Which May Manifest as Headache

Brain abscess
Brain tumor
CO_2 poisoning
Cranial arteritis[a] (temporal arteritis)
Glaucoma[a]
Hypertension
Meningitis[a]
Pheochromocytoma[a]
Polycythemia vera
Sepsis
Subarachnoid hemorrhage[a]
Subdural hematoma[a]
Trigeminal neuralgia[a] (tic douloureux)

[a] Commonly associated with headache.

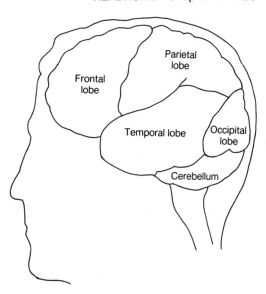

Figure 40.1.   Brain topography.

described as a specific time length or in less precise terms such as continuous, cyclical, short, intermittent, or others. Vascular headaches (e.g., migraine or hypertensive or due to fever) tend to be pulsatile and throbbing. Cluster headaches (so-named because sufferers will have several or many in a short period and then be headache-free for months or years) are intense, steady or boring and deep. Tension headaches due to muscle contractions are usually bilateral and can originate in the neck, forehead or with a hatband distribution. They commonly are a dull ache that can last for days.

The *intensity* of headaches is not of consistent diagnostic importance, but it can be useful in judging therapy success. For example, trigeminal neuralgia may produce the most severe head pain, but diagnosis is based on other characteristics; cluster headaches are very severe, but it is their pattern and accompanying autonomic symptoms that are diagnostically important. *Location* can be important in distinguishing two separate headache types in the same patient. Similar headaches usually affect the same location each time. See Fig. 40.1 for an anatomic map of the common descriptors of headache pain. Finally, it can be important for both diagnosis and treatment to know what, if any, other symptoms accompany the headaches.

There are several categories of pain-sensitive structures in the head, several broad natural mechanisms for causing head pain, and many combinations of these that may produce headaches. Table 40.2 lists the structures in and on the skull which are sensitive to pain

and might be sources of headache. Table 40.3 lists the general mechanisms by which the pain might be caused in those structures. Table 40.4 expands that material further into a classification of major headache types, modified from that prepared by the American Medical Association's Ad Hoc Committee on Classification of Headache (7).

Despite this apparent diagnostic complexity, there is evidence that routine clinic patients with headache can be accurately diagnosed and successfully treated by using a protocol that accommodates only four categories of headaches: muscular headaches, acute sinusitis, chronic sinusitis and migraine (8). These categories included almost 92% of the patients; more than 70% of the patients got partial or complete relief from their headaches. Further, a recent report suggests that the answers to 3 to 7 questions by non-physician care providers can indicate the "correct" headache diagnosis in approximately 85% of cases. In the study, the correct diagnosis was that rendered later by an internist using each patient's entire medical record (9). It is clear that, while the causes of headache may be many, the diagnosis need not be complicated in all cases and therapy generally can be successful when administered by non-physicians with physician support.

The great majority of headaches can be treated successfully with relatively few drugs. Important concepts are:

Table 40.2.
Cranial Structures Sensitive to Pain

1. External coverings: skin, subcutaneous tissue, muscle, arteries, periosteum of the skull
2. Sensory organs: eyes, ears, nose
3. Internal veins and venous sinuses
4. Internal coverings in direct contact with the brain and their arteries
5. Nerves: trigeminal, glossopharyngeal, vagus, and the first three cervical nerves

Table 40.3.
General Head Pain Mechanisms

1. Spasm or inflammation of cranial or cervical muscles or tissues
2. Displacement or traction of large intracranial veins or venous sinuses
3. Dilatation or traction of intracranial and extracranial arteries
4. Inflammation or traction or compression of cranial nerves with sensory components or of cervical nerves

Table 40.4.
Classification of Headache

1. Vascular headache
   a. Classic migraine
   b. Common migraine
   c. Cluster headache
   d. Hemiplegic and ophthalmic migraine
2. Muscle contraction (tension) headache
3. Combined headache: vascular and muscle contraction
4. Headache of nasal vasomotor reaction
   a. Allergy
   b. Infection
5. Headache of delusional, conversion, or hypochondriacal states
6. Nonmigrainous vascular headaches
   a. Systemic infections
   b. Caffeine withdrawal
   c. Postconvulsion
   d. "Hangover" reaction
   e. Early morning hypertensive headache
7. Traction headache
   a. Malignant tumors
   b. Hematomas
   c. Abscesses
   d. Lumbar puncture
8. Headaches due to disease of eyes, ears, nose and sinus, throat and teeth
9. Cranial neuralgias

1. The more information known about a patient's headaches, the better able one will be to classify, treat and monitor those headaches;

2. The classification and understanding of headaches does not require sophisticated patient assessment skills nor elaborate diagnostic tests—most care is provided to patients on the basis of the patient's history;

3. The active treatment of headaches is a dynamic process requiring the trial of medication with subsequent reassessment and modification of the regimen; and

4. In patients with headaches that are treated largely with medication (that is, the great majority of patients), pharmacists are well suited as disease and therapy monitors.

There is, however, a small group of patients with headaches that are difficult to control with the usual drugs. These patients require treatment with exotic drugs (perhaps not usually used for headache) or high doses of narcotic analgesics. This is a group of patients whom pharmacists and physicians alike hesitate to treat due to the special demands on time and therapeutic ingenuity. Often these patients are directed to the neurologist who deals especially with problem headache patients. They are infrequent enough to be outside the scope of this practical discussion. In addition, there is a group of patients in whom headache is but a symptom of another, perhaps

more serious, disease. Table 40.1 lists diseases which may cause headache. It has been estimated that approximately 0.4% of headache patients seen by a generalist have a serious underlying organic disorder as the cause (9). It is the specter of these disorders that may cause well-intentioned pharmacists to refrain from counseling patients for fear of delaying definitive treatment of the underlying headache cause. While it is well to keep these possibilities in mind, they are only rare causes of headache.

PRINCIPAL VARIETIES OF HEADACHE

Described below are some important categories of headaches that may be encountered in general practice. Appreciation of their major differences can be important to pharmacists who make recommendations to these patients or who follow patient progress during treatment. Table 40.5 describes the important characteristics of the three most common types of headache. There are opinions that absolute distinction of headaches into discrete types is possible only in classic cases; most headaches can best be described as falling into a continuous spectrum, each related to every other (10, 11). Figure 40.2 illustrates such a spectrum. Nevertheless, current convention still uses mutually exclusive titles for headache syndromes (12). In a discussion of therapy, this has some merit: it can offer structure and guidance for initial treatment without preventing the discussion of the drugs for other headache types. Headache therapy here will be discussed in terms of tension, migraine and cluster headaches with the understanding that a given patient with a particular headache may receive, at some time, therapy more often used for another headache type. It is common for patients to report headaches that are not classed easily as one single type. Many patients will have headaches of more than one kind. In these situations it is most important to realize the multiple nature of the complaint. Therapy often can be begun with the more severe or more frequent headache in mind. The expectations for therapy success must be modified but, occasionally, different headaches will respond to the same therapy.

Tension (muscle contraction) *headache* is the most common headache reported today. The pain is usually bifrontal but may also be occipital or in the neck and shoulders. It may begin by being dull, persistent and steady and progress in severity until it pulsates. Patients may describe a feeling of tightness, pressure or a band around the head. Some patients will have almost daily headaches or complain of never being pain-free.

Studies of behavioral treatment of tension headache (see below) have raised questions about the actual origin of the headache (13). While relaxation and depressant drugs often bring relief from the headache, it may not follow that the pain is due solely or primarily to increased muscle tension. Still, as a working description, classification of these headaches as tension or muscle contraction pain is justifiable, if not mechanistically correct.

Migraine headaches are renowned for their severity and accompanying constitutional symptoms. They are vascular headaches, i.e., accompanied by changes in the permeability and caliber of cranial blood vessels, but also may be combined with muscle contraction pain. Because of this, there is a growing suspicion that migraine and tension headaches are related. There are two major categories of migraine: common migraine (comprising 80%

of all cases) and classic migraine. It has been postulated that common migraine is the response to mild precipitating vasospasm and cerebral ischemia and classic migraine is the response to stronger precipitants. Only one research group has been fastidious in studying solely classic or common migraineurs. They have reported evidence of a reduced cerebral blood flow (CBF) during the prodrome of classic migraine but no change in blood flow before common migraine (14, 15). If corroborated, this mechanistic distinction between common and classic migraine may have therapy consequences. The major symptomatic differences are (a) the neurologic prodrome, which occurs only in classic migraine, and (b) the duration, which may be longer (up to days) with common migraine.

The accepted vascular mechanism for classic migraine is two-phased. The initial phase is one of arterial constriction and ischemia to areas of the brain. The first phase is thought to produce the transient prodrome in classic migraine. Some feel that the prodrome is the basic phenomenon of the disorder. The following headache is an over-reactive compensation (16). The prodrome is usually visual (e.g., scotomas or scintillations), which may be due to the special sensitivity of the occipital lobe to ischemia (17), and may be relieved by inhalation of isoproterenol (18). It also can manifest as ataxia, dysarthria and perioral numbness. It abates as the headache enters the second phase: rebound vasodilation follows the vasoconstriction. This vasodilation, a local sterile inflammation and lowered pain threshhold are responsible for the painful throbbing that is seen in about half of migraines.

Detailed biochemical research now strongly implicates altered platelet function in the mechanisms of migraine (19). Normally, platelets in blood are in constant equilibrium between aggregation (an initial step toward thrombus formation) and disaggregation. This balance is maintained by two products of prostaglandin metabolism: thromboxane A_2 is manufactured in platelets and stimulates aggregation; prostacyclin is manufactured in blood vessel wall cells to prevent platelet aggregation on those walls. In addition, thromboxane A_2 is a potent vasoconstrictor and prostacyclin is a potent vasodilator. Between them, the equilibrium is stable. Platelets of migraineurs have increased tendency to aggregate between headaches and during a headache

Table 40.5.
Characteristics of the Major Headache Types[a]

Headache	Prevalence	Frequency	Quality	Duration	
				Time (hr)	Frequency (%)
Tension	65% of population (197) 72% are women (198)	Daily—50% (199) Weekly—15%	Dull; throbbing; pressure	0–1 1–12 24–72 Constant	Rare (199) 33 20 20
Migraine	9.1% of men 16.1% of women (200)	Variable	Pulsatile—47% Pressing—2% (201)	0–4 4–24 24–48 Over 48	27 (61) 40 11 22
Cluster	Less than 1% (2) 90% are men	Daily during cluster	Boring; burning; nonpulsatile	0–½ ½–2 2–3 3–6 Over 6	11 (202) 50 17 13 9

[a] Numbers in parentheses are references.

prodrome (20–22). During the headache phase, the platelet aggregability decreases. This hyperaggregability is proposed to cause microemboli which, with local vasoconstriction, decrease cerebral blood perfusion and produce the prodromal symptoms of classic migraine. The microemboli might be the cause of permanent neurologic deficits in "complicated migraine" (23), but there has been no general correlation between the platelet hyperaggregability and migraine severity (24).

When platelets aggregate, they release serotonin (or 5-hydroxytryptamine, 5-HT) from intracellular storage granules. This 5-HT release also can be precipitated by epinephrine, reserpine or tyramine (25, 26). Platelets of migraineurs release their 5-HT more readily than those of normal persons (27). Since platelets are probably the only source for 5-HT in the blood, 5-HT concentrations are taken as evidence of platelet aggregation. Plasma 5-HT concentrations increase during the migraine prodrome (20, 28, 29). Serotonin is an arteriolar constrictor which may contribute to the decreased cerebral blood flow of the prodrome. Further, it increases the sensitivity of pain receptors and increases vessel permeability, allowing pain-producing kinins to escape into

the tissues surrounding the cerebral vessels (30). As the prodrome progresses, the blood concentration of 5-HT decreases (perhaps due to its metabolism in vessel wall cells) (20, 28, 29). This permits relaxation of the cranial arteries and the pulsatile pain characteristic of the headache phase. This scheme is simplified in Figure 40.3 and includes the proposed sites of action of many drugs used to treat migraine. Table 40.6 lists drugs that may be effective against headaches by their effects on platelet function.

Migraine pain is usually unilateral, but can occur on both sides. Unilateral headaches may occur on either side, even in the same patient. They often begin with painful throbbing in the temporal, orbital or frontal regions and progressively become less severe to a dull, nonthrobbing ache. Other associated symptoms include nausea, abdominal cramping, vomiting and anorexia. These may interfere with the patient's willingness to take oral medication or ability to keep it in the stomach, or even interfere with absorption.

Cluster headaches are relatively rare (about 1 sufferer in 1000 persons) (2), but are notable for their unique presentation and problems of treatment. They are vascular headaches; in

| Intensity | Location | | Improved by | Worsened by | Other Symptoms | |
	Area	Frequency (%)			Complaint	Frequency (%)
Mild to moderate	Unilateral Bilateral	10 (199) 90	Sedation; vasodilators	Stress; noise; glare; vasoconstrictors	Depression	
Severe—68% Medium—30% Mild—2% (201)	Hemicranial Whole head Bifrontal Unifrontal	44 (201) 22 14 13	Sleep; lying still; vasoconstrictors	Rapid head motion; coughing; alcohol; reserpine	Nausea Photophobia Dizziness Scalp tenderness Vomiting	86 (201) 87 (61) 49 82 72 69 65 47 56
Severe	Unilateral Ocular Temporal Half-face	90 (202) 62 12 14		Nitroglycerin Alcohol— 5–50% Stress— 12–54% Amyl nitrite (203)	Ipsilateral: red eye tearing nasal block rhinorrhea ptosis Nausea	(202) 45 62 37 7 17 21

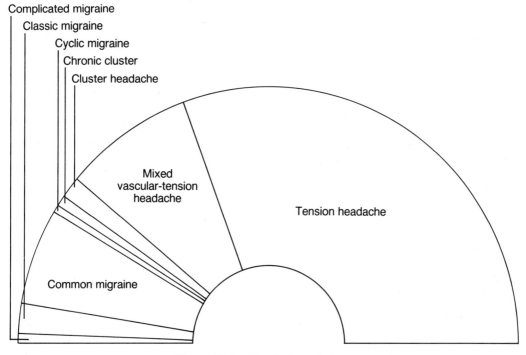

Figure 40.2.   Headache spectrum.

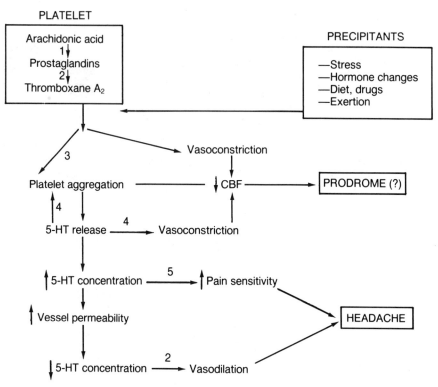

Figure 40.3. Possible migraine mechanisms (*1*) blocked by aspirin, nonsteroidal antiinflammatory agents, glucocorticoids. (*2*) Blocked by propranolol, timolol, metoprolol, atenolol (?). (*3*) Blocked by amitriptyline, desipramine, imipramine, nortriptyline. (*4*) Blocked by cyproheptadine, ergotamine, methysergide. (*5*) Blocked by narcotic analgesics.

that regard, they are similar to migraine headaches. The pain is abrupt in onset, always on the same side behind the eye and relatively brief in duration. The pain progresses rapidly and often brings nasal congestion, tearing and a bloodshot appearance to the eye. The pain is pulsatile; the affected side of the face may perspire as the pain spreads to the temple or jaw. The attacks tend to occur regularly at the same time of day or night and produce intolerable pain. They commonly occur in the morning hours and may last from ½ to 2 hours. The term "cluster" comes from the peculiar pattern of headaches often occurring daily for 4 to 10 weeks; the attacks diminish rapidly and then cease altogether. The patient may remain headache-free (except for isolated headaches of other types) until the next cluster, often months or years later. Vasodilator drugs such as alcohol, nitroglycerin and amyl nitrite exacerbate the headache and may precipitate headache in a symptom-free individual.

Hypertension headache probably does occur

Table 40.6.
Headache Drugs That Disturb Platelet Function[a]

Amitriptyline (229)	Lithium (190)
Aspirin (230)	Methysergide (64)
Chlorpromazine (229)	Metoprolol (128)
Cyproheptadine (147)	Naproxen
Desipramine (229)	Nortriptyline (229)
Ergotamine (64)	Propranolol (125)
Glucocorticoids (230)	Timolol (128)
Ibuprofen	Tolfenamic acid
Imipramine (229)	Zomepirac
Indomethacin (230)	

[a] Numbers in parentheses are references.

in patients with diastolic blood pressures above 120 to 130 mm Hg (31). Below that level, however, there appears to be no correlation between blood pressure and headache (32–34). When headache does occur due to high blood pressure, it is said to occur in the morning upon arising and to subside during the day. In spite of the infrequency of this headache type, the importance of hypertension detection and control make it notable for pharmacists. Successful control of the hypertension will eliminate the headaches. In one study, all of the patients whose headaches did not subside with control of their blood pressures were found to have cervical spondylosis (31).

Menstrual headache is the term applied to headache associated with menstruation. As many as 55% of women who suffer from headaches notice an association between their headaches and menstruation (35), with vascular, tension and mixed headaches occurring approximately equally (36). The mechanism appears to be the falling plasma concentration of estrogen (37). There are a few reported cases of headache due to estrogen deficiency that have responded to hormone replacement (38). Headache related to oral contraceptive use is a companion issue that has been well studied. It is clear that estrogen-containing oral contraceptives do initiate or aggravate headache occurrence (39), and they cause the platelets of estrogen users to aggregate more readily (a possible cause of headache) (40). When estrogen therapy is stopped, headache frequency (41), severity (39) and platelet aggregability (40) decrease.

Occasionally, drugs can be the cause of headaches. These *drug-induced headaches* usually have a vascular mechanism. Vasodilators (e.g., alcohol, nitroglycerin) produce a vascular situation similar to that found in the headache phase of migraine. Adrenergic agents (e.g. amphetamine, fenfluramine) may cause headache by blood pressure elevation. Table 40.7 lists agents that may cause headache in a patient due to the presence or withdrawal of the drug. Included in the table are drugs which cause benign intracranial hypertension, a symptom of which is headache. Readers interested in drug-induced headache should consult a recent review (42).

THERAPY OF HEADACHE

The selection of therapy (Tables 40.8 and 40.9) is based on the characteristics of the headache gathered in the history: quality, duration, intensity, frequency and precipitating and ameliorating factors. Refinement of that therapy is based upon associated symptoms and specific patient characteristics. Discussion here primarily will concern drug therapy. Nevertheless, non-drug treatments that have been tried with success include, chiropractic,

Table 40.7.
Drugs Which May Cause Headaches[a]

Alcohol	Griseofulvin (204)
Amphetamine	Hydralazine
Amyl nitrite	Indomethacin
Arsenic poisoning	Isoniazid (212)
Barbiturates (204)	Isosorbide dinitrate
Bromocriptine (205)	Ketoprofen (217)
Caffeine (172)	Lead poisoning
Caffeine withdrawal	Loxapine (218)
(172)	Mazindol (219)
Cannabis (206)	Mefenamic acid
Carbachol (207)	Mercury, ammon-
Carmustine (207)	iated, topical (220)
Corticosteroid, oral	Nalidixic acid (221)
(208)	Naproxen (222)
Corticosteroid, with-	Nitrofurantoin (223)
drawal (209)	Nitroglycerin (203)
Corticosteroid, topical,	Oral contraceptives
withdrawal (210)	(39)
Digitalis (211)	Pentaerythritol tetra-
Dopamine (212)	nitrate
Ergotamine withdrawal	Phenylbutazone
(192)	Reserpine (153)
Erythrityl tetranitrate	Retinoic acid, oral
Estrogen	(224)
Estrogen withdrawal	Rifampin (225)
(213)	Tamoxifen (226)
Fenfluramine (214)	Tetracycline (227)
Flurazepam (215)	Theophylline (228)
Glutethimide with-	Vitamin A
drawal (216)	

[a] Numbers in parentheses are references.

yoga, acupuncture, physiotherapy, exercise, psychotherapy, hypnosis, relaxation, transcendental meditation, biofeedback and cryosurgery (43).

Tension Headache

While severe muscle contraction or tension may not be the actual mechanism of this headache type, teleological treatment with sedation, muscle relaxation and analgesics has proved the most successful. Non-drug treatments are becoming increasingly popular. Biofeedback therapy for headache has been the subject of two reviews (13, 44). Biofeedback has some effect in tension headache but no more than simple relaxation training. Drug therapy is divided into treatment of the acute attack and its prevention.

Acute Attack. Treatment depends on mild to moderate analgesics and sedatives (45, 46). Aspirin or acetaminophen can be useful if taken early in the headache. The use of these

Table 40.8.
Drugs for Acute Headache Attacks[a]

Drug	Disorder	Dose Range	Route	Serum Concentration (μg/ml)	$t_{1/2}$ (hr)	t_{max}	Side Effects	Ref.
Acetaminophen	Tension, Migraine, Cluster	325–975 mg/ha	PO	10–20	2	30–60 min	Rash	194
Aspirin	Tension, Migraine, Cluster	325–975 mg/ha	PO	150–300	0.25[b]	2 hr	gi	194
Codeine	Tension, Migraine, Cluster	30–120 mg/ha	PO		2.5	2 hr	gi, Constipation, sedation	194
Dihydroergotamine	Migraine, Cluster	0.5–1 mg/ha	IV	0.001–0.01	20	5 min	gi, Diarrhea, dizziness	66, 194
			IM	0.001–0.01		30 min		66,67,194
Ergotamine	Migraine, Cluster	2–6 mg/ha nte 10 mg/wk	SL	0.0005–0.001	21		gi, Diarrhea	66, 194
		0.36–1.8 mg/ha	INH		21		gi;	66, 78
		1–6 mg/ha nte 10 mg/wk	PO	0.0005–0.001	21	1–2 hr	gi, Diarrhea, ha	67, 194
		0.25–1 mg/ha	IM/SC	0.001–0.01	21	30 min	gi	67, 194
		1–6 mg/ha nte 10 mg/wk	PR	0.0001–0.001	21	1 hr	gi	67, 194
Indomethacin	Chronic Paroxysmal Hemicrania	75–150 mg/d	PO	0.5–3	2.5		gi, ha	194
Isometheptene compound	Tension, Migraine, Cluster	2–5 cap/ha	PO				Sedation, dizziness	92, 94
Methysergide	Cluster	3–8 mg/d	PO	0.009–0.06	10		gi, Sedation, inflammatory fibrosis	194, 195
Metoclopramide	Migraine	10–20 mg/ha	PO		4	40–120 min	Sedation, dry mouth	72, 73, 196
Prednisone	Cluster	10–80 mg/d 21d taper	PO		3.6		Cushing's syndrome	180–182, 194

[a] Abbreviations: cap, capsules; d, day; gi, gastritis, nausea; ha, headache; hr, hour(s); IM, intramuscular; INH, inhaler; IV, intravenous; min, minute(s); nte, not to exceed; PO, oral; PR, rectal; SC, subcutaneous; SL, sublingual; wk, week(s).
[b] $t_{1/2}$ for salicylic acid is dose-dependent, range = 2.4–19 hours.

Table 40.9.
Drugs Used to Prevent Headache[a]

Drug	Disorder	Dose Range (mg/d)	Serum Concentration	$t_{1/2}$ (hr)	t_{max}	Side Effects	Ref.
Amitriptyline	Tension Migraine	50–150	0.16–0.24 μg/ml	57		Sedation, dry mouth	194
Aspirin	Migraine	650				gi	97, 98
Atenolol	Migraine	100	~0.0013 μg/ml	6.3		Sedation	112, 194
Chlorpromazine	Cluster	70–700	0.03–0.35 μg/ml	30		Sedation, dry mouth	185, 194
Clonidine	Migraine	0.05–0.15	~0.001 μg/ml	8.5		Fatigue, constipation	
Cyproheptadine	Migraine Cluster	12–32				Sedation, weight gain	45
Ergonovine	Migraine	0.4–2			30 min	gi	45
Lithium	Cluster Cyclic migraine	900–1200	0.4–1.2 mEq/L	22	2–4 hr	Edema	180, 187, 194
Propranolol	Migraine	40–320	~0.02 μg/ml	3.9		Fatigue	45, 194
Timolol	Migraine	20				Fatigue	117, 194

[a] Abbreviations as in Table 40.8. PO administration for all drugs.

agents in combination with codeine is common and effective. A combination of acetaminophen, butalbital and caffeine (Fiorinal) also can be effective (45). Diazepam 15 mg daily was effective in 16 of 19 patients in one study (47). The use of zomepirac in tension headache has been reported. One study was inconclusive as to its effect in tension headache, although the 100-mg dose was superior to placebo (48). Two reports of the same patients showed the 100-mg dose to be superior to placebo in the first headache episode but statistically indistinguishable from the 50-mg dose and placebo in subsequent headaches (49, 50). Ibuprofen also has been used with some success (51). With all drug treatments of tension headaches, success can be increased with concomitant relaxation.

Prophylactic Therapy. While several agents may be effective in preventing tension headache, amitriptyline appears to be the drug of choice (52–54). Amitriptyline acts, at least peripherally by inhibiting the reuptake of serotonin released from presynaptic neuronal endplates. It is the most selective of the tricyclic antidepressants for serotonin reuptake inhibition (55). Amitriptyline is also the most sedative of the tricyclic antidepressants. For patients who cannot tolerate that side effect, even when dosed at bedtime, desipramine or imipramine seem to be reasonable alterna-

tives, despite the selectivity of desipramine for norepinephrine reuptake inhibition (54, 56). When used alone in mixed headache, amitriptyline was more effective than propranolol or biofeedback (57). Amitriptyline plus propranolol was more effective than any single treatment mode and amitriptyline plus propranolol plus biofeedback was the most successful (57). The combination of amitriptyline and propranolol produced no adverse reactions in the 141 patients studied (57). The safety of this combination has been reported before (58). Doxepin in one study decreased headache severity and analgesic use without decreasing the number of headaches (59). Side effects were prominent, but tolerable.

Migraine Headache

Vascular headaches are the most easily recognized due to their usual pulsatile character. They often are very severe, occur during times of relaxation after stress, are aggravated by alcohol and do not respond readily to the usual doses of nonprescription analgesics. Into this group fall migraine, cluster and mixed headaches, which generally are treated in two ways. The first approach is to treat each headache with specific therapy when it threatens. When headaches occur with sufficient frequency, the second approach is to consider prophylactic treatment to prevent them. In general, treatment which decreases the frequency of headaches also decreases the duration and intensity of those headaches that do occur.

Acute Attack. Because the pain is due partly to vasodilation, the migraine headache usually will respond to vasoconstrictor *ergot drugs*, if given in adequate dose (60). Almost half of patients will have their headaches abolished and another third report partial relief (61). This may occur without an alteration in cerebral blood flow (62, 63). Ergots also may affect platelet aggregation (64). If the ergot is given too late during the attack, it may have little or no effect. There is some thought that by giving a vasconstrictor drug during the prodrome of classical migraine, cerebral ischemia might be made worse. This is of theoretical consequence, but may not be significant in practice.

Ergot products are available for every route of administration: oral, sublingual, inhalation, intramuscular, intravenous and rectal. Oral tablets are the slowest acting, but they are convenient and may be sufficient for some patients. After a single oral dose, the time to peak plasma concentration is approximately 2 hours (65–68). This is not altered by the addition of caffeine to the product but the absorption is increased, perhaps by the formation of soluble ergot complexes (69), and the peak plasma ergotamine concentration can be increased by one third (65). Ergotamine concentrations in cerebrospinal fluid parallel those in plasma (67). The elimination half-life is approximately 21 hours (66) but, because of the generally low concentrations, ergotamine usually is undetectable in plasma 24 hours after a 2-mg dose. Paradoxically, the plasma levels may increase after that (with no added doses) and may surpass the initial peak in 48 hours (67). This unexplained prolonged presence of the drug in plasma is corroborated by decreases in peripheral systolic blood pressure for at least a day after a single intravenous dose of ergotamine (70). The long plasma half-life and duration of activity explain the occurrence of chronic ergotism with relatively low doses (see below).

For the headache that is accompanied by nausea and vomiting, oral medication may not be suitable; ergots are all irritating to the stomach and can produce nausea and gastric distress. Ergotamine tartrate is worse in this regard than ergonovine maleate, but ergotamine also is more effective against the headache.

Parenteral administration does not solve this problem because nausea is even more pronounced with injectable drugs. To combat the nausea of migraine and of ergot preparations, antiemetic agents have been used. Unfortunately, agents which have anticholinergic properties slow gastric emptying, prolong the nausea and inhibit drug absorption. Recently, metoclopramide has been released for use in the United States. The drug enhances gastrointestinal motility and appears to be the antiemetic of choice in migraine (71). It can relieve nausea in up to 86% of patients with migraine (72) and enhances the effect of ergotamine (73). The usual oral dose is 20 mg. One nonsteroidal antiinflammatory agent, tolfenamic acid, has been shown as effective as ergotamine for the acute migraine attack (74). It has the advantage of producing less gastrointestinal distress. A trial of a similar agent, flufenamic acid, gave inconclusive results (75) and indomethacin was no better than placebo (76).

Oral ergotamine tartrate is available in 1-mg tablets and, more commonly, in combination with other agents designed to combat the headache or associated symptoms. The usual regimen is to start with 1 to 2 mg at the first hint of a headache and follow with additional 1-mg doses half-hourly to a maximum of 6 mg per attack or 10 mg per week. The most common ingredient added to ergotamine is caffeine, for its additional vasoconstrictive effect and its effect to increase gastrointestinal absorption of ergotamine (65). Also combined are belladonna alkaloids or antiemetic agents to treat the nausea that commonly accompanies severe headache (or which may be due to the ergot). Hypnotic agents may be included to induce relaxation or sleep, which often can alleviate the headache. The combination oral products usually are dosed according to their ergotamine content as described above.

Another common route of administration for ergotamine in the acute attack is sublingual. The drug can enter by this route and be distributed first to the cerebral circulation without dilution into the general circulation and metabolism by the liver. Patients should be instructed to keep the sublingual tablet in place under the tongue and to avoid chewing movements that may stimulate salivation. A practical problem is the production of saliva caused by the presence of an object under the tongue. As the fluid accumulates, the patient will be tempted to swallow it. Some neurologists recommend spitting out the saliva rather than swallowing it. Ergotamine in the stomach is eratically absorbed and will contribute to the patient's nausea. Patients should keep the saliva in their mouths as long as possible, spreading it to all buccal surfaces with the tongue. The absorption of ergotamine through buccal surfaces is influenced by pH, but there seems to be little current application for that knowledge (77).

Ergotamine is also available in a metered pressurized inhaler for acute attacks (78). Forty-seven percent of attacks can be aborted or diminished with this product. Patients should understand how to use the device before it is needed. There is evidence that closing the mouth around the mouthpiece causes the drug to be impacted on the back of the throat and then swallowed (79). The intent of an inhaler is to introduce drugs into the pulmonary circulation and then into the cerebral blood. Buccal absorption from improper inhaler technique may be as effective, but swallowing the drug is not beneficial. The patient needs to be instructed to hold the inhaler close to the open mouth, to begin a deep inhalation after complete exhalation and to press the device to produce the puff once the flow of inward air is established. The patient should continue the inhalation to maximum capacity and hold it as long as possible. The breath may be released slowly through semiclosed lips. If no headache relief results within 5 min, the dose may be repeated. Further doses rarely give additional relief, but do produce nausea.

Rectal suppositories are not a particularly convenient dosage form for storage or use by patients, but this route of administration has advantages similar to the buccal route: rapid absorption and initial bypassage of the general circulation. When combined with caffeine, ergotamine is rapidly absorbed from a rectal suppository and plasma ergotamine concentrations peak at 1 hour (67). Plasma concentrations after rectal administration are slightly higher than those after oral administration. Suppositories prevent the gastric effect of ergotamine which cause nausea. The suppositories available are combination products with caffeine and ergotamine and a sedative or anticholinergic or analgesic included. The dosage regimen begins with an initial dose of one half suppository, followed at intervals by additional doses to a maximum.

Parenteral ergotamine and dihydroergotamine are available for intramuscular and subcutaneous administration. The ergotamine parenteral dose should be one fourth the oral dose to produce comparable plasma concentrations (66, 67). Dihydroergotamine produces less nausea than ergotamine and can be given IM in a 0.5- to 1-mg dose (66), repeated no more than twice.

The most important side effect of ergots is ischemia due to vasoconstriction (80, 81). Ergotism probably occurred historically as a result of ingestion of the natural product on contaminated grain. Chronic ergotism has been reported as early as the ninth century, again in the eleventh century and most recently in 1952 (82). Chronic ergotism may have been responsible for the Salem witchcraft trials in 1692 (83). Despite the common knowledge among health professionals of this side effect, and many reports in professional literature (82, 84–89) patients still develop toxicity due to inattentive monitoring by practitioners and overzealous treatment by pained patients. Chronic toxicity may develop, usually as increasing headache, in patients taking as little as 7 to 10 mg of ergotamine weekly. Nausea, malaise and cold extremities are other common signs. Central nervous system involvement occurs with high doses, producing confusion, drowsiness and hemiplegia (90). Conversely with low doses, subclinical ergotism in the form of low systolic blood pressures may occur (82). Severe vasospasm due to ergotism may require immediate reversal to avoid permanent damage or death. The most effective treatment appears to be with nitroprusside (91).

Isometheptene mucate is the other oral agent that may be useful in treating acute attacks of headache. The marketed product contains 65 mg of isometheptene (a sympathomimetic), dichloralphenazone 100 mg (a sedative) and acetaminophen 325 mg. It has been found to be more effective than acetaminophen alone in treating vascular headaches (92). When isometheptene is used alone, however, it is only slightly more effective than placebo (93). The sedative and analgesic components are definitely important to the combination product. The recommended dosage is 2 capsules at the start of a headache, followed by 1 capsule every hour until relief or up to 5 capsules within 12 hours. It may be most useful in patients intolerant to the side effects of ergot (94).

Even though the abortive therapy for migraine headaches primarily is based on the use of ergot derivatives, more than 80% of patients have had experience using *mild nonprescription analgesics* (43). Aspirin and acetaminophen are available to patients for self-medication and one or both have been tried by the time the patient reaches formal medical care and prescription drugs. While success with these drugs in severe headaches may be hampered by low patient expectations, their effectiveness may be surprising for several reasons. First, patients who suffer from severe headaches also may experience lesser head pain. Acetaminophen and aspirin can be effective against mild to moderate head pain. The attenuation of a moderate headache might be mistaken for great success against an anticipated severe migraine. Second, headache is only the most prominent of the several features of migraine, including the prodrome, nausea, vomiting and dizziness. Each feature contributes to the patient's discomfort. Aspirin may be as effective as ergotamine in the migraine without gastric upset (95). Conversely, the effect of aspirin is diminished by impaired absorption during the migraine (71). This is related to the severity of the headache, not the duration, and occurs even in the absence of nausea. It is due to decreased gastrointestinal motility and rate of gastric emptying (71). To combat this, coadministration of an antiemetic drug that can also increase gastrointestinal motility, metoclopramide, has been studied. While the drug has no analgesic effect of its own (72), it can potentiate the effect of aspirin (95), acetaminophen (72) and ergotamine (73). When administered with metoclopramide and diazepam, aspirin and acetaminophen seem to be equipotent and effective against common and classic migraine (96). Finally, patients may ingest aspirin, even unknowingly, in a huge number of products for a variety of complaints. Since the platelet effect of aspirin is permanent and continues until new platelets are manufactured, aspirin taken for other reasons may decrease headache frequency or effects caused by platelet hyperaggregability. Two studies have shown favorable results from using aspirin in migraine prophylaxis (97, 98).

Narcotic analgesics are often necessary to treat the severe migraine that has escaped prophylactic and abortive measures. Because of their adverse effect on motor function and mentation and because of their abuse potential, they should not be used for mild-to-moderate headaches or before abortive therapy has been tried. During prophylactic therapy, analgesics may inhibit the prophylactic effect (see below) (53). Nevertheless, many headache patients, perhaps as many as 70% (43), regularly use prescription analgesics for migraine attacks.

Within the central nervous system, pain is modulated by a dynamic endorphin-mediated analgesia system. In migraine, serum endorphin concentrations are normal during headache-free periods, slightly decreased during the headache, but significantly elevated by the end of the attack (99). Headache is thought to be an expresison of endorphin deficiency (100) and opiates stimulate endorphin production or bind to the endorphin receptor to ease pain. Codeine, 30 to 60 mg in combination with aspirin or acetaminophen, is a common analgesic for migraine. Propoxyphene combinations can be effective treatment of migraine (101), but dangerous side effects can occur (102).

Prophylactic Therapy. When headaches occur as frequently as once each week, preventative therapy should be considered. If the patient has been taking ergots for the acute attacks, the maximum safe weekly dose probably has been reached. Further, the headaches undoubtedly have become disruptive to the patient's life and predictable enough to warrant prevention. Prophylactic therapy can have a significant effect on the frequency and severity of headaches (103). It is in the area of preventative therapy that great progress has been made in drug treatment. There are now many unexpectedly effective agents which provide additional insight to the possible mechanisms of vascular headache.

β-Adrenergic blocking agents without intrinsic sympathomimetic activity are currently the most effective drugs to prevent migraine (57). While propranolol is the prototype and the most studied (104–116), atenolol (112) and timolol (117) have produced success. Other similar agents, i.e., alprenolol (118), oxprenolol (119), pindolol (119–121), acebutolol (122) and practolol (112), are not of consistent value. The property apparently associated with prophylaxis success is the lack of intrinsic sympathomimetic activity (123).

While the exact mechanism of action is not known, there are a number of general explanations. The β-blockade prevents the vasodilation which could aggravate migraine. The drugs also reduce platelet aggregation (124) and inhibit the lipolysis which might reduce prostaglandin synthesis. Recently, it has been shown that propranolol doses of 160 to 640 mg daily can inhibit thromboxane A_2 synthesis to prevent platelet aggregation (125). Further, d-propranolol (with only 2.5% of the β-blocking activity of racemic propranolol) is equally effective (125). This substantiates an earlier study showing the effectiveness of d-propranolol in preventing migraine (126). Propranolol is able to block thromboxane A_2 synthesis without blocking prostacyclin synthesis (127). Timolol and metoprolol appear to have the same inhibitory properties on thromboxane A_2 synthesis and platelet aggregation (128).

The effective daily dosage of propranolol is 60 to 320 mg, with therapy beginning low and increasing weekly until success, side effects or maximum dose. The propranolol regimen is usually four times daily, but the success of twice daily dosing in hypertension may suggest a trial of that regimen for headache prophylaxis. The usual precautions for the use of β-blocking agents in patients with diabetes mellitus, congestive heart failure and asthma must be observed. Two recent cases have associated complicated migraine (with permanent neurologic damage) with the use of propranolol (129, 130) and one case of neurologic deficit following propranolol dose reduction (131). There is one report of paradoxical headache due to combined propranolol-ergotamine vasoconstriction (132). Several other studies reported no such problem (106, 110, 111, 126).

Ergot preparations may be effective for migraine prophylaxis. Ergonovine is approved only for use against pospartum or post-abortive uterine bleeding and has a greater effect on uterine contraction than does ergotamine. The basis for the use of ergonovine in migraine has been the smaller degree of nausea and gastrointestinal distress (45). With time, the drug is well tolerated by most patients. It is logical to continue a patient taking chronic ergots for headache prevention if sporadic ergots worked against acute attacks. Patients begin taking one 0.2-mg tablet 3 times daily. They increase that dose in 3 to 4 days (as soon as they can tolerate the mild stomach distress) to 2 tablets, 3 times daily. The dose is increased every 3 to 4 days until the headaches subside or a maximum of 2.4 mg daily is reached. The contraindications for chronic ergot use are the same as for acute use. Patients should not use ergots if they have peripheral vascular disease, atherosclerosis, coronary artery disease, hypertension or are

pregnant. Patients with diabetic vascular disease should be watched closely.

Nonsteroidal antiinflammatory agents have been used to prevent migraine. Indomethacin, because of its success in other rare headache types, has been studied most often with mixed results. It is useful in a type of cluster headache (see below). Ketoprofen has been tried with moderate success (133). While patients with migraine preferred naproxen treatment to placebo in one study, more objective results were not found (134). Zomepirac and ibuprofen have been used for the treatment of tension headache (see above).

Methysergide maleate is an ergot derivative with very little vasoconstrictor activity. It is a serotonin antagonist. The drug can be effective in up to 65% of patients (135), but it has been less effective than propranolol (113). Its usefulness is limited by the occurrence of adverse effects in about 36% of patients (113). The most serious of these side effects is a reversible inflammatory fibrosis that can involve the kidneys, lungs, heart or penis. Fortunately, this effect can be minimized by scheduling patients for a 1-month drug-free period every 5 months. The drug must be tapered over 2 to 3 weeks to avoid rebound headaches. During that methysergide holiday, the patient should have access to abortive ergot drugs or begin another prophylatic agent. Dosage of methysergide is 2 mg, 3 to 4 times daily. If the headaches have not responded after 3 weeks of therapy, it is unlikely that they will.

Amitriptyline, a tricyclic antidepressant, can bring some relief to as many as 70% of patients (136–138). The drug, however, is generally more effective against tension or mixed headache. One survey found that 40% of patients had tried "tranquilizers and mood elevators" at some time against their migraines (43). The dose range is broad, 25 to 150 mg at bedtime, but most patients require 75 to 100 mg. Many patients have heard that amitriptyline is used to treat depression and may feel that success with this therapy is evidence of an underlying depression. Some patients have even refused to begin therapy with that argument. There are at least 2 studies that refute that the antimigraine effect is related to the drug's antidepressant effect (137, 138). The onset of headache relief is usually 10 days to 2 weeks, half of the time needed for antidepressant effect.

Clonidine has been well-studied for migraine prophylaxis with mixed results; the best studies failed to show significant, long-term effect against migraine (139–143). Nevertheless, a recent comparison found no statistically significant difference between clonidine and propranolol (144). The doses used have ranged from 0.1 to 0.2 mg daily.

Pizotifen has found wide success in preventing migraine in Europe but is not available in this country (116, 145). Pizotifen is a serotonin antagonist similar to, but more effective than, cyproheptadine (146). *Cyproheptadine* can prevent migraine, presumably by serotonin inhibition, but has limited use due to side effects such as sedation and increased appetite (146). It also inhibits platelet aggregation (147). *Phenelzine* is used occasionally, apparently for its monoamine oxidase (MAO) inhibitory effect, which prevents the drop in serum serotonin and the resulting vasodilation of the headache phase in migraine (148). Diet interactions and drug interactions make close monitoring mandatory. Other drugs that have been used successfully to prevent migraine are papaverine (149–151), heparin (152), reserpine (153) (despite its indictment as a frequent precipitant of migraine), chlorpromazine (12), flunarizine (154), lisuride (155, 156), tryptophan (157, 158), Divascan (159), phenytoin (160, 161), primidone (161), bromocriptine (162), and chenodeoxycholic acid (163). Hydroxytryptophan has had positive (157, 164) and negative (165) results.

Drugs that have been studied with adverse effect or no effect on migraine prophylaxis include cimetidine (166, 167), lithium (168) and carbamazepine (169).

Diet Therapy. Diet has long been thought to trigger or contribute to the vascular headaches of some patients. Foods included here are those that contain nitrites (170) and nitrates, which are used to impart a smoked flavor or pink color: smoked fish, bacon and ham, corned beef and pastrami, and sausages (bologna, frankfurters, salami and pepperoni). Monosodium glutamate can act as a vasodilator and produce headache after consumption of Asian-style food (171), instant soups and gravies, some dry-roasted nuts and potato chips, gourmet seasonings and TV dinners. Caffeine can cause headaches and is found in coffee, tea, chocolate and cola drinks (172). Tyramine-induced headache has been controversial, but a recent literature review suggests that some patients do have headaches precipitated by tyramine and can be helped by avoidance of tyramine (173). Because of similarities between dietary migraine and food allergy, the role of allergy in migraine has been investigated (174). Elevated serum concentrations of immunglobulins pertinent to atopy are found no more often in patients with migraine, cluster or tension headaches than in patients without such chronic headaches. Nevertheless, food allergy may play a role in the headaches of certain patients (175). One apparent food precipitant of migraine, ice cream, actually produces headache by its cold temperature on the roof of the patient's mouth (176). Patient's may be asked to try a diet free of any or all of these things in order to rid themselves of the headache (175, 177). Finding the cause and eliminating it would be much simpler and less expensive than chronic medication.

Cluster Headache

Because of their pulsatile nature and rarity in the population, cluster headaches often are treated in a manner similar to migraine. There may be some overlap (178) but, generally, they are distinct headaches with a response to certain drugs that is very different than the response of migraine (179). A current review of therapy finds some antimigraine treatments to be effective, but several newer treatments appear to benefit cluster headache specifically. Drug treatment is divided into acute and preventative therapies.

Acute Attack. Ergotamine is the drug of choice for acute cluster headache (180). It is dosed as for migraine. The use of glucocorticoids to abort clusters appears to be very successful (180–182). Seventy percent of patients can show marked improvement given doses of 40 mg daily, tapered over 21 days (180). Some patients may even respond to a single 30-mg dose (181). Other useful agents include oxygen inhalation (183, 184), chlorpromazine (185), isometheptene (184) and indomethacin (1986). Narcotic analgesics also are useful.

Prophylactic Therapy. Currently lithium carbonate, 900 to 1200 mg daily, is the most useful agent (180, 187). It can be effective both for chronic and episodic clusters (188) and against a similar disorder, cyclic migraine (189). The effect may be due to the drug's effect on platelet count, platelet serotonin or platelet histamine concentrations (190). The drug can be effective in patients who are not depressed, which speaks against "antidepression" as its mechanism of action (188).

Other drugs useful for prevention of attacks

are methysergide (180), prednisone (181), ergotamine (184), cyproheptadine (183), indomethacin (183) and propranolol (183).

DRUG DEPENDENCE

It is reasonable to try to treat headaches with as specific a therapy as possible. This generally suggests the use of vasoactive agents for vascular headache and muscle relaxants or removal of stress for muscle contraction headaches. Among persons who treat headache patients there is a desire to avoid narcotic analgesics when they are not required because they generally treat the symptom, not the cause, and they are drugs of potential abuse. Headache patients initially have the most legitimate of needs for analgesic drugs, but it is not surprising that a high (35%) proportion of them may use more drugs than recommended (191). What may be more surprising is the finding that ergots (192) and propranolol (193) also may be overused by patients with severe headache.

A provocative study has been done in 200 patients with chronic tension headache (53). Patients were treated with or without amitriptyline prophylaxis and, within those two groups, with or without analgesics. At the end of the 1-month study, headaches were most improved in the group that received amitriptyline without analgesics. The second best response was in the no amitriptyline, no analgesic group. Then came the amitriptyline plus analgesic group and, finally, the analgesics only group. The results, of course, speak well for the effectiveness of amitriptyline, but two other points are important. First, the restriction of all analgesics improved headache indices in all patients, with or without amitriptyline. This would suggest that chronic analgesic use somehow sustains the chronic occurrence of headache (not unlike the situation wherein increased headache is the most common symptom of chronic ergot abuse). Second, the result that patients taking both amitriptyline and analgesics did less well than those taking amitriptyline alone suggests that analgesic use may have inhibited the prophylactic effect of the amitriptyline. The lesson here is important.

Analgesic use for the acute sporadic headache can be warranted. Patients should have access to analgesics that can control the headache that eludes prophylaxis and surmounts abortive therapy. In contrast, chronic analgesic use (analgesic abuse) can be dependence-forming, can support the chronic pain syndrome and can antagonize the effect of prophylactic drugs.

The fact remains that headache pain is a tremendous incentive for the overuse of effective medication. Despite our efforts, patients will continue to protect themselves from pain with increasing doses of analgesic without realizing their own perpetration of the chronic pain syndrome.

References

1. Nikiforow R, Hokkanen E: An epidemiological study of headache in an urban and a rural population in Northern Finland. *Headache* 18:137–145, 1978.
2. Ekbom K, Ahlborg B, Schele R: Prevalence of migraine and cluster headache in Swedish men of 18. *Headache* 18:9–19, 1978.
3. Bass M: The pharmacist as a provider of primary care. *Can Med Assoc J* 112:60–64, 1975.
4. Porter S: Your money: do-it-yourself medical care. San Francisco *Chronicle*, April 20, 1982.
5. Adams RD, Victor M: *Principles of Neurology*, ed 2. New York: McGraw-Hill, 1980.
6. Larson EB, Omenn GS, Lewis H: Diagnostic evaluation of headache: impact of computerized tomography and cost-effectiveness. *JAMA* 243:359–362, 1980.
7. Ad Hoc Committee on Classification of Headache: Classification of headache. *JAMA* 179: 717–718, 1962.
8. Greenfield S, Komaroff AL, Anderson H: A headache protocol for nurses. *Arch Intern Med* 136:1111–1116, 1976.
9. Diehr P, Wood RW, Barr V, et al: Acute headaches: presenting symptoms and diagnostic rules to identify patients with tension and migraine headache. *J Chronic Dis* 34:147–158, 1981.
10. Medina JL, Diamond S: Cyclical migraine. *Arch Neurol* 38:343–344, 1981.
11. Nappi G, Bono G: Headaches and transient cerebral ischemia. *Adv Neurol* 33:41–44, 1982.
12. Caviness VS, O'Brien P: Headache. *N Engl J Med* 302:446–450, 1980.
13. Nuechterlein KH, Holroyd JC: Biofeedback in the treatment of tension headache: current status. *Arch Gen Psychiatry* 37:866–873, 1980.
14. Olesen J, Larsen B, Lauritzen M: Focal hypersemia followed by spreading oligemia and impaired activation of rCBF in classic migraine. *Ann Neurol* 9:344–352, 1981.
15. Olesen J, Tfelt-Hansen P, Henriksen L, et al: The common migraine attack may not be initiated by cerebral ischaemia. *Lancet* 2:438–440, 1981.
16. Graham JR: Migraine headache: diagnosis and management. *Headache* 19:133–141, 1979.
17. Russell RWR, Bharucha N: The recognition and prevention of border zone cerebral ischaemia during cardiac surgery. *Q J Med* 47:303–323, 1978.

18. Kupersmith MJ, Hass WK, Chase NE: Isoproterenol treatment of visual symptoms in migraine. *Stroke* 10:299–305, 1979.
19. Gawel MJ, Rose FC: Platelet function in migraineurs. *Adv Neurol* 33:237–242, 1982.
20. Lance JW, Anthony M, Hinterberger H: The control of cranial arteries by humoral mechanisms and its relation to the migraine syndrome. *Headache* 7:93–102, 1967.
21. Hilton BP, Cummings JN: 5-Hydroxytryptamine levels and platelet aggregation responses in subjects with acute migraine headache. *J Neurol Neurosurg Psychiatr* 35:505–509, 1972.
22. Couch JR, Hassanein RS: Platelet aggregability in migraine. *Neurology* 27:843–848, 1977.
23. Kalendovsky Z, Austin JH: "Complicated migraine": its association with increased platelet aggregability and abnormal plasma coagulation factors. *Headache* 15:18–35, 1975.
24. Ryan RE Sr, Ryan RE Jr: The use of platelet inhibitors in migraine. *Adv Neurol* 33:247–252, 1982.
25. Curzon G, Barrie M, Wilkinson MIP: Relationship between headache and amine changes after administration of reserpine to migrainous patients. *J Neurol Neurosurg Psychiatry* 32:555–561, 1979.
26. Ghose K, Coppen A, Carroll JD: Intravenous tyramine response in migraine before and during treatment with indoramin. *Br Med J* 1:1191–1193, 1977.
27. Dalsgaard-Nielsen T, Genefke IK: Serotonin (5-hydroxytryptamine) release and uptake in platelets from healthy persons and migrainous patients in attack-free intervals. *Headache* 14:26–32, 1974.
28. Deshmukh SV, Meyer JS: Cyclic changes in platelet dynamics and the pathogenesis and propylaxis of migraine. *Headache* 17:101–108, 1977.
29. Anthony M, Hinterberger H, Lance JW: The possible relationship of serotonin in the migraine syndrome. *Res Clin Stud Headache* 2:29–59, 1969.
30. Sicuteri F, Fanciullaci M, Franchi G, et al: Serotonin-bradykinin potentiation of the pain perception in man. *Life Sci* 4:309–316, 1965.
31. Badran RHA, Weir RJ, McGuiness JB: Hypertension and headache. *Scott Med J* 15:48–51, 1970.
32. Waters WE: Headache and blood pressure in the community. *Br Med J* 1:142–143, 1971.
33. Weiss NS: Relation of high blood pressure to headache, epistaxis, and other selected symptoms. *N Engl J Med* 287:631–633, 1972.
34. Bauer GE: Hypertension and headache. *Aust NZ J Med* 6:492–497, 1976.
35. Nattero G: Menstrual headache. *Adv Neurol* 33:215–226, 1982.
36. Kashiwagi T, McClure JN Jr, Wetzel RD: The menstrual cycle and headache type. *Headache* 12:103–104, 1972.
37. Somerville BW: The influence of progesterone and estradiol upon migraine. *Headache* 12:93–102, 1972.
38. Chaudhuri TK, Chaudhuri ST: Estrogen therapy for migraine. *Headache* 15:139–141, 1975.
39. Dalton K: Migraine and oral contraceptives. *Headache* 15:247–251, 1976.
40. Hanington E, Jones RJ, Amess JAL: Platelet aggregation in response to 5-HT in migraine patients taking oral contraceptives. *Lancet* 1:967–968, 1982.
41. Kudrow L: The relationship of headache frequency to hormone use in migraine. *Headache* 15:36–40, 1975.
42. Allain HJ, Weintraub M: Drug induced headache. *Rational Drug Ther* 14/7:1–6, 1980.
43. Parnell P, Cooperstock R: Tranquilizers and mood elevators in the treatment of migraine: an analysis of the migraine foundation questionnaire. *Headache* 19:78–89, 1979.
44. Jessup BA, Neufeld RWJ, Merskey H: Biofeedback therapy for headache and other pain: an evaluative review. *Pain* 7:225–270, 1979.
45. Raskin NH, Appenzeller O: *Headache.* Philadelphia: W. B. Saunders, 1980.
46. Ziegler DK: Tension headache. *Med Clin North Am* 62:495–505, 1978.
47. Weber MB: The treatment of muscle contraction headaches with diazepam. *Curr Ther Res* 15:210–216, 1973.
48. Ryan RE Sr, Ryan RE Jr: Symptomatic treatment of tension headache. *Ear Nose Throat J* 58:29–34, 1979.
49. Diamond S: Zomepirac in the symptomatic treatment of muscle contraction headache. *J Clin Pharmacol* 20:298–302, 1980.
50. Diamond S, Medina JL: A double-blind study of zomepirac sodium and placebo in the treatment of muscle contraction headache. *Headache* 21:45–48, 1981.
51. Ryan RE Sr: Motrin—a new agent for the symptomatic treatment of muscle contraction headache. *Headache* 16:280–283, 1977.
52. Diamond S, Baltes BJ: Chronic tension headache with amitriptyline—a double blind study. *Headache* 11:110–116, 1971.
53. Kudrow L: Paradoxical effects of frequent analgesic use. *Adv Neurol* 33:335–341, 1982.
54. Lance JW, Curran DA: Treatment of chronic tension headache. *Lancet* 1:1236–1239, 1964.
55. Maas JW: Clinical and biochemical heterogeneity of depressive disorders. *Ann Intern Med* 88:556–563, 1978.
56. Tyler GS, McNeely HE, Dick ML: Treatment of posttraumatic headache with amitriptyline. *Headache* 20:213–216, 1980.
57. Mathew NT: Prophylaxis of migraine and mixed headache. A randomized controlled study. *Headache* 21:105–109, 1981.
58. Dexter JD, Byer JA, Slaughter JR: The concomitant use of amitriptyline and propranolol in intractable headache. *Headache* 20:157, 1980.
59. Morland TJ, Storli OV, Mogstad TE: Doxepin in the prophylactic treatment of mixed "vascular" and tension headache. *Headache* 19:382–383, 1979.
60. Edmeads J: Management of the acute attack of migraine. *Headache* 13:91–95, 1973.
61. Selby G, Lance JW: Observations on 500 cases of migraine and allied vascular headache. *J Neurol Neurosurg Psychiatry* 23:23–32, 1960.
62. Simard D, Paulson OB: Cerebral vasomotor pa-

ralysis during migraine attack. *Arch Neurol* 29:207–209, 1973.

63. Hachinski V, Norris JW, Edmeads J, et al: Ergotamine and cerebral blood flow. *Stroke* 9:594–596, 1978.

64. Hilton BP, Zilkha KJ: Effects of ergotamine and methysergide in blood platelet aggregation responses of migrainous subjects. *J Neurol Neurosurg Psychiatry* 37:593–597, 1974.

65. Schmidt R, Fanchamps A: Effect of caffeine on intestinal absorption of ergotamine in man. *Eur J Clin Pharmacol* 7:213–216, 1974.

66. Aellig WH, Nuesch E: Comparative pharmacokinetic investigations with tritium-labeled ergot alkaloids after oral and intravenous administration in man. *Int J Clin Pharmacol* 15:106–112, 1977.

67. Ala-Hurula V, Myllyla VV, Arvela P, et al: Systemic availability of ergotamine tartrate after oral, rectal and intramuscular administration. *Eur J Clin Pharmacol* 15:51–55, 1979.

68. Ala-Hurula V, Myllyla VV, Arvela P, et al: Systemic availability of ergotamine tartrate after three successive doses and during continous medication. *Eur J Clin Pharmacol* 16:355–360, 1979.

69. Zoglio MA, Maulding HV Jr, Windheuser JJ: Complexes of ergot alkaloids and derivatives; I. The interaction of caffeine with ergotamine tartrate in aqueous solution. *J Pharm Sci* 58:222–225, 1969.

70. Tfelt-Hansen P, Eickhoff JH, Olesen J: The effect of single dose ergotamine tartrate on peripheral arteries in migraine patients: methodological aspects and time effect curve. *Acta Pharmacol Toxicol* 47:151–156, 1980.

71. Volans GN: Migraine and drug absorption. *Clin Pharmacokinet* 3:313–318, 1978.

72. Tfelt-Hansen P, Olesen J, Aebelholt-Krabbe A, et al: A double blind study of metoclopramide in the treatment of migraine attacks. *J Neurol Neurosurg Psychiatry* 43:369–371, 1980.

73. Hakkarainen H, Allonne H: Ergotamine vs. metoclopramide vs. their combination in acute migraine attacks. *Headache* 22:10–12, 1982.

74. Hakkarainen H, Vapaatalo H, Gothoni G, et al: Tolfenamic acid is as effective as ergotamine during migraine attacks. *Lancet* 2:326–328, 1979.

75. Vardi V, Rabey IM, Streifler M, et al: Migraine attacks: alleviation by an inhibitor of prostaglandin synthesis and action. *Neurology* 26: 447–450, 1976.

76. Anthony M, Lance JW: Indomethacin in migraine. *Med J Aust* 1:56–57, 1968.

77. Sutherland JM, Hooper WD, Eadie MJ, et al: Buccal absorption of ergotamine. *J Neurol Neurosurg Psychiatry* 37:1116–1120, 1974.

78. Crooks J, Stephen SA, Brass W: Clinical trial of inhaled ergotamine tartrate in migraine. *Br Med J* 1:221–224, 1964.

79. Connolly CK: Method of using pressurized aerosols. *Br Med J* 3:21, 1975.

80. Robb LG: Severe vasospasm following ergot administration. *West J Med* 123:231–235, 1975.

81. Merhoff GC, Porter JM: Ergot intoxication: historical review and description of unusual clin-

ical manifestations. *Ann Surg* 180:773–779, 1974.

82. Dige-Petersen H, Lassen NA, Noer I, et al: Subclinical ergotism. *Lancet* 2:65–66, 1977.

83. Caporael LR: Ergotism: the satan loosed in Salem? *Science* 192:21–26, 1976.

84. Hokkanen E, Waltimo O, Kallanranta T: Toxic effects of ergotamine used for migraine. *Headache* 18:95–98, 1978.

85. Andersson PG: Ergotamine headache. *Headache* 15:118–121, 1975.

86. Wolpaw JR, Brottem JL, Martin HL: Tongue necrosis attributed to ergotamine in temporal arteritis. *JAMA* 225:514–515, 1973.

87. Rowsell AR, Neylan C, Wilkinsson M: Ergotamine induced headaches in migrainous patients. *Headache* 13:65–67, 1973.

88. Ala-Hurula V, Myllyla VV, Hokkanen E, et al: Tolfenamic acid and ergotamine abuse. *Headache* 21:240–242, 1981.

89. Evans PJD, Lloyd JW, Peet KMS: Antonomic dysaesthesia due to ergot toxicity. *Br Med J* 281:1621, 1980.

90. Senter HJ, Lieberman AN, Pinto R: Cerebral manifestations of ergotism. *Stroke* 7:88–92, 1976.

91. Andersen PK, Christensen KN, Hole P, et al: Sodium nitroprusside and epidural blockade in the treatment of ergotism. *N Engl J Med* 296:1271–1273, 1977.

92. Diamond S: Treatment of migraine with isometheptene, acetaminophen, and dichloralphenazone combination: a double-blind, crossover trial. *Headache* 15:282–287, 1976.

93. Diamond S, Medina JL: Isometheptene—a nonergot drug in the treatment of migraine. *Headache* 15:211–213, 1975.

94. Yuill GM, Swinburn WR, Liversedge LA: A double-blind crossover trial of isometheptene mucate compound and ergotamine in migraine. *Br J Clin Pract* 26:76–79, 1972.

95. Parantainen J, Jakkarainen H, Vapaatalo H, et al: Prostaglandin inhibitors and gastric factors in migraine. *Lancet* 1:832–833, 1980.

96. Tfelt-Hansen P, Olesen J: Paracetamol (acetaminophen) versus acetylsalicylic acid in migraine. *Eur Neurol* 19:163–165, 1980.

97. O'Neill BP, Mann JD: Aspirin prophylaxis in migraine. *Lancet* 2:1179–1181, 1978.

98. Masel BE, Chesson AL, Peters BH, et al: Platelet antagonists in migraine prophylaxis: a clinical trial using aspirin and dipyridamole. *Headache* 20:13–18, 1980.

99. Della Bella D, Carenzi A, Casacci F, et al: Endorphins in the pathogenesis of headache. *Adv Neurol* 33:75–79, 1982.

100. Sicuteri F: Natural opioids in migraine. *Adv Neurol* 33:65–74, 1982.

101. Hakkarainen H, Quiding H, Stockman O: Mild analgesics as an alternative to ergotamine in migraine: a comparative trial with acetylsalicylic acid, ergotamine tartrate, and a dextropropoxyphene compound. *J Clin Pharmacol* 20:590–595, 1980.

102. Editorial: Dangers of propoxyphene. *Br Med J* 1:668, 1977.

103. Raskin NH, Schwartz RK: Interval therapy of

migraine: long-term results. *Headache* 20:336–340, 1980.

104. Weber RB, Reinmuth OM: The treatment of migraine with propanolol. *Neurology* 21:404–405, 1971.

105. Malvea BP, Gwon N, Graham JR: Propranolol prophylaxis in migraine. *Headache* 12:163–167, 1973.

106. Brogesen SE, Lanng-Nelson J, Moller LE: Prophylaxis of migraine with propranolol. *Acta Neurol Scand* 50:651–656, 1974.

107. Wideroe T, Vigander T: Propranolol in the treatment of migraine. *Br Med J* 2:699–701, 1974.

108. Ludvigsson J: Propranolol used in prophylaxis of migraine in children. *Acta Neurol Scand* 50:109–115, 1974.

109. Nair KG: A pilot study of the value of propranolol in migraine. *Postgrad Med J* 21:111–113, 1975.

110. Diamond S, Medina JL: Double blind study of propranolol for migraine prophylaxis. *Headache* 16:24–27, 1976.

111. Forsmann B, Henriksson KG, Johannsson V, et al: Propranolol for migraine prophylaxis. *Headache* 16:238–245, 1976.

112. Stensrud P, Sjaastad O: Comparative trial of Tenormin (atenolol) and Inderal (propranolol) in migraine. *Headache* 20:204–207, 1980.

113. Behan PO, Reid M. Propranolol in the treatment of migraine. *Practitioner* 224:201–204, 1980.

114. Bekes M, Matos L, Rausch J, et al: Treatment of migraine with propranolol. *Lancet* 2:980, 1968.

115. Wykes P: The treatment of angina pectoris with coexistant migraine. *Practitioner* 200:702–704, 1968.

116. Forssman B, Henriksson KG, Kihlstrand S: A comparison between BC-105 and methysergide in prophylaxis of migraine. *Acta Neurol Scand* 48:204–212, 1972.

117. Briggs RS, Millac PA: Timolol in migraine prophylaxis. *Headache* 19:379–381, 1979.

118. Ekbom K: Alprenolol for migraine prophylaxis. *Headache* 15:129–132, 1975.

119. Ekbom K, Zetterman M: Oxprenolol in the treatment of migraine. *Acta Neurol Scand* 56:181–184, 1977.

120. Sjaastad O, Stensrud P: Clinical trial of a beta-receptor blocking agent (LB46) in migraine prophylaxis. *Acta Neurol Scand* 48:124–128, 1972.

121. Ekbom K, Lundberg PO: Clinical trial of LB-46 an adrenergic beta-receptor blocking agent in migraine prophylaxis. *Headache* 12:15–17, 1972.

122. Nanda RN, Johnson RH, Gray J, et al: A double blind trial of acebutolol for migraine prophylaxis. *Headache* 18:20–22, 1978.

123. Fozard JR: Basic mechanisms of antimigraine drugs. *Adv Neurol* 33:295–307, 1982.

124. Weksler BB, Gillick M, Pink J: Effect of propranolol on platelet function. *Blood* 49:185–196, 1977.

125. Campbell WB, Johnson AR, Callahan KS, et al: Antiplatelet activity of beta-adrenergic antagonists: inhibition of thromboxane synthesis and platelet aggregation in patients receiving long-term propranolol treatment. *Lancet* 2:1382–1384, 1981.

126. Stensrud P, Sjaastad O: Short-term clinical trial of propranolol in racemic form (Inderal), d-propranolol and placebo in migraine. *Acta Neurol Scand* 53:229–232, 1976.

127. Callahan KS, Campbell WB, Johnson AR: Antiplatelet activity of propranolol: interaction with PGI_2 and endothelial cells. *Fed Proc* 39:392, 1980.

128. Campbell WB, Callahan KS, Johnson AR, et al: Mechanism of the antiplatelet activity of the beta-adrenergic antagonists. *Int J Clin Pharmacol* (in press).

129. Prendes JL: Considerations on the use of propranolol in complicated migraine. *Headache* 20:93–95, 1980.

130. Gilbert GJ: An occurrence of complicated migraine during propranolol therapy. *Headache* 22:81–83, 1982.

131. Cohen RJ, Taylor JR: Persistent neurologic sequelae of migraine: a case report. *Neurology* 29:1175–1177, 1979.

132. Blank NK, Rieder MJ: Paradoxical response of propranolol in migraine. *Lancet* 2:1336, 1973.

133. Stensrud P, Sjaastad O: Clinical trial of a new antibradykinin, antiinflammatory drug, keto-profen (19.583 R.P.) in migraine prophylaxis. *Headache* 14:96–100, 1974.

134. Lindegaard K, Ovrelid L, Sjaastad O: Naproxen in the prevention of migraine attacks: a double-blind placebo-controlled cross-over study. *Headache* 20:96–98, 1980.

135. Graham JR: Methysergide for prevention of migraine: experience in five hundred patients over three years. *N Engl J Med* 270:67–72, 1964.

136. Couch JR, Ziegler DK, Hassanein RS: Amitriptyline in the prophylaxis of migraine: effectiveness and relationship of antimigraine and antidepressant effects. *Neurology* 26:121–127, 1976.

137. Couch JR, Hassanein RS: Amitriptyline in migraine prophylaxis. *Arch Neurol* 36:695–699, 1979.

138. Gomersall JD, Stuart A: Amitriptyline in migraine prophylaxis: changes in pattern of attacks during a controlled clinical trial. *J Neurol Neurosurg Psychiatry* 36:684–690, 1973.

139. Stensrud P, Sjaastad O: Clonidine (Catapresan)—double-blind study after long-term treatment with the drug in migraine. *Acta Neurol Scand* 53:233–236, 1976.

140. Mondrup K, Moller CE: Prophylactic treatment of migraine with clonidine: a controlled clinical trial. *Acta Neurol Scand* 56:405–412, 1977.

141. Boisen E, Deth S, Hubbe P, et al: Clonidine in the prophylaxis of migraine. *Acta Neurol Scand* 58:288–295, 1978.

142. Ryan RE, Ryan RE Jr: Clonidine—its use in migraine therapy. *Headache* 14:190–192, 1975.

143. Ryan RE, Diamond S, Ryan RE Jr: Double blind study of clonidine and placebo for the prophylactic treatment of migraine. *Headache* 14:202–206, 1975.

144. Kass B, Nestbold K: Propranolol (Inderal) and clonidine (Catapressan) in the prophylactic

treatment of migraine. *Acta Neurol Scand* 61:351–356, 1980.

145. Nelson RF: BC-105—a new prophylactic agent for migraine—four years' experience in seventy-five patients. *Headache* 13:96–103, 1973.

146. Lance JW, Anthony M, Somerville B: Comparative trial of serotonin antagonists in the management of migraine. *Br Med J* 2:327–330, 1970.

147. Ambrus JL, Ambrus CM, Thurber L: Study of platelet aggregtion in vivo; V. Effect of the antiserotonin agent cyproheptadine. *J Med* 8:317–320, 1977.

148. Anthony M, Lance JW: Monoamine oxidase inhibition in the treatment of migraine. *Arch Neurol* 21:263–268, 1969.

149. Poser CM: Papaverine in prophylactic treatment of migraine. *Lancet* 1:1290, 1974.

150. Vijayan N: Brief therapeutic report: papaverine prophylaxis of complicated migraine. *Headache* 17:159–162, 1977.

151. Sillanpaa M, Koponen M: Papaverine in the prophylaxis of migraine and other vascular headache in children. *Acta Paediatr Scand* 67:209–212, 1978.

152. Thonnard-Neumann E: Migraine therapy with heparin: pathophysiologic basis. *Headache* 16:284–292, 1977.

153. Nattero G, Lisino F, Brandi G, et al: Reserpine for migraine prophylaxis. *Headache* 15:279–281, 1976.

154. Louis P: A double-blind placebo-controlled prophylactic study of flunarizine (sibelium) in migraine. *Headache* 21:235–239, 1981.

155. Hermann WM, Horowski R, Dannehl K, et al: Clinical effectiveness of lisuride hydrogen maleate: a double-blind trial versus methylsergide. *Headache* 17:54–60, 1977.

156. Somerville BW, Herrmann WM: Migraine prophylaxis with lisuride hydrogen maleate—a double blind study of lisuride versus placebo. *Headache* 18:75–79, 1978.

157. Sicuteri F: The ingestion of serotonin precursors (L-5-hydroxytryptophan and L-tryptophan) improves migraine headache. *Headache* 13:19–22, 1973.

158. Kangasniemi P, Falck B, Lanvik VA, et al: Levotryptophan treatment in migraine. *Headache* 18:161–166, 1978.

159. Osterman PO: Divascan in migraine prophylaxis: open trial with three different doses. *Headache* 18:225–228, 1978.

160. Millichap JG: Recurrent headaches in 100 children: electroencephalographic abnormalities and response to phenytoin (Dilantin). *Child Brain* 4:95–105, 1978.

161. Swanson JW, Vick NA: Basilar artery migraine: 12 patients with an attack recorded electroencephalographically. *Neurology* 28:782–786, 1978.

162. Hockaday JM, Peet KMS, Hockaday TDR: Bromocriptine in migraine. *Headache* 16:109–114, 1976.

163. Levy VG, Nusinovici V, Rosner D, et al: Chenodeoxycholic acid in the prevention of migraine. *N Engl J Med* 298:630, 1978.

164. Bono G, Criscuoli M, Martignoni E, et al: Sero-

tonin precursors in migraine prophylaxis. *Adv Neurol* 33:357–363, 1982.

165. Mathew NT: 5-Hydroxy tryptophane in the prophylaxis of migraine: a double blind study. *Headache* 18:111, 1978.

166. Anthony M, Lord GDA, Lance JW: Controlled trials of cimetidine in migraine and cluster headache. *Headache* 18:261–264, 1978.

167. Nanda RN, Arthur GP, Jonson RH, et al: Cimetidine in the prophylaxis of migraine. *Acta Neurol Scand* 62:90–95, 1980.

168. Peatfield RC, Rose FC: Exacerbation of migraine by treatment with lithium. *Headache* 21:140–142, 1981.

169. Anthony M, Lance JW, Somerville B: A comparative trial of pindolol, clonidine, and carbamazepine in the interval therpay of migraine. *Med J Aust* 1:1343–1346, 1972.

170. Henderson WR, Raskin NH: "Hot dog" headache: individual susceptibility to nitrite. *Lancet* 2:1162–1163, 1972.

171. Schaumburg HH, Byck R, Gerstl R, et al: Monosodium L-glutamate: its pharmacology and role in the chinese restaurant syndrome. *Science* 163:826–828, 1969.

172. Anon: Headaches and coffee. *Br Med J* 2:284, 1977.

173. Kohlenberg RJ: Tyramine sensitivity in dietary migraine: a critical review. *Headache* 22:30–34, 1982.

174. Medina JL, Diamond S: Migraine an atopy. *Headache* 15:271–274, 1976.

175. Monro J, Brostoff J, Carini C, et al: Food allergy in migraine. *Lancet* 2:1–4, 1980.

176. Raskin NH, Knittle SC: Ice cream headache and orthostatic symptoms in patients with migraine. *Headache* 16:222–225, 1976.

177. Speer F: Allergy and migraine: a clinical study. *Headache* 11:63–67, 1971.

178. Medina JL, Diamond S: The clinical link between migraine and cluster headaches. *Arch Neurol* 34:470–472, 1977.

179. Ekbom K: Clinical aspects of cluster headache. *Headache* 13:176–180, 1974.

180. Kudrow L: Comparative results of prednisone, methysergide, and lithium therapy in cluster headache, in Greene R: *Current Concepts in Migraine Research*. New York: Raven Press, 1978, pp 159–163.

181. Jammes JL: The treatment of cluster headaches with prednisone. *Dis Nerv Syst* 36:375–376, 1975.

182. Couch JR, Ziegler DK: Prednisone therapy for cluster headache. *Headache* 18:219–221, 1978.

183. Kudrow L: Cluster headache: diagnosis and management. *Headache* 19:142–149, 1979.

184. Diamond S: Cluster headache: relation to and comparison with migraine. *Postgrad Med* 66:88–91, 1979.

185. Caviness VS, O'Brien P: Cluster headache: response to chlorpromazine. *Headache* 20:128–131, 1980.

186. Mathew NT: Indomethacin responsive headache syndromes. *Headache* 21:147–150, 1981.

187. Ekbom K: Lithium for cluster headache: review of the literature preliminary results of long-term treatment. *Headache* 21:132–139, 1981.

188. Mathew NT: Clinical subtypes of cluster headache and response to lithium therapy. *Headache* 18:26–30, 1978.
189. Medina JL: Cyclic migraine: a disorder responsive to lithium carbonate. *Psychosomatics* 23:625–637, 1982.
190. Medina JL, Fareed J, Diamond S: Lithium carbonate therapy for cluster headache: changes in number of platelets, and serotonin and histamine levels. *Arch Neurol* 37:559–563, 1980.
191. Medina JL, Diamond S: Drug dependency in patients with chronic headaches. *Headache* 17:12–14, 1977.
192. Lucas RN, Falkowski W: Ergotamine and methysergide abuse in patients with migraine. *Br J Psychiatry* 122:199–203, 1973.
193. Klimek A, Pozniak-Patewicz E: The phenomenon of "drug dependency" in the treatment of migraine with propranolol. *Headache* 17:75, 1977.
194. Gilman AG, Goodman LS, Gilman A (Eds): *The Pharmacological Basis of Therapeutics*, ed 6. New York: Macmillan, 1980.
195. Meier J, Schreier E: Human plasma levels of some anti-migraine drugs. *Headache* 16:96–104, 1976.
196. Anon: Metoclopramide (Reglan). *Med Lett* 24:67–69, 1982.
197. Philips C: Headache in general practice. *Headache* 16:322–329, 1977.
198. Jerrett WA: Headaches in general practice. *Practitioner* 222:549–555, 1979.
199. Friedman AP, vonStorch TJC, Merritt HH: Migraine and tension headaches. *Neurology* 4:773–788, 1954.
200. Goldstein M, Chen TC: The epidemiology of disabling headache. *Adv Neurol* 33:377–390, 1982.
201. Olesen J: Some clinical features of the acute migraine attack. An analysis of 750 patients. *Headache* 18:268–271, 1978.
202. Sutherland JM, Eadie MJ: Cluster headache. *Res Clin Stud Headache* 3:92–125, 1972.
203. Ekbom K: Nitroglycerine as a provocative agent in cluster headache. *Arch Neurol* 19:487–493, 1968.
204. Dukes MNG (Ed): *Side Effects of Drugs*. Amsterdam: Excerpta Medica, 1975, vol 8.
205. Farrar DJ, Pryor JS: The effect of bromocriptine in patients with benign prostatic hypertrophy. *Br J Urol* 48:73–75, 1976.
206. Ames F: A clinical and metabolic study of acute intoxication with *Cannabis sativa* and its role in the model psychoses. *J Ment Sci* 104:972–999, 1958.
207. Dukes NMG (Ed): *Side Effects of Drugs*. Amsterdam: Excerpta Medica, 1977, annual 1.
208. Cohn GA: Pseudotumor cerebri in children secondary to administration of adrenal steroids. *J Neurosurg* 20:784–786, 1963.
209. Dees SC, McKay HW: Occurrence of pseudotumor cerebri (benign intracranial hypertension) during treatment of children with asthma by adrenal steroids. *Pediatrics* 23:1143–1151, 1959.
210. Roussounis SH: Benign intracranial hypertension after withdrawal of topical steroids in an infant. *Br Med J* 2:564, 1976.
211. Batterman RC, Gutner LB: Hitherto undescribed neurological manifestations of digitalis toxicity. *Am Heart J* 36:582–586, 1948.
212. Dukes MNG (Ed): *Side Effects of Drugs*. Excerpta Medica, Amsterdam: 1978, annual 2.
213. Somerville BW: Estrogen-withdrawal migraine. *Neurology* 25:239–244, 1975.
214. Sicuteri F, Del Bene E, Anselmi B: Fenfluramine headache. *Headache* 16:185–188, 1976.
215. Greenblatt DJ, Shader RI, Koch-Weser J: Flurazepam hydrochloride, a benzodiazepine hypnotic. *Ann Intern Med* 83:237–241, 1975.
216. Good MI: Catatonialike symptomatology and withdrawal dyskinesias. *Am J Psychiatry* 133:1454–1456, 1976.
217. Fossgreen J: Ketoprofen. *Scand J Rheumatol Suppl* 14:7–32, 1976.
218. Chouinard G, Annable L, De Montigny C, et al: Loxapine succinate in the treatment of newly admitted schizophrenic patients. *Curr Ther Res* 21:73, 1977.
219. Evans ER, Wallace MG: A multicentre trial of mazindol (Teronac) in general practice in Ireland. *Curr Med Res Opin* 3:132–137, 1975.
220. Young E: Ammoniated mercury poisoning. *Br J Dermatol* 72:449–455, 1960.
221. Boreus LO, Sundstrom B: Intracranial hypertension in a child during treatment with nalidixic acid. *Br Med J* 2:744–745, 1967.
222. Smith RD: Experience with naproxen in a rheumatology practice. *Curr Ther Res* 21:415, 1977.
223. Mushet GR: Pseudotumor and nitrofurantoin therapy. *Arch Neurol* 34:257, 1977.
224. Stuttgen G: Oral vitamin A acid therapy. *Acta Dermatol Venereol* 55 (Suppl 74):174–179, 1975.
225. Mangi RJ: Reactions to rifampin. *N Engl J Med* 294:113, 1976.
226. Ward HWC: Anti-oestrogen therapy for breast cancer; a trial of tamoxifen at two dose levels. *Br Med J* 1:13–14, 1973.
227. Ohlrich GD, Ohlrich JG: Papilloedema in an adolescent due to tetracycline. *Med J Aust* 1:334–335, 1977.
228. Shapiro GG, Bamman J, Kanarek P, et al: The paradoxical effect of adrenergic and methylxanthine drugs in cystic fibrosis. *Pediatrics* 58:740–743, 1976.
229. Packham MA, Mustard JF: Platelet reactions. *Semin Hematol* 8:30–64, 1971.
230. Packham MA, Mustard JF: Clinical pharmacology of platelets. *Blood* 50:555–573, 1977.

CHAPTER 41

Attention Deficit Disorder

ROBERT W. PIEPHO, Ph.D., F.C.P.
DICK R. GOURLEY, Pharm.D.
JOHN W. HILL, Ph.D.

The term "attention deficit disorder" (ADD) is one of the many terms that have been used to describe a cognitive/ behavioral disorder of childhood. Other synonyms for this disorder include: minimal brain dysfunction, postencephalitic behavior disorder, hyperkinesis, hyperactivity, hyperkinetic syndrome, minimal brain damage, and minimal cerebral dysfunction (MCD). The term "ADD" will be used to describe this syndrome in this chapter, as it is the least objectionable term, since it implies no specific etiology, no pathognomonic signs, and no particular similarity in cause, course of the disease, or treatment (1, 2).

ADD was first described in the 1920s, when its occurrence was noted as a sequelae to von Economo's encephalitis. The recognition of the disorder has increased over the past 50 years, and ADD is now recognized as a disorder of considerable clinical importance. Although the diagnostic criteria are not always uniform, a fairly consistent prevalence rate for this disorder is usually noted between studies, viz. 5 to 10%. It is at least twice as common in males. In clinics that are involved with treatment of psychiatrically disturbed children of primary school age, a diagnosis of ADD is noted in approximately 50% of cases referred (1).

Although often described as a disease of childhood, some symptoms of ADD, such as impulsive personality traits, may persist into adult life (3). The "adult hyperkinetic" may be diagnosed via the use of the childhood medical history (meeting the criteria for diagnosis of ADD as defined in DSM-III) and the "Utah Criteria" described by Wender et al. (4).

PATHOGENESIS

The actual causative factors in ADD have remained a mystery since its initial definition in the 1920s. Most pathological studies have attempted to correlate prenatal or perinatal events with ADD. In a 1974 study by Hart and co-workers (5), 15% of children defined as scholastic underachievers were found to have perinatal complications that could have affected the CNS. Other studies have found a slightly higher incidence of prenatal or perinatal CNS insult, but there is still not a conclusive link between medical history and presence of ADD (6). Lesions or abnormalities that have been postulated to be responsible for the symptomatology of ADD are noted in Table 41.1.

DIAGNOSTIC AND CLINICAL FINDINGS

The clinical delineation of ADD is not well defined; many sets of symptomatology have been described in the scientific literature, but it is impossible to define a checklist of symptoms for a cerebral disorder that manifests itself in a heterogenous group of school age children. The actual diagnosis of ADD is usually made on the basis of medical and sociopsychological history. The historical material is generally obtained from the child's family members, teachers and counselors, since physical examination of the child is often of little use by itself. In one study, approximately 75% of children referred for ADD displayed no hyperactive behavior in the physician's office, indicating that the hyperactive child that is usually disruptive in the classroom setting will not manifest this behavior in the one-to-one setting. Although there is not a critical diagnostic test for ADD, it is important to attempt to rule out other syndromes such as borderline schizophrenia or reactive difficulties. The schizophrenic child will usually appear more fearful, will have pronounced phobic symptomatology, and will avoid social contact while exhibiting undue preoccupation with violent or sexual matters. The child with social or

Table 41.1.
Postulated Causative Factors in Attention Deficit Disorder (ADD) (5, 6, 8)

Prenatal or perinatal insult
Brain damage
Neurochemical lesions
Congenital physical anomalies
Low CNS arousal level
Genetic disorders
Exposure to environmental toxins

Table 41.2.
Clinical Manifestations of Attention Deficit Disorder (ADD) (1,7)

Behavioral Alterations
Increased level of motor activity
Impaired coordination
Short attention span
Excessive impulsiveness
Interpersonal problems
Lability of emotion
Perceptual-Cognitive Difficulties
Impaired spatial orientation
Difficulty in auditory and visual memory
Difficulty in transferring information between sensory modalities
Scholastic underachievement (with normal IQ)
Minor Neurological Abnormalities
Impaired fine motor coordination
Visual/motor difficulties
Problems in speech articulation

reactive difficulties can usually be defined on the basis of recent disruption in the familial environment, but psychoenvironmental trauma of this type still doesn't totally rule out the concomitant presence of ADD (1).

Over 100 clinical manifestations have been attributed to ADD in various descriptions found in the neuropsychiatric literature. The two major areas of dysfunction in ADD are the areas of *behavior* and *perception/cognition*. Some of the more commonly noted symptoms of ADD are listed under these two headings in Table 41.2. Many ADD victims exhibit learning difficulties in spite of normal intelligence and a reasonably healthy family background. The reason for their scholastic underachievement (usually noted in reading, spelling, or arithmetic) can usually be attributed to either the behavioral problems with attention span or the cognitive deficits in processing of didactic information. Two thirds of nonretarded adolescent underachievers have been shown to have had typical manifestations of ADD in their early childhood, thus reemphasizing the importance of early recognition of this syndrome (1, 7).

GENERAL MEASURES OF TREATMENT

The treatment of the child with ADD must be specifically tailored to meet the needs of each individual case. Obviously, since the pathogenesis of the disorder is not defined, therapy must be symptomatic and is quite empirical. The four main approaches in the treatment of the disease are: (a) education of the family with appropriate counseling, (b) remedial education for the affected child, (c) psychotherapy for the child, and (d) pharmacotherapy. *Education* of the family is extremely important for their understanding of the problem and for their cooperation in compliance with the medication regimen. *Specialized remedial education* for the child is essen-

tial, so that the child, once treatment has been initiated, can erase his academic deficits and attain the academic level of his peers. Special education techniques should include: (a) the establishment of baseline data; (b) the recognition and reinforcement of on-task desirable behaviors; (c) modification of instructional sequences; and (d) parent counseling. *Psychotherapy* is indicated for the child, so that he can learn to cope with his family and friends now that he is in a recuperative phase. The child is often acclimated to censure from his teachers and parents along with abuse from his peers, resulting in the formation of many psychological scars. These problems must be ameliorated with adequate psychotherapy as most of the medications currently used can only relieve the immediate symptoms of ADD, but they will not aid the child in coping with the indirect consequences of his former behavior on other individuals (1).

PHARMACOTHERAPY

Many pharmacotherapeutic approaches have been taken in the tretment of ADD. The use of medications in these children is most likely to be effective when utilized as an adjunctive therapy to the aforementioned academic behavioral interventions. The use of selected drugs, such as dextroamphetamine or methylphenidate, is considered an acceptable therapy for managing specific inappropriate motor activity behaviors of children with learning disabilities, particularly where the hyperactivity is neurologically and not anxiety based (9). However, medications do not cure learning disabilities. They only make the child more available to the learning experience. The likelihood that medications will be effective is enhanced when there is an interdisciplinary diagnostic approach and when there is complete cooperation and communication between the physician and the child's home and school where he is most likely to be at odds with his parents and school authorities because of distractibility, short attention span and impulsiveness (10). Perhaps the greatest difficulty in drug usage is that children are often put on medications before any specific inappropriate behaviors are identified and documented. Without this baseline information from home and school, changes in behavior become difficult to evaluate. Furthermore, with pinpointed behaviors, other forms of behavior management such as positive reinforcement and modified curriculum can be instituted once the child becomes available to learning, with the ultimate goal being the gradual withdrawal of the drugs. When drugs are prescribed, counseling is always necessary (11).

Drugs that have been used include amphetamine and amphetamine-like compounds, antipsychotic agents, tricyclic antidepressants, antianxiety agents and sedatives, anticonvulsants, caffeine, deanol, antihistamines, lithium salts, penicillamine, calcium disodium edetate and vitamins.

Centrally Acting Sympathomimetics

The primary agents utilized in the treatment of ADD are the centrally acting sympathomimetics, viz. methylphenidate, dextroamphetamine, and magnesium pemoline. The use of this therapeutic approach began in 1937, but actual definition and characterization of this indication in pediatric psychopharmacology had not been popularized nor revived until the late 1960s (12). Dextroamphetamine was initially used in 1937 and continued to be the agent of choice until the late 1960's, when methylphenidate usage increased in association with reports of a lower incidence of side effects with the latter drug. It would appear that these reports of greater safety with methylphenidate are of questionable clinical significance (8). There are also studies attesting to the greater clinical efficacy of methylpheni-

date (13) over dextroamphetamine by some authorities that prefer use of the former drug, while proponents of dextroamphetamine indicate that, in their hands, it has comparable clinical efficacy at a lower cost (14).

Methylphenidate is the primary agent for pharmacotherapy of ADD. It is given orally in doses of 0.3 to 1.5 mg/kg twice daily (in the morning and at noon, in order to avoid the potential iatrogenic insomnia that can ensue from the drug). Most patients respond well at 10 to 20 mg b.i.d. and daily dosage should be limited to 80 to 120 mg maximum. A study with single dose methodology for methylphenidate revealed that a morning dose of 20 mg had similar clinical efficacy to a multiple dosage form of dextroamphetamine. However, 15% of the children did not retain a therapeutic response for the entire school day (15). In addition, children will often experience decreased blood levels in the "play" hours after school and social conflicts may develop. Our current approach with methylphenidate therapy is to use a "twice daily" dosing pattern with morning and noon dosing times; this approach has provided good control in our patients with a minimum of problematic side effects (16, 17).

Methylphenidate is of value (72 to 85% response rate) in therapy of ADD, as it appears to reduce hyperactivity and restlessness, prevent distraction, and increase the attention span. These factors all aid in making the child more available for the learning environment, so that a secondary, but important effect of the drug is to increase learning ability. Motor ability and coordination are also enhanced by the drug (18).

The usage of methylphenidate in children with ADD can also be marked by certain undesirable side actions. Suppression of growth has been reported with both weight and height decrements being noted (19); however, when medication was discontinued over vacations, a spurt in growth returned the treated children to control levels (20, 21). A more recent study in 100 patients has revealed "no stunting of growth from the long term use of methylphenidate, dextroamphetamine, or imipramine/desipramine in children" (22). It appears that a temporary decrease in rate of growth in weight/height occurs during the first few years of therapy, dependent upon both dosage and use of drug holidays. However, there does not appear to be any effect on adult height or weight (23). Our current treatment approach is to allow the child to remain drug-free, if pragmatically possible, over weekends and vacations in order to both prevent any transient growth decrement and allow for continual re-evaluation of the need for pharmacotherapy (16). If a child's hyperactive behavior is pronounced at home as well as school, drug-free holidays may pose difficult patient compliance issues in the absence of behavioral and counseling therapies. The child whose hyperactive behavior was primarily a school referral is a better candidate for intermittent drug therapy.

Cardiovascular side effects, usually either increased diastolic blood pressure or tachycardia, have been reported. Insomnia and anorexia (resulting in weight loss) have been reported, but may occur less commonly than with other amphetamine derivatives. Methylphenidate is also reported to inhibit hepatic drug metabolism and the half-life of several substances, viz. ethyl biscoumacetate, desipramine and phenytoin may be prolonged resulting in potential toxicity. It is particularly important to consider the potential interactions with the anticonvulsant drugs, as these are often used concurrently in the child with ADD, and there have been several reports of ataxia in patients on phenytoin/methylphenidate combination regimens (18).

Dextroamphetamine is used similarly to methylphenidate in treatment of ADD, and although some studies indicate similar clinical efficacy (14), most of the clinical literature surveyed indicates an approximately 10 to 15% higher symptom improvement rate with methylphenidate (13, 19). The use of dextroamphetamine in ADD rather than usage of levoamphetamine or racemic amphetamine mixtures is based on the established superiority of the former agent in various clinical trails (24). The usual dosing pattern for dextroamphetamine is 5 to 20 mg twice daily, morning and at noon, or the sustained release dosage forms that are available can be used in a single morning dose. The use of 5-mg tablets will allow for greater latitude in dosage adjustment and better evaluation of clinical response on a time course basis (16). The time course of dextroamphetamine action in the ADD child is only slightly shorter than that of methylphenidate, with peak effect being noted 1 to 2 hours after dosing and a duration of action of 4 to 6 hours. Dosage is generally titrated from an initial dose of 5 mg b.i.d. up to an effective level by increasing the dose by 5 mg per dose every 2 to 3 days until either the symptoms are ameliorated or side effects are noted.

Side effects reported with dextroamphetamine are similar to those indicated for methylphenidate, and usually tend to decrease a few weeks after initiation of therapy. Persistence of insomnia may be treated with a mild hypnotic agent such as diphenhydramine (25 mg) or can be occasionally alleviated by taking the child off dextroamphetamine and initiating therapy with methylphenidate. When this type of a change in stimulant therapy is attempted, a 24-hour period should elapse prior to initiation of therapy with the new stimulant drug (14).

The question of potential abuse of psychostimulant drugs by children previously treated with these agents has been one of concern to many health professionals. However, at present, there are studies that indicate that abuse of drugs in later life is not a sequelae to amphetamine therapy in childhood (8, 25, 26).

Magnesium pemoline has also been used in children with ADD. This drug is a CNS stimulant with similar psychostimulant actions to dextroamphetamine. It has been shown to possess similar beneficial actions to those of dextroamphetamine as well as similar side effects, with insomnia and anorexia being most prevalent. Pemoline has a slower onset of action than the other CNS stimulants (2 to 4 hours), but a longer duration of action (8 to 12 hours). It may be given as a single morning dose or in two divided doses (morning/after school), depending upon patient response. Initial dosage should be 37.5 to 75 mg/day, with incremental increases of 18.75 mg/day at weekly intervals until maximal therapeutic response is attained. Maximum recommended dose is 112.5 mg/day (27). Magnesium pemoline does not give as rapid a clinical response as dextroamphetamine, but after 8 weeks of treatment with either drug, a similar clinical response can be anticipated. This drug may be considered as an alternate agent in those patients that cannot tolerate either of the stimulants previously discussed (28).

Antipsychotic Agents

A variety of other agents have been used in attempts to treat cases of ADD that are nonresponsive to or inappropriate for psychostimulant therapy. Several antipsychotic drugs have been utilized, including chlorpromazine, thioridazine, haloperidol and reserpine. Chlorpromazine has been reported to be significantly effective in treatment of hyperactivity as compared to placebo, and in some studies, it has equivalent efficacy to that of dextroamphetamine (which is generally effective in approximately 55 to 70% of cases). However, the psychostimulants have a broader spectrum of action in ADD, as chlorpromazine was found to control hyperactivity, but failed to result in significant attentional improvement (29). Studies with thioridazine have provided results essentially similar to those described for chlorpromazine (29). A report of haloperidol usage on cognitive behavior in children with hyperactivity indicated that methylphenidate and low-dose haloperidol (0.025 mg/kg) both facilitated cognitive performance, while high dose haloperidol (0.05 mg/kg) appeared to cause a slight deterioration of performance (30). Reserpine has been shown to give improvement in 34% of children with ADD, and this limited success rate negates its use in this disorder (13). Thus, the antipsychotic agents may be useful occasionally in therapy of ADD, but they are capable of depressing the higher CNS functions of attention, and more importantly, cognition. These latter concerns coupled with the multiple autonomic and extrapyramidal side effects associated with the antipsychotic agents preclude their use as primary agents. They can be viewed as an alternate choice of therapy only in those patients that are poor candidates for psychostimulant therapy.

Tricyclic Antidepressants

Many reports have indicated that the tricyclic antidepressants, usually imipramine, may be of benefit in the treatment of the child with ADD. However, while most studies have indicated their superiority over placebo, they are still not as effective as the psychostimulants. Further drawbacks to their use include the development of tolerance in some children and the numerous deleterious side effects of these agents (1). Side effects may be somewhat limited by the maximum daily dose approved by the FDA (5 mg/kg/day), but autonomic effects, weight loss, gastrointestinal irritation, fine tremors, hyperirritability, and mood alterations must be continually evaluated. In addition, the more severe effects on the CNS, e.g. seizures, and the cardiovascular system must

be monitored, but these are usually not seen if the practitioner adheres to the FDA recommendation. Thus, although the tricyclic antidepressants are useful in the child with ADD, their usage at this point is experimental and precautions must be taken if they are to be used (8, 31).

Other Therapeutic Approaches

Many other therapeutic approaches have been used in an attempt to find the ideal drug for therapy of ADD. Antianxiety agents have been evaluated on a limited basis and appear to be of little use. The benzodiazepines appear to be of no value in therapy (32), while phenobarbital is similarly not useful and has been reported to worsen the child's behavior (8, 33). Therefore, usage of these agents should be avoided in the child with ADD. Similarly, anticonvulsant drugs (8, 33), caffeine (34), antihistamines (35), lithium salts (36) and deanol (37) are either unacceptable for therapy or inadequately evaluated. A more thorough discussion of these therapies have been previously published (16). Similarly, further evaluation of the potential therapeutic benefit of levodopa in adults with ADD is needed. An initial report indicates the positive aspects of therapy with this agent in three patients (38).

There are several indications that chronic low level lead exposure can result in subtle CNS damage and hyperactivity. In one reported study, 13 hyperkinetic children with blood and urinary lead levels that were elevated, but in a "nontoxic" range, were treated with the lead chelating agents, penicillamine or calcium disodium edetate. Six of the children had positive medical history of perinatal or developmental CNS insult and did not respond, while the other seven ADD children that had unremarkable histories and a potential lead-induced hyperactivity showed marked improvement. The authors concluded that lead may play an important role in etiology of ADD, and measurements of blood and urinary lead levels may become a part of the standard workup in cases of ADD with no previous history of CNS insult (39).

There have also been isolated reports on the use of megavitamin therapy in ADD (40). The use of this approach is to be discouraged due to the potential toxic effects of vitamins A and D (41, 42); however, it is important to ensure adequate nutrition in the child with ADD via monitoring of appropriate dietary measures.

Food Additives

In 1973 an allergist postulated that hyperactivity was caused by food additives (43). Subsequent studies have failed to demonstrate any benefit of dietary regulation deleting food additives in treatment of children with ADD (44, 45). As mentioned previously, the causes of ADD are not definable and may be multiple, and therefore the success of the Feingold diet should be viewed with some pessimism until more definitive studies are performed to validate its purported benefits. While there are individual testimonials as to the positive outcomes of dietary treatment of hyperactivity, studies carried out by numerous investigators over a five year period provide "sufficient evidence to refute the claim that artificial food colorings, artificial flavorings, and natural salicylates produce hyperactivity" (45).

THERAPEUTIC CONSIDERATIONS

From the previous discussion of pharmacotherapy, it is evident that the psychostimulants (methylphenidate or dextroamphetamine) are the drugs of choice in this disorder. When these drugs are not effective, magnesium pemoline, chlorpromazine or thioridazine are the second agents to consider followed by consideration of tricyclic antidepressants. If none of these agents are successful, the use of deanol or caffeine might be attempted in hope for a response. Appropriate doses for commonly used agents are given in Table 41.3.

Table 41.3.
Daily Dosage Ranges of Drugs Useful in Therapy of Attention Deficit Disorder (ADD)

Drug	Dosage Range (mg)
Psychostimulants	
1. Methylphenidate	5–120
2. Dextroamphetamine	2.5–60
3. Pemoline	56.25–75
Phenothiazines	
1. Chlorpromazine	10–1000
2. Thioridazine	20–600
Tricyclic Antidepressants	
1. Imipramine	25–200
2. Desipramine	25–200
Miscellaneous Agents[a]	
1. Caffeine	100–200
2. Deanol	250–500

[a] Agents in this group are of questionable value in treatment of ADD.

It should be kept in mind that the child and his family will need supportive counseling to ensure compliance with the medication regimen as well as to ensure therapeutic success. As mentioned previously, counseling, remedial education, and psychotherapy may all be indicated in addition to pharmacotherapy. The pharmacist can play an important role in the assurance of total therapy for the ADD patient, as it has been shown that pharmacists have the knowledge and attitudes required to become more actively involved in monitoring the medications and behaviors of children with learning disabilities. Utilizing this expertise could help physicians, teachers and parents lead children toward a goal of ideal therapy (46).

A question is often raised by parents in regard to the duration of therapy. This is a difficult inquiry to answer, because duration of therapy is somewhat empirical based on the response of the child during drug-free periods such as weekends and vacations. A number of children with ADD will continue to show characteristics of the disorder into adult life, and therapy of some type may be needed for the remainder of the patient's life. Some clinicians have treated patients into the fourth decade of life and, interestingly, these patients do not appear to become tolerant to the effects of the psychostimulant drugs, and they do not become dependent upon the psychological attraction of their euphoric actions (1, 26). However, there may be concern for patients who view drugs as responsible for the control of their behavior without a corresponding increase in the development of personality skills such as constructive encountering and modification of goals.

PROGNOSIS

The prognosis for the ADD child is questionable. It is generally assumed that ADD is a benign psychiatric disorder that is outgrown by puberty or in early adolescence; however, ADD has been casually linked to a variety of serious psychiatric disorders in adult life. Hyperactivity usually disappears at puberty, but the secondary characteristics of the disorder are not always lost. Academic underachievement, impulsive character disorders, sociopathy, schizophrenia, and other recognized psychiatric disorders may then become the diagnosis. It is difficult with the present medical evidence to give an adequate prognosis in light of limited followup data. To ensure the most favorable prognosis, follow-up on at least a twice yearly basis is mandatory. In the words of Dr. Bernard Fox of the National Institute of Neurological Diseases and Stroke, "the symptoms of MBD may be less obvious in the young adult than in the school child because of changing behavioral demands—some jobs, for example, may not penalize the diverting of attention—or, if an adult has repeated car accidents, they usually are not attributed to MBD."

In summary, it should be remembered that ADD is a common disorder of primary grade school children that can remain into adult life. The cardinal features involve behavioral difficulties and academic deficiencies in the presence of normal intelligence. Treatment with psychostimulants will be effective in approximately 75 to 80% of affected children for amelioration of behavioral symptoms, but the cognitive disability of the disorder will rarely be totally alleviated by drug therapy and other nonpharmacological psychotherapeutic measures must be used hand in hand with these agents. When all of these approaches are effectively utilized, there is no reason for the quality of life of these patients to be any different from that of the rest of the populace.

References

1. Wender PH: The minimal brain dysfunction syndrome. *Annu Rev Med* 26:45–62, 1975.
2. Schmitt BD: The minimal brain dysfunction myth. *Am J Dis Child* 129:1313–1318, 1975.
3. Weiss G, Hechtman L, Perlman T, et al: Hyperactives as young adults. *Arch Gen Psychiatry* 36:675–681, 1979.
4. Wender RP, Reimkerr FW, Wood DR: Attention deficit disorder (minimum brain dysfunction) in adults. *Arch Gen Psychiatry* 38:449–456, 1981.
5. Hart Z, Rennick PM, Klinge V, et al: A pediatric neurologist's contribution to evaluations of school underachievers. *Am J Dis Child* 128:319–323, 1974.
6. Haller JS: Minimal brain dysfunction syndrome. *Am J Dis Child* 129:1319–1324, 1975.
7. Wender PH: Minimal brain dysfunction in children. *Pediatr Clin North Am* 20:187–202, 1973.
8. Werry JS: Medication for hyperkinetic children. *Drugs* 11:81–89, 1976.
9. Silver LB: Acceptable and controversial approaches to treating the child with learning disabilities. *Pediatrics* 55:408, 1975.
10. Safer DJ, Allen RP: *Hyperactive Children: Diagnosis and Management.* Baltimore: University Park Press, 1976, pp 225–233.
11. Brutten M, Richardson SO, Mangel C: *Something's Wrong with My Child.* New York: Harcourt Brace Jovanovich, 1973, p 83.
12. Sprague RL, Sleator EK: Effects of psychopharmacologic agents on learning disorders. *Pediatr Clin North Am* 20:719–735, 1973.
13. Millichap JG: Drugs in management of hyperkinetic and perceptually handicapped children. *JAMA* 206:1527, 1968.
14. Winsberg BG, Yepes LE, Bialer I: Pharmacologic management of children with hyperactive/aggressive/inattentive behavior disorders. *Clin Pediatr* 15:471–477, 1976.
15. Safer DJ, Allen RP: Single daily dose methylphenidate in hyperactive children. *Dis Nerv Syst* 34:325–328, 1973.
16. Piepho RW, Gourley DR, Hill JW: Current therapeutic concepts: minimal brain dysfunction. *J Am Pharm Assn* 17 (NS):500–504, 1977.
17. Barkley RA, Cunningham CE: Stimulant drugs and activity level in hyperactive children. *Am J Orthopsychiatry* 49:491–499, 1979.
18. Fischer KC, Wilson WP: Methylphenidate and the hyperkinetic state. *Dis Nerv Syst* 32:695–698, 1971.
19. Safer DJ, Allen RP: Factors influencing the suppressant effect of two stimulant drugs on the growth of hyperactive children. *Pediatrics* 51:660, 1973.
20. Safer DJ, Allen RP, Barr E: Growth rebound after termination of stimulant drugs. *J Pediatr* 86:113, 1975.
21. Satterfield JH, Cartwell DP, Schnell A, et al: Growth of hyperactive children treated with methylphenidate. *Arch Gen Psychiatry* 36:212–217, 1979.
22. Gross MD: Growth of hyperkinetic children taking methylphenidate, dextroamphetamine, or imipramine/desipramine. *Pediatrics* 58:423–431, 1976.
23. Roache AF, Lipman RS, Overall JE, et al: The effects of stimulant medication on the growth of hyperkinetic children. *Pediatrics* 63:847–850, 1979.
24. Arnold LE, Huestis RD, et al. Levoamphetamine vs. dextroamphetamine in minimal brain dysfunction. *Arch Gen Psychiatry* 33:292–301, 1976.
25. Laufer MW: Long-term management and some follow-up findings on the use of drugs with minimal cerebral syndromes. *J Learn Disabil* 4:55, 1971.
26. Charles L, Schain RJ, Guthrie D: Long-term use and discontinuation of methylphenidate with hyperactive children. *Dev Med Child Neurol* 21:758–764, 1979.
27. AMA Drug Evaluations: *Drugs Used in Nonpsychotic Mental Disorders,* ed 4. Chicago: American Medical Association, 1980, p 222.
28. Connors CK, Taylor E, Meo G, Kurtz MA, Fournier M: Magnesium pemoline and dextroamphetamine: a controlled study in children with minimal brain dysfunction. *Psychopharmacologia* 26:321–336, 1972.
29. Klein-Gittelman R, Klein DF, Katz S, Saraf K, Pollack E: Comparative effects of methylphenidate and thioridazine in hyperkinetic children. *Arch Gen Psychiatry* 23:1217–1231, 1976.
30. Werry JS, Aman MG: Methylphenidate and haloperidol in children. *Arch Gen Psychiatry* 32:790–795, 1975.

31. Werry JS, Aman MG, Diamond E: Imipramine and methylphenidate in hyperactive children. *J Child Psychol Psychiatry* 21:27–35, 1980.
32. Greenblatt D, Shader R: *Benzodiazepines in Clinical Practice.* New York: Raven Press, 1974.
33. Erenberg G: Drug therapy in minimal brain dysfunction: a commentary. *J Pediatr* 81:359–365, 1972.
34. Huestis RD, Arnold LE, Smeltzer DJ: Caffeine vs. methylphenidate and d-amphetamine in minimal brain dysfunction; a double blind comparison. *Am J Psychiatry* 132:868–870, 1975.
35. Connors C: Pharmacotherapy, in Quay HC, Werry JS: *Psychopathological Disorders of Childhood.* New York: John Wiley & Sons, 1972, pp 316–347.
36. Greenhill LL, Reider RO, Wender PH, Buchsbaum M, Zahn TP: Lithium carbonate in the treatment of hyperactive children. *Arch Gen Psychiatry* 28:636–640, 1973.
37. Lewis JA, Young R: Deanol and methylphenidate in minimal brain dysfunction. *Clin Pharmacol Ther* 17:534–540, 1975.
38. Reimken FW, Wood DR, Wender PH: An open clinical trial of L-dopa and carbidopa in adults with minimal brain dysfunction. *Am J Psychiatry* 137:73–75, 1980.
39. David OJ, Hoffman SP, Sverd J, Clark J, Voeller K: Lead and hyperactivity; behavioral response to chelation: a pilot study. *Am J Psychiatry* 133:1155–1158, 1976.
40. Shaywitz BA, Siegel NJ, Pearson HA: Megavitamins for minimal brain dysfunction. *JAMA* 238:1749, 1977.
41. White PL: The lid is off (editorial). *JAMA* 238:1761, 1977.
42. Vaisrub S: Vitamin abuse (editorial). *JAMA* 238:1762, 1977.
43. Feingold BF: Hyperkinesis and learning disabilities linked to artificial food flavors and colors. *Am J Nurs* 75:797–803, 1975.
44. Wender EH: Food additives and hyperkinesis. *Am J Dis Child* 131:1204–1206, 1977.
45. Lipton MA, Wender EH, et al: National Advisory Committee on Hyperkinesis and Food Additives, Final Report of the Nutrition Foundation. The Nutrition Foundation, Inc., Washington, D.C., October 16, 1980.
46. Hill JW, Kimberlin CL, Gourley DR, et al: Pharmacist's knowledge and attitudes regarding monitoring the behaviors of children with learning disabilities. *Am J Hosp Pharm* 35:300–303, 1978.

CHAPTER 42

Pain Management

ARTHUR G. LIPMAN, Pharm.D.

Pain is one of the most common complaints for which patients seek advice and help from health professionals. A contemporary definition of pain (*Dorland's Illustrated Medical Dictionary*, W. B. Saunders Co., 1974) is "a more or less localized sensation of discomfort, distress or agony resulting from the stimulation of specialized nerve endings. It serves as a protective mechanism insofar as it induces the sufferer to remove or withdraw from the source."

This definition is accurate and useful for most cases of acute pain. But pain is not as simple or as easily described as its definition suggests. Pain is complex—in fact, it is not one phenomenon, but several. An understanding of the etiology, natural history and pathophysiology is necessary for any pharmacist who provides advice or participates in the treatment of pain.

HISTORICAL PERSPECTIVE

The English word pain is derived from the Greek *poine* and Latin *poene* meaning penalty or punishment. Ancient Greeks and Romans interpreted pain as a price paid for offending the gods. It was believed to be an occurrence more of the spirit than of the body.

Over 2000 years ago, Aristotle described pain as an emotion, the opposite of pleasure. A few years later, Epicurus described pain as the absence of pleasure. These Greek philosophers saw pain as an affective disorder, i.e., arising from and influencing emotions. We now know that affect is an important part of pain. But it is only one part.

In the post-renaissance period, pain was considered to be a physical event. The specificity theory of pain, which was described by Descartes in 1644, is illustrated in Figure 42.1. While the anatomical pathways described by Descartes do not fully conform to current knowledge, some of the concept is useful. According to the specificity theory, for each unit of pain stimulus, a patient experiences one

unit of perceived pain. The specificity theory is useful in describing the ascent of pain impulses from peripheral nerve endings (nociceptors) via specialized nerve pathways in the spinal cord to the cerebral cortex. But this theory does not address the role of affect and past experience of pain. Therefore, it is incomplete.

Recognizing that previous pain experiences influence current pain perceptions, many noted physiologists, psychologists and philosophers debated the origin of pain and developed several pain theories during the past 300 years. They attempted to integrate physical and psychological components of pain into one model. None have succeeded fully to date. However, the recent description of the gate control theory and our rapidly increasing understanding of the biochemical basis of pain has begun to allow us to more fully understand this common human process.

PATHOPHYSIOLOGY

In 1965, Melzack and Wall (1) described the gate control theory of pain. This theory integrates the anatomical pain pathways which have been identified and several previous psychological pain models. It proposes that a neural mechanism in the dorsal horn of the spinal cord acts like a gate which can block or allow the transmission of pain impulses from the periphery to the brain.

We now know that the nociceptors are not specialized pain receptors. They are simply bare nerve endings in the periphery. According to the gate control theory, pain signals are carried from the nociceptors to the spinal cord via two types of nerve fibers. These are small, unmyelinated fibers and large myelinated fibers. The small fibers transmit impulses slowly (0.5 to 2 m/sec) and are associated with dull pain such as burning and aching. Visceral pain is an example. The large fibers transmit pain impulses at 3 to 20 m/sec and are associated with acute, sharp, pricking type pain. These

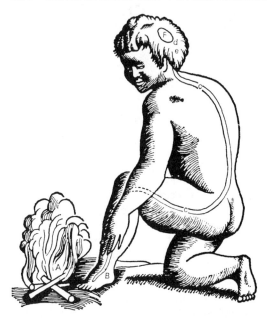

Figure 42.1. Descartes' (1644) concept of the pain pathway. He writes: "If for example fire (*A*) comes near the foot (*B*), the minute particles of this fire, which as you know move with great velocity, have the power to set in motion the spot of the skin of the foot which they touch, and by this means pulling upon the delicate thread (*cc*) which is attached to the spot of the skin, they open up at the same instant the pore (*de*) against which the delicate thread ends, just as by pulling at one end of a rope one makes to strike at the same instant a bell which hangs at the other end."

fibers are widely distributed in the skin, arterial walls, periosteum, joint surfaces and parts of the cranial vault. While large fiber stimulation produces initial pain, small fiber stimulation produces pain which can become worse with time. Sharp pain causes the subject to withdraw from the source and the sharp pain ceases. The dull sensation which comes later, is often severe and lasting.

As shown in Figure 42.2, the two types of nerve fiber impulses can be antagonistic. Indeed, mild stimulation of large fibers can greatly diminish the pain felt due to stimulation of the small fibers. An example is the effect of rubbing one's elbow (stimulating large fibers) to ameliorate the pain caused by banging it on a door frame (stimulating small fibers). This spinal gate effect also helps to explain the efficacy of topical counterirritants and electrical and physical pain treatment modalities.

The gate control theory helps to explain the pain states addressed by most earlier pain theories. Autonomic nervous system involvement

in pain is explained by the fact that afferent fibers from the sympathetic chain ganglia connect with the same spinal cord cells that receive inputs that influence the spinal gating mechanism. The gate control theory still remains only a theory. The T cell which is central to this theory has not yet been demonstrated. However, this theory helps us to understand many of the processes associated with pain.

Our current understanding of pain has been greatly enhanced by two recent pharmacological discoveries. For decades, pharmacologists have postulated that opioid receptors exist in the central nervous system. If that is the case, logically there should be an endogenous opioid agonist which attaches to those receptors. Only in the 1970s were sterospecific opioid receptors and endogenous opiates demonstrated (2). These "endogenous morphine-like" substances are termed endorphins. Several endorphins have now been identified in the central nervous system of man. Endorphin is a generic term used for all of these substances, including the enkephalins.

When a painful stimulus occurs, the nociceptors initiate transmission of the pain impulse. The nociceptors may be stimulated by compression, stretching or by physical or chemical insult. Noxious chemicals such as bradykinin result from inflammation, anoxia, or other pain-inducing stimuli, and are probably involved in initiating the pain impulses. Prostaglandins are involved in the sensitizing of nociceptors.

The pain signals are transmitted from the periphery via the A-delta and C fibers to the dorsal horns of the spinal cord. Substance P, a polypeptide, appears to be the neurotransmitter at this site. Spinal gating is postulated to occur in the region of the dorsal horns known as the substantia gelatinosa. Opioid receptors may be occupied by endorphins at the spinal level thus blocking pain transmission (Fig. 42.3). Pain impulses are modified in the central nervous system by chemical mediators including norepinephrine and serotonin (5-hydroxytryptamine). In the dorsal roots of the spinal cord, the pain fibers interconnect with ascending nerve cells which cross to the contralateral side of the column as they ascend. The pain impulse terminates in the brain at the thalamus where conscious pain perception may be localized, and the cerebral cortex where the pain is recognized and interpreted. The limbic system, which is anatomically close to these

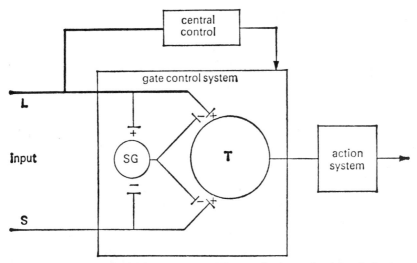

Figure 42.2.   Schematic diagram of the gate control theory of pain mechanisms: L, the large diameter fibers; S, the small diameter fibers. The fibers project to the substantia gelatinosa (SG) and first central transmission (T) cells. The inhibitory effect exerted by SG on the afferent fiber terminals is increased by activity in L fibers and decreased by activity in S fibers. The central control trigger is represented by a line running from the large fiber system to the central control mechanisms; these mechanisms, in turn, project back to the gate control system. The T cells project to the entry cells of the action system; +, excitation; −, inhibition. (Reproduced with permission from R. Melzack and P. D. Wall: *Science*, 150:971, 1965 (1).)

structures and this part of the central nervous system, appears to be responsible for the emotional component of pain at this level. Past pain experiences, belief about pain and other outcomes of the patient's socialization influence the patient's response to pain at the cerebral level. There are two related anatomical pathways. The reticular and limbic systems comprise the pathway largely responsible for motivational and affective functions. The thalamic and neocortical structures are associated with discriminative capacity (Fig. 42.4).

Several subsets of opioid receptors have been suggested and differentiated. Effects have been suggested for three of these types of receptors (Table 42.1). Impressive advances are being made in the identification of biochemical pathways involving pain. With the increasing understanding of the pharmacology and biochemistry of pain, some clinically useful information is also becoming available. There is increasing documentation that acute and chronic pain occur in somewhat different biochemical environments.

PAIN ORIGIN

Pain is commonly categorized as being either somatic or visceral. Somatic pain is initiated in the skin or musculoskeletal system.

Visceral pain is initiated in the abdomen or thorax. Highly localized visceral damage does not necessarily cause severe pain. Visceral pain is often difficult to localize and is frequently associated with referred pain sites, e.g., pain from angina pectoris radiating down the left arm.

As with any other complaint, pain should not be treated as a nonspecific disorder when a specific etiology can be identified and treated. Headache is one of the most common types of pain. Most headaches are managed with nonspecific analgesics, but headache may be a symptom of severe, underlying disease. Therefore, chronic headache should be evaluated by a clinician experienced in this area. Tension headaches may require therapy which includes relaxation techniques and possibly anxiolytic drugs. Ischemic type headaches, e.g., migraine and cluster headaches, usually require specific treatments which affect the hemodynamics of the area. Sinus headache commonly responds better to decongestants than to analgesics alone (see Chapter 40, "Headache").

Inflammatory processes of the bones and joints normally require aggressive antiinflammatory therapy rather than simple analgesics. Treatment of these diseases with analgesics which do not reduce inflammation, e.g., acet-

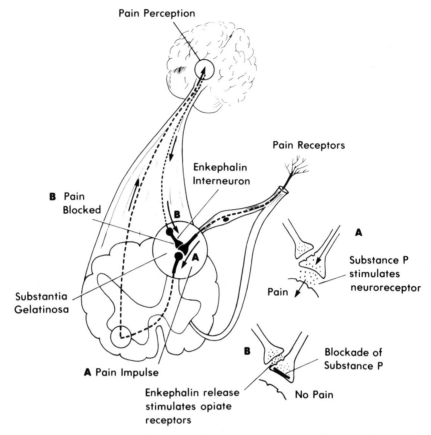

Figure 42.3. Current biochemical theory of pain stresses role of brain opiate receptors and endogenous opioids. Presence of specific binding sites in the limbic system and in substantia gelatinosa suggests that endogenous narcotics are active in both brain and spinal cord. Details (*A* and *B*) hypothesize how endogenous narcotics may operate to block pain perception. Intrinsic and extrinsic discrepancies in neurotransmissions are held to account for individual differences in psychophysiologic response to painful stimuli. (Reproduced with permission from J. M. Luce, T. L. Thompson II, C. J. Getto, and R. L. Byyny: New concepts of chronic pain and their implications. *Hospital Practice*, 14:113–123, 1979.)

aminophen, opiates, may lead to painless destruction of the joints (see Chapter 33).

Many other examples of specific causes of pain could be identified. Surgical, medical, or drug treatments other than analgesics may be more appropriate in such cases.

PAIN PERCEPTION

The common organic pain model assumes that pain is a defense mechanism against noxious stimuli. While this is frequently true, it is not always the case. Pain associated with a functional process is termed organic pain. In such cases, pain is indeed a warning sign—at least in the early stages of the process—and can be a useful clinical monitoring parameter. Conversely, pain can be a symptom of an emotional process or a response to conditioning in which the patient receives attention or some other desired outcome in response to complaints of pain. Such pain is commonly termed psychogenic. Although a specific, physical etiology may not exist, such pain does constitute a pathological syndrome which requires treatment. For psychogenic pain, analgesic therapy is rarely indicated and may contribute to the pain problem. Rather, psychological care is appropriate. Patients who seek continuous drugs, surgeries, or other therapies with no relief and for whom no physical cause of pain can be identified, should be evaluated by a clinical psychologist or other psychiatric clinician with training in pain control. Psychogenic pain hurts. It requires appropriate treatment.

The differentiation between organic and

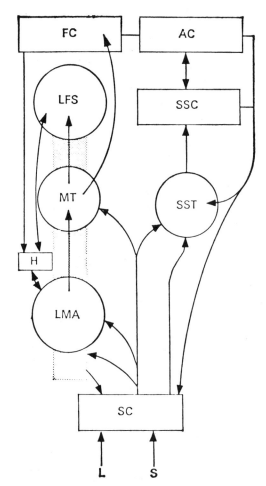

Figure 42.4. Schematic diagram of the major relationships among structures in the central nervous system that are related to pain. *On the right:* thalamic and neocortical structures subserving discriminative capacity. *On the left:* reticular and limbic systems subserving motivational-affective functions. Ascending pathways from the spinal cord (*SC*) are: (1) the dorsal column-lemniscal and dorsolateral tracts (right ascending arrow) projecting to the somatosensory thalamus (*SST*) and cortex (*SSC*), and (2) the anterolateral pathway (left ascending arrow) to the somatosensory thalamus via the neospinothalamic tract, and to the reticular formation (*stippled area*), the limbic midbrain area (*LMA*) and medial thalamus (*MT*) via the paramedial ascending system. Descending pathways to spinal cord originate in somatosensory and associated cortical areas (*AC*) and in the reticular formation. Polysynaptic and reciprocal relationships in limbic and reticular systems are indicated. Other abbreviations: *FC*, frontal cortex: *LFS*, limbic forebrain structures (hippocampus, septum, amygdala, and associated cortex); *H*, hypothalamus. (Reproduced with permission from R. Melzack and K. L. Casey: Sensory, motivational and central control determinants of

psychogenic categories is not always clear. Pain behavior is governed by factors in the patient's environment. Thus, a patient's support group, life-style and other environmental factors should also be evaluated. Organic disorders which cause pain often cause emotional change. Increased reports of hypochondriasis, depression and hysteria occur in pain of both organic and psychogenic origin.

But even when due to a clearly identifiable cause, pain is a highly suggestive experience. Some people are very voluble about their pain; they appear to have low pain tolerance. Others are stoic and accepting. Patients' socialization processes, parenteral and peer examples and past pain experiences greatly influence their reactions to pain. Good communications between patients and care givers is important in the planning and monitoring of treatment of the pain.

Patients' personal philosophy and religious beliefs may also influence their response to pain. Many religions value pain as a sign of atonement. Some persons with chronic pain may not seek pain relief due to the belief that pain is necessary for their spiritual well-being. Others refuse to admit to pain due to their not wanting to inconvenience other persons. An important part of the initial interaction with pain patients is for the clinician to ascertain the patient's feelings and belief about the pain.

Reactive and emotional aspects of pain are normal secondary components of the pain process. The more severe or chronic the pain, the more pronounced the secondary component is apt to become. Effective clinicians expect and anticipate these aspects and are prepared to address them when these reactions occur.

ACUTE AND CHRONIC PAIN

Acute pain is a phenomenon that almost all persons have experienced. It presents, it hurts, and it goes away (3). Most of us learned about this type of pain when we were very young. Typically, youngsters who hurt themselves are told by their parents to "be a big kid—it will be better in a minute." As part of our socialization process, we are taught to be stoic and accepting of pain. In most cases the parental advice is appropriate. The pain does go away. But when pain does not resolve rapidly, a

pain: a new conceptual model, in D. Kenshalo: *The Skin Senses.* Charles C Thomas, Springfield, Ill., 1968.)

Table 42.1.
Summary of the Action of Prototypical Agonists, Antagonists, and Agonist-Antagonists at Hypothetical Subtypes of Opioid Receptor[a]

Compound	Receptor Types[b]		
	μ	κ	σ
Morphine	Agonist	Agonist	—
Naloxone	Antagonist	Antagonist	Antagonist
Pentazocine	Antagonist	Agonist	Agonist
Nalorphine	Antagonist	Partial agonist	Agonist
Buprenorphine	Partial agonist		—
Propiram	Partial agonist		—
N-Allylnormetazocine	Antagonist		Agonist

[a] From J. H. Jaffe and W. R. Martin: Opioid analgesics and antagonists, in A. G. Gilman, L. S. Goodman and A. Gilman: *The Pharmacological Basis of Therapeutics*, ed. 6. New York: Macmillan, 1980, p. 521.
[b] The μ receptor is thought to mediate supraspinal analgesia, respiratory depression, euphoria, and physical dependence; the κ receptor, spinal analgesia, miosis, and sedation; the σ receptor, dysphoria, hallucinations, and respiratory and vasomotor stimulation.

complex clinical problem may result. When this occurs, stoic acceptance is neither feasible nor appropriate.

Classical studies of pain have demonstrated that when pain is associated with positive outcomes, it hurts less. Beecher, in 1959, demonstrated that soldiers severely wounded in battle complained little of pain from their wounds. The wounds meant that they were out of combat (4). A little later in the hospital, the same men complained of discomfort from venipuncture. To them, that process had no perceivable positive outcome. Similarly, athletes often experience massive trauma with few pain complaints when the pain is associated with a perception of positive outcome.

In 1979, Wall (5) described three phases of pain. He described pain as more of an awareness-of-a-need state like hunger than an awareness-of-an-event state like seeing. Pain is not necessarily linked to an injury. Rather, it is linked to a need. Therefore, injury will not always generate pain or pain be associated with injury. A pain stimulus may be difficult to localize, and the cause may not be discernible. When injury occurs, the first or immediate phase presents. The impulse is to withdraw from the source and pain is not experienced. Other priorities such as escape or protection from the source of the injury occupy the subject. The second or acute phase occurs when one can concentrate on caring for the injury. This phase is dominated by anxiety. When the cause of the pain is under control of the subject—such as hitting one's thumb with a hammer, the acute phase is the first phase experienced. When the cause is out of the subject's control, such as when one is being attacked, the acute phase occurs when the attack is over or the subject has escaped or overcome the attacker. The third or chronic phase of pain is associated with overcoming the effects of the injury. Most subjects are quiet and withdrawn in the chronic phase, and they overcome their pain. However, a chronic pain syndrome may occur when pain does not abate with the resolution of the effects of the injury or when the injury does not resolve as in chronic diseases. Then, intractable pain, behavior changes and depression often occur.

The body's endogenous pain control system—the endorphins and opioid receptors—provide protection against pain in the immediate and acute phases. However, there is some evidence that endorphins do not provide protection against chronic pain of physical origin. In such situations the endorphins may be activated and may occupy opioid receptors, but pain relief may not occur. The reasons for this are not clear. Chronic pain must be treated very differently from acute pain.

Acute pain is commonly described as mild, moderate or severe (6). Drugs are usually effective and can be taken as needed (p.r.n.) to manage the symptoms. Reflecting back on childhood experiences with acute pain, we expect the pain to resolve. Reflecting also on a societal ethic to use drugs sparingly and only when truly needed, we usually take analgesics (especially narcotics) for acute pain only when the pain is severe. That is fine; we get pain relief when needed, and in a few hours to days the pain resolves. The anxiety associated with acute pain usually resolves rapidly as the pain lessens. Physical or psychological sequelae are seldom seen.

Most patients cope well with acute pain because it can be understood and rationalized. The pain is understood in the context of a particular event or injury. It is often rationalized by patients as a part of the healing process and by health care personnel as a clinical monitoring parameter. And with time, as expected, it lessens and resolves. Chronic pain is far more complex. When the pain remains for an extended period of time, it can no longer be rationalized. Such pain becomes the central focus of the patient's existence. Patients in severe chronic pain frequently do not communicate effectively, have minimal social interactions and exhibit behavior that differs greatly from when they were not in pain. Severe, chronic pain does not conform to the mild-moderate-severe continuum used to describe acute pain. Chronic pain is better described as a circular continuum from aching to agony (Fig. 42.5). At times, the patient is in agony and is unable to focus on subjects other than the pain. At other times, the pain is present but bearable and the patient can function in a more normal manner. Frequently, the patient will go from ache to agony for no discernible reason. The nature of severe, chronic pain is that it is frequently unpredictable.

Chronic pain appears to have multiple dimensions (Fig. 42.6). The physical cause of the pain comes first. As the duration of the pain increases, the other dimensions may appear. When the pain is not managed in a few hours to days, the second or psychological dimension is frequently seen. This dimension commonly presents as anxiety and depression. When the pain continues for days to weeks, the third or social dimension may be seen. Here, the patient's behavior changes. Hostility and anger are common.

Severe, chronic pain does not present as a single problem. Rather, it presents as a symptom complex (Fig. 42.7). The initiation of the complex is the injury or disease that first causes the pain. The physical pain, anxiety and depression are interrelated biochemically and are associated with shifts in cellular levels of neurohumoral transmitters in the central nervous system.

ACUTE PAIN MANAGEMENT

Acute pain is most commonly treated with simple analgesics. Aspirin remains unsurpassed by other nonopiate analgesics. In a double-blind, crossover, single dose study of mar-

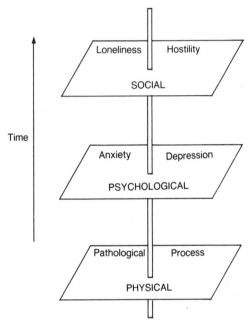

Figure 42.6. Dimension of severe, chronic pain. (Adapted with permission from A. G. Lipman: *Cancer Nursing*, 2:39, 1980 (6).)

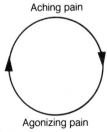

Figure 42.5. The circular continuum of severe, chronic pain.

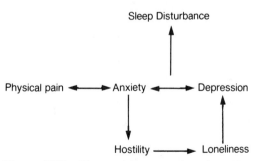

Figure 42.7. The symptom complex of severe, chronic pain. (Adapted with permission from A. G. Lipman: *Cancer Nursing*, 2:39, 1980 (6).)

keted analgesics published in 1972 by Moertel et al. (7), aspirin was shown to be equal to or better than eight other analgesics. This study was conducted in 57 patients with mild to moderate pain due to unresectable cancer (Table 42.2). Two years later, Moertel et al. (8) published a controlled evaluation of eight analgesics in combination with aspirin, aspirin alone and placebo (Table 42.3). In that study, only combinations of aspirin with codeine, oxycodone and pentazocine were shown to be more effective than aspirin alone. The second study involved 100 ambulatory patients with mild to moderate, chronic or recurrent pain due to cancer.

Some drugs, such as propoxyphene, which were shown to be less effective than aspirin in these and other controlled studies, enjoy reputations among many laymen and some health professionals as being more effective than aspirin (9). Indeed, many patients insist that propoxyphene is far superior to aspirin. If a patient believes that a placebo is an effective analgesic, that patient may well exhibit an elevated level of circulating endorphins following a dose of placebo. Therefore, it may be appropriate to continue an analgesic of questionable efficacy if a patient reports a good effect. This is not an advocacy of initiating analgesic therapy with such an agent unless the patient reports a strong desire to use the drug due to excellent past experience with it. This finding

has obvious implications in counseling patients about analgesics. The efficacy of an analgesic may be enhanced by positive, suggestive counseling. Severe, acute pain is often most appropriately managed with narcotic analgesics. However, these drugs are commonly used in too low doses. In 1973, Marks and Sachar (10) reported underdosing of narcotic analgesics, especially meperidine, in one third to two thirds of medical inpatients at a New York hospital. Narcotics are often used in too low doses and not administered as often as necessary to provide pain relief. A questionnaire survey of 102 housestaff physicians in two New York teaching hospitals showed considerable misinformation about narcotics.

There is a common misplaced fear of treatment-induced addiction. In 1980, Porter and Jick (11) of the Boston Collaborative Drug Surveillance Program reported that addiction is

Table 42.2.
Relative Therapeutic Effect of Oral Analgesics According to Mean Percentage of Relief of Pain Achieved in 57 Patients[a]

Analgesic Agent	Dose (mg)	Relief of Pain (%)	
Aspirin	650	62	
Pentazocine	50	54	
Acetamino-phen	650	50	Significantly superior to placebo ($p <$ 0.05)
Phenacetin	650	48	
Mefenamic acid	250	47	
Codeine	65	46	
Propoxy-phene	65	43	
Ethohepta-zine	75	38	Significantly inferior to aspirin ($p <$ 0.05)
Promazine	25	37	
Placebo	—	32	

[a] From C. G. Moertel et al.: *New England Journal of Medicine*, 286:814, 1972 (7).

Table 42.3.
Comparative Therapeutic Effect of Analgesic Preparations as Reported by 100 Patients[a]

Analgesic Preparation	Therapeutic Effect[b]	
	Mean percent pain relief	Rank sum
Codeine sulfate, 65 mg + aspirin, 650 mg	63 (S)	429 (S)
Oxycodone, 9.76 mg + aspirin, 650 mg	63 (S)	430 (S)
Pentazocine hydrochloride, 25 mg + aspirin, 650 mg	59 (S)	490 (B)
Propoxyphene napsylate, 100 mg + aspirin, 650 mg	55 (NS)	511 (NS)
Promazine hydrochloride, 25 mg + aspirin, 650 mg	51 (NS)	556 (NS)
Pentobarbital sodium, 32 mg + aspirin, 650 mg	50 (NS)	581 (NS)
Caffeine, 65 mg + aspirin, 650 mg	48 (NS)	603 (NS)
Ethoheptazine citrate, 75 mg + aspirin, 650 mg	48 (NS)	619 (NS)
Aspirin, 650 mg	51 (NS)	554 (NS)
Placebo	33 (I)	726 (I)

[a] From C. G. Moertel et al.: *Journal of the American Medical Association*, 229:55, 1974 (8).
[b] Letters in parentheses indicate significance: S, significant superiority to aspirin alone ($p <$ 0.05); B, borderline superiority to aspirin alone ($p \approx$ 0.05); NS, no significant difference from aspirin alone; I, significant inferiority to all other preparations ($p <$ 0.05).

rare in patients treated with narcotics. Of 39,941 hospitalized patients who were consecutively monitored, 11,882 received at least one narcotic preparation. Only four cases of addiction were documented in patients with no previous history of addiction. The addiction was considered major in only one of these four patients.

Another exaggerated fear with narcotic analgesics is that of respiratory depression. While this effect does occur, the respiratory center is low in the central nervous system. Depression of the central nervous system proceeds from the highest centers (thought processes) to the lowest centers. Thus, if the dose of narcotic is not causing clouded thinking and obtundation, respiratory depression risk is minimal.

Many health professionals mistakenly think that there is an upper limit to the appropriate dose of a narcotic analgesic. This is not true. Effective pain control usually requires titration to response. Some patients will require much higher doses than others (12).

Analgesics provide symptomatic relief. They do not correct any underlying disorder which causes or contributes to the pain. Analgesics may mask pain, fever, inflammation or other symptoms while the disease progresses. However, short-term use of analgesic drugs in the management of acute pain usually has a favorable risk to benefit ratio.

Aspirin is the drug of choice for mild to moderate acute pain. Aspirin can be manufactured by an inexpensive process in which water is used to make the granulation necessary for tablet compression, or by an anhydrous method which requires two compression processes and thus is more expensive. When the former process is utilized, water is hydrogen bonded to the aspirin molecules. This residual water favors hydrolytic cleavage of the acetylsalicylic acid ester with time. However, fresh aspirin made by either method which has not been exposed to excesses of heat or humidity should be acceptable. Any aspirin exposed to water will degrade. Aspirin with a very strong vinegar odor or excessive loose powder in the bottom of the bottle will produce less clinical effect and may cause more gastritis than fresh drug. Pharmacists should advise patients to purchase amounts of aspirin that will be used up within about a year. This is to help assure that fresh drug is taken. Bottles should be tightly capped between uses and protected from excesses of moisture and heat. Many bathroom medicine cabinets do not meet these criteria. Aspirin-induced gastritis occurs partly due to unionized particles of drug contacting the gastric mucosa. Dissolution can be accelerated resulting in more rapid ionization if the aspirin tablets are taken with about 8 ounces of water. This technique is often as effective as substituting the much more expensive buffered aspirin tablets to decrease the incidence of stomach upset associated with aspirin.

Many combination products containing aspirin and other nonprescription analgesics are commercially available. These combinations are no more effective than the equivalent dose of the ingredients as aspirin alone (8). Acetaminophen is the aspirin substitute of choice for most cases in which a simple analgesic is desired and aspirin is contraindicated. Contraindications to aspirin include peptic ulcer disease, pregnancy—especially approaching term, blood clotting disorders, concurrent use of oral anticoagulants, and aspirin allergy. Aspirin allergy presents as asthma-like bronchospasms or rash. Gastrointestinal upset is not indicative of allergy to aspirin. Relative contraindications include bronchial asthma and gastric upset.

Acetaminophen is as effective as aspirin in simple pain. But much pain for which aspirin is used also has an inflammatory component and acetaminophen does not produce clinically useful antiinflammatory activity. Acetaminophen is generally more expensive than aspirin. If an antiinflammatory agent is needed by a patient in whom aspirin is contraindicated, any of the nonsteroidal antiinflammatory agents might be used. In addition to their antiinflammatory activity, these drugs are excellent analgesics. In dysmenorrhea, the nonsteroidal antiinflammatory agents appear to be more effective than aspirin. Available nonsteroidal antiinflammatory agents are listed in Table 42.4.

Combinations of aspirin and phenacetin are generally believed to be more nephrotoxic than aspirin alone when used chronically. Since these combinations offer no therapeutic advantage over aspirin alone, their use should be discouraged. Combinations of aspirin and acetaminophen have recently been introduced with anecdotal claims of advantages over aspirin alone. Data from controlled studies to support these claims are lacking.

Pharmacists should advise patients that

Table 42.4.
Nonsteroidal Antiinflammatory Agents[a]

	Aspirin (various)	Fenoprofen (Nalfon)	Ibuprofen (Motrin)	Meclofenamate Sodium (Meclomen)	Mefenamic Acid (Ponstel)	Naproxen (Naprosyn)
Peak blood levels (hr)	0.66 fasting; 1.66-2 normal meal	1–2	1–2	0.5–1	2–4	2–4
Plasma half-life (hr)	Aspirin 20 min; salicylic acid: 3–6	3	2 (1.6–2.5)	2 3.3 hr with multiple doses	2	13 (12–15)
Excretion	10% free as salicylic acid	5% free, 90% in 24 hr	1% free, complete in 24 hr	⅓ in urine, ⅔ in feces most as glucuronide conjugates	67% excreted unchanged in urine, 20–25% in feces	10% free, 95% eliminated in 5 days
Protein binding (%)	Aspirin very slight; salicylic acid: 50–80	99	99	99	91–97	99
Dosage range (mg/day)	4500–7500	2400–3200	1200–2400	200–400	1250	500–750
Dosage forms	325 mg tablets, and suppositories	200 mg white (Dista H76) and 300 mg yellow (Dista H77) capsules and 600 mg yellow (U59) tablets	300 mg (Upjohn 733) white, 400 mg (Upjohn 750) orange and 600 mg (Upjohn 742) peach tablets	50 mg peach (PD-268) and 100 mg beige (PD-269) tablets	250 mg capsules (PD 540)	250 mg yellow (Syntex 272) and 375 mg peach (Syntex 273) tablets
Relative contraindications	Pregnancy, bleeding disorders, impaired renal function	Upper GI disease, impaired renal function pregnancy nursing	Pregnancy, impaired liver function	Upper GI disease, pregnancy, nursing	Impaired renal function, upper GI disease, diarrhea, late pregnancy, nursing	Pregnancy, nursing, oral anticoagulants, impaired renal function, congestive heart failure (CHF), bleeding disorder
Adverse reactions: GI tract	GI upset, abdominal pain, ulceration, anorexia, hepatomegaly with chronic use. Fecal blood loss of 6 ml/day at 3600 mg/day	Dyspepsia, constipation, abdominal pain, anorexia, blood in stool	Diarrhea, GI upset (4–15.9%), bleeding, ulcers, nausea (3–9%) heartburn (3–9%)	Diarrhea 10–33%, nausea 11%, other GI disorders 10%, abdominal pain 11%. Fecal blood loss of 2.3 ml/day at 400 mg/day	Diarrhea 5%, nausea, abdominal pain	Abdominal pain, GI upset, diarrhea, cholestatic jaundice
Skin	Pustular acneiform eruptions after continued use	Rash, pruritis (10%) urticaria sweating	Rash, 3–9%, pruritus	Rash, urticaria, pruritus	Urticaria, rash, facial edema	Rash, echymoses, pruritus, sweating

Naproxen Sodium (Anaprox)	Sulindac (Clinoril)	Tolmetin Sodium (Tolectin)	Zomepirac Sodium (Zomax[b])	Piroxicam (Feldene)	Benoxaprofen (Oraflex[c])
1–2	2–3	0.5–1	1–2	3–5	1.5–8
13	7	1	4 hr; 9.6 hr with multiple doses	30–86	25–32
95% in urine as free drug	2.7 free, 66% in 24 hr	10% free, 90–95% in 24 hr	Primarily excreted in urine	5% unchanged in urine; metabolized by hydroxylation and glucuronide conjugation	Primarily in urine; 90% as glucuronide conjugate
Same as naproxen	93, metabolites 95–98	99	98	Approximately 99	98 in urine
550–1100	200–400	600–1800	200–600	10–20	400–1000
275 mg blue tablets equivalent to 250 mg naproxen base	150 mg yellow (MSD 941) and 200 mg yellow (MSD 942) scored tablets	200 mg white tablets marked 200 and McNeil and 400 mg orange capsules	Tablets scored 100 mg marked McNeil Zomax	Capsules 10 mg; maroon and blue, marked Pfizer 322; 20 mg, maroon, marked Pfizer 323	Tablets 40 mg, 600 mg
Same as naproxen	Upper GI disease, CHF pregnancy nursing	Upper GI disease, bleeding disorders, CHF, nursing, pregnancy	Upper GI disease, chronic use, pregnancy, nursing, CHF, hypertension	Upper GI disease, CHF, liver disease, systemic lupus erythematosus (SLE), asthma	Upper GI disease, CHF, hypertension, renal disease
Same as naproxen	GI upset, constipation transient LPT elevation	GI upset (16%), abdominal pain, heartburn (2%), ulceration, constipation (1.6%), nausea (4%)	Nausea (6–12%), GI distress, flatulence, gastritis, anorexia	GI upset, abdominal and epigastric pain, ulceration, nausea, vomiting, melena, hematemesis	Peptic ulceration, GI bleeding, nausea, dyspepsia, abdominal pain, vomiting, flatulence, constipation, diarrhea
Same as naproxen	Rash pruritus	Rash (3%) pruritus (2%)	Rash, pruritus, skin irritation, sweating	Rash, pruritus	Photosensitivity, onycholysis, rash, pruritus, urticaria
Same as naproxen	Dizziness headache nervousness vertigo	Dizziness (4%), lightheadedness (4%), drowsiness (2%), nervousness (2%), headache (7%)	Dizziness, insomnia, drowsiness, paresthesia, anxiety, depression	Dizziness, somnolence, vertigo	Headache, vertigo, sleep disturbance, asthenia and malaise, nervousness
Same as naproxen	Tinnitus	Tinnitus (2.5%)	Tinnitus, taste charge	Tinnitus	Tinnitus, hearing decrease, vision disturbance
Same as naproxen	Mild edema	Mild edema (2.5%)	Mild peripheral edema	Hypertension	Edema, hypertension, heart failure

Table 42.4. (Continued)

	Aspirin (various)	Fenoprofen (Nalfon)	Ibuprofen (Motrin)	Meclofenamate Sodium (Meclomen)	Mefenamic Acid (Ponstel)	Naproxen (Naprosyn)
Central nervous system	Headache, dizziness, mental confusion	Tremor, dizziness, drowsiness (14%), confusion, insomnia headache (14%)	Headache, dizziness (3–9%), lightheadedness, depression, fatigue	Malaise, fatigue, paresthesia, insomnia, depression	Drowsiness, dizziness, nervousness, headache, insomnia	Headache, drowsiness, dizziness, light-headedness, vertigo
Sensory effects	Tinnitus hearing loss	Tinnitus (10%), blurred vision, hearing loss	Blurred vision (<1%) colored vision (<1%), tinnitus (<3%)	Blurred vision, taste dysfunction	Eye irritation, ear pain, blurred vision reversible loss of color vision	Tinnitus, visual and hearing disturbance
Cardiovascular system	—	Palpitations (4%)	Fluid retention	Edema	Nephropathy, renal failure, palpitations	Edema, dyspnea, palpitations
Laboratory test effects	May alter urine glucose determinations with glucose oxidase reagent (Testape) and cupric sulfate reagent (Clinitest)	Anemia, abnormal liver function tests (LFTs) BUN elevation	Abnormal LFTs, WBC counts, BUN elevation	Decreased hemoglobin and hematocrit. Elevated SGOT and transaminase in 4% of patients	Prolonged prothrombin time, false (+) urinary bile (diazo tablet test	Abnormal LFTs, prolonged bleeding time, interference with 5-HIAA assays

three 325-mg aspirin tablets provide the same degree of analgesia as one 1000-mg "maximum strength" tablet. Caffeine has not been shown to be a useful adjunct to aspirin. Effervescent formulations often contain quantities of sodium that should be avoided in patients with hypertension, congestive heart failure or other conditions in which sodium intake should be restricted. Examples of some commercially available nonprescription combination analgesics are listed in Table 42.5. Generally, these products have no advantage over simple aspirin. Several analgesics require prescriptions and are actively promoted as agents for moderate pain and are much more expensive than aspirin and usually no more effective than aspirin as indicated in Tables 42.2 and 42.3.

There are only three levels of analgesia which can be achieved pharmacologically (3). Aspirin provides good relief for mild to moderate pain. Combinations of aspirin with codeine, oxocodone or pentazocine provide greater pain relief. These three agents alone are usually no more potent than aspirin. Morphine and the other narcotic analgesics (except codeine and oxycodone) provide the most profound analgesia. Only one drug which is not chemically related to the opiates has been reported to provide analgesia comparable to morphine. That drug is methotrimeprazine (Levoprome). Unfortunately, this drug is not available in an oral form and it induces severe orthostatic hypotension and drowsiness. Therefore, its use is limited to bedfast patients.

CHRONIC PAIN MANAGEMENT

Chronic pain is a far more complex clinical event than acute pain (13). A determination must be made of the etiology of the pain; whether it is psychogenic or organic. This distinction may be blurred due to similar presentation of psychogenic and organic pain. Several organic pain etiologies, notably low back injury, are difficult to document. There may be a psychogenic component to organic pain. Therefore, psychological evaluation is useful for most chronic pain patients. Identification of those factors that influence pain is important.

Naproxen Sodium (Anaprox)	Sulindac (Clinoril)	Tolmetin Sodium (Tolectin)	Zomepirac Sodium (Zomax[b])	Piroxicam (Feldene)	Benoxaprofen (Oraflex[c])
Same as naproxen	Elevated alkaline phosphatase	Slight decrease in hematocrit, hemoglobin without GI bleeding, granulocytopenia	Prolonged bleeding time, elevated BUN and serum creatinine	Slightly elevated BUN, alkaline phosphatase and serum creatinine; slight decline in hemoglobin and hematocrit	Transient LFT abnormalities, elevated bleeding time

[a] Modified from A. G. Lipman: Drug actions and interactions. *Modern Medicine*, 50 (August): 1982. (Trade names are given in parentheses.)

[b] Withdrawn from the market in 1983. May be introduced at a later date with amended warnings and recommended doses.

[c] Withdrawn from the market in 1982. May be introduced at a later date with amended warnings and recommended doses.

A broad range of modalities is useful in the management of chronic organic pain. Table 42.6 lists a variety of methods utilized in treating chronic pain of various etiologies. General surgical procedures may alter hormonal balance which influences pain in certain cancers. Hypophysectomy has been demonstrated to increase the level of circulating endorphins. Neurosurgical procedures which interrupt the pain pathways often provide only temporary relief. Alternate pathways often allow pain to return in a few months. Therefore, these procedures are used primarily for patients with advanced, irreversible disease and intractable pain which fails to respond to other therapies. About a third of patients with tic douloureux who fail to respond to drugs require neurosurgical treatment to control their pain. Bony metastases of cancer are major sources of pain.

Local irradiation of these lesions often provides rapid pain relief. Reversible nerve blocks with local anesthetics are useful in determining the nerves involved in pain processes, determining the prognosis of treatment and in providing temporary pain relief (14). Irreversible neurolytic blocks with alcohol or phenol may provide long lasting relief. Such blocks do carry risk of diminished motor function. Myofascial trigger point injections are being used increasingly to provide relief from localized and regional pain (15). Such procedures have been useful in pain associated with causalgias, reflex sympathetic dystrophy syndromes, injury induced vasospasm, and abdominal visceral disease. Local anesthetics injected into the trigger point provide relief for several days to weeks—time periods greatly exceeding the duration of drug activity. Trigger point injec-

Table 42.5.
Examples of Commercially Available Nonprescription Aspirin Containing Analgesics (Oral Route)

Combination Products	Average Dose Range	Comments
Aspirin, buffered (Bufferin) Aspirin 324 mg with aluminum glycinate and magnesium carbonate	2–3 tabs q3–4h	Dissolves more easily than some acetylsalicylic acid, may produce somewhat less GI upset; much more expensive than plain aspirin
Anacin Aspirin 400 mg Caffeine 32.5 mg	2 tabs q3–4h	No distinct advantage over aspirin; caffeine withdrawal may cause severe headaches
Alka-Seltzer Aspirin 324 mg Calcium phosphate Citric acid Sodium bicarbonate	1–2 tabs dissolved in water	rapid absorption; may cause gastric perforation; high sodium content may exacerbate congestive heart failure
APC Aspirin 225 mg Phenacetin 162 mg Caffeine 32 mg	2 tabs q3–4h	No advantage over aspirin and more nephrotoxic with chronic use
Excedrin Aspirin 194.4 mg with 129.6 mg, acetaminophen 97 mg and caffeine 64.8 mg	2 tabs q4h	Salicylamide is a less effective salicylate than aspirin

tions appear to affect sympathetic pathways but the exact mechanism is unclear.

Physical procedures are useful in several types of pain. The effectiveness of acupuncture and acupressure may be partially explained by release of endorphins and partially by the gate control theory of pain (16). Clinical results with these modalities are variable. Electrical stimulation has been reported useful in from 10 to 70% of subjects (17). Transcutaneous electrical nerve stimulation (TENS) is the most common form. A TENS unit is approximately the size of a package of cigarettes. The electrodes are placed in the same locations as trigger points or acupuncture points. These may be direct or referred pain foci. Transcutaneous nerve stimulation is most commonly successful in spinal pain, post-herpetic neuralgia, amputation stump pain, phantom limb pain and pain due to peripheral nerve injury. The method exploits the gate control therapy by mildly stimulating the large nerve fibers leading to the substansia gelatinosa in the dorsal horns of the spinal cord. Other forms of electrical stimulation which have been useful are electrode implantation, dorsal column stimulators with radiofrequency implanted devices, and percutaneous epidural stimulation. The usefulness of electrical stimulation procedures will probably continue to increase

with improved technology. Physical therapy is also a useful modality in the management of much chronic pain. Such therapy is particularly useful in injuries resulting in changes in posture or gait. Correction of physical deformities through physical therapy often produces pain relief. Strengthening muscles often helps patients to overcome functional deficits induced by pain.

Several psychological procedures are useful in pain management (4). These procedures become increasingly important as the psychogenic component of the pain becomes more dominant. In 1953, Skinner (4) described how a pain behavior can become an operant. Operants are actions or responses potentially subject to voluntary control and mediated by striated muscle. They may be elicited by antecedent stimuli but are subject to influence by consequences. Operant conditioning is a process by which behavior is changed or influenced through manipulation of consequences. Operant conditioning can be a major modality in managing chronic pain. Behavior modification is generally reserved for patients with chronic pain which is not associated with physical disorders that induce severe pain. Behavior modification requires the participation of both the patients and their families. This modality is often useful when the cause

Table 42.6.
Modalities Useful in Chronic Pain
Management

Surgery
  Adrenolectomy
  Hypophysectomy
Neurosurgery
  Dorsal rhizotomy
  Cordotomy
  Tractotomy
  Thalamotomy
  Psychosurgery
Palliative irradiation
  (for bony metastases of cancer)
Anesthesiology procedures
  Nerve blocks
  Trigger point injections
Physical procedures
  Physical therapy
  Transcutaneous electrical nerve stimulation
    (TENS)
  Electrode implantation
  Acupuncture and acupressure
Psychological procedures
  Operant conditioning
  Psychotherapy
  Relaxation techniques
  Hypnosis
  Biofeedback
Drug Therapy
  Endocrine agents
  Psychotropic agents
  Glucocorticosteroids
  Analgesics

may be useful. Psychotropic drugs are sometimes useful to treat anxiety or depression associated with pain (18). Tricyclics antidepressants are also being used experimentally to treat chronic pain due to their ability to reduce the central nervous system reuptake of serotonin and to block dopaminergic receptors. These drugs have been useful in treating trigeminal neuralgia and other peripheral neuropathies and post herpectic neuralgia. Tricyclic antidepressants are sometimes used in combination with a phenothiazine or butyrophenone with some suggestion of increased efficacy. Frequently, however, sedating and anticholinergic side effects of psychotropic drugs outweigh their potential benefits. They should be used only when the affective components of the pain are major problems.

In cancer and some other diseases in which glucocorticosteroids are used, reduced analgesic requirements have been noted when the steroids were introduced (3). This effect appears to be related to the effect of the steroids on calcium metabolism and inflammatory processes. While steroids may lower analgesic requirements, the use of steroids as analgesics is not supported by available data.

Chronic, psychogenic pain is usually most effectively managed with psychotherapeutic measures; behavior modification, operant conditioning and other psychological interventions (4). Use of psychotropic or analgesic drugs is occasionally indicated, but such pharmacotherapy may induce undesirable conditioning leading to chronic drug use or abuse.

Chronic, organic pain requires attention to appropriate target symptoms. The chronic pain symptom complex illustrated in Figure 42.7 includes several symptoms commonly seen in such patients (6). Unfortunately, many health professionals fail to recognize these symptoms as a complex. Patients experiencing this complex are sometimes considered hypochondriacs due to their many complaints when in fact they are suffering from a predictable set of interrelated problems. Due to frustration over the multiple symptoms and the patients' seeming failure to respond to therapy, many health professionals and lay people tend to withdraw from such patients. The patients' perception of decreased caring can exacerbate the symptom complex.

The symptom complex depicted in Figure 42.7 begins with the physical cause of the pain. The pain induces anxiety and the anxiety in-

of the pain cannot be eliminated. Relaxation techniques, including biofeedback, hypnosis and other psychotherapeutic modalities are frequently useful in management of psychogenic pain. Electromyographic biofeedback provides a visual or audio signal as muscle tension increases. It is useful in teaching autonomic and somatic control because it provides immediate feedback of muscular tension levels. This technique is most useful in treating tension headaches, neck pain and other pain syndromes associated with excessive muscle tension. Hypnosis has been used in a variety of pain problems. It may be effective in chronic organic pain but may be ineffective in relieving functional pain. In the latter case, hypnosis carries the risk of providing operants for which hypnotherapy offers no alternative.

Drug therapy is usually the major modality used in treating chronic organic pain. In hormone dependent cancers, endocrine agents creases the pain perception. Likewise, the anxiety and depression are interrelated. Hostility results from the anxiety, loneliness from the hostility and the loneliness reinforces the depression. Insomnia, or less commonly, hypersomnia, are common sequelae of depression and anxiety. It is common, but usually inappropriate, to treat each component of this complex as an independent symptom. Such attempts often result in polypharmacy; drugs used to treat one symptom induce further undesirable side effects for which additional drugs are used. For effective treatment, it is usually more appropriate to address the two major components of the complex. These are physical pain and anxiety. Other parts of the symptom complex usually resolve once the pain and anxiety lessen. Therefore, drugs usually should not be initiated for the other parts of the complex during the early part of the therapy. For severe, chronic pain of a physical origin, potent analgesics are indicated. Antianxiety drugs are of only limited value. It is more effective to determine the causes of the patients' anxiety and address those causes. With severe, chronic pain, the continual recurrence of the pain is the most common cause of anxiety. Each dose of analgesic provides pain relief, but within a few hours, pain returns. This continual pattern of pain relief-pain return causes the patient to become anxious about when the pain will return. Chronic pain consists of current pain, remembered pain, and anticipated pain. The memory of pain, even after the current pain has been relieved, results in anticipated pain. This anticipated pain induces anxiety about the return of the pain. When patients are very anxious, they usually require much higher doses of analgesics than they would need if the anxiety were not contributing to the pain problem.

To break this pattern of pain relief-pain return, analgesics should be given to prevent the return of pain rather than to treat the pain once it recurs. To accomplish this, the analgesic should be given on a regular schedule, by the clock rather than p.r.n. Preventing pain return results in markedly decreased anxiety about pain. Within a day or two of being relatively pain free, patients' anticipation of pain usually diminishes.

Various antianxiety drugs have been used to treat the anxiety component of the symptom complex. In a double-blind, controlled pilot study of a phenothiazine, a benzodiazepine, hydroxyzine and placebo, taken in addition to regularly scheduled analgesics by patients in the oncology clinic, no clear benefit was obtained from the antianxiety agents (unpublished data, University of Utah).

Antidepressant medications may be helpful in 10 to 15% of patients whose depression does not resolve once the pain and anxiety are controlled. These may be the same patients who have a genetic predisposition to depression. Most patients' depression appears to be linked to the pain and anxiety. Potential side effects of the antidepressant agents mediate against their being used routinely as initial therapy.

The major causes of insomnia are the pain itself and the affective components of the chronic pain complex. Persons in pain usually cannot sleep. Insomnia is a common occurrence for anxious and depressed patients. Therefore, management of the pain and anxiety is the most effective treatment of the insomnia. Analgesic doses at bedtime are sedating. There have been suggestions that barbiturates may increase pain perception. Hypnotic drugs generally are not indicated.

For severe, chronic pain of physical origin, narcotic analgesics are usually indicated (3). Dosing may either be started low and increased until an effective level is reached or started high with the objective of titrating downward to the appropriate dose. The latter method is preferred. An initial low dose which is not effective may cause the patient to become anxious about the failure of the drug to work. Anxiety is also exacerbated by the patients' fear that there is nothing stronger, and many patients have inappropriate concerns about addiction liability. Therefore, an initial mild overdose is preferred to an initial underdose.

A suggested dose titration for severe, chronic pain due to degenerative disease is pictured in Figure 42.8. The goal is to reach the optimal dose—the lowest dose that provides a reasonable level of comfort. Complete elimination of pain is often not possible. But appropriate dosing of analgesics will allow the patient to experience a reasonable level of comfort. If the initial dose exceeds the upper limit of the effective range, the patient is apt to sleep. Sleep following a dose of narcotic is common due to the sleep deficit accumulated prior to the patient becoming comfortable enough to sleep. Therefore, sleep is not necessarily indicative of overdose.

If the initial dose provides effective analge-

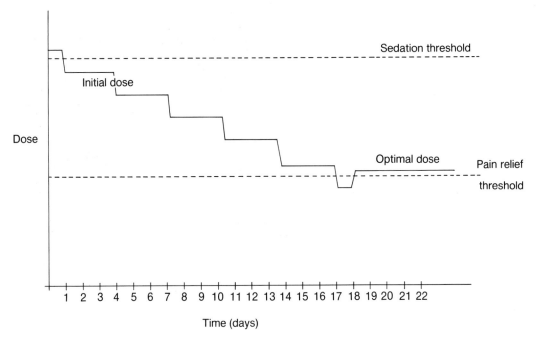

Figure 42.8. Narcotic dose titration. (Adapted with permission from A. G. Lipman: *American Journal of Hospital Pharmacy*, 32:270, 1978 (3).)

sia, the dose should be titrated downward until either the patient experiences return of pain or the patient no longer requires the analgesic. If pain recurs, the last effective dose and the less-than-effective dose can be averaged to determine the maintenance dose. Commonly, this dose can be maintained with good effects. As disease progresses, increasing analgesic doses may be needed. Tolerance is not regularly seen in patients with severe chronic pain of physical origin who are dosed with narcotics by this method. Doses should be reduced only after the drug has reached steady state serum levels. Therefore, the doses are gradually given in decremental amounts. Appropriate reductions are 20% of the total daily dose every 2 days for morphine and every 3 days for methadone. If the initial dose is too low, the dose should be increased rapidly. Doses may be increased by 25 to 33% at each dosing interval. When pain relief is not experienced with the initial dose, anxiety about the failure to obtain pain relief increases. As anxiety increases, the narcotic requirement increases. Thus, as the time necessary to obtain initial pain relief increases, the dose needed for pain relief often increases. Titration to response is necessary. Interpatient dose requirements vary greatly. Attempts at reducing the dose should be undertaken every 7 to 14 days. Doses should be increased as necessary.

Any of the narcotic analgesics with the exception of codeine and oxycodone provide equivalent analgesia at appropriate doses. Codeine and oxycodone appear to have a multiphasic dose response curve (Fig. 42.9). Other narcotic analgesics appear to have a relatively straight line dose response curve. Therefore, as the dose of morphine, methadone or most other narcotic analgesics increases, the effectiveness increases accordingly. While this is true at low doses of codeine and oxycodone, these drugs appear to provide smaller analgesic increments with dose increments at doses above average. This change appears to occur at a dose exceeding 30 to 60 mg of codeine every 3 hours or 2 oxycodone compound tablets (e.g., Percodan, Percocet, Tylox) every 3 hours.

Narcotics provide analgesia at a dose lower than is necessary for anesthesia. Not infrequently, severe pain patients will alternate between pain and somnolence. This is usually indicative of inappropriately high serum levels of drug alternating with too low levels. This effect seldom occurs with regularly scheduled doses. If the patient continues to experience severe, chronic pain while receiving regularly scheduled doses which are highly sedating, the clinician should consider causes of anxiety other than the pain itself. It is usually necessary to identify and alleviate the anxiety to

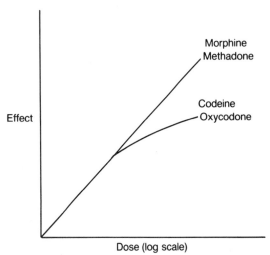

Figure 42.9. Relative dose response curves (clinical observation).

Table 42.7.
Narcotic Analgesics: Approximate Equianalgesic Doses in Severe, Chronic Pain of Physical Origin with Regularly Scheduled Administration

Drug	Route	Dose (mg)	Dosing Frequency (hr)
Morphine sulfate	IM, SC	10	4–6
	PO	20–30	4–6
Methadone	IM, SC	10	6–8
	PO	12.5	6–8
Meperidine	IM, SC	75–100	2½–3½
	PO	150	2½–3½
Levorphanol	IM, SC	2	6–8
	PO	2–3	6–8
Hydromorphone	IM, SC	2–3	4–6
	PO	2–3	4–6
	PR	3–6	4–6
Oxymorphone	IM, SC	1–2	4–6
	PR	2–5	4–6

obtain pain relief. Psychological consultation is often indicated.

The approximate equinanalgesic doses of several commonly used narcotic analgesics are listed in Table 42.7. These equivalences are for regularly scheduled doses. The commonly accepted oral to parenteral dose ratio for morphine is 6 to 1. That ratio is appropriate for single or intermittent doses. The 6-fold difference is largely due to the first pass phenomenon. When morphine is taken orally, the drug is absorbed from the gastrointestinal tract and passes through the liver where it is largely inactivated before reaching the central nervous system where it acts. When given by injection, the drug reaches the central nervous system before being inactivated through conjugation in the liver. After several regularly scheduled doses of morphine, the conjugation system appears to become somewhat saturated and higher levels of the drug reach the central nervous system. If a patient is changed from a regularly scheduled parenteral dose of morphine to 6 times that dose orally, severe sedation will usually occur.

The initial dosing interval for morphine is normally 4 hours. After pain control is obtained, this interval can usually be extended to 6 hours. The initial interval for methadone and levorphanol is 6 hours. That time can often be extended to 8 hours. These latter two drugs usually should not be administered any more frequently than every 6 hours. More frequent dosing can lead to gradual accumulation as pictured in Figure 42.10. Such accumulation produces gradual onset sedation in a few days. In such cases it is difficult to maintain pain relief while lowering the dose sufficiently to overcome the sedation. This problem is more common in older patients due to their decreased kidney elimination capability.

When narcotics are administered on a regularly scheduled basis, there is no advantage to their being administered parenterally (12). The sole advantage of parenteral administration is a more rapid therapeutic response. If the doses are administered in anticipation of the return of pain, that advantage is obviated. Intravenous administration of narcotic analgesics is appropriate for patients who cannot take drugs orally or rectally and who do not have sufficient muscle mass for intramuscular or subcutaneous injections. When high intravenous doses of narcotic analgesics are used, continuous infusion with an infusion pump provides the most consistent serum levels. However, intravenous administration is usually not necessary.

Pentazocine was the first of a series of opioid agonist-antagonist agents to be used clinically as analgesics. When first introduced, this drug was thought to have little or no abuse potential due to its opioid antagonist activity. Unfortunately, this is not the case. Dependence and tolerance do occur with the drug. Furthermore, due to the agonist activity of the drug on the sigmoid opioid receptor, the incidence of hallucinations, dysphoria and vasomotor stimulation with pentazocine is higher than

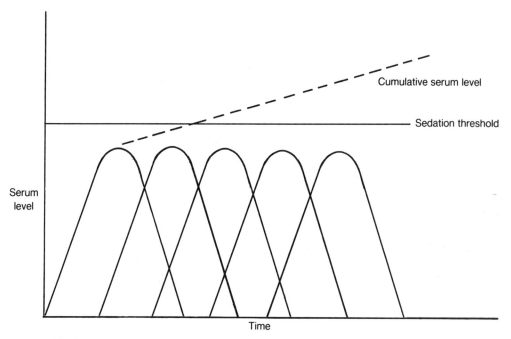

Figure 42.10. Accumulation toxicity dose response curves that occur with too frequent dosing.

with morphine. Butorphanol and nalbuphine are related agonist-antagonist agents. The clinical usefulness of these agents is limited by these side effects. These drugs have little usefulness in managing chronic pain.

NEW ADMINISTRATION METHODS

Recently, intrathecal and epidural administration of low doses of morphine has been shown to provide excellent pain relief for 2 to 4 times the duration expected with oral or intramuscular administration (19). Intraventricular administration through an Ommaya reservoir has also been shown to be useful in selected advanced cancer patients with severe pain. Direct spinal or supraspinal administration into the central nervous system provides immediate and prolonged analgesia with relatively few systemic effects. Such procedures have not yet been fully refined.

Patient controlled analgesia has also been shown to be an effective method of administering narcotics for pain (20). This procedure has been used with good results in postsurgical pain. Patients receive a predetermined dose of drug via an intravenous catheter. The drug is administered by a syringe pump that is programmed to inject the dose no more frequently than the time interval preset on the pump. The drug is administered on demand when the patient presses a button. Early reports indicate that patients taper their doses resulting in lowered risk of dependence and tolerance, and that patients are able to maintain normal sleep-wake cycles while experiencing good pain relief.

As the intensity of chronic pain varies, analgesic requirements change. Therefore, pharmacists involved in pain management should be aware of methods for evaluating pain longitudinally. Visual analog scales, on which patients indicate their pain level, are useful (Fig. 42.11) (21). Melzack developed a pain rating scale which uses six terms for which interpatient reliability has been established (Table 42.8). Standardized pain rating instruments should be used to determine patients' relative discomfort over time.

PAIN IN TERMINAL DISEASE

Pain can be a major problem in cancer and other advanced, irreversible diseases. Over 300,000 Americans die of cancer annually. About two thirds of these, over 200,000 persons, experience severe pain in the terminal stages of their disease.

Today, over 90% of severe cancer pain is manageable with modalities currently available. The daily doses of narcotics that are appropriate and necessary for some of these

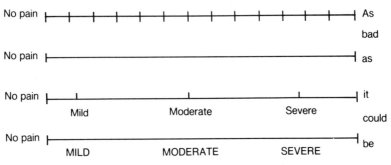

Figure 42.11. Visual analog scales for rating pain.

patients are equivalent to hundreds of milligrams, and in some cases greater than a gram of morphine. Yet patients receiving these doses remain awake and alert. Other patients require only tens of milligrams of morphine per day. The interpatient variance is very high.

Much of the progress in controlling pain due to advanced, irreversible disease has been associated with hospice programs. Hospice programs for the care of the ill originated in the Middle Ages. Contemporary hospice programs, which fully integrate medical and psychosocial care, originated in 1967 with the opening of St. Christopher's Hospice in London, England. Over 1,200 hospices now exist in the United States. Most are home care programs. The goals of hospice care are to provide interdisciplinary, palliative care for patients who have advanced irreversible disease, and whose life expectancy is measurable in weeks or months as opposed to years. The cornerstone of hospice care is symptom control and pain is one of the major symptoms addressed. The cornerstone of symptom control is drug therapy.

In the late 1960s and early 1970s, Dame Cicely Saunders and Dr. Robert Twycross, two leading British hospice physicians, advocated the use of heroin as an analgesic of choice in pain due to terminal illness. Furthermore, they advocated the use of the Brompton cocktail as the oral liquid narcotic analgesic dosage form of choice. More recent studies conducted in England, Canada, and the United States have conclusively demonstrated that morphine, methadone and other narcotic analgesics are equal in effectiveness to heroin (22). The only potential advantage of heroin over morphine sulfate is that heroin is far more soluble in water (12). Therefore, it can be formulated in a more concentrated solution for intramuscular injection into a patient with a wasted mus-

Table 42.8.
McGill Pain Questionnaire Pain Rating Scale

0 — None
1 — Mild
2 — Discomforting
3 — Distressing
4 — Horrible
5 — Excruciating

cle mass. However, dilaudid is also far more soluble than morphine sulfate. In 1984, a concentrated dilaudid dosage form became available for parenteral administration. This advantage of heroin is now obviated. The Brompton cocktail is a solution originally formulated at the Brompton Hospital for Chest Diseases in 1896 for the management of post-thoracotomy pain. The original solution contained morphine (heroin was later substituted), cocaine, alcohol and chloroform water as a flavoring agent. Twycross demonstrated in a controlled study that the cocaine is noncontributory to the analgesic or mood effects; it may cause dysphoria (23). Cocaine was added to the original formulation as a local anesthetic for the throat pain caused by intubation. Its use in a simple analgesic formulation is irrational. The alcohol simply adds to the central nervous system depressant activity of the formulation. It provides no advantage (24). Both Dame Cicely and Dr. Twycross now use simple oral morphine solution as their analgesic of choice.

The vast majority of hospice patients have cancer. However, other chronic, degenerative diseases, such as end stage organ failure, stroke, multiple sclerosis, and amyotrophic lateral sclerosis which require symptom control, meet the admission criteria for hospice care. Many pharmacists are now actively involved as staff members, consultants, and members of the boards of directors of hospice programs. With rapid progress in control of pain and other symptoms in recent years, symptom control increasingly is becoming a regular component of clinical oncology meetings and other medical and pharmaceutical specialty meetings.

INTERDISCIPLINARY CARE

Multidisciplinary pain clinics are becoming increasingly common in university and community hospitals. Such programs frequently have inpatient services as well. The objective of pain clinics is to provide multidisciplinary evaluation of severe and chronic pain, to help establish the etiology and complicating factors and to plan and provide appropriate treatment of the pain. Pharmacists are frequently involved in such services. Drugs play a central role in pain management and are often implicated in the cause and complications of chronic pain. The existence and growth of these clinics is a testimony to the advantages of interdisciplinary care in the management of difficult pain problems. Pain management is an area of growing interest and potential for clinically oriented pharmacists.

Effective control of pain requires good diagnosis and identification of the factors which contribute to the pain. When drugs are indicated, titration to effect is important. Severe obtundation or wide swings in pain control can usually be avoided through appropriate dosing. With regularly scheduled drugs, the oral route of administration usually can be used effectively. A major component of chronic pain which must be addressed for effective pain control is anxiety. When drugs are used in control of severe chronic pain, they often must be used very aggressively. However, drugs should only be used when they are clearly indicated. Frequently, the risk to benefit ratio of adjunctive symptomatic agents is unfavorable. It is common for a patient with severe pain of long duration to be taking a large variety of drugs. One of the first steps often necessary in controlling the pain is to eliminate most of those drugs.

Pharmacists involved in pain control programs and those who counsel pain patients have good reason to be optimistic about available pain management modalities. This optimism should be shared with patients. Both health professionals and the public subscribe to many misconceptions about pain and analgesics, especially narcotics. Patient education may be necessary to convince some patients to take their regularly scheduled analgesics before the pain returns. New technology including infusion pumps, patient controlled analgesia devices and equipment needed for the new routes of administration directly into the central nervous system are areas in which pharmacists' expertise is useful. Increasing pharmacist involvement in pain clinics and hospice programs is needed. There are several new analgesics currently in development and pharmacists should be influential in determining which of these drugs will provide meaningful therapeutic advantages.

References

1. Melzack R, Wall PD: Pain mechanisms: a new theory. *Science* 150:971, 1965.
2. Snyder SH: Opiate receptors and internal opiates. *Sci Am* 236:44, 1977.
3. Lipman AG: Drug therapy in terminal illness. *Am J Hosp Pharm* 32:270, 1975.
4. Skinner BF: *Science and Human Behavior.* New York: Macmillan, 1953.
5. Wall PD: On the relationship of injury to pain. *Pain* 6:253, 1979.
6. Lipman AG: Drug therapy in cancer pain. *Cancer Nurs* 2:39, 1980.
7. Moertel CG, Ahmann DL, Taylor WF, et al: A comparative evaluation of marketed analgesic drugs. *N Engl J Med* 286:813, 1972.
8. Moertel CG, Ahmann DL, Taylor WF, et al: Relief of pain by oral medications. *JAMA* 229:55, 1974.
9. Miller RR, Feingold A, and Paxionos J: Propoxyphene hydrochloride: a critical review. *JAMA* 213:996, 1970.
10. Marks RM, Sachar EJ: Undertreatment of medical inpatients with narcotic analgesics. *Ann Intern Med* 78:173, 1973.
11. Porter J, Jick H: Addiction rare in patients treated with narcotics (letter). *N Engl J Med* 302:123, 1980.
12. Twycross RG: Clinical experiences with diamorphine in advanced malignant disease. *Int J Clin Pharmacol* 9:184, 1974.
13. Revler JB, Girard DE, Nardone DF: The chronic pain syndrome: misconceptions and management. *Ann Intern Med* 93:588, 1980.
14. Bonica JJ: Introduction to nerve blocks, in Bonica JJ, Ventafridda V: *Advances in Pain Research and Therapy.* New York: Raven Press, 1979, vol 2.
15. Wyant GM: Chronic pain syndromes and their treatment; II. Trigger points. *Can Anaesth Soc J* 26:216, 1979.
16. Ulett GA: Acupuncture treatments for pain relief. *JAMA* 245:768, 1981.
17. Magora F, Aladjemoff L, Tannenbaum J, et al: Treatment of pain by transcutaneous electrical

stimulation. *Acta Anaesthesiol Scand* 22:589, 1978.

18. Clarke IMC: Amitryptyline and perphenazine in chronic pain. *Anaesthesia* 36:210, 1981.

19. Leavans ME, Hill CS, Cech CA, et al: Intrathecal and intraventricular morphine for pain in cancer patients: initial study. *J Neurosurg* 56:241, 1982.

20. Tamsen A, Hartvig P, Dahlstrom B, et al: Patient controlled analgesic therapy in the early postoperative period. *Acta Anaesthesiol Scand* 23:462, 1974.

21. Melzack R: *The Puzzle of Pain.* New York: Basic Books, 1973.

22. Kaiko RF, Wallenstein SL, Rogers AG, et al: Analgesic and mood effects of heroin and morphine in cancer patients with postoperative pain. *N Engl J Med* 304:1501, 1981.

23. Twycross R: Value of cocaine in opiate-containing elixirs (letter). *Br Med J* 2:1348, 1977.

24. Melzack R, Mount BM, Gordon R: The Brompton mixture versus morphine solution given orally: effects on pain. *Can Med Assoc J* 120:435, 1971.

SECTION 11
Diseases of the Eye

CHAPTER 43

Glaucoma

DICK R. GOURLEY, Pharm.D.
ROBERT J. IGNOFFO, Pharm.D.
THEODORE G. TONG, Pharm.D.

Glaucoma is a disease of the eye that is characterized by an increase in intraocular pressure (IOP). More than 3 million Americans have glaucoma and approximately 15% of them have varying degrees of blindness caused by damage to the optic disk and visual field changes which are secondary to glaucoma. Open-angle glaucoma is the second leading cause of blindness and unfortunately over 1 million Americans have glaucoma which is undiagnosed. Glaucoma usually manifests itself after the age of 35, but can occur in younger people as well. Glaucoma screening is a part of routine eye examinations because of this. One to two percent of the population over 40 years of age and 5 to 9% over 65 years of age suffer from glaucoma.

This disease is insidious in onset and often produces only minor symptoms of discomfort, such as headache or "tired eyes." A large number of patients do not seek medical attention until the disorder is well established due to the lack of symptoms. Some patients will exhibit much higher IOP, but with a lack of symptoms. Fortunately, optic nerve and retinal damage are late findings of end-stage disease. Symptoms such as persistent headache and eye pain will usually prompt patients to seek medical assistance before these serious consequences develop (1).

PATHOGENESIS

The IOP is physiologically determined by the relative production and elimination of aqueous humor. An increased IOP can result only from either increased production of aqueous, decreased elimination, or both. The major cause of increased IOP is decreased elimination.

There are more than 40 different types of glaucoma. The two major types of glaucoma are angle-closure and open-angle. The more acute type is the angle-closure glaucoma. It occurs in only 5% of all cases, compared to 90% for the open-angle type. Both types can be further classified into primary and secondary glaucoma. A third type is congenital glaucoma which results from developmental ocular abnormalities and occurs in less than 2% of cases. Table 43.1 lists the classifications of glaucoma.

The familial relationship of glaucoma has been well established; whether the hereditary pattern is one consistent with a dominant or recessive autosomal trait remains equivocal. Particular attention to factors which contribute to greater risk of developing this disease should be paid for any patient with a familial history of glaucoma. Although there are more males with primary open-angle glaucoma, sex predilection for the disease is not clinically significant. Primary open-angle glaucoma is a relatively more common disorder in Caucasians and blacks than American Indians and Asians. Although many patients may present with unilateral involvement initially, it can be anticipated that the other eye will be involved within 5 years. Myopia has been suggested to be a high risk factor in predisposition to glaucoma. Although it is more common to find open-angle glaucoma in patients with myopia, especially in the younger age group, the evidence of association between the two factors remains equivocal (2).

PATHOPHYSIOLOGY

There are several anatomic factors associated with acute-closure glaucoma: (a) small hyperopic (farsighted) eyes, (b) tautness of the iris and large pupils, (c) anterior lens dislocations, (d) swollen hypermature lens, and (e) posterior or anterior synechiae (fibrous scars).

Farsighted individuals are particularly at risk for angle closure since the tissue of their eyeballs are relatively compacted and the lens is shifted anteriorly.

Table 43.1.
Classification of Glaucomas[a]

I. Primary Glaucoma
  A. Primary open-angle glaucoma; synonyms: chronic open-angle glaucoma; chronic simple glaucoma; glaucoma simplex
  B. Low tension glaucoma
  C. Primary closed-angle glaucoma; synonyms: primary angle-closure glaucoma; narrow-angle glaucoma; iris-block glaucoma; acute congestive glaucoma
    1. Acute angle-closure glaucoma
    2. Chronic angle-closure glaucoma (may also be secondary to other ocular diseases)
    3. Intermittent angle-closure glaucoma
    4. Superimposed on chronic open-angle glaucoma (combined mechanism)
II. Variants of Primary Glaucoma
  A. Pigmentary glaucoma
  B. Exfoliation glaucoma; synonyms: pseudoexfoliation of the lens capsule; glaucoma capsulare
III. Developmental Glaucoma
  A. Primary congenital glaucoma
  B. Infantile glaucoma with associated defects such as Axenfeld's and Reiger's anomalies
  C. Glaucoma associated with hereditary or familial diseases such as aniridia, encephalotrigeminal hemangiomatosis (Sturge-Weber syndrome), neurofibromatosis, oculocerebrorenal (Lowe's) syndrome
IV. Secondary Glaucoma
  A. Inflammatory glaucoma
    1. Uveitis of all types
    2. Fuchs' heterochromic iridocyclitis
  B. Phacogenic glaucoma
    1. Angle-closure glaucoma with mature cataract
    2. Phacoanaphylactic glaucoma secondary to rupture of lens capsule
    3. Phacolytic glaucoma caused by phacotoxic meshwork blockage
    4. Subluxation of lens
  C. Glaucoma secondary to intraocular hemorrhage
    1. Hyphema
    2. Hemolytic glaucoma (erthroclastic glaucoma)
  D. Traumatic glaucoma
    1. Traumatic recession of chamber angle
    2. Postsurgical glaucomas
      a. Aphakic pupillary block
      b. Ciliary block (malignant) glaucoma
  E. Neovascular glaucoma (especially in diabetic patients)
  F. Drug-induced glaucoma
    1. Corticosteroid-induced glaucoma
    2. Postoperative ocular hypertension from use of α-chymotrypsin
  G. Glaucomas of miscellaneous origin
    1. Associated with intraocular tumors
    2. Associated with retinal detachments (rare)
    3. Secondary to severe chemical burns of the eye
    4. Associated with essential iris atrophy
V. Absolute Glaucoma

---

[a] Reprinted with permission from *Clinical Symposia.*

    In individuals with significant lack of tautness of the iris diaphragm (usually in large pupils), a bulging iris (bombé) may occur because of increased iridotrabecular contact.

    Two conditions which lead to anterior lens dislocation are ocular trauma or a severe blow to the eye, both of which may lead to pupillary blockage or direct obstruction of the angle. Similarly, a swollen lens, as in inflammatory conditions (uveitis), produces pupillary blockage.

    Posterior synechiae can form in the eyes of patients with uveitis and in the presence of sufficient numbers of them to occlude the pupil. An increase in IOP may then result. Anterior synechiae can form after long standing iritis and produce adhesion of the anterior portion of iris to the trabecular meshwork. The outflow of aqueous humor is further obstructed, increasing IOP.

As mentioned previously the damage from either type of glaucoma is primarily due to the inhibition of aqueous humor outflow. Aqueous humor formation occurs at a rapid rate (approximately 1 ml/min) and is dependent on several interacting mechanisms within the ciliary processes. The aqueous humor is secreted by the ciliary processes into the posterior chamber of the eye (Fig. 43.1), where it flows to the anterior chamber and then to the trabecular meshwork and finally out through the canal of Schlemm. Since a decrease in the outflow facility of aqueous humor is the primary mechanism for producing an increase in IOP, the anatomical changes in open angle and angle closure will be discussed (2).

In *open angle glaucoma* a physical blockage occurs within the trabecular meshwork which retards elimination of aqueous humor. The obstruction is presumed to be located between the trabecular sheet and the episcleral veins, into which the aqueous ultimately flows.

The impairment of aqueous drainage elevates the IOP to between 25 and 35 mm Hg (normal 10 to 20 mm Hg), indicating the obstruction is usually partial. This increase in IOP is sufficient to cause progressive cupping of the optic disk and eventual visual field defects. As the trabecular spaces become more involved, detachment of the cornea and formation of bullae may develop. In addition, scotomas (blind spots) may develop. Since visual acuity remains largely unaffected until late in the disease, presence of scotomata must be regarded as a major indication for the institution of medical therapy.

In *angle-closure glaucoma* increased IOP is caused by pupillary blockage of aqueous outflow. In contrast to open-angle, the blockage to outflow is more severe. The basic requirements leading to an acute attack of angle closure are (a) a pupillary block, (b) a narrowed

anterior chamber angle, and (c) a convex iris (iris bombé). The sequence of events leading to increased IOP is depicted in Figure 43.2. When a patient has a narrow anterior chamber (Fig. 43.2A) or a pupil that dilates to a degree where the iris comes in greater contact with the lens (Fig. 43.2B), there is interference with the flow of aqueous humor from the posterior to the anterior chamber. Since aqueous humor is continually secreted, pressure from within the posterior chamber forces the iris to bulge forward (Fig. 43.2C). This may progress to complete blockage (Fig. 43.2D).

The pathologic complications of angle-closure and open-angle glaucoma include the formation of cataracts, peripheral anterior synechiae, atrophy of the optic nerve, retina and absolute glaucoma (complete blockage of aqueous outflow). The development of cataracts can increase existing pupillary block and the degree of angle closure.

ETIOLOGY

Drugs which have autonomic effects produce several types of ocular changes. Of great importance is the effect of anticholinergic agents on angle-closure glaucoma. The section on drugs contraindicated in glaucoma gives more detail on this subject. Several factors appear to be associated with drug-induced glaucoma. They are listed in Table 43.2.

In addition to drugs, glaucoma can occur as a secondary manifestation of systemic disorders or trauma. A list of systemic disease associated with increased IOP is given in Table 43.3.

Congenital glaucoma is a rare disorder in

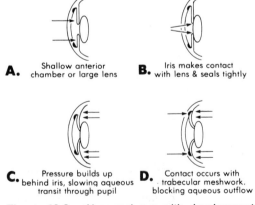

A. Shallow anterior chamber or large lens

B. Iris makes contact with lens & seals tightly

C. Pressure builds up behind iris, slowing aqueous transit through pupil

D. Contact occurs with trabecular meshwork, blocking aqueous outflow

Figure 43.2. Abnormal eye with development of pupillary block.

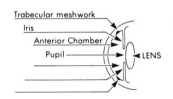

Figure 43.1. Normal eye anatomy.

Table 43.2.
Factors Implicated in Potential Drug Induction of Angle-Closure Glaucoma

1. Age—usually over 30
2. History—familial, genetic basis
3. Race—usually Caucasian
4. Sex—usually female
5. Anterior chamber angle—shallow and narrow
6. Vision—hyperopia, hypermetropia
7. Convexity of the iris—flattened
8. Dose and duration of the offending drug used
9. Duration of effect on the eye—longer duration
10. Route of administration—topical more than systemic

Table 43.3.
Systemic Conditions Associated with Glaucoma (Secondary)[a]

Congenital rubella
Diabetes mellitus
Down's syndrome
Hallermann-Streiff syndrome
Homocystinuria
Idiopathic infantile hypoglycemia
Lowe's syndrome
Marfan's syndrome
Melanoma (intraocular tumors)
Neurofibromatosis (von Recklinghausen's)
Turner's syndrome
Uveitis (secondary)

[a] Modified from Scheie et al. (135).

which the IOP is increased as a result of developmental abnormalities of the ocular structures in the newborn. It may occur in association with other congenital abnormalities and anomalies such as homocystinuria and Marfan's syndrome. Congenital glaucoma should be considered in those newborns who have sensitivity to light, excessive tearing or spasm of the eyelids.

DIAGNOSIS AND CLINICAL FINDINGS

The common signs of open-angle glaucoma may be marginal and will not appear immediately. As time progresses the signs become more marked until they finally restrict vision. In some cases there may be a total absence of signs. The common signs are: (a) increased IOP, (b) visual field loss, (c) optic disk changes, (d) decreased outflow facility, (e) gonioscopically open angles, and (f) positive provocative tests (3).

An increased IOP can have several interpretations. Most normal individuals have pressures of 21 mm Hg or less. However, there is a small group of patients who may sustain glaucomatous damage even with pressures under 20 mm Hg (3). In general, pressure readings in the high 20s are suspicious and those above 30 are cause for serious concern. Patients between the age of 50 and 75 with pressures above 30 as the only sign of glaucoma should be treated medically because decreased vascular perfusion in older people can endanger the optic nerve. In the younger patient with similar readings, it may only be necessary to assess for changes in the optic disk or visual fields at frequent intervals (1).

In the early stage of chronic (open-angle) glaucoma, symptoms of pain or visual field loss are usually not present (Table 43.4). It is estimated that 50% of patients do not know they have the disorder.

Acute angle-closure glaucoma usually presents with signs and symptoms of blurred vision (often with colored halos around light), severe ocular pain, and nausea (occasional vomiting) (4). The eye appears red, the cornea cloudy, the pupil mid-dilated, the anterior chamber is narrow, and the IOP is frequently above 50 mm Hg.

Visual acuity is reduced because of corneal changes or edema. Bullae may be present on the cornea if the acute attack is prolonged. Colored halos result from diffraction of light by the edematous cornea.

Ocular pain may vary from moderate to severe. The oculovagal reflex is thought to produce nausea, vomiting, bradycardia, and sweating which may accompany an acute attack.

With very high IOPs, the pupil may become fixed in mid-dilation and eventually damaged. In severe cases, the pupil changes from a round to an oval shape and may resist contriction by topical parasympathomimetic agents.

Chronic angle closure is a less severe form of glaucoma than acute angle closure; the symptoms may range from none to intermittent and severe ocular pain along with halo formation and/or ocular congestion. Synechiae do not form without ocular congestion, which may be evident only with moderately high pressure readings.

With both major types of glaucoma several diagnostic procedures are available to evaluate visual field loss, optic disk changes, outflow facility, angle measurements and provocative

Table 43.4.
Clinical Findings and Symptoms of Primary Glaucomas

Glaucoma	Onset	Early Findings and Symptoms	Late Findings and Symptoms
Open-angle	Insidious	Asymptomatic slight rise in intraocular pressure; decrease rate of aqueous humor outflow, optic disk changes (symptoms may be marginal or even at times absent)	Gradual loss of peripheral vision (over months to years); persistent elevation of intraocular pressure; optic nerve degeneration; retinal nerve atrophy; edema of the cornea; cataracts; trabecular meshwork degeneration
Angle-closure	Sudden	Blurred vision; severe ocular pain and congestion; conjunctival redness; cloudy cornea; moderately dilated pupil; poor pupil response to light; intraocular pressure markedly elevated; nausea and vomiting	Complete blindness in 2–5 days

tests, but their discussion is beyond the scope of this chapter. A brief tabulation of these tests and procedures is provided in Table 43.5.

DRUGS CONTRAINDICATED IN GLAUCOMA

Specific classes of drugs such as anticholinergics, adrenergics and corticosteroids have been implicated in inducing glaucoma. Any drug with atropine-like side effects can produce pupillary dilation and paralysis of accommodation for near vision. Concern for this iatrogenic complication has prompted Food and Drug Administration requirements for warnings on the systemic use of anticholinergics in the presence of glaucoma.

One must distinguish between open-angle and angle-closure glaucoma in arriving at a therapeutic decision because drug effects are different in the two cases. Drugs that dilate the pupil, for instance, may precipitate an acute attack of angle closure glaucoma but usually do not produce harmful effects in open angle cases. Dilation of the pupil in angle closure may cause the peripheral iris to bulge forward, blocking the trabecular meshwork. The aqueous humor is prevented from reaching the outflow channels and, therefore, results in an increase in IOP. Since excessive resistance to outflow in open angle glaucoma is caused primarily by changes within the trabecular outflow channels, dilation of the pupil usually will not exacerbate the IOP.

Since *topical* administration of some drugs (Table 43.6) is known to elevate IOP in some patients with glaucoma, it has been assumed that *systemic* administration of such medications will have a similar effect. If this assumption is correct, then glaucoma patients should probably not use anticholinergics, antihistamines, psychotropic agents, antiparkinson drugs, certain cardiovascular drugs, or glucocorticoids. In patients with mild or controlled glaucoma it may be unwarranted to prohibit the use of systemic sympathomimetics, anticholinergics, and other atropine-like drugs because the evidence that they exacerbate the condition is not well documented (5). The evidence for lack of adverse effect of these agents is discussed in their specific sections.

Anticholinergics

In patients with normal eyes, topically instilled anticholinergics (6) such as atropine, scopolamine and cyclopentolate produce no significant elevations in IOP. However, in patients over 30 years of age who have abnormally shallow anterior chambers, there is a significant risk of precipitating acute attacks of angle-closure glaucoma. The incidence has been estimated to be nearly 1 in 4000 (7). Atropine and scopolamine have a profound effect on the eye because of their longer duration of action than other agents with anticholinergic effects, i.e., phenothiazines, tricyclic antidepressants and antihistamines. These locally instilled agents cause mydriasis and cycloplegia which may persist for as long as 2 weeks. In some open angle patients, the agents can produce a slight rise of IOP (less than 6 mm Hg) when instilled into the eyes (8). Other mydriatics, however, do not appear to have this effect.

Conventional doses of atropine systemically

Table 43.5.
Diagnostic Studies for Glaucoma

Procedures	Comments
Tonometry	Measures intraocular tension; routinely used for mass screening studies; diurnal variations of intraocular tension in open-angle glaucoma should be considered; repeated readings should be done before definite diagnosis; between acute attacks of angle-closure glaucoma, the intraocular tension may be normal, applanation tonometry measures the force applied per unit area while indentation tonometry uses a plunger to produce a pit in the cornea, which serves as a measure of intraocular pressure
Gonioscopy	Differentiates the type of glaucoma; gonioscopic appearance of narrowed anterior chamber angle is usually diagnostic of angle closure glaucoma
Tonography	May reveal impaired facility of aqueous humor outflow; early open angle glaucoma can be detected by this technique; tonometer is applied to the eye and the resultant reduction in the intraocular tension is measured as an indicator of outflow facility
Water-drinking test	Rise in intraocular tension after rapid ingestion of a quart of water is significant indication of glaucoma; positive result occurs in 30% of open angle glaucoma cases; negative result does not rule out glaucoma. Tonography and water-drinking test will reveal open angle glaucoma with 90% reliability
Ophthalmoscopy	Glaucomatous excavation or cupping of the optic dish is found in chronic primary open angle and congenital glaucomas; glaucomatous changes of optic dish and/or occlusion of the central retinal vein in absence of elevated intraocular tension should arouse suspicion of glaucoma in early stage
Visual field examination	Isolated areas of impaired vision surrounded by normal areas in a visual field is indicative of open angle glaucoma; visual field changes are irreversible and parallel optic disk changes
Corticosteroid instillation	Striking differences in ocular tension (between primary open-angle glaucoma patients and normal subjects) are produced by topically instilled corticosteroids; steroid provocative test is used to evaluate genetic predisposition to glaucoma; response of primary angle-closure glaucoma to corticosteroid instillation is much more similar to normal subjects
Dark room test	Intraocular tension is assessed in patient before and after being placed in a dark room; in chronic angle closure glaucoma, a considerable rise in the intraocular tension is observed after being in the dark

administered for preanesthesia have little ocular effect; in contrast, equivalent therapeutic doses of scopolamine can cause definite pupillary dilation (9, 10). Belladonna, of which atropine is the main component, has been reported to exacerbate preglaucomatous eyes, although this is rare (11). Prolonged use of anticholinergics can exacerbate open-angle glaucoma to some extent, but studies have shown that oral atropine at a dose of 0.6 mg every 4 hours for 1 week produced only slight elevations of IOP (12). In another study, the administration of proprietary cold remedies containing 0.2 mg of belladonna alkaloids (given twice daily for 4 days) caused no changes in IOP in 27 normal volunteers and 37 patients with glaucoma (including 18 patients with chronic angle closure) (13).

Propantheline, a commonly used anticholinergic, has been shown to produce no significant elevation in IOP in either normal or angle closure patients (14). Anticholinergics, in fact, can deepen the anterior chamber by inhibiting the contraction of the ciliary body and produce cycloplegia which widens rather than narrows the anterior chamber angle making angle closure less likely to occur (15). No recent reports of exacerbations of glaucoma with diazepam or amitriptyline have appeared in the literature, although the manufacturers of these drugs contraindicate their use in patients with the disorder (16). Very high doses of phenothiazines given for schizophrenia have reportedly been observed to produce slight elevations of IOP (16). Treatment with miotics easily overcame the effect.

In summary, withholding systemic anticholinergics for fear of inducing open angle glaucoma probably is not justified. This is true especially with regard to the use of parenteral atropine or scopolamine given preoperatively prior to general anesthesia. Sensitivity of the

Table 43.6.
Ability of Drugs to Induce Glaucoma

Drug	Route	Open angle	Angle closure
Anticholinergics			
Atropine	Topical	Rarely	Frequently
Scopolamine	"	"	"
Belladonna	"	"	"
Propantheline	Systemic	Rarely	Rarely
Adrenergics			
Phenylephrine 10%[a]	Topical	Never	Occasionally
Epinephrine	Systemic	Never	Rarely
Miotics			
Pilocarpine 4–8%	Topical	Never	Occasionally
Echothiophate	"	"	"
Isoflurophate	"	"	"
Carbonic anhydrase inhibitors			
Acetazolamide	Systemic	Never	Rarely
α-Chymotrypsin[b]	Topical	Rarely	Occasionally
Antihypertensives[c]	Systemic	Never	Never
Prochlorperazine[b]	Systemic	Never	Never
Promethazine[b]	Systemic	Never	Rarely
(high doses)			
Corticosteroids (at equipotent doses)			
Betamethasone	Topical	Frequently	Never
Dexamethasone	"	"	"
Hydrocortisone	Topical	Occasionally	Never
Prednisolone	"	"	"
Triamcinolone	"	"	"
Dexamethasone	Systemic	Occasionally	Never
Hydrocortisone	"	"	"
Prednisolone	"	"	"

eye to systemic drugs is relatively low (15, 16). Although these agents can induce angle closure in rare instances, the concomitant use of parasympathomimetic miotics will prevent any of the IOP effects. However, ocularly instilled potent anticholinergics, such as atropine, scopolamine, cyclopentolate and homatropine should not be used in patients diagnosed or predisposed to having angle-closure glaucoma (17).

Sympathomimetics

Adrenergic agents commonly found in appetite suppressants, bronchodilators, central nervous stimulants and vasoconstrictors produce slight pupillary dilation. No adverse effects on open-angle glaucoma have been experienced. The incidence of deleterious effects on angle-closure glaucoma has been extremely small after systemic administration (18). Adrenergic agents such as epinephrine and phenylephrine have been used ocularly to treat open-angle glaucoma. It is important to note, however, that these agents will elevate the

IOP by narrowing the anterior chamber angle when instilled into eyes of angle closure patients (5, 19, 20).

General anesthetics producing parasympathetic and sympathetic imbalance may cause pupillary block. Topical pilocarpine 1% may be instilled into the eye 1 hour prior to inducing anesthesia to prevent this complication (5, 15, 16).

Cardiovascular Drugs

There is no convincing evidence that vasodilators significantly can aggravate glaucoma despite the fact that subconjunctival injection of strong vasodilators such as isoxsuprine and tolazoline can induce transient elevations in IOP, particularly in chronic open-angle glaucoma (5). Nitrates, nitrites, aminophylline, nylidirin and cyclandelate can be used safely in glaucoma (5, 7, 21). Antihypertensives will decrease intraocular blood flow which can lead to loss of small visual fields in the patient with a high IOP. Therefore, it is probably best to decrease blood pressure gradually in angle closure patients. If it is necessary to decrease blood pressure rapidly, one should either increase the patient's miotic medication or simultaneously lower the IOP rapidly with an agent such as acetazolamide.

Miscellaneous Agents

Amphetamines, tricyclic antidepressants, monoamine oxidase inhibitors, indomethacin and cocaine (22) produce slight degrees of mydriasis, but the likelihood of inducing angle closure with these drugs is very low (23). Strong miotics such as pilocarpine 4 to 8% and the indirect acting nonreversible cholinesterase inhibitors may lead to pupillary block and inhibition of aqueous humor outflow and increase vascular congestion of the peripheral part of the iris so that the swollen iris becomes opposed to the cornea (5, 9, 15, 24, 25).

Polarizing neuromuscular blocking agents such as succinylcholine used as adjuvants to general anesthesia can cause a marked rise in IOP if the patient is not adequately anesthetized (26). They should not be used in glaucomatous patients. A nondepolarizing neuromuscular blocking agent such as gallamine is effective in preventing the rise in IOP (16).

An acute transient myopia has occurred following vaginal absorption of AVC cream which contains sulfanilamide, complicated by retinal edema, shallowing anterior chambers and acute angle closure (27). Similar reactions have occurred involving carbonic anhydrase inhibitors (28), tetracycline (29), prochlorperazine and promethazine (30). A few of these may be responsible for ocular hypertension, but more commonly they act to increase retinal fluid production. These reactions can be classified as idiosyncratic phenomena.

Patients who have received α-chymotrypsin while undergoing cataract extraction characteristically show an increase in IOP 2 to 5 days after surgery for 1 week or more (31). Deep anterior chambers and open angles are seen, differentiating α-chymotrypsin from pupillary block-induced glaucoma. The induced ocular hypertension appears to be dose-related and self-limiting (32).

Corticosteroid-induced Glaucoma

Corticosteroid-induced glaucoma is well documented (5, 15–17, 33–44). This form of glaucoma is usually without pain, physical findings in the eye, or visual field defects. The lesion produced probably occurs in the trabecular meshwork which severely decreases the outflow facility. Systemically or topically administered corticosteroids produce decreased outflow facility accompanied by a corresponding increase of IOP. After topical therapy, the glaucomatous change occurs in that eye instilled with the drug. This ocular hypertensive effect is usually fully reversible within 1 month after the discontinuation of the steroid.

The increase in IOP is approximately 10 mm Hg for patients with preglaucomatous anterior chambers and 5 mm Hg in normal persons (36). In some cases irreversible eye damage occurs if ocular tension persists for 1 to 2 months or even longer. In addition, cupping of the optic disk and defects of visual field may develop a few months after topical administration of corticosteroids is begun. Patients on chronic topical steroid therapy should, therefore, have tonometric examination performed every 2 months.

The degree of rise in pressure appears to be associated with the antiinflammatory potency of the agents involved and is most marked with dexamethasone and betamethasone. Equivalent doses of ophthalmic prednisolone and triamcinolone use 4 times daily gave similar elevations of IOP to betamethasone instilled only once daily. Duration of corticosteroid treatment and the age of the patient influence the degree of ocular hypertension that is experienced. In some instances, topical epinephrine or systemic carbonic anhydrase inhibitors can maintain the ocular tension within normal limits. On other occasions, it may be necessary to reduce the frequency of administration or substitute a less potent steroid. Withdrawal of the drug may even be necessary to return ocular tension to normal levels.

Steroids administered systemically can make preexisting open-angle glaucoma more difficult to control, but their effect on IOP is much smaller than topically applied steroids. Ocular hypertension may occur during prolonged systemic therapy, usually over a period of 1 year or more, in patients with such conditions as rheumatoid arthritis or disseminated lupus erythematosus. This complication, however, should not deter one from using systemic corticosteroids in situations where they are appropriate.

The ocular hypertensive effect induced by steroids has been categorized into three patient groups in the general population who do not have diagnosed glaucoma. Two-thirds of the general population (Group 1) respond with an average rise in pressure of 1.6 mm Hg after 4 weeks of 0.1% dexamethasone 3 times daily (45). A second group (29%) responds with an average rise of 10 mm Hg. Finally, a third group (5%) responds with a rise greater than 16 mm Hg. For each group, the rate of IOP increase differs significantly. The clinical implication is that patients who are receiving corticosteroids for at least 1 month who have tonometric pressures below 21 mm Hg are unlikely to have glaucomatous complications. In addition, since approximately one third of the general population will have a Group 2 or Group 3 response to topical steroids, tonometric monitoring should be performed on a monthly basis.

Summary of Drug-induced Glaucoma

Table 43.6 lists those drugs which can induce glaucoma. It is important to consider the following factors when appraising a problem of drug-induced glaucoma. Topically administered drugs will induce glaucoma more frequently than those given systemically; acute angle-closure glaucoma should be regarded as an emergency; and any agent which might precipitate an attack must be used cautiously. A diagnosed case of angle-closure glaucoma should be a contraindication to the use of such drugs. Conditions under which any drugs are contraindicated should be made specific. Seldom, if ever, in a package insert or other form of information available to the pharmacist does a recommendation against the use of a particular agent in glaucoma indicate which type of glaucoma is meant.

In general remarkably few drugs, other than those used to treat glaucoma, worsen existing or preeminent glaucoma (5, 15). The literature suggests that it is probably unwarranted to absolutely contraindicate the systemic use of anticholinergics or sympathomimetics in patients with chronic or uncomplicated glaucoma.

THERAPY

The goal of treatment of glaucoma is the immediate and sustained reduction of IOP to prevent deterioration of the optic nerve and loss of visual function. Drugs used in the treatment of glaucoma may be divided conveniently into those that increase the elimination of aqueous humor or decrease its formation.

Parasympathomimetic miotic agents act by removing the obstruction to the outflow channels thereby facilitating the elimination of aqueous humor (1, 2). Sympathomimetic mydriatic agents lower elevated IOP by decreasing the rate of aqueous humor formation (1, 2). The β-blockers such as timolol increase outflow; however, the mechanism of action is not clearly understood (46–56). Secretion and inflow of aqueous humor is most effectively decreased by the carbonic anhydrase inhibitors (57). Hyperosmotic agents reduce the IOP by increasing the osmolarity of the plasma relative to the aqueous and vitreous humor (58). Ocularly instilled parasympathomimetic miotics, sympathomimetic mydriatics, and orally administered carbonic anhydrase inhibitors find their greatest clinical application in primary open angle glaucoma. The management of acute angle closure glaucoma and congenital glaucoma is essentially surgical. Medical treatment is limited to preparing the patient for surgery. Treatment of secondary glaucoma should be directed at correcting the underlying cause as well as the elevation of IOP. Table 43.7 summarizes the basis of medical treatment of glaucoma.

Miotics

Miotics are cholinergic agents which facilitate the outflow of aqueous humor from the anterior chamber of the eye (Table 43.8). This is accomplished primarily by their action on the musculature of the iris and the ciliary body. The exact mechanisms of improved fluid drainage remains poorly understood. The contraction of the ciliary musculature appears to be a primary mechanism by which the IOP is reduced. It is widely held that the trabecular meshwork and veins peripheral to the canal of Schlemm also become dilated, thereby facilitating the outflow of aqueous humor. This action is independent of the pupillary constriction or miosis produced by the cholinergic miotic since outflow has been demonstrated to be unaffected in its absence. Miotics can directly lower IOP by stimulating the post-functional effector cells innervated by the cholinergic fibers. Structurally these agents are similar to acetylcholine, the endogenous mediator of nerve impulses which produce miosis and facilitate the outflow of aqueous fluid through the canal of Schlemm. Cholinergic miotics are therapeutically beneficial for treatment of open-angle glaucoma and preoperative

Table 43.7.
Basis of Medical Treatment for Glaucoma[a]

Because elevated intraocular pressure is responsible for glaucomatous damage in the majority of patients, therapeutic measures are directed at:

1. Increase the rate of outflow of aqueous humor via the drainage system
   Drugs: Parasympathomimetics
   Sympathomimetics
   β-Blockers
2. Decrease formation of aqueous humor by the ciliary processes
   Drugs: Sympathomimetics
   Carbonic anhydrase inhibitors
3. Reduction of volume of aqueous humor in anterior chamber
   Drugs: Hyperosmotics

[a] From I. H. Leopold (46).

Table 43.8.
Miotic Drugs Used in the Management of Glaucoma

Drug	Dosage[a]	Comment
Parasympathomimetics:		
Pilocarpine hydrochloride Pilocarpine nitrate	0.25–10% instilled 1 or 2 drops in affected eye from every 6–8 hr to as often as every 4 hr	Most commonly used. Onset of intraocular pressure lowering effect rapid with 4–8 hr duration. Although strengths above 4% are available, there is little if any advantage to using any strength above 4%
Carbachol	0.75–3% instilled 1 or 2 drops in affected eye every 8–12 hr to as often as every 4 hr	Response varies with dose. May require frequent administration for weaker solutions than usually suggested. A suitable alternative when other miotics cannot be used due to allergy or side effects. Poor corneal penetration. Contraindicated in presence of corneal injury
Short acting anticholinesterases:		
Physostigmine salicylate Physostigmine sulfate	0.25–0.5% instilled 1 or 2 drops in affected eye every 6–12 hr; 0.25% ointment applied at bedtime	Onset of intraocular pressure lowering effect similar to pilocarpine. Considered to be stronger miotic than pilocarpine. Aqueous solutions unstable. Decomposition on exposure to light
Neostigmine bromide	3–5% instilled 1 or 2 drops in affected eye every 4–6 hr	More stable and less irritating than physostigmine. Less effective due to poor corneal permeability.
Long acting anticholinesterases:		
Echothiophate iodide	0.03–0.25% instilled 1 drop in affected eye no more frequently than every 12 hr	Potent, long acting. Maximum effects in 10–20 hr and may persist for several days. Unstable in solution. Should be used when shorter acting miotics are inadequate. Contraindicated prior to filtering surgery. Not used prior to cataract extraction
Demecarium bromide	0.125–0.25% instilled 1 or 2 drops in affected eye every 12 hr to once or twice weekly	Potent, long acting. Should be used only when shorter acting miotics do not give desired result. Duration of miosis is prolonged
Isoflurophate	0.025% instilled 1 or 2 drops in affected eye every 12–24 hr or longer	Potent, long acting. Should be used when shorter acting miotics are inadequate. Unstable. Ointment supposedly most stable and less irritating. Blurring of vision common complaint with ointment.

[a] For open-angle glaucoma.

preparation for surgery in narrow angle. Their disadvantage is their short duration of action requiring frequent administration.

Acetylcholine is not used in glaucoma therapy because of its poor corneal penetration upon ocular instillation and rapid inactivation by cholinesterase. Pilocarpine is the most common drug used for initial and maintenance therapy of chronic primary open-angle glaucoma (3, 4, 46, 59, 60). Pilocarpine penetrates the cornea after ocular instillation with miosis and fall in IOP reaching their maximum levels in 30 to 40 min (61–63). It is employed in solution strengths varying from 0.25 to 10% (although there appears to be little if any therapeutic advantages in the use of concentrations above 4%). The duration of IOP lowering 4 to 8 hours. The usual frequency of instillation is 2 to 3 times daily but it may be given as often as every 2 hours. The Ocusert system is an innovative method of pilocarpine administration. Slightly larger than a contact lens and containing pilocarpine solution in its core, it is worn in the eye where the drug diffuses out at a constant rate. It is available as Pilo-20 or Pilo-40 and releases 20 and 40 μg of pilocarpine per hour (64). Patients previously using 0.5 or 1% drops are controlled with Pilo-20; those using 2 to 4% drops require the Pilo-40. The Ocusert is replaced every 7 days. Advantages of the Ocusert include a constant rate of drug released and improved compliance. Disadvantages of the Ocusert include expense, and irritation which occasionally results in the patient having to return to pilocarpine drops (64).

Carbachol is a synthetic derivative of choline with a direct action like that of pilocarpine or parasympathetic receptors. It is more resistant to inactivation by cholinesterase and therefore is considered to be more effective than pilocarpine in comparable strengths for IOP control. The solution is available in strengths of 0.75 to 3%. In the treatment of open-angle glaucoma 1 drop is instilled usually 2 or 3 times daily. Response has been shown to vary with the dose and weaker strength solutions may require more frequent administration than usually suggested (65). In circumstances where pilocarpine and other miotics cannot be used owing either to allergy or intolerable side effects, carbachol may be a suitable alternative. However, if the glaucoma is uncontrollable with pilocarpine, it is doubtful that carbacol would yield much, if any, therapeutic improvement.

Diurnal fluctuations of IOP have been shown to be more effectively diminished by carbachol than by pilocarpine. The major disadvantage of carbachol is its poor corneal penetration. In addition, it must be prepared in a vehicle such as methylcellulose to ensure prolonged contact with the cornea or with a wetting agent such as benzalkonium chloride in an effort to enhance corneal permeability. In the treatment of nonedematous glaucoma an ointment of carbachol applied locally twice daily causes blurring of vision, a disadvantage of an ophthalmic ointment.

Methacholine bromide pharmacologically is very similar to acetylcholine with the exception of being very resistant to cholinesterase. However, poor corneal penetration and instability in solution makes it an unsuitable miotic for clinical use in glaucoma.

The anticholinesterase miotics act by inhibiting the cholinesterase enzyme, thereby permitting the accumulation of acetylcholine and prolonging the parasympathetic activity on the effector end organs of the eye.

IOP is reduced by facilitating aqueous outflow. Cholinesterase inhibitors used in the management of glaucoma, such as physostigmine and neostigmine, are relatively short acting. Organophosphate compounds, such as demecarium, echothiophate, isoflurophate, have long durations of action. The essential pharmacologic difference between these compounds is the relative reversibility or permanency of their parasympathomimetic activity. Although the direct and indirect acting parasympathomimetic miotics pharmacologically act on different sites of action, their clinical effects on lowering elevated IOP in glaucoma are quite similar (61, 66).

Anticholinesterase miotics are therapeutically beneficial for the treatment of primary open-angle glaucoma; they are not advised for the treatment of angle-closure glaucoma or congenital glaucoma. Since these agents act indirectly by inhibiting cholinesterase, activity prolonging the effects of endogenous acetylcholine, parasympathetic activity of the fibers to the pupil must be functional. They are not effective if given after retrobulbar injections of anesthesia such as during cataract extraction since liberation of acetylcholine is impaired.

Physostigmine lowers IOP by facilitating the outflow of aqueous humor. It has a longer duration of action and is considered to be a stronger miotic than pilocarpine. Physostigmine can be given in strengths of 0.25 to 0.5% every 4 to 6 hours. The onset of reduction in IOP usually occurs within 10 to 30 min, reaching its maximal effect within 1 to 2 hours, and lasting 4 hours or more after instillation. The miotic effects, however, may persist much longer. Aqueous solutions of physostigmine are unstable. Decomposition occurs with pH changes and upon exposure to light. This is detected by the presence of progressive darkening of the solution. Decomposition products of physostigmine solutions are quite irritating and therapeutically ineffective. Physostigmine ointment should perhaps be reserved for bedtime use since the intense miosis produced soon after application would be less discomforting for the patient while asleep. The prolonged duration of increased aqueous humor outflow facilitation is ideal and convenient since the patient need not be interrupted from his sleep to administer miotics.

Neostigmine is more stable but less effective than physostigmine because of poorer corneal permeability. It is less irritating and has fewer unpleasant side effects than physostigmine. Ocular instillation of 3 to 5% aqueous solutions of neostigmine can be given every 4 to 6 hours alone or on an alternating schedule with pilocarpine. Demecarium is chemically similar to neostigmine with comparable miotic and IOP lowering activity to that of echothiophate and isoflurophate. In contrast to the organophosphates, the inhibition of cholinesterase activity by demecarium 0.06 to 0.25% instilled every 12 to 48 hours will give beneficial effects on IOP lasting from 12 hours to several days. In open-angle glaucoma, maximal reduction of IOP with demecarium is seen in 24 to 36 hours. The rapidity of the onset and duration of miosis is directly related to the concentrations used. Tolerance and refractoriness to demecarium occurs earlier than reportedly for echothiophate and isoflurophate.

Echothiophate is a slow onset but long acting cholinesterase inhibitor (67, 68). Aqueous solutions of 0.03 to 0.25% instilled 1 drop every 12 to 24 hours for open-angle glaucoma can produce miosis within 10 to 15 min, although maximal effect on lowering IOP is not seen until 10 to 20 hours later and may persist as long as 96 hours. Instillation of 0.25% solution more often than twice daily does not appear to enhance the effectiveness on the reduction of IOP (69).

The advantage of echothiophate is its long duration of action requiring fewer instillations and better control of the IOP on a diurnal basis. The intense miosis can produce a pupillary block and resultant shallowing of the anterior chamber of the eye. Therefore, in the presence of subacute narrow angles or angle closure glaucoma, echothiophate should not be used. Aqueous solutions of echothiophate are unstable and must be prepared just prior to dispensing. Storage under refrigeration for no more than 6 months should be recommended to the patient.

Isoflurophate possesses more potent and longer duration of action than physostigmine. A drop of 0.025 to 0.1% concentration once or twice daily produce effects on IOP similar to those of echothiophate in open-angle glaucoma. Miosis is maximally experienced within 15 to 20 min. IOP is maximally reduced within 24 hours after instillation. Instillation of 0.1% solution more than twice daily yields very minimal additional therapeutic benefit.

A direct and short acting miotic such as pilocarpine can produce local conjunctival irritation as a result of frequent instillations. Allergic sensitivity or refractoriness to pilocarpine has developed after prolonged use. Frequent instillation of the short acting miotics can exacerbate chronic allergic conjunctivitis or blepharitis.

Discontinuation of the offending agent will most often eliminate the symptoms and other miotics can be tried. Miotics may stimulate progressive deterioration of the visual field defect associated with glaucoma. Poor vision in dim light and blurring of vision from pupillary constriction and accommodative myopia is particularly troublesome for some patients. It is likely that the elderly patient already has diminished visual acuity and therefore should be made aware of the effect of the drug. This problem can be further complicated in those aged patients who have cataracts in addition to impairment of visual function.

Miotics can produce annoying side effects such as transient headaches, ocular and periorbital pain, twitching of the eyelids, ciliary congestion and spasms.

The indirect long acting anticholinesterase miotics produce the most severe symptoms including discomfort associated with bright lights and closeup work. The affected eye is extremely sensitive to efforts in accommodating to light and is extremely myopic. It is particularly intense in younger patients who have active accommodation and are myopic to begin with. Patients should be reassured that these difficulties will usually diminish within a week or so. Severe fibrinous iritis can be induced by miotics and is most likely to occur with the long and indirect acting cholinesterase inhibitors. After intense and prolonged administration of the stronger miotics pupillary cyst production is likely to occur (70). These are seen more commonly in children but the reason is not known.

Anticholinesterase miotics may also produce vitreous hemorrhaging, contact dermatitis and allergic conjunctivitis. Retinal detachment and cataracts have been associated with use of anticholinesterase miotics; however, their role is probably as a contributing factor secondary to underlying retinal pathology.

Glaucoma secondary to ocular inflammation may be exacerbated by these agents as a result of further vascular disruption. Lens opacities have been reported in patients treated with anticholinesterase miotics (71–76). The incidence of cataractogenic lens changes appears related to the drug, the concentration the patient is receiving and the duration of treatment. Cataract formation does not appear to be directly associated with glaucomatous eyes; patients not receiving treatment with anticholinesterase miotics are less likely to develop lens opacity. The lens changes may be partly reversible when the drug is discontinued. Progressive worsening of the cataract may occur, however, necessitating surgical extraction.

Systemic absorption of antiglaucoma drugs following ocular instillation may result in undesirable stimulating effects (77–79). These are seen more commonly after administration of the indirect and longer acting anticholinesterase agents. Gastrointestinal disturbances, i.e., nausea, diarrhea, abdominal pain, muscle spasm and weakness, sweating, lacrimation, salivation, hypotension, bradycardia, bronchial constriction and respiratory failure are systemic effects that have been experienced (78, 80). Most systemic effects rapidly reverse after discontinuation of the drug. In severe cholinergic toxicity, atropine sulfate 2 mg or pralidoxine chloride 25 mg/kg intravenously or subcutaneously can be given without affecting the control of the glaucoma. Caution with the use of any potent long acting miotic agent should be exercised when a patient has bronchial asthma, parkinsonism, peptic ulcer or other gastrointestinal disease, or cardiac disease since anticholinesterase systemic effects can exacerbate their clinical course.

There is evidence that echiothiophate can traverse the placental barrier, therefore its use should be dictated by considerations for the potential risks and benefits during pregnancy (81).

When known sensitivities to these agents exists, they should not be used. Considerable inhibition of plasma cholinesterases can be produced by prolonged topical anticholinesterase therapy (82, 83). A patient who is receiving these agents must be closely monitored for prolongation of apnea when given succinylcholine chloride during surgery (84).

Patients who may be exposed to organophosphate pesticides should be made aware of the potential problem and risks associated with prolonged topical anticholinesterase exposure. There is an additive and cumulative effect on the parasympathetic nervous system. Systemically administered cholinergic agents such as ambenomium, neostigmine, physostigmine used in disorders such as myasthenia gravis can potentiate the action of the anticholinesterase miotics.

The long acting, irreversible anticholinesterase miotics should be reserved for use in chronic primary noncongestive glaucomas and secondary glaucomas when the shorter acting miotics or β-blockers have not successfully reduced the IOP. Undesirable side effects from these agents can also be minimized by instillation of their lowest effective concentrations at reasonable intervals.

β-Blockers

The use of β-blockers in the treatment of glaucoma has been investigated for several years (85). The reason for the initial clinical trials with these agents was due to the reduction of β-adrenergic activity which seems to be beneficial in the reduction of IOP. These agents reduce or abolish β-adrenoreceptor stimulation due either to catecholamines released from sympathetic nerve endings or the adrenal medulla, or from injected sympathomimetic agents (85). There are several β-blockers which have been and are being used in the treatment of open angle glaucoma including timolol maleate (46–56), propranolol (86, 87), pindolol (88), and atenolol (89). This discussion will be limited to timolol.

Timolol is a nonselective β-blocker (85). It was approved for use in the fall of 1978. The ocular hypotensive effect may be due to suppressing aqueous formation (90). An exact mechanism is not known at this time. Timolol is available as a 0.25 and 0.5% solution. The usual starting dose is 1 drop of 0.25% in the affected eye(s) twice a day. If this does not control the glaucoma, the dosage may be increased to 0.5% solution, 1 drop twice a day (47). Timolol may be used alone or in combination with other agents such as epinephrine, pilocarpine, carbachol or acetazolamide (46, 85). Addition of timolol to the therapy of patients on these agents demonstrated a significant reduction in IOP (91). Conflicting reports concerning the reduction of IOP when timolol and epinephrine are combined has been clarified by Cyrlin et al. (92). They determined that there is a significant reduction in IOP due to the additive effect of timolol and epinephrine. This study confirms that the two agents must be given at appropriate times. The recommendation is that epinephrine be administered 3 hours after timolol.

Studies by Daily et al. (93) suggest that the effects of acetazolamide and timolol are similar in reducing IOP. However, the combination of these two agents is significantly more effective than either drug alone. This study utilized acetazolamide 250 mg and timolol 0.5%.

When adding timolol to a patient's therapy (i.e., 1 drop of 0.25% solution), the other agent should be continued as well. The other agents may be discontinued on the following day or dosage adjusted depending on the therapeutic response of the patient. Stabilization of timolol therapy may take several weeks. A reevaluation should take place at 2 and 4 weeks after therapy is begun. If the IOP is maintained, the schedule may be decreased to 1 drop once a day due to the diurnal variations in IOP. Tonometer readings should be done at different times of the day (47–51, 53–56). If 1 drop of timolol (0.5% solution) twice a day is not effective, then increasing the dosage alone will not be effective (47). Concomitant therapy with other agents would then be warranted.

Side effects of timolol include burning or pain after instillation (most common), blurring of vision, dilated pupils with timolol-epinephrine combination. Systemic side effects include cardiovascular problems (bradycardia, palpitations, hypertension, congestive heart failure (CHF), CNS disturbances (headaches, dizziness, drowsiness, anxiety and depression), and pulmonary system side effects which have been limited to exacerbation of existing asthma (47–51, 53–56). Patients with diabetes should use timolol with caution.

Contraindications of timolol include use in patients with bronchospasm (including bronchial asthma or severe chronic obstructive pulmonary disease) and in patients who have experienced cardiac failure (94). Timolol should not be used alone in patients with angle-closure glaucoma (use with pilocarpine) (47, 48).

Sympathomimetics

Reduction of IOP in open-angle glaucoma may be accomplished successfully by ocular instillation of sympathomimetic mydriatics. The mechanism of their action is not fully understood but the main effects appear to be decreasing the rate of aqueous humor secretion and increasing its outflow.

Epinephrine, 1 to 2% solutions instilled every 8 to 24 hours, can reduce IOP in open-angle glaucoma. The rate of aqueous secretion is initially decreased probably through or by means of adrenergic stimulation at receptor sites in the ciliary epithelium. Improved facility of outflow is not immediate but may be seen after several months of epinephrine therapy. The probable mechanism suggested is β-adrenergic response to epinephrine at the trabecular meshwork. The pressure lowering by epinephrine of 3 to 15 mm Hg occurs in 6 to 8 hours and lasts from several hours to days. Patient response appears to be highly variable from individual to individual. Epinephrine is seldom used alone for open-angle glaucoma but usually with miotics (95, 96). Epinephrine does not disturb accommodation and is especially beneficial in overcoming the disabling miosis induced by the parasympathomimetics. When used in combination, it should be given 5 to 10 min after the miotic has been instilled. Comparative effects of epinephrine bitartrate 2% and epinephrine borate 1% have been studied and no statistical differences in ability to reduce IOP in glaucomatous eyes can be found between individual preparations (95). The commercial borate salt is buffered to enhance corneal penetration and is perhaps better tolerated than the others (97).

Phenylephrine has not proven to be any more effective than epinephrine in lowering IOP. A 10% solution of phenylephrine is used primarily in assisting with ophthalmoscopic examination as it is without disturbing cycloplegic effects (98). Guanethidine interferes with sympathetic transmission by interrupting normal release or synthesis of norepinephrine at sympathetic nerve endings (99, 100). Its major clinical use is as an antihypertensive agent. When 2, 5 and 10% solutions are instilled ocularly the reduction in IOP is relatively minor. The onset of effect occurs within 1 hour and duration varies widely from 3 to 24 hours. Its action has been considered comparable to a 1% solution of pilocarpine. Propranolol is a β-adrenergic blocker used in the management of angina and cardiac arrhythmias. It has been demonstrated that a dose of 20 mg given orally is able to reduce IOP in open-angle glaucoma quite effectively. However, in many cases, the dose had to be increased with time to maintain effective reduction of IOP. The fall in systemic blood pressure and potential for cardiac difficulties attendant with the use of propranolol makes it very unlikely that widespread use is warranted.

Isoproterenol in 5% solution produce comparable effects to those of epinephrine with maximal reduction of IOP in 6 hours persisting for 12 to 60 hours. The widespread use of iosproterenol for ocular instillation is militated against by the common occurrence of systemic side effects such as tachycardia and palpitation (101).

Appreciable local and systemic side effects are experienced by patients who use ocular sympathomimetics for long periods of time (102, 103). Local side effects include melanin deposits on the conjuctiva and cornea, hyperemia and corneal edema and allergic blepharoconjunctivitis (104–106). Headache, periobital pain, and lacrimation with intermittent visual blurring and distortion are not uncommon complaints. Although the incidence is relatively low, cardiac irregularities and elevations of blood pressure after ocular administration of epinephrine have been reported (107). Side effects, both local and systemic, are promptly relieved after the epinephrine is discontinued. Close supervision and caution should be exercised for patients who are receiving anesthetics in preparation for surgery since the reported incidence of systemic side effects of the ocular sympathomimetics is higher in such cases. Sympathomimetics are contraindicated in angle-closure glaucoma prior to peripheral iridectomy. Gonioscopic examinations must be advised before the ocular instillation of sympathomimetic mydriatics

in order to rule out the existence of asymptomatic or subacute angle-closure glaucoma. After the iridectomy is performed, ocular epinephrine can be useful, especially, if aqueous humor outflow is impaired. It should not be used, however, if IOPs can be adequately managed by miotics alone.

A relatively new agent in the treatment of glaucoma is dipivefrin. It is a prodrug of epinephrine. It differs from epinephrine by being more lipophilic and therefore increasing its corneal penetration. Once administered it is hydrolyzed to epinephrine. An advantage of dipivefrin over epinephrine is achieving the desired therapeutic effect with fewer side effects. A 0.1% solution of dipivefrin given twice a day will produce decreases in intraocular pressure equal to 1–2% epinephrine. Side effects which are similar to those of epinephrine have been reported and in some cases have been significant enough to cause discontinuation of the drug (106a, 106b).

Carbonic Anhydrase Inhibitors

The lowering of IOP can be achieved by systemic administration of carbonic anhydrase inhibitors (Table 43.9) (57, 93, 108). These agents are of particular value where control of glaucoma is unobtainable with parasympathomimetic miotics. Carbonic anhydrase is a widely distributed enzyme in the body that catalyzes the reversible reaction of water and carbon dioxide to form carbonic acid and subsequently the bicarbonate ion (109). In the eye, large concentrations of carbonic anhydrase are found in the ciliary process and retina. The mechanism of action of the carbonic anhydrase inhibitor on the IOP is not clearly understood (110). Acetazolamide has been found to increase the outflow of aqueous fluid in some glaucoma patients. While a decrease in outflow has also been reported to occur in normal eyes and in eyes with very early glaucoma. The lowering of the intraocular volume is not dependent upon its diuretic effect and cannot be explained simply as a depletion of the bicarbonate ion content. It is probable that the buffer system necessary for maintaining secretory functions in the ciliary epithelium is impaired or inhibited thus reducing aqueous formation. Only slight, if at all, changes in IOP is experienced in normal tensive eyes when carbonic anhydrase inhibitors are administered. There is no effect on the IOP when

Table 43.9.
Carbonic Anhydrase Inhibitors Used in the Management of Glaucoma

Drug	Daily Dosage	Comment
Acetazolamide	125 mg to 1.0 g	Used in short term therapy for primary and secondary glaucoma especially if refractory or uncontrollable by miotics. Used with miotics and hyperosmotics in emergency treatment of primary angle closure glaucoma. Fair success with long term use in open angle glaucoma. Failures frequently due to side effects. Carbonic anhydrase inhibitor of choice in management of glaucoma
Methazolamide	100–300 mg	50 mg is equivalent to 250 mg of acetazolamide. Little significant difference from acetazolamide with exception of side effects and slower onset of action. Drowsiness, fatigue, malaise with minimal gastrointestinal disturbance are common. Main indication for chronic glaucoma insufficiently controlled by miotics or acetazolamide
Dichlorphenamide	25–150 mg	Metabolic acidosis occurs less frequently with dichlorphenamide than other carbonic anhydrase inhibitors. Patient intolerant or refractory to acetazolamide. Anorexia, nausea, paresthesias, dizziness, or ataxia and tremor should alert one of the possibility of toxicity
Ethoxozolamide	60–600 mg	125 mg is equivalent to 250 mg of acetazolamide. Therapeutic effects achieved essentially the same with acetazolamides. Side effects are similar. Patients intolerant to acetazolamide may not be to ethoxozolamide

carbonic anhydrase inhibitors are instilled locally. These drugs are concomitantly employed with cholinergic miotics and hyperosmotic agents for the emergency treatment of primary angle closure glaucoma. The prompt and vigorous reduction of IOP to normal levels prior to peripheral iridectomy is necessary for a better postoperative prognosis.

A single dose of oral or intravenous acetazolamide can maintain reduced IOP for 4 to 6 hours. The maximum effect is seen in about 2 hours after oral administration. Following intravenous administration the maximum effect is attained within 20 min. The rarely seen hypersecretion glaucoma can respond to treatment with carbonic anhydrase inhibitors alone. In chronic primary glaucoma where control has been difficult to obtain with miotics or during acute exacerbations, addition of a carbonic anhydrase inhibitor to cholinergic and sympathomimetic agents may produce satisfactory ocular tension control. Carbonic anhydrase inhibitors are useful in the short-term management of glaucomas secondary to trauma or uveitis and in the preoperative management of congenital glaucoma. Their use in chronic angle-closure glaucoma should be discouraged since symptoms of progressive angle narrowing can easily be obscured. The prognosis for a successful iridectomy may be compromised by the severity of involvement when surgical intervention is the remaining alternative.

Long-term use of carbonic anhydrase inhibitors is frequently unsuccessful due to their side effects. Patients differ in their ability to tolerate the various carbonic anhydrase inhibitors. However, the side effects produced are similar with variations in severity and intensity. The gastrointestinal effects are a common cause of discomfort for the patient and often become so severe that their use is discontinued. Nausea, vomiting, intestinal colic, diarrhea and anorexia, paresthesis of the face and extremities are common side effects experienced. Transient myopia is an unusual and rare occurrence. Long-term treatment with a carbonic anhydrase inhibitor does not appear to deplete intracellular potassium, although, when treatment with the agent is begun, there may be marked depletion of electrolytes, including potassium (111). Careful monitoring of serum potassium levels and clinical manifestation of cellular potassium depletion should be undertaken (112). However, the routine supplementation of potassium for glaucoma patients receiving carbonic anhydrase inhibitors is not encouraged and is of doubtful value in the absence of depletion.

Acetazolamide reportedly can produce a significant hyperglycemia in prediabetics and diabetics receiving oral hypoglycemic agents. Hyperuricemia has occurred following treatment with carbonic anhydrase inhibitors. Prolonged use of these drug inhibitors can lead to production of urinary and renal colic secondary to formation of calcium calculi (113, 114). Alkalinization of the urine by acetazolamide results in an enhanced renal tubular reabsorption of drugs such as quinidine, amphetamine and the tricyclic antidepressants which may magnify their desired and undesired effects. Alkalinization of the urine can also significantly decrease the acid-dependent and antibacterial activity of methenamine. Ex-

foliative dermatitis secondary to these agents is similar to those dermatologic reactions encountered with the sulfonamides. Rare occurrences of idiosyncratic reactions such as cholestatic jaundice, drug fever, blood dyscrasias including thrombocytopenia, agranulocytosis and aplastic anemia have been reported. Carbonic anhydrase inhibitors are not recommended in patients with hemorrhagic glaucoma, hepatic or renal dysfunction, adrenocortical hypofunction or a history of prior sensitivities to the drug.

Hyperosmotic Agents

Hyperosmotic agents lower the IOP by creating an osmotic gradient between the plasma and aqueous humor from the anterior chamber of the eye (Table 43.10) (115, 116). Given systemically these agents induce withdrawal of fluids from the anterior chamber of the eye to the plasma. Hyperosmotic agents are most useful in the preoperative management of primary acute angle closure glaucoma. The degree of IOP lowering depends upon the tension ele-

Table 43.10.
Hyperosmotic Agents Used in the Management of Glaucoma

Drug	Dosage (g/kg of body weight)	Comment
Mannitol	1.0–2	Given intravenously. Requires larger volumes than other hyperosmotics. Rapid diuresis produced. Not metabolized. Can be used in the diabetic. Less irritating and free of tissue necrosis when solution extravasates. Not contraindicated in patients with renal disease. Monitor for cellular dehydration, hypokalemia, cardia irregularities, urinary output and chest pain. More effective for glaucoma with inflammation than urea or glyceria. Avoid excessive hydration or therapeutic effect diminishes
Urea	1.0–1.5	Given intravenously over 30 min. Unstable, sloughing, phlebitis, acute psychosis, severe headaches, nausea, vomiting hemolysis, "rebound diuresis." Contraindicated in nephrotic patients. Caution in hepatic impairment. Use freshly made solutions only. Maximal effect in 1 hr
Ascorbic acid	0.4–1.0	Given intravenously or orally. Gastric distress and diarrhea follows oral administration. Seldom used since more effective agents are available
Glycerol	0.7–1.5	Given orally. Nausea, vomiting, hyperglycemia can occur. Caution in diabetic patients. As effective as intravenous hyperosmotic agents. Less diuresis produced
Isosorbide	1–2	Investigational. Given orally. Can be given to diabetic. Effects on intraocular tension comparable to intravenous hyperosmotics. Diarrhea, nausea and vomiting less frequently experienced
Ethyl alcohol	0.8–1.5	Given orally. Pressure reduction slower than other hyperosmotics. Can produce nausea, vomiting, central nervous systems effects, potential drug-drug interactions. Rarely used since more effective agents are available

vation and the osmotic gradient induced. The greatest effect of rapid changes in plasma osmolarity is on the eye with very profound pressure elevations. The most commonly used hyperosmotics are mannitol, urea and glycerol (117).

Mannitol can effectively reduce acutely elevated IOPs when given slowly by intravenous route in a 20% solution to adults and a 10% solution to children (118–122). The ocular hypotensive effect is produced in 30 to 60 min and lasts from 4 to 6 hours. The degree of effectiveness of the hyperosmotic agents depends upon rate of administration and amount absorbed. Mannitol is preferred in the management of secondary glaucomas accompanied by hyperemia or uveitis since it less readily penetrates the eye which is particularly of advantage where inflammatory processes are active. Agents which enter the eye rapidly produce less osmotic gradient and shorter duration of action than those which do so slowly or not at all. Inflammation greatly increases the ocular permeability of agents such as urea. Therefore, it is less desirable under those circumstances. There is relatively less local tissue irritation, thrombophlebitis and necrosis occurring with mannitol than urea when either is given intravenously. Renal disease does not contraindicate the use of mannitol.

Excessive thirst is a common sensation experienced by patients following infusion of hyperosmotic agents. However, these patients should not be given fluids during the period of osmotic dehydration. Secondary rises in IOP will occur following administration of fluids, diminishing the therapeutic effects of the hyperosmotics. Headache is also a common occurrence but can be minimized simply by bed rest. Monitoring for symptoms of cellular dehydration, hypokalemia, and cardiac irregularities secondary to mannitol therapy should be carried out. Since mannitol is not absorbed orally, it is not effective when given by that route. On rare occasions disorientation and severe agitation may be observed. Pulmonary edema and congestive heart failure may be precipitated in the elderly especially with mannitol infusions. Potassium deficiency is a complication which can accompany diuresis following hyperosmotic infusion and cautious monitoring of cardiac patients, or patients with cardiac hepatic or renal disorders should be routinely maintained.

Urea given by intravenous route as a 30%

solution will reduce elevated IOP within 30 to 40 min (123–125). Miotics and carbonic anhydrase inhibitors are used concomitantly with urea in the management of acute glaucoma prior to surgery. Nausea, vomiting, confusion, disorientation and anxiety are seen. Severe headache is a common complaint and can begin soon after initiation for the duration of the intravenous infusion. The patient's head should not be elevated during this time.

Although urea produces less cellular dehydration because of its ease of penetrability into the cell a "rebound phenomenon" can occur as the plasma level of the hyperosmotic agent drops below that of the vitreous fluid. As the urea is cleared from the circulation rapidly with diuresis the osmolality of the blood will decline. The hyperosmotic vitreous in turn induced the entrance of fluid into the eye resulting in an increased IOP or pressure "rebound" effect.

Ascorbic acid has been shown to successfully reduce IOP in glaucoma patients (126). It has been claimed that in cases of refractoriness to acetazolamide and miotics, ascorbic acid given intravenously was able to lower the ocular hypertension. A 20% solution of sodium ascorbate at a pH of 7.2 to 7.4 can produce normal ocular tensions in 60 to 90 min.

Oral hyperosmotic agents will effectively reduce elevated IOP and are useful where the rapid action infused preparations are not required. Glycerol is a convenient hyperosmotic agent when given as a 50 or 75% solution. The ocular penetration of glycerol is poor, therefore a substantial osmotic gradient can be produced between the plasma and aqueous humor. IOP reduction is considered as effective as hyperosmotic agents given by intravenous infusion. IOPs normally return to pretreatment levels within 5 to 6 hours. Hyperglycemia and glycosuria can occur following glycerol and should be used with particular caution in labile diabetics. There have been reports of acute diabetic acidosis, ketosis being experienced following treatment with glycerol (127). Nausea, diarrhea and headache are also common complaints following oral glycerol (120, 121, 128).

The reduction of IOP with isosorbide is comparable to that of intravenous mannitol, urea or oral glycerol. Given as a 50% solution orally its absorption is rapid and primarily unchanged upon excretion in the urine. Effective reduction in IOP occurs within 30 min following ingestion and remains for 1 to 2 hours or more depending on dosage. Side effects include transient headaches and diarrhea. Other gastrointestinal disturbances such as nausea are usually less of a problem with isosorbide than glycerol (129, 130).

MEDICAL MANAGEMENT

Conservative medical management can successfully control the majority of cases of chronic open-angle glaucoma. Consideration for the stage or severity of the disease as evidenced by the condition of the optic disk and quality of the visual field should be the major influence for the choice of treatment implemented. Mild elevations of IOP (less than 30 mm Hg) in the presence of a normal optic disk and visual field is not an absolute indication for therapy. These patients should have routine periodic follow-ups in order to detect any optic disk changes which may occur since such changes can be detected long before permanent visual field impairment will be experienced. There is no absolute level of IOP that must be maintained in order to be assured of therapeutic success. The IOP should be maintained at the level where further deterioration of the optic disk and impairment of visual field is prevented. If the disk on gonioscopic examination is normal, IOP in the high 20s is not as clinically significant as one with concurrent disk involvement or abnormal visual field. The former situation may warrant only close periodic following while in the latter appropriate medical treatment should deserve immediate consideration. If there is the slightest indication of disk pathology, the IOP should be preferably maintained at 20 mm Hg or even lower by medical management. In cases of considerable disk degeneration and visual field loss, vigorous treatment should be undertaken to attain a level of 15 mm Hg or lower.

In situations where advanced cupping of the optic disk and visual loss is not apparent in the presence of high IOP (greater than 30 mm Hg) medical therapy should be considered a priority. The aim of therapy is to lower the IOP adequately to interrupt the course of the disease. One should always keep in mind problems common to antiglaucoma therapy before proceeding to reduce IOP with drugs. The expense and inconvenience of the medication used should be considered as well as whether the side effects and toxicities of the drugs

constitute a greater risk to the patient than the increased level of IOP.

For primary open-angle glaucoma a miotic agent should be given at its lowest effective concentration and at intervals no more frequent than necessary to maintain a satisfactory level of IOP. Generally pilocarpine 1% or its equivalent is tried first. The IOP should be measured prior to beginning therapy. The effects of therapy on the IOP can be determined within a week or so. If the reduction of IOP is not satisfactory the concentration of miotic agent should be increased, keeping in mind, however, that there is little advantage for use of concentrations of pilocarpine solutions greater than 4% or its equivalent.

Refractiveness following prolonged use of cholinergic miotics often occurs. Rather than increase the frequency of instillation or strength used, the selection of an alternative agent should be considered. Responsiveness to the cholinergic miotics often is restored following their replacement for a brief period of time by an anticholinesterase miotic. Various combinations of glaucoma medications are often given together with the intention of potentiating their therapeutic effects. Not all combinations, however, produce an additive pharmacologic response.

Epinephrine or phenylephrine may be added to miotic therapy provided that gonioscopic examination has failed to demonstrate excessive narrowing of the anterior chamber angle if IOP control is inadequate (131). There is evidence suggesting that greater activity is produced when pilocarpine and epinephrine are separately applied rather than in combination (132, 133). Combinations of anticholinesterase miotics can reduce rather than potentiate the effectiveness of each other. Prior instillations of physostigmine or demecarium will reduce the activity of subsequently instilled echothiophate or isoflurophate by a competitive inhibition of the acetylcholinesterase. Pretreatment with either echothiophate or isoflurophate will enhance only slightly the activity of physostigmine or demecarium. However, the action of physostigmine and demecarium is additive rather than competitive regardless of their order of instillation. Differences in the duration of action and type of cholinesterase inhibiting activity inherent with each miotic given in combination contribute to these predictable responses. Concomitant instillation of miotics, particularly those that act indirectly, offer very few advantages and should not be encouraged in attempts to treat difficult to control open angle glaucoma.

Timolol therapy alone is being used as much as pilocarpine as the drug of choice. Also combinations of timolol with pilocarpine, epinephrine or acetazolamide have also been used effectively as previously discussed. The use of other agents when glaucoma is refractory to the cholinergic miotics may be seen; however, timolol should be selected first due to less side effects and its effectiveness.

Addition of an agent from another class of antiglaucoma drugs is preferred to substitution or addition of an agent from the same group. Deterioration of the glaucomatous condition should always be ruled out. The pharmacist should inquire into the storage condition of the medication, expiration date, and method of administration when a patient experiences diminished effects from the eye drops. The patient's physician should then be made aware of the situation and consulted on whether increasing the frequency of instillation or strength of the patient's medication or substitution with another agent would be appropriate.

SURGICAL MANAGEMENT

Surgical management of open angle glaucoma should be reserved for situations in which maximal efforts utilizing miotics, sympathomimetics and carbonic anhydrase inhibitors have been unsuccessful in maintaining an acceptable level of IOP and preventing progressive changes of the optic disk or the visual field. The surgical procedure involves creating a collateral drainage from the anterior chamber. An acute angle-closure glaucoma attack must receive prompt and intensive attention in order to avoid irreparable damage to the eye. Pilocarpine 1 to 4% or an equivalent cholinergic miotic is instilled into the affected eye at frequent intervals until the IOP is reduced to levels at which surgery can be performed. The surgical procedure is a peripheral iridectomy which allows for the anterior chamber to communicate with the posterior chamber. Table 43.11 summarizes the basis of surgical treatment of glaucoma. Cholinesterase-inhibiting miotics should be avoided. Concurrent administration of intravenous or oral carbonic anhydrase inhibitors or hyperosmotic agents to an acutely dilated pupil not respon-

Table 43.11.
Basis of Surgical Treatment for Glaucoma

A. Re-establish circulation between posterior and anterior chamber
   Procedures—Peripheral iridectomy
B. Create new outflow channels
   Procedures—Iridencleisis
   Trephine with iridectomy
   Sclerectomy
   Cyclodialysis
   Cyclodiathermy
   Cyclocryosurgery
   Goniotomy

sive to the miotic agent may be required. Control of an attack should be established within 1 to 2 hours following the initiation of this intensive treatment. Experience has suggested that the incidence of subsequent involvement in the unaffected eye is significantly reduced when pilocarpine is given as a prophylactic measure (134). Instillation of pilocarpine at normal intervals into the unaffected eye following an episode of acute angle-closure glaucoma is considered appropriate. The use of the laser to create a small opening in the iris without surgery is a recent development. Treatment of secondary glaucomas should be directed at the underlying and contributory factors. Medical treatment of congenital glaucoma may lower IOP levels but this disorder can be successfully corrected only by surgery.

CONCLUSION

The successful outcome of treatment in glaucoma is greatly dependent upon the patient's proper use of medications. It is not unreasonable to suspect that an asymptomatic patient who does not understand why he must continue to use eyedrops both expensive and inconvenient to administer will be less inclined to use them according to prescribed instructions. The blurring of vision and occasional discomfort associated with the use of these medications further enhances the likelihood of noncompliance. As a consequence, visual function is often irreversibly impaired and therapeutic intervention no longer influences the clinical course of the disease. It is vital that the glaucoma patient be given an understanding of the nature of his disorder and appropriate expectations of the therapeutic measures being employed against it. A pharmacist can make significant contributions to reducing the incidences of therapeutic failures by virtue of his accessibility to the glaucoma patient. Conscientious monitoring of patient adherence to a prescribed therapeutic regimen, increasing the patient's awareness of the nature of glaucoma and participating with the patient's physician in evaluating the effectiveness of therapy should be responsibilities of a pharmacist. Success at this formidable task can be achieved only if the pharmacist understands the nature of the disease and is aware of the capabilities and limitations of available therapeutic approaches.

References

1. Newell FW: The glaucomas, in *Ophthalmology: Principles and Concepts*. St. Louis: C. V. Mosby, 1982, chap 20.
2. Paton D, Craig JA: Glaucomas: diagnosis and management. *Clin Symp* 28:20, 1976.
3. Portney GL: *Glaucoma Guidebook*. Philadelphia: Lea & Febiger, 1977, p 7.
4. Vaughan D, Asbury T: Glaucoma, in *General Ophthalmology*, ed 9. Los Altos, Calif.: Lange Medical Publications, 1980, pp 166–183.
5. Fraunfelder FT: *Drug-Induced Ocular Side Effects and Drug Interactions*. Philadelphia: Lea & Febiger, 1976.
6. Kitazawa Y: Primary angle-closure glaucoma. *Arch Ophthalmol* 84:724, 1970.
7. Grant WM: Ocular complications of drugs-glaucoma. *JAMA* 207:2089, 1969.
8. Harris LS: Cycloplegic-induced intraocular pressure elevations. *Arch Ophthalmol* 79:242, 1968.
9. Leopold, IH, Comroe JH Jr: Effect of intramuscular administration of morphine, atropine, scopolamine and neostigmine on the human eye. *Arch Ophthalmol* 40:285, 1948.
10. Mehra KS, Chandra P, Khare BB: Ocular manifestations of parenteral administration of scopolamine (hyoscine). *Br J Ophthalmol* 49:557, 1965.
11. Ullman EV, Mossman FD: Glaucoma and orally administered belladonna. *Am J Ophthalmol* 33:757, 1950.
12. Lazenby GW, Reed JW, Grant WM: Anticholinergic medications in open-angle glaucoma. *Arch Ophthalmol* 84:719, 1970.
13. Mulberger RD: Effect of a common cold product containing belladonna on intraocular pressure. *Eye Ear Nose Throat Month* 47:61, 1968.
14. Hiatt RL, Fuller IB, Smith L, et al: Systemically administered anticholinergic drugs and intraocular pressures. *Arch Ophthalmol* 84:735, 1970.
15. Spaeth GL: General medications, glaucoma and disturbances of intraocular pressure. *Med Clin North Am* 53:1109, 1969.
16. Bryant JA: Effects of systemic drugs on intraocular pressure. *Hosp Formulary Mgmt* 4:15, 1969.
17. Roberts W: Rapid progression of cupping in glaucoma. *Am J Ophthalmol* 66:520, 1968.
18. Grant WM: Systemic drugs and adverse influence on ocular pressure, in Leopold IH: *Symposium on Ocular Therapy*. St. Louis: C. V. Mosby, 1968, vol 3, p 57.
19. Ballin N, Becker B, Goldman ML: Systemic effects of epinephrine applied topically to the eye. *Invest Ophthalmol* 5:125, 1966.
20. Becker B, Cage T, Kolker AE, et al: The effect of phenylephrine hydrochloride on the miotic-treated eye. *Am J Ophthalmol* 48:313, 1959.
21. Whiteworth CG, Grant WM: Use of nitrate and nitrate vasodilators by glaucomatous patients. *Arch Ophthalmol* 71:492, 1964.
22. Peczon JD, Grant WM: Sedatives, stimulants, and intraocular pressure in glaucoma. *Arch Ophthalmol* 72:188, 1964.
23. Willetts GS: Ocular side effects of drugs. *Br J Ophthalmol* 53:252, 1969.
24. Drance SM: The effects of phospholine iodide on the lens and anterior chamber depth, in Leopold IH: *Symposium on Ocular Therapy*. St. Louis: C. V. Mosby, 1969, vol 4, p 25.
25. Zeckman TH, Syndacker D: Increase intraocular pressure produced by di-isopropyl fluorophosphate (DEP). *Am J Ophthalmol* 36:1709, 1953.
26. Lincoff HA, Ellis EH, DeVoe GA, et al: The effect of succinylcholine on intraocular pressure. *Am J Ophthalmol* 40:501, 1955.
27. Maddalena MA: Transient myopia associated with acute glaucoma and retinal edema following vaginal administration of sulfanilamide. *Arch Ophthalmol* 80:186, 1968.
28. Galin MA, Baras I, Zweifach P: Diamox-induced myopia. *Am J Ophthalmol* 54:237, 1962.
29. Edwards TS: Transient myopia due to tetracycline. *JAMA* 186:69, 1963.
30. Bard LA: Transient myopia associated with promethazine therapy. *Am J Ophthalmol* 58:682, 1964.
31. Jocson VL: Tonograph and gonioscopy—before and after cataract extraction with alpha-chymotrypsin. *Am J Ophthalmol* 60:318, 1965.
32. Havener WF: Alpha-chymotrypsin, in Havener WF: *Ocular Pharmacology*, part 1, ed 4. St. Louis: C. V. Mosby, 1978, p 46.
33. Armaly MF: Inheritance of dexamethasone hypertension and glaucoma. *Arch Ophthalmol* 77:747, 1967.
34. Armaly MF: Effect of corticosteroids on intraocular pressure and fluid dynamics; I. The effect of dexamethasone in the normal eye. *Arch Ophthalmol* 70:482, 1963.
35. Armaly MF: Effect of corticosteroids on intraocular pressure and fluid dynamics; II. The effect of dexamethasone in the glaucomatous eye. *Arch Ophthalmol* 70:492, 1963.
36. Becker B, Mills DW: Corticosteroids and intraocular pressure. *Arch Ophthalmol* 70:500, 1963.
37. Becker B, Hahn KA: Topical corticosteroids and heredity in primary open-angle glaucoma. *Am J Ophthalmol* 57:543, 1964.
38. Bernstein HN, Schwartz B: Effects of long-term systemic steroids on ocular pressure and tonographic values. *Arch Ophthalmol* 68:742, 1962.
39. Bernstein HN, Mills DW, Becker B: Steroid-induced elevation of intraocular pressure. *Arch Ophthalmol* 70:15, 1963.

40. Burde RM, Becker B: Steroid-induced glaucoma and cataracts in contact lens wearers. *JAMA* 213:2075, 1970.

41. Kolker AE, Becker B, Mills DW: Topical corticosteroids in secondary glaucoma. *Arch Ophthalmol* 72:772, 1964.

42. Romano J: Anterior chamber depth in medically-treated open-angle glaucoma. *Br J Ophthalmol* 52:361, 1968.

43. Smith CL: Corticosteroid glaucoma—a summary and review of the literature. *Am J Med Sci* 252:239, 1966.

44. Spiers F: A case of irreversible steroid-induced rise in intraocular pressure. *Acta Ophthalmol* 13:419, 1965.

45. Havener WH: Corticosteroid therapy, in Havener WF: *Ocular Pharmacology*, part 1, ed 4. St. Louis: C. V. Mosby, 1978, p 347.

46. Leopold IH: Glaucoma drug therapy, in *Monograph IV—New Developments in Clinical Practice*. Laguna Beach, Calif.: Allergan Pharmaceuticals, 1981.

47. Anon: *Timoptic in the Management of Chronic Open-Angle Glaucoma*. West Point, PA.: Merck Sharp and Dohme Publish., 1979, vol II.

48. Willcockson J, Willcockson T: Long-term use of timolol in open-angle glaucoma. *Curr Ther Res* 27:545, 1980.

49. Anon: Timolol maleate—A new drug for glaucoma. *Med Lett* 20:109, 1978.

50. Anon: Beta blockers for glaucoma. *Lancet* 1:1064, 1979.

51. Boger WP III, et al: Clinical trial comparing timolol ophthalmic solution to pilocarpine in open-angle glaucoma. *Am J Ophthalmol* 86:8, 1978.

52. Moss AP, et al: A comparison of the effects of timolol and epinephrine on intraocular pressure. *Am J Ophthalmol* 86:489, 1978.

53. Phillips CI, et al: Penetration of timolol eye drops into human aqueous humor. *Br J Ophthalmol* 65:593, 1981.

54. LeBlanc RP, Krip G: Timolol: Canadian multicenter study. *Ophthalmology* 88:244, 1981.

55. Lin LL, et al: Long-term timolol therapy. *Surv Ophthalmol* 23:377, 1979.

56. Obstbaum SA, Galin MA, Katz IM: Timolol: effect on intraocular pressure in chronic open-angle glaucoma. *Ann Ophthalmol* 10:1347, 1978.

57. Ellis PP: Carbonic anhydrase inhibitors: Pharmacologic effects and problems of long-term therapy, in Leopold IH: *Symposium on Ocular Therapy*. St. Louis: C. V. Mosby, 1969, vol 4, p 32.

58. Peczon JC, Grant WM: Diuretic drugs in glaucoma. *Am J Ophthalmol* 65:680, 1968.

59. Atchoo PD, Vogel HP: Phospholine iodide (0.03%) in the therapy of glaucoma. *Am J Ophthalmol* 62:1044, 1966.

60. Klayman J, Taffet S: Low-concentration phospholine iodide therapy in open-angle glaucoma. *Am J Ophthalmol* 55:1233, 1963.

61. Drance SM: Comparison of action of cholinergic and anticholinesterase agents in glaucoma. *Invest Ophthalmol* 5:130, 1966.

62. Fenton RH, Schwartz B: The effect of two percent pilocarpine on the normal and glaucomatous eye; I. The time response of pressure. *Invest Ophthalmol* 2:289, 1963.

63. Durkee DP, Bryant BG: Drug therapy reviews; drug therapy glaucoma. *Am J Hosp Pharm* 35:682, 1978.

64. Pearson D: Complications with the use of Ocusert (letter). *Arch Ophthalmol* 94:168, 1976.

65. Flindall RJ, Drance SM: Dose response of intraocular pressures of single installations of carbaminoylocholine chloride. *Can J Ophthalmol* 1:292, 1966.

66. Leopold IH: Ocular cholinesterase and cholinesterase inhibitors: the Friedenwald memorial lecture. *Am J Ophthalmol* 51:885, 1961.

67. Kellerman L, King AC: Echothiophate iodide in glaucoma. *Am J Ophthalmol* 62:278, 1966.

68. Wahl JW, Tyner GA: Echothiophate iodide. *Am J Ophthalmol* 60:419, 1965.

69. Harris LS: Dose response analysis of echothiophate iodide. *Arch Ophthalmol* 86:502, 1971.

70. Chin NB, Gold AA, Breinin GM: Iris cysts and miotics. *Arch Ophthalmol* 71:611, 1964.

71. Axelsson U, Holmberg A: The frequency of cataracts after miotic therapy. *Acta Ophthalmol* 44:421, 1966.

72. DeRoetth A Jr: Lens opacities in glaucoma patients on phospholine iodide therapy. *Am J Ophthalmol* 62:619, 1966.

73. Drance SM: The effects of phospholine iodide on the lens and anterior chamber depth, in Leopold IH: *Symposium on Ocular Therapy*. St. Louis: C. V. Mosby, 1969, vol 4, p 25.

74. Harrison R: Bilateral lens opacities associated with use of di-isopropylfluorophosphate eye drops. *Am J Ophthalmol* 50:153, 1960.

75. Levene RZ: Echothiophate iodide and lens changes, In Leopold IH: *Symposium on Ocular Therapy*. St. Louis: C. V. Mosby, 1969, vol 4, p 45.

76. Shaffer RN, Hetherington J: Anticholinesterase and cataracts. *Am J Ophthalmol* 62:613, 1966.

77. Ellis PP: Systemic effects of locally applied anticholinesterase agents. *Invest Ophthalmol* 5:146, 1966.

78. Humphreys JA, Holmes JH: Systemic effects of echothiophate iodide in treatment of glaucoma. *Arch Ophthalmol* 69:737, 1963.

79. Leopold IH: Cholinesterases and the effects and side effects of drugs affecting cholinergic systemic. *Am J Ophthalmol* 62:771, 1966.

80. Hiscox PEA, McCulloch C: Cardiac arrest occurring in a patient on echothiophate iodide therapy. *Am J Ophthalmol* 60:425, 1965.

81. Birks DA, Prior VJ, Silk E: Echothiophate iodide treatment of glaucoma in pregnancy. *Arch Ophthalmol* 79:283, 1968.

82. DeRoetth A Jr, Wong A, Wolf-Dietrich D, et al: Blood cholinesterase activity of glaucoma patients treated with phospholine iodide. *Am J Ophthalmol* 62:834, 1966.

83. Eilderton TE, Farmati O, Zsigmond EK: Reduction in plasma cholinesterase levels after prolonged administration of echothiophate iodide eyedrops. *Can Anaesth Soc J* 15:291, 1968.

84. Gesztes T: Prolonged apnea after suxamethonium injection associated with eyedrops containing an anticholinesterase agent. *Br J Anaesth* 38:408, 1966.

85. Katz IM: Beta blockers and the eye: an overview. *Ann Ophthalmol* 10:847, 1978.

86. Wettrell K, Pandolfi M: Early dose response analysis of ocular hypotensive effects of propranolol in patients with ocular hypertension. *Br J Ophthalmol* 60:680, 1976.

87. Ohrstrom A, Pandolfi M: Long-term treatment of glaucoma with systemic propranolol. *Am J Ophthalmol* 86:340, 1978.

88. Smith SE, Smith SA, Reynolds F, et al: Ocular and cardiovascular effects of local and systemic pindolol. *Br J Ophthalmol* 63:63, 1979.

89. Elliot MJ, Cullen PM, Phillips CI: Ocular hypotensive effect of atenolol (Tenormin, I.C.I.). *Br J Ophthalmol* 59:296, 1975.

90. Coakes RL, Brubaker R: The mechanism of timolol in lowering intraocular pressure. *Arch Ophthalmol* 96:2045, 1978.

91. Keates EU: Evaluation of timolol maleate combination therapy in chronic open-angle glaucoma. *Am J Ophthalmol* 88:565, 1979.

92. Cyrlin MN, Thomas JV, Epstein DL: Additive effect of epinephrine to timolol therapy in primary open-angle glaucoma. *Arch Ophthalmol* 100:414, 1982.

93. Daily RA, Brubaker RF, Bourne WM: The effects of timolol maleate and acetazolamide on the rate of aqueous formation in normal human subjects. *Am J Ophthalmol* 92:232, 1982.

94. Anon: Additions to timoptic contraindications. *FDD Drug Bull* 11:1, 1981.

95. Becker B, Petitt TH, Gay AJ: Topical epinephrine therapy in open-angle glaucoma. *Arch Ophthalmol* 66:219, 1961.

96. Briswick VG, Drance SM: Epinephrine salts and intraocular pressure. *Arch Ophthalmol* 75:768, 1966.

97. Vaughan G, Shaffer R, Riegelman S: A new stabilized form of epinephrine for treatment of open-angle glaucoma. *Arch Ophthalmol* 66:232, 1961.

98. Becker B, Gage T, Kolker AE, et al: The effect of phenylephrine hydrochloride on the miotic-treated eye. *Am J Ophthalmol* 48:313, 1959.

99. Bonomi L, DiComite P: Effect of guanethidine and other sympatholytic drugs. *Am J Ophthalmol* 61:544, 1965.

100. Sneddon JM, Turner P: The interactions of local guanethidine and sympathomimetic amines in the human eye. *Arch Ophthalmol* 81:622, 1969.

101. Ross RA, Drance SM: Effects of topically applied isoproterenol on aqueous dynamics in man. *Arch Ophthalmol* 83:39, 1970.

102. Aronson SB, Yamamoto EA: Ocular hypersensitivity to epinephrine. *Invest Ophthalmol* 5:75, 1966.

103. Ballin N, Becker B, Goldman ML: Systemic effects of epinephrine applied topically to the eye. *Invest Ophthalmol* 5:125, 1966.

104. Corwin ME, Spencer WH: Conjunctival melanin depositions—side effects of topical epinephrine therapy. *Arch Ophthalmol* 69:317, 1963.

105. Mooney D: Pigmentation after long-term topical usage of adrenaline compounds. *Br J Ophthalmol* 54:823, 1970.

106. Reinecke RE, Kuwabara T: Corneal deposits secondary to topical epinephrine. *Arch Ophthalmol* 70:170, 1963.

106a. Cebon L, West RH, Gillies WE: Experience with dipivalyl epinephrine, its effectiveness, alone or in combination, and its side effects. *Aust J Ophthalmol* 11:181–183, 1983.

106b. Theodore J, Liebowitz HG: External ocular toxicity of dipivalyl epinephrine. *Am J Ophthalmol* 88:1013, 1979.

107. Lansche RK: Reaction to epinephrine and phenylephrine. *Am J Ophthalmol* 61:95, 1966.

108. Gallin MA, Harris LS: Acetazolamide and outflow facility. *Arch Ophthalmol* 76:493, 1966.

109. Maren TH: Carbonic anhydrase: chemistry, physiology and inhibition. *Physiol Rev* 47:595, 1967.

110. Thomas RP, Riley MW: Acetazolamide and ocular tension: notes concerning the mechanism of action. *Am J Ophthalmol* 60:241, 1965.

111. Draeger J, Gtuttner R, Theilmann W: Avoidance of side-reactions and loss of drug efficacy during long-term administration of carbonic anhydrase inhibitors by concomitant supplement electrolyte administration. *Br J Ophthalmol* 47:457, 1961.

112. Spaeth GL: Potassium, acetazolamide, and intraocular pressure. *Arch Ophthalmol* 78:578, 1967.

113. Parfitt AM: Acetazolamide and sodium bicarbonate induced nephrocalcinosis and nephrolithiasis. *Arch Intern Med* 124:736, 1969.

114. Peyes MB: Acetazolamide and renal stone formation. *Lancet* 1:837, 1970.

115. Becker B, Kolker AE, Krupin T: Hyperosmotic agents, Leopold IH: in *Symposium on Ocular Therapy*, St. Louis: C. V. Mosby, 1968, vol 3, p 42.

116. Galin MA, Davidson R, Schachter N: Ophthalmological use of osmotic therapy. *Am J Ophthalmol* 62:629, 1966.

117. Kronfeld PC: The efficacy of combinations of ocular hypotensive drugs. *Arch Ophthalmol* 78:140, 1967.

118. Adams RE, Kirschner RJ, Leopold IH: Ocular hypotensive effect of intravenously administered mannitol. *Arch Ophthalmol* 69:55, 1963.

119. Spaeth EW, Spaeth EB, Spaeth PG, et al: Anaphylactic reaction to mannitol. *Arch Ophthalmol* 78:583, 1967.

120. Drance SM: Effect of oral glycerol on intraocular pressure in normal and glaucomatous eyes. *Arch Ophthalmol* 72:491, 1964.

121. Virno M, Cantore P, Bietti C, et al: Oral glycerol in ophthalmology—a valuable new method for the reduction of intraocular pressure. *Am J Ophthalmol* 55:133, 1963.

122. Weiss DI, Shaffer RN, Harrington DD: Treatment of malignant glaucoma with intravenous mannitol infusion. *Arch Ophthalmol* 69:154, 1963.

123. Davis M, Duehr P, Javid M: The clinical use of urea for reduction of intraocular pressure. *Arch Ophthalmol* 65:526, 1961.

124. Galin MA, Aizawa R, McLean JM: Urea as an osmotic ocular hypotensive agent in glaucoma. *Arch Ophthalmol* 62:347, 1959.

125. Hill K, Whitney J, Trotter R: Intravenous hy-

pertonic urea in the management of acute angle-closure glaucoma. *Arch Ophthalmol* 65:497, 1961.

126. Suzuki Y: Studies on the effect of ascorbic acid on the intraocular pressure of rabbits. *Acta Ophthalmol* 75:201, 1966.

127. D'Alena P, Ferguson W: Adverse effects after glycerol orally and mannitol parenterally. *Arch Ophthalmol* 75:201, 1966.

128. McCurdy DK, Schneider B, Scheic HG: Oral glycerol: the mechanism of intraocular hypotension. *Am J Ophthalmol* 61:1744, 1966.

129. Barry KG, Khoury AH, Brooks MH: Mannitol and isosorbide. *Arch Ophthalmol* 81:695, 1969.

130. Krupin T, Kolker AE, Becker B: A comparison of isosorbide and glycerol for cataract surgery. *Am J Ophthalmol* 69:373, 1970.

131. Becker B, Morton RW: Topical epinephrine in glaucoma suspects. *Am J Ophthalmol* 62:272, 1966.

132. Becker B: Round table discussion, in Armaly MF: *Fifteenth Annual Session of the New Orleans Academy of Ophthalmology,* St. Louis, C. V. Mosby, 1967, vol 1, p 239.

133. Swan KC: Problems in the use of combinations of drugs in ophthalmology, in Leopold IH: *Ocular Therapy—Complications and Management.* St. Louis: C. V. Mosby, 1967, vol 2, p 29.

134. Winter FG: The second eye in acute primary shallow-chamber angle glaucoma. *Am J Ophthalmol* 40:557, 1955.

135. Scheie HG, Edwards DL, Yanoff MC: Clinical and experimental observations using alpha chymotrypsin. *Am J Ophthalmol* 59:469, 1965.

SECTION 12
Skin Diseases

CHAPTER 44

Skin Diseases

C. A. BOND, Pharm.D.

ACNE VULGARIS

Acne is a self-limiting disease primarily affecting adolescents, with over 90% of all teenagers affected to some degree. Acne lesions usually clear during the early 20s but may occasionally persist for many years. Acne is almost exclusively limited to seborrheic or oily areas of the skin, including the face, ears, neck, upper back and occasionally the upper arms. Unfortunately, acne affects adolescents at a time when they are undergoing tremendous growing stress, and, as a consequence, the disease can have profound social and psychological effects on these patients which may permanently affect their personality.

Etiology

The exact cause of acne is not well understood. Hereditary and environmental factors play a role in determining susceptibility; and it is well documented that rising androgen levels seem to trigger the onset of the disease at adolescence (1, 2). The exact source of the female androgenic substance is unknown. Current theories suggest that it may be secreted by ovarian tissue or possibly the adrenal glands (3, 4). Also, it is believed by some that progesterone may be metabolically converted in the body to an androgenic substance. Androgens have been shown experimentally to increase sebaceous gland activity and thus increase sebum production with males affected to a greater extent than females. Severe forms of acne are 10 times more likely to occur in males than females. It has been estimated that up to 15% of males may develop severe acne (4, 6).

The highest incidence of acne occurs between the ages of 14 and 20, but the disease can be found from the neonatal period through the 8th decade of life. When very young or very old patients present with acne, or when there is a sudden appearance of symptoms, endocrine abnormalities or the possibility of drug-induced acne must be considered. When acne is drug-induced, the lesions are identical to those seen in common acne except there is usually an absence of comedones and they appear to be at the same stage of development. Preexisting acne may be made worse by certain drugs, including those found in Table 44.1 (5).

Pathogenesis

The basic lesion of acne is an inflammation of the pilosebaceous follicles of the skin manifested as comedones, papules, pustules, nodules, or cysts, depending on the severity of the disease. With most hair follicles, the size of the sebaceous gland is roughly proportional to the size of the hair (2); however, in the areas of the body where acne occurs, large sebaceous glands are present with small or rudimentary hairs. This combination is much more favorable for the development of acne, which explains why acne occurs on the face but only rarely on the scalp.

At puberty, under the influence of androgens, the sebaceous glands increase in size and activity and the follicular walls hypertrophy. When this increase in keratinization occurs, the flow of sebum to the outside skin becomes mechanically blocked (2, 6, 7). The pilosebaceous follicle starts to dilate and becomes filled with entrapped sebum and cellular debris. At this point the lesion is known as a comedo or blackhead. The follicular orifice of the blackhead usually remains partially open and allows varying amounts of sebum to reach the outside skin, but can close off completely which is known as a whitehead.

When the comedo forms, growth of organisms which are normally present on the skin and in the follicular canal is favored because of the nutrient-rich environment. Organisms most often found are the acid-producing bacteria *Corynebacterium acnes*, *Staphylococcus albus* and the fungi *Pitrysporum ovale* (2, 8). Of these *C. acnes* and, to a lesser extent, the

Table 44.1.
Drugs Reported to Induce Acneiform Eruptions

ACTH	Phenytoin
Androgens	Quinine
Bromides	Scopolamine
Chloral hydrate	Thiouracil
Cod liver oil	Thiourea
Disulfiram	Trimethadione
Iodides	Vitamin B_{12}
Isoniazid	

Table 44.2.
Acne Classification and Treatment

Type	Symptoms	Treatment
Mild	Comedones only	Topical
Moderate	Many comedones, few papules and pustules	Topical
Severe	Many comedones, inflammatory pustules, abcesses, cysts, scarring may be present	Topical and systemic therapy

other organisms produce lipolytic enzymes (6, 9). These enzymes convert the sebum, which is normally composed of esterified long chain fatty acids, into short chain free fatty acids. It has been shown that free fatty acids, especially those of carbon chains between 8 and 14, have the ability to provoke a nonspecific type of inflammatory response. Thus, while these bacteria do not take an active role in producing acne, they act as mediators or catalysts in the inflammatory response (6).

As the free fatty acid content of the entrapped sebum builds up, an inflammatory reaction occurs with characteristic leukocytic infiltrates. As this process continues, bacterial by-products and dead leukocytes cause the walls of the sebaceous gland and follicular canal to become thinner and more brittle. Trauma to this area can cause the follicle to rupture, spilling its contents into the surrounding dermis, causing a foreign body reaction and cyst formation. At this point, the hair follicle is usually destroyed and will not regenerate (2). Sometimes these cysts will rupture repeatedly, forming larger cysts. When a large number of cysts occur in any given area, they can form interconnecting channels (4). This type of acne is known as *acne conglobata* and is a very severe form of the disease. Systemic therapeutic agents should be used with this type of acne to lessen the chance of scarring, which may otherwise occur.

Diagnosis

The diagnosis of acne is relatively easy. Since 90% of the adult population has had the disease during adolescence, the lay public is familiar with its signs and symptoms. Only when acne occurs very suddenly or at ages where it is not generally seen should the clinician suspect underlying endocrine dysfunction or drug-induced types of acne. Table 44.2 lists the diagnostic criteria for classifying the severity of acne.

The most severe side effect of acne for most patients is the psychic trauma it can induce. Unfortunately, the disease occurs during a period of emotional, physical and social upheaval, and it tends to complicate preexisting problems. It is not uncommon to see a patient's personality dramatically affected. It is often beneficial, therefore, to give these patients counseling regarding their disease and to have a sympathetic attitude when explaining proper therapy. The physical complications of acne are limited to the scarring that sometimes remains after the acne has cleared. Seborrhea or dandruff is also related to increased sebum production and thus both diseases often occur together.

Topical Therapy

The goal of topical acne therapy is to interrupt the degeneration of the pilosebaceous follicles so that cysts do not form and scarring will not occur (Table 44.3). Treatment is directed toward keeping the skin clean and to the peeling of skin so that the follicular orifices are kept open and draining properly. The role of soaps or other cleansing agents has been somewhat overplayed (4). As one can see from the discussion on the pathology of the disease, acne lesions occur beneath the skin, and soaps, regardless of their ingredients, affect only the surface of the skin. Since sebum and bacteria on the skin do not play an active role in the pathogenesis of acne, any usefulness of soap lies in its ability to remove sebum from the skin and thus help promote a state of dryness. For this purpose it is recommended that the patient wash his face 2 to 3 times a day with soap and a wash cloth.

Table 44.3.
Agents Commonly Used to Treat Acne (3, 4, 6, 7, 10–13, 21)

Abrasives:	
1. Polyethylene granules	
2. Aluminum oxide	
Mild to moderate keratolytics:	Concentrations most often employed:
1. Sulfur	3–12%
2. Resorcinol	2–10%
3. Salicylic acid	0.5–3%
Potent keratolytic or peeling agents:	Concentrations most often employed:
1. Benzoyl peroxide	5–10% cream or gel
2. Tretinoin	0.05–0.1% solution, cream, gel
Drying agents:	Concentrations most often employed:
1. Alcohol	10–70%
2. Acetone	Varying concentrations
3. Phenol	0.5–2%
Topical antibiotics:	Concentrations most often employed:
1. Clindamycin	1–2%
2. Tetracycline	0.22%
3. Erythromycin	2%
Systemic agents:	Dosage:
1. Hydrochlorothiazine (or equivalent)	25–100 mg/day
2. Prednisone (or equivalent)	20–30 mg with gradual withdrawal over 1 month
3. Interlesional steroids, triamcinolone (or equivalent)	1 mg or less
4. Tetracyline	250 mg q.i.d. decreasing to the minimal effective dose over 3–4 weeks
5. Erythromycin	Dosing similar to tetracycline
6. Minocycline	100 mg b.i.d. decrease to minimal effective dose over 3–4 weeks
7. Estrogens:	
a. Ethinylestradiol	0.1 mg/day
b. Mestranol	0.1 mg/day
c. Equivalent estrogen substance	
8. Isotretinoin	1–2 mg/kg/day

For mild to moderate cases of acne, only topical therapy is usually required to control the symptoms. Two classes of compounds are used in proprietary acne preparations; the mild keratolytic agents and the potent keratolytic or peeling agents (4, 6, 10, 11). The mild keratolytic agents are often used for initial treatment. These agents have both keratolytic and keratoplastic properties depending on the concentration of each individual agent. In the treatment of acne it is important to maximize the keratolytic effects and minimize the keratoplastic properties. Preparations containing sulfur in a concentration of 3 to 12% are used, with the higher concentrations producing a more intense effect. The use of sulfur-containing preparations is somewhat controversial since it has recently been reported that sulfur is comedogenic. Another popular agent is salicylic acid, which is used in concentrations of 0.5 to 3%. Salicylic acid has keratoplastic properties below 2% and keratolytic effects above this concentration. Resorcinol is also used in many proprietary preparations in concentrations of 2 to 20%. It is not uncommon to find several keratolytic agents used in combination in the same product. In this way, the concentration of each agent can be lowered while still maintaining an adequate keratolytic effect (6, 7, 21).

The second class of compounds used in the topical treatment of acne are the potent keratolytic or peeling agents. These agents are designed to remove the skin from around the comedones and that covering superficial acne pustules. This helps to keep sebaceous follicles patent and draining properly (7, 10). Benzoyl peroxide is generally considered to be the most effective over-the-counter (OTC) product for the treatment of mild to moderate acne (6). It is converted to hydrogen peroxide on the skin and acts as an oxidizing agent to promote peeling. The drug also has antiseptic properties, thereby reducing bacterial flora concentrations on the skin and has been shown to decrease free fatty acids on the skin by as much as 60% after 2 weeks of therapy (6).

Tretinoin has proved to be very effective in promoting peeling despite its high irritant properties (14). While the exact mechanism of action of tretinoin is not understood it is thought to work by decreasing the cohesiveness of horny cells which helps to loosen and expel existing comedones. Additionally, tretinoin prevents the formation of new comedones. The product is usually applied at night since it may cause some degree of photosensitization. The patient should also be cautious to avoid applying the drug immediately after washing since this markedly increases its irritant properties, and should avoid applying the drug around the eyes, lips, or nose since it is quite irritating to these areas of the face. Hydrated skin (recently washed) seems to increase the irritancy of tretinoin, thus this preparation must be applied at least 15 min after washing. Frequently the patient may experience a worsening of the acne in the first 3 weeks before improvement is noted. Optimum results with tretinoin may take up to 3 months to be seen. Occasionally, benzoyl peroxide and tretinoin therapy are combined to synergistically treat resistant acne. The benzoyl peroxide is usually applied in the morning and the tretinoin at bedtime. When tolerated, this type of therapy has been quite effective with results comparable to systemic antibiotics (6, 20).

Ultraviolet light treatments are sometimes used to produce mild peeling. They act by producing a mild burn which then causes peeling. There are also several types of mechanical peeling agents available. These agents contain an abrasive compound, usually a fine sand or small plastic balls, and are used to produce peeling and to help keep the skin clean. When using any of the peeling agents, there should be a mild, tolerable level of irritation produced. There is considerable variance from patient to patient in the amount of peeling agent tolerated. For example, some patients can tolerate up to four applications of tretinoin daily while other patients may not be able to use the agent at all because of the severe irritation produced. It is often necessary, therefore, to individualize treatment regimens when using these agents.

Topical antibiotics may be used when other topical therapy produces too much irritation or has been ineffective. Topical clindamycin has generally received the most study and is considered by most authorities to be the most effective topical antibiotic preparation (6, 13, 15–17). The onset of beneficial effects with topical antibiotic therapy is often delayed for three to four weeks and allergic sensitization may occur. Generally, other topical therapies are not used if topical antibiotics are used.

Systemic Therapy

The use of systemic agents in the management of acne should be reserved for more severe forms of the disease. Antibiotics are the most commonly used systemic agents and are used for their suppressive effects on the bacteria responsible for producing the lipolytic enzymes in the sebum. Tetracycline (18) is most often used, but erythromycin, clindamycin, minocycline and trimethoprim-sulfamethoxazole are all equally effective (6, 21). Clindamycin should not be used systemically to treat acne because of its ability to cause a potentially life threatening pseudomembranous colitis. Minocycline is generally reserved for patients who do not respond to other agents due to its increased cost and the relatively common gastrointestinal side effects and dizziness. Due to limited study, the role of trimethoprim-sulfamethoxazole in treating acne remains unclear. When initiating antibiotic therapy, a normal dosing regimen should be employed. After several weeks of therapy, the dosage should be tapered gradually until the minimal effective dose is found. In the case of tetracycline, initiate treatment with 250 mg 4 times a day tapering to a maintenance dosage of 250 to 500 mg per day. The bacteria responsible for producing the free fatty acids are uniformly sensitive to antibiotics, thus sensitivity tests are not necessary. The epithelium lining the pilosebaceous follicle is considered to be an effective barrier against the penetration of these antibiotics. It is thought that they produce their effect by sequestering in cells surrounding the sebaceous follicle and then being shed into the sebum. Such a sequestering process would explain why such low doses of antibiotics are effective and also the lag time observed between initiation of treatment and observance of therapeutic effects (6, 21).

X-ray therapy is quite effective because it reduces the size of the sebaceous glands. However, due to the dangers involved with repeated x-ray treatments, this therapeutic modality is used only infrequently and usually in cases that are refractory to other types of therapy. Estrogen therapy sometimes is employed in women and is usually very effective. Oral contraceptive agents are the most commonly used agents for this purpose and have been shown to decrease sebum production by as much as 40% in some patients. The use of sedative agents in selected anxious patients is controversial (6, 7, 19). Anxiety increases sebum production and in these patients antianxiety agents may be beneficial.

Diuretics seem to produce improvement in some patients, especially those women who have premenstrual flares of their acne. If diuretics are to be used for this purpose, they should be given 5 to 7 days prior to menses and continued during the menstrual period (4). When acne is very severe, systemic corticosteroids may be employed. The rationale for using these drugs is to interrupt the inflammatory reaction and thus hopefully reduce the chance of scarring. Unfortunately, once steroid therapy is started, it often has to be continued to maintain its beneficial effect (4, 11). The side effects of these drugs must be weighed against the therapeutic benefits. For this reason, corticosteroids usually are reserved for very severe cases of acne when other therapeutic modalities have failed.

Recently approved isotretinoin (Accutane) will probably become the therapy of choice in treating moderate to severe forms of acne. When taken orally at doses averaging 2 mg/kg/day most patients (92%) with severe acne had complete clearing of their acne. The remaining patients in this study had a 75% improvement in their disease (22). Prolonged remissions, in some cases lasting as long as 20 months, were observed after discontinuation of therapy. Side effects appear to be primarily limited to the skin, are dose dependent, and reversible after discontinuation of the drug. While the mechanism of action is unknown it is thought to have a direct inhibitory effect on the sebaceous gland (22).

Surgery

Surgical procedures are often employed by the dermatologist. These include the sterile rupturing of the comedones, pustules and cysts to allow proper drainage. Usually scarring will not result from this procedure unless the le-

sion is very deep and requires extensive cutting. Dermabrasion is a surgical procedure employed to remove acne scars. This procedure involves freezing the skin and then abrading it with a high speed rotating wire brush. After dermabrasion, the patient should be instructed to avoid excessive sunlight for 6 to 8 weeks to reduce the chances of hyperpigmentation of the area (6).

Diet

The role of diet as a means of acne therapy has been exaggerated, and opinions on the usefulness of diet vary greatly from practitioner to practitioner. There is no evidence to support the value of eliminating various dietary items in helping the course of disease (3, 4, 7, 11). Some patients, though, insist they have flareups of their disease from certain foods. In these cases, despite no evidence to support the role of diet in acne, the patient should be cautioned to avoid those foods which worsen the condition.

Prognosis

The prospects for recovery from acne vulgaris are very favorable. In most cases, the disease will undergo spontaneous remission. The only major sequela is scarring, and with proper treatment early in the course of the disease, this can often be minimized. When treating acne, it is extremely important to discuss the disease and the proper treatment completely with the patient, emphasizing that only full compliance will produce the hoped-for results.

Conclusion

While there is no specific cure for acne, many of the physical symptoms can be made more tolerable by the use of various topical and systemic medications. Generally speaking, acne certainly cannot be considered a threat to the physical well being of the emerging adolescent, but it is important to remember that the most severe problems may penetrate deeper than the lesions of the skin, causing severe emotional problems. An appreciation of the impact that acne can have on the psyche of the adolescent is paramount in establishing a successful therapeutic regimen.

PSORIASIS

Psoriasis as a disease state has been mentioned in the literature for thousands of years, although it has often been confused with other disease states, such as leprosy and syphilis. The first well documented description of the disease was made early during the 19th century in England, but most knowledge, and the development of effective treatments have been limited to the last 20 years (23). The disease is estimated to occur in 2 to 3% of the population of the United States when all stages of the disease are included (24, 25). Psoriasis does not affect all populations equally. It is rarely seen in North and South American Indians, and Eskimos. The disease is also rare in American blacks, probably because this racial group has ancestral origins in West Africa where the disease is extremely rare (4). There is no difference in incidence with respect to sex, although women generally develop symptoms of the disease earlier in life than do men (24).

Etiology and Pathogenesis

The exact cause of psoriasis is not known. While hereditary factors play a role in determining susceptibility, environmental factors also seem to influence the occurrence of the disease. Although the cause is unknown, a great deal of work has been done with regard to the pathogenesis of the disease (26). The basic lesion of psoriasis is due to a loss of control over the normal growth-regulating mechanisms in the epidermis (27). The normal turnover time for a cell to proceed from the generative layer of the skin to the point where it sloughs off is 27 days. In the psoriatic, the turnover time is decreased to 3 or 4 days. With this shortened transit time, the cells do not mature and keratinization fails to reach completion (4, 28, 29). The epidermis becomes thickened because of the increase in mitotic activity of the generative layer. Along with the increased cell turnover, there is also a corresponding increase in nucleoprotein synthesis as well as an increase in certain enzymes responsible for growth. Vascular changes are noted as the blood vessels become dilated and tortuous, extend further up into the skin than normal and cause bleeding when the lesions are subjected to trauma. Inflammation with leukocyte infiltrates into the skin is also seen to varying degrees and is a secondary process to the underlying psoriatic lesion.

Diagnosis

Psoriasis is classified as one of the papulosquamous dermatoses (4). The common feature among these types of dermatoses is a scaling papule. With psoriasis this papule is erythematous and is topped by a silvery scale which is loosely adherent. When this scale is removed, several bleeding sites are usually noted (called Auspitz signs). These signs, while not entirely diagnostic of psoriasis, are strongly suggestive of this disease. The primary lesions may coalesce to form large plaques which can lead to significant cosmetic disfigurements involving the extremities and trunk areas. The individual lesions are usually symmetrical and can occur on any part of the body, although some areas are more prone to developing lesions than others. The most common sites of involvement are the knees and elbows. Often the scalp is affected and lesions here are often confined to this area. Mucous membrane involvement can occur, but is rare. Nail involvement often provides considerable assistance in establishing the diagnosis. The nails may have brownish yellow discoloration, an uplifting of the front of the nailbed, and a cracking of the edge of the nails. There is usually a characteristic pitting of the nails associated with psoriasis.

The clinical course of psoriasis is extremely variable. The mean age at onset of the disease is 27 years, but generally the earlier the appearance of symptoms, the more severe it is (24). Psoriasis is characterized by remissions and exacerbations. People who have been in remission for years may suddenly have explosive exacerbations for unknown reasons. Others who have had only slight involvement for decades may suddenly develop severe psoriasis. Injury or trauma to the skin (known as "Köbner's" response), cold weather and psychic upsets can all trigger exacerbations while hot weather, sunlight and, sometimes, pregnancy are factors which have been associated with improvement of the condition (24). Remissions have been shown to occur in approximately 40% of males and 60% of females sometime during the course of the disease (24).

Complications

Approximately 25% of patients afflicted with psoriasis have arthritis (30). Although it mimicks rheumatoid arthritis, this condition is actually a separate clinical entity with females usually having a higher incidence than males. Rheumatoid factor tests are usually negative. Another complication that can arise with psoriasis is an exfoliative dermatitis which can be precipitated by withdrawal of systemic corticosteroid therapy, use of synthetic antimalarial drugs, overuse of topical therapy, or systemic infection. This can be a life-threatening situation, as the patient is severely ill, complicated by large amounts of fluid loss. Severe secondary bacterial infections may also occur. Occasionally, increases in serum uric acid levels and steatorrhea may be present, but this is rare. Diabetes mellitus and an elevation in serum lipids and cholesterol have been reported to occur in psoriatics, but well controlled studies indicate no increases over a normal population (4, 28).

Treatment

A variety of treatments are available to combat psoriasis. Two well established methods for topical treatment of hospitalized patients are the Goeckerman and the Ingram techniques. The Goeckerman regimen employs coal tar or its derivatives and ultraviolet light. A coal tar ointment is applied to each plaque several times a day and removed after 24 hours followed by exposure to ultraviolet light. In addition, a coal tar bath is given at least once a day. With successive daily treatments, the exposure to ultraviolet light is increased. This regimen is particularly effective, resulting in a complete clearing in up to 80% of patients treated (4, 31). Remissions often last 6 to 18 months after clearing has occurred. The Ingram regimen differs in that an anthralin paste is applied to each plaque instead of the coal tar ointment (4, 32). Many patients find anthralin difficult to use since it often stings and stains skin, hair, nails, and clothes. This regimen is very effective but requires close supervision. Many variants of these two regimens may be employed, such as the addition of topical corticosteroids, or systemic therapy. When steroid creams and ointments are used, a prompt response is usually seen. When there is scalp involvement, the steroid is suspended in a propylene glycol vehicle and then applied. The corticosteroids, in addition to having antiinflammatory actions, also depress mitotic activity, which is very beneficial. To facilitate penetration of steroids into the skin, an occlusive dressing is often applied from 8 to 24 hours at a time (4, 23). Either Saran Wrap or a plastic suit are commonly used. Intralesional steroid injections are sometimes employed, especially where only small lesions exist. Unfortunately, there is often atrophy of the subcutaneous tissue which can lead to a depression in the skin that may take months to resolve. While intralesional steroids are initially quite effective, the lesions usually reappear within a short time and other therapy must be initiated.

TARS

There are many different tar-containing products available in oil or water-soluble bases (10, 25). Their frequency of use is second only to corticosteroids. Tar-containing products have keratoplastic and keratolytic properties in addition to mild antiinflammatory and antipruritic effects. It has been proposed that these agents increase the skin's sensitivity to ultraviolet light, which in turn decreases mitotic activity, thus improving the conditions. However, this mechanism has never been proven, despite intensive study. Other mechanisms which have yet to be elucidated may also be involved. While the majority of psoriatics see improvement from tars and ultraviolet light, some psoriatics are made worse by sunlight, and tars are definitely contraindicated in these patients.

ANTHRALIN (4, 25, 32)

Anthralin, incorporated into Lassar's paste stiffened with paraffin, is extremely effective in the treatment of psoriasis (4, 25, 32). Salicylic acid is usually added to the mixture. The paste is applied only to the psoriatic plaques, as it is very irritating to unaffected skin. While anthralin treatments are very effective in producing remission, they are messy, irritating, and the relapse rate approaches 100%.

METHOTREXATE

Most of the drugs used in systemic therapy are used for their suppressive activity on rapidly proliferating skin. Methotrexate is the most often used systemic agent. Side effects are similar to other antimetabolites, i.e. blood dyscrasias, gastrointestinal tract ulceration and hepatotoxicity. There are three dosing schedules commonly utilized with methotrexate:

1. Large doses (10 to 25 mg, occasionally as much as 37.5 mg) administered weekly by the oral, intramuscular or intravenous route. As the dose is increased, more frequent blood counts are indicated.

2. A large weekly dose administered over a 36-hour period, usually 2.5 to 5 mg given orally

every 12 hours for 3 doses or every 8 hours for 4 doses. The total dose should be exceed 37.5 mg/week.

3. Low oral doses given daily with rest periods. Usually 2.5 mg are given daily for 5 days followed by a minimum 2-day rest period; a second 5-day course is followed by a rest period of at least 7 days.

The use of this drug by the IV or IM route is not recommended, as it is more toxic by these routes, and it is no more effective when compared with the oral route (28, 33). When the cellular kinetics of psoriasis are considered, schedule 2 is most appropriate (33). This regimen is probably also the least toxic (34, 35). All dosage regimens should be tailored to the individual patient. The goal of methotrexate therapy is not to cure psoriasis, but to achieve a tolerable level of disease activity with the lowest possible dose. Response rates to methotrexate varies from 67 to 78%.

Methotrexate is normally 50% bound to plasma proteins, and this bound form can be displaced from its binding sites by a number of drugs, thus potentiating its toxic effects (25). Among these are: aspirin, p-aminosalicylic acid (PAS), sulfonamides and sulfonylureas. Methotrexate is contraindicated in patients with a history of liver disease, peptic ulcer disease, renal disorders and in patients who are pregnant (10). Since liver toxicity can occur, it is prudent to monitor liver function tests and to take liver biopsies at regular intervals. It is extremely important to obtain regular blood counts to determine the suppressive effect of the drug on bone marrow and blood elements. Psoriasis treatment with methotrexate generally clears or improves fairly rapidly, and may be followed by prolonged periods of remission or marked suppression of the lesions in about 70% of patients (24, 25). However, methotrexate is only suppressive, not curative, and the beneficial effects of this treatment must be weighed against the life-threatening side effects of the drug.

METHOXSALEN

Recently there have been several studies documenting the efficacy of methoxsalen, an oral photosensitizing agent, in combination with long wave ultraviolet light (36–38) (UV-A 320 to 400 nm). This drug and light combination has been termed PUVA (psoralen and UV-A). These initial studies (36–38) indicate PUVA treatment to be remarkably effective with up to 90% of the patients achieving complete clearing. At present there appears to be a very low incidence of short-term side effects but there may be a risk of carcinogenesis with long-term therapy. Generally about 25 treatments, taken 2 to 3 times per week, are required for remission. Follow-up treatments are required to maintain remission. The FDA has recently approved DUVA therapy for treating psoriasis. This form of treatment will become the standard treatment of psoriatics with moderate to severe forms of the disease and replace methotrexate which is probably more toxic and less effective.

MISCELLANEOUS AGENTS

Various other agents are used topically. Keratolytics such as salicylic acid are used to remove scales. Nitrogen mustards are rarely used topically. Although effective in treating psoriasis, these compounds lead to a very high rate of sensitization and thus cannot be used by most patients. Topical therapy is the mainstay in the treatment of psoriasis. Systemic therapy usually is employed only in severe cases of psoriasis where topical therapy has proved inadequate in controlling the disease and it affects more than 25% of the body.

Other systemic agents that have been employed in the treatment of psoriasis include: hydroxyurea, busulfan, mycophenolic acid, and azaribine (25, 39). Systemic corticosteroids, while very effective in treating psoriasis, are generally not used because there is often a severe rebound of the disease after they are tapered or stopped (4). The side effects of systemic corticosteroids also greatly limit their long-term use.

Prognosis

Since psoriasis follows such an unpredictable course, it is difficult to make any statement regarding its prognosis. The disease is characterized by spontaneous remissions as well as severe exacerbations. In most cases, the patient must "learn to live with it" and carry on his life as normally as possible.

Conclusion

Although the medical literature contains reports proclaiming the discovery of the cause of psoriasis, the actual origin of the disease is still obscure. Treatment to date has largely been aimed at suppression of the disease, rather than producing a cure. At present, toxicity greatly limits many of the drugs which would be very effective in treating psoriasis, and when antimetabolite therapy is employed, the patient must be closely monitored. Although remissions do occur for long periods of time, exacerbations are common, therefore treatment is directed toward suppression of the disease to the point where the psoriatic can live comfortably and interact reasonably well with their environment. Looking to the future, drugs must be developed to maximize their effects on tissue that is proliferating abnormally without interfering with normal tissue growth. Methoxsalen may prove to be one of these agents.

DRUG ERUPTIONS

Drug eruptions present one of the most difficult diagnostic problems that a clinician might encounter. Statistics regarding the incidence of drug eruptions in the community are almost nonexistent, but it has been shown that between 1 and 5% of hospitalized patients will experience a drug-induced skin eruption. Clinically recognizable adverse drug reactions are seen more often in the skin than in any other organ or organ system (40, 41). The statement has often been made that any drug can produce any type of eruption; however, drug eruptions are rarely described accurately (41–44), and, in most cases, adverse reactions involving the skin are described only as a "rash." Accurate statistics on the type and incidence of drug eruptions have been kept only recently. Thus, statistical inference with regard to drug eruptions is difficult, except in those cases where large numbers of specific reactions have been reported.

Another problem in accurately documenting most drug eruptions is the lack of test procedures available. Generally, all one can do to prove a drug hypersensitivity is to withdraw therapy, wait for the lesions to clear and rechallenge the patient with the suspected agent. This type of challenge-testing procedure obviously is not practical. Drug eruptions also have a remarkable ability to mimic other types of dermatitis, but can be differentiated by the fact that they generally occur quite suddenly and are usually symmetrical and widespread.

Many mechanisms have been offered to explain drug eruptions, but true allergy probably accounts for a majority of cases (4, 43, 45). However, allergic mechanisms rarely are demonstrable; in most cases drugs act as haptens and not as complete antigens. In addition, the drug itself may not be the causative agent, and the eruption may be due to a metabolite or an impurity in the formulation. Allergic skin responses generally are classified in two ways. The first is an immediate reaction in which urticaria, angioneurotic edema or anaphylaxis may occur—serum antibodies often are demonstrable and desensitization is possible. The second type of response, and the one to which most drug eruptions belong, is the delayed or tuberculin-type reaction. With this type of eruption, serum antibodies cannot usually be demonstrated. Desensitization is usually not possible in these types of reactions (4, 11, 40, 41, 46, 47).

Drug eruptions usually are limited to the skin. In rare instances, other organs may be involved. The time interval between the first dose of the drug and the appearance of the rash is determined by the state of sensitivity. Most drug eruptions appear soon after drug therapy is begun, but in some cases, eruptions may appear months after the drug is discontinued. A good history is paramount when a drug eruption is suspected. In some cases, preexisting lesions can be made worse by the use of certain drugs. It has been shown that patients with acne are more susceptible to acneiform eruptions caused by iodides, bromides, androgens and other corticosteroids; persons with purpuric and hemorrhagic conditions may be more susceptible to purpuric lesions caused by barbiturates, arsenicals, gold salts, sulfonamides and salicylates. Patients who are susceptible to the development of urticarial eruptions are more likely to experience such reactions from salicylates, iodides, and bromides. It should be pointed out that large doses or prolonged therapy may be necessary to elicit an eruption, but once it appears, small doses of the offending agent at a much later date may cause a recurrence. It has been suggested that if the same agent is used both systemically and topically, there appears to be an increased chance of a drug eruption occurring (4, 40–42). Drugs that are often associated with causing eruptions may be found in Table 44.4 (48–50).

Exanthematic Eruptions

Exanthematic eruptions are subdivided into two groups: scarlatiniform and morbilliform. Most drug eruptions fall within one of these two groups. Scarlatiniform eruptions are ery-

Table 44.4.
Drugs Most Often Causing Drug Eruptions (50)

Drug	Incidence (%)[a]
Trimethoprim/sulfamethoxazole	5.9
Ampicillin	5.2
Semisynthetic penicillins	3.6
Corticotropin	2.8
Erythromycin	2.3
Sulfisoxazole	1.7
Gentamicin	1.6
Penicillin G	1.6
Practolol	1.6
Cephalosporins	1.3
Quinidine	1.2
Nitrofurantoin	0.91
Heparin	0.77
Trimethobenzamide	0.66
Barbiturates	0.5
Indomethacin	0.44
Chlordiazepoxide	0.42
Diazepam	0.38
Propoxyphene	0.34
Isoniazid	0.3
Guaifenesin	0.29
Chlorothiazide	0.28
Furosemide	0.26
Phenytoin	0.11
Flurazepam	0.05
Chloral hydrate	0.02

[a] Percent of patients receiving medication who developed an allergic skin reaction.

Table 44.5.
Exanthematic Eruptions

Allopurinol	Meprobamate
Ampicillin	Mercury compounds
Antihistamines	Morphine
Antipyrine	Novobiocin
Arsenic	Nitrofurantoin
Aspirin	PAS
Atropine	Penicillin
Barbiturates	Phenothiazines
Bismuth	Phenylbutazone
Carbamazepine	Phenytoin
Chloral hydrate	Quinacrine
Chloramphenicol	Quinidine
Codeine	Quinine
Digitalis	Salicylates
Gold salts	Streptomycin
Gentamicin	Sulfonamides
Griseofulvin	Sulfonylureas
Hydantoins	Tetracycline
Isoniazid	Thiazides
Insulin	Thiouracil

thematous and usually involve extensive areas (4, 11). They are differentiated from scarlet fever by the lack of other diagnostic signs and laboratory studies. Morbilliform eruptions usually begin as discrete, reddish brown macules which may coalesce to form a diffusion rash. Likewise, morbilliform eruptions are differentiated from measles by the lack of other diagnostic signs and laboratory studies (4, 50). In either type of exanthematic eruption, pruritus may or may not be present. Generally this type of eruption will appear within 1 week after the causative drug has been started and will completely clear within 7 to 14 days after stopping it. Drugs reported to have caused these types of reactions are found in Table 44.5.

Urticaria

Urticarial eruptions usually appear as sharply circumscribed, edematous and erythematous plaques with an abrupt onset. In most cases, the lesions disappear within a few hours and are associated with an intense itching, stinging or prickling sensation. Urticarial eruptions are commonly called hives and are frequently associated with certain drugs, foods, psychic upsets and serum sickness. Rarely, parasites or neoplasms may precipitate hives (51–53). Angioneurotic edema, a variation of urticaria, can be explained best as a more severe form where giant hives predominate. Drugs associated with the development of urticarial and angioneurotic edema reactions may be found in Table 44.6).

Erythema Multiforme Eruptions

As the name implies, erythema multiforme eruptions take on a variety of morphological forms. The lesions are discrete and sharply circumscribed and usually are arranged symmetrically. They appear as acute, polymorphous, bright or dark red macules, papules, vesicles, or bullae; however, only one type of lesion usually predominates in a given patient. Erythema multiforme is more common in children and young adults. Sometimes malaise, a low grade fever, and itching or burning may be seen with this type of eruption. Etiological factors associated with erythema multiforme include drugs, infections, deep x-ray therapy, foods and sometimes neoplasms. Sulfonamides are the drugs most often implicated in erythema multiforme eruptions (11, 40, 48). Other drugs implicated in causing this eruption may be found in Table 44.7.

Stevens-Johnson Syndrome

The Stevens-Johnson syndrome is probably the most common type of severe drug eruption (54). It is classified as a serious variant of bullous erythema multiforme. In addition to what has been described earlier, the Stevens-Johnson syndrome usually involves the mucous membranes and includes constitutional symptoms of fever and malaise. The skin can become hemorrhagic and pneumonia and joint pains may occur. Serious ocular involvement is common and can culminate in partial or complete blindness. Besides drugs, this syndrome has been associated with infections, pregnancy, foods, deep x-ray therapy and neoplasms. Mortality is estimated to be in the range of 5 to 18% (54, 55). The duration of the syndrome is usually 4 to 6 weeks. The long acting sulfonamides are most often implicated.

Table 44.6.
Urticarial Eruptions

ACTH	Meperidine
Adrenalin (possibly from chlorbutanol)	Meprobamate
	Mercury Compounds
Allopurinol	Morphine
Aminopyrine	Nalidixic acid
Antitoxins	Nitrofurantoin
Arsenic	Novobiocin
Aspirin	Penicillin
Barbiturates	Penicillamine
Bismuth	Phenacetin
Bromides	Phenolphthalein
Chlordiazepoxide	Phenothiazines
Chloral hydrate	Phenylbutazone
Chloramphenicol	Pilocarpine
Chlorpropamide	Pituitary extracts
Codeine	Procaine
Dextran	Propxyphene
Digitalis	Pyribenzamide
Ephedrine	Quinine
Erythromycin	Saccharin
Fluorides	Streptomycin
Gold salts	Sulfonamides
Griseofulvin	Tartrazine
Heparin	Tetanus toxoid
Hydantoins	Tetracycline
Imipramine	Thiamine
Insulin	Tragacanth
Iodides	Tuberculin skin test
Isoniazid	Vaccines
Liver extracts	Warfarin

Other drugs associated with causing Stevens-Johnson syndrome may be found in Table 44.8.

Erythema Nodosum Eruptions

Drug-induced erythema nodosum is quite rare. It appears as red, tender nodules usually located around the shins, but they can occur elsewhere. Occasionally, there may be mild constitutional symptoms, but there is usually no mucous membrane involvement. Etiological factors associated with the development of erythema nodosum are drugs, rheumatic fever, leprosy, certain bacterial infections and systemic fungal infections. Usually the lesions heal slowly over several weeks after the offending agent is removed (4, 40). Drugs that have been reported to cause this type of eruption may be found in Table 44.9.

Fixed Drug Eruptions

This eruption, unlike the others mentioned, is caused exclusively by drugs. The lesions are erythematous, sharply bordered and have a tendency to be darker than the surrounding, unaffected skin. They also may be eczematous, urticarial, vesicular, bullous or nodular. Because these lesions have a marked propensity to recur at the same location, the word "fixed" is applied (40, 56). Although the eruptions heal

Table 44.7.
Erythema Multiforme Eruptions

Acetazolamide	Phenothiazines
Chlorpropamide	Phenylbutazone
Furosemide	Phenytoin
Gold salts	Propranolol
Griseofulvin	Salicylates
Iodides	Smallpox vaccine
Mechlorethamine	Sulfonamides
PAS	Thiazides
Penicillin	Tolbutamide
Phenolphthalein	

Table 44.8.
Stevens-Johnson Syndrome

Antipyrine	Phenobarbital
Aspirin	Phensuximide
Carbamazepine	Phenylbutazone
Chloramphenicol	Phenytoin
Chlorpropamide	Smallpox vaccine
Hydralazine	Sulfonamides
Measles vaccine	Tetracycline
Penicillin	Trimethadione

Table 44.9.
Erythema Nodosum Eruptions

Aspirin
Bromides
Codeine
Gold
Iodides
Oral contraceptives (progestagens)
Penicillin
Streptomycin
Sulfonamides
Tuberculin skin test

Table 44.10.
Fixed Drug Eruptions

Acetaminophen	Iodine
Acetanilid	Ipecac
Aminopyrine	Mandelic acid
Amphetamine	Meprobamate
Anthralin	Mercury compounds
Antihistamines	Methenamine
Antimonial com-	Morphine
pounds	PAS
Aspirin	Penicillin
Barbiturates	Pentaerythritol tetrani-
Belladona alkaloids	trate
Bismuth	Pentazocine
BSP	Phenacetin
Chloral hydrate	Phenolphthalein
Chlordiazepoxide	Phenothiazines
Chloramphenicol	Phenylbutazone
Chloroquine	Phenytoin
Codeine	Progestagens
Dapsone	Quinacrine
Diethylstilbestrol	Quinine
Digitalis	Reserpine
Disulfiram	Saccharin
Ephedrine	Salicylates
Ergot	Streptomycin
Ethchlorvynol	Sulfonamides
Gold salts	Tetracyclines
Griseofulvin	Vermouth
Hydralazine	

after withdrawal of the causative drug, there usually is a marked hyperpigmentation of the area which may take months to resolve. The mechanism by which fixed drug eruptions occur has not been elucidated but is believed to be allergic in nature (41, 57). It can be described figuratively as islands of hypersensitivity, one area of the skin having the ability to evoke an allergic response and other areas lacking this ability. Drugs that have been reported to cause this type of eruption may be found in Table 44.10.

Purpura

Purpuric lesions are characterized as hemorrhages into the skin. They are purplish, sharply bordered and have a tendency to become brownish as they get older. These lesions may or may not be associated with thrombocytopenia. Etiological factors other than drugs that are associated with purpura are: vitamin C deficiency, snake bites and infections. The mechanism by which these lesions are produced is not known, but they have a tendency to recur with reexposure to the causative agent. Sometimes purpura may develop from other types of eruptions, such as erythema multiforme. It is worth noting that a clot retraction test is available to document quinidine-induced purpura. Although not commonly associated with drugs, purpuric lesions have been observed following therapy with the drugs listed in Table 44.11.

Acneiform Eruptions

Acneiform eruptions appear very much like common acne (58). They may be differentiated from acne by their sudden occurrence, the absence of comedones in affected areas and the fact that they can occur on any part of the body. Eruptions can also occur during any

Table 44.11.
Purpuric Eruptions

Antitoxins	Isoniazid
Aspirin	Insulin
Barbiturates	Indomethacin
Bromides	Iodides
Carbromal	Meprobamate
Chloral hydrate	Penicillin
Chloroform	Phenothiazines
Chlorpromazine	Phenylbutazone
Corticosteroids	Propranolol
DDT	Quinidine
Diethylstilbestrol	Quinine
Ephedrine	Sulfonamides
Ergot	Tetracycline
Fluoxymesterone	Thiazides
Furosemide	Thiouracils
Gold salts	Warfarin
Griseofulvin	

period of the patient's life and, thus, acne that appears in age brackets where it does not appear normally may be suspected of being caused by drugs (5, 58). Someone who already has acne may have the existing lesion made worse. Table 44.12 lists the drugs that have been reported to cause this type of lesion.

Photosensitive Eruptions

These eruptions require the presence of both drug and light source to occur. Photosensitive eruptions are divided into two subtypes based on different mechanisms of action. The first type is called photoallergic and requires the presence of light to alter the drug so that it becomes an antigen or acts as a hapten (59, 60). Photoallergic eruptions require previous contact with the offending drug, are not dose-related, exhibit cross sensitivity with chemically related compounds, and may appear as a variety of lesions including urticaria, bullae, and sunburn. These lesions are usually secondary to the use of topical agents. The second type of photosensitive eruption is known as phototoxic reaction in which the light source alters the drug to a toxic form, resulting in tissue damage independent of allergic response. This eruption may occur on first exposure to a drug, is dose-related, usually has no cross sensitivity, and almost always appears as an exaggerated sunburn. In some instances, a drug may produce both photoallergic and phototoxic reactions (61). Drugs that have been reported to cause photosensitive eruptions may be found in Table 44.13 (61, 62).

Lichen Planus-like Eruptions

These lesions appear as flat-topped papules which have a distinctive sheen. Pruritus is usually quite pronounced and any part of the body may be affected, including mucous membranes. The lesions are sometimes confused with fixed eruptions but can easily be differentiated histologically. Drugs reported to cause lichen planus eruptions may be found in Table 44.14.

Toxic Epidermal Necrolysis

This type of eruption was first described by Lyell in 1956 and may be preceded by a prodrome characterized by malaise, lethargy, fever and occasionally throat or mucous membrane soreness (63). Epidermal changes follow and consist of erythema and massive bullae formation which easily rupture and peel. The skin appears to be scalded. Hairy parts of the body are usually not affected, but mucous membrane involvement is common. Approximately 30% of the patients with toxic epidermal necrolysis succumb, often within 8 days after bullae appear (54). The usual cause of death is infection complicated by massive fluid and electrolyte loss. Even though the skin takes on a very grave appearance, healing occurs within 2 weeks in about 70% of patients, usually with no scarring (4, 11). In addition to drugs, certain bacterial infections and foods

Table 44.12.
Acneiform Eruptions

ACTH
Androgens
Anovulatory agents (although preexisting acne may improve with anovulatory agents)
Bromides
Chloral hydrate
Cod liver oil
Corticosteroids
Disulfiram
Iodides
Isoniazid
Phenobarbital
Phenytoin
Quinine
Scopolamine
Thiouracil
Thiourea
Trimethadione
Vitamin B_{12}

Table 44.13.
Photosensitive Eruptions

Antimalarials	Norethynodrel
Barbiturates	Phenothiazines
Chlordiazepoxide	Protriptyline
Chlorpromazine	Psoralens
Chlorothiazide	Quinethazone
Diphenhydramine	Quinine
Gold salts	Smallpox vaccine
Griseofulvin	Sulfonamides
Isoniazid	Sulfonylureas
Mestranol	Tetracyclines
Nalidixic acid	Thiazides

Table 44.14.
Lichen Planus-like Eruptions

Chloral hydrate
Chlordiazepoxide
Chloroquine
Gold salts
Meprobamate
Mercury
PAS
Phenytoin
Propylthiouracil (PTU)
Quinacrine
Quinidine
Thiazides

are believed to cause this type of eruption. Most cases of toxic epidermal necrolysis in children are due to infection: *Staphylococcus aureus* has been implicated. Drugs thought to cause toxic epidermal necrolysis are listed in Table 44.15.

Exfoliative Dermatitis

Exfoliative dermatitis, as the name would imply, is characterized by large areas of skin becoming scaly and erythematous and then sloughing off. Hair and nails are sometimes lost. In most patients, a generalized systemic toxicity also accompanies the eruption. Secondary bacterial infections may occur and most fatalities are due to infections. Exfoliative dermatitis also may follow other drug eruptions; thus, a less severe eruption may culminate with an exfoliative dermatitis (40, 53). This type of eruption may take weeks or months to resolve, even after withdrawal of the offending agent. Drugs implicated in causing this type of eruption may be found in Table 44.16 (64, 65).

Bullous Eruptions

Bullous lesions may occur in combination with other drug eruptions, such as erythema multiforme or toxic epidermal necrolysis, or by themselves. The lesions may be round or irregular in shape and contain a clear, serous fluid. The fluid-filled sacs may be either tense or flaccid and can occur on mucous membranes as well as the skin. Table 44.17 lists the drugs that have been reported to cause these eruptions.

Miscellaneous Drug Eruptions

Pigmentary changes usually are not allergic in nature but are classified as idiosyncratic reactions. Examples of drugs that cause pigmentary disorders are: ACTH, bismuth, corticosteroids, mesantoin, phenolphthalein, phenothiazines, quinacrine and silver compounds (11, 66). Drug-induced tumor-like lesions involving the skin are extremely rare; a few cases have been reported with iodides, bromides and arsenic compounds. Eczematous lesions are seen more often with contact sensitizers than with internally administered compounds. However, drugs that can produce this type of reaction after ingestion are chloramphenicol, meprobamate, penicillin and tetracyclines. Although alopecia is not a true drug eruption, hair may occasionally be lost when such reactions occur. Eruptions which may lead to alopecia are exfoliative dermatitis and erythema multiforme. Hair loss may be attributed to a toxic action of a drug, such as an antimetabolite, or to an interference with the normal growth phases of hair, as can be seen with warfarin (65–68). Drugs reported to cause alopecia may be found in Table 44.18.

Table 44.16.
Exfoliative Dermatitis

Actinomycin D	Methantheline
Allopurinol	Methylphenidate
Antimony compounds	Nitrofurantoin
Arsenic	PAS
Barbiturates	Penicillin
Boric acid (internally)	Phenacemide
Carbamazepine	Phenolphthalein
Chloroquine	Phenothiazines
Chlorpropamide	Phenylbutazone
Codeine	Phenytoin
Diethylstilbestrol	Quinacrine
Gold salts	Quinidine
Iodides	Streptomycin
Isoniazid	Sulfonamides
Mercury compounds	Tetracycline
Mesantoin	Vitamin A

Table 44.15.
Toxic Epidermal Necrolysis

Acetazolamide	Nitrofurantoin
Aminopyrine	Penicillin
Atropine	Phenolphthalein
Barbiturates	Phenylbutazone
Brompheniramine	Phenytoin
Chloramphenicol	Poliomyelitis vaccine
Chlorpromazine	Promethazine
Chlorpropamide	Sulfonamides
Dapsone	Tetanus antitoxin
Diphtheria	Tetracycline
inoculations	Tolbutamide
Gold salts	

Table 44.17.
Bullous Eruptions

Acetazolamide	Iodides
Aminopyrine	Licorice
Arsenicals	Mercury compounds
Atropine	Mesantoin
Barbiturates	Penicillin
Bismuth	Phenolphthalein
Bromides	Phenylbutazone
Chloral hydrate	Phenytoin
Digitalis	Promethazine
Ergot	Sulfonamides
Gold salts	

Table 44.18.
Drugs Causing Alopecia

Antimetabolites
Cytotoxics
Dextran
Heparin
Quinacrine
Thiouracil
Trimethadione
Warfarin

Treatment

Diagnosis is very important in determining adequate therapy. For the more severe eruptions, early diagnosis and prompt treatment may modify the severity and eventual course of the eruption. The treatment of drug eruptions is mostly supportive. After withdrawal of the causative compound, most drug eruptions improve in a matter of days, with complete resolution of most drug eruptions occurring within 7 to 14 days. For less severe cases, topical therapy may be all that is needed. This usually includes a topical corticosteroid cream and/or antipruritic lotion or cream. If the lesions are weeping, a wet dressing or soak utilizing normal saline or Burow's solution diluted 1:20 to 1:40 should be employed until the area can be dried (2 to 4 days).

For more severe generalized eruptions, the patient should be given 60 to 100 mg of prednisone (or equivalent). As the reaction subsides the dose of prednisone can be decreased fairly rapidly. Most patients can be managed with a 10- to 14-day course of prednisone although some patients may require longer treatment. Supportive care includes decreasing the frequency of bathing, using nonabrasive soaps or cleansing agents, eliminating harsh or abrasive clothing and avoiding high temperatures and humidity. The use of a wet dressing may be used to help sooth inflamed skin. For more severe eruptions, systemic corticosteroids should be used to control symptoms. Antihistamines also may be beneficial. In lesions where large amounts of fluid are lost, parenteral replacement is mandatory. Although patients with severe drug eruptions are more prone to infection, the prophylactic use of antibiotics is not warranted, and they should be used only when an infection occurs.

CONTACT DERMATITIS

Contact dermatitis is one of the most commonly encountered dermatologic problems seen today. It has been estimated that 20 to 30% of all patients seen by a dermatologist suffer from this disease (4, 69). Patient susceptibility to contact sensitization is apparently independent of sex, race, or geographical variables. Generally, a person is more prone to develop contact dermatitis between the second and fourth decades of life, although this may represent sociological or occupational factors rather than age, since studies using experimental sensitizers show little variation with respect to the age of the subject. The capacity to become sensitized to an allergen varies considerably from patient to patient and is believed to be under genetic control. It has not been proven that atopic individuals (those with asthma, hay fever, and atopic dermatitis) are more susceptible to contact sensitization, nor does it appear that any other preexisting disease states would predispose to contact dermatitis (70). In fact, patients suffering from certain diseases of the immune system (lymphomas) or who are receiving cancer chemotherapy often lack the ability to respond to a contact sensitizer (71–73).

Contact dermatitis includes those inflammations of the skin which are caued by external agents, and is seen in patients exposed to chemical allergens, irritants, toxins and mechanical agents. Most contact dermatitis is eczematous in nature, initially appearing as fine, superficial, erythematous papules and vesicles, with pruritus. Later, the lesions may weep, ooze, or crust as the vesiculation and inflammation continues. Rarely, contact dermatitis may present as a urticarial of granulomatous reaction. The lesions originate in the area of contact, reflecting localization of exposure. An example is poison ivy/oak dermatitis where a characteristic linear pattern is found, caused when the leaf of the plant comes in contact with and brushes over the exposed skin area.

Different areas of the body are more or less susceptible to contact dermatitis. The skin covering the top of the hands, eyelids, and around the eyes is most sensitive, while the palms of the hands, soles of the feet and scalp are areas of least sensitivity (74). Generally, the thicker the skin the less chance there is of developing contact sensitization at that site.

Types of Contact Dermatitis

Contact dermatitis can be divided into two types based on the mechanism by which the adverse reaction occurs (75). The first type, primary irritant dermatitis, includes all contact dermatitis resulting from nonimmunologic or allergic mechanisms and represents the vast majority of all cases seen. The second type includes those reactions which are immunologic or allergic in nature. In some instances a substance may cause an irritant dermatitis in some patients and an allergic reaction in others. The type of reaction is determined primarily by the concentration of the substance exposed to the skin and/or the patient's individual sensitivity to the offending substance.

IRRITANT CONTACT DERMATITIS

Irritant contact dermatitis can be caused by exposing the skin to a chemical substance or by subjecting the skin to a mechanical irritant. Mechanical irritation occurs when the skin is exposed to a coarse, scratchy substance, the most common example being clothing containing wool (76). Wool has also been reported to cause an allergic reaction in a small number of patients (due to lanolin or the dye used), but most cases of wool dermatitis are secondary to the mechanical scratchiness of the cloth. Patients suffering from atopic dermatitis seem to be particularly sensitive to wool, and in most cases should be advised to avoid clothing made of this fabric. Fiberglass is another common cause of mechanical irritation (77). Although most cases of mechanical irritation are minor in nature and self-limiting, pruritus is quite common, and patients soon learn to avoid certain substances which cause such a reaction. Skin which is mechanically irritated will become more sensitive to other irritating chemicals.

Chemical irritants account for the largest number of cases of nonallergic contact dermatitis. In addition to the primary irritation produced, burns or erosive lesions may be seen in all patients if the chemical is sufficiently concentrated, or with chronic exposure. The most common chemical irritants are water, and alkali-containing soaps. Water by itself is not an irritant, but with prolonged exposure painful maceration will occur. In addition the skin loses some of its barrier function, enhancing the penetration of other chemicals such as soaps or solvents. Occlusive dressings, applied over topical corticosteroids to achieve an enhanced steroid effect, are an example of a therapeutic use of this phenomenon. Chronic

exposure to water can also promote yeast infections.

Many soaps are mildly irritating due to their alkalinity, as well as their ability to remove oils from the skin. If an eczematous reaction occurs secondary to use of an alkaline soap, the pH of the skin tends to become more alkaline, resulting in an impairment of the skins neutralization ability. This in turn results in further skin damage from the soap (4, 74).

Biological irritants frequently produce contact dermatitis after prolonged skin contact. Diaper dermatitis is a common example. Sensitization is probably due to exposure to urine and feces rather than the ammonia which is produced by coliform bacteria acting upon urea in the urine (78). This type of dermatitis is seen more commonly in babies whose parents do not change diapers frequently after soilage, use plastic pants, or when the baby has an intestinal disturbance. In intestinal disturbance, the high pH of the liquid feces may be the underlying cause.

A list of common irritating substances that can cause contact dermatitis may be found in Table 44.19 (76, 79). Most cases of irritant dermatitis appear earlier than allergic contact dermatitis, and may appear as dry, red, scaly, or pustular lesions, rather than eczematous. Areas of the skin which have been burned or which have had a prior eczematous reaction may be hypersensitive to irritating substances. This hypersensitivity can remain for several months after the lesions heal. Some patients chronically exposed to irritating substances actually seem to develop a type of tolerance.

Table 44.19.
Common Causes of Irritant Contact Dermatitis

Asbestos	Isopropanol
Acetone	Paint thinner
Benzene	Phenol
Cement	Plaster
Cutting oils	Potassium permanganate
Detergent	Sand
Ethanol	Sawdust
Feces	Soap (alkaline)
Fiberglass	Solvents
Formaldehyde	Tars
Gasoline	Urine
Gentian violet	Water (prolonged exposure)
Hair dyes	Wool
Hair permanents (thioglycolates)	

In these cases, patients notice an improvement of their dermatitis despite continued contact with the irritating substance. At present, there is no explanation for this phenomenon.

ALLERGIC CONTACT DERMATITIS

Allergic contact dermatitis is usually eczematous in nature and may be caused by an almost endless list of potential sensitizers; however, the mechanism of action in all cases remains the same. This delayed hypersensitivity reaction is identical to the tuberculin or homograft reaction. The sensitizers or allergens are small molecules, since they must possess the ability to cross the stratum corneum. Larger molecules, even though they may possess the ability to cause a delayed hypersensitivity reaction, generally do not, because they are too large to penetrate into the skin. A potential sensitizer must also have a reactive chemical group, capable of combining with proteins in the skin, since the small molecule by itself cannot cause a delayed hypersensitivity reaction.

Once the molecule has combined with a protein in the skin, it forms a larger complex capable of eliciting an allergic reaction. This complex is activated in the skin so as to instruct an information-bearing compound, or more likely cell, which then carries this information to a regional lymph node, where the sensitization process proceeds. The allergen-protein complex may also be transferred to a regional lymph node through the lymphatic drainage system. Once in the regional lymph node, the information bearing compound, cell, or the allergen-protein complex sensitizes lymphocytes, so that if the person comes in contact with the allergen again an eczematous reaction occurs at the site of contact. Because the thymus gland is involved in the activation of lymphocytes capable of causing delayed hypersensitivity, they are referred to as T lymphocytes. Another type, referred to as B lymphocytes, is involved in forming immunoglobulins and does not play an active role in contact dermatitis (80–82). The sensitization process takes between 5 and 21 days. Once the sensitization process is completed, all areas of the skin should be considered potentially reactive as the sensitized T lymphocytes are carried by the blood, and may react with the sensitizing agent wherever it contacts the skin.

Why some people react to certain substances and others do not is unknown at present. It is believed to be influenced by genetic factors, as well as the concentration and frequency of exposure to the antigenic substance. As the concentration of allergen, and frequency of contact increase, the likelihood of an allergic reaction also increases (83, 84). There appears to be a threshold level for reaction in many patients, that is, a certain concentration of allergen must be present to elicit the initial allergic reaction, but once reached, subsequent reactions may require only very small concentrations. This type of reaction is often seen in patients who have contact dermatitis to jewelry. It is not unusual for such a person to have worn the offending jewelry for years without problems, but who is not unable to do so because of the resultant dermatitis. Upon questioning, the patient will usually admit to wearing a new piece of jewelry approximately 10 days earlier which probably contained a higher percentage of the allergen, sufficient to overcome the threshold, and cause the allergic reaction.

The severity of an allergic contact dermatitis is quite variable from patient to patient; however, once a reaction has occurred, chances of developing additional contact sensitivity reactions increases. There also appears to be an increased risk involved if a patient is under stress or has just gone through a stressful period (74). Cross sensitivity to chemically similar compounds can occur, but is unpredictable. If a medication must be applied to a patient who is known to be sensitive to chemically similar products, a patch test (see below) using the new medications should be employed to rule out a cross sensitivity reaction.

Once sensitization occurs, any repeated contact with the same agent will elicit a reaction at the site of contact. The reaction usually occurs within 12 to 48 hours, but may be seen from 4 to 72 hours. Individual patient sensitivity determines the length of time needed for the reaction to occur, with patients with a high state of sensitivity reacting earlier than others. Most patients will retain this sensitivity for the remainder of their lives, although some may lose their sensitivity over a period of years. Resensitization requires 10 days in the latter group. Some common sensitizers are listed in Table 44.20 (4, 85, 86).

Diagnosis

Diagnosis is extremely important, since the condition usually will not improve unless the

Table 44.20.
Common Sensitizers

Adhesives	p-Aminobenzoic acid
Antihistamines (topical)	Parabens
Benzalkonium	Paraphenylenediamine
Chromates	Penicillin
Cobalt	Poison Ivy/oak (rhus)
Cosmetics (usually the perfuming agent)	Resorcinol
Ethylenediamine	Rubber compounds
Formaldehyde	Soaps containing halogenated aromatic chemicals
Hydroxquinolines	Steptomycin
Lanolin	Sulfonamides
Local anesthetics (especially benzocaine)	Tars
Mercury	Tolnaftate
Nickel	Turpentine
Neomycin	

cause of the reaction is eliminated. The differential diagnosis often includes atopic dermatitis (eczema), and occasionally, a systemic drug eruption. A lack of a family history of atopic disorders will often eliminate atopic dermatitis as the cause of the reaction. Also, the areas often affected with atopic dermatitis—antecubital and popliteal fossas—generally are not affected in contact dermatitis, since it is less likely that these areas would have come in contact with the allergen. Systemic drug eruptions rarely cause eczematous reactions, nor is the reaction limited to a specific area, as with contact dermatitis. In addition, drug-induced systemic eczematous reactions appear more erythematous, and extend deeper into the skin than contact dermatitis. A list of drugs reported to cause eczematous reactions may be found in Table 44.4.

Once the diagnosis of contact dermatitis has been made, a careful history of exposure to new products or allergens must be taken in order to determine the cause. Often the site of the dermatitis can give a clue as to the type of allergen which is causing the reaction. Table 44.21 lists some of the common offenders of various areas of the body. If the cause cannot be determined from the history and confirmation is required, a patch test may be employed. The procedure involves the application of suspected chemicals to the patient's back, covering for 48 hours with a patch or tape. At the end of this time, the covering is removed and the test is read. If the area is red or eczematous, allergy to the chemical is assumed, and the patient is instructed to avoid contact with products containing that substance. Patch testing requires considerable

Table 44.21.
Contact Dermatitis and Site of Eruption

Site	Causative Agent
Face	Cosmetics, hair dyes, hair sprays, soaps
Ears	Earrings, perfumes
Eyelids	Cosmetics, nail polish
Nose	Glasses, or spectacle supports
Lips	Lipstick, toothpaste, mouthwash
Neck	Perfumes, clothing
Axillae	Deodorants
Trunk	Metal clasps, clothing
Breasts	Elastic, rubber, metal buckles
Perianal areas	Medications (hemorrhoidal)
Arms-legs	Poison ivy/oak
Thighs	Material carried in pants-coins
Wrists	Jewelry-watches
Hands	Detergents, cleansers, gloves
Feet	Shoes (rubber), medications

skill and experience, and should be performed only by those thoroughly familiar with the technique.

Treatment

The most important step in treating contact dermatitis is to determine the cause of the dermatitis and eliminate it. If this is not done, the dermatitis will continue despite adequate therapy. If elimination of the causative agent cannot be done the skin should be protected from the causative agent. This can be accomplished by having the patient wear heavy duty vinyl gloves (if hands are affected) or have the patient use barrier protective creams like Kerodex.

Topical therapy is employed for minor reactions, and is intended to reduce itching and inflammation, and prevent scratching. Selection of topical therapy is determined by whether the dermatitis is in the acute or chronic stage, as well as by the severity of the reaction. In the acute stage, when the skin is pruritic, oozing, and there is extensive vesiculation, cold, wet dressings are usually quite soothing. A typical regimen would consist of 15- to 20-min soaks 3 to 6 times a day, using cold normal saline. Burow's solution diluted 1:20 or 1:40 may also be used. This solution can be prepared by dissolving 1 to 2 Domeboro tablets in a pint of water, which should be discarded after the soak. If lesions are small a clean cloth soaked in the solution (lightly wrung out) may be applied to the lesions. The soaked cloth should be left in place for no more than 15 min when it should be resoaked and reapplied. The patient may repeat this procedure for 30 min to 2 hours, 3 to 4 times a day. A sitz bath using tap water may be helpful if the lesions are extensive, or on parts of the body that cannot be easily soaked. The addition of 2 cupfuls of colloidal oatmeal to the sitz bath may provide an additional soothing effect. Generally, the colder the soak, the more antipruritic it will be. It is believed that the same nerves which carry the itch sensations also carry heat and cold sensations. Cold may be able to partially block the itch sensation generated from the contact dermatitis. Heat should not be used since a rebound phenomenon is often seen, and there is also a chance of scalding or burning the patient. If the involved area is small, ice cubes may be used alone or added to a soak to decrease pruritus. Care should be taken not to add ice cubes to soaks if large areas of the body are to be immersed to avoid chilling. During the acute stage most topical medications are useless, since they will be washed away by the oozing. Shake lotions (calamine, starch, or zinc oxide) are an exception, and may be applied at night or where wet dressing cannot be used.

After the acute phase has subsided, or during the chronic phase of the dermatitis, topical corticosteroid preparations have been proven to be beneficial. The choice of which preparation to use is probably less important than the vehicle (76, 87). If the lesions are dry, and not in intertriginous areas or on the hands, an ointment base should be used. For areas where ointment cannot be used due to locations or patient acceptability, a cream can be used to reduce inflammation. Bathing, and exposure to soaps or cleansers should be avoided during this stage of the dermatitis since additional drying and increased irritation may result. When bathing is necessary, fat-containing soaps (Lowila or Dove) should be used, since they are less irritating than most other soaps or cleansers.

Topical products containing local anesthetics or antihistamines should be avoided due to their sensitizing potential and very short duration of action. If they are used it is best to use them only when a short duration of anesthesia is required (trying to get to sleep at night). Many patients suffering from pruritus respond favorably to systemic antihistamines. Their major benefit is probably due to their sedative effects rather than their antihistamine effects. There is considerable disagreement concerning which antihistamines or antiserotonin agents are most efficacious in treating pruritus (88, 89). It has recently been reported that hydroxyzine was more effective than diphenhydramine and cyproheptadine, but additional study is required to confirm these findings (90, 91). Cotton gloves may be used at night to protect the patient from the adverse effects of excessive scratching.

If the lesions are extensive or quite severe systemic corticosteroids should be employed, provided there are no contraindications. If used, oral corticosteroids must be continued for 3 weeks on a tapering dosage regimen in order to avoid "rebound" of the dermatitis. Initially, up to 80 mg/day of prednisone or equivalent can be used. The initial dose can usually be tapered to one half to one fourth the original dose by the end of the first week with continual gradual reduction over the next 2 weeks (92).

Hyposensitization, while possible, has met with variable responses, and sensitivity returns after the process is stopped. The mechanism of hyposensitization is not totally understood. Progressively larger systemic doses of a sensitizer is given to a patient in hopes of reducing the severity of a future contact sensitivity by quantitative neutralization. Complete desensitization is often not possible due to the massive doses of sensitizer required. The goal of treatment is a decrease in the state of sensitivity so that the patient will not react as severely when he comes into contact with the suspected sensitizer. The process is not without the risk of a generalized dermatitis. Only patients who must come into contact with a known sensitizer and who have had severe reactions to that sensitizer should be considered for hyposensitization. Most hyposensitization to contact allergens has been done with poison ivy/oak extracts. The reader is referred to the work done by Kligman in this area for additional information (93, 94).

References

1. Cunlis WJ, Shuster S: Pathogenesis of acne. *Lancet* 1:685, 1969.
2. Freinkel RK: Pathogenesis of acne vulgaris. *N Engl J Med* 280:1161, 1969.
3. Andrews CC: Acne vulgaris. *Med Clin North Am* 49:737, 1965.
4. Fitzpatrick TB: *Dermatology in General Medicine*, ed 2. New York: McGraw-Hill, 1979.
5. Hitch JM: Acneform eruptions induced by drugs and chemicals. *JAMA* 200:878, 1967.
6. Arndt K: *Manual of Dermatologic Therapeutics*, ed 2. Boston: Little Brown, 1978.
7. Frank SB: *Acne Vulgaris*. Springfield, Ill.: Charles C Thomas, 1971.
8. Scehadeh NH, Kligman AM: The bacteriology of acne. *Arch Dermatol* 88:829, 1963.
9. Reisner RM, Silver S, Puhvel M, et al: Lipolytic activity of corvnebacterium acne. *J Invest Dermatol* 51:190, 1968.
10. Anon: *American Hospital Formulary*. Washington, D.C.: American Society of Hospital Pharmacists, 1972.
11. Domonkas AN: *Andrews' Diseases of the Skin*, ed 6. Philadelphia: W. B. Saunders, 1971.
12. Freinkel RK, Strauss J, Yip S, et al: Effect of tetracycline on the composition of sebum in acne vulgaris. *N Engl J Med* 273:850, 1965.
13. Reisner RM: Systemic agents in the management of acne. *Calif Med* 106:28, 1967.
14. Kligman EM, Fulton JE, Plewig G: Topical vitamin A acid in acne vulgaris. *Arch Dermatol* 99:469, 1969.
15. Resh W, Stoughton RB: Topically applied antibiotics in acne vulgaris. *Arch Dermatol* 112:182, 1976.
16. Stoughton RB, Resh W: Topical clindamycin in the control of acne vulgaris. *Cutis* 17:551, 1976.
17. Algra RJ, Bear J, King G, et al: Topical clindamycin in acne vulgaris. *Arch Dermatol* 113:1290, 1977.
18. Ashurst PJ: Tetracycline in acne vulgaris. *Practitioner* 200:539, 1968.
19. Strauss JS: Effect of cyclic progestin estrogen therapy on sebum and acne in women. *JAMA* 190:815, 1964.
20. Kraus SLJ: Stress, acne and skin surface free fatty acids. *Psychosom Med* 32:503, 1970.
21. Melski J, Arndt K: Topical therapy for acne. *N Engl J Med* 302:503, 1980.
22. Peck G, et al: Prolonged remissions of cystic and conglobate acne with 13-cis-retonic acid. *N Engl J Med* 300:329–333, 1979.
23. Farber E, McClintock R Jr: A current review of psoriasis. *Calif Med* 108:440, 1968.
24. Farber E, Bright RD, Nall ML: Psoriasis—a questionnaire survey of 2,144 patients. *Arch Dermatol* 98:248, 1968.
25. Farber E: *International Symposium on Psoriasis*. Stanford University Press, Stanford, Calif., 1971.
26. Shuster S: Research into psoriasis, the last decade. *Br J Med* 3:236, 1971.
27. Sidi E, Zagula-Mally Z, Hincky M: *Psoriasis*. Springfield, Ill.: Charles C Thomas, 1968.
28. Farber E: Studies on the nature and management of psoriasis. *Calif Med* 114:1, 1971.
29. Van Scott EJ, Ekel TM: Kinetics of hyperplasia in psoriasis. *Arch Dermatol* 88:363, 1963.
30. Reed WB, Becker SW, Rohde R, et al: Psoriasis and arthritis. *Arch Dermatol* 83:541, 1961.
31. Perry H, Soderstrom C, Schulze R: The Goeckerman treatment of psoriasis. *Arch Dermatol* 78:176, 1968.
32. Comaish S: Ingram method of treating psoriasis. *Arch Dermatol* 92:56, 1965.
33. Weinstein GD, et al: Methotrexate for psoriasis. *Arch Dermatol* 103:33, 1971.
34. Almeyda J, et al: Drug Reactions; XV. Methotrexate, psoriasis, and the liver. *Br J Dermatol* 85:302, 1971.
35. Dali MD: Methotrexate hepatotoxicity in psoriasis, comparison of different dosage regimens. *Br J Dermatol* 1:654, 1972.
36. Parish JA: Treatment of psoriasis with long-wave ultraviolet light. *Arch Dermatol* 113:1525, 1977.
37. Parish JA, et al: Photochemotherapy of psoriasis with oral methosalen and long wave ultraviolet light. *N Engl J Med* 291:1207, 1974.
38. Wolff K, et al: Photochemotherapy for psoriasis with orally administered methoxsalen. *Arch Dermatol* 112:943, 1976.
39. McDonald CJ: Chemotherapy of psoriasis. *Br J Dermatol* 14:563, 1975.
40. Baer RL, Harris H: Types of cutaneous reactions to drugs. *JAMA* 192:189, 1965.
41. Coleman WP: Unusual cutaneous manifestations of drug hypersensitivity. *Med Clin North Am* 51:4, 1969.
42. Kirshbaum BA, Beerman H, Stahl EB: Drug eruptions; a review of some of the recent literature. *Am J Med Sci* 240:512, 1960.
43. Kopf A, Andrade R: *Year Book of Dermatology*. Chicago: Year Book Medical Publishers, 1969, p 146.
44. Sternberg TH, Biermiau SM: Unique syndromes involving the skin induced by drugs, food additives and environmental contaminants. *Arch Dermatol* 88:779, 1963.
45. Baer RL, Witten VH: Drug eruptions: a review of selected aspects of an age old, but always timely and fascinating subject. In *Year Book of Dermatology*. Chicago: Year Book Medical Publishers, 1961, p 9.
46. Newbold PC: Drug eruptions. *Calif Med* 113:23, 1970.
47. Rostenberg A: Mechanism of cutaneous drug reactions. *JAMA* 154:211, 1954.
48. Torok H: Dermatitis medicamentosa: a ten-year study. *Dermatol Int* p 57 (April-December), 1969.
49. Burrows D, Shanks RG, Stevenson CJ: Adverse reactions in a dermatology ward. *Br J Dermatol* 81:391, 1969.

50. Arndt K, Hershel J: Rates of cutaneous reactions to drugs. *JAMA* 235:918, 1976.
51. Tatro DS: Drug induced cutaneous eruptions. *Alta Bates Newsletter* Vol. 11, No. 7, July, 1970.
52. Tatro DS: Drug induced cutaneous eruptions. *Alta Bates Newsletter* Vol. 11, No. 9, September, 1970.
53. Tatro DS: Drug induced cutaneous eruptions. *Alta Bates Newsletter* Vol. 11, No. 10, October, 1970.
54. Rostenberg A, Fagelson HJ: Life threatening drug eruptions. *JAMA* 194:660, 1965.
55. Bianchine J, Macareg P, Lasagna L, et al. Drugs are etiologic factors in Stevens-Johnson syndrome. *Am J Med* 44:390, 1968.
56. Derbes VJ: The fixed eruption. *JAMA* 190:765, 1964.
57. Savin JA: Current causes of fixed drug eruption. *Br J Dermatol* 83:546, 1970.
58. Weary PE, Russell CM, Butler HK, et al: Acneform eruptions resulting from antibiotic administration. *Arch Dermatol* 100:179, 1969.
59. Pillsbury DM, Baro WA: The increasing problem of photosensitivity. *Med Clin North Am* 50:1295, 1965.
60. Sams WM: Photosensitizing therapeutic agents. *JAMA* 174:2043, 1960.
61. Dickey RF, Hartmen DL: Photodermatitis induced by drugs. *Skin* 3:169, 1964.
62. Baer R, Harber L: Photosensitivity induced by drugs. *JAMA* 192:189, 1965.
63. Baïley G, Rosenbaum JM, Anderson B: Toxic epidermal necrolysis. *JAMA* 191:979, 1965.
64. Meyler L, Herxheimer A: *Side Effects of Drugs.* Baltimore: Williams & Wilkins, 1968, vol 2, p 320.
65. Shelley WB: *Consultations in Dermatology.* Philadelphia: W. B. Saunders, 1972.
66. Santanouf J: Pigmentation due to phenothiazines in high and prolonged dosages. *JAMA* 191:263, 1965.
67. Crounse R, Van Scott E: Changes in scalp hair roots as a measure of toxicity from cancer chemotherapeutic drugs. *J Invest Dermatol* 35:83, 1960.
68. Simister JA: Alopecia and cytotoxic drugs. *Br Med J* 2:1138, 1966.
69. Fregert S: *Manual of Contact Dermatitis.* Copenhagen: Munksgaard Publications, 1974.
70. Bandman HJ, et al: Dermatitis from applied medicaments. *Arch Dermatol* 106:335, 1972.
71. Schier WW, et al: Hodgkin's disease and immunity. *Am J Med* 20:94, 1956.
72. Rostenberg A: Etiologic and immunologic concepts regarding sarcoidosis. *Arch Dermatol* 64:385, 1951.
73. Johnson MW, et al: Skin reactivity in patients with cancer. *N Engl J Med* 284:1255, 1971.
74. Moschella S, et al: *Dermatology.* Philadelphia: W B. Saunders, 1975.
75. Wilkinson DS, et al: Terminology of contact dermatitis. *Acta Dermatol* 50:287, 1970.
76. Fisher AA: *Contact Dermatitis,* ed 2. Philadelphia: Lea & Febiger, 1973.
77. Heisel BB, Hunt FE: Further studies in cutaneous reactions to glass fibers. *Arch Environ Health* 17:705, 1968.
78. Leyden JJ, et al: Urinary ammonia and ammonia producing microorganisms in infants with and without diaper dermatitis. *Arch Dermatol* 113:1678, 1977.
79. Baer RL: Allergic eczematous sensitization in man. *J Invest Dermatol* 43:223, 1964.
80. Samter M: *Immunological Diseases,* ed 2. Boston: Little, Brown, 1971.
81. Craddock CG, et al: Lymphocytes and the immune system. *N Engl J Med* 285:324, 1971.
82. Parker CW: Control of lymphocyte function. *N Engl J Med* 295:1180, 1976.
83. Calnan CD: The climate of contact dermatitis. *Acta Dermatol* 44:34, 1964.
84. Kligman A: The identification of contact allergens by human assay. *J Invest Dermatol* 47:369, 375, 393, 1966.
85. Baer RL, Witten VH: Allergic eczematous contact dermatitis: A review of selected aspects for the practitioner (Part I). In: *Year Book of Dermatology.* Chicago: Year Book Medical Publishers, 1956–57.
86. Baer RL, Witten VH: Allergic eczematous contact dermatitis: A review of selected aspects for the practitioner (Part II). In: *Year Book of Dermatology.* Chicago: Year Book Medical Publishers, 1957–58.
87. Sulzberger MB, et al: *Dermatology Diagnosis and Treatment,* ed 2. Chicago: Year Book Medical Publishers, 1961, p 164.
88. Anon: Cyproheptadine (Periactin) for allergic and pruritic dermatoses. *Med Lett* 9:28, 1967.
89. Fischer RW: Comparison of antipruritic agents administered orally; a double blind study. *JAMA* 203:418, 1968.
90. Baraf CS: Treatment of pruritus in allergic dermatoses; an evaluation of the relative efficacy of cyproheptadine and hydroxyzine. *Curr Ther Res* 19:32, 1976.
91. Rhoades RB, et al: Suppression of histamine induced pruritis by three antihistamine drugs. *J Clin Immunol* 55:180, 1975.
92. Fisher A, Maibach H: Poison ivy: are you up to date on steroid therapy? *Patient Care* p. 18, 1971.
93. Kligman AM: Poison ivy (rhus) dermatitis. *Arch Dermatol* 77:149, 1958.
94. Kligman AM: Hyposensitization against rhus dermatitis. *Arch Dermatol* 78:47, 1958.

SECTION 13
Neoplastic Diseases

CHAPTER 45

The Acute Leukemias

DOUGLAS G. CHRISTIAN, B.S.Pharm., M.B.A.
WILLIAM A. CORNELIS, Pharm.D.
CLARENCE L. FORTNER, M.S.

The leukemias are a group of related malignant diseases characterized by quantitative and morphological alterations in the peripheral blood white cells and in the precursors of the affected white cell series in the bone marrow. Anemia, granulocytopenia and thrombocytopenia develop secondary to infiltration of the bone marrow by leukemic cell growth and competition with normal myeloid elements. Untreated, the acute leukemias are uniformly and rapidly fatal due to infection, hemorrhage, or other complications associated with progression of the disease. The American Cancer Society estimated that 23,500 new cases of leukemia were reported for 1982; 40% of which were "acute" leukemia. The incidence of leukemia is 6.5 cases per 100,000 population (1). Sixteen thousand deaths will result this year from the various leukemias.

Generally, an "acute" and a "chronic" form of leukemia can be associated with each of the five main types of white cell, although some leukemias involve mixed cell types. The varying characteristics and clinical courses of these diseases allow that each form may have a slightly different pathogenesis. While the etiology of most leukemia cases is obscure, scattered reports can be cited to implicate infective (viral) agents, genetic factors, chemical (or environmental) inducers, and iatrogenic causes. High dose radiation exposure has been confirmed as a causative agent, although a threshold between "safe" and "leukogenic" doses of radiation has not been determined. If every exposure of a person to radiation accumulates to some threshold level, radiation may prove to be a major causative factor for leukemias. However, the link has been demonstrated only in cases where there were unusually high level exposures to radiation (examples: survivors of the atomic blasts at Hiroshima and Nagasaki; radiologists in practice before the need for protective measures was noted; persons treated with high dose irradiation for previous malignant disease). It has also been demonstrated (2, 3) that chemotherapeutic drugs, especially alkylating agents, given for prior malignant disease (Hodgkin's disease, carcinoma, multiple myeloma) or inflammatory collagen vascular conditions (rheumatoid arthritis, polyarteritis nodosa, chronic glomerulonephritis, scleroderma) were the probable cause of acute leukemias which developed later in certain patients. Unfortuantely, these cases were also refractory to further chemotherapy. Ionizing radiation, alkylating drugs and other postulated causes of leukemia seem to have as a common feature the possible alteration of genetic structure of hematopoietic stem cells. Cell growth kinetic studies suggest acute leukemia is a monoclonal disease, evolving from an event which transforms one cell or a small group of cells at one time from normal to abnormal leukemic stem cells which, if they proliferate, result in the disease.

The terms "acute" and "chronic" leukemia became common early in the clinical description of these diseases, in reference to expected rate of progression of the condition if left untreated. It was later discovered that length of survival after diagnosis is closely related to the maturity of the white cell which predominates the blood and bone marrow cell population. In general, the less mature the predominating cell type, the worse the prognosis. "Acute" leukemias demonstrate a high percentage of very immature forms of the white cell series involved, in both peripheral blood and bone marrow. In "chronic" leukemias, the predominating cell type is a more mature form.

There has been significant progress in the diagnosis, understanding and treatment of acute leukemias in both children and adults. Mortality of childhood leukemias has dropped 50% in the 10 years since the first edition of *Clinical Pharmacy and Therapeutics* was printed. While there is frustration regarding treatment failures, and known aggressive therapies produce disagreeable side effects, therapy available today holds sufficient promise that no patient should be denied the opportunity for proper care. Utilizing theories and methods described below, specialized cancer treatment centers (often in partnership with a patient's local physician and hospital) regularly prolong the useful and symptom-free life of leukemia victims for periods many times the expected survival if the leukemia is left untreated. Approximately 15 to 20% of aggressively treated acute leukemia patients have been free of relapse of their disease for 5 or more years. Some of these persons should be considered cured.

CLASSIFICATION OF LEUKEMIAS

Besides the early division of leukemias into "acute" and "chronic" categories based on the natural clinical course, further description of the diseases in terms of white cell morphology and histology became helpful as it was observed that the various white cell types responded differently to treatment. Naegeli in 1900 had described the myeloblast and divided the blastic leukemias into myelocytic and lymphocytic varieties. The monocytic variety was described a decade later.

There are five series of white blood cells (lymphocytes, monocytes, neutrophils, basophils, and eosinophils) and each follows a similar pathway of maturation, deriving from a "blast" cell (itself arising from a "stem cell" located in the bone marrow) and progressing through histologically defined stages to the mature form which is then released into the blood stream (Figure. 45.1). The normal percentage distribution of the white cell types in peripheral blood is described in Table 45.1.

In circumstances of physiological stress, it is not uncommon for the less mature leukocyte forms to appear in the peripheral blood. The very primitive "blast" stage of white cell, however, should not be present in the peripheral blood, and its appearance introduces clinical suspicion of leukemia.

Acute lymphocytic leukemia (ALL), as shown in Figure 45.1, is defined by proliferation within the lymphocytic series. ALL is the most common childhood leukemia, although it does occur in adults. In children aged 2 to 10 years, ALL has begun to yield to therapeutic advances.

Acute myelocytic leukemia (AML), involving the precursors of the three types of granulocytes, or polymorphonuclear leukocytes, is the most common acute leukemia in adults.

Acute nonlymphocytic leukemia (ANLL) is a group term used when referring to the clinical similarities of AML along with acute monocytic leukemia (AMOL), acute myelomonocytic leukemia (AMML), acute progranulocytic leukemia, and acute erythroleukemia. These diseases have been considered as a group when discussing prognosis, treatment and complications. It can be said that ANLL has responded much less dramatically to therapeutic attempts than ALL. However, subtle differences have been identified in the profile of complications, effectiveness of therapy and prognosis associated with several subgroups of the "nonlymphocytic" acute leukemias. While the ANLL designation is used extensively in the literature the need was obvious for more precise terminology.

In 1976, the French-American-British (FAB) Cooperative Group proposed a system of standard nomenclature and classification now used widely in the literature to describe morphologic subgroups of acute leukemias, their further characterization and treatment. The FAB system is summarized in Table 45.2.

Additionally, various subgroups of leukemia may now be described in terms of their reaction with histochemical stains such as peroxidase, Sudan black, several esterases, and periodic acid-Schiff (PAS). Immunofluorescent stains can identify an enzyme, deoxynucleotidyl terminal transferase (TdT) which exists in the nuclear material of lymphoblasts in 95% of patients with ALL. Cell surface markers on lymphoblasts serve to distinguish T-cell and B-cell varieties, and chromosomal studies are used to show relationship to some leukemias to other genetic anomalies.

The ultimate importance of classifying the leukemias by these finite means is in correlating sensitivity of the subclasses to therapy, and in defining prognostic signs for remission of long-term survival. While this process continues, further subclassification is part of the process of cataloging knowledge for a more precise diagnosis.

CLINICAL COURSE OF ACUTE LEUKEMIAS

The presenting symptomatology of patients with acute leukemia varies greatly but usually

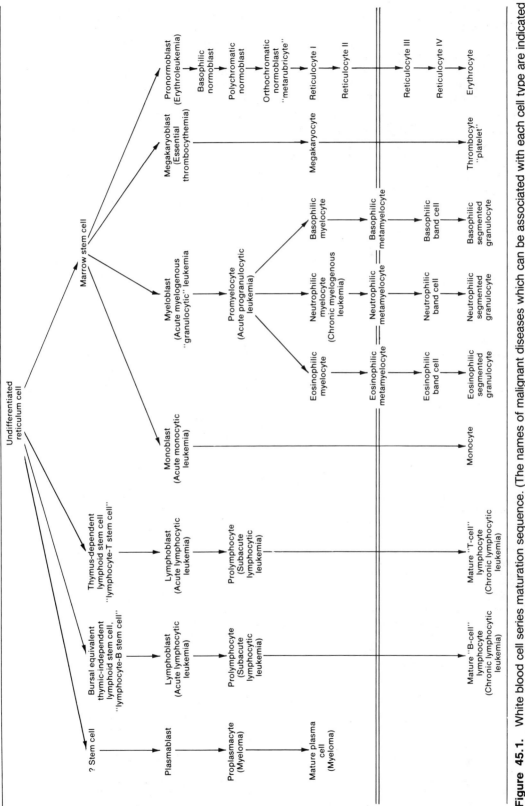

Figure 45.1.   White blood cell series maturation sequence. (The names of malignant diseases which can be associated with each cell type are indicated in parentheses.) *Note:* The double horizontal line represents the marrow/blood barrier, and the cell types listed below it would be found in the normal peripheral blood. (See Table 45.1 for normal percentage distributions.)

can be referred to the underlying disorders of the disease. Displacement of normal elements from the bone marrow by neoplastic cells leads to anemia, thrombocytopenia and granulocytopenia. Symptoms referrable to these conditions would include the possibilities listed in Table 45.3. Fever and weight loss can be ascribed to increased metabolic activity of the bone marrow tissue. Many signs of organ infiltration are absent in the acute forms of leukemia, but lymphadenopathy and splenomegaly are not uncommon.

These clinical findings are vague at best, and diagnosis always must be based as mentioned on complete evaluations, including bone marrow studies. Because the patients can often

relate these symptoms to more benign disorders they have previously experienced, tentative diagnosis of leukemia often is made upon blood studies drawn for less specific purposes.

Whichever cell type is prevalent, there are many factors which will influence the clinical course of a patient with an acute leukemia. At diagnosis, these factors include the age and general condition of the patient, cytogenetic or immunologic features of the involved cell line, presence or absence of other underlying conditions such as diabetes mellitus, cardiovascular disease, impaired renal or hepatic function, or a prolonged symptomatic interval preceding diagnosis. Occurrence of septicemia, while the patient's immune response is compromised, and sensitivity of the patient to side effects of the vigorous treatment regimen will greatly affect the progress of treatment.

However, the most critical factor in prolongation of life is whether or not treatment successfully brings about and then maintains "complete remission" status, wherein all symptoms of the disease, including peripheral blood and bone marrow appearance, are normalized (4). The treatment leading to remission status from clinical disease is termed "induction." Although undetectable by current methods, leukemic stem cells linger even when the patient is in complete remission. In some protocols, treatment continues after remission is achieved, using moderate doses of the same drugs which caused remission. This is called "cytoreductive therapy" or "consolidation." Periodic treatment during remission

Table 45.1.
The Normal Differential White Blood Cell Count[a]

Blood Cell	Differential (%)
Total neutrophils	50–70
Segmented neutrophils (polys)	50–70
Band cells	3–5
Metamyelocytes	0–1
Lymphocytes	20–40
Monocytes	0–7
Eosinophils	0–5
Basophils	0–1
Blasts (of any type)	0–0

[a] Total white cell count is in the range of 5,000 to 10,000/cu mm, with considerable normal variation. Of this number, the above percentage distribution of cell types is normal in the peripheral blood.

Table 45.2.
The French-American-British (FAB) Cooperative Group Classification of Acute Leukemias

FAB Designation	Common Terms (Abbreviations) for Leukemic Subgroups	Predominating Cell Type
L-1	Acute lymphocytic leukemia, childhood (ALL)	Microlymphoblasts
L-2	Acute lymphocytic leukemia, adult (ALL)	Mixed lymphoblasts, prolymphocytes
L-3	Burkitt's-type leukemia	Lymphocytes[a]
M-1	Acute myelocytic leukemia, undifferentiated; acute myelogenous, acute granulocytic (AML)	Myeloblasts
M-2	Acute myelocytic leukemia, differentiated	Mixed myeloblasts, promyelocytes
M-3	Acute progranulocytic leukemia	Hypergranular promyelocytes
M-4	Acute myelomonocytic leukemia (AMML)	Mixed myelocytes, monocytes
M-5	Acute monocytic leukemia (AMOL)	Monocytes
M-6	Erythroleukemia	Mixed erythroblasts, erythrocytes, myelocytes

[a] Distinguished from L-1 and L-2 in that L-3 lymphocytes carry membrane-bound immunoglobulins, which characterizes them immunologically as deriving from B-cell lines (see also Fig. 45.1).

Table 45.3.
Clinical Symptoms from Leukemic Replacement of Normal Bone Marrow Elements

Anemia	Thrombocytopenia	Granulocytopenia
Fatigue	Conjunctival and fundal hemor-	Infection (fever and/or chills)
Pallor	rhages	"Flu" symptoms; frequent or prolonged
Shortness of	Gingival hemorrhages	colds
breath	Gastrointestinal bleeding (eme-	
Headache	sis or melena)	
Tachycardia	Renal hemorrhages (blood in	
	urine)	
	Petechiae; ecchymosis	
	Purpura	
	Subarachnoid hemorrhages	

with lowered doses of the induction drugs, or with different drugs, in an attempt to destroy newly activating leukemic cells is termed "maintenance." "Reinduction" courses will be necessary to treat each successive relapse, or return of active disease, which is recognized by return of symptoms and of "blasts" in the peripheral blood. In both ALL and ANLL, duration of each succeeding remission tends to be progressively shorter. Complete remission status implies functional as well as morphological normalization, and the patient in remission no longer is subject to abnormal hemorrhagic risk or the greatly lowered resistance to infection. Increased survival beyond the natural course of the disease was established early to be closely comparable to the total time a patient spends in complete remission (4).

As will be discussed later, drugs known effective in suppressing lymphocytic cell proliferation are not necessarily active against the myelocytic (granulocytic) cell lines. Therefore, induction of remission in ALL produces granulocytopenia to a lesser extent than in AML. Drugs effective in suppressing myelocytic cell lines, however, produce a prolonged and profound marrow aplasia affecting thrombocytic and lymphocytic precursors as well. Induction therapy for ANLL thus infers a more rigorous procedure which exposes the patient to relatively prolonged periods of risk to hemorrhage and infection. While ALL can often be treated in general medical hospitals, the intensive supportive therapy required by the ANLL patient during the granulocytopenic/thrombocytopenic phases of induction therapy is usually only available in the specialized cancer treatment center.

Almost all acute leukemia occurring in persons under 15 years of age is ALL. Presently available treatment can reliably produce com-

plete remission in 90% of cases, with median survival among childhood ALL patients achieving at least one complete remission now averaging 36 months. Survival beyond 5 years is now common, and some knowledgeable observers speak in terms of cures. Approximately 15% of acute leukemias in adults are FAB-classifiable as ALL. In contrast to childhood ALL, however, these cases respond poorly to therapy.

The acute leukemias classified as nonlymphocytic, ANLL, primarily affect adults. Intensive therapy, with sophisticated medical support, now regularly induces remission in 60 to 70% of cases, with median survival among patients achieving remission now averaging up to 24 months. Some patients have survived longer than 5 years, and survivals beyond 2 years are not uncommon.

While leukemic cell infiltration of body organs and tissues outside the bone marrow (bowel, liver, spleen, lymph nodes, kidneys, and subcutaneous lesions) is a major problem in chronic leukemias, infiltration presents little morbidity in acute varieties of leukemia, if the leukemic cell line is responsive to therapy.

However, central nervous system (CNS) leukemic infiltration is a serious and not uncommon development. The CNS can apparently serve as a reservoir and pharmacologic sanctuary for leukemic cells (not reached by lipid-soluble therapeutic agents which cannot cross the blood-brain barrier). Cells later emerging from the CNS may rise to systemic relapse.

Leukemic infiltration of the meninges is a serious complication which can occur independently of bone marrow condition and indeed may arise and progress while the patient is in bone marrow and peripheral blood remission. This complication has become more prevalent in all varieties of leukemia as their respective survival times have lengthened. Meningeal leukemia is most successfully treated early in remission before there is overt or symptomatic meningeal involvement, by intrathecal administration of methotrexate or cytosine arabinoside and/or external irradiation of the spinal column and brain. Radiation is usually administered at a rate of 200 rads daily for a total exposure of 2400 rads. Chemotherapy given in conjunction with radiation is usually administered in 5 divided doses over 6 weeks (5). Neurological manifestations of CNS leukemia may be minimal or flagrant, but symptoms of increased intracranial pressure and cranial nerve palsies are reason for concern.

Leukemic cells which have infiltrated or proliferated in the CNS can be identified by lumbar puncture and cerebrospinal fluid (CSF) sampling. CSF samples as well as bone marrow and peripheral blood sample become important in monitoring progression of the disease as well as success of treatment.

Leukemic cell infiltration of intracerebral alveolar structures (rather than the meninges and subarachnoid space) may occur in ANLL, and occasionally ALL, especially when peripheral blast counts exceed 200,000 cells per mm^3. Intracerebral intravascular plugging (leukostasis) with increased local pressure on vessel walls is a life threatening situation predisposing to intracranial hemorrhage, and it must be treated vigorously. Small doses of radiation (300 to 600 rads) should be administered immediately to resolve leukostatic foci, followed by hydroxyurea, given in a single oral dose of 50 to 100 mg/kg daily until the blast cell count drops below 100,000/mm^3. Often one dose is effective within 72 hours (6). Allopurinol should be given concurrently and serum uric acid levels should be monitored. Alkalinization of the urine should be considered and adequate hydration should be maintained to minimize possibility of urate nephropathy due to the large-scale cell lysis.

AVAILABLE MODALITIES OF TREATMENT

In all malignant conditions, therapeutic options incude the use of one or more of the following agents: surgery, ionizing irradiation, immunotherapy or chemotherapy. In leukemias, surgical excision of the tumor tissue is impossible, which relegates this modality to a minor supportive role.

Irradiation also has a supportive role in antileukemic therapy, particularly in reducing the size of an infiltrative leukemic mass. This is useful when functional impairment of some organ or vessel has occurred, or when pain is the result of marrow hyperactivity (i.e., sternal tenderness) or leukemic infiltration in an area such as a joint. Irradiation also is used to decrease numbers of proliferating leukemic cells when they occur in the CNS, and is used to obliterate functional bone marrow in preparation of a patient to receive bone marrow transplant.

Immunotherapy has received some attention in recent years with the demonstration of specific tumor antigenic sites in two cancerous states, Burkitt's lymphoma and choriocarcinoma. Data have suggested that immunotherapy is effective only when the tumor burden is "small" (less than 10^5 cells). An ANLL patient may have 10^{10} or 10^{12} leukemic cells at the time of diagnosis and symptomatic disease. It is postulated that 10^8 leukemic cells may remain, undetectable by current means, when the patient is in complete remission. Investigators have been prompted to explore use of immunotherapy as an adjunct to cytoreductive or maintenance chemotherapy because patients almost invariably break out of chemotherapeutically induced remission, and become increasingly refractory to further chemotherapy. For immunotherapy to be effective, we must assume (a) that leukemia-specific or leukemia-associated antigens exist, (b) that the leukemic patient retains the capability to develop immune responses to specific stimuli, and (c) that this immune response will favorably affect the balance of conditions which suppress emergence of the fulminant disease process and prolong remission. Specific agents (attenuated or killed allogeneic leukemic cells, cell-free extracts or cultured cell lines) and nonspecific agents (BCG vaccine, MER—methanol extraction residue of BCG) have been evaluated, with some positive results in use of both specific and nonspecific immunotherapy to prolong remission in ANLL. Evidence does not yet support routine use of immunotherapy to treat acute leukemias, but work continues on this intriguing approach (7).

Bone marrow transplantation in leukemia is based on the premise that the disease marrow can be destroyed and replaced by normal bone marrow (8). The procedure is limited in application by the fact that a suitable allogeneic marrow donor (HLA-matched sibling) is available in only 20% of potential candidates. When an isogeneic (identical twin) donor is available, reducing the occurrence of graft-versus-host disease, 2-year survival rates after transplantation reach 30%. With an allogeneic donor, 2-year disease-free survivals are achieved in 15 to 20% of recipients. This survival rate compares favorably to the most aggressive experimental ANLL chemotherapeutic protocols but probably represents a slightly different group of candidates. Autologous bone marrow (obtained from the ANLL patient while in remission and cryopreserved for later reinfusion) has been considered attractive since graft-versus-host complications could theoretically be reduced. A major reservation with using this approach is that even if obtained during remission, such marrow contains leukemic stem cells which would be reimplanted with the graft. Other problems remain with bone marrow transplantations, including relapse due to inadequate pretreatment "conditioning" of the patient. The relapse rate following conditioning with cyclophosphamide plus total body irradiation is 70%. Intensive conditioning regimens with cytosine arabinoside, 6-thioguanine, daunorubicin and cyclophosphamide in combination with total body irradiation reduced the post-conditioning relapse rate to only 24%. However, patients relapsing from such a regimen are usually refractory to further chemotherapy. The conditioning regimens themselves are highly toxic, and the combination of disease and conditioning results in a period of 10 to 20 days without marrow function during which the patient needs intensive supportive protection and therapy. After implantation it takes 2 to 3 months for hematologic values to return to normal. Recurrent leukemia, graft-versus-host disease, interstitial pneumonitis and persistent immunodeficiency are other problems with bone marrow transplantation, where solutions will undoubtedly be aggressively researched because the alternatives are so few.

To date, successful treatment of the acute leukemias has rested almost entirely on chemotherapy. The history of antileukemic chemotherapy is short, having begun with demonstration of the lympholytic properties of adrenocortical steroids in 1947 and application of this effect to treat acute leukemia with prednisolone in 1949. Development of antineoplastic drugs has been steady since that time. Attrition has left us with fewer than 10 drugs presently in common use against leukemias.

Many of the basic pharmacologic and pharmacokinetic/pharmacodynamic characteristics of these are still being investigated, while clinical use of the agents has produced therapeutic advances. We have mentioned that science has not yet elucidated the external agent or biological errors which cause leukemias. Because of this, many theories, proposals and models of antileukemic chemotherapy were developed in an empiric manner. Progress to date represents refined extrapolation of the original principles, plus a tremendous effort to demonstrate in well-controlled clinical trials the added benefit or toxicity of each proposed improvement, whether in drug moiety or schedule of drug administration.

CONCEPTS RELATIVE TO CHEMOTHERAPY

Modern growth-kinetic studies have disproved the concept of the leukemic cell population as a runaway prolific body. Analogous to growth of a bacterial colony, as the leukemic cell population expands, rate of growth seems to "plateau." The abnormal immature cells accumulate in the bone marrow, leading to failure of normal hematopoiesis by mechanisms that are unclear, but are more complicated than simple replacement or crowding of normal elements. Contrary to notions held by many in the recent past, and though it is obvious that leukemic stem cells demonstrate some metabolic advantage permitting growth at the expense of normal tissue, the rate of replication of leukemic cells has not been demonstrated to be faster than that of the surrounding normal formed element precursors. Henderson (5) has thus described leukemic cell populations as "self-renewal systems which, though they march to a different drummer, depend upon external stimuli and internal mechanisms similar to other living tissue."

It is worthwhile to review the cell cycle as it is depicted by Figure 45.2. This description applies to both normal and malignant cells. The portion of the cycle labeled "D" represents cellular division (mitosis). "G_1" (which may also be referred to as "G_0" in chemotherapy literature) is a resting phase, until recently considered to be relatively quiescent. The "S" phase is that of active deoxyribonucleic acid (DNA) synthesis, which is followed by "G_2," another resting phase. The S, G_2 and D phases are relatively fixed periods of time for a given cell population, and if rate of division (length

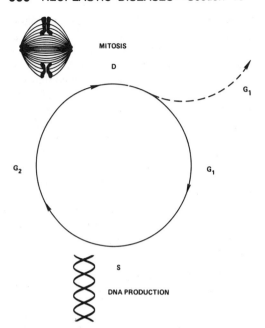

Figure 45.2. The mitotic cell cycle.

of the average cell cycle) varies, it is usually the G_1 phase which accommodates. When cells stop proliferating and come to rest, they do so in the G_1 phase, and when proliferative activity is high, the G_1 may become very short. Certain aspects of ribonucleic acid (RNA) production are known to occur during the G_1 phase, but it is not known how a cell receives the biological message to proceed to DNA synthesis (9).

In a malignant body of cells, the immediately premitotic event of spindle formation and the cell division, as well as the S phase of DNA replication necessary for reproduction of the cell line, have been the specific targets of antineoplastic chemotherapy. Drugs which act at these or some other defined phase of cell life are called "cycle-specific." Drugs are also in effective use, however, for which no phase specificity has been demonstrated and these are designated "cycle-nonspecific." The classification of the action of a drug on this basis is weak, however the terms are used widely in the literature.

Antileukemic chemotherapeutic approaches evidently take advantage of very subtle differences in rate of growth and cellular metabolism between the leukemic cell population and the patient's normal tissues. Both irradiation and chemotherapeutic drugs are basically toxic or injurious to all cells. Selec-

tivity of response to drugs depends on the relative vulnerability of malignant versus normal cells during the period of exposure to active drugs.

Cycle-specific drugs tend to be more effective in rapidly proliferating tissues, where their incorporation into disruptive cytotoxic events will kill the maximal number of tumor cells. Predictably, toxic manifestations of most antineoplastic drugs are borne by normal tissues (i.e., the bone marrow, alimentary canal mucosa, reproductive system germinal cells, and hair follicles) in which the percent of cells in division approaches or exceeds that of the malignant tissue under treatment. In antileukemic chemotherapy, toxicity to certain elements of the bone marrow is the object of treatment, but the need for careful titration of dosage is obvious.

Recalling the mechanism of drug activity above, remission induction involves disruption and lysis of the many immature leukocytes present in the peripheral circulation and bone marrow. Maintenance phases are designed to suppress leukemic stem cells newly proliferating (in an otherwise normal hematological state) before they cause relapse to clinical disease. Though exceptions exist, cell cycle-specific drugs are generally used in induction while cell cycle-nonspecific drugs have been most effective in maintenance.

The timing of sequential doses of chemotherapeutic agents to catch larger numbers of neoplastic cells in their susceptible phase is of clinical importance. Like normal tissues, leukemic cell lines do not exhibit synchronized division. That is, at a given moment, different cells within the leukemic cell population are in different phases of their individual cycle. As such, only a percentage will be vulnerable to the effects of a cycle-specific drug while that drug is present in an active form in the body. Attempts to synchronize the cellular division of the leukemic cell population in order to increase overall susceptibility to cycle-specific drugs have not been successful.

As stated recently in a review by Chang and Wiernik (10), "without a sensitive method to predict what combinations, sequencing, and order will achieve maximal cell kill with the minimum of side effects, most regimens are empiric and tend to be rather complex."

The experience to date has shown that combinations of drugs which produce qualitatively different toxicities can produce additive and perhaps synergistic increases in remission induction rate and remission duration. The administration of combinations of antineoplastic drugs in some cancers has two cytotoxic objectives. The first is to combine drugs which act at different points of the cell cycle and thus expose a larger percentage of the cancerous cells to the drug when those cells are in a susceptible state. The second (analogous in many respects to theories of antimicrobial therapy) is to expose susceptible cancer cells to toxic effects by as many mechanisms as possible to suppress selective emergency of cell strains which are resistant to further therapy. Again, from the perspective of Chang and Wiernik, "since none of these therapies has yet been uniformly successful, no standard treatment regimens have really been established, and investigators are still trying to improve upon current results with comparative clinical trials" (10). With the addition of each drug to a proposed combination regimen, many questions should be considered: Is the tumor type uniformly and reliably susceptible to one drug, or does resistance to repeated therapy occur? Does the proposed combination produce additive toxicity to particular normal tissues, or are the combined expected toxicity spread to different organs of the body? Is an effective dose of one drug (or all drugs) in the combination influenced by concomitant or subsequent administration of the other drugs? Is the effective dosage schedule of one drug (or all drugs) in the combination altered by administration of the other drugs? As can be seen, complexity of the variables involved in formulating new, more effective combination antineoplastic chemotherapy dictates that experimentation be undertaken by physicians with the clinical background and sufficient laboratory and supportive facilities to monitor results of drug administration.

One exception to those drugs which act by some interference with cell division is that of L-asparaginase (L-ASP). Development of this agent followed the discovery that some leukemic cells did not have the capacity to synthesize their own requirements of the amino acid, L-asparagine. These cells utilized circulating asparagine produced by other cells. It was postulated that sensitive leukemic cells could be starved out if endogenous asparagine were eliminated, and it was shown that the enzyme asparaginase from bacteria (especially *Escherichia coli*) inhibits replication of suscep-tible leukemic cells in vitro and in vivo. This is an apparent effect of catalyzing hydrolysis of L-asparagine in the blood and extracellular fluid. Asparaginase thus exploits a difference in metabolic requirements between leukemic and normal cells. Theoretically, L-ASP should be the most specific cytotoxic drug available to date and less toxic to normal tissues, especially those of the hematopoietic system. Because of this potential for relative marrow-sparing specificity, it was investigated in combination chemotherapy with myelotoxic drugs.

Unfortunately, the specificity of the drug does not appear as great as postulated. Evidence has accumulated to suggest that some leukemic cells can produce sufficient asparagine for survival and that normal tissue may, in contrast, be damaged. Allergic reactions including anaphylaxis are frequent and should be of particular concern. Pancreatitis has occurred during and following therapy and may be the limiting factor of treatment with L-ASP. The drug has proven more effective in ALL than AML and those complete remissions induced by L-ASP have been of relatively short duration. Asparaginase is used as a component of ALL induction in combination with prednisone and vincristine sulfate.

ANTILEUKEMIC DRUGS IN USE

ALL can be effectively treated when it occurs in preadolescent children. The leukemic lymphoblast cell population in these patients is lysed by chemotherapeutic drugs which in effective doses cause relatively little suppression of granulocytic and thrombocytic cell lines. As a result, induction therapy required to achieve complete remission (CR) in childhood ALL is less rigorous than in AML where the leukemic myeloblasts are the target of therapy. Chemotherapeutic drugs effective in AML lead to 4- to 6-week periods of profound agranulocytosis necessitating reverse isolation and other complications of therapy. Other acute leukemias of the ANLL group as well as ALL occurring in adults are similarly resistant to chemotherapy, with higher early mortality during induction therapy than childhood ALL.

In childhood ALL, the combination of vincristine sulfate (VCR) with prednisone (PRED) reliably induces CR in 80 to 90% of patients. Several three- and four-drug combinations have been tried which do not measurably improve CR rates over those obtainable with the constituent drugs used alone. Other drugs with activity against childhood ALL produce the following CR rates: L-ASP, 45%; daunorubicin (daunomycin, DMN), 40%; 6-mercaptopurine (6-MP), 35%; and methotrexate (MTX), 31 to 100% (the last on a schedule of intermittent high dose infusion). MTX administered daily, cyclophosphamide (CTX), and cytarabine (ARA-C) are less effective but do demonstrate some activity.

A three-drug combination of PRED, VCR and DMN or L-ASP has been reported to produce CR rates up to 95%. The four-drug combination known as "POMP" (PRED, Oncovin or VCR, MTX and Purinethol or 6-MP) also produces complete remissions in 95% of childhood ALL patients. Many cancer centers, however, elect to use the VCR and PRED induction regimen, to avoid the greater risk of toxicity of additional drugs. The limited toxicity and long-term clinical experience with this regimen often permit childhood ALL induction therapy to be conducted at a patient's local hospital; sometimes on an outpatient basis. Patients who do not achieve CR on the VCR/PRED regimen can be treated successfully with more aggressive regimens.

ALL in adults is significantly more resistant to therapy. The VCR and PRED regimen effective in 80 to 90% of childhood ALL cases induces CR in only 50 to 60% of adults with ALL. A more acceptable CR rate of 70 to 80% is attainable using a four-drug combination consisting of VCR (2 mg IV weekly for 3 doses, beginning on Day 1), PRED (40 mg/m² PO daily for 21 days, beginning Day 1, then tapered to zero over 7 days), DMN (45 mg/m² IV daily for 3 doses, on Day 1 through Day 3), and L-ASP (500 IU/kg/day IV daily for 10 doses, on Day 22 through Day 32). More myelosuppressive as well as more complex to administer, this regimen requires adult ALL patients to be hospitalized for induction therapy.

ANLL, as mentioned, is resistant to drugs effective in other leukemic conditions. CR rates achievable in ANLL with several chemotherapeutic drugs used singly are as follows: PRED, 15%; VCR, 10%; 6-MP, 11%; MTX, 10%. CTX and L-ASP show limited activity. The POMP ALL induction regimen produced CRs in 25% of ANLL patients treated. ARA-C, developed in the 1960s, was a major new drug breakthrough, able to induce CRs in 30% of ANLL patients. Using ARA-C in combination with 6-thioguanine (6-TG) or with CTX, VCR and PRED, or with CTX and MTX, remissions could be induced in 50% of patients. Daunomycin (DMN), which became available shortly after cytarabine, produced CR rates up to 50% when used singly, depending on dose and schedule of administration. Adriamycin (ADR), an anthracycline similar to DMN was nearly as effective in producing CR but was found to produce higher levels of toxicity to gastrointestinal mucosal lining. To date, DMN remains the most effective single agent in the treatment of ANLL. Also, most drug combinations have not demonstrated greater efficacy than DMN used alone. However, a two-drug combination of DMN (45 mg/m² IV daily for 3 doses beginning Day 1) with ARA-C (100 mg/m² IV continuous infusion, Day 1 through Day 7) produces CR in over 65% of patients treated. This is presently the most accepted ANLL induction regimen. A combination of VCR, ARA-C and PRED (OAP) has produced CR rates of up to 50% (11). The addition of DMN (DOAP), CTX (COAP), and Adriamycin (Ad-OAP) to OAP has produced similar results. A high dose induction regimen consisting of 6-thioguanine, ARA-C and DMN (TAD) has been reported to produce CRs in 82% of cases (12). With proper supportive care, and use of one of the above regimens, a majority of ANLL patients may now be expected to achieve a complete remission. This represents tremendous progress over the situation just 10 years ago.

However, with all acute leukemias including childhood ALL, relapse from complete remission has been an absolute clinical certainty. Over several years, greater experience permitted manipulation of the drugs, doses and schedules of drug administration in induction therapy to result in first remissions of progressively longer duration for each variety of acute leukemia. Additionally, consolidation, maintenance and intensification regimens have been developed to prolong duration of the first remission and thus disease-free survival. Of undisputed benefit in prolonging initial CR in childhood ALL, the benefit of consolidation or maintenance therapy in adult ALL and ANLL has not been conclusively demonstrated (13).

In ALL, 6-MP and MTX given consistently, with reinforcing doses of VCR and PRED every 4 to 12 weeks and prophylactic CNS therapy has kept children in first remission for over 5 years. There is no concensus on an appropriate period after which it may be safe to discontinue therapy.

In ANLL, there have been few randomized controlled studies which discern whether any reported extraordinary prolongations of first remissions were due to the induction regimen, or to consolidation or maintenance regimens employed. However, several regimens are under active investigation. Peterson and Bloomfield (14) reported median remission durations up to 16.5 months using weekly maintenance chemotherapy of oral 6-TG on 4 successive days with intramuscular ARA-C on Day 5. This approach is typical in that an attempt is made to keep prolonged treatment to the outpatient setting and minimally disruptive to the patient's life. "Late intensification" regimens have also been reported in which patients still in remission after several months are retreated with intensive induction-like protocols as if they had relapsed. More recently, the use of androgens in addition to chemotherapy has been proposed to prolong ANLL remissions (15). While effectiveness of consolidation, maintenance or late intensification therapy has not been conclusively demonstrated in ANLL, such therapy will continue to be evaluated because duration of first CRs is still unacceptably short (24 to 36 months at best) and because of the relative difficulty in obtaining second and third CRs in ANLL.

Reinduction therapy, to take the patient from relapse into a second or successive remission, usually requires different drugs from those employed in the original induction regimen.

In childhood ALL, combination chemotherapy using VCR, PRED, DMN and L-ASP may yield second CR rates up to 80%, though such remissions are of very short duration.

Adult ALL is less responsive to reinduction, and no regimen has received wide acceptance. However, "MOAD" (MTX 100 mg/m^2 IV push, Day 1; Oncovin 2 mg IV push, Day 2; L-ASP 500 IU/kg IV, Day 2; Dexamethasone 6 mg/m^2 PO daily, Day 1 through Day 10) has been reported to induce remission in 70% of previously treated/relapsed adult ALL patients.

Although several approaches have been tried, the induction of a second remission in ANLL remains difficult. As a single agent, 5-azacytidine (investigational) may be effective in 20% of patients. The podophyllin derivative VP-16-213, etoposide (investigational), produces 15% second CRs, with better responses in the monocytic acute leukemia variants. Approximately 25% of patients may achieve a second remission with a combination of ARA-C and 6-TG, or DMN. The leukemia often develops resistance to drugs previously given.

Acute leukemias which are refractory to more common therapy may be treated with 5-azacytidine or amsacrine (AMSA). AMSA (investigational) is now available on a Group C protocol from the National Cancer Institute for refractory adult AML. This drug used as a single agent, has induced CR in up to 30% of patients who were unresponsive to DMN and ARA-C (16, 17).

Pharmacological mechanisms, commonly encountered toxicities and the clinical applications of current antileukemic drugs are listed briefly in Table 45.4. As the knowledge base is growing at a very rapid pace, current information regarding the uses, doses, dosage schedules and combination therapy should be obtained from recent review articles on the subject drug(s) or treatment of the subject variant of acute leukemia. Therapeutic trends are difficult to detect in the primary literature, as virtually every report introduces a new building block in the critical foundation of understanding of these diseases, and the potent agents used to combat them.

SUPPORTIVE THERAPY

Supportive therapy has been developed to treat complications both of disease progression and side effects of therapy.

CNS leukemic infiltration and CNS leukostasis are serious developments, treatments of which were discussed earlier.

Hyperuricemia and obstructive urate nephropathy can result from the increased nucleoprotein production of large numbers of neoplastic cells. The problem is compounded when chemotherapy produces lysis of large numbers of tumor cells and release of their contents. Degradation of the purine by-products of these nucleoproteins to the final metabolite, uric acid, is mediated by the enzyme, xanthine oxidase. Administration of the xanthine oxidase inhibitor, allopurinol, interferes with the process at this point, leaving purine degradation products in the form of xanthines, which are more soluble metabolic precursors of uric acid. Prevention of hyperuricemia, a nearly inevitable consequence of the leukemia and its treatment, is much more satisfactory

Table 45.4.
Drugs in Current Use against Leukemias

Drug Name	Pharmacologic Category	Cycle Specificity	Mechanism of Action	Outstanding Toxicities and Side Effects	Application in Acute Leukemias
Amsacrine	Synthetic aminoacridine	Specific	Inhibition of RNA and DNA synthesis	Nausea and vomiting; myelosuppression, mucositis, alopecia	ANLL remission induction
L-Asparaginase	Enzyme	Unknown	Depletion of endogenous extracellular asparagine	Multiple defects in protein synthesis; clotting abnormalities; hypoalbuminemia hepatic and pancreatic toxicities; allergic response	Acute lymphocytic leukemia (ALL) remission induction only
Cyclophosphamide	Polyfunctional alkylating agent	(?)Nonspecific	Requires in vivo activation; believed to act by cross-linking macromolecules including DNA	Nausea and vomiting; myelosuppression; chemically induced sterile hemorrhagic cystitis; alopecia	ALL remission induction
Cytarabine (cytosine arabinoside)	Pyrimidine analog	Specific	Interferes with conversion of cytidylic to deoxycytidylic acid; inhibits DNA synthesis	Nausea and vomiting; myelosuppression; hepatic dysfunction; esophagitis	Acute myelocytic leukemia (AML) and ALL remission induction and maintenance; intrathecal use in CNS, leukemic infiltration
Daunorubicin (daunomycin; rubidomycin)	Antibiotic	Specific	Inhibition of RNA and DNA synthesis	Nausea and vomiting; myelosuppression; cardiotoxicity; alopecia	AML and ALL remission induction
Doxorubicin	Antibiotic	Specific	Inhibition of RNA and DNA synthesis	Nausea and vomiting; alopecia; myelosuppression; cardiotoxicity; stomatitis	AML and ALL remission induction
6-Mercaptopurine	Purine analog	Specific	Inhibition of purine synthesis; inhibition of DNA synthesis	Nausea and vomiting; myelosuppression; stomatitis; diarrhea; hepatic dysfunction	ALL remission induction and maintenance
Methotrexate	Folic acid antagonist	Specific	Inhibits activity of enzyme dihydrofolate reductase; interferes with synthesis of tetrahydrofolic acid, a coenzyme necessary in metabolic transformations in the production of DNA	Myelosuppression; oral and gastrointestinal ulceration; hepatic dysfunction alopecia; dermatitis	AML and ALL remission induction and maintenance; intrathecal use in CNS leukemic prophylaxis and treatment

Prednisone, prednisolone	Adrenocortical steroids	(?)Nonspecific	Direct lysis of lymphoid tissue; (?)inhibition of DNA synthesis	Psychoses; acute hypertension; peptic ulcer; fluid retention; immunosuppression, etc.; osteoporosis	ALL remission induction; (?)ALL maintenance
6-Thioguanine	Purine analog	Specific	Inhibition of purine synthesis; inhibition of DNA	Nausea and vomiting; myelosuppression; hepatic dysfunction; stomatitis; diarrhea	ALL and AML remission induction and maintenance
Vincristine SO$_4$	Vinca alkaloid	Specific	Disruption of mitotic spindle formation; inhibition of RNA and DNA synthesis	Peripheral neuropathies; paralytic ileus; alopecia	ALL remission induction; (?)ALL maintenance

than treating urate nephropathy once it occurs. Additional measures utilized in prevention and treatment of hyperuricemia, with differing degrees of success, include adequate hydration of the patient and alkalinization of the urine with sodium bicarbonate or acetazolamide to favor solubility of uric acid. Routine use of allopurinol, recognizing its possible untoward effects, can circumvent the problem in most cases.

Anemia, as a result of leukemic crowding of red cell precursors in the marrow, chemotherapeutically induced aplasia, or hemorrhage can be treated by transfusion of packed red cells or whole blood. Packed cells are preferable because they introduce a smaller antigenic load, having been separated from the other cellular elements and plasma proteins. The goal of transfusion is to keep the hematocrit above 25 volumes percent since anemia may also predispose the patient to bleeding.

Hemorrhage is more often a result of thrombocytopenia. Severe thrombocytopenia is less common in ANLL than in ALL, though chemotherapy may certainly induce it in either ANLL or ALL. The risk of hemorrhage increases when the platelet count drops below 20,000 per mm^3.

As recently as 1959, hemorrhages were responsible for nearly 67% of deaths from acute leukemias. Many of these were generalized (systemic) hemorrhages, although the greatest percentage were pulmonary hemorrhages associated with pneumonias. Other difficulties included bleeding into the subarachnoid space and into the GI tract. Freshly collected platelets obtained from whole blood or plasmapheresis techniques are able to maintain effective levels of circulating platelets when given by transfusion. Initially, random donor HLA-mismatched platelets are used to restore hemostasis. If alloimmunization and refractoriness develops, HLA-matched or single-donor platelets may restore function. Platelets are usually titrated to patient response rather than to a predetermined number of units. Half-life of transfused platelets is approximately 24 to 48 hours in the thrombocytopenic recipient. Repeated infusions are thus necessary as dictated by circulating platelet levels for the several weeks until the patient's marrow regains the ability to sustain platelet counts on its own above a hemostatic level. Adequate blood-banking facilities with relatively large platelet sources are required to support such treatment. Since this procedure became available in 1961, the percentage of hemorrhagic deaths in acute leukemias has dropped from 67% to 37% of the total mortality, as discussed by Hersh et al. (18). The category most greatly affected has been that of generalized (systemic) hemorrhage.

ANLL patients, particularly those with acute progranulocytic leukemia, seem predisposed to another severe hemorrhagic complication known as disseminated intravascular coagulation (DIC) which is characterized by thrombocytopenia, hypofibrinogenemia, decreased levels of factor V and increased levels of fibrin split products. Low dose heparin (50 to 70 units/kg every 6 hours) has been found to cause improvement within 24 to 48 hours.

Infections in the granulocytopenic patient continue to be a serious problem. Because progression of a septicemia or pneumonia is so rapid in the neutropenic patient, and because many clinical signs of systemic infection (induration, purulence) are absent in granulocytopenic patients, vigorous antibiotic therapy should be instituted at the first sign of fever. The accepted approach in the management of the febrile granulocytic cancer patient for the past decade has been the combination of a carboxy-penicillin (carbenicillin or ticarcillin) with an aminoglycoside (gentamicin, tobramicin or amikacin). These drugs were chosen for their differing modes of action and synergistically overlapping spectra to minimize the risk that resistant bacteria might develop. Piperacillin and mezlocillin, new broader-spectrum penicillin derivatives, possess greater activity than carbenicillin/ticarcillin against *Pseudomonas aeruginosa*, plus activity against *Klebsiella pneumoniae* and *Serratia marcescens*. Moxalactam, a third generation synthetic cephalosporin, has a similarly broad spectrum. Clinical efficacy of piperacillin plus amikacin and moxalactam plus amikacin has been recently evaluated against ticarcillin plus amikacin (19, 20) producing similar results, with the potential for fewer adverse effects including resistance by Gram-negative organisms. One of these newer combinations may represent a clinically significant improvement, particularly if optimal blood levels of the aminoglycoside are maintained through monitoring and dosage adjustment. Cultures of most likely suspected sites of infection plus blood, urine, stool, nose, gingiva and axilla are taken at the time the antibiotics are begun. Once the cultures from a patient become available, drugs

can be altered to suit the sensitivities as determined by disk and tube-dilution methods; or discontinued if infection is ruled out as source of the fever. Most clinicians feel safer continuing the antibiotic for 10 to 14 days, or until granulocyte levels rise to normal even if infection cannot be documented. Addition of amphotericin may also be considered. The number of leukemic deaths precipitated by infection has remained about 70%. Since deaths due to hemorrhage have been reduced in proportion to the total over the past few years, it is reasonable that figures for infections may have been inflated in spite of the numerous advances in antibacterial chemotherapy during the same period. Owing to effective suppression of some species, the pattern of infective organisms involved has been altered quite drastically. With the use of penicillinase-resistant antibiotics, incidence of fatal staphylococcal infection dropped from 23.5 to 3.1% of those deaths due to infection (19). Decrease in prevalence of this organism has been supplanted in turn by *P. aeruginosa*, *E. coli* and *Klebsiella* sp., *Enterobacter* sp., and group D *Streptococcus*. Systemic fungal infections with *Candida* sp. (monilia), aspergillosis and mucormycosis are rising in incidence, while available methods of managing fungal therapy are less than optimal. Treatment of infections in the acute leukemic patient promises to continue as a therapeutic challenge.

Effective prophylaxis against infection would provide more reasonable therapeutics than treating infections when they occur. Investigation along this line has evaluated reverse isolation (isolating the patient from contact with bacteria from exogenous sources) in programs at several institutions with the aim of protecting the patient from nosocomial microorganisms as well as protecting him prophylactically from opportunistic invasion by his own normal flora. The latter frequently occurs with GI lesions, including hemorrhoids, as the portal of entry.

A very stringent approach employs laminar air flow (LAF) rooms which place the patient in a virtually sterile environment. Supplies are sterilized before being passed to patients confined in these units, foods (especially vegetables) must be well cooked, and contamination from all sources (including drug products) must be considered. In addition, topical flora of the patient's body is suppressed by rigid hygienic efforts and flora of the GI tract is suppressed by administration of oral antibiotics. A 1975 study from the Baltimore Cancer Research Center (BCRC) (21) evaluates (a) LAF room reverse isolation plus oral nonabsorbable antibiotic prophylaxis versus (b) ward care plus oral antibiotics versus (c) ward care and no oral antibiotics. Their observation was that LAF plus oral antibiotic protection offered significantly decreased incidence of total infection, bacteremias, pneumonias, rectal abscesses, urinary tract infections, and pharyngitis. Infectious deaths were also reduced in this group. Ward care patients who regularly ingested the oral antibiotics had a reduction in infections almost as good as the LAF group, but those who could not tolerate the antibiotics used at that time (oral vancomycin, gentamicin and nystatin) had an incidence of infection comparable to regular leukemic ward patients. More recent work (22) from BCRC indicates the sulfamethoxazole/trimethoprim oral tablets plus nystatin suspension is better tolerated by patients and may be as effective as the oral gentamicin/nystatin suspension (vancomycin was dropped from the regimen several years ago).

Another rational measure against infection in granulocytopenic patients would seem to be the transfusion of granulocytes from donors. Elaborate selective centrifuging techniques have only recently been successful in yielding great enough numbers of granulocytes to transfuse effectively. Red cells and platelets can be obtained in pure fractions for transfusion because their specific gravities and other physical characteristics allow successful filtration, sedimentation and centrifugation procedures. Leukocytes are relatively few in number in the prospective donor (red cells: platelets:leukocytes = 500:20:1) and are intermediate in specific gravity. Thus, collected leukocytes generally have been contaminated with the other two formed elements. Selective granulocyte centrifugation is only available at larger treatment centers which utilize sophisticated cell separation machines. At present, sufficient evidence has accumulated which justifies recommending granulocyte transfusions in neutropenic patients with Gram-negative bacteremias. Side effects are serious and frequent enough to preclude prophylactic granulocyte transfusion.

PHARMACIST CLINICAL MONITORING OF CHEMOTHERAPY

Having noted the clinical course of acute leukemias, the concepts relative to antineo-

plastic chemotherapy and supportive therapy, it is obvious that this patient population requires intensive surveillance efforts by all health professionals concerned with their care. The drug therapy each patient receives is the specific end result of diagnostic procedures, clinical evaluations and efforts to minimize toxicities, side effects and complicating secondary problems. The pharmacist, utilizing support of current medication profiles and accurate dispensing records (including intravenous drugs and fluids), is in an excellent position to advise on such relevant matters as effective suppression of treatment-related nausea, solve problems relative to optimal oral dosage forms, and to review and be aware of all aspects of the patient's status.

Surveillance efforts relative to chemotherapy are directed at the emergence of toxic effects, side reactions and drug interactions of clinical significance and adherence to rational utilization of antineoplastic drugs. "Rational utilization" is an evolving concept in this instance, since the optimal doses, dosage schedules and the complete indications for most of the antineoplastic drugs are not fully known yet. Also, these drugs are not completely selective for neoplastic cells, and exhibit a narrow therapeutic margin. The effectiveness of many antineoplastic agents is measured by appearance of their toxic effects, and the doses prescribed are often titrated against "tolerable" levels of adverse effects, especially against hematopoietic tissues. With respect to drug interactions, this delicate balance assumes special significance. If the biological availability of antineoplastic agents is enhanced, or their metabolism or excretion inhibited, the danger of increased toxicity should be readily apparent.

To date, few reported drug interactions involving cancer chemotherapeutic agents have been well documented (23). A working understanding of the pharmacology of the drugs involved and the mechanisms which are plausible for a suspected potential interaction is invaluable to the pharmacist, who would expect to do some extrapolation from those principles. The pharmacist who is interested in monitoring effects of these drugs in patients will have to be familiar also with laboratory indices, especially those concerning bone marrow function, peripheral blood counts and coagulation parameters. Additionally, hepatic and renal function can be reviewed. With respect to renal function in leukemic patients it should be remembered that as systemic infection occurs, several antibiotics (including all those of the aminoglycoside class) might be needed and can, themselves, produce acute tubular necrosis. When decreased renal function is noted, doses of aminoglycosides should be adjusted on the basis of serum drug levels. Evaluation of the clinical situation might suggest similar alterations for other drugs the patient is taking which normally are excreted in active forms in the urine. Electrolytes and acid-base balance can be monitored as indicated.

In addition to their leukemia, these patients present a normal cross-section of other medical problems, including hypertension, diabetes, congestive heart failure, etc. Treatment for these conditions must continue, but the patient should be observed carefully for adverse response in the face of chemotherapy. Steroids used to lyse neoplastic lymphoid tissue, for example, may aggravate or precipitate a diabetic condition. Drugs used for treating underlying problems will have their contraindications and toxicities, and adequate monitoring can avoid additive complications of these and the antineoplastic drugs.

CONCLUSION

The acute leukemias are malignancies of the white blood cell-forming tissue of bone marrow. Chemotherapy, administered in sequential or concomitant doses of combinations of toxic drugs, may prolong the useful life of the victim if complete remission of the disease is achieved and can be maintained. Side effects of the treatment regimen and complications of the disease are severe, and success in achieving remission status is variable. Nearly 95% of children with ALL and approximately 50 to 60% of adults with ANLL will achieve a complete remission, extending their useful life up to 10 years and 2 years, respectively. Thus, significant progress has been noted and hopeful avenues of research have been opened to investigation. More selective cytotoxic drugs or more sophisticated dosage regimens, improved techniques to limit infection as a complication of treatment, bone marrow transplantation techniques and approaches utilizing specific active immunotherapy will be goals of future development.

It is anticipated that, for several years to come, effective induction therapy of acute nonlymphocytic leukemias will, of necessity,

be restricted to specialized treatment centers where supportive facilities can adequately serve the needs of the patient. Well-evaluated therapeutic regimens and more complete appreciation for possible complications allow the successful chemotherapy of acute lymphocytic leukemia in children in conventional medical facilities.

Through multifaceted surveillance efforts, assurance of an accurate and well-documented drug delivery system and constant involvement in the clinical area with patients, physicians and nurses, the pharmacist can serve a vital function in the direct care of those patients being treated for acute leukemia.

References

1. Anon: Cancer statistics, 1982. CA 32:15–42, 1982.
2. Kapadia SB, Krause JR, Ellis LD et al: Induced acute non-lymphocytic leukemia following long-term chemotherapy. Cancer 45:1315–1321, 1980.
3. Sheibani K, Bukowski RM, Tubbs RR, et al: Acute nonlymphocytic leukemia in patients receiving chemotherapy for nonmalignant diseases. Hum Pathol 11:175–179, 1980.
4. Henderson E: Treatment of acute leukemia. Semin Hematol 6:273–297, 1969.
5. Henderson E: Acute leukemia, in Williams WJ et al: Hematology, ed 2. New York: McGraw-Hill, 1977, p 998.
6. Grund FM, Armitage JO, Burns CP: Hydroxyurea in the prevention of the effects of leukostasis in acute leukemia. Arch Intern Med 137:1246–1247, 1977.
7. Gale RP: Advances in the treatment of acute myelogenous leukemia. N Engl J Med 300:1192, 1979.
8. Dabich L: Adult acute nonlymphocytic leukemias. Med Clin North Am 64:692, 1980.
9. Cline MJ, Haskell CM: Cancer Chemotherapy, ed 2. Philadelphia: W.B. Saunders, 1975, p 3.
10. Chang P, Wiernik PH: The leukemias, in Tice F: Practice of Medicine. Hagerstown, Md.: Harper & Row, 1978, vol VI, ch 29, p 12.
11. Hewlett J, Balcerzak S, Gutterman J, et al: Remission induction in adult acute leukemia by 10-day continuous intravenous infusion or ARA-C, plus Oncovin and prednisone: maintenance with and without BCG. Proc Am Assoc Cancer Res and Am Soc Clin Oncol 16:234, 1975.
12. Gale RP, Foon KA, Cline MJ, et al: Intensive chemotherapy for acute myelogenous leukemia. Ann Intern Med 94:753–757, 1981.
13. Foon KA, Gale RP: Controversies in the therapy of acute myelogenous leukemia. Am J Med 72:966, 1982.
14. Peterson BA, Bloomfield CD: Prolonged maintained remissions of adult acute nonlymphocytic leukemia. Lancet 2:158–160, 1977.
15. Hollard D, Sotto JJ, Berthier R, et al: High rate of long-term survivals in AML treated by chemotherapy and androgentherapy—a pilot study, Cancer 45:1540–1548, 1980.

16. Grove WR, Fortner CL, Wiernik PH: Review of amsacrine, an investigational antineoplastic agent. *Clin Pharm* 1:320–325, 1982.

17. Lawrence HJ, Ries CA, Reynolds RD, et al: AMSA—a promising new agent in refractory acute leukemia. *Cancer Treat Rep* 66:1475–1478, 1982.

18. Hersh EM, Bodey GP, Niles BA, et al: Causes of death in acute leukemia. *JAMA* 193:99, 1965.

19. Wade JC, Schimpff SC, Newman KA, et al: Piperacillin or ticarcillin plus amikacin. *Am J. Med* 71:983–990, 1981.

20. DeJongh CA, Wade JC, Schimpff SC, et al: Empiric antibiotic therapy for suspected infection in granulocytopenic cancer patients. *Am J Med* 73:89–96, 1982.

21. Schimpff S, Greene W, Young V, et al: Infection prevention in acute nonlymphocytic leukemia. *Ann Intern Med* 82:351–358, 1975.

22. Wade JC, Schimpff SC, Hargadon MT, et al: Comparison of trimethoprim-sulfamethcoxazole plus nystatin with gentamicin plus nystatin in the prevention of infections in acute leukemia. *N Engl J Med* 304:1057–1062, 1981.

23. Hansten PD: *Drug Interactions*, ed 4. Philadelphia: Lea & Febiger, 1979, pp 183–191.

CHAPTER 46

Hodgkin's Disease

WILLIAM A. CORNELIS, Pharm.D.
DOUGLAS G. CHRISTIAN, B.S.Pharm., M.B.A.
CLARENCE L. FORTNER, M.S.

The malignant lymphomas and lymphatic (lymphocytic) leukemias are lymphoreticular malignancies. Both are derived from lymphatic tissue and at times the lymphatic leukemias may resemble the lymphocytic lymphomas ((1) p. 944). The lymphatic leukemias affect the bone marrow with resulting peripheral blood abnormalities associated with leukemic infiltration of the spleen, liver, lymph nodes and other tissue. In contrast, the malignant lymphomas may originate either as extensive involvement of tissue or as localized involvement to one or more lymph nodes in a single anatomic region or a solitary extranodal site ((1) p. 1026).

The differences between the malignant lymphomas are found in microscopic examination of diseased tissue where characteristic cellular composition will distinguish them. Hodgkin's disease is a malignant lymphoma and like all other malignant lymphomas it is termed a lymphoreticular disorder.

Hodgkin's disease was first described in 1832 by the British physician Thomas Hodgkin in his paper "On Some Morbid Appearances of the Absorbent Glands and Spleen" after he had made some initial anatomical investigations of patients who had this disease of their lymphoreticular system. Another British physician, Sir Samuel Wilks, had independently described several cases of the same disease and had reassessed Hodgkin's paper; several years later Wilks named the disease after Hodgkin in another paper. The later work of two pathologists, Carl Sternberg (1898) and Dorothy Reed (1902), led to the subsequent naming of the Sternberg-Reed cell, the cell which is considered the actual malignant cell of Hodgkin's disease.

For many years there existed a great deal of controversy concerning whether Hodgkin's disease was a true neoplastic disease or an infectious disease of microorganismal etiology. The proponents of the microbial etiology of the disease argued that the afflicted nodes resembled granulomatous changes found in the lymph nodes of patients with tuberculosis, brucellosis and a variety of systemic fungal infections. In addition, some of the symptoms of Hodgkin's disease such as lymphadenopathy, fever and night sweats were also impressive clinical features which suggested an infectious process. Various workers even cultured brucella organisms, diphtheroids, *Histoplasma capsulatum*, *Cryptococcus neoformans* and avian strains of mycobacteria from the lymph nodes of patients with Hodgkin's disease, though later studies and follow-up work found these microorganisms to be contaminants in the tissue culture. Studies investigating possible viral etiology have been performed with inconclusive results.

The histopathology of a lymph node invaded with Hodgkin's disease reveals that the number of Sternberg-Reed cells is remarkably sparse when compared to the great number of neoplastic cells in other malignancies. In the past this finding cast further doubt on the neoplastic nature of Hodgkin's disease.

The support for the neoplastic basis of Hodgkin's disease comes from the metastatic nature of Hodgkin's disease (characteristic of all untreated malignancies) with eventual disease infiltration into organs. Also the typical infectious disease spreads via horizontal transmission from one person to the next, but to date this has never been proven conclusively for Hodgkin's disease. Studies have been conducted in certain geographical areas where the incidence of Hodgkin's disease among the resident population has been unusually high (2). These studies suggest a possible infectious etiology of Hodgkin's disease but concrete evidence to support the implications of these studies is still lacking. Hodgkin's disease is presently considered a malignant neoplastic process and associated therapy is conceived along the same lines as therapy for other malignant diseases.

PATHOLOGY

Lymph nodes are discrete nodules of lymphatic tissue anatomically located along lymphatic vessels. Lymphatic tissue is not uniquely found in lymph nodes, for lymphatic aggregates are also found in intestinal submucosa, bone marrow, bronchi, spleen and thymus. As distinct structures, the lymph nodes have a fibrous capsule from which connective tissue forms a framework by radiating throughout the node. The capsule is perforated by afferent lymphatic vessels which lead to a peripheral sinus. Branches of the sinus extend throughout the node and finally terminate at the hilus where efferent lymphatic vessels emerge. The lymph vessels within the node are lined with reticuloendothelial cells. The lymph nodes have the following three functions: formation of lymphocytes, production of antibodies and filtration of the lymph.

Diagnosis of Hodgkin's disease can be made only by microscopic examination of biopsied tissue from a suspicious lymph node or organ invaded by the disease. The presence of the Sternberg-Reed cell, in the appropriate cellular picture, will confirm the diagnosis. The diagnosis of suspected tissue can at times be difficult due to the relative paucity of Sternberg-Reed cells within diseased tissue. Microscopic examination of a diseased node not only reveals Sternberg-Reed cells, but predominant cellular elements may also include normal lymphocytes, histiocytes, occasional eosinophils, plasma cells, polymorphonuclear leukocytes, a hyperplasia of reticulum cells and varying degrees of collagen deposits. As Hodgkin's disease progresses, the normal nodal architecture is destroyed and concurrent disease infiltration of the node capsule occurs.

The histopathology of lymph nodes invaded by Hodgkin's disease can be classified into four distinct tissue types: lymphocyte predominant, nodular sclerosis, mixed cellularity and lymphocyte depleted. The differences between each tissue type are described in Table 46.1. Tissue type is one factor which determines the prognosis and course of the disease. Lymphocyte-predominant type offers the best prognosis with the nodular sclerosing type offering the second best prognosis. Mixed cellularity type is considered to have a poor prognosis and lymphocyte-depleted type has the poorest prognosis (3). Histology can be correlated with the stage of the disease.

The establishment of Hodgkin's disease as a neoplastic process brought about questions as to whether the disease was unicentric or multicentric in origin. Some cases suggested a unicentric origin because the disease could be localized to a single lymph node or lymph node

Table 46.1.
Histologic Subtypes Found in Hodgkin's Disease

1. *Lymphocyte predominance*
   A. Lymphocytic and/or histiocytic diffuse: sinusoids of lymph nodes become filled with lymphocytic cells and general normal architecture of the lymph node becomes obscured; this picture does not occur uniformly throughout the node and normal foci may be found; the lymph node capsule is not invaded by lymphocytes in early stages of the disease
   B. Nodular proliferative type: this form differs little from the diffuse form except for the tendency of the lymphocytic cells to be placed into poorly defined large and closely arranged nodules
2. *Nodular sclerosis*
   This tissue type is characterized by formation of bands of connective tissue which intercommunicate and separate the cellular and necrotic areas into islands
3. *Mixed cellularity*
   Presents a picture between lymphocyte predominance and lymphocyte depleted and characterized by having a variable number of lymphocytes and the presence of neutrophils, eosinophils and plasma cells
4. *Lymphocyte depleted*
   A. Diffuse fibrosis: characterized by widespread disorderly fibrosis with depletion of lymphoid cells and eventually of all other cellular elements
   B. Reticular type: lesions in this category have no significant characteristics other than a predominance of Sternberg-Reed cells to distinguish them from other diffuse, fibrotic, mixed or even nodular sclerotic lesions

chain. Other cases suggested a multicentric origin since some patients presented with involvement of virtually all lymph nodes. It is now agreed that Hodgkin's disease is probably unicentric in origin and spreads via contiguous lymph node chains and hematogenous routes. The natural course of the disease can be followed rather well and it has been observed that the disease generally spreads caudad rather than cephalad, suggesting a spread against the normal direction of lymph flow. Characteristically, 60 to 80% of the patients present with complaints of unilateral lymphadenopathy either in the cervical or supraclavicular region. The disease may spread in a retrograde fashion from cervical and supraclavicular regions to adjacent nodes in the ipsilateral axilla. If unchecked the disease may eventually spread to lymph nodes in the chest or abdomen, including the spleen. This may open a portal for the disease to invade such visceral organs as the liver as well as invasion of the bone marrow. There are some cases of Hodgkin's disease where spread of the disease is in a noncontiguous fashion and as the disease progresses, certain contiguous lymph node chains are skipped and remain uninvolved. These cases of noncontiguous dissemination probably reflect hematogenous spread and represent a poor prognosis since the anatomic involvement of the disease cannot be predicted.

STAGING

After Hodgkin's disease has been diagnosed and the cell type established, the patient must be staged; that is, the anatomical extent of the disease must be determined. Just as the histopathology is one factor in determining prognosis, so too is staging. Staging is important in order to identify and treat all involved areas, since untreated areas may continue to serve as a source for the dissemination of the disease. There are four stages of Hodgkin's disease: I, II, III and IV. Each stage is further subdivided into two categories, A and B (Table 46.2). As the disease progresses from Stage I to Stage IV, the prognosis becomes poorer. The categories A and B indicate if the patient is asymptomatic (A) or symptomatic (B). The presence of symptoms within the individual stages of Hodgkin's disease reflects a poorer prognosis than if no symptoms are present. The clinical symptoms of Hodgkin's disease are general rather than specific; they are unexplained weight loss of

Table 46.2.
Ann Arbor Classification for the Staging of Hodgkin's Disease[a]

Stage I: Disease involvement of a single contiguous lymph node region (I) or of a single localized extralymphatic organ or site (I$_E$) on the same side of the diaphragm

Stage II: Disease involvement of two or more contiguous lymph node regions on the same side of the diaphragm (II) or localized involvement of an extralymphatic organ or site and of one or more lymph node regions on the same side of the diaphragm (II$_E$). An optional recommendation is that the number of node regions involved be indicated by a subscript (e.g., II$_3$)

Stage III: Disease involvement of lymph node regions on both sides of the diaphragm (III) which may also be accompanied by localized involvement of an extralymphatic organ or site (III$_E$) or by involvement of the spleen (III$_S$), or both (III$_{SE}$)

Stage IV: Diffuse or disseminated disease involvement of one or more extralymphatic organs or tissues with or without associated lymph node enlargement. The extralymphatic sites of involvement should be identified by symbols.

[a] Each stage subdivided into A (asymptomatic) and B (symptomatic). Symptoms are (a) weight loss greater than 10% of body weight, (b) unexplained fever with temperature above 38°C (100.4°F), and (c) night sweats.

more than 10% of the body weight, unexplained fever with temperature above 38°C (100.4°F) and night sweats. A patient may experience additional symptoms such as pruritus or alcohol-induced pain, but they do not correlate with severity of disease and therefore are not considered in the staging evaluation.

The anatomical landmark which has key significance in the staging of Hodgkin's disease is the diaphragm, which is the reference point from which the extent or stage of Hodgkin's disease is measured. If the disease is confined to lymph nodes only on one side (above or below) of the diaphragm, the disease is considered to be localized and the prognosis is better than if the disease were more disseminated and present on both sides of the diaphragm.

Clinical staging (CS) involves an intensive compilation of data obtained from the patient's history, physical examination and results of laboratory tests and procedures, the purpose of which is to determine the "clinical" extent of disease short of diagnostic laparotomy. A detailed patient history is obtained making note of the presence or absence of unexplained fevers, night sweats and weight loss. A complete and thorough physical examination must be performed giving particular attention to areas of bone tenderness, and the size of the liver and spleen.

The laboratory tests and procedures which are conducted are designed to detect any clinical abnormality which may implicate a specific organ or organ system invaded by Hodgkin's disease. The necessary laboratory tests are as follows: a complete hematologic workup consisting of a white blood cell count and differential, platelet count, hemoglobin and/or hematocrit; evaluation of renal function including routine urinalysis, serum creatinine, blood urea nitrogen and creatinine clearance; evaluation of liver function by measuring albumin, bilirubin, lactic dehydrogenase, serum glutamic oxaloacetic transaminase, and alkaline phosphatase (elevated alkaline phosphatase may also imply bone disease and require further workup). Radiological studies which are advised consist of: chest x-ray with posteroanterior and lateral views and tomograms if the chest x-ray is suspicious; views of skeletal system to include thoracic and lumbar vertebra, the pelvis, proximal extremities, and other areas of bone pain tenderness; a bilateral lower extremity lymphogram for visualization of deeper lymph nodes in the abdomen which may be diseased; an intravenous pyelogram if indicated, for visualization of the renal system and detection of any obstruction or organ displacement.

Required evaluation procedures in the presence of suspected organ involvement with Hodgkin's disease include scintiscans of osseous tissue, liver, and spleen, and one marrow biopsy by needle or open surgical method. Other laboratory tests and diagnostic procedures are indicated if involvement of Hodgkin's disease is suspected in other organs (4, 5).

Clinical staging therefore, serves only as a means of estimating disease extent by identifying organs or organ systems in which disease is suspected, but it does not serve to diagnose Hodgkin's disease within organs. Positive diagnosis can only be made by tissue biopsy and subsequent identification of Sternberg-Reed cells within lymphatic or nonlymphatic tissue.

Pathological staging (PS) serves as a scheme to diagnose Hodgkin's disease in various tissues which have been implicated by the clinical staging procedure. Pathological staging involves biopsy and examining microscopically lymphatic tissue, organs, and other tissue clinically evidenced as being diseased. Exploratory laparotomy is one surgical procedure employed if management decisions depend on identification of abdominal disease. During laparotomy, various biopsies of abdominal lymph nodes, bone, liver and spleen are performed in detail.

Adequate tissue biopsies are important since tissue diagnosis of Hodgkin's disease depends on the presence of the sparse Sternberg-Reed cells and tissue which is clinically evidenced as diseased will not always show pathological evidence of disease.

The abdominal lymph nodes which should be biopsied include: an upper periaortic node; a splenic hilar node (located on the fissure of the gastric surface of the spleen where vessels and nerves enter); an iliac node (located on the expansive superior portion of the pelvis); a porta hepatis node (located on the transverse fissure of the visceral surface of the liver where portal vein and hepatic artery enter and hepatic ducts leave) and a mesenteric node. It is important that a porta hepatis node and a mesenteric node be biopsied because lymph nodes in these two regions cannot be clinically evidenced as diseased (they are not visualized in a lower extremity lymphogram), and later radiation therapy normally does not include these anatomical areas within radiation fields or "ports." If Hodgkin's disease is present in these areas, the radiation ports may have to be extended to include them or chemotherapy used instead, if appropriate ports cannot be designed.

Tissue sampling of the liver should include two needle biopsies (one in each lobe of the liver) and a wedge biopsy where a 2-cm cube of a hepatic tissue is excised. Bone marrow biopsy, if indicated, is performed on the iliac crest region of the pelvis by obtaining a core of osseous tissue via a needle biopsy or an open surgical biopsy where an actual piece of bone is removed.

In addition to the various biopsies, a splenectomy is also performed during the laparotomy procedure. There are three reasons for removal of the spleen; disease involvement of the spleen may be impossible to determine grossly and may only be found if the spleen is carefully sectioned; a histologically proven negative spleen is of prognostic significance since such patients essentially never have hepatic Hodgkin's disease; and the spleen overlies the left kidney and is adjacent to the left lung; if radiation therapy to the spleen were necessary, this would increase the risk of radiation-induced nephritis and/or pneumonitis.

Staging laparotomies initially were begun to investigate a more accurate method of staging patients with abdominal disease. However, today laparotomies are not routinely performed nor should they be. Laparotomy and splenectomy should be performed only if management decisions are related to abdominal disease since therapy advances and more sophisticated diagnostic tools have become available. Computerized axial tomography (CAT) and sonography in conjunction with lymphography may be sufficient to replace laparotomy. In addition, peritoneoscopy may be used to obtain liver biopsies. These procedures are certainly associated with less morbidity than a laparotomy and should be considered prior to laparotomy. Thus, pathologic staging can be accomplished in patients by less invasive procedures.

The findings from pathological staging procedures are subscripted by symbols indicating the tissue sampled. The results of the histopathological examination are indicated by + when positive for Hodgkin's disease and by − when negative. The recommended abbreviations used in the pathological staging procedure are as follows:

N+ or N− For lymph node positive or negative for disease by biopsy.

H+ or H− For liver positive or negative by liver biopsy.

S+ or S− For spleen positive or negative following splenectomy.

L+ or L− For lung positive or negative by biopsy.

M+ or M− For bone marrow positive or negative by biopsy or smear.

P+ or P− For pleura positive or negative by biopsy or cytological examination.

O+ or O− For osseous tissue positive or negative by biopsy.

D+ or D− For dermal tissue positive or negative by biopsy.

Examples of staging classification utilizing re-

sults of CS and PS procedures are given in Table 46.3.

The data collected over the past several years have revealed some interesting statistics regarding the correlation of clinical stage of Hodgkin's disease with histological tissue type. Review of the literature has shown that patients presenting with the lymphocyte predominant variety have a strong association with clinical stages I and II while the lymphocyte depleted variety is seen mainly in patients presenting with clinical stages III and IV. The mixed cellularity variety occurs in all clinical stages of the disease without any strong correlations. The nodular sclerosis variety is seen primarily in patients presenting with clinical stage II disease and is the one histologic subtype which presents with a distinctive anatomical pattern of distribution, namely a predilection to involve the lower cervical lymph nodes and mediastinum (6). The lymphocyte-predominant, lymphocyte-depleted and mixed cellularity varieties exhibit a variable propensity for anatomical involvement when compared within the same clinical stage. In contrast to the other three histological subtypes, nodular sclerosis occurs primarily in females within all age groups.

CLINICAL COURSE AND COMPLICATIONS

Hodgkin's disease usually manifests itself initially with patients noting lymphadenopa-

Table 46.3.
Staging Classification Examples

CS IA PS I$_{S-H-N-M-}$
Implies clinical Stage I without symptoms and pathological Stage I without disease involvement of the spleen, liver, additional lymph nodes and bone marow

CS IIA$_3$ PS III$_{S+N+H-M-}$
Implies clinical Stage II without symptoms and three lymph node regions involved; pathologic Stage III with spleen and additional lymph nodes positive for disease; liver and bone marrow negative for disease

CS IIIB PS IV$_{H+M-S-}$
Implies clinical Stage III with symptoms; pathologic Stage IV with liver positive for disease; bone marrow and spleen negative for disease

CS IVB$_{LH}$PS IV$_{H+M-}$
Implies clinical Stage IV with symptoms and clinical evidence for lung and liver disease; pathologic Stage IV with liver positive for disease and bone marrow negative for disease. Lung involvement was only documented clinically, but not pathologically

thy and occasionally with Hodgkin's disease symptoms of fever, night sweats and weight loss. Patients presenting with these symptoms will many times receive a short course of antibiotic therapy since some infectious process will frequently be suspected by the attending physician. Since the symptoms will not subside with antibiotic therapy, patients may be hospitalized and further workup will reveal Hodgkin's disease as the underlying problem. Routine chest x-rays may show an enlarged mediastinum with some displacement or obstruction of the trachea and/or esophagus due to an impinging mass. The patient may be symptomatic and may complain of dysphagia or coughing.

The lymphadenopathy of Hodgkin's disease is usually a painless enlargement of peripheral lymph nodes (cervical, axillary, inguinal) presenting with or without additional symptoms. Rapid enlargement of the lymph nodes, however, may cause them to become tender. In the early stages of the disease, the affected lymph nodes are discrete and easily palpable, but as the disease progresses, these nodes may become matted. If the lymphadenopathy is present initially above the diaphragm, the disease, if unchecked, can be expected to spread to areas below the diaphragm by dissemination via contiguous lymphatics. Disease presentation below the diaphragm, if unchecked, will in most cases remain below the diaphragm since dissemination to areas above the diaphragm would suggest a cephalad spread which is not generally characteristic for Hodgkin's disease.

It has been postulated that the fever may be a consequence of some immune response to the disease and may be brought about by pyrogens released from lysed granulocytes involved in the immune mechanism. Whatever the cause, the fever is fluctuating in nature and frequently responds to salicylates or acetaminophen. In refractory cases, indomethacin has been found effective in reducing the fever of patients who do not respond to the usual antipyretics (7). The etiology of the weight loss and night sweats remains unclear, but it is noted that the night sweats can, at times, be so profuse as to warrant the changing of bed clothes several times during the night. There is one unique symptom experienced by a minority of the patients, and this is alcohol-induced pain. This phenomenon is characterized by severe pain localized in anatomical

areas of active disease after the patient has ingested alcohol; the pain eventually subsides as the alcohol is metabolized (8). The alcohol intolerance syndrome has remained an enigma, for no etiology has been found.

Advanced Hodgkin's disease is characterized by invasion of the disease into various organs or organ systems culminating in a variety of complications and clinical problems. Pleural effusions are a frequent physical and radiographic finding, most commonly caused by mediastinal adenopathy and lymphatic obstruction. This causes the pleural tissue to leak fluid into the pleural cavity and results in accumulation of fluid known as pleural effusion. The patient complains of difficult or labored breathing (dyspnea) and has severe dyspnea on exertion. Treatment involves repeated removal of this pleural fluid (thoracentesis). If the fluid continues to accumulate, this may necessitate the intrapleural instillation of sclerosing agents such as mechlorethamine, bleomycin, or tetracycline (9–11).

Invasion of osseous tissue may cause local destruction of bone (osteolytic lesions) or may cause local osseous reactions characterized by the formation of new bone tissue (osteoblastic lesions). This bone destruction and local attempts at repair will alter the clinical chemistry of the patient by causing an elevation of serum alkaline phosphatase. Bone involvement may lead to severe bone pain in the patient, and palliative relief can be obtained by local radiation.

Hepatic involvement is not uncommon in stage IV of Hodgkin's disease. A notable observation found in staging procedures is that hepatic presence of Hodgkin's disease is almost always found with attendant disease in the spleen but the converse is not true (12).

Some disease involvement may occur in the gastrointestinal (GI) tract and renal system, but is rare; symptoms can be related to organ displacement or obstruction. Neurologic complications occur in 12% of the cases and consist mainly of spinal cord compression, peripheral nerve palsies and cranial nerve palsies.

One notable finding that has been reported is that some Hodgkin's disease patients may be free of their disease for several years only to present again with a diagnosis of leukemia (13). Initially, this observation stirred some debate. It was uncertain whether the leukemia was a normal manifestation of the disease, being noted due to longer survival rates of Hodgkin's disease patients, or if the leukemia was induced by prior radiation or drug therapy. However today, there is persuasive evidence that combined modality therapy increases the risk of a second malignancy in Hodgkin's disease patients. It is known that high dose radiation can induce leukemia, but to accuse radiation therapy as the sole cause of subsequent leukemia is still conjectural.

Infectious complications have a high incidence in Hodgkin's disease patients, especially in the later stages of the disease. These patients have a great tendency toward infections because, as a manifestation of their disease, they are immunologically deficient. This deficiency is not clearly understood but it has been noted that some of these patients are unable to react to various intradermal antigens such as mumps and chemical agents such as dinitrochlorobenzene (DNCB); patients unable to react to dermal antigens are termed anergic. A patient with Hodgkin's disease may even have active tuberculosis but may be unreactive to a tuberculin skin test. This finding shows that there exists some cellular immunological deficiency, since a delayed immunological reaction (characteristic of dermal antigens) is mediated by cells, unlike an immediate immunological response which is mediated by antibodies. Normal antibody formation is found in Hodgkin's disease except in the terminal stage. Also important to note is that this delayed immunologic reactivity may be present in early stages of the disease but may disappear as the disease progresses.

Tuberculosis was the major infection associated with Hodgkin's disease patients, but is to a lesser degree now because of improved drug therapy of tuberculosis. Bacteria still remain the most common cause of infection but recently viruses such as herpes zoster, herpes simplex and cytomegalovirus (CMV) have been recognized to cause infections in these patients. Systemic fungal infections such as actinomycosis, nocardiosis, histoplasmosis, cryptococcosis, candidiasis, aspergillosis, pneumocystis and the protozoal infection toxoplasmosis also have an unusually high incidence of infecting Hodgkin's disease patients.

THERAPY

The treatment of Hodgkin's disease centers mainly around radiation therapy and/or chemotherapy. Surgery, although useful in the management of some other malignancies, does not directly play a role in the treatment of Hodgkin's disease and is primarily employed in staging and diagnostic procedures. Therapy of Hodgkin's disease is aimed at eliminating all clinical signs and symptoms of the disease. If all symptomatic and objective parameters for monitoring the disease resolve (approach normal), the disease is considered inactive and the patient is considered in "remission." If all symptoms or abnormal objective parameters recur, the disease is considered again present and the patient is said to be in "relapse." More effective therapy of Hodgkin's disease is still under investigation and several research centers around the country are evaluating radiation therapy, chemotherapy and various combinations of both in the treatment of the different stages of Hodgkin's disease.

Stages I and II disease are very amenable to radical radiation therapy (radical implying high doses of radiation with curative intent) because in these stages the disease is present in a few well defined focal areas, not disseminated, and can be effectively treated with radiation of involved nodes and uninvolved adjacent lymph nodes at high risk for occult disease. Some investigators, however, are subjecting stages I and II patients initially to radiation therapy followed by chemotherapy and have found these patients to have a lesser incidence of relapse than those patients treated with radiation alone (14).

The therapy of stage III patients is not well defined and debatable among clinicians. Accepted therapy has been to treat all stage III patients with radical radiation therapy. However, findings reported by some researchers have shown that patients with stage IIIB disease should be treated like stages I or II disease utilizing radiation therapy alone or radiation therapy followed by chemotherapy, and that stage IIIB disease should be treated like stage IV disease using chemotherapy with palliative doses of radiation therapy (14, 15 (p. 1382), 16).

Stage IV disease is not well suited for radiation therapy since sites of the disease in this stage may be so numerous and diffuse that localized radiation cannot be effectively carried out. Parenchymal organs cannot tolerate curative doses of radiation and the presence of Hodgkin's disease in these areas precludes the use of radical radiation. Stage IV disease is therefore treated primarily with systemic chemotherapy which has access to all sites of disease. "Spot" radiation is also used in stage

IV disease for palliative treatment to anatomical areas of disease involvement not responding to chemotherapy and causing pain, tenderness or obstruction.

RADIATION THERAPY

The use of radiation has been employed in treating Hodgkin's disease since the early 1900s when it was shown that the disease responded to small doses of x-irradiation, although a response of only temporary benefit. These early attempts were rather crude since the radiation did not penetrate to the tumor but delivered its maximum effect on the skin. The 1950s brought about advances in equipment (use of ^{60}Co and linear accelerators for clinical use) so that megavoltage radiation could be given increasing the penetration and dose rate of radiation with skin-sparing effect. These devices allow the practical use of large fields, exposing entire lymph nodes to radiation in the range of 3500 to 4000 rads ("rad" stands for radiation absorbed dose and equals 100 ergs/g tissue). Radiation therapy essentially has the same effect on cellular biochemistry as do the alkylating agents employed in chemotherapy. Deoxyribonucleic acid (DNA) replication is prevented by interfering with cross links necessary for the double helix integrity of the DNA molecule. Proliferating tissue, characteristic of malignancies, is especially radiosensitive owing to constant DNA production necessary for cell division. The epithelial lining of the GI tract also is rapidly dividing tissue and frequently encountered side effects with radiation therapy are radiation-induced pharyngitis, esophagitis and gastroenteritis. The rapid production of cells in the bone marrow also makes this site very susceptible to radiation-induced bone marrow suppression. It is, therefore, important that vital, uninvolved organs and viscera be shielded during radiation therapy to minimize radiation-induced toxicities.

In stages I and II disease, tumoricidal doses of radiation are given to diseased nodes over a period of 4 to 6 weeks and radiation also is administered prophylactically to adjacent lymph node areas uninvolved with disease. Extended field radiation therapy involves irradiating all localized areas of disease and all involved adjacent areas. Total nodal irradiation involves treating all lymph node regions above the diaphragm (cervical, supra- and infraclavicular, axillary, mediastinal) and all lymph node regions below the diaphragm (periaortic, retroperitoneal, inguinal and splenic regions) with tumorcidal doses. Irradiation of all lymph nodes, contiguous or not, above the diaphragm in the presence of stage I or II disease is known as radiation to the upper mantle. Stage I or II disease below the diaphragm is treated by irradiating all abdominal and inguinal nodes. This technique is known as an inverted "Y," due to the anatomical pattern formed by the lymph nodes below the diaphragm. Therefore, total nodal radiation therapy involves irradiating all lymph node bearing areas which would include the upper mantle plus the inverted "Y" as mentioned above.

In general, stage I and II disease above the diaphragm would be treated with the upper mantle technique including the high periaortic nodes and splenic pedicle nodes. Stage II disease below the diaphragm would be treated with the inverted "Y" technique. Stage IIIA is considered local disease and would receive irradiation to all lymph node bearing areas. Stages IIIB and IV are disseminated and therefore combination chemotherapy is the primary and initial treatment.

CHEMOTHERAPY

Malignant growths are characerized by proliferating tissue which synthesize and assimilate DNA quickly for cell division and growth. Chemotherapy may not be selective against malignant growth in all cases because cytotoxic effects may also be exerted against normal tissue whose rates of proliferation parallel those of the malignancy: bone marrow elements, GI epithelial cells and hair follicles. The search for effective chemotherapy is in large part a search for increased selectivity of effect against tumors.

The use of chemotherapy in the treatment of Hodgkin's disease relies upon using combinations of drugs. This approach is true for many malignancies. Combination chemotherapy employs drugs with different mechanisms of action which attack proliferating cells at different stages of cell replication. The resulting toxicities are selective due to the different drugs employed ((17) p. 44).

Combination chemotherapy also minimizes the emergence of resistant malignant cell lines which are refractory to drug therapy. A number of cellular mechanisms may be involved in drug resistance—altered drug metabolism, cell impermeability to the active compound, elevations of drug inhibitory enzymes and increased activity of cellular repair ((17) p. 33). Drugs in combination attack the malignant cell at different stages of the cell cycle making it more difficult for the cell population to acquire multiple drug resistance than if only a single drug were used (this concept is analogous to antibiotic therapy utilizing combinations to prevent emergence of resistant bacterial strains) ((17) p. 42).

The scheduling of combination chemotherapy is important. Drug doses ideally should be administered at a time when malignant cells are actively synthesizing and assimilating DNA components so that maximum cell kill can occur. Chemotherapy should continue at specified time intervals to destroy any newly formed malignant cells and keep the total number of malignant cells at a level where clinical signs of disease are not evident.

The drug combination which has been very successful in obtaining the induction of remissions in Hodgkin's disease is MOPP (mechlorethamine or Mustargen, vincristine or Oncovin, prednisone, and procarbazine). First pioneered by DeVita et al. (18), MOPP therapy has endured and remains the mainstay of initial chemotherapy for Hodgkin's disease (19, 20). MOPP therapy is given in cycles which repeat every 28 days; at least six such cycles are given, provided a complete remission is obtained prior to administration of the last two cycles. Should toxicities occur during a MOPP cycle, appropriate dosing adjustments are indicated before the next cycle is begun (see Table 46.4). There has been some controversy in the past regarding the use of MOPP as maintenance therapy after remission induction. This issue now appears resolved in that numerous reports have concluded no prolongation of remission when MOPP or other combinations of drugs are used for maintenance ((15) p. 1376). Therefore, MOPP treatment should be discontinued after remission is attained.

Alternatives to MOPP therapy are available and are employed when MOPP remission induction fails. Some of these alternates keep prednisone and procarbazine in the regimen but substitute mechlorethamine with another alkylating agent such as cyclophosphamide, chlorambucil, lomustine (CCNU), carmustine (BCNU) or substitute vinblastine for vincristine. Additionally some regimens may add or substitute bleomycin, doxorubicin, dacarbazine or streptozocin (investigational) or their combinations as salvage treatments for MOPP failures. These unique combinations all are identified with acronyms which identify the component drugs: CVPP (cyclophosphamide, vinblastine, procarbazine, prednisone); SCAB (streptozocin, CCNU, doxorubicin (Adriamycin), bleomycin); ABVD (doxorubicin, bleomycin, vinblastine, dacarbazine) ((15) p. 1378). Other drug combinations currently being evaluated include new combinations of established chemotherapeutic agents and newer investigational drugs.

Table 46.4.
MOPP Regimen with Dosing Adjustments

Mechlorethamine	6 mg/m² IV	Day 1 and 8
Vincristine (Oncovin)	1.4 mg/m² IV	Day 1 and 8
Procarbazine	100 mg/m² PO	Day 1 through 14
Prednisone[a]	40 mg/m² PO	Day 1 through 14, cycles 1 and 4 only

Repeat cycle every 4 weeks
Six cycles minimum

WBC Count	Platelet Count	Dose Adjustment
4000/mm³	100,000/mm³	100% all drugs
3000–4000/mm³	100,000/mm³	100% vincristine 50% procarbazine and mechlorethamine
2000–3000/mm³	50,000–100,000/mm³	100% vincristine 25% procarbazine and mechlorethamine
1000–2000/mm³	50,000/mm³	50% vincristine 25% procarbazine and mechlorethamine
1000/mm³	50,000/mm³	No therapy

[a] No dosage adjustment required.

Antineoplastic Drugs

The classes of antineoplastic drugs used in the treatment of Hodgkin's disease are outlined in Table 46.5. The mechanisms of action of the various antineoplastic agents are as follows:

ALKYLATING AGENTS

These drugs attack functional groups on the purine base guanine, interfering with necessary cross-linking between the two strands of

DNA. This prevents DNA replication and transcription of ribonucleic acid (RNA).

VINCA ALKALOIDS

Two alkaloids, vincristine (VCR) and vinblastine (VLB), isolated from the periwinkle plant (*Vinca rosea*) have been used in combination chemotherapy of Hodgkin's disease. VCR has a similar spectrum of clinical activity as VLB but one important distinction between these two drugs is that Hodgkin's disease ap-

Table 46.5.
Drugs Currently Used in Treatment of Hodgkin's Disease

Pharmacological Class	Drug Name	Mechanism of Action	Side Effects and Outstanding Toxicities
Alkylating agents	Mechlorethamine	Attacks functional groups on guanine interfering with cross-linking between DNA strands; Interferes with DNA replication and RNA transcription	Nausea and vomiting, alopecia, myelo-suppression
	Dacarbazine (DTIC)	Requires in vivo activation by hepatic enzymes; mechanism of action is same as for mechlorethamine	Nausea and vomiting, myelosuppression
Antibiotics	Doxorubicin (Adriamycin)	Binds to DNA preventing DNA replication and RNA transcription	Nausea and vomiting, alopecia, myelo-suppression, cardio-myopathy
	Bleomycin	Same as Doxorubicin	Mucocutaneous reaction pulmonary fibrosis
Vinca alkaloids	Vincristine	Unknown exactly; observed to disrupt mitosis by interfering with spindle formation in metaphase	Neurotoxicity causing peripheral neuropathy and constipation, alopecia
	Vinblastine	Same as vincristine	Myelosuppression, neurotoxicity (but less than vincristine)
Adrenocortico-steroids	Prednisone, prednisolone	Unknown exactly; observed to have lympholytic effects and interference with mitosis	Fluid retention, electrolyte imbalance, ulcerogenic, adrenal dysfunction, psychoses
Methylhydrazines	Procarbazine	Unknown exactly; believed to auto-oxidize with formation of hydrogen peroxide which exerts cytotoxic effects	Nausea and vomiting, myelosuppression, central nervous system toxicities, dermatitis
Nitrosoureas	Carmustine	Inhibits both DNA and RNA synthesis	Nausea and vomiting, delayed myelo-suppression, burning at site of injection
	Lomustine	Same as carmustine	Same as carmustine
	Streptozocin (investigational)	Inhibits DNA synthesis	Nausea and vomiting, proteinuria, glycosuria

pears not to have cross-resistance between them. VCR has relatively little myelosuppression, its outstanding side effect being neurotoxicity manifested by peripheral paresthesias and numbness, loss of deep tendon reflexes and constipation due to autonomic nervous neuromuscular toxicity. Because of this last side effect patients who receive VCR therapy should be maintained on stool softeners.

The mechanism of action of the vinca alkaloids is unknown, but they have been observed to cause an arrest of cell division during metaphase; this arrest of cell division is also characteristic of colchicine and its derivatives.

ADRENOCORTICOSTEROIDS

Drugs in this class are employed in very high doses (for prednisone, 40 mg/m^2 of body surface area per day or higher) when used in the treatment of Hodgkin's disease. The mechanism of action of these drugs in Hodgkin's disease therapy is unknown but may reside in lympholytic effects and the ability to suppress mitosis. Side effects observed are typical of corticosteroid therapy (e.g., fluid retention, electrolyte imbalance, ulcerogenic possibilities).

METHYLHYDRAZINE DERIVATIVES

Procarbazine is the sole drug in this class of antineoplastic agents which has found application in the treatment of Hodgkin's disease. The mechanism of action is not clearly understood but the drug is believed to undergo autooxidation in vivo resulting in the formation of hydrogen peroxide. The hydrogen peroxide then presumably interacts with DNA preventing cross-linkage. The drug is also a weak monoamine oxidase inhibitor. Therapeutic incompatibilities with alcohol similar to disulfiram-type reactions have been observed.

ANTIBIOTICS

Doxorubicin and bleomycin are two antibiotics which have been employed in the chemotherapy of Hodgkin's disease. All drugs in this class have the ability to bind to DNA. This prevents DNA replication and RNA transcription.

The notable toxicity seen with doxorubicin is cardiomyopathy evidenced in two types. An acute form exists where ST-T segment changes and arrhythmias occur that can be demonstrated in the ECG. This situation is usually transient and generally not a cause for concern. A later, chronic form of cardiomyopathy also occurs and is manifested as congestive heart failure unresponsive to digitalis therapy. This chronic toxicity is generally seen when cumulative doses of doxorubicin exceed 550 mg/m^2 although it may also be seen at lower cumulative doses.

Toxicity of bleomycin is related to mucocutaneous reactions (stomatitis, ulceration, vesiculation) and pulmonary toxicity characterized by fibrosis. In contrast to other antineoplastic agents, bleomycin causes minimal myelosuppression.

NITROSOUREAS

Carmustine and lomustine are generally considered to act as alkylating agents. Their mechanism has not been completely elucidated. Both agents are thought to inhibit both DNA and RNA synthesis. The most outstanding toxicity is delayed myelosuppression which usually occurs in 4 to 6 weeks. Thrombocytopenia usually occurs prior to leukopenia by approximately 1 week.

Streptozocin is investigational in treating neoplastic diseases. It is a nitrosourea antibiotic which is thought to have a primary effect on inhibition of DNA synthesis. Its acute toxicities include nausea and vomiting with delayed toxicities of proteinuria, glycosuria and an increase in serum creatinine.

PROGNOSIS

Hodgkin's disease was once a rapidly fatal disease. However, recent advances in the treatment of Hodgkin's disease have produced results that should provide many patients with a normal life span. Institutions engaged in the research and treatment of Hodgkin's disease are consistently reporting longer survival rates for patients in all stages of their disease following treatment. Stage IA patients are remaining disease-free and are apparently cured. Data has shown that 95 to 100% of patients with stages IIA and IIIA disease will remain disease-free 5 years or more. The prognosis of stages IIIB and IV disease has also improved to the point where survival in 50% of the patients can be expected for 10 years and beyond. Advances in therapy have allowed many patients to remain clinically free of their disease for years and have decreased relapse rates during the first 5 years after initial therapy. It has also been observed that 90% of patients who do relapse will do so within 3 to 4 years after initial therapy and only infrequently does disease recur after 5 years of freedom from clinical signs of the disease.

Cure for Hodgkin's disease sometimes is discussed in the literature, but this does not imply a state where all microscopic foci of disease are eradicated. Cure as discussed in the literature relates to a "statistical cure" which states that after a certain period of time—perhaps a decade—there remains a population of patients whose death rate from all causes is similar to that of a normal population of the same age and sex (21).

CONCLUSION

Hodgkin's disease is a malignant lymphoma which originates in the lymphoreticular system, disseminates via contiguous lymphatics and possibly the blood stream to other lymph nodes, and if unchecked, will eventually invade organ systems and bone marrow. The prognosis and treatment of the disease are related to the histopathology of diseased lymph nodes and the anatomic extent of the disease determined by staging procedures. Available therapy relying on radiation therapy and chemotherapy or judicious combinations of both has greatly improved the outlook and length of survival for patients, but 1600 deaths per year in the United States are still attributed to Hodgkin's disease (22).

Therapeutic concepts of Hodgkin's disease involve an understanding of the diagnostic and staging procedures and the rationale behind the available modes of treatment. Prospects for the future include new chemotherapeutic agents and combinations of both new and old antineoplastic drugs with minimization of attendant toxicities. Advances in diagnostic procedures promise to locate disease presence more accurately and efficiently. Improvements in radiation therapy and therapeutic plans employing radiation therapy and combination chemotherapy also promise more effective treatment. The future holds a better understanding and insight into the nature of Hodgkin's disease itself.

Acknowledgments. The authors would like to express their gratitude to Dr. Peter H. Wiernik, University of Maryland Cancer Center, and Dr. Robert Esterhay, Baltimore Cancer Research Program, NCI, NIH, for their thoughtful comments in reviewing the manuscript.

References

1. Williams WJ, Beutler E, Erslev AJ, et al (eds): *Hematology*, ed 2. New York: McGraw-Hill, 1977, p 944.
2. Vianna NJ, Greenwald P, Brady J, et al: Hodgkin's disease; cases with features of a community outbreak. *Ann Intern Med* 77:169, 1972.
3. Lukes RJ, Butler JJ, Hicks EB: Natural history of Hodgkin's disease as related to its pathologic picture. *Cancer* 19:317, 1966.
4. Carbone PP, Kaplan JS, Musshoff K, et al: Report of the committee on Hodgkin's disease staging classification. *Cancer Res* 31:1860, 1971.
5. Harris JM, Tang DB, Weltz MD: Diagnostic tests and Hodgkin's disease: a standardized approach to their evaluation. *Cancer* 4:2388, 1970.
6. Berard C, Thomas LB, Axtell LM: The relationship of histopathological subtype to clinical stage of Hodgkin's disease of diagnosis. *Cancer Res* 31:1776, 1971.
7. Goodman LS, Gilman A: *The Pharmacological Basis of Therapeutics*, ed 6. New York: Macmillan, 1980, p 706.
8. Isselbacher KJ, Adams RD, Braunwald E, et al (eds): *Harrison's Principles of Internal Medicine*, ed 9. New York: McGraw-Hill, 1980, p 1635.
9. Manufacturer's Package Insert: Mustargen. Merck Sharp & Dohme, 1979.
10. Paladine W, Cunningham T, Sponzo R, et al: Intracavitary bleomycin in the management of malignant effusions. *Cancer* 38:1903, 1976.
11. Bayly T, Kisner D, Sybert A, et al: Tetracycline and quinacrine in the control of malignant pleural effusions. *Cancer* 41:1188, 1978.
12. Kadin ME, Glastein E, Dorfuran RF: Clinicopathologic studies of 177 untreated patients subject to laparotomy for the staging of Hodgkin's disease. *Cancer* 27:1277, 1971.
13. Borum K: Increasing frequency of acute myeloid leukemia complicating Hodgkin's disease: a review. *Cancer* 46:1247, 1980.
14. Wiernik PH, Gustafson J, Schimpff SC, et al: Combined modality treatment of Hodgkin's disease confined to lymph nodes. Results eight years later. *Am J Med* 67:183, 1979.
15. DeVita VT, Hellman S, Rosenberg SA (eds): *Principles and Practice of Oncology*, Philadelphia: J.B. Lippincott, 1982, p 1382.
16. Glatstein E: Radiotherapy in Hodgkin's disease: past achievements and future progress. *Cancer* 39 (2 suppl):837, 1977.
17. Haskell CM: *Cancer Treatment*. Philadelphia: W.B. Saunders, 1980, p 44.
18. DeVita VT, Serpick A, Carbone P: Combination chemotherapy in the treatment of advanced Hodgkin's disease. *Ann Intern Med* 73:881, 1970.
19. Frei E, Luce JK, Gamble JE, et al: Combination chemotherapy in advanced Hodgkin's disease: induction and maintenance of remission. *Ann Intern Med* 79:376, 1973.
20. DeVita VT, Simon RM, Hubbard SM, et al: Curability of advanced Hodgkin's disease with chemotherapy: long-term follow up of MOPP treated patients at NCI. *Ann Inter Med* 92:587, 1980.
21. Frei E, Gehan EA: Definition of cure for Hodgkin's disease. *Cancer Res* 31:1828, 1971.
22. Anon: Cancer statistics, 1982. *CA* 32:23, 1982.

CHAPTER 47

Carcinoma of the Breast

WILLIAM R. GROVE, M.S.
CLARENCE L. FORTNER, M.S.

Breast cancer has become the most common malignancy among women in the United States, with an estimated 112,900 new cases to be diagnosed in 1982. During this same year, approximately 37,300 women of all ages will die of this disease (1). Both the incidence and the mortality per 100,000 have remained essentially constant over the last 50 years, indicating that there has been little improvement in prognosis in this disease which claims more female victims between the ages of 40 and 44 than any other single disease. Notable advances have been made in recent years, however, which may result in the improved management and prolonged survival of patients with breast cancer. These advances have been in the areas of improved methods of diagnosis, increased public awareness, investigation of the adjuvant chemotherapy approach to primary management, and the identification of the role of hormone receptor proteins in endocrine therapy. In addition, studies are in progress evaluating new surgical and radiotherapeutic techniques and new chemotherapeutic agents used singly and in combination to improve both cosmesis and survival in patients with breast cancer.

INCIDENCE

The risk of a woman developing breast cancer in the United States is about 1 in 15 during her lifetime. Several factors have been identified, however, which influence one's chances of developing breast cancer. The two risk factors considered most significant are a family history of breast cancer and a personal history of breast cancer. There is a familial component involved in developing breast cancer, thereby imparting a greater risk to relatives, especially daughters and sisters, of patients who have breast cancer. If the lifetime risk in the general American female population is approximately 7%, then the development of breast cancer in the following relatives imparts a corre-

spondingly higher risk to any individual: sister—9.5%, second degree relative—18.5%, mother—40% (2). Further evidence of this familial tendency is reflected in the fact that daughters of women who have breast cancer develop it 10 to 12 years earlier than their mothers. The second factor accepted as an increased risk factor is a past history of breast cancer. Women who are treated for breast cancer are candidates for developing a second lesion at a rate 7 times the expected incidence. The cumulative risk of a new primary breast cancer is 4% at 5 years and steadily increases to 13% at 20 years after the initial diagnosis. There is a histologic component to the risk of bilaterality, with a 50 to 60% incidence for patients with lobular carcinoma.

A definite pattern is evident when age at diagnosis is compared against incidence. Breast cancer occurring under the age of 30 is rare and is nearly unheard of under the age of 15. Over 30, however, the incidence rises sharply with age, never reversing this trend, so that a woman in her 70s or 80s continues to be at increased risk.

Several other variables have been identified which appear to place certain women in a higher risk category. The longer the total menstrual life is, the greater the tendency for developing malignant breast disease. Women whose menstrual life is surgically ended through an oophorectomy years prior to their expected natural menopause develop breast cancer at a much reduced rate. There is a reduced risk if the age at first pregnancy is less than 19 years old. Menopausal estrogen use may be associated with an increased risk of breast cancer, particularly when high-dose preparations or prolonged therapy is involved (3, 4). Finally, higher socioeconomic levels are associated with an increased incidence.

There was some initial concern that the widespread use of oral contraceptives would result, after an appropriate lag time, in an increased incidence of breast cancer in users. There has not been, with over 10 years of use, any increased risk of breast cancer demonstrated in studies of women who have used oral contraceptives for varying periods of time. In fact, there has been a decrease in the incidence of certain nonmalignant breast conditions. At best, these results are encouraging. It will, however, require long term follow-up studies, for perhaps as long as 20 years, before the question can be absolutely resolved (5).

ETIOLOGY

Understanding the relationships between hormonal, environmental, dietary and genetic risk factors will help in understanding the etiology of breast cancer.

DIAGNOSIS

Approximately 95% of all patients with breast cancer first detect some breast abnormality themselves. The most frequent sign (75 to 80%) is a mass, or lump, and is usually found accidentally while bathing or dressing. Occasionally (10%) the presenting symptom may be a stabbing or aching pain. Other symptoms which are noticed less frequently are nipple retraction (most notable when the arms are raised), spontaneous nipple discharge, or dimpling. Breast tissue undergoes cyclic hormonally influenced changes during the menstrual cycle. A breast mass which appears prior to menstruation and disappears afterward is most likely not a malignancy, but rather normal breast tissue. For this reason, women who practice breast self-examination should do so at approximately the same phase of their menstrual cycle each month.

Women who practice breast self-examination (BSE) are more likely to have localized disease present at the time of diagnosis, compared to women who do not practice BSE. In a study of over 2000 women with newly diagnosed breast cancer, 30% of those who practiced BSE had early disease compared to 19% of those who did not practice BSE ($P < 0.001$) (6). In addition, only 16% of woman who practiced BSE had advanced disease compared to 36% of those who did not practice BSE ($P < 0.001$). A similar study revealed that 48% of women who practiced BSE monthly had their diagnosis confirmed prior to axillary lymph node involvement, compared to 38% of those who practiced BSE rarely and 33% of those who never practiced BSE ($P < 0.001$, each

comparison) (7). Increased public awareness of breast cancer has resulted in less patient delay in seeking medical attention and is responsible for the increased percentage of patients presenting with earlier stages of disease.

The initial approach to evaluate a possible breast cancer is a careful and complete history and physical examination. Certain characteristics of a mass such as size, shape, firmness, movability and tenderness can be determined by palpation. These findings may be sufficient to suspect carcinoma, but confirmation rests on biopsy. Further diagnostic procedures may be performed, however, which can provide additional more specific information. It is important to realize that these additional methods work best when they complement each other. They are meant to identify areas of clinical suspicion which should be biopsied to obtain a histologic diagnosis.

Mammography is a commonly used diagnostic procedure which employs X-rays to detect areas of increased density in breast tissue. It is much more sensitive than palpation and may detect densities which are yet undetectable by palpation. Properly done mammography may detect a cancer up to 2 years before it becomes clinically palpable (8). Mammography has a true positive accuracy of 85 to 90%, i.e., correctly detecting a malignant lesion. The false positive and false negative rates are 10 to 15%. A refinement of conventional mammography, xeromammography, allows greater resolution of detail and may improve the results obtained by conventional mammography. For either of these two procedures, the breasts are positioned on a table to allow tangential x-ray exposures to be taken from various angles without exposing the rest of the body to radiation. The films are then interpreted for the presence of any abnormality.

Under the clinical assumption that early detection of breast cancer correlates with an improved prognosis, the National Cancer Institute and the American Cancer Society sponsored the Breast Cancer Detection Demonstration Project (BCDDP), starting in 1973. This project involved an initial screening of asymptomatic women, and then yearly follow-up evaluations for 5 years. Approximately 280,000 women were evaluated in the 27 diagnostic centers using physical examination and mammography. Greater than 2700 breast cancers had been detected as of February 1978. Positive mammography alone (negative physical examination) was responsible for 44% of these cases which were referred for biopsy. A positive physical examination together with a positive or suspicious mammogram was responsible for an additional 48% of these cases which were referred for biopsy. Thus, 92% of the patients who were diagnosed as having breast cancer had a positive or suspicious mammogram (9). In those patients diagnosed as having breast cancer, 26% had noninfiltrating lesions and 15% were infiltrating, but with a tumor size less than 1 cm. Also, 70% of these newly diagnosed patients had negative axillary lymph nodes. These two favorable prognostic signs, small tumor size and negative axillary nodes, suggest a very favorable outcome for these women, due to early detection (9).

However, the BDCCP is not without controversy. The yearly radiation exposure, particularly to women under age 50, has been theoretically calculated to increase the patient's risk of developing breast cancer. One estimate of the significance of this risk, accepting several assumptions about the extrapolation of data from high-dose radiation exposure, reveals that approximately 2.2 new cases of breast cancer per one million women screened per year would result from standard screen-film mammography (10).

The "Working Group for the Evaluation of the BCDDP" concluded that mammography should be used in the routine screening of asymptomatic women in the following categories: (a) age 50 years or greater; (b) age 40 to 49 years, with personal history of breast cancer or positive history in a first degree relative; and (c) age 35 to 39, with personal history of breast cancer (9). In this population of women, the benefit from early detection outweighs the risk from the cumulative effects of mammography.

This discussion of the pros and cons of screening mammography should not be misinterpreted to detract from the unquestionable benefit of mammography in evaluating masses in symptomatic women. In symptomatic women, mammography is an extremely useful and reliable diagnostic tool.

Another aid has been developed for the detection of breast cancer. Thermography is an entirely innocuous procedure which involves no radiation exposure and is based upon the detection of minute differences in temperature patterns in the skin overlying the breast. Un-

fortunately, several nonmalignant conditions, such as fibrocystic disease, acute inflammation, abcesses and other benign masses may produce a false positive thermogram. Similarly, a high false negative rate has been reported, which is the most serious drawback to thermography as a screening tool. The initial enthusiasm for thermography has not been sustained, due to this unacceptably high rate of false negatives.

These diagnostic aids mentioned are meant to select patients for biopsy who have some breast abnormality suggestive of a carcinoma. Microscopic examination of biopsy material is the only method of absolutely diagnosing a breast malignancy.

Once the diagnosis of breast cancer is confirmed, the patient should undergo a diagnostic evaluation to detect the presence of distant metastases. This is important in determining the stage of disease at initial presentation to eliminate the need for surgery in patients who already have disseminated disease.

STAGING

The greatest single factor determining the fate of a patient with breast cancer is the extent of involvement, specifically the axillary lymph node status, at the time of diagnosis. Breast cancer metastasizes from the primary tumor site by two routes. Tumor cells escape into the circulation and lodge in distant sites, resulting in skeletal, liver, lung and less frequently brain metastasis, among others. These tumor emboli may be present in the blood stream by the time the disease is first clinically evident, as demonstrated by Handley (11). The competency of the patient's defense mechanisms responsible for the destruction of these cells may be a critical factor in their ability to survive. The second route of tumor spread is through the lymphatic drainage of breast tissue to two primary lymph node chains, the axillary and the internal mammary lymph nodes. Theoretically, tumor cells reaching these lymph nodes should be filtered and destroyed by the body's defense mechanism. They may, however, proliferate in these nodes rather than be destroyed. When this process has occurred for a sufficient period of time the nodes become enlarged and clinically palpable.

The location of the primary tumor has a direct anatomic relationship to the nodes which are likely to become involved. Thus, the internal mammary nodes are more likely to be involved if they are responsible for a greater proportion of the lymphatic drainage from the area of the primary tumor. The presence of involved lymph nodes at surgery serves as a prognostic indicator of survival. A steady fall in 5-year survival rates, as shown by the American College of Surgeons 1978 Survey (Table 47.1), demonstrates the significance of lymph node involvement (12). Another factor that also bears prognostic significance is the size of the primary lesion. The larger the presenting tumor mass is, the greater the chance of nodal involvement. All of these interrelated factors concerning the size of the primary lesion and the presence and the extent of lymph node involvement serve to emphasize the importance of early diagnosis and treatment.

Recently it has been established that most breast cancers are already disseminated at the time of diagnosis, with micrometastatic foci of disease present in distant sites. With this understanding, the involvement of axillary lymph nodes can be viewed as representing one manifestation of disseminated disease, rather than a progression from local disease to regional disease.

Documentation of extensive local breast involvement is important in the clinical staging of breast cancer, as it conveys a poor prognosis. This may be evidenced by several clinically apparent signs. Extensive edema of the skin of the breast (called peau d'orange because of its characteristic orange skin-like pitting), is caused by tumor emboli blocking lymphatic drainage of the skin and subcutaneous tissues.

Satellite nodules are multiple skin lesions resulting from direct infiltration of the tumor from the primary lesion which has spread along lymphatic channels to reach the skin. Skin ulceration is caused by direct growth of the primary lesion through breast tissue to the surface of the skin. This locally advanced stage is preceded by immobility of the skin over the tumor and localized erythema. Immobile fixation of the tumor to the chest wall is another sign of extensive local tumor involvement.

These criteria of lymph node involvement and extensive local disease are characteristics important in staging breast cancer. The course of therapy most beneficial to each patient is dependent upon the extent of disease at the time of diagnosis. For example, radical surgery would not be indicated in a patient presenting with evidence of distant metastases, as it could not possibly provide a "cure." From a research standpoint, staging is necessary to standardize collection of data, evaluation of therapy and to allow uniform end-results reporting.

Several staging systems have been developed based on clinical and/or pathological findings. The most widely used clinical staging system is the one adopted by both the International Union against Cancer (UICC) and the American Joint Commission in Cancer Staging and End Results Reporting (AJC) (Table 47.2).

TREATMENT

Once the patient is properly diagnosed and staged, treatment may be begun. Great variations exist in the characteristics of breast cancer from patient to patient, especially factors of growth rate and hormonal sensitivity, and require that each patient's course of therapy be individually planned. Following initial treatment for localized disease, breast cancer may lie dormant and undetectable for 5, 10, or 20 years in some patients, and then recur locally or with distant metastases. Other patients may not be so fortunate, experiencing disease recurrence within months of initial therapy. A third, and most fortunate group, are those whose disease never recurs following initial treatment. For this reason, the standard disease-free interval of 5 years, which is spoken of as a "cure" for many other malignancies, is invalid when discussing breast cancer. A more realistic figure of 10 years has been accepted and, realizing exceptions do occur, is the disease-free interval required to be considered "cured" of breast cancer.

Table 47.1.
Five-Year End Results in 20,547 Patients with Breast Cancer According to Number of Pathologically Positive Axillary Lymph Nodes (12)

No. of Positive Axillary Lymph Nodes	5-Year Survival (%)	5-Year Recurrence (%)
0	71.8	19.4
1	63.1	32.9
2	62.2	39.9
3	58.8	43.0
4	51.9	43.9
5	46.9	54.2
6–10	40.7	63.4
11–15	29.4	71.5
16–20	28.9	75.1
21+	22.2	82.2

Table 47.2.
UICC-AJC Clinical Staging of Breast Cancer

T: Primary Tumor

T1 Tumor 2 cm or less in its greatest dimension
T2 Tumor more than 2 cm in size but not more than 5 cm in its greatest dimension
T3 Tumor more than 5 cm in its greatest dimension
T4 Tumor of any size with direct extension to chest wall or skin

N: Regional Lymph Nodes

N0 No palpable homolateral axillary nodes
N1 Movable homolateral axillary nodes
   a. Nodes not considered to contain growth
   b. Nodes considered to contain growth
N2 Homolateral axillary nodes that are fixed to one another or to other structures
N3 Homolateral supraclavicular or infraclavicular nodes or edema of the arm

M: Distant Metastases

M0 No distant metastases
M1 Distant metastases present
These descriptions are then combined to define four stages:
Stage I: T1/N0 or N1a/M0
Stage II: T1/N1b/M0; T2/N0 or N1/M0
Stage III: T1 or T2/N2/M0; T3/N0, N1 or N2/M0
Stage IV: T4/any N/any M
         Any T/N3/any M
         Any T/any N/M1

The main factor which determines the initial treatment approach in most patients is the extent of disease. Patients whose workup indicates minimal local disease only are considered candidates for surgery. Patients presenting with advanced disease (distant metastases or primary tumors with fixation to the chest wall or skin) do not have surgically curable disease and are considered for any of the various other modalities of treatment including radiotherapy, hormonal therapy, antineoplastic chemotherapy or combinations of these.

SURGERY

Surgery is the standard therapy for early breast cancer. Once a patient has been selected for surgery the extent of the operation to be performed must be decided.

The pioneer in the area of mastectomy was William Steward Halsted who designed the classical radical mastectomy. His first paper on this subject was published in 1894. The procedure has become the standard surgical approach against which all other procedures have been compared. It is a disfiguring operation, however, requiring removal of the entire breast, pectoral muscles and an en bloc resection of the axillary contents. Several alternative operations have been proposed since that time, differing in their purpose from improving cure rates to improving cosmesis. The important fact to remember is that the purpose of surgery is to cure the patient by removing all disease present while retaining appearance and function as close to normal as possible.

The most limited operation performed is the removal of the primary lesion and breast tissue immediately surrounding the mass. This method (lumpectomy or tylectomy) produces the least disfigurement, as, frequently only a dimple in the normal breast contour is detectable and there is no loss of function or mobility.

A simple (total) mastectomy involves removal of the breast tissue with preservation of the pectoral muscles and no axillary intervention.

A modified radical mastectomy is a further attempt at compromise between a less extensive operation (lumpectomy or simple mastectomy) and the radical mastectomy. Nearly all breast tissue is removed and the lower ¾ of the axillary contents are resected to remove axillary lymph nodes for histologic examination. The pectoral muscles are preserved, giving the patient an improved appearance with the normal pectoral fold.

Operations more extensive than the radical mastectomy include the extended radical mastectomy where the internal mammary nodes are excised, and the superradical mastectomy which includes dissection of the supraclavicular lymph nodes. Neither of these two procedures have shown to improve survival, and in fact, may worsen prognosis.

Which operative procedure is the "treatment of choice"? Many studies are in progress to determine the optimal surgical procedure. Preliminary information from several studies has indicated that a more conservative approach than the radical mastectomy has not compromised the patient's chance of cure and has improved the cosmetic result (13). This approach may reap secondary benefits by promoting more prompt medical attention in those women whose delay is caused by fear of a disfiguring, mutilating operation.

The specific approach with any particular patient should be based on individual variables, such as the size of the lesion, presence of clinically positive axillary nodes, location of the lesion in the breast, duration of symptoms, age, etc. The procedure most commonly performed today is the modified radical mastectomy with full axillary dissection, which has essentially replaced the radical (Halstead) mastectomy. Table 47.3 shows the results of comparative surveys in 1972 and 1977 by the American College of Surgeons, demonstrating this trend toward less aggressive surgery (14).

One explanation why these various surgical approaches may not significantly alter survival is the fact that, in most patients, breast cancer has already disseminated as micrometastatic disease at the time of discovery of the primary lesion (15). Therefore, even though local control is desirable, distant metastases, the most significant factor affecting survival, may already be present although not clinically detectable by the time of initial management. Recent advances in two areas of breast cancer management indicate that the primary evaluation should include: (a) tissue from the primary lesion be sent for assay of hormone receptor protein content, and (b) axillary lymph node dissection should be performed to determine if adjuvant chemotherapy should be recommended to the patient (discussion to follow).

Whatever operation is performed, the surgeon must be acutely aware of the psychological impact a mastectomy may have. He must be prepared to support both the emotional and medical needs of the patient. A physician-patient relationship based on trust and understanding is crucial toward achieving an uncomplicated adjustment and adaptation to postmastectomy life. The American Cancer Society's "Reach to Recovery Program," where a previous mastectomy patient visits and counsels the new patient, has been very successful in this emotional and physical transition period.

A major postoperative complication of radical mastectomy is edema of the arm due to partial obstruction of lymphatic drainage. There is usually some edema immediately postoperatively. This should disappear within 1 month with the development of collateral lymphatics to provide adequate drainage. Approximately 5% of the patients develop permanent edema, which may be massive and severely debilitating in some cases. This is directly due to the surgical technique and may be aggravated by infectious complications. A secondary delayed edema may occur at any time following mastectomy when an infection of the hand or arm occurs. This may result in permanent edema in some patients. Mastectomized patients are susceptible to this complication for the rest of their lives and must be very cognizant of what may appear to be only a minor infection on the limb of the affected side. An active program of rehabilitation and patient education is encouraged to regain maximal function and mobility and minimize unnecessary morbidity.

The frequency and degree of postoperative edema appears directly related to the extent of axillary dissection performed during the procedure. A super-radical mastectomy is accompanied by a more frequent and greater degree of edema than a more limited operation. Patients who receive postoperative radiation to the axilla also have greater problems with edema due to the development of fibrosis causing restricted lymphatic drainage.

RADIOTHERAPY

Radiation therapy for breast cancer has been an important method of treatment both as a single modality and in combination with surgery. Just as there is much controversy among surgeons concerning the operation to be performed, radiotherapists differ in opinion as to when and how radiotherapy should be employed in the treatment of primary breast cancer.

Patients who are not candidates for surgery because of the presence of locally advanced disease may receive radiotherapy to the primary lesion and to local areas likely to be involved, such as the axillary and internal

Table 47.3.
Changes in Surgical Management of Breast Cancer (14)

Type of Surgery	Incidence (%)	
	1972	1977
None	3.4	3.3
Wedge excision	3.3	3.7
Total mastectomy only	11.4	6.5
Total mastectomy with low axillary dissection	6.3	5.6
Modified radical mastectomy with full axillary dissection	26.8	59.1
Radical (Halstead) mastectomy	47.3	21.0
Extended radical and super-radical mastectomies	1.5	0.8

mammary lymph node chains. This produces results approximately equal to that achieved from radical mastectomy in these advanced stages. Radiotherapy, however, should not be recommended as the sole initial treatment of patients with limited local involvement, unless surgery is contraindicated for other medical reasons or is refused by the patient.

Radiotherapy has been combined with surgery in an attempt to improve the results achieved with mastectomy. Both pre- and postoperative radiation have been used. The theory behind administering preoperative radiation is that it prevents viable tumor cell dissemination during surgery. The physical manipulation of excising breast tissue, including lymphatic and circulatory drainage routes, may liberate tumor cells into the circulation. Disadvantages credited to the use of preoperative radiation are that it delays the surgery 6 to 8 weeks; it increases the incidence of postoperative complications, specifically edema, and it renders many lymph node specimens removed during surgery falsely negative.

Postoperative radiation has been used extensively following all of the various surgical techniques previously described. Some physicians feel less extensive surgery may be performed if postoperative radiotherapy is employed. Several disadvantages have been attributed to the use of postoperative radiotherapy. First, the majority of women will remain locally free of disease after the surgical procedure alone, never needing this radiation exposure to achieve local control of their disease. Thus, the side effects and complications associated with radiation exposure such as skin reactions, pulmonary fibrosis, and potential carcinogenicity are unwarranted. Secondly, although prophylactic postoperative radiotherapy has been proven to lower the incidence of local recurrences, studies have demonstrated that the survival rate may be lower in these women compared to women treated by surgery alone (16). This is due to the earlier appearance of distant metastases as the first evidence of recurrent disease in these women. A summary of 10 available controlled clinical trials of postoperative radiation reveals eight trials which demonstrate an increased mortality of 1 to 10% in the radiotherapy treated groups at 4 to 5 years (17). The mechanism of this disadvantage to radiated women is thought to involve interference with the immunologic mechanisms of surveillance and

destruction of tumor cells. For these reasons, neither preoperative nor prophylactic postoperative radiotherapy is recommended. The trend away from primary therapy using radical surgery plus radiotherapy is confirmed by the results of the surveys conducted by the American College of Surgeons, which showed that 12% of all patients treated in 1977 received this combined modality approach, compared to 26% of all patients treated in 1972 (14).

ADJUVANT CHEMOTHERAPY

Considering all of the various surgical and radiotherapy techniques employed for the primary treatment of breast cancer, the fact remains that approximately 25% of women with negative axillary nodes and 75% with positive axillary nodes at the time of surgery will present with recurrent disease within 10 years after treatment. It is becoming more evident that this failure rate is due to most, if not all, patients having occult disseminated disease at the time of diagnosis.

Because of these considerations, a "new" approach to the treatment of primary breast cancer was begun in 1972 under the direction of the National Surgical Adjuvant Breast Project (NSABP) for the purpose of determining the potential role of prolonged adjuvant chemotherapy in lengthening the disease-free interval. Patients with histologically proven breast cancer involving one or more positive axillary lymph nodes were randomized to receive either L-phenylalanine mustard (L-PAM, melphalan) or a placebo, beginning within 4 weeks after radical mastectomy. Patients assigned to L-PAM received 0.15 mg/kg/day for 5 consecutive days every 6 weeks until there was documented evidence of recurrent disease, or for 2 years, whichever occurred first. Single agent chemotherapy was chosen, rather than combination chemotherapy, as the logical starting point for determining the effectiveness of the concept of adjuvant therapy and because of the understandable desire to use what was anticipated to be a minimally toxic regimen in these otherwise healthy women.

A summary of results at 4 years of follow-up, when stratified on the basis of age and axillary lymph node status at the time of surgery (1 to 3 positive nodes vs. ≥4 positive nodes), indicated a certain subgroup of women who appeared to benefit from the L-PAM therapy. Compared with their corresponding controls, women ≤49 years old with 1 to 3 positive axillary lymph nodes experienced a marked benefit in terms of disease-free survival ($P = 0.006$). Women ≤49 years old with 4 or more positive axillary nodes as well as women greater than 49 years old did not show a statistically significant benefit from this adjuvant chemotherapy [18].

In a separate study by Bonadonna begun in 1973, the three-drug combination of cyclophosphamide, methotrexate and 5-fluorouracil (CMF) was administered for 12 monthly cycles to patients with positive axillary lymph nodes. Therapy was started within 4 weeks after radical mastectomy. These patients were compared to a concurrent control group who received no therapy following surgery. The early 5-year results of this study revealed several significant findings. Total survival as well as total disease-free survival were significantly improved for premenopausal women, as shown in Table 47.4. In addition, a greater percentage of premenopausal women with 1 to 3 positive axillary nodes at the time of surgery remained disease-free at 5 years, compared to those with more than 3 nodes [19].

In contrast, overall results in postmenopausal patients did not show any positive benefit from CMF, compared to surgical controls (56.0% disease-free survival vs. 51.5% respectively). However, when the data was examined with respect to total dose actually received, a therapeutic benefit was seen for those postmenopausal women who received greater than 85% of the expected total dose, compared to those who received lower doses of chemotherapy, as shown in Table 47.5 [20].

The weight of evidence from these and other studies of adjuvant chemotherapy for breast cancer favors its continued study in women with one or more positive axillary nodes at the

Table 47.5.
Relationship of Disease-Free Survival at Five Years vs. Dose Level of Adjuvant CMF Received, Postmenopausal Patients (20)

Dose Level Received (%)	% Disease Free Survival
>85	75
65–84	56
<65	49

time of surgery. A real benefit in terms of disease-free survival as well as overall survival has emerged, particularly in premenopausal women and in patients who receive maximally scheduled doses of chemotherapy. The acute toxicities are tolerable and reversible for most patients [21]. The delayed or long-term complications of adjuvant chemotherapy continue to be studied. Additional studies are in progress to determine the optimum drugs, doses, and duration of therapy to be used.

One explanation offered for the beneficial effects from adjuvant chemotherapy in premenopausal women is that the drugs are inducing a "chemical oophorectomy." This theory has been disproven through studies which fail to show an association of disease-free survival with depression of ovarian function [18, 19].

RECURRENT DISEASE

Once a patient has received primary treatment for localized breast cancer, there is usually a disease-free interval. Approximately one-half of all such patients will remain clinically free of disease. The other half, however, will develop recurrent disease anywhere from a few months to over 20 years after the initial treatment. For this latter group of patients, several therapeutic options are available, depending upon factors particular to each case.

Many patients have their disease recur locally. These lesions most frequently occur along the suture sites of the previous mastectomy and are probably due to failure to remove all viable tumor cells during surgery. They generally respond well to local radiation.

Disease appearance in the opposite breast may be either a metastatic lesion or a second primary malignancy, and if not accompanied by involvement elsewhere, may be treated by the same therapy that was used for the initial presentation. Breast cancer may also recur in remaining axillary or internal mammary lymph nodes after surgery. Treatment of these nodes is also with radiation.

Table 47.4.
Early Five-Year Results of Adjuvant CMF[a] (12 Cycles) in Premenopausal Patients (19)

	Surgical Controls (%)	Surgery + CMF (%)	P
Total disease-free survival			
1–3 nodes	51.3	82.2	0.0001
>3 nodes	28.8	39.7	<0.01
Total survival			
1–3 nodes	68.3	90.0	0.008
>3 nodes	46.5	78.9	0.05

[a] CMF = cyclophosphamide, methotrexate and 5-fluorouracil.

One additional group of patients are those whose disease recurs not locally, but metastasizes to some distant organ. For these women, this signals the beginning of a series of palliative therapeutic attempts to halt the progression of a disease which is generally considered beyond the curable stage.

HORMONAL THERAPY

In the patient who develops recurrent, but not immediately life-threatening disease, consideration should be given to hormonal therapy. It has been well demonstrated that changing the hormonal environment affects the growth of hormone-sensitive tissues. This provides a variety of therapeutic approaches for the patient with breast cancer. An advancement in the approach to treating recurrent disease has been the discovery that determination of the hormone-receptor status allows for prediction of response to hormonal management (22).

The estrogen receptor protein (ERP) refers to the presence of a specific cytoplasmic protein in a biopsy of malignant breast tissue (or from a site of metastatic disease) which binds to estrogen that enters a cell. This steroid-receptor complex then migrates to the nucleus of the cell where it initiates the biochemical actions characteristic of estrogen stimulation.

The value of the ERP lies in its correlation with response to hormonal therapy. Overall, approximately 30% of unselected patients respond to some appropriate method of hormonal therapy. When this result is stratified on the basis of ERP status, the responses are found to occur in approximately 50 to 60% of ERP positive patients and only 5 to 10% of ERP negative patients (23).

Although it is helpful to be able to select patients who would have a 60% chance of responding to any particular therapy, the most significant value of the ERP determination is to identify those patients who would have virtually no chance of responding to hormonal manipulation, and allow them to be promptly treated with chemotherapy. This spares them the unnecessary side effects and consequences of hormonal therapy for which there would be no predictable benefit and eliminates a delay in the time before potentially effective therapy could begin.

In the absence of an ERP determination, women who have an initial disease-free interval of greater than two years are in a group which favors a beneficial effect from a hormonal manipulation.

Assay of the progesterone receptor protein (PRP) content of malignant tissue is currently being investigated as a method to improve the predictability of hormone receptor assay. Preliminary information indicates the ERP positive patients who are also PRP positive would have approximately a 75 to 85% chance of responding to some method of hormonal manipulation. The ERP positive patients who are PRP negative are less likely to respond. Therefore, the current status of the usefulness of hormone receptors lies in the predictable failure of hormonal manipulation in ERP negative patients and the predictable response in ERP positive plus PRP positive patients (24).

Women who are premenopausal or within 1 year postmenopausal may undergo surgical removal of the ovaries (oophorectomy) to remove the ovarian source of estrogenic hormones. This produces objective regression of disease in 30% of premenopausal women unselected for ERP status with advanced breast cancer and also serves as an indicator of the hormonal responsiveness of the tumor. Women who respond to castration are said to have a hormonally responsive tumor and are candidates for future hormonal manipulations. Some additional method of endocrine manipulation will be attempted in most women who relapse following a response to oophorectomy, because a tumor which initially was responsive to this mode of therapy will be responsive to additional hormonal changes in approximately 40 to 50% of the cases. Premenopausal women who fail to respond to castration historically experience little chance of responding to subsequent hormonal therapy and may proceed to antineoplastic chemotherapy. The duration of response to therapeutic castration averages 10 to 14 months.

Disease recurrence in postmenopausal women is frequently treated initially with estrogens or androgens. Generally reserved for women 5 or more years postmenopausal, additive hormonal therapy produces regressions in about 20% of cases with androgens and 30% with estrogens, the chance of improvement increasing with age and ERP positive status. It is most effective in patients with pleural effusions, skin lesions, nodular pulmonary disease and bone metastases, and least effective in brain and liver metastases. An expected survival of several months is optimal, since 6 weeks or more may be required to demonstrate a response to hormonal therapy. In general, estrogens are preferred to androgens because of the distressing virilizing side effects of androgens and the greater effectiveness of estrogens.

Alternative hormonal management in postmenopausal women may involve techniques designed to remove the end-organ effect of endogenous biologically active compounds, either through ablative surgical procedures, such as adrenalectomy or hypophysectomy, or through chemical means, such as aminoglutethimide or tamoxifen. Adrenalectomy removes a significant extraovarian source of estrogen and would be indicated only after ovarian function has stopped, either naturally or artificially. Hypophysectomy abolishes the secretion of several factors arising from the pituitary, including ACTH, growth hormone, prolactin, thyroid-stimulating hormone and posterior pituitary hormone. Of these, the removal of the first three is considered significant in the treatment of breast cancer. Elimination of ACTH secretion results in adrenal atrophy, giving a therapeutic effect similar to that of adrenalectomy, with the exception of preservation of the zona glomerulosa, that area of the adrenals responsible for aldosterone production. The response rate in unselected patients approximates 30% for either adrenalectomy or hypophysectomy, with a much higher response rate occurring in those patients who initially responded to castration or who are ERP positive (45%) compared to those who initially failed castration or who are ERP negative (<10%).

Endocrine replacement therapy is necessary following either of these ablative procedures. Following adrenalectomy, glucocorticoid and occasionally mineralocorticoid replacement is required. Following hypophysectomy, replacement therapy would include glucocorticoid, thyroid hormone and posterior pituitary hormone. In either case, requirements must be individually determined and reevaluated frequently to adjust for changing conditions of stress and environment.

Aminoglutethimide has recently been investigated for the therapy of postmenopausal patients with advanced breast cancer, as an alternative to adrenalectomy. Those patients whose disease characteristics make them suitable candidates for adrenalectomy appear to do at least as well with the "chemical adrenalectomy" produced by aminoglutethimide, showing an overall response rate of 31% in unselected patients (25). Its use in women who are estrogen receptor positive results in response rates of approximately 50% (26). The proposed mechanism of action is by inhibiting the biosynthesis of adrenal steroids and by blocking the conversion of androgens to estrogens in peripheral tissues. Because of the impaired biosynthesis of adrenal steroids, a compensatory rise in ACTH levels sufficient to override the metabolic block will result. For this reason suppressive doses of hydrocortisone must be administered. Therapy is maintained as long as the patient continues to demonstrate a response. The duration of complete responses averages 29 months; partial responses 13 months (27). Side effects associated with aminoglutethimide include lethargy, skin rash, ataxia, and orthostatic dizziness. The metabolic block is readily reversible when the drug is discontinued.

The currently preferred approach to additive hormonal therapy in postmenopausal women with breast cancer became commercially available in 1978 with the introduction of the oral antiestrogen tamoxifen. By inhibiting the binding of estrogen to the ERP in the cytoplasm of the target tissues, the formation of the active mediator, the estrogen-ERP complex, is inhibited with the ultimate effect being reduction of DNA synthesis. Because of this proposed mechanism, a therapeutic effect from tamoxifen would be expected only in those patients whose tumor tissue contains estrogen receptor protein.

Overall, 50 to 60% of patients who are ERP positive respond to tamoxifen compared to 0 to 10% of ERP negative patients. As was presented above, progesterone receptor analysis may significantly increase the response rate by selecting those patients who are most likely to respond, those who are both ERP and PRP positive.

As with other methods of hormonal therapy, there may be a delay in the observance of the maximum response for several months. In fact, the average time to achieve a response in those patients who do respond is 72 days. For this reason, patients with life-threatening disease (i.e., visceral metastases) are not candidates for hormonal therapy. The reason for this delayed response is not known but may be related to the different mechanism of cellular destruction involved compared to the rapid cell lysis associated with chemotherapy or radiotherapy.

Patients whose disease actively stabilizes or improves should remain on tamoxifen until evidence of disease progression appears.

There does not appear to be a clear dose/response relationship with tamoxifen. Increasing from the lower recommended dose of 10 mg twice a day to 20 or 30 mg twice a day does not produce a corresponding increase in response rates.

In general, the adverse effects from tamoxifen are mild, rarely requiring therapy be discontinued. Most frequently reported effects are hot flashes, nausea and vomiting. Less common reactions include bone pain, hypercalcemia, anorexia, vaginal discharge, vaginal bleeding, and transient leukopenia or thrombocytopenia which frequently reverses in the face of continued therapy.

Since the side effects from tamoxifen or aminogluthethimide are better tolerated than some of the other methods of hormonal therapy, both surgical and replacement, they should be considered in the initial approach to hormone therapy in those postmenopausal patients with a favorable hormone receptor status.

ANTINEOPLASTIC CHEMOTHERAPY

The field of antineoplastic chemotherapy has been explored in recent years with the hope of finding agents effective in breast cancer. Chemotherapy has generally been reserved for patients who have either failed or relapsed on hormonal therapy or patients with life-threatening visceral involvement in whom hormonal therapy would not be appropriate due to the long treatment time which may be required to demonstrate a response, as previously discussed.

Thus, most patients treated with chemotherapy have had far advanced disease, often with poor performance abilities, poor nutritional status and an enormous tumor burden. Faced with these circumstances, the fact that approximately 60% of patients with recurrent disease treated with combination chemotherapy show an improvement in both quality and duration of life, should not be viewed as a discouraging figure. Rather, with increased understanding of the concepts of tumor biology, as demonstrated by the design of adjuvant chemotherapy trials, prolonged survival time and the possibility that a potential "cure" of

breast cancer may occur with a future shift toward earlier use of antineoplastic drugs is very encouraging (28). Nevertheless, there will always be patients who develop metastatic breast cancer requiring chemotherapeutic agents for the purpose of palliation. For these patients, we must be aware of specific drugs, combinations, doses, toxicities, etc. to enable us to most effectively treat the patient with metastatic breast cancer.

The premise behind administering antineoplastic drugs is that the cells incorporate the drug into their cell metabolism where the drug exerts it cytotoxic effect, killing the cell. Unfortunately, since this drug effect is not specific to malignant cells, certain normal rapidly dividing tissues, such as bone marrow, gastrointestinal epithelia and hair follicles receive cytotoxic quantities of these drugs as well. Consequently, the primary toxicities of antineoplastic drugs as a class are granulocytopenia, thrombocytopenia, anemia, stomatitis, gastrointestinal ulceration and alopecia. Specific agents differ in their tendency to produce one or more of these toxicities, in addition to other more specific individual toxicities.

The chemotherapeutic approach to malignant disease began with the investigation of single agents to determine which drugs demonstrated an antitumor effect. These agents were then studied in various combinations to find the optimum drug combination and dosage schedule. All classes of antineoplastic agents have been tried in breast cancer with some measure of success being demonstrated by one or more members of each class.

Table 47.6 summarizes the single agent response rates for several agents in advanced breast cancer (29).

Combinations of chemotherapeutic agents have resulted in dramatic advances in the treatment of several malignancies, including Hodgkin's disease, childhood acute lymphocytic leukemia, testicular cancer and others. In general, the improvement in response with combination chemotherapy over single agent chemotherapy is measured by four parameters: increased overall response rate, increased percent of complete responses obtained, prolonged duration of remission, and improved survival. Combination chemotherapy of breast cancer has demonstrated improved results compared to single agent therapy.

In combining agents effective against a cer-

Table 47.6.
Single Agent Therapy in Advanced Breast Cancer: Response Rate

Drug	Response Rate (%)
Alkylating agents:	
Mechlorethamine	35
Cyclophosphamide	34
Thiotepa	30
Melphalan	23
Chlorambucil	20
Antimetabolites:	
Methotrexate	34
5-Fluorouracil	26
6-Mercaptopurine	14
Cytosine arabinoside	9
Mitotic inhibitors:	
Vincristine	21
Vinblastine	20
Antibiotics:	
Mitomycin C	38
Doxorubicin	37
Miscellaneous:	
Hexamethylmelamine	28
Dibromodulcitol	27
Carmustine	21
Prednisone	20
Lomustine	12

tain malignancy, one must bear in mind two factors. Each agent employed should work through a different mechanism of action, i.e., as an alkylating agent, a pyrimidine analog, a folic acid antagonist, etc. Secondly, the dose and schedule of each agent should be chosen to avoid overlapping common toxicities within the combination.

There have been literally hundreds of studies of chemotherapeutic combinations in metastatic breast cancer. Most have attempted to modify various regimens by adjusting dosages, or substituting other agents to maximize the response rate and minimize the toxicities. An overall view of these various studies indicates that a plateau has been reached in the chemotherapeutic management of advanced breast cancer. The following summary reflects response parameters achieved by combination chemotherapy studies in advanced breast cancer (25, 28):

Overall response rate	50–60%
Complete response rate	15–25%
Duration of response	8 months
Survival of responders	20 months
Survival of nonresponders	7 months

The potential for future improvements in the field of chemotherapy of breast cancer lies in the development of new agents and their corresponding combinations, the exploration of combined modality therapies such as chemotherapy with hormonal therapy, and the continued investigation of the use of chemotherapy in earlier stages of disease.

SUMMARY

Certain risk factors have been identified which increase a woman's chance of developing breast cancer. Of these, a positive family history and a previous breast malignancy in the patient in question are most significant. The overall risk for a woman in the United States is about 7% during her lifetime.

Information derived from studies of tumor cell growth indicates that a malignant process has been developing for many years by the time a diagnosis of breast cancer is made. During this period, the disease may have disseminated from the primary lesion and established clinically occult micrometastases. A change in the therapeutic approach away from the idea that breast cancer is initially a local disease has significantly contributed to improvement in treatment results.

The treatment of breast cancer utilizes four disciplines: surgery, radiotherapy, endocrine manipulation and antineoplastic chemotherapy. Several surgical procedures of varying magnitude have been proposed. Radiotherapy may be employed and considered as primary initial therapy for patients unable or unwilling to undergo surgery. Reports of adjuvant chemotherapy after primary surgery, utilizing both single agent and combination chemotherapy have demonstrated a significant reduction in disease recurrence and an increase in survival in certain groups of women, particularly when maximally scheduled doses are administered.

Hormonal manipulation may produce gratifying results in patients who relapse from primary therapy, especially in those patients who are ERP positive (and PRP positive). Depending on the menopausal status of the patient, either an oophorectomy, tamoxifen, aminoglutethimide or estrogen therapy may be used. Subsequent hormonal manipulation is frequently beneficial in those patients who initially responded to hormonal therapy, and then relapsed.

Chemotherapy is reserved for patients who

have failed all other forms of treatment, patients whose disease is rapidly progressing, patients who are hormone receptor negative, and patients with life-threatening visceral metastases. Single agents which have been shown to be relatively effective in breast cancer include doxorubicin, cyclophosphamide, methotrexate, 5-fluorouracil, vincristine and prednisone. Research to identify other effective single agents, as well as effective drug combinations, is in progress.

Acknowledgment. The authors wish to acknowledge Arlene Forastiere, M.D., for her valuable comments and review of this manuscript.

References

1. Anon: Cancer statistics. *CA* 32:15–31, 1982.
2. Anderson D: Genetics and the etiology of breast cancer. *Breast* 3:37–41, 1977.
3. Ross RK, Paganini-Hill A, Gerkins VR, et al: A case-control study of menopausal estrogen therapy and breast cancer. *JAMA* 243:1635–1639, 1980.
4. Brinton LA, Hoover RN, Szklo M, et al: Menopausal estrogen use and risk of breast cancer. *Cancer* 47:2517–2522, 1981.
5. Fechner R: Influence of oral contraceptives on breast cancer. *Cancer* 39:2764–2771, 1977.
6. Huguley CM, Brown RL: The value of breast self-examination. *Cancer* 47:989–995, 1981.
7. Feldman JG, Carter AC, Nicastri AD, et al: Breast self-examination, relationship to stage of breast cancer at diagnosis. *Cancer* 47:2740–2745, 1981.
8. Galante M: Minimal breast cancer: a surgeon's dilemma. *Cancer* 28:1516, 1971.
9. Smart CR, Oliver HP: Breast cancer screening results as viewed by the clinician. *Cancer* 43:851–856, 1979.
10. Dodd GD: Radiation detection and diagnosis of breast cancer. *Cancer* 47:1766–1769, 1981.
11. Handley RS: A surgeon's view of the spread of breast cancer. *Cancer* 24:1231, 1969.
12. Nemoto T, Vana J, Bedwani RN, et al: Management and survival of female breast cancer: results of a national survey by the American College of Surgeons. *Cancer* 45:2917–2924, 1980.
13. Fisher B, Montague E, Redmond C, et al: Comparison of radical mastectomy with alternative treatment for primary breast cancer. *Cancer* 39:2827–2839, 1977.
14. Vana J, Bedwani R, Mettlin C, et al: Trends in diagnosis and management of breast cancer in the U.S. *Cancer* 48:1043–1052, 1981.
15. Gullino P: Natural history of breast cancer. Progression from hyperplasia to neoplasia as predicted by angiogenesis. *Cancer* 39:2697–2703, 1977.
16. Stjernsward J: Decreased survival related to irradiation postoperatively in early operable breast cancer. *Lancet* 2:1285, 1974.
17. Stjernsward J: Adjuvant radiotherapy trials in breast cancer. *Cancer* 39:2846–2867, 1977.
18. Fisher B, Sherman B, Rockette H, et al: 1-Phenylalanine mustard (L-PAM) in the management of premenopausal patients with primary breast cancer. *Cancer* 44:847–857, 1979.
19. Bonadonna G, Rossi A, Tancini G, et al: Adjuvant combination chemotherapy for operable breast cancer. Trials in progress at the Instituo Nazionale Tumori of Milan. *Cancer Treat Rep* 65(suppl 1):61–65, 1981.
20. Bonadonna G, Valagussa P: Dose-response effect of adjuvant chemotherapy in breast cancer. *N Engl J Med.* 304:10–15, 1981.
21. Glass A, Wieand HS, Fisher B, et al: Acute toxicity during adjuvant chemotherapy for breast cancer: the national surgical adjuvant breast and bowel project (NSABP) experience from 1717 patients receiving single and multiple agents. *Cancer Treat Rep* 65:363–376, 1981.
22. McGuire W: Current status of estrogen receptors in human breast cancer. *Cancer* 36:638–644, 1975.
23. Byar DP, Sears ME, McGuire WL: Relationship between estrogen receptor values and clinical data in predicting the response to endocrine therapy for patients with advanced breast cancer. *Eur J Cancer* 15:299–310, 1979.
24. Bloom ND, Tobin EH, Schreibman B, et al: The role of progesterone receptors in the management of advanced breast cancer. *Cancer* 45:2992–2997, 1980.
25. Henderson IC, Canellos GP: Cancer of the breast, the past decade. *N Engl J Med* 302:17–30 and 78–90, 1980.
26. Santen RJ, Worgul TJ, Lipton A, et al: Aminoglutethimide as treatment of postmenopausal women with advanced breast carcinoma. *Ann Intern Med* 96:94–101, 1982.
27. Santen RJ, Misbin RI: Aminoglutethimide: review of pharmacology and clinical use. *Pharmacotherapy* 1:95–120, 1981.
28. Carbone P, Bauer M, Band P, et al: Chemotherapy of disseminated breast cancer; current status and prospects. *Cancer* 39:2916–2922, 1977.
29. Broder L, Tormey D: Combination chemotherapy of carcinoma of the breast. *Cancer Treat Rev* 1:183–203, 1974.

Index

Page numbers in *italics* denote figures; those followed by "t" or "f" denote tables or footnotes, respectively.